BSAVA Textbook of
Veterinary Nursing
4th edition

Editors

Dick Lane BSc FRAgS FRCVS
York, UK

Barbara Cooper VN Cert Ed Lic IPD DTM Hon Assoc RCVS
Principal, The College of Animal Welfare, London Road
Godmanchester, Huntingdon, Cambs PE29 2LJ

Lynn Turner MA VetMB MRCVS
St David's Farm & Equine Practice, Nutwell Estate
Lympstone, Exmouth EX8 5AN

Consulting Editor – Exotics

Simon J. Girling BVMS (Hons) DZooMed CBiol MIBiol MRCVS
RCVS Recognised Specialist in Zoo & Wildlife Medicine
Vets Now Ltd, 2B Hutchison Crossways, Edinburgh EH14 1RR

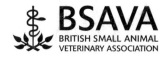
BSAVA
BRITISH SMALL ANIMAL
VETERINARY ASSOCIATION

Published by:

British Small Animal Veterinary Association
Woodrow House, 1 Telford Way,
Waterwells Business Park, Quedgeley,
Gloucester GL2 2AB

A Company Limited by Guarantee in England.
Registered Company No. 2837793.
Registered as a Charity.

First published 1994
Second edition 1999
Third edition 2003
Reprinted 2004
Fourth edition 2007
Reprinted 2008

The publishers and contributors cannot take responsibility for information
provided on dosages and methods of application of drugs mentioned in this
publication. Details of this kind must be verified by individual users from the
appropriate literature.

Printed by: Replika Press Pvt. Ltd, India

Contents

Contributors

Wendy Adams VN
Guide Dogs for the Blind,
Tollgate House,
Banbury Road,
Bishops Tachbrook,
Leamington Spa,
Warwickshire CV33 9QJ

Davina Anderson MA VetMB PhD DSAS(ST) DipECVS MRCVS
Anderson Sturgess Veterinary Specialists,
The Granary,
Bunstead Barns,
Poles Lane,
Hursley,
Winchester,
Hampshire SO21 2LL

Victoria Aspinall BVSc MRCVS
Director of Abbeydale Vetlink Veterinary Training Ltd,
Gloucester

Trudi Atkinson VN DipAS(CABC) CCAB
Bradford-on-Avon,
Wiltshire

Amanda Boag MA VetMB DipACVIM DipACVECC MRCVS
Department of Veterinary Clinical Science,
Royal Veterinary College,
Hawkshead Lane,
Hatfield,
Hertfordshire AL9 7TA

David C. Brodbelt MA VetMB PhD DVA DipECVA MRCVS
Royal Veterinary College,
Hawkshead Lane,
Hatfield,
Hertfordshire AL9 7TA

Elizabeth Bryan BSc (Hons) VN
Kingston Upon Hull,
East Yorkshire HU5 4BJ

Ray Butcher MA VetMB MRCVS
Upminster,
Essex RM14 1UY

Melanie Cappello (O'Reilly) BSc (Hons) PGCE VN
Clinical Skills Centre,
Royal Veterinary College,
Hawkshead Lane,
Hatfield,
Hertfordshire AL9 7TA

Sharon Chandler VN DAVN (Surg) DAVN (Med)
Queens Veterinary School Hospital,
University of Cambridge,
Madingley Road,
Cambridge CB3 0ES

Carole Clarke MA VetMB CVPM MRCVS
Mill House Veterinary Surgery and Hospital,
20 Tennyson Avenue,
King's Lynn,
Norfolk PE30 2QG

Ruth Dennis MA VetMB DVR DipECVDI MRCVS
Animal Health Trust,
Lanwades Park,
Kentford,
Newmarket,
Suffolk CB8 7UU

Elizabeth Earle TD BA RN
Royal College of Veterinary Surgeons,
London SW1P 2AF

Jonathan Elliott MA VetMB PhD CertSAC DipECVPT MRCVS
Professor of Veterinary Clinical Pharmacology,
Royal Veterinary College,
University of London,
Royal College Street,
London NW1 0TU

Gary England BVetMed PhD DVetMed DVR DVRep DipECAR DipACT ILTM FRCVS
School of Veterinary Medicine and Science,
University of Nottingham,
College Road,
Loughborough,
Leicestershire LE12 5RD

Maggie Fisher BVetMed CBiol MIBiol MRQA DipEVPC MRCVS
Shernacre Enterprise,
Shernacre Cottage,
Lower Howsell Road,
Malvern,
Worcestershire WR14 1UX

Robyn Gear BVSc DipECVIM-CA DSAM MRCVS
Department of Veterinary Medicine,
University of Cambridge,
Madingley Road,
Cambridge CB3 0ES

Simon J. Girling BVMS (Hons) DZooMed CBiol MIBiol MRCVS
Vets Now Ltd,
2B Hutchison Crossways,
Edinburgh EH14 1RR

Carol Gray BVMS MRCVS PGCert MedEd
University of Liverpool,
Veterinary Teaching Hospital,
Leahurst,
Chester High Road,
Neston,
South Wirral CH64 7TE

John Helps BVetMed CertSAM MRCVS
Intervet UK,
Walton Manor,
Walton,
Milton Keynes,
Bedfordshire MK7 7AJ

Susan Howarth VN Cert Ed DAVN (Surg) DAVN (Med)
The College of Animal Welfare,
Mypetstop,
Topcliffe Close,
Capitol Park,
Tingley,
West Yorkshire WF3 1BU

Andrea Jeffery MSC Cert Ed DipAVN (Surg) VN
Division of Companion Animals,
University of Bristol,
Langford House,
Langford,
Bristol BS40 5DU

Philip Lhermette BSc(Hons) CBiol MIBiol BVetMed MRCVS
Elands Veterinary Clinic,
Station Road,
Dunton Green,
Sevenoaks,
Kent TN13 2XA

Susan E. Long BVMS PhD DipECAR MRCVS
Canine Reproduction Referrals,
Clarendon Veterinary Centre,
2 Clarendon Road,
Weston-super-Mare,
North Somerset BS23 3EF

Donald Mactaggart BVM&S CertSAD MRCVS
Thistle Veterinary Health Centres,
Clovenstone,
Edinburgh EH14 3BF

Sandra McCune VN BA PhD
Waltham Centre for Pet Care and Nutrition,
Freeby Lane,
Waltham-on-the-Wolds,
Melton Mowbray,
Leicestershire LE14 4RT

Dawn McHugh VN BA (Hons) DAVN EVN
65 High Street,
Stetchworth,
Newmarket,
Suffolk CB8 9TH

Daniel S. Mills BVSc PhD ILTM CBiol MIBiol DipECVBM-CA MRCVS
University of Lincoln,
Department of Biological Sciences,
Riseholme Park,
Lincoln LN2 2LG

Louise Monsey Cert Ed VN
The College of Animal Welfare,
Cambridge PE29 2LJ

Helen Moreton BSc (Hons) PhD
Royal Agricultural College,
Cirencester,
Gloucestershire GL7 6JS

Kate Nichols VN DAVN (Surg)
Senior Nurse,
Intensive Care Unit,
Queen Mother Hospital,
Royal Veterinary College,
Hawkshead Lane,
Hatfield,
Hertfordshire AL9 7TA

Amanda Rock BVSc MRCVS
The Veterinary Hospital,
Colwill Road,
Estover,
Plymouth,
Devon PL6 8RP

Jennifer Seymour Cert Ed VN
Lecturer in Veterinary Nursing,
19 Wheatcroft Close,
Penkridge,
Staffordshire ST19 5JS

Kendal Shepherd BVSc CCAB MRCVS
Finedon,
Wellingborough,
Northamptonshire NN9 5NA

Jenny Smith DAVN (Surg) VN
Queens Veterinary School Hospital,
University of Cambridge,
Madingley Road,
Cambridge CB3 OES

Cedric Tutt BSc Agric BVSc (Hons) MMed Vet (Meds) MRCVS
Cape Animal Dentistry Service,
Cape Animal Medical Centre,
78 Rosmead Avenue,
Kenilworth 7708,
Cape Town,
South Africa

Caroline van der Heiden VN
Aberlour,
Banffshire AB38 9NQ

Sue Vranch VN
Petdent Ltd,
Veterinary Dentistry and Oral Surgery Referrals,
58 Hampton Lane,
Blackfield,
Southampton,
Hampshire SO45 1WN

Vicky Walsh VN
Hartpury College,
Gloucester GL19 3BE

Anne Ward BSc VN DipAVN (Surg)
Lecturer in Veterinary Nursing,
College of Animal Welfare,
Royal (Dick) School of Veterinary Studies,
1 Summerhall Square,
Edinburgh EH9 1QH

Elizabeth Welsh PhD BVMS MRCVS
West Linton,
Peebleshire EH46 7HQ

Anna Williams BSc (Hons)
Animal Health Trust,
Lanwades Park,
Kentford,
Newmarket,
Suffolk CB8 7UU

Foreword

When, in 1965, the Royal College of Veterinary Surgeons made their momentous decision to establish a Register of Animal Nursing Auxiliaries, a major milestone in the development of British small animal practice was reached. A new professional group was created who, by passing examinations leading to the qualification, enabled their names to be entered on the Nurses' Register.

This action created a need for a comprehensive text and reference book for the guidance of both trainees and teachers at the approved training practices and colleges. The Council of the BSAVA acted quickly and directed their Publications Committee to produce a book based on the recommended course of tuition.

A deadline had to be worked to: we were fortunate in being able to assemble the talents of 14 authors, to cover the diverse syllabus, and in 1966 the first edition of this book appeared, known then as *Animal Nursing*.

I was privileged to act as editor for that book and re-read with pleasure a paragraph from my Editorial Foreword – 'It is hoped that this will be the first of many editions of this work which will grow and improve as the A.N.A. course develops and matures with the growth in small animal practice that it is designed to assist.'

Now, 40 years later, it is illuminating to look back on four decades of change and progress. The RANA qualification has moved on to Registered Veterinary Nurse, with both an associated upgrading in status and a progressive evolution of professional qualifications. Most importantly, this progression has meant an extension and expansion of the required learning process, well demonstrated by this 4th edition of *Veterinary Nursing*.

The subject coverage of this book, compared with that of the 1966 edition, reflects the demands of the enlargement not only of the syllabus but also of the required knowledge base. The core subjects remain, now expressed in a more explicit 'hands-on' manner, together with the inclusion of the newer specialties: genetics, animal behaviour, dentistry.

The inclusion of health and safety and legal and ethical aspects reflects current demands, but most importantly the chapter on client communication and practice organization illustrates the now well recognized role of the nurse in providing a vital interface with both the veterinary surgeon and the client.

The editors and the production team have succeeded in drawing together contributions from 41 authors that are elegantly presented, easy to read and to learn from, in a well displayed and illustrated text. Above all, this book is also a reflection of the growth of small animal veterinary nursing from what was a bold concept into a well trained, knowledgeable profession. The BSAVA continues to lead its chosen and most important role as an educator.

Bruce V. Jones
November 2006

Preface

This is a new edition in a long line stretching back to *Animal Nursing* (Parts 1 and 2) edited for the BSAVA by Bruce Jones and published in 1966 – in essence it is the ninth edition of the BSAVA's core textbook for veterinary nursing.

This new edition again covers the whole range of veterinary nursing in small animal practice, with all chapters revised or rewritten. New features include: extensive integrated coverage of exotic and small mammal care; expanded clinical nutrition; a new separate chapter on dentistry; coverage of alternative therapies; and extended coverage of animal behaviour problems. Recent advances in training and in the nursing profession are reflected in the inclusion of brand new sections on communication and on the process and models of veterinary nursing. The need for evidence-based medicine is shown in the introduction of care plans and this new edition emphasises professional standards.

The introduction of full colour illustrations, specially commissioned line drawings, and highlighted tables will aid the reader, many of whom will be using the book while studying to pass examinations.

In addition to students of veterinary nursing, qualified veterinary nurses will use this book as a comprehensive reference source.

A total of 41 contributors have been involved in this edition, either updating or writing completely new chapters. They and we have endeavoured to produce a modern and comprehensive text that will ensure the best in patient care.

Dick Lane
Barbara Cooper
Lynn Turner
November 2006

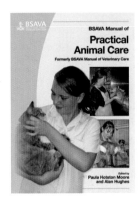

BSAVA Manual of Practical Animal Care

Editors: Paula Hotston Moore and Alan Hughes

- For animal care assistants, veterinary nurses and students
- Replaces *BSAVA Manual of Veterinary Care*

- Practical approach
- Updated and reorganized
- New chapter on Communications skills
- Features Exotic pets
- Illustrated throughout in full colour
- *Due Summer 2007*

Contents: Introduction to the veterinary profession; General care and management of the cat; General care and management of the dog; General care and management of exotic pets and wildlife; Introduction to veterinary care; Management of an animal ward; Use of medicines; Animal first aid; Communicating with clients; Veterinary terminology; Index

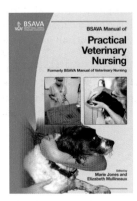

BSAVA Manual of Practical Veterinary Nursing

Editors: Marie Jones and Elizabeth Mullineaux

- For veterinary nurses and students
- Replaces *BSAVA Manual of Veterinary Nursing*

- Practical approach
- Completely reorganized and rewritten
- Includes new elements such as Nursing models
- Geared to the National Occupational Standards
- *Due Summer 2007*

Contents: Responsibilities of the veterinary nurse; Client communication; Practical pharmacy for veterinary nurses; Management of clinical environments, equipment and materials; Management of the inpatient; General principles of veterinary nursing; Triage and emergency nursing; Practical fluid therapy; Medical nursing; Practical laboratory techniques; Diagnostic imaging; Anaesthesia and analgesia; Surgical nursing; Wound management, dressings and bandages; Index

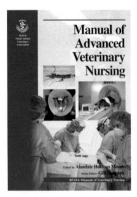

BSAVA Manual of Advanced Veterinary Nursing

Editor: Alasdair Hotston Moore

- For veterinary nurses and diploma candidates

Contents: Advanced medicine and medical nursing; Advanced surgery and surgical nursing; Advanced anaesthesia; Management of a critical care unit; Advanced radiography; The practice laboratory; General practice management; Small animal, exotic and wildlife nursing; Equine nursing; Index

'... written to be easily read... excellent tables throughout each chapter that are easy to understand and could definitely be used as a quick reference... an excellent addition to the veterinary nursing literature. It should be required reading for all and especially any veterinary nurse who works in a practice that performs any advanced procedures.'
Veterinary and Comparative Orthopaedics and Traumatology

For information on these and all BSAVA publications please visit our website: www.bsava.com

Chapter 1

Principles of health and safety

Ray Butcher

Learning objectives

After studying this chapter, students should be able to:

- Identify the legislation that pertains to veterinary practice
- Describe the key features of Health and Safety management
- Discuss the procedure for dealing with first aid and accident reporting
- Describe how to carry out a risk assessment
- List the categories of hazards in a veterinary practice
- Understand the safe use of common equipment
- Appreciate the Health and Safety implications of carcass disposal following euthanasia
- Describe the safe handling, storage and disposal of anaesthetic agents

The laws relating to occupational health

The very nature of veterinary practice means that staff, clients and visitors can be exposed to potential hazards such that accidents are possible. The Health and Safety legislation attempts to make the workplace as safe an environment as possible, by ensuring that practices examine their working procedures and adapt them to reduce to a minimum the risk of exposure to hazardous materials or circumstances in which accidents can occur. Even so, accidents will happen and practices should draw up contingency plans to deal with them. The legislation also makes provision for the recording and reporting of diseases and injuries that occur in the workplace (Reporting of Injuries, Diseases and Dangerous Occurrences Regulations 1995 (**RIDDOR**)).

It is important that veterinary nurses are familiar with Health and Safety legislation, not only because they have specific obligations as employees but also because they may become involved in formulating the practice policy or ensuring that other staff adhere to it. The two most important general pieces of legislation are the Health and Safety at Work etc. Act 1974 (**HSW Act**) and the Management of Health and Safety at Work Regulations 1999 (**MHSW Regulations**). The Royal College of Veterinary Surgeons (**RCVS**) Practice Standards Scheme incorporates all this legislation within its Core Standards (these standards are relevant to all veterinary practices) and inspectors will check that practices are complying with the legal requirements (see Chapter 2).

Health and Safety at Work etc. Act 1974

The HSW Act applies to all businesses, however small, and relates to all persons in the workplace, whether employers, employees or visitors. It sets out the specific duties of both employers and employees, and indicates that the ultimate responsibility rests with the partners or principal of the practice.

The general provisions of the Act dictate that every employer should ensure that:

- Proper provision is made to establish safe systems of work. These should be written down as 'Local Rules' and displayed on Health and Safety notice boards at the appropriate workstations
- All equipment is adequately maintained to the manufacturer's specification
- The premises (including vehicles) should be kept in a good state of repair and adequate attention given to providing safe access or exit in times of emergency
- All articles and substances used within the practice should be handled, stored and transported in a safe manner
- Information, instruction and supervision of employees should be carried out regularly
- All appropriate protective clothing is provided free of charge
- A satisfactory working environment is maintained with adequate facilities and arrangements for employees' welfare at work. This should include adequate washing and toilet facilities as well as a separate hygienic area for rest and refreshment

- Appropriate first aid facilities are available. All accidents should be recorded, and the more serious ones reported to the Health and Safety Executive (**HSE**).

Any employer with five or more employees must prepare, and when necessary revise, a written Health and Safety Policy Statement. This must outline the general policy of the practice, as well as list the general duties of all members of the practice. It is necessary to appoint (in writing) individual members of staff to jobs with special responsibilities (e.g. practice safety officer, fire officer, first aid officer), providing written job specifications for these posts. It is essential that this statement, and any revision, is brought to the attention of all employees. The HSE document *Starting Your Business – Guidance on Preparing a Health and Safety Policy Document for Small Firms* provides a useful template with blanks that can be completed by the individual practice to ensure that it is complying with the law.

The Act highlights the responsibilities of all employees, who must:

- Take reasonable care for the health and safety of themselves and of other persons who may be affected by their acts or omissions
- Cooperate with the employer so far as it is necessary to enable any duty or requirement under the Act to be performed or complied with
- Not interfere, recklessly or intentionally, with anything provided in the interests of health, safety and welfare.

These broad guidelines to the Act are highlighted on a poster and leaflet produced by the HSE entitled *Health and Safety Law – What You Should Know*. The poster should be displayed on the practice notice board and the leaflets should be provided to all staff.

Management of Health and Safety at Work Regulations (amended 1999)

The MHSW Regulations build on the HSW Act and include duties to assess risks and ensure that the arrangements for Health and Safety are effective. It requires the following steps:

- Planning
- Organization
- Control
- Monitoring
- Review.

These regulations stress the requirements for health surveillance. The essential element of the effective management of Health and Safety is a thorough Risk Assessment (see below).

Additional legal requirements for specific health risks at work

Although the HSW Act and the MHSW Regulations provide the overall framework, there are some specific laws that relate to particular risks and also the Special Waste Regulations 1996 (as amended). The requirements of these laws must be incorporated in the overall Health and Safety management plan for the practice.

In addition to these major regulations, a number of others have relevance to the practice of Health and Safety and some of these are considered in Chapter 2.

Specific health and safety legislation of relevance to veterinary practice

- Special Waste Regulations (as amended) 1996
- Hazardous Waste (England and Wales) Regulations (**HWR**) 2005
- Fire Precautions Act 1971
- Control of Pollution Act 1974
- First Aid at Work Regulations 1981
- Ionizing Radiation Regulations 1985
- Electricity at Work Regulations 1989
- Environmental Protection Act 1990
- Manual Handling Operations Regulations 1992
- Health and Safety (Display Screen Equipment) Regulations 1992
- Reporting of Injuries, Diseases and Dangerous Occurrences Regulations (**RIDDOR**) 1995
- Chemicals (Hazard Information and Packaging for Supply) Amendment Regulations 2002 (**CHIP** 96)
- Control of Substances Hazardous to Health (**COSHH**) Regulations 2002
- Fire Precautions (Workplace) (Amendment) Regulations 1999
- Personal Protective Equipment at Work (**PPE**) regulations 1992

Ionizing Radiation Regulations 1985

These apply specifically to the hazards associated with radiography and are dealt with in Chapter 20.

Control of Substances Hazardous to Health (COSHH) Regulations 2002

The COSHH Regulations were introduced specifically to cover the management of risks associated with hazardous substances and relate to all pharmaceutical products and chemicals used in veterinary practice. Manufacturers should supply COSHH Hazard Data Sheets with all such products to help the practice to formulate its COSHH Assessment. This is part of the Risk Assessment demanded by the MHSW Regulations (see later).

Hazardous Waste (England and Wales) Regulations (HWR) 2005

The HWR came into force in 2005, replacing the Special Waste Regulations 1996. The HWR regulate the correct segregation, storage, transfer and eventual destruction of waste products produced at the surgery. It is now mandatory for all premises producing hazardous waste, unless exempt, to be registered with the Environment Agency on an annual basis. An appropriate *Premises Code* is then issued, which is essential before a licensed contractor can remove the waste. In summary, the provisions of the Act state the following:

- Hazardous waste is defined as having properties that are hazardous to health or to the environment. These properties are listed in the European Commission's Hazardous Waste Directive. Hazardous waste includes fluorescent tubes, cathode ray tubes (computer monitors, TV screens), fridges, radiograph developer chemicals, infectious materials, and certain pharmaceuticals such as cancer chemotherapeutic agents

- Hazardous waste must be segregated and kept separate from non-hazardous waste
- The Environment Agency will have greater powers to monitor waste producers and issue fixed penalty fines
- Hazardous waste producers must keep detailed records of the wastes they produce.

Non-hazardous waste acceptable for domestic rubbish collection (e.g. handtowels, disposable masks, etc. that have not been contaminated with pharmaceuticals, blood or infectious contaminants) can go into domestic black bags. Non-hazardous waste that is acceptable for domestic rubbish collection but may be classed as 'offensive' waste by the local authority may include kennel waste and bedding. The local authority may request that this waste is collected into black and yellow striped ('wasp') bags.

If a practice is unsure how to classify particular items of waste, it should check with the registered carrier, the licensed waste management company or the Environment Agency prior to disposal.

Clinical waste

The hazardous waste produced at veterinary practices includes that classified as clinical waste.

Hazardous clinical waste consists wholly or partly of animal tissues, blood or other body fluids, excretions, drugs or pharmaceutical products that are likely to be hazardous to health. Such waste should be collected and stored in approved colour-coded plastic sacks (yellow, with the words 'Clinical waste' and the name of the practice clearly printed on the outside) (Figure 1.1).

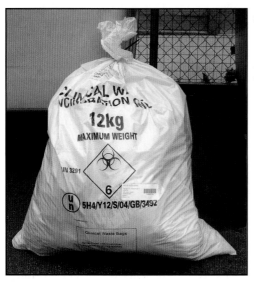

1.1

Disposable bag for clinical waste.

Non-hazardous clinical waste is theatre waste, blood-stained dressings and non-identifiable body parts that are deemed not to be a hazard to human beings. This is collected in orange bags and pre-treated before disposal, which is cheaper than incineration.

'Sharps'

'Sharps' are a special category of clinical waste that includes used needles, scalpel blades or other sharp instruments. These should be discarded, immediately after use, into special yellow plastic tubs that can be sealed once full (Figure 1.2). 'Sharps' used to deliver cancer infusion therapies must be segregated into a container with a purple or black lid.

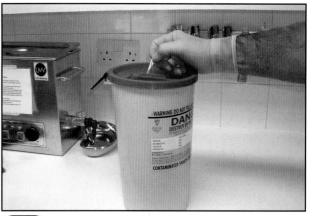

1.2   'Sharps' bin.

Bottles and vials

Bottles and vials contaminated with pharmaceutical products should be stored in specific yellow plastic bins prior to appropriate disposal.

Cadavers

The final category of clinical waste is cadavers, which are currently handled via local pet crematoria and pet cemeteries or can be released for home burial. Strict interpretation of the law would preclude owners from burying their pets in the garden, but the Government has made an exception in this case (*The Department of Environment Management Paper No. 25*).

Cadavers must be collected by a licensed carrier and disposed of at a licensed plant. Prior to collection, they are stored within the practice in some form of cold storage facility in sealed yellow plastic sacks. If, in the future, cadavers are brought within the Hazardous Waste Regulations, then animals dying of infectious disease would be deemed hazardous and would have to be incinerated by a specialist contractor, and ashes would not then be returnable.

There may be additional Health and Safety implications in the case of those animals euthanased while suffering from zoonotic disease or those receiving certain types of therapy. In these circumstances the body fluids and secretions may pose a special threat and care must be taken to clean the surrounding area thoroughly and avoid contamination of the outside of the plastic sack. Protective clothing should be worn and this should be specified in the appropriate practice Standing Operating Procedure (SOP).

Segregation and storage within the practice

The practice must have a strict policy on the segregation of waste. To be practical this must allow for the immediate disposal of material after use and hence there must be sufficient receptacles to allow for segregation at each workstation. This should also apply to practice vehicles. Prior to collection, clinical waste should be stored in a secure place within the practice.

Transport and disposal

Hazardous waste must be collected by a registered carrier in a 'dedicated' vehicle, licensed specifically for the transport of such waste. It is transferred to a licensed plant, where final disposal is achieved. (In the case of clinical waste this is preferably by high-temperature incineration.) Each collection (or batch of collections) should be accompanied by the appropriate certification, copies of which should be kept by the practice.

The HWR 2005 place a duty of care on the producers of hazardous waste to ensure that, from production to ultimate disposal, the waste is dealt with according to the law. The practice itself is responsible for checking that both the carrier and the waste management company have the appropriate licences and ideally should keep photocopies for its own records.

General maintenance of buildings and equipment

It is important that all buildings are kept in a good state of repair, especially with regard to electrical or gas installations and fittings. All equipment (e.g. X-ray machines, anaesthetic machines, autoclaves) should be regularly serviced according to the manufacturer's recommendations and service records should be kept.

Electricity at Work Regulations 1989

These regulations state that all systems should be maintained so as to prevent, as far as is reasonably practicable, all dangers. HSE guidelines on maintaining portable electrical equipment in offices and other low-risk environments recommend a regular visual inspection and recording system. The frequency of inspection depends on the type of equipment, with suggestions ranging from every 6 months for hand-held equipment to every 2 years for static equipment (e.g. photocopiers).

Fire precautions

Adequate precautions should be taken to avoid or combat fires. Very valuable advice can be obtained from the local Fire Prevention Officer. The legislation includes the following and the practice should appoint a fire officer to oversee these provisions.

Fire Precautions Act 1971

This Act involves:

- The provision of adequate fire-fighting equipment (advice needs to be taken on the correct extinguishers for different workstations and these should be checked regularly)
- An alarm system, regularly maintained
- Well signposted emergency exits (Figure 1.3)
- Emergency lighting
- Clear local rules stating what to do in case of fire (these should be posted in strategic places and reinforced by regular fire practices)
- Care in the storage of inflammable and explosive material
- The provision of fire doors where appropriate.

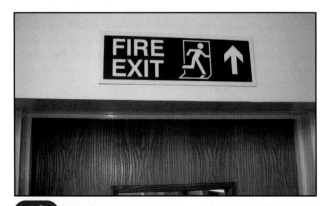

1.3 Fire exit sign.

Fire Precautions (Workplace) (Amendment) Regulations 1999

These further specify requirements for:

- Competent assistance to deal with general fire safety risks
- Providing employees with information on fire provisions
- Employers and self-employed people in a shared workplace to cooperate and coordinate with others on fire provisions and to provide outside employers with comprehensive information on fire provisions.

Oxygen cylinders and other flammable substances

The HSE document *Safe Working with Flammable Substances* (1997) highlights the following five principles ('VICES') when considering working safely with flammable substances:

- Ventilation
- Ignition
- Containment
- Exchange
- Separation.

Special consideration should be given to the transport and storage of oxygen cylinders. Ideally, they should be stored in a locked construction away from the main building.

Protection of the person against physical attack

Unfortunately, veterinary practices are not immune from the attention of criminals. Nurses or veterinary surgeons 'on call' at night and weekends are especially vulnerable and it might be worth incorporating personal 'panic buttons' into the practice alarm system. The local Crime Prevention Officer may give useful advice on this matter.

It is wise to have a practice policy of noting names, addresses and phone numbers of clients being visited. Staff members should never go out on a visit without informing other staff of their whereabouts.

First aid and reporting accidents

First aid

Despite every precaution, accidents happen. The First Aid at Work: Approved Code of Practice and Guidelines 1997 states the requirement for a suitably stocked accessible first aid box and the appointment of a nominated first aider. There are no hard and fast rules about the contents of the first aid box, but it must reflect the number of staff and the type of hazards encountered.

The personnel responsible for first aid include:

- A First Aid Appointed Person – responsible for taking charge when someone is injured or falls ill, including calling an ambulance if required. They are also responsible for maintaining and stocking the first aid box and ensuring that accidents are recorded in the accident book. They should not attempt to administer first aid

- A qualified first aider – this person must have attended an HSE-approved training course and hold a current First Aid at Work Certificate.

The recommended number of first aid personnel for a 'medium risk' business is given in Figure 1.4. The availability of staff during different shifts should be taken into account, as well as the fact that clients attending the clinic may significantly increase the number of people at risk at any one time.

Number of employees	Suggested first aid staff
< 20	At least one appointed first aid person
20–100	At least one qualified first-aider for every 50 employees (or part thereof)
> 100	One additional qualified first-aider for every additional 100 persons

 Recommended numbers of first aid personnel for 'medium risk' businesses.

Discussion of the principles of human first aid is beyond the scope of this chapter. However, the regulations described above make it clear that there must be someone trained on the staff who is able to assess human casualties and provide basic life support. In addition, they should be able to manage emergency situations such as fractures, wounds and burns.

Recording accidents

It is the duty of the practice to record all accidents and injuries that occur involving either employees or clients. An accident book approved by HSE (Form B1 510) is available from HMSO. The information that is to be recorded includes:

- The full name, address and occupation of the person who had the accident
- The signature (with date) of the person filling in the book (this must also include their address and occupation if they are not the one who had the accident
- When and where the accident happened
- Details about the cause of the accident (record details of any personal injury)
- An indication of whether the injury needs to be reported under RIDDOR.

Reporting accidents

Under the provisions of the Reporting of Injuries, Diseases and Dangerous Occurrences Regulations (RIDDOR) 1995, the practice is obliged to report certain serious events direct to the HSE via the incident contact centre website www.riddor.gov.uk. The appropriate forms can be downloaded from this site. Serious events are classified as:

- Major or fatal accidents
- 'Three-day' accidents
- Dangerous occurrences and near misses.

Fatal accidents include those instances where a fatality occurs within 1 year as a result of an original accident at work. **'Three-day' accidents** relate to absences from work for a minimum of 3 days as a result of an accident at work. **Major accidents** are defined as:

- A fracture of the skull, spine or pelvis
- A fracture of a long bone of the limb
- Amputation of a hand or foot
- Loss of sight of an eye
- Any other accident that results in an injured person being admitted into hospital as an inpatient for more than 24 hours, unless only detained for observation.

Major or fatal accidents must be reported as soon as possible by telephone, followed by written confirmation within 7 days on Form 2508.

There is a list of dangerous occurrences that should be reported to the HSE (Form F2508) whether or not an injury occurs. These include:

- Explosion from a gas cylinder or sterilizer
- Uncontrolled release of substance (including gases, vapours and X-rays) liable to be hazardous to health
- Any escape of substances that might result in problems due to inhalation or lack of oxygen
- Any cases of acute ill-health that could have resulted from exposure to pathogens in infected material
- Any unintentional ignition or explosion.

(See also Chapter 17 for dangerous occurrences in the laboratory.)

Manual handling procedures

More than a quarter of the accidents reported each year to the enforcing authorities are associated with manual handling, i.e. the transporting or supporting of loads by hand or body force. Indeed, statistics published by the HSE indicate that this may be as high as 55% for those working in medical, veterinary and other health services. Sprains and strains arise from the incorrect application or prolongation of bodily force. Poor posture and excessive repetition of movement can be important factors in their onset. Many manual handling injuries are cumulative, rather than being truly attributable to any single handling incident.

The Manual Handling Operations Regulations 1992 expand on the general provisions of the HSW Act in this regard. The HSE booklet *Manual Handling – Guidance on Regulations* clearly outlines the requirements and application of these regulations. The general provisions highlight a hierarchy of measures:

1. Avoid hazardous manual handling operations so far as is reasonably practicable
2. Assess any hazardous manual handling operations that cannot be avoided
3. Reduce the risk of injury so far as is reasonably practical.

Assessment of manual handling procedures

The HSE Guidelines give some practical help, but the regulations set no specific requirements such as weight limits. The importance of an ergonomic approach to the assessment of each procedure is stressed – giving consideration to the task, the load, the working environment, the individual's capability and the relationship between them. The intention is to fit the operation to the individual, rather than the other way around.

Factors to be considered in making an assessment are fully explained in the HSE Guidelines and specific references are made to some problems in veterinary practice. When carrying animals, for example, the load lacks rigidity, there is a concern on the part of the handler to avoid damaging the load, and sudden movements of the load add an element of unpredictability. All these factors serve to increase the likelihood of injury compared with handling an inanimate load of similar weight and shape.

An individual's physical capability varies with age, the risk of injury being higher in the teens or above the age of 50 years. Pregnancy also has significant implications for the risk of manual handling injuries. Hormonal changes can affect the ligaments, increasing the susceptibility to injury, and postural problems may increase as pregnancy progresses. Particular care should also be taken for women who may handle loads during the 3 months following a return to work after childbirth.

Display screen equipment

Possible hazards associated with the use of display screens are those leading to musculoskeletal problems, visual fatigue and stress. The likelihood of experiencing these is related mainly to the frequency, duration, intensity and pace of spells of continuous use on the display screen equipment.

The HSE booklet entitled *Display Screen Equipment Work – Guidance on Regulations* clearly outlines the provisions and requirements of the regulations (e.g. the provision of appropriate eye and eyesight tests for designated 'operators' and 'users').

In general it is very unlikely that many staff working in a veterinary practice would be classified as 'operators' or 'users' under the provisions of the regulations, since most of the display screen work is intermittent. However, the guidelines do give some useful points to consider in relation to the physical layout of the workstation (e.g. lighting, correct posture, layout of screen and keyboard). Such considerations would be part of the normal Health and Safety assessment irrespective of whether the specific Display Screen Equipment Regulations apply.

Risk assessments

The Management of Health and Safety at Work Regulations require that all employers and self-employed people assess the risks to workers and any others who may be affected by their work or business. Moreover, those who employ five or more employees should record the significant findings of that risk assessment. A separate risk assessment is required for the employment of young persons (under 18 years of age). The five basic stages that are required are outlined:

1. Identify what the hazards are
2. Identify who might be harmed and how
3. Evaluate the risks from the identified hazards
4. Record
5. Review and revise.

Hazards and risks

The essence of Health and Safety management is to identify all the hazards to which the staff are exposed and then to develop work protocols that reduce the risks from these hazards to a minimum.

- **Hazard** – anything with the potential to cause harm.
- **Risk** – the likelihood of the hazard's potential being realized.

The HSE *Health Risk Management Guide* identifies the broad categories of hazard as:

- Hazardous chemicals
- Sprains, strains and pains
- Noise
- Vibration
- Ionizing radiation
- Extremes of temperature, pressure and humidity
- Hazardous microorganisms
- Stress.

The range of potential hazards within a veterinary practice is vast, and the author has found the following list to be of practical use in making his own risk assessment.

Suggested categories of hazard in veterinary practice

Chemical agents:
- Dispensed drugs
- Laboratory chemical reagents
- Cleaning materials
- Inhalation of dust and fumes
- Explosive/flammable agents
- Radiographic processing chemicals
- Miscellaneous non-laboratory solvents

Biological agents:
- Non-specific organisms
- Specific zoonotic infectious agents
- Non-zoonotic infectious agents
- Animal tissues – allergens
- Unidentified allergens

Traumatic injuries:
- 'Sharps'
- Manual lifting
- Direct injury inflicted by animals
- Burns and scalds
- Accidental falls
- Accidents in the car park and entrance

Hazards from using equipment:
- Electrocution
- Burns and scalds
- Eye strain from visual display screens
- Repetitive strain injuries
- Back injuries from poorly adjusted seating

Hazards from poor environmental control:
- Heating/air conditioning
- Humidity
- Ventilation
- Contamination of water supply
- Noise
- Radiation

Warning labels and CHIP

All hazardous chemicals have clear warnings on the bottle (see Chapter 17) and are classified as either toxic, highly flammable, corrosive, harmful or irritant. A more complex numerical code system employed for the purposes of the classification and labelling of hazardous chemicals was introduced as a result of the Chemicals (Hazard Information and Packaging for Supply) Amendment Regulations 1996 (CHIP 96). This classification includes data relating to the potential risks and safety precautions required for these chemicals. Although much is of little relevance to veterinary practice, the veterinary nurse should be aware of its existence. The HSE has produced an explanatory booklet called *The Complete Idiot's Guide to CHIP*.

Risk assessment and development of management plan

In making the risk assessment, the first three steps involve:

1. Identifying the hazards
2. Identifying who might be at the greatest risk
3. Assessing the nature of the risk.

In the case of hazardous substances, some may have specific maximum exposure limits (**MELs**) while others may have occupational exposure standards (**OESs**). The MEL of a hazardous substance is assessed in relation to a specific reference period when calculated by a method approved by the Health and Safety Commission. Exposure should not exceed this level. Where an OES has been approved for an inhalation agent, control can still be regarded as adequate if the level is exceeded and yet the employer identifies the reasons and takes the appropriate action to remedy the situation as soon as is reasonably practical. Thus, when considering a particular hazard consideration should be given to:

- **Nature of the hazard**. What symptoms are seen if exposure occurs? Is there a published MEL or OES? Is there an available COSHH Hazard Data Sheet, or does the material carry a specific warning label?
- **Route of exposure**. Remember that there may be more than one for each substance, and that accidents may result in unexpected routes of exposure (e.g. injectable drugs could enter the body by accidental self-injection, but also via the skin or eyes if the bottle is broken)
- **First aid**. Are there any specific first aid measures if accidental exposure occurs? Such information should be included in the COSHH Hazard Data Sheet
- **Preventive measures**. Does this particular substance need to be used or is a safer alternative available? Will strict Standard Operating Procedures (SOPs), possibly involving the use of protective clothing, greatly reduce the risk?
- **High-risk staff**. Are there any members of staff who may be at a greater risk (e.g. those with known allergies or at risk during pregnancy)? In this regard it is important that staff feel able to notify the practice safety officer or senior partner in confidence if they consider there is any chance of being pregnant, or if they have any disease or condition that might increase the risks when working in a particular environment
- **Recording of exposure**. Are there any monitoring schemes available to record exposure? This would include dosimetry for X-ray radiation exposure and any monitoring for halothane, isoflurane and nitrous oxide.

Many of the individual hazardous substances can be grouped together since the hazards are similar.

Standard operating procedures (SOPs)

Having identified the types of hazard, those at particular risk and the nature of the hazard, the Health and Safety management system should develop working protocols to make the hazards as low risk as possible. This generally requires the production of written SOPs that cover the full range of all work performed at the surgery. They must above all be clear and concise, and be tailored to the work protocols of each individual practice. Copies should be posted at the appropriate workstations, so that the group of SOPs in that area forms the basis of the Local Rules as required by the general Health and Safety legislation. A pictorial component would give more impact to SOPs posted on notice boards. The actual SOPs required by each practice may vary, but suggested topics (some of which are discussed in greater detail in relevant chapters of this book) are given in the following list.

Suggested list of standard operating procedures (SOPs)

- Radiation protection
- Accidents and first aid
- Health surveillance
- Laboratory procedures
- Postage of laboratory specimens
- Safe prescribing and handling of medicines
- Injections
- Restraint of animals
- Spillages
- The dental scaler
- Waste disposal
- Disinfectants and floor cleaning
- Kennel management
- Bathing animals
- Anaesthetic gases – scavenging and monitoring
- Fire precautions
- The mortuary/postmortem examinations
- X-ray film processing
- Sterilizers
- Visits to kennels, farms or stables/the practice vehicle/farms or stables
- Manual handling/lifting
- Display screens
- Refreshments/the staff kitchen
- Staff children and pets

Practical risk assessment at each workstation

This builds on the information collated above and is basically a critical look at the safety of each workstation within the practice. At each workstation (or room or department) the assessment involves the methodical listing of:

- **Hazards** that may be encountered in that area. For each one the practice must assess the degree of risk and allot a hazard code (H = high; M = moderate; L = low; N = negligible)
- If the substance has a **known MEL or OES**, this too should be recorded

- All the **members of staff** present in this area. This should include their gender, official job title and a brief summary of their involvement in this area. A note should be made if the member of staff is at particular risk (e.g. pregnant, under 18 years of age)
- All the **practice SOPs** that may be of relevance in this area
- The **control measures** in use in the area. This may simply require reference to specific SOPs
- **Safety clothing** provided and used.

Having completed this stage of the assessment, it is important to record a comment that represents an **overview** of the exposure and actual risks in that area. It is possible that various deficiencies are highlighted. These should be listed and a note made when they have been corrected.

An important part of the assessment is to ascertain where further staff **training** or instruction is required. This too should be planned and a note made when completed. Finally, the **date** of the next assessment should be set (at least annually). The risk assessment is therefore an ongoing process promoting continual improvements to the practice's safety standards.

General points
Many items covered by SOPs will be common to all parts of the practice (e.g. first aid, fire precautions, floor cleaning and disinfectants) and will not be mentioned below. In all work areas where hands are likely to become contaminated, it is worth considering the use of elbow taps on sinks and disposable towels.

Waiting room/reception
Probably the major potential hazard in this area is injury from unrestrained animals. The practice is liable for injuries sustained by any person on their premises, so it is important that clients are made aware (ideally by a sign outside the building) that all animals must be suitably restrained. Leads and cat baskets should be available in reception for clients who arrive without them and reception staff should give a verbal reminder to clients arriving with unrestrained animals.

Recently washed floors must be dried well or 'wet floor' warning notices displayed.

Should an accident occur, whether it involves a member of staff or a client, it is important that it is recorded in the accident book.

The consulting room
A special consideration here is the potential hazard of children becoming injured by contact with 'sharps' or pharmaceutical products. Ideally, drugs should be stored outside the consulting room. Where this is not practical, they must be kept well out of reach of children.

Clinical waste, including 'sharps', should be disposed of in the appropriate manner immediately after use.

The dispensary
The correct storage and dispensing of drugs (as recommended by the RCVS), including special provisions for controlled drugs, is an important factor and is discussed fully in Chapter 9.

Care must be taken when dispensing drugs that can be absorbed through the skin (e.g. cytotoxic drugs). Some individuals show skin hypersensitivity to antibiotics and so disposable gloves should be considered when handling tablets. The use of automatic tablet counters avoids direct handling altogether. Care must also be taken when dispensing small quantities of

powdered material that could be a hazard if inhaled. Face masks should be worn. Similarly, precautions may be needed if dispensing small volumes of liquid from a larger stock solution.

Stores
In most practices, space is at a premium and so storage often involves high shelving. Full consideration of the provisions of the Manual Handling Regulations should be made. Avoid putting heavy material on the highest shelf and provide non-slip stools in each room where they may be required (Figure 1.5). Where heavy items need to be transported within the practice (e.g. trays of petfood or anaesthetized dogs), a trolley should be available to avoid back injury. It is important to keep corridors free from stored material as this could impede rapid exit in the case of fire.

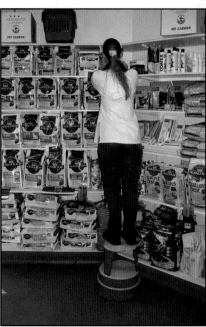

1.5
A non-slip stool should be used to reach higher shelves.

The practice laboratory
There are many potential hazards in the practice laboratory and strict attention to SOPs is required. This is considered in more detail in Chapter 17. In practices without a laboratory, it is important to adhere to the regulations for the postage of pathological specimens (Figure 1.6).

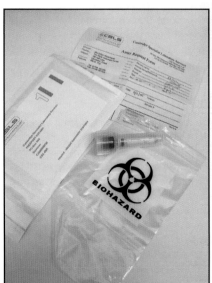

1.6
Equipment for safe postage of pathological specimens.

The X-ray room

The problems associated with radiation hazards (Figure 1.7) are discussed fully in Chapter 20. It is worth considering here the problems of disposing of spent developer and fixer solutions. The appropriate protective clothing should be worn when dealing with these chemicals and good ventilation is essential to avoid inhalation of fumes. Spent developer and fixer should not be discharged into the normal waste water supply, but stored in appropriate containers and removed by a licensed agent.

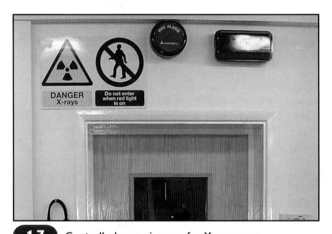

1.7   Controlled area signage for X-ray room.

The preparation area

The problems related to anaesthetic gas scavenging and monitoring are of significance in this area (Figure 1.8). In addition, the amount of animal hair should be reduced to a minimum, not only to improve general hygiene but also to reduce the risk of hypersensitivity reactions in some individuals.

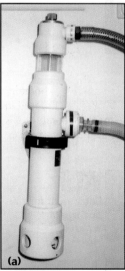

1.8   (a) Anaesthetic scavenger – Barnsley receiver. (b) Checking the scavenger.

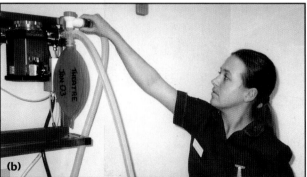

Dental scalers are often used in this area, and an SOP should be formulated to cover the use of masks and eye protection. In practices using oscillating saws to remove plaster casts, thought should be given to the control of the amount of dust, which could be hazardous if inhaled.

The operating area

There are no specific problems here not already dealt with elsewhere but it is worth considering the transport of animals to and from the theatre using trolleys and providing hydraulic tables to avoid excessive heavy lifting of animals.

The level of waste anaesthetic gases in the recovery area may be high as the animals exhale it on recovery. To keep this problem to a minimum, it is desirable to keep the animal connected to the anaesthetic circuit for as long as possible to make use of the scavenging system (ideally until extubation) (see Figure 1.8). Nevertheless, good ventilation is still essential in this area. Personal monitoring of exposure to anaesthetic pollutants is required and there are occupational exposure standards for the agents used.

Hospital kennels and catteries

Thought should be given to hygienic kennel protocols that reduce the risk of infection from zoonotic agents. The practice might consider the provision of isolation facilities (see Chapter 12) in cases where there is a known risk of zoonoses and there should be a written policy for dealing with cases where there is a known risk.

There should also be clear instructions to staff relating to the handling of animals and their transport within the building to avoid physical injury from bites and scratches, as well as from manual lifting procedures.

Safe handling, storage and disposal of anaesthetic agents

- The anaesthetic agents may be volatile liquids or injectable solutions. Each will have an individual COSHH Data Sheet outlining the potential hazards of exposure, the symptoms that might be seen following accidental exposure, and the recommended actions to be taken.
- The safe use of injectable anaesthetics involves storage, safe methods of injection, disposal of 'sharps', and the ultimate disposal of the empty bottles or vials.
- Consideration should also be given to how best to deal with accidental exposure following breakage of bottles.
- Volatile anaesthetics can cause pollution of the working environment and there are published maximum exposure limits (MELs).
- The level of pollution should be monitored on a regular basis and records kept.
- The level of pollution can be reduced by an efficient scavenging system, which may be active (using powered suction pumps) or passive. It is important that the equipment is well maintained and without leaks. It is also recommended that the vaporizers should be topped up at the end of the day in a well ventilated area.

Mortuary

Correct protective clothing and disinfection regimes are essential in this area. Special thought should also be given to precautions taken if postmortem examinations are to be performed on parrots, since there is the additional risk of the inhalation of the agent causing psittacosis from feather debris.

Staff rest room

Adequate rest room facilities should be provided to allow refreshments to be enjoyed away from the working areas. A sink should be provided specifically for the supply of drinking water and for washing up crockery.

Office

This is an area of the practice that is often ignored from the Health and Safety point of view. Hazards do occur, and further information can be obtained from the HSE booklet *Officewise*. There are guidelines relating to the minimum temperatures and lighting conditions for the workplace. The use of display screen equipment has been referred to above.

Car park/entrance

The Health and Safety legislation extends to the limit of the practice boundaries. Adequate lighting should be provided at night and consideration should be given to providing bins for the disposal of dog faeces.

Practice vehicles

Within vehicles, ensure that all drugs are stored safely and securely. Also make provision for the immediate disposal of clinical waste and 'sharps'. The habit of bringing trays of used syringes and needles back to the surgery for others to dispose of greatly increases the risk of accidental self-injection (which is especially important in relation to drugs such as prostaglandins).

On the farm

The same principles of Health and Safety apply when working on the farm. Many potential hazards relate to zoonotic infections. Farmers also have responsibilities under the Health and Safety at Work Act and the COSHH Regulations, and the veterinary surgeon's advice is very important in helping farmers to formulate their own SOPs with regard to zoonotic infections. Biosecurity also has to be considered where staff and vehicles are entering/leaving farm premises.

Using and managing equipment

The section above describing the range of potential hazards in veterinary practice identified the following in connection to using equipment:

* Electrocution
* Burns and scalds
* Eye strain from visual display screens
* Repetitive strain injuries
* Back injuries from poorly adjusted seating.

Each type of equipment will have its own range of hazards, but by considering first principles it is possible to draw up guidelines for their safe use. These should be incorporated into the practice SOPs. In addition, all equipment should be maintained according to the manufacturer's recommendations, and records of such services should be kept. Equipment can also be damaged, rendering it unsafe to use. There should be a procedure in place to report such damage and contingency plans to avoid use until repaired.

Further reading

HSE (1997) *First Aid at Work – Approved Code of Practice and Guidance.*

HSE (1998) *Five Steps to Risk Assessment.*

HSE (1998) *Manual Handling Regulations 1992 – Guidance on Regulations.*

HSE (1999) *COSHH – A Brief Guide to the Regulations.*

HSE (1999) *Essentials of Health and Safety at Work.*

HSE (1999) *RIDDOR Explained.*

HSE (2000) *First Aid at Work – Your Questions Answered.*

HSE (2000) *Management of Health and Safety at Work Regulations 1999 – Approved Code of Practice and Guidance.*

NOAH (1990) *The Safe Storage and Handling of Animal Medicines.*

RCVS Guidelines (1988) *Dispatch of Pathological Specimens by Post.*

Websites:
HSE   www.hse.gov.uk
RIDDOR   www.riddor.gov.uk

Chapter 2

Client communication and practice organization

Carol Gray and Carole Clarke

> ### *Learning objectives*
>
> After studying this chapter, students should be able to:
>
> - **Describe the basic skills involved in verbal and non-verbal communication**
> - **Recognize the structure of a consultation**
> - **Describe informed consent**
> - **List admission and discharge procedures for inpatients**
> - **Describe the legal and ethical responsibilities of veterinary nurses**
> - **Describe the principles of good record-keeping and organization**
> - **Describe the principles of handling appointments and reception duties, including processing payments and debt control**
> - **Consider all the relevant issues when controlling stock and ordering supplies**
> - **Describe the aims and basic organization of common nursing clinics**

Principles of communication

- True communication is a two-way process – someone sends a message and another person receives it.
- In fact, communication is based on a helical model: feedback from the receiver will strongly influence the sender of the message, and cause the sender to adapt the message or to reinforce it, to add further information or to stop transmission.

It is accepted that 93% of the meaning of a message is transmitted non-verbally, i.e. by means other than the actual words chosen.

Non-verbal communication consists of:

- Facial expression (including eye contact)
- Posture (including position of the two participants and any barriers between them, e.g. the examination table)
- Hand gestures (used to emphasize verbal communication)
- Proxemics (personal space – what is acceptable varies between cultures)
- Haptics (touch)
- Appearance (a professional appearance reinforces trust and confidence).

In fact, 55% of meaning is transmitted by facial expression or body language, with 38% by vocal tone. Only 7% of the meaning of a message is transmitted by the actual words spoken. This highlights the difficulty of talking on the telephone, or communicating in writing (including email communication). Communication by telephone or email is fraught with difficulty; with so much of a message being conveyed by body language and facial expression, how do we make sure that our written or spoken words mean what we intended when they reach their destination? Both methods allow the receiver to feed back – but how quickly, and do we pick up immediately what they are trying to tell us?

One-way communication

The ultimate vehicle for one-way communication is the written word. Brochures, flyers, websites, advertisements – they all rely on the meaning of the words used being unambiguous. They have to say exactly what they want the reader to receive. There is no margin for error. This is why proofreading is essential for all written material that is prepared for public scrutiny, both for spelling and grammar and for meaning. The content should also be tested on members of the target audience.

Public information about a veterinary practice must be accurate. Information about the practice is also transmitted by interpersonal communication, and disgruntled clients are likely to tell more people about their experiences than are satisfied clients.

Two-way communication

Telephone calls are a more severe test of communication skills. Why is the receiver reacting like this? Have we missed an important cue (it is more difficult to pick up verbal cues than non-verbal ones)? Does the receiver understand the sender correctly? Telephone communication can be practised by sitting with your back to another person and talking.

Email communication is like a slow-motion version of the telephone call. It takes longer to rectify an incorrect interpretation by the receiver, and you have to wait until the end of the message to question any difficult points.

Communicating with clients

It is useful to have a structure for client interviews, whether as part of a consultation in a nurse clinic, or when discharging an animal, or when dealing with an emergency that has been rushed in to the practice.

The veterinary consultation model has been adapted from the Calgary–Cambridge Observation Guide for medical interviews (Figure 2.1). It provides a framework for good practice, but can also be used to evaluate communication skills.

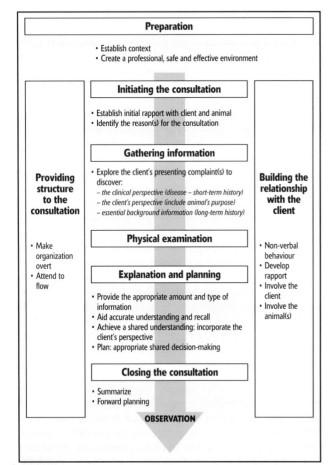

2.1 A guide to the veterinary consultation, based on the Calgary–Cambridge Observation Guide.

Preparation

Preparation is an integral part of the process. This involves ensuring that both the environment (e.g. the consulting room) and the person involved (i.e. the nurse) are ready.

Preparation of the room

- Privacy (no interruptions, no phone calls put through, no-one using the room as a thoroughfare).
- Safety (windows and doors closed to ensure safety of patient, chairs available if necessary for clients, clean and tidy environment).

Personal preparation

- Knowledge of patient's history (patient's medical records available and read, any extra information to hand).
- Mental (brain 'in neutral', especially if previous work was emotionally demanding).
- Appearance (professional, clean and tidy uniform, facial expression).

Opening the interview

It is essential that the first few seconds of the encounter go well; this is when the client decides whether they like the nurse and can trust them. How can you make a difference to their opinion? It is useful to open the interview with some general conversation. This is important because it puts the client at ease. Many people forget that taking an animal to a veterinary practice is actually quite stressful, and this can affect a client's behaviour and response. Some comments about the weather, or how hard it is to get parked near the surgery, or about the animal, can go a long way to easing the stress at the start. Of course, there are some cases where it is inappropriate to spend time chatting about other topics, e.g. with an emergency case or a planned euthanasia.

In nearly all cases, the first question that should be asked is an open question such as: 'What has been happening with Scamp?' or 'How has he been since the last time we saw him?'. The client should be allowed to reply, without interruption.

Gathering information

The process of gathering information involves tactical use of summarizing and screening, and making use of **open questions** (those that can have a number of possible answers) and **closed questions** (those that have a more defined answer).

Example: A client with a diabetic dog has come in for a regular check-up

Nurse: 'How's Scamp been since we last saw him?'

Client: *'Well, I've been quite pleased with him, but he didn't eat his breakfast one day last week, so I didn't give him his injection. He was a bit quiet that day, but the next day he was eating really well again so we went back to his normal routine. He doesn't seem to be drinking as much, and he has definitely got more energy. I worry about hurting him when I inject him, but I suppose he's quite used to it now.'*

Nurse (Summarizing): 'So, in general things are going well, but you had a problem when he didn't eat his breakfast. He seems to be better in himself, but you are concerned about the injections hurting him.'

Nurse (Screening): 'Is there anything else you need to discuss?'

Client: *'We go on holiday in two months' time. I'm not sure if we can put him in kennels or if I need to teach someone else in the family to inject him.'*

Use of closed questions can investigate this new information further:

Nurse: 'Is there someone else in the family who could look after him?'

So the basic principle is to start with open questions, then move to closed questions for specific bits of information. Other types of question may be useful, such as **multiple choice** if the client does not seem to understand what is being asked. For example, 'What is Scamp's reaction to the injection – does he squeal, or turn round, or just flinch slightly?'

It is important *not* to use **leading questions**, such as 'He's not drinking nearly so much now, is he?' where the phrasing of the question suggests the correct answer, or the answer that the questioner wants to hear.

Giving information

Information is best given in small pieces, regularly making sure that the client understands ('chunking and checking'). It is best to ask if the client has any questions about the information given, rather than asking if they understand what they have been told. Retention of information is increased if the client receives written or visual aids. It is important to determine the client's level of knowledge before embarking on an explanation, and to pitch language appropriately. In most cases, it is best to avoid the use of scientific or medical terminology ('jargon'), unless the client has indicated that they have specialized knowledge. Similarly, if the client's first language is not English, then explanations have to be carefully worded to avoid ambiguity. It is especially important to avoid the use of colloquial terms if language difficulties exist (e.g. 'put him down', 'knock him out', 'put him to sleep').

Closing the interview

It is important that the end of the interview is structured to provide a clear way forward and to delineate responsibilities. The client should feel adequately supported by the practice, and should have a named person to contact with any queries. If a return visit is needed, the client should be asked to return on a specific day and to make sure they see the same nurse. If you have agreed to telephone the client, or have asked the client to telephone you, decide on a day and a time and enter this in the diary so that you are available at that time.

Picking up cues

Clients will often signal when they are feeling a particular emotion. This signal may be verbal or non-verbal. Most people will ignore the signal. With training, nurses can learn to pick up on cues (signals) and respond appropriately to them. It is not difficult to learn this technique, and it can avoid escalation to extreme displays of emotion (where the signals become more obvious until you *have* to react to them).

It is perhaps easiest to start with non-verbal cues. The client may look worried when the nurse gives them a particular piece of information, or when they are telling them what has been happening with their animal. Going back to the diabetic dog, the client gave a cue that she was worried about giving injections. This could be picked up and acknowledged at the time: 'You said that you are worried about the injections hurting Scamp. Perhaps we can go through your injection technique again?' This could prevent the problem escalating to eventual non-compliance, where the client is so worried about the injections that he/she stops giving them.

Other causes of non-compliance can be identified and dealt with. For example, if a client has financial concerns about continuing treatment for a chronic condition, a discussion with the veterinary surgeon regarding choice of treatment and cheaper alternatives can be arranged. Or if a client cannot give the medication to the patient, offering supervision for the first few occasions or, in some cases, giving the treatment at the practice can alleviate this concern. Perhaps the client is not convinced that the treatment will help. Again, picking this up at an early stage and describing other similar, successful cases may deal with this concern. In each of these cases, it is vital to pick up cues from the client at an early stage, to ensure that the patient receives the treatment.

Most responses to cues will be empathic responses. For example, the client looks very concerned when the nurse is describing aftercare following surgery. This can be picked up on by saying, 'I can see that you are concerned about this. Is there anything in particular that is worrying you?'

Dealing with bereavement or breaking bad news

Empathy is particularly useful for dealing with a bereaved client, or when breaking bad news to a client. The classical processes of grief (shock/denial, guilt/anger, bargaining, acceptance) do not happen in every case, nor in that particular order. Identifying the client's emotional response correctly allows the nurse to use empathy in an appropriate way.

For example, if a client has just been told that their cat is positive for feline leukaemia virus, their response may be to question whether these are the correct results for their cat (denial). If the nurse can spot why this is happening, he/she can use empathy to try to help the client to move forward: 'I can see that this news is a great shock to you, and with his being so young, it's difficult to take it in. I'm so sorry that the result is positive.'

Appropriate use of silence is very important when breaking bad news. If the client is very upset, it is pointless to carry on talking, as they will not hear a word that you say. It is something that can be practised. Silences always seem awkward to the person who is breaking the bad news, but not to the client.

The nurse should always be prepared to deal with tears. A box of tissues, handed to the client at the right moment, signifies that 'it's all right to cry'. Silence is, again, an important part of dealing with a distressed client.

It is always difficult to decide whether touch can be used in this situation. If you have to think about it, don't do it. It is said that a light touch on the upper arm is the safest form, but with a client that the nurse knows well, a hug may be appropriate.

You should bear in mind the possibility of touch being misinterpreted by an emotionally distressed person, particularly if they are of the opposite sex.

Euthanasia

Clients require the most sensitive communication skills from professionals when they have decided to opt for euthanasia of their animal. This may be due to incurable disease, lack of finance to pay for treatment, because it is a kinder option for the patient, or for some other reason. The first thing to remember is how the client is feeling. If they are unable to afford treatment, they may be feeling guilty, or angry that they have been put in this position. In most cases, however, the predominant feeling is grief and overwhelming sadness. It is important that the nurse learns to deal with this, as he/she will meet it frequently. Skills that can be used include:

- Giving the client time to think, speak, show emotion
- Showing empathy
- Making sure that the procedure itself goes smoothly.

It is very distressing for clients to see their pet struggle, or for the procedure to go wrong. This possibility needs to be minimized. If you can see that the animal is distressed, it may be sedated first. Some veterinary surgeons will insert an intravenous catheter to minimize the chance of failure and this also allows the client to hold the animal while the injection is given.

Dealing with the financial aspect at the time of euthanasia is always difficult. The nurse should be guided by the practice policy. If it is a client unknown to the practice, they should be asked to settle the payment beforehand. Whilst some clients do prefer to settle their bill at the time, for many others dealing with the money at a later date is preferable and allows the client to be left with the animal afterwards, with all the time in the world to say goodbye. Sending the request for payment should not be combined with sending a sympathy card.

Euthanasia should always be adequately planned for, with a double appointment booked, or at the end of surgery. It also helps if there is a dedicated room in the practice, or at least a separate exit, to avoid the client having to go back through the waiting room.

Clients vary in their responses to grief. If a client seems to be severely affected, it may be advisable to contact friends or relatives (and, if possible, the client should not be sent home on their own). Bereavement counsellors are available in most areas and their numbers should be available at reception in each practice. Remember that you are not a trained counsellor, and should not take on areas beyond your expertise.

Dealing with anger

It is important to realize the reasons for a client's anger, to acknowledge these reasons, and to let the client know that you have acknowledged them. The main skill used in dealing with anger is empathy. You must also remain calm. Remaining seated while the client paces about is very difficult, but also highly effective. Keep your tone of voice much softer than the client's. Don't react to personal insults. An angry person needs a reaction to fuel the anger.

A checklist for dealing with anger may look like this:

- Remain outwardly calm
- Keep your voice low and even
- Try to stay at a lower level than the client (but see section on personal safety below)
- Use empathy ('I can see that you are very angry, and you have had an upsetting experience')
- Try to move things forward ('I am sorry that this has happened. How can we try to put it right?').

Personal safety

When dealing with anger, personal safety may be compromised. In this case, there should be some method of raising the alarm (e.g. panic buttons in consulting rooms) and an escape route. If a client has a history of anger, it would be sensible practice policy to ensure that no-one is left alone with them, or they should be asked to send another member of the family with the patient. It is essential to have a practice protocol on personal safety. Remember that a client with a grudge may pose a risk to every member of staff. If there are genuine concerns about the safety of practice staff, the local police should be informed.

Dealing with assertive clients

This seems to be the type of client who strikes fear into everyone's heart, but dealing with assertive clients can be less intimidating if a few golden rules are followed.

- **Acknowledge their expertise.** Most assertive clients feel that they have specialist knowledge about their animal and its condition. Treat them as if they know more than the average client. If they bring in pages printed out from the internet, take these from them and thank them for doing the research, telling them that the practice team will read the articles to increase their knowledge of the condition.
- **Involve them in the decision-making process.** All clients appreciate being part of a team involved in healthcare delivery, but assertive clients will react particularly positively to this strategy.
- **Do not dismiss their ideas for treatment.** Acknowledge that they could be right, although current research would suggest an alternative method is better. Perhaps you could try their method if the first method fails? You will have to put up with 'I told you so!' but you can admit that they were correct.
- **Do not be afraid to admit that you do not know.** It can be difficult if a client is demanding a particular method of care, but if you have no experience of this method, then say so. Refer the client to the veterinary surgeon in charge of the case.

Attitudes to animals

The main factors influencing an individual's attitudes to animals are:

- Culture and religion
- Socioeconomic status
- Health status.

Culture and religion

Religion is the basis for an ethical code for many people. Judaism and Christianity have promoted kindness to animals from a standpoint of the negative effect of cruelty to animals on the perpetrator and on the animal owner. Animals are regarded as possessions in the UK and in most Christian nations. Damage to someone else's property is not allowed either in law, or from a religious standpoint. There is also growing evidence of links between animal abuse and violence against other humans.

Many eastern religions, such as Buddhism, Hinduism and Jainism, give an intrinsic value to animals' lives, and belief in reincarnation means that cruelty to animals (or ending their lives) could be interfering with a fellow human in one of his other incarnations. Such religions will not allow euthanasia under any circumstances.

The Islamic faith has identified certain animals, for example the pig and the dog, as 'unclean' and many Muslims would never keep a dog in the house. They may have a guard dog, which is kept outside, and it is important that their religious beliefs are acknowledged when discussing care of this animal.

Socioeconomic status

People may attempt to use animal ownership to elevate their status socially (e.g. ownership of large aggressive dogs). It is often agreed that the UK's high level of animal welfare is a luxury that many poor countries cannot afford. However, in those countries a family's wealth is often dependent on the health and welfare of their animals. The UK is a relatively wealthy country and clients need to be allowed to decide for themselves how they wish to spend their money, and have all of the options for healthcare presented without any preconceptions about wealth.

Health status

Just as the family in a poor country might depend on their animals for their income, the assistance animal provides more than companionship alone. Assistance animals include guide dogs for blind people, hearing dogs for deaf people, assistance dogs for disabled people, dogs that alert epileptic owners to imminent fits, and even companion dogs that can help people with mental health problems to lead as normal an existence as possible. The effect on the client of illness or planned surgery on such dogs is enormous, and must be borne in mind when communicating risk and aftercare. If the dog is unable to work for a while, it is important to remember the effect this will have on the client's life.

It should also be remembered that animals can have a negative effect on human health. For example, people with asthma may refuse to rehome their pets and continue to live with a chronic disease rather than without their pets. Pets may potentially cause illness or injury to people on long-term medication, such as those on warfarin or immunosuppressants. Also, the risks of zoonotic diseases, such as ringworm, toxocariasis and toxoplasmosis, should be conveyed to pet owners.

How to improve your communication skills

- **Set up** a suitable encounter – this could be an actual conversation with a client (you must get consent from the client if you do this), or a role play with a colleague (Figure 2.2) or with a professional actor.
- **Video** this encounter.
- **Analyse** the encounter, describe what happened, the effect this had on the communication, and evaluate your skills (this can be done either on your own or with a few colleagues).
- **Reflect** on the exercise – what have you learned and how will you use this?
- **Start** again – changes in behaviour are effected by rehearsal.

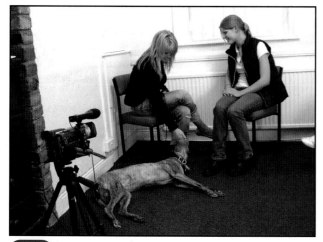

2.2   Role playing to improve communication skills.

Communicating with colleagues

A team works well when each member knows exactly where they fit into the team, what is expected of them, and how they can raise concerns or suggest improvements. A line management system that delineates responsibility, but also values and rewards initiative, will help to keep the team together and lead to greater employee satisfaction. Job descriptions and line management structure should be set out in contracts of employment. However, this ethos still requires effective communication between members of the team for it to work.

Regular formal communication is best achieved by holding team meetings. It can be difficult to arrange a time when everyone can attend. Meetings should be held at a fixed frequency and time, so that all members of the team know when they can next air their views. Some practices have a suggestion box that allows team members to post their concerns or comments anonymously. This can be a good idea, though it is better for the person with the concern to maintain responsibility for it until it is resolved.

The increasing use of email communication can allow members of the team to be given information and to comment on it, bearing in mind the limitations of this form of communication. This requires all members of the team to have access to a computer and to have their own email addresses.

Rewarding good performance by the team is vital. If the practice has had a particularly good month, then a message of congratulations, or even a celebratory party, is a real boost.

Appraisal

Most practices will monitor the performance of individual team members via the appraisal system, and this can be a worthwhile learning experience for both the appraiser and the appraised. However, the appraisal system only works if it is regarded as important enough to warrant protected time for meetings, and if the appraisal is seen as a reflective tool (known as a 360-degree appraisal in human healthcare). The person being appraised should be asked to evaluate their own performance first, and to suggest areas for improvement or training required. The appraiser then goes through a similar list and discusses any points of contention. Eventually both should reach consensus.

Not all appraisals go well or are seen as a positive experience. It is part of human nature to dislike criticism and to become defensive, to blame someone else, or to experience a delayed reaction that can manifest itself in odd behaviour (e.g. displacement activity, when the person involved cannot deal with the negative feelings of failure and so will spend hours on a seemingly trivial task). It is obviously much better if those involved realize their own failings and bring these to appraisal meetings, ready to discuss remedial action. Reflection is a vital aspect of professional life. Individuals must take responsibility for their actions, and must be able to be honest with themselves and to work out a plan for remedying any deficiencies. If reflection becomes part of the team ethos, with everyone willing to assess and evaluate what they do continually, then appraisals become a formal part of that cycle. A key professional skill is practising self-appraisal and being aware of personal strengths and weaknesses. For many people, this requires practice.

One way to do this is to look at 'critical incident analysis': choose one major event in which you are involved each day; reflect on it from the perspective of all people involved (including yourself). Soon, this will become a natural strategy for reflecting on your own practice.

Ethics and accountability: clinical audit

Practice teams can take the reflective ethos a stage further and investigate all areas of veterinary care on a regular basis. This requires someone to take responsibility for an area of practice, to investigate how this works in the practice and to compare the results with the evidence available on 'best practice'. This is known as clinical audit. Veterinary nurses can play an important part in this cycle by developing and investigating particular areas of interest.

Practices should implement a system of clinical governance, where important areas of the practice are subject to regular clinical audit. The areas selected will vary from one practice to another, depending on the type of work carried out, but should include both surgical and medical examples. The example below gives a rough idea of what is involved in a clinical audit.

Example: Clinical audit to review the nursing care of 'small pets' perioperatively

1. Decide on which species will be included (e.g. rabbits, rodents).
2. Consider what this practice does to care for small pets, i.e. what is the normal protocol (a) preoperatively, (b) during the operation itself, and (c) postoperatively.
3. Look at the mortality rate for small pets undergoing surgery in this practice over the past year. This will require access to case records and operating lists. There will be variable factors, such as different types and duration of anaesthesia, and these should be taken into account.
4. Consider how this compares with reported studies (research the literature).
5. Ask whether there is anything that the practice could change to improve its mortality rates (search the literature for 'best practice').
6. Implement changes.
7. Monitor results over the next year.
8. Repeat the exercise.

Areas of responsibility of the veterinary nurse

Surgical and medical admissions

Responsibility for admitting animals for surgical or medical interventions is likely to be delegated to the veterinary nurse. It is important to realize that this is an area where misunderstandings can develop. The veterinary nurse should be able to refer any difficult clients or situations back to a veterinary surgeon.

Identification

First of all, correct identification of the animal must be considered. There have been many horror stories of mix-ups; for example, the champion stud dog booked in for dental treatment that was mistakenly castrated in place of another dog of the same breed in the neighbouring kennel.

If the animal is microchipped or tattooed, mistakes are less likely to happen (provided that the chip or tattoo is read immediately before the operation). However, most animals will be brought in with only a collar for identification purposes (or

often, in the case of cats, no means of identification at all). How can the practice come up with a more foolproof method of identification? One idea, adapted from human hospitals, is to use disposable lightweight collars (tab band collars) for every inpatient. The collar should be marked with the patient's name and the procedure for which they have been admitted, written clearly. The name and telephone number of the practice must also be included (these can be pre-printed) in case of escape. These collars can be used for dogs, cats and rabbits.

Inpatient cards

An inpatient card for every surgical patient is common practice. Two cards are best: one card can accompany the patient into theatre, to be used for intraoperative checks and monitoring, while the other is left on the kennel to ensure that each animal is returned to the same kennel. The inpatient card should contain the following information: identity of patient, procedure, description, temperament, any special requirements (e.g. medication, fluids) and observation records. Accommodation should be clearly identified.

Admission health check

The admission procedure should also include a full health check. This allows assessment of temperament (this is useful before the patient is put in a kennel), investigation of feeding regime (when last fed and watered) and detection of any clinical abnormalities. At the very least, the patient should have a physical health check that includes TPR (temperature, pulse and respiration) observations. Some practices will offer preanaesthetic blood tests to surgical patients, to check hepatic and renal function. This may be offered to all surgical patients, or only to those undergoing non-elective procedures. It is important to conform to practice protocol in this area.

Isolation

Isolation cages should be available for both dogs and cats. Any animal showing signs of an infectious disease, whether likely to be contagious or not, should be isolated, with special guidelines for nursing. If the animal is booked for an elective procedure, it should be checked by a veterinary surgeon, as the surgery may need to be postponed and the animal sent home. Particular care must be taken with potential zoonotic diseases, such as ringworm. All staff must be made aware of the risks to their health if such animals are admitted.

Possessions

Many practices refuse to take in clients' possessions when admitting animals but sometimes it is necessary to accept them (e.g. collars and leads, cat baskets). These should be clearly labelled with the names of the client and the patient. Similarly, any other possessions taken in must be clearly labelled, with a note on the inpatient card of what has been left. When discharging the patient, the person responsible should sign to indicate that the possessions have been returned to the client.

Admission procedure
1. Check patient identification.
2. Check client identification.
3. Check when last fed/watered.
4. Complete patient ID tag/collar.
5. Complete inpatient cards.
6. Make a health check.
7. Gain client consent.
8. Label possessions.
9. Advise on time to phone or time to collect.

Informed consent

Consent for any surgical procedure on an animal (including admission for blood sampling and radiography) must be obtained from the owner or their representative (Figure 2.3). Under English law, animals are regarded as property and owners have the ultimate sanction over what happens to their animals.

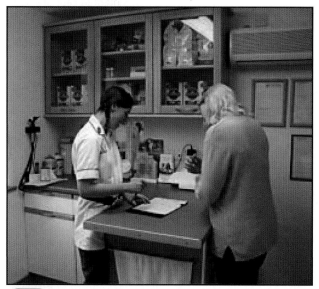

2.3   Obtaining consent from a client.

Informed consent requires:

- A detailed description of exactly what is going to be done to the animal
- Any side effects or risks of death or injury that are associated with the procedure
- Any alternative treatments or diagnostic options available.

The person seeking to obtain the owner's consent should be appropriately trained (and qualified) to give a full explanation of the procedure. Reliance on written consent forms should be minimal; the detail of the form should be explained verbally, with any scientific jargon simplified. In human medicine, informed consent includes information on who is going to perform the procedure, but this is not usually included for veterinary practice. The main exception to this is when a veterinary nurse undertakes minor surgery under Schedule 3 of the Veterinary Surgeons Act, in which case the owner should be told that a veterinary nurse will perform the surgery.

Consent is usually obtained in writing, which makes it easier for any subsequent complaints to be investigated. There are exceptions, such as telephone consent for euthanasia while an animal is anaesthetized. In this case, two people should obtain verbal consent from the owner and this should be written in the case notes as soon as possible. Many veterinary surgeons do not ask owners of terminally ill animals to sign consent forms if they have been involved in the treatment along the way. However, it is sensible practice to get written consent for euthanasia in most instances.

Financial estimates

The consent issue also falls under the law of contract. That is why it is important to give financial estimates for the treatment. Estimates are a rough guide to cost. If they are going to be exceeded, the owner must be kept informed of this. Some elective procedures will have fixed costs; these are then quotes rather than estimates, and must be adhered to if the surgery proceeds normally.

Should financial information be included on a consent form? It can prevent the client from considering the other aspects of consent. It would be better practice to use two forms: one for consent to the procedure, and one for consent to financial obligations.

Legal age of consent

In order to be party to a financial contract (which is what is essentially being described here), the person signing the form must be at least 18 years of age. However, the age for legal medical consent is 16. It would be possible for a 16-year-old to give consent for the surgical procedure, but there would be no guarantee that the bill would be paid. That is why most practices insist on a minimum age of 18 for signing consent forms.

Discharging inpatients

If given responsibility for returning an animal to a client (Figure 2.4), it is important to know the full facts about the case or procedure, so that any questions that the client may have can be answered.

- Remember the 'chunking and checking' technique for giving information, and allow the client time to think about questions they may want to ask.
- Make sure that both you and the client know what happens next, and reassure them that there is a 24-hour service available for emergencies.

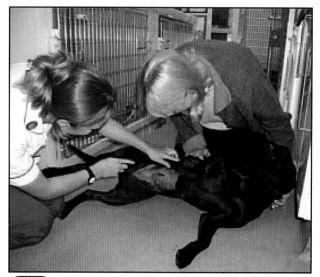

2.4   Discharging a patient postoperatively.

Discharge procedure

1. Check patient identification.
2. Check client identification.
3. Prepare discharge sheet (pre-printed for common procedures?).
4. Prepare medication.
5. Explain procedure/aftercare to client.
6. Collect/check possessions left with patient.
7. Bring patient through from ward.
8. Arrange next visit.

Legal and professional aspects of veterinary nursing

Veterinary nurses must comply with legal and professional guidelines. This topic is explored further in Chapter 3.

Criminal law

Criminal law involves 'crimes' against the State, i.e. breaking the law of the land as written in its legislation (Acts of Parliament), which exists to protect society. For veterinary nurses, legal accountability in criminal law involves compliance with the terms of the Veterinary Surgeons Act 1966, which governs the practice of veterinary surgery. It also involves abiding by the laws that concern animal welfare, such as the Protection of Animals Act 1911, the main anti-cruelty legislation in the UK. This will soon be updated by the Animal Welfare Bill, when it becomes law.

Veterinary Surgeons Act 1966

The Veterinary Surgeons Act sets out lists of those who are allowed to treat animals, restricting most veterinary treatment to qualified veterinary surgeons and approved veterinary students. Exemptions from this restriction are listed in Schedule 3.

Paragraph 6, added in 1991, allows qualified veterinary nurses to carry out medical and minor surgical procedures under the direction of a veterinary surgeon. A 2002 amendment allows student veterinary nurses to carry out medical and surgical procedures under supervision.

For correct interpretation of this important piece of legislation, it is necessary to clarify the terms used in Schedule 3 and its amendments. Paragraphs 6 and 7 refer to exemptions from restrictions on practise – treatment and operations that may be given or carried out by unqualified persons, specifically qualified and student veterinary nurses (see Chapter 3).

- **Direction** means that the veterinary surgeon has given the responsibility for carrying out the procedure to the veterinary nurse, but does not necessarily have to be present when the procedure is carried out.
- **Supervision** means that the veterinary surgeon or veterinary nurse is present throughout, and watches as the trainee veterinary nurse performs the procedure.

Civil law

Veterinary nurses also have accountability in civil law. Civil law protects an individual from the harm caused by another individual (or company). Although this individual or company may not have committed a crime, the person who has been caused harm can try to remedy the situation by taking the case to a civil court. In many cases, the person caused harm (the plaintiff) is awarded damages, a sum of money as compensation for the harm they have suffered. This brings in the idea of **duty of care**, a phrase that is used to decide many civil cases. Does the person being sued have a duty of care to the plaintiff? If so, has that duty of care been breached? If so, has this resulted in loss, damage or injury? If so, the plaintiff may be entitled to damages, a sum of money to compensate for the loss.

Veterinary nurses owe a duty of care to a client whose animal is in for treatment.

Example

While the nurse is leading the animal through from the kennels to the X-ray room, the animal escapes from the practice via a door that has been left open. The animal is never seen again.

The client can sue the veterinary nurse for damages as a result of negligence.

If the court feels that a reasonable person with the veterinary nursing qualification would not have allowed the animal to escape, it may find the nurse to be liable and award damages to the owner.

Alternatively, the client could sue the practice for not having a system in place that prevented escape of an animal.

Legal responsibility for owner injury when handling animals

It is recognized that the veterinary surgeon is in charge of risk assessment when an animal is presented for treatment at the surgery, or when visiting the client at home. It is important that the animal does not injure the client. There have already been a few cases in the UK where clients have received severe injuries during the course of their animal's receiving veterinary treatment, and have successfully claimed against the veterinary surgeon's indemnity insurance. It is sensible that an experienced nurse should handle any animal likely to cause injury, using all the restraint aids that are available. In the USA, most practices have signs advising clients that technicians (the American equivalent of veterinary nurses) will always handle animals for examination and treatment.

Professional accountability

To whom are veterinary nurses accountable? This depends on who is governing the profession. At the moment, all veterinary nurses have accountability to their employers. They are therefore governed by the regulatory system described in the Veterinary Surgeons Act, and any misdemeanours by veterinary nurses will result in disciplinary action by the Royal College of Veterinary Surgeons (RCVS) against their employers.

The setting up of the Veterinary Nurses Council heralded a change in the way that the nursing profession may regulate itself in future. Professional accountability will be laid down by Council, in the form of guidance on professional conduct, and any misdemeanours may then be dealt with directly by Council. From January 2007, a voluntary scheme will allow veterinary nurses who qualified before 2003 to choose to become registered. All recently qualified veterinary nurses will be registered automatically.

As an example of how things may change, let us consider the following case. A veterinary surgeon is reported to the RCVS for allowing a veterinary nurse to carry out dental extractions. In fact, the veterinary surgeon was not even on the premises at the time. The RCVS decides that the veterinary surgeon is guilty of disgraceful professional conduct and decides to strike the surgeon's name from the Register. At the moment, in such a case there is no mechanism for disciplining the veterinary nurse, who was carrying out illegal acts of veterinary surgery beyond the limits of the nurse's responsibility. Should the profession start to regulate itself, the veterinary nurse in this case would be reported to the VN Council and would have to explain why this happened. The VN Council would then decide how to deal with the nurse.

Royal College of Veterinary Surgeons

The RCVS is given the powers of regulation of the veterinary profession via the Veterinary Surgeons Act. It produces a *Guide to Professional Conduct* for veterinary surgeons and also a separate professional conduct guide for qualified veterinary nurses. It is responsible for the registration of qualified veterinary surgeons and listing of qualified veterinary nurses, and maintains the standards of veterinary education through regular visits to veterinary schools in the UK. It took over responsibility for veterinary nurse training from the BVNA, and approves Veterinary Nursing Assessment Centres and Training Practices.

In 2005 the RCVS Practice Standards Scheme was introduced. Practices can be accredited in different categories, depending upon the nature of the practice. The scheme includes Core Standards (comprising mainly legal and Health and Safety requirements), species-specific standards (e.g. Small Animal, Farm Animal, Equine) and Small Animal or Equine Hospital standards. There are additional standards for Emergency Service Clinics. All practices within the scheme are inspected regularly. Details of these standards, the inspection process, fees and how to apply are available from the RCVS. Accredited practices can use the approved logos available for each type of practice.

Guide to Professional Conduct

All individual veterinary surgeons must comply with the requirements set out in the *RCVS Guide to Professional Conduct*, which is distributed to every registered veterinary surgeon. It is regularly updated to keep abreast of changes in practice. It provides guidance on such areas as **supersession** and **referrals** (see later).

Professional ethics

This covers the way that members of the profession deal with colleagues, both veterinary nurses and veterinary surgeons. It is unethical to criticize a colleague in front of a client; not only is it bad for the colleague, but it is bad for the profession too. If a colleague has admitted doing something that is unethical, the correct procedure is to report this to the employer (in the first instance), or to the profession's governing body if the employer is unwilling to deal with it. 'Whistle-blowing', or reporting cases of unprofessional behaviour, can lead to unpleasantness at work, but the 'whistle-blower' cannot be dismissed for reporting their concerns.

Personal ethics

Whereas a code of professional ethics will be composed by the profession's governing body, each individual has a code of personal ethics – a sense of what is right and what is wrong, even if some things that they regard as wrong are legal. For example, a veterinary nurse might think that euthanasia of healthy animals is wrong, whatever the circumstances. The nurse could discuss the problem with the employer, and come to an arrangement that suits both parties, such as the nurse being allowed to refuse to assist with such euthanasia procedures.

Important animal-related legislation

Veterinary nurses need to be aware of important legislation pertaining to the keeping of animals (see also Chapter 3). Legislation is changing constantly and it is a good idea to keep up to date with animal-related legislation by visiting the DEFRA (Department for Environment, Food and Rural Affairs) website at www.defra.gov.uk. DEFRA now has responsibility for all animal health and welfare-related legislation, except for the Animals (Scientific Procedures) Act 1986, which protects animals used for research. This is still monitored by the Home Office.

Dangerous animals

People may require licences for keeping certain types of animal (e.g. dangerous wild animals, zoo animals, endangered exotic animals, dogs used for breeding). Owners of certain breeds of dog may need to register them under the Dangerous Dogs Act 1991. This Act deals with dogs of breeds that are regarded as 'dangerous' and allows a destruction order to be imposed after one biting incident.

Cruelty to animals

The Protection of Animals Act, the main law preventing cruelty to animals, has been in force since 1911 but anti-cruelty laws may soon be updated. The proposed new Animal Welfare Act brings together all the current anti-cruelty legislation and also introduces the concept of preventing poor welfare, allowing owners to be prosecuted if the way in which they are keeping animals is not in the interests of the animals' welfare. According to the *RCVS Guide to Professional Conduct*, the usual obligations to client confidentiality can now be broken in cases where animal abuse is suspected.

Wildlife

The Wildlife and Countryside Act 1981 protects native species of animals and plants. Certain non-native species of wild animal cannot be re-released into the wild after being found injured and treated; this list includes the grey squirrel and the Canada goose.

Spread of animal disease

The Animal Health Act 1981 allows legislation to be passed to prevent the spread of serious animal diseases, including zoonoses such as rabies. Companion animals may be subject to a variety of controls in such an outbreak, ranging from a complete curfew (cats) or a requirement to be muzzled and kept on leads (dogs), to being banned from certain areas (dogs, horses).

Practice organization

Duties and rights

In employment

Every employee should have a contract of employment or a written statement of particulars of employment that sets out full details of the employment, including job title, pay, hours, location, holiday entitlement, pensions, sickness, and disciplinary procedures. Ideally, this should be agreed and signed before starting work but, if not, should be in place within two months.

- **Employers** have a duty to provide a safe workplace, to expect employees to work within the Working Time Directive unless opted out, and to offer the statutory employment rights in force at any time.
- **Employees** have a duty to work within the contract and also to abide by any rules the employer may make, such as dress and behaviour codes, specific ways of working, and Health and Safety codes of practice.

- Employers should **consult** with employees over certain areas of work (e.g. Health and Safety – see Chapter 1).

Employees have statutory employment rights, which may vary according to length of service and to their specific contracts. All pregnant employees are entitled to statutory maternity leave according to current regulations and time off for antenatal appointments and parenting classes. Statutory paternity leave is also an entitlement after a minimum length of service. Unpaid time off for emergency leave is also an entitlement and definitions are available on the ACAS website (www.acas.org.uk) and the Department of Trade and Industry website (www.dti.gov.uk).

Discrimination at work must be avoided and there is specific legislation to deal with this. It is illegal to discriminate against people at work on the grounds of age, gender, disability, race, religion or belief or sexual orientation. Not only must employers take care not to discriminate, but employees must ensure that they do not discriminate in their daily work or if in a supervisory capacity.

Bullying and harassment must be avoided. If an employee is uncertain of their rights or is unhappy about their or anyone else's treatment at work, it is advisable to seek professional advice. As well as its excellent website, ACAS has a free helpline (08457 474747) and the British Veterinary Nursing Association (BVNA) will also be able to advise.

Discussing the issues informally with an employer is always best but if that is impossible the grievance procedure should be used. If a workplace does not have a grievance procedure, the grievance should be put in writing to the employer and a response should be received in due course. If this is not done, it may be difficult to argue the case if it goes to an employment tribunal. This is a very complex area and further information is available on the above websites for ACAS and the Department of Trade and Industry.

In relation to clients and colleagues

In addition to the rights and duties outlined above, nurses have a duty to maintain confidentiality in relation to clients and colleagues, and to treat everyone they meet at work with respect and courtesy and without discrimination. These issues are covered elsewhere in this chapter.

It is the duty of the employee to take responsibility for their own safety at work and that of their colleagues (see Chapter 1). This means working to safe codes of practice and using personal protective equipment where required. Veterinary nurses are in a good position to check the condition of such equipment, ensure that it is used correctly and alert senior staff to any shortcomings. Unsafe working practices must always be brought to the attention of senior staff. The safety of clients and contractors is paramount when on practice premises, and nurses should advise clients not to take risks when handling their pets in the practice (see later). To ensure the safety of other visitors to the practice a risk assessment should be made (see Chapter 1) and the visitors should be properly briefed on health and safety issues.

Keeping and organizing records

Efficient record-keeping is essential for maintaining good communication within the practice. Accurate records aid patient care, protect the practice from legal challenges and are vital for proper financial control. Records may be paper-based and electronic or include other media.

Types of records a practice might keep

- Client records with contact information
- Supplier records
- Medical records, including ward or hospitalization notes, anaesthetic charts, laboratory results, slides, radiographs, digital images and recordings
- Personnel records, including salary records, recruitment records, application forms and staff appraisals
- Financial records, bank statements and invoices
- Payment records, electronic payment slips
- Health and Safety records, accident records, risk assessments and local rules
- Training records, NVQ assessments, internal verifier reports, portfolio tracking records
- Monitoring, e.g. closed circuit television (CCTV) tapes, or recordings of telephone conversations
- Correspondence.

Practices that keep personal records of staff or clients must comply with the Data Protection Act 1998 (DPA). This requires that anyone holding information about living individuals in electronic format, and in some cases on paper, must follow the eight data protection principles of good information handling.

Personal information must be:

- Fairly and lawfully processed
- Processed for specific purposes
- Adequate, relevant and not excessive
- Accurate and, where necessary, kept up to date
- Not kept for longer than is necessary
- Processed in line with the rights of the individual
- Kept secure
- Not transferred to countries outside the European Economic Area unless there is adequate protection for the information.

The DPA requires that data users, including some veterinary practices, must notify the Information Commissioner if they wish to use records for particular purposes. Practices can complete a simple checklist at www.informationcommissioner.gov.uk, where full guidance on the Act and need for notification is easy to access. Notification is straightforward with a standard fee in 2005 of £35.00. The DPA also gives all individuals certain rights, including the right to see information that is held about them and to have it corrected if it is wrong. Clients may request access to their records under the Act.

Clarity and accuracy

Accurate record-keeping will increase the confidence that clients have in the practice. Clarity, legibility and accuracy are vital; poorly spelt names, untidy writing or an inability to read a colleague's notes do not present a good impression.

Records should be easy to understand by anyone required to access them (Figure 2.5). This may include referral clinicians, practice staff, clients, or a new practice if the client moves house. Only commonly understood abbreviations should be used, and developing a standard list for the practice will help with this and in training junior staff. Records should be kept of every clinical examination and should include: presenting signs, history, results of the physical examination, clinical findings, differential diagnoses and treatment plan. It is good practice to outline any conversations with the client, including notes on decision-making and whether a client declines a recommended treatment.

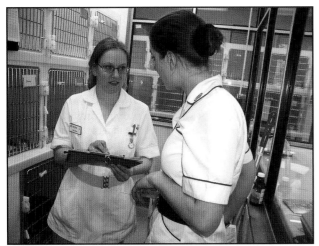

2.5 Clear and comprehensive records are essential when handing over cases to colleagues.

Financial information (e.g. fees, drugs and consumables costs, payments and balance outstanding) may be kept on the clinical record. It can also be kept on a separate system, though auditing of charging can then be more difficult.

Both financial and clinical records should be written up at the time or as soon as possible afterwards. Contemporaneous notes (those made at the time) are particularly valuable in solving any disputes about what was said, and are generally more accurate than notes written up later.

Medical and financial records should never be altered. If editing is necessary, a note should be included explaining why, and the alteration should be clear. Computer systems should either forbid editing or should maintain an audit trail of any editing that has taken place.

Records should be objective – based on observation and factual information, with subjective opinions included only where they are relevant, perhaps where a risk assessment has influenced decision-making or where a diagnosis is unclear. Never should anything personal be written about a client, particularly disparaging comments or tongue-in-cheek notes. At any time, the records could end up in a court of law and the practice needs to be happy with their quality. Particular care should be taken not to write any false or defamatory statements about a person (libel), or make any malicious, false or injurious spoken statements about anyone (slander). Information about a person's character or financial situation should never be taken outside the practice, and it is good practice never to talk disparagingly about a client or another member of staff within the practice either.

If records are computerized, there should be a supply of temporary paper record sheets, price and data guides for use if there is a loss of power. Records can be input later when power is restored.

Filing

Records should be stored conveniently near where they are needed, using an appropriate filing system. Rarely used files can be stored away from the clinical areas, with commonly used ones in reception or close to where they are needed.

Alphabetical filing

Clients' paper or card records are generally filed alphabetically. In veterinary practice, where different members of the family may bring pets in at different times, a system based on surname and house number or pet name may be preferable to

surname and initials. Computerized records can search on a number of parameters, including pet name, owner name and address, and reduce the drudgery and error of manual filing.

Chronological filing

Other records, such as dental charts, radiographs, ECGs and laboratory reports, can be filed in date order and cross-referenced on the client record. This chronological filing is much quicker to maintain than alphabetical filing, as each new record can be filed on top of the last one. Archiving old records is also simpler with this system and saves the continual file expansion required in an alphabetical system.

Electronic storage

It is now possible for laboratory results to be emailed into the practice and attached directly to client computer records, for ECG tracings and radiographs to be stored digitally, and for records to be shared between veterinary surgeons via the internet. This saves storage space and makes retrieval much faster. As electronic storage increases, however, practices will need to review their back-up systems to include the increasing number and size of files.

Labelling

All files should have a standard labelling system, whether in hard copy or electronic format. This will generally include the owner and animal name plus a reference number and date. Radiographs should be permanently identified at the time of exposure.

File markers

Non-electronic files should always be returned to their files after use – a marker can be inserted into the space as the file is removed to aid replacement (Figure 2.6). The marker can be useful if a file remains missing: staff can be alerted to chase up its return.

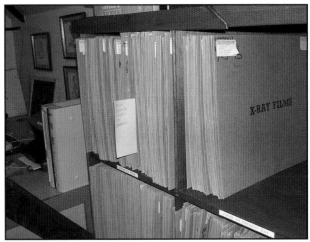

2.6 Marking where an X-ray file has been removed makes correct replacement simpler and also alerts staff that the file is missing in the meantime.

Security

Records should be recorded on permanent material, such as good quality paper or other media. Paper records should be stored securely, under lock and key if necessary.

Computers

Magnetic media such as back-up tapes or floppy discs should be stored in a clean dry place away from possible sources of radiation or magnetism. Compact discs and DVDs should be kept in protective cases and clearly identified. Computer records should be regularly backed up on to storage media, and these back-ups should be verified so that the data are reliable for restoring on to the system should the need arise. A minimum of daily backing up is recommended for medical records and financial information, and weekly for less sensitive records. Back-up files should be stored off-site or in secure fireproof safes. Many computer networks now include automatic back-up, with duplicate hard drives to take over if one fails, and some are web-based with central holding of data. Practices should verify the integrity and security of data if stored remotely by a third party.

Computers should be protected by using uninterruptible power supplies to allow controlled shut-down in the event of power loss, and by using surge protectors. It is best not to install computers in dirty areas, such as where animals are clipped or where there are high moisture levels. If this is unavoidable, regular vacuum cleaning around them will prevent dust and hair from building up, and keyboard covers should be used to protect against spills and contamination.

Records may be stolen and so hard copies should not be left out on reception desks or in other public areas. Computers, particularly laptops, are very attractive to casual thieves; locking devices to fix them down and alarms are recommended. Computers should never be left in vehicles, and care should be taken if staff take laptops home with practice data on them. Protection of data with secure passwords is essential so that unauthorized personnel cannot gain access.

Purging, archiving and disposal

To reduce size and to comply with the DPA, old or unused files should be archived or discarded regularly. There are no legal limits on document storage times, but in general:

- **Financial, tax and PAYE records** should be kept for 6 years after the financial year end
- **Medical records, radiographs, etc.** should be kept for at least 6 years in case of legal claims, and longer if deemed necessary by the clinician
- **Practice insurance records** for employer liability should be kept indefinitely, and it may be prudent to keep Health and Safety records and staff appraisal records of current staff as long as practicable
- **Recruitment records**, such as application forms and references from unsuccessful candidates, should not be kept longer than 6 months.

Archived records should be stored securely until destroyed. Garden sheds and outhouses are not suitable; secure storage should be available. Computers should be disposed of only after permanently erasing any sensitive data. Paper records should be destroyed by shredding or burning, or by using a professional confidential waste contractor.

Access and ownership of records

RCVS guidance recognizes that clients who now have access to their own medical records are likely to seek similar access to their pets' records. In such cases it may be helpful, on the direction of a veterinary surgeon, for a client to be offered sight of the records at the surgery by appointment at a mutually convenient time.

Case records including radiographs and similar documents are the property of, and should be retained by, veterinary surgeons in the interests of animal welfare and for their own protection. Copies with a summary of the history should be passed on request to a colleague taking over the case. Where a client has been specifically charged and has paid for radiographs or other reports, the client is legally entitled to them. However, the practice may choose to make it clear that they are charging not for the radiographs but for diagnosis or advice only. In appropriate circumstances they may be prepared also to provide copies of the radiographs. Practices should consider clarifying their position on ownership of and access to diagnostic material in their standard terms of business document.

Disclosure of records may be ordered in disciplinary or court hearings, and the RCVS may request copies of case records routinely in the course of investigating a complaint.

Confidentiality

The veterinary nurse must maintain the confidentiality of client and practice information at all times, and should not discuss professional or privileged information outside the practice.

RCVS Guide to Professional Conduct guidance on confidentiality:

- The veterinary surgeon/client relationship is founded on trust, and in normal circumstances a veterinary surgeon must not disclose to any third party any information about a client or their animal either given by the client or revealed by clinical examination or by postmortem examination. This duty also extends to associated support staff
- In circumstances where the client has not given permission for disclosure but the veterinary surgeon believes that animal welfare or public interest are compromised, the RCVS may be consulted before any information is divulged. (See 'Important animal-related legislation' above)
- Permission to pass on confidential information may be express or implied. Express permission may be either verbal or in writing, usually in response to a request. Permission may also be implied from circumstances, for example in the making of a claim under a pet insurance policy, when the insurance company becomes entitled to receive all information relevant to the claim and to seek clarification if required
- Registration of a dog with the Kennel Club permits a veterinary surgeon who carries out surgery to alter the natural conformation of a dog to report this to the Kennel Club.

If there is any doubt about the disclosure of any information, confirmation should be sought from a practice veterinary surgeon or from the RCVS. In particular, giving out details over the telephone to any third party is not recommended, due to the difficulty in identifying the parties involved. People may not be who they say they are. Where it is considered that client information should be divulged on animal welfare or public interest grounds, the severity and urgency of the issues should be considered carefully, as should the options to resolve the issue without disclosure. Involving a third party may destroy the veterinary surgeon/client relationship and make resolution of the problem more difficult.

Receptionist duties

Every client will make contact with the practice initially by telephoning or dropping into reception, and the welcome and response they receive may make or break the practice/client relationship. If possible, the nurse or receptionist on the front desk should not be distracted by other duties. Every client should be greeted immediately and needs full attention. It is the receptionist's job to find out why the client has made contact, and to ascertain their needs and priorities, before ensuring that these needs are met, the client's questions are answered and any action required is followed up efficiently so that expectations are not just met, but exceeded.

The nurse in reception must:

- Feel confident and in control
- Have a well organized tidy area to work in
- Understand all the relevant practice processes and protocols
- Know how to make and record appointments
- Know which personnel are available and when
- Know how to prioritize appointments so that urgent cases are seen quickly, and be able to offer interim advice to the client
- Know how much time to allow for each appointment so that the clinical staff do not 'run behind'
- Have a good rapport with the clients and a professional and friendly manner that puts clients at their ease
- Know when and where to ask for assistance
- Be able to handle sales transactions and process payments.

Working on reception can be more stressful than working behind the scenes, for two main reasons. First, the nurse is 'on show' and may be worried about how much they know and how they come across to others. Secondly, on reception it is more difficult to control the flow of work, and there will be busy and slack periods. Clients with difficult queries or complaints never come into an empty reception area! If you are a student nurse, it may help to explain that you are learning and ask people to bear with you if you are not working as quickly as your colleagues. Clients are usually supportive if they know that someone is new to the job, particularly if they ask for help appropriately. In quieter periods, the nurse can chat to the clients and patients and get to know them – this helps the nurse to relax and can build relationships that may last a whole career. Filing and tidying can be done along the way.

Confidence on reception and on the telephone comes with experience and practice. The more confident the nurse becomes, the more they will enjoy interacting with the clients and their pets (Figure 2.7).

Most practices have a sales area in reception and the nurse must be familiar with all the products and how they are used so that they can recommend them to clients. It is important to understand the practice's protocols for selling and approving prescription-only medicines.

Keeping reception and the waiting area clean and neat means walking around regularly, removing out-of-date notices and other clutter, making sure that children's toys are clean and tidy and that magazines look inviting. Plants or flowers should be fresh and healthy.

Confidence and respect will be gained from having appropriate, neat and clean uniform or clothes, polished shoes and tidy hair. If you have just been working in the clinical areas, check that you have no splashes of blood or clumps of hair on your clothing.

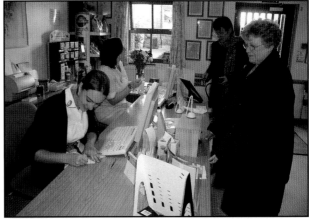

2.7 A busy reception area. Confidence comes with experience.

Handling appointments

Although many veterinary practices still hold open surgeries, where clients are seen in the order they arrive, most now have at least some appointment-only surgeries. Depending on the practice's policy, appointments may be made just for a specific time, or also to see a specific veterinary surgeon or nurse. Diaries may be in book or loose-leaf form or may be on computer. The advantage of a computerized diary is that it can be linked to the records themselves, is easier to change and can often be accessed anywhere in the building, even remotely.

Appointments may be for a set time, e.g. 10 minutes, or may be run on a flexible basis. For example, 5-minute slots may be used, with puppy vaccinations being allowed 20 minutes, suture removals 5 minutes, repeat prescription checks 10 minutes, and so on.

Most people telephone for an appointment or make one on the previous visit. It is vital to ensure that the owner's and animal's names have been recorded accurately. If the appointment is for a new client, a telephone number should be taken so that they can be contacted if necessary.

Priorities

Often, the practice will have quiet and busy periods. The quieter times should be offered first, leaving the popular times for those who have no option but to come in then. When prioritizing appointments, consideration should be given to the urgency of the case, the preference of the owner, available staff and the possibility that the client may be able to book elsewhere. Clients may be looking for a particular time or day rather than a particular veterinary surgeon, and losing the appointment to a neighbouring practice may mean losing the lifetime value of that pet to the practice – a substantial sum of money.

Emergencies and delays

Recognition of emergencies is covered elsewhere but emergency cases should be seen as soon as possible and may have to take priority over existing appointments. The situation should be explained to those waiting – most will be happy to wait. If possible, due clients should be telephoned and asked to rebook or warned that there will be a wait. The veterinary nurse should never say, 'We are running behind,' or, 'The vet is busy,' but should always give as much information as permitted about the nature of the emergency or difficult case without identifying animal or owner (clients are always interested in what is going on behind the scenes). For long waits, clients should be updated on the situation at least every 10 minutes or given an option to return later or rebook. The veterinary surgeons and nurses should be consulted on difficult days to decide how to handle the list. As clients with appointments arrive, they should be seen in the order of appointment rather than order of arrival, unless someone is late.

Second opinions and supersession

New clients should always be asked whether the animal is currently under treatment. It is not unusual for clients to seek a second opinion or to try a new veterinary surgeon during a course of treatment. In these situations, all veterinary surgeons must follow the guidelines in the *RCVS Guide to Professional Conduct*. The client is free to choose whichever veterinary practice they wish, and veterinary surgeons should not obstruct a client from changing to another veterinary practice, nor should they discourage a client from seeking a second opinion. If a veterinary surgeon sees an animal that has been treated elsewhere for its current problem, the previous veterinary surgeon should be contacted as soon as possible to obtain details of the case and medications prescribed. This guidance is given in the interests of the patient, but informing a colleague of a consultation with their former client is also professional courtesy and helps them to know what has happened with the case.

The taking over of a patient in this way is termed **supersession**. Occasionally a client will be embarrassed about changing practices and may attempt to withhold details of their previous veterinary surgeon. A gentle explanation that the history is important for the health of their pet usually helps them to understand why it is necessary to talk to the previous veterinary surgeon. In an emergency it is acceptable to make an initial assessment and administer any essential treatment before contacting the original veterinary surgeon.

Veterinary surgeons may also advise clients to seek a second opinion, particularly where there may be doubt about the diagnosis. In this situation, the veterinary surgeon will arrange for the second practitioner to see the case and will expect to take back responsibility for the case after the consultation.

Referral

Where further expertise or equipment is required to make a diagnosis or treat an animal, **referral** to another veterinary surgeon may be considered. The referral veterinary surgeon usually holds further qualifications or RCVS Specialist Status in a particular field of activity. A referral letter is written, outlining the progress of the case so far and the reasons for referral, and the results of diagnostic tests may be sent, such as radiographs or laboratory reports. Following the referral consultation, a referral report is sent to the referring veterinary surgeon, who may take over responsibility of the case again. Owners should be made aware of the level of expertise of the referring veterinary surgeon, and the probable costs. Referrals may also be made to behaviourists and alternative therapy practitioners.

Processing payments

When a practice provides a service for a client, it usually makes a charge, which may be explained orally or by producing an invoice. An itemized invoice should always be produced if the client asks for one. This may be broken down item by item, or split into categories, e.g. surgery, consultations, medication, food.

VAT

Value added tax (VAT) is payable on veterinary services and on most medications, except for those that are 'zero rated' for VAT. This should be indicated on the invoice, with the net amount (fees without VAT), the VAT and the total listed. VAT is usually paid quarterly to HM Customs and Excise, and the practice can reclaim VAT it has spent on overheads and purchases for resale.

When quoting fees in companion animal practice, the inclusive price should be given. Many farm and equine practices, who deal with other businesses, may state their fees exclusive of VAT and then add the VAT to the invoice. Invoices and receipts should include the practice's VAT registration number.

Checking and recording payments

When taking payments, it is important to ensure that the bill has been properly calculated, that all charges are included, and that if treatment has been given to more than one animal these are also included in the total. It may be difficult to collect payment later for money that was not asked for at the time the client paid.

Payments may be recorded in a day book, a receipt book, or, as in most practices, through a till or computer system. Electronic systems will produce a receipt automatically. All clients should receive a receipt for money paid.

Cash and electronic payment slips must be kept secure and it is important that clients' personal card details are not easily stolen – these may be printed in full on the payment slip.

Methods of payment

Payment may be made by cash, cheque, credit card or debit card. Practices will have their own policies regarding accepted methods of payment, each of which costs different amounts to administer. Many banks charge to deposit cash and cheques, and most charge for change. Card-handling services charge a set fee for each debit card transaction and a percentage of the payment for a credit card transaction. Cash and electronic payments are credited to the practice account immediately they are banked; cheques may take a few days to clear. Practices may have policies regarding minimum payments accepted on cards or by cheque. Taking payments is a serious responsibility and should never be rushed.

Cash

When taking cash, the amount tendered should be confirmed to the client, particularly if the practice's till does not have a 'sum tendered' key. Clients may occasionally claim to have tendered a higher sum, and mistakes are less likely if cash changing hands is counted out loud. Nurses unused to handling cash and giving change should practise before taking money in a busy reception area.

Cheques

Cheques should only be accepted if guaranteed with a cheque guarantee card. This will limit the amount the cheque can be made out for, and electronic card payment may be more secure.

Credit and debit cards

Credit and debit card payments may require authorization and it is important to know the procedure for this and what to do if a payment is refused. Some practices allow credit or debit card payment over the telephone and may allow payment direct into bank accounts using the BACS system. In the latter case, the practice's bank details may be included on the invoice and clients can make payments direct from their bank accounts.

Reconciliation

Reconciliation is the process of balancing up the total payments taken in a period with the amounts recorded. By reconciling the totals, errors can be spotted early on, e.g. payments not recorded against the client's records. Proper reconciliation is vital to protect the practice against fraud, and to spot errors straight away so that clients' accounts are accurate.

Insurance

Clients with pet insurance may pay as they go and claim fees back, but some practices will accept direct payment terms with certain insurance companies, sending their accounts for payment direct to the company. In these cases, clients will still be required to pay an 'excess' (a minimum amount towards the cost of each course of treatment).

Many practices have leaflets about insurance, and these can be displayed and handed out. General insurance is regulated by the Financial Services Authority, which stipulates that unless a person or organization is regulated by the FSA, they cannot carry out certain activities. These include:

- Giving advice on insurance, except in very general terms, or recommending particular policies or offering inducements for people to take out a particular insurance
- Assisting clients to complete proposal forms
- Collecting insurance payments.

A practice that is an Appointed Representative or Introducer Appointed Representative may specifically recommend an insurer. For more information, see www.fsa.gov.uk or contact the relevant veterinary fee insurers.

Financial control

Veterinary practices are businesses, and attracting and keeping clients is essential for the practice to survive, as is adequate cash flow. Money earned by the business is used to pay the costs of running it (premises, salaries, overheads, loan interest, etc.) and to purchase stock for sale. Money remaining is the profit, and a proportion of this will be used to improve the practice, to purchase equipment and vehicles, to pay off any loans, and to give the practice owners an adequate return for their investment.

Good financial control and effective budgeting are very important for the financial health of a practice and the job security of its staff. This area is usually the responsibility of the practice owner(s) and a practice manager or administrator. Fees should be set at levels that provide a sufficient return for the work done, and stock and drugs should be priced competitively but so that income covers the costs of purchase, storage and handling. Regular reviews and close monitoring of costs and stock invoices is essential.

As well as ensuring that the fees and prices are appropriate, it is important to ensure that clients are charged the correct fees, and that charges are not missed or forgotten, or stock given away. The veterinary nurse can monitor and audit records to ensure that clients are charged correctly for everything they have received, but this is often neglected in practice. Consumables, medications for inpatients and hospitalization fees may all be missed from time to time, and a simple method of writing up cases as they progress will help to reduce missed fees.

Debt control

Speed of payment can have a huge impact on the financial health of the practice, for two reasons. First, prompt payment is essential for healthy cash flow; and with many practices running a bank overdraft or with substantial loans, cash in the bank will reduce interest charges and can be used for the business. Secondly, the longer a debt is outstanding, the less likely it is that it will be paid.

Most small animal practices work on a pay-as-you-go basis: the client is invoiced and pays at the time of treatment. Referral, mixed and equine practices may have a high level of account clients, who may be sent a regular invoice for payment within a specified period of time, generally 30 days. Discounts may be given for prompt payment, to encourage clients to pay early. Offering payment by credit and debit card as well as by cash or cheque is helpful in encouraging prompt payment. There will, however, always be some who are slow to pay or who do not pay at all.

Successful debt collection depends on prompt reminders and requests for payment, prompt follow-up of any queries or complaints, and positive action if the debt is not paid. An outline of the procedure should be included in the practice's term of business. Methods that may be used include debt collection agencies, court proceedings (usually through the Small Claims Court) and writing to the client after a predetermined time to inform them that they must seek treatment for their animals elsewhere in future if the account is not settled. Some clients will pay when they receive this last letter, having ignored all other requests.

Avoiding a debt building up in the first place is always the best option. Good estimating, noting estimates on consent forms, clear terms and conditions of business issued to all clients, and making it clear that you expect to be paid, all help to avoid debts occurring.

If a debt is impossible to collect, it can be written off after 6 months for VAT. This means that the practice can reclaim the VAT due on the debt if it is using the accrual basis of accounting, and include the fee as a cost in the practice overheads.

Security

The safety of people at work is paramount (see also Chapter 1) and the security of the premises and its contents is vital for the business.

People and premises

Premises must be secure, with no opportunity for people to enter areas unseen, e.g. through an unlocked back door. The public should not be permitted access to the pharmacy or patient areas, unless supervised.

Valuable items should never be left on show or where they can be easily picked up. Computer equipment, cash, personal belongings, charity boxes, stock and drugs with a value 'on the street' are all easy targets for thieves.

Particular attention should be paid to ground floor windows and any upstairs windows or doors with access over a flat roof or other structure. Where alternative ventilation is available, windows are best kept closed and locked. At the end of the working day, a routine security check should ensure that all locks are in place, whether the premises are left unattended or if duty staff will be working, and particularly if one person will be left alone.

Alarm systems

Security alarms can be set to cover doors and windows while still allowing staff to work within the building. Personal alarm buttons can be integrated into the alarm system and may be helpful for reception areas and for lone workers. Security and fire alarms should be serviced and tested regularly and ideally should alert a remote centre or responsible person via a telephone dialler.

Lone workers

Lone workers should at all times have access to telephone support in an emergency. If they are away from the premises (e.g. on a visit) they should follow a set safety procedure, which should include:

- Carrying out a risk assessment for the visit before agreeing to attend
- Ensuring that they know exactly where they are going
- Letting another person know where they are going and when they are expected back
- Checking in on return.

Very often, the nurse will be the contact person when a veterinary surgeon is out on a call. Lone workers include night staff on call and any veterinary surgeon or nurse out on a visit at any time of the day. Callers should be identified before being let into the practice, and any practice safety guidelines followed. Excellent guidance and information on personal safety is available from the Suzy Lamplugh Trust website (www.suzylamplugh.org).

Cash

Cash should always be kept securely in a locked place and minimum sums kept in till drawers or cash tins. A counter cache is useful for storing notes securely away from the till, and secure safes are essential if large sums of money are stored before banking. A till should never be left with the keys in place, nor positioned where it is easy to reach in and grab cash. Tills should be left empty with open drawers at night to deter opportunist thieves (Figure 2.8).

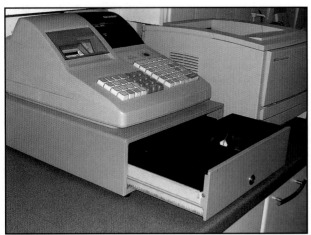

2.8   To deter thieves, tills should be left with drawers open after hours.

Cash should never be counted in a public area; counting should be done out of sight. When cash is taken to the bank:

- Vary the time of day that it is taken
- Do not carry a bank cash bag, but carry cheques and traceable items in a bag and notes close to the person
- If challenged and asked to hand over the bag, do not put yourself at risk – hand over what is asked for.

Patients

Security of inpatients is of the utmost importance.

- Always try to have two doors between the patient and outside to prevent escape.
- If windows are used for ventilation, they should be fitted with stays to prevent them opening wide, or grilles or netting to prevent escape.
- Small pets, such as birds and rodents, should be handled with care in a secure area, with no nooks and crannies they can fly or creep into.
- Check that animals cannot get behind units and cupboards; furniture should be either fixed and sealed or movable.
- All animals should be moved around the practice with approved restraint. In particular, check that dog collars fit snugly (many owners keep collars too loose) and always replace slip leads and choke chains with collars and leads. This is especially important if walking patients out of an enclosed area. Be careful not to release quick-release buckles when holding collars or muzzles.
- Cats and other small pets should always be transported in secure baskets, with locking catches. Patients should be transferred to secure practice baskets if owners' carriers do not look secure.
- Always double-check that cage doors are securely shut and use a locking system if pets can work catches free by themselves.
- Never underestimate an animal's ability to escape from any accommodation.
- Take particular care when more than one animal is in an area at a time: dogs chase cats and rabbits, and in the ensuing panic, escape or injury may be a real possibility.
- Know where animal handling equipment is stored and how it is used, so that it can be accessed quickly in an emergency.

Controlled drugs

Controlled drugs require special handling under the Misuse of Drugs Act 1971 and the Misuse of Drugs Regulations made under the Act in 1985. Controlled drugs are divided into five schedules:

- **Schedule 1** includes drugs such as LSD that have no therapeutic use
- **Schedule 2** drugs include pethidine, morphine, cocaine and fentanyl. They should be kept in a locked cabinet, fixed securely to the premises, and their purchase and use recorded in a bound register. They can only be purchased from a supplier with a signed requisition. The locked cabinet should only be opened by a veterinary surgeon or a person authorized by the veterinary surgeon
- **Schedule 3** drugs include buprenorphine and pentobarbital. They should be kept securely, but their use does not have to be recorded in a register
- **Schedule 4** includes anabolic substances and the benzodiazepines. In normal veterinary practice use, they are exempt from most controlled drugs restrictions
- **Schedule 5** includes certain preparations of cocaine, codeine and morphine that contain less than a specified amount of the drug and so are exempt from the Controlled Drugs requirements
- In addition, **ketamine**, as a drug of potential misuse, should be kept locked away and its use recorded in an informal register.

Stock

Practice stock will include:

- Drugs used within the practice, such as anaesthetics, sedatives, antibiotics, intravenous fluids, topical treatments, injectable drugs, vaccines
- Consumables used in the course of treatments, such as cotton wool, syringes and needles, disposable gloves, gowns and drapes
- Suture materials, bandages and dressings
- Drugs dispensed in the course of treatment, such as tablets and topical treatments (e.g. ear drops, shampoos)
- Food for hospitalized patients
- X-ray film and processing chemicals
- Dispensing items such as child-proof tablet bottles, boxes, dispensing bags and carriers
- Items for general sale such as pet carriers, grooming equipment, leads, toys, pet foods and supplements
- Stationery, such as headed paper, computer paper, envelopes, business cards
- Cleaning materials, disinfectants, washing powder
- Tea, coffee and milk.

Practices use their own systems to ensure adequate supplies, but maintaining stocks of medicines and items for sale will be the particular concern of the veterinary nurse.

Most practices buy their main supplies from one source, generally a veterinary wholesaler. Different manufacturers supply the wholesaler, who fills the practice's order, often breaking down bulk boxes ('outers') into individual units. Other items may be purchased locally or from mail order suppliers. A list of suppliers' details and the items ordered should be kept accessible.

Practices are required to audit their purchases, sales and stocks of prescription-only medicines at least annually and to record any discrepancies. Practices are also required to record the batch numbers and expiry dates of all medicines received and when each batch was first used. The aim is that, should a batch need to be recalled, practices should be able to determine to whom that batch has been dispensed. For food animals, batch numbers of all medicines used must be recorded on the clinical record and this is good practice for small animal work too.

Ordering stock

Methods will vary from practice to practice, but the principles are the same. The aim is to keep adequate stock levels for the day-to-day and emergency needs of the practice without tying up excessive resources. The value of stock on the shelf can be substantial, and losses can be considerable if items go out of date. If stock levels fall too low the practice may run out of items, possibly jeopardizing an animal's treatment or forcing a client to buy elsewhere.

Manual ordering

Stock is ordered when it is felt that it is needed. Either a note of ideal stock levels is made on the shelf, or an experienced staff member checks daily and 'has a feel' for when to reorder items. This can work well in small practices where stock is kept in one place and the experienced member never goes on holiday, but it is time-consuming and not particularly accurate. Alternatively, staff may note on an order pad when they sell a certain quantity of an item, so that it is reordered. This is not a reliable system and only works well for large items – not items where many small transactions are made through the day.

Computerized stock control

Hand-held computers are popular and may be supplied by the wholesaler. They hold a database of the drugs and items used and may hold stock level information. The list can often be set so that products are listed in the order in which they are stored on the shelf. The nurse can enter the product code, or scan a bar code from the product or a shelf label, to bring up that item and set either the quantity in stock (from which the computer calculates the number to order) or the quantity to order. The complete order can then be sent electronically to the supplier. Some systems can incorporate seasonal stock requirements and automatically adjust stock levels to usage.

The most sophisticated systems are those that use the practice's main computer records system. Set up properly, this can be an extremely effective method of stock control, as each time a product is used it is taken from the stock quantity and when the stock level reaches the present reorder level it is added to the order. The system may take time to set up and must be used accurately without being overridden to be successful. Orders are generated electronically and minimum stock levels can be automatically calculated according to usage, increasing as an item is used more. The system can generally handle part-quantities such as individual tablets and volumes of injectable drugs, and can be extremely accurate if used properly. It is, however, only as good as the data it is given: if products are not charged for or de-stocked, there will be no reorder.

Computerized systems help greatly with stock auditing and reconciliation, as well as with batch number recording. Tracking stock discrepancies will show where stock is short, which may be due to stocking-on or de-stocking errors, pilfering, undercharging and unnoticed errors in deliveries, so is well worthwhile.

Placing the order

How a stock order is placed will depend on the system used by the veterinary wholesaler or supplier. Small suppliers may be happy taking a phone order, but written or faxed confirmation is ideal. Individual orders can be written in an order book; supplier details and contact numbers can be kept at the front, and orders checked off when they arrive. Suppliers often ask for an order number. Use your name or initials and the date if you do not have a purchase order system. Wholesalers may require faxed orders but most take electronic orders, either from their own computer systems or directly from a practice management system. Price lists, price updates and details of stock delivered can all be transmitted back to the practice computer.

The timing of ordering can be crucial for reliable delivery. Wholesalers have a cut-off time after which orders cannot be accepted and so it is vital to be in good time, as there are always interruptions and distractions on a busy day to take you past the deadline! Daily ordering is now commonplace and useful for keeping stock levels low and for last-minute items. Less frequent ordering, though, can be more efficient as larger quantities are handled at once, saving staff time. Interim orders can be used to top up in between.

Receiving stock

Practices should ensure that delivered goods only arrive during opening hours where possible, so that goods remain secure and can be dealt with as soon as possible.

Delivery notes

When products arrive they are generally accompanied by a delivery note (not to be thrown away with the packaging). This will detail the items supplied and may also show the price. The goods delivered should always be carefully checked, both against the delivery note and against the original order, and it is a good idea to initial the delivery note so that if there is a query everyone knows who unpacked and checked the order (Figure 2.9).

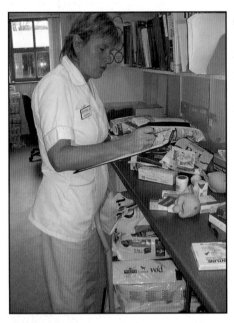

The condition of the goods and their packaging should be examined to ensure that there are no breakages or damage to the product that may make it unusable or difficult to sell. Any problems or shortages must be notified to the supplier as soon as possible; a specific time period may be stated in their terms and conditions.

For parcels delivered by courier and requiring signature, it should always be stated that the item is 'unexamined' if it is not possible to unpack and check it immediately (which would not be popular with the waiting delivery driver). If someone in the practice has signed that the goods were in good condition on receipt, it may be difficult to complain about damage later.

'Stocking-on'

If automatic computerized stock control is in operation, the items will need to be 'stocked on', i.e. added to the quantity held in stock on the computer. This can be done manually, or automatically across a modem or by scanning in a bar code on the delivery note. Stock should only be 'stocked on' if it has actually arrived.

Unpacking

Great care should be taken not to cut hands or damage the contents when opening boxes with a sharp blade or scissors, and to be aware of the hazards of metal staples, sharp wrapping tape and sharp paper edges. Special cutting tools for boxes are available and are recommended.

Order of unpacking and storing

Perishable items or those requiring special storage conditions should be unpacked and dealt with first. Vaccines, some laboratory diagnostics and insulin all need to be kept refrigerated

and should arrive in insulated packaging, often with cold packs. They should be checked and placed in the appropriate refrigerator immediately. If there has been a delay in delivery, prolonged storage at too high a temperature will make them unusable and they should be rejected.

The rest of the order should be put away as soon as possible, using good stock rotation practice (see below) and ensuring that the delivery and any packaging do not obstruct fire exits and access ways in the practice nor present a trip hazard.

Particular care should be taken in handling heavy items. Trolleys should be used where possible to move large items such as food bags (Figure 2.10) and heavy boxes should not be lifted on to high worktops. Many wholesalers use reusable packing cases that can be collected on the next delivery. Other packaging should be disposed of responsibly, recycling where possible.

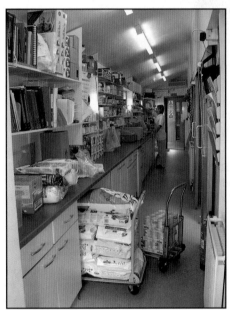

Returns

Goods to be returned should be stored safely for collection or packed securely for return. Suppliers will have their own systems for returns and the practice should ensure that the return is expected and use the correct documentation, a copy of which should be kept for reconciling to a credit note later.

Organizing and maintaining stock

Poor stock organization, handling and human error will limit the effectiveness of any ordering system. Stock levels should be altered according to seasonal changes (generally more flea and tick treatments are sold during summer and autumn), introduction of new products, and changes in prescribing habits in the practice. Involving the clinical team in controlling stock is essential.

Stock may be stored according to therapeutic category (antibiotics; steroids; non-steroidal anti-inflammatories) or product group (topicals; injectables; oral fluids; tablets) and alphabetically.

Quality control

Stock must be easy to find and access and should be stored so that older stock is used first. Newly delivered items must be put behind or under older items, expiry dates of products should be checked so that the oldest are used first, and items that are short-dated (will expire shortly) should be rejected on delivery or used up first.

Gravity-fed sloping shelving can be useful in rotating stock. Dispensary shelving should be clearly labelled and designed so that stock fits well and can be stored with labelling clearly visible and the right way up.

Drug stock in the practice and in cars should be checked regularly for expiry dates and for general condition. Multi-dose injection bottles should be marked with the date of broaching (when the first dose was extracted) and discarded after the time period indicated in the data sheet (Figure 2.11).

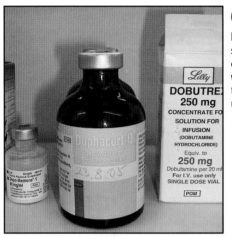

2.11
Broached vials should be clearly labelled with the date they were first used.

Environmental control

Refrigerated products generally should be kept at 2–8°C and provision must be made for products that need to be kept away from light. Drug storage areas, including cars, should have maximum and minimum temperature recording to ensure that the temperature stays within the required range stated on the drug packaging or in its data sheet (Figure 2.12). If drugs are taken on visits, insulated cool boxes with temperature recording should be used and minimal stock carried. Cars become very cold in winter and very hot in summer, and drugs should not be left in them overnight or on non-working days. Protection from extremes of humidity is also important.

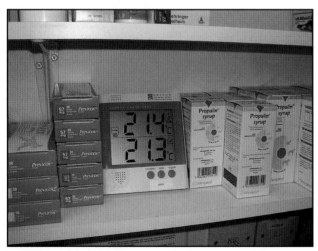

2.12 Digital thermometer. Maximum and minimum temperatures should be recorded in all areas in which drugs are stored.

Drug storage and preparation areas should be kept clean, dry and free of vermin. They should have impermeable work surfaces, and facilities for hand washing and disinfection. Food and drink should not be permitted where drugs are stored or dispensed.

Security is paramount, particularly when away from the practice. The public should not have access to the practice pharmacy or any area where drugs are stored. Where drugs are used in consulting rooms, it is vital that children cannot access them or any syringes or sharps.

Nurse clinics

More and more nurses are finding that running their own clinics in specific delegated areas can be very rewarding, can benefit the practice financially, and offers clients a service they really appreciate.

Popular areas for nurse clinics

- Puppy and kitten advice (Figure 2.13)
- Flea and worm control
- Dental home care
- Support for pets who need to lose weight
- Help and advice for senior pets
- Advice on some behavioural problems
- Puppy classes.

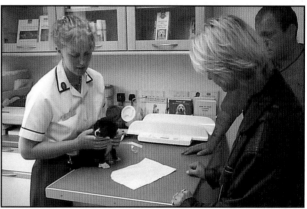

2.13 Correct advice from the start of a pet's life is one of the benefits of nurse clinics.

Nurses can also offer support for owners of pets with chronic conditions, such as diabetes mellitus, arthritis, urinary tract problems and allergic skin disease. Ensuring compliance with chronic treatment regimes can improve a pet's quality of life and help to reduce stress for an owner who may find giving medication difficult. Nurses can train owners to administer medications correctly and help them to gain in confidence, e.g. with insulin injections. Clients also often ask the nurse questions which they would not 'bother the vet with' but which are nonetheless important for the pet's health.

Deciding when to see clients can be problematical, particularly in a busy practice with limited consulting room space. Ideally, clients should be seen in a consulting room, or dedicated 'nurses room', but areas of reception are used in some practices. Clients can be seen by appointment at particular times, but it is a good idea for the nurse to be available at the request of the consulting veterinary surgeon so that clients identified as needing a nurse consultation can be referred immediately.

Protocols should be agreed for each type of consultation, so that veterinary surgeons and nurses know exactly which areas will be discussed and can avoid duplication of effort. Checklists are helpful. The veterinary nurse should have received adequate training and be confident to cover the areas expected. All consultations and advice should be recorded in the clinical notes.

Examples of protocols for nursing consultations

Dental homecare

- Discuss current homecare
- Examine the mouth, use disclosing solution to show plaque
- Discuss diet
- Demonstrate and discuss tooth brushing and other preventative measures
- Make recommendations for dental homecare
- Make appointment for follow-up visit

Obesity clinic

- Weigh pet
- Work out ideal weight and target weight
- Discuss current feeding, exercise, treats, etc.
- Make sure pet is healthy (veterinary surgeon to check if unsure)
- Agree action plan and proposed dietary and exercise changes; issue weight chart
- Arrange next appointment to check progress

It is helpful to have information supporting your advice, for the client to take away. This can be produced in-house, or you can make use of the literature provided by the suppliers of products you are recommending, and personalise it with your own and your practice details.

Puppy classes

Puppy classes (see Chapter 11) can be run as single sessions or as a course and can include general care issues, nutrition, parasite control, early puppy training and, most importantly, socialization. Approximately six puppies and their families are regarded as the optimum number, though some practices run larger groups quite successfully.

Location may be a problem, as many reception areas are not suitable. Good hygiene is essential, particularly if puppies are coming before completing their primary vaccination. A dedicated room is ideal, but just a dream for many nurses.

Further reading

Anonymous (2005) *The Ultimate Puppy Toolkit*. Urban Puppy Inc., Toronto, Canada/Premier Pet Products, Richmond, VA (www.premier.com)

Bower J, Gripper J, Gripper P and Gunn D (1998) *Veterinary Practice Management, 2nd edn*. Blackwell Science, Oxford

Chapman MJ and Scott PW (1997) *BVA Code of Practice on Medicines*. BVA, London (also available online at www.bva.co.uk)

Gray C and Pullen S (2006) *Ethics, Law and the Veterinary Nurse*. Elsevier Science, Oxford

Kurtz SM, Silverman JD and Draper J (2004) *Teaching and Learning Communication Skills in Medicine, 2nd edn*. Radcliffe Medical Press, Oxford

Radford AD (2003) *Development Teaching and Evaluation of a Consultation Structure*. LTSN-01 project report, available online (www.medev.ac.uk/newsletter/01.3.html)

Radford M (2001) *Animal Welfare Law in Britain – Regulation and Responsibility*. Oxford University Press, Oxford

RCVS (2006) *Guide to Professional Conduct*. RCVS, London (also available online at www.rcvs.org.uk)

Shilcock M and Stutchfield G (2003) *Veterinary Practice Management, A Practical Guide*. WB Saunders, Philadelphia

Silverman JD, Kurtz SM and Draper J (2004) *Skills for Communicating with Patients, 2nd edn*. Radcliffe Medical Press, Oxford

Chapter 3

Legal and ethical aspects of veterinary nursing practice

Elizabeth Earle

Learning objectives

After studying this chapter, students should be able to:

- **Discuss the roles and responsibilities of the veterinary team**
- **Outline the legal accountability of the veterinary nurse**
- **Describe the differences between civil and criminal law**
- **Outline the concept of informed consent**
- **Describe the legal and ethical requirements for record keeping**
- **Describe the legal scope of veterinary nursing practice**

Introduction

Veterinary practice, like other professions and businesses, operates within the framework of the law. The role of the veterinary nurse has expanded with the provisions laid down within Schedule 3 of the Veterinary Surgeons Act 1966 and continues to evolve. This chapter provides a background to the legal obligations of the veterinary nurse as a member of the veterinary team. Ethical issues often arise in relation to the law; these are highlighted where they are important.

The veterinary team

Veterinary practices vary widely in their size, focus and the composition of their staff. Whilst the range of practices encompasses large hospitals, corporate multi-branch businesses and single practitioners, the majority of practices remain small privately owned businesses with an average of five to six veterinary surgeons (RCVS, 2006b). Practices accordingly employ a variable mix of staff in order to address the needs of their business.

Members of the veterinary team

- Veterinary surgeons (partners, principals, assistants and locums)
- Listed veterinary nurses
- Unlisted veterinary nurses
- Student veterinary nurses
- Practice managers
- Other staff (clerical, kennel assistants, cleaners, etc.)

The *clinical* work of a veterinary practice is regulated by law through the Veterinary Surgeons Act 1966. This Act of Parliament (Statute) defines veterinary surgery and the role of veterinary surgeons and sets out who may provide treatment for animals.

Veterinary surgeons

Veterinary surgeons are the only individuals who may practise veterinary surgery in the UK. In order to practise, they must be registered on the Royal College of Veterinary Surgeons (RCVS) Register of veterinary surgeons.

What is veterinary surgery?

The Veterinary Surgeons Act defines veterinary surgery as 'the art and science of veterinary surgery and medicine and, without prejudice to the generality of the foregoing, shall be taken to include–

(a) the diagnosis of diseases in, and injuries to, animals including tests performed on animals for diagnostic purposes;
(b) the giving of advice based upon such diagnosis;
(c) the medical or surgical treatment of animals; and
(d) the performance of surgical operations on animals.'

Whilst other members of the veterinary team may be involved in the care, and in some cases treatment, of animals, the overall management of each case is always led by a veterinary surgeon who is professionally accountable for diagnosis and treatment, whether carried out personally or delegated to another member of the veterinary team.

Veterinary nurses

The primary role of veterinary nurses is to provide supportive nursing care to animals receiving veterinary treatment. They may also undertake a number of technical functions in support of veterinary diagnosis and treatment, such as diagnostic imaging (radiography), laboratory testing and the monitoring of anaesthesia. Whilst a recognized qualification and registration process exists for veterinary nurses, this is not yet required by law and there are therefore four 'types' of veterinary nurse that may be encountered in practice.

Listed veterinary nurses

Listed veterinary nurses are qualified to the nationally agreed standard in the UK and are registered on the RCVS List of Veterinary Nurses. Listed nurses are recognized within the Veterinary Surgeons Act and may undertake certain delegated *acts of veterinary surgery* under veterinary direction.

Student veterinary nurses

Student veterinary nurses are trainee nurses enrolled on the RCVS database of student veterinary nurses. They are also recognized within the Veterinary Surgeons Act and may undertake certain delegated *acts of veterinary surgery* under veterinary supervision in the course of their training.

Unlisted veterinary nurses

Unlisted veterinary nurses are qualified nurses who are not currently registered on the RCVS List.

Veterinary nursing assistants

Veterinary nursing assistants are nursing staff who have not completed professional veterinary nurse training and are not qualified to register on the RCVS List. Nursing assistants may, however, have undertaken basic training courses and be very experienced in supporting the veterinary team. Neither unlisted nurses nor veterinary nursing assistants are legally recognized (within the Veterinary Surgeons Act) and they are consequently not entitled to carry out any care or treatment that is defined as an *act of veterinary surgery*. As the legal definition of veterinary surgery is broad, this means that the clinical work of unlisted and unqualified nurses is restricted to the provision of supportive nursing care only. The scope of veterinary nursing is discussed later in this chapter and in Chapter 2.

Practice managers

Practice managers are employed by many larger practices to manage the business operations of the veterinary practice, leaving the veterinary surgeons and nurses free to concentrate on the provision of clinical care. The role of practice managers varies according to the nature of the particular business, but they are usually involved in the management of practice accounts and client billing, maintenance of the premises and clinical resources, and the management of human resources. They are also often involved in the marketing of a practice and the development of client relations. Practice managers may have a veterinary or veterinary nursing background but increasingly are specialists in business management.

Other support staff

Practices, especially larger establishments, may employ a variety of staff in support of clinical care. These may include kennel assistants, stable assistants, technicians and domestic staff. They are all members of the veterinary team and, when engaged in any clinically related work or supportive care, work under the direction of a veterinary surgeon.

Suitably qualified persons

The Veterinary Medicines Regulations 2005 allow for certain categories of medicines to be prescribed by a trained individual who is nether a veterinary surgeon nor a pharmacist. Such an individual is termed a suitably qualified person (SQP). POM-V (prescription-only medicine – veterinarian) products, however, must be prescribed by a veterinary surgeon and can only be dispensed by a veterinary surgeon or pharmacist.

As the supply of veterinary medicines is a major element of the business of most veterinary practices, it is likely that some practices will employ SQPs to supply many of the routine pharmaceuticals to clients. It is also likely that, by virtue of their established role and qualifications, veterinary nurses will form a large group of those seeking to work in this role.

SQPs must achieve the qualifications stipulated by the Veterinary Medicines Directorate (VMD) and must be registered with that body in order to practise. The premises from which they work must also be registered with the VMD. Current regulations and information may be found on the VMD website (www.vmd.gov.uk).

Non-veterinary clinicians

Veterinary surgeons may ask certain qualified health professionals in the human field to undertake the treatment of animal patients. This provision is very specific and relates to doctors, dentists and physiotherapists (and the related manipulative therapies such as osteopathy and chiropractice). Whilst a veterinary surgeon may undertake complementary therapies (such as acupuncture or homeopathy) if appropriately qualified, it remains illegal for a complementary therapist qualified in the human field to treat animals, whether under veterinary direction or not (see *RCVS Guide to Professional Conduct*).

The legal system in which the veterinary team works

Members of the veterinary team operate within the framework of the law. Whilst the details of the legal system will be peripheral to the routine daily work of most veterinary professionals, it is very important to understand how the law works in order to recognize and avoid some common potential problems. The legal system comprises two main branches: criminal and civil law.

Criminal law

Criminal law is concerned with the punishment of offences by the State. It exists in order to protect the individual and prevent harm to others. Generally speaking, the State intervenes only where there is a real justification for interfering with the liberty of others in the public interest and avoids areas of private morality where there is no clear consequence of harm to others. Criminal prosecutions are usually brought by the police through the Crown Prosecution Service. In any criminal case the **prosecution** is always brought by the State (the Crown) and the accused person is always known as the **defendant**.

Civil law

Civil law is concerned with addressing harm or loss to an individual brought about by another person or organization. The types of civil action most likely to affect a veterinary practice are **breach of contract** and actions in **tort**. A tort is a civil, rather than a criminal, wrong and the law of tort provides protection for a person's personal security, property and reputation. For example, a person could bring an action for negligence if they suffered injury as a result of poor medical practice, or an action for defamation if someone published information which damaged their reputation.

The person bringing the action is called the **claimant** and the person or organization alleged to have caused the harm or loss is the **defendant**. If a claimant wins a civil case, the court may award compensation for injury or financial loss or may award an injunction to prevent the defendant from causing further harm.

Public law and judicial review

Government organizations and other public bodies often exercise their own internal regulations granted by statute. Examples are government departments (such as the Department for Work and Pensions), universities and professional regulatory bodies such as the RCVS.

Sources of law

Law originates from **Statutes** (Acts of Parliament) and from the **Common Law**, based on the precedents of case law decided in the courts. This means that the decisions of the courts in important cases guide judges in subsequent similar situations. Some precedents are especially binding, for example those set in the Court of Appeal or the House of Lords.

Statutes are Acts of Parliament. These are developed from **Bills** presented to both Houses of Parliament. A Bill must proceed through three **readings** in the House of Commons and House of Lords. It must then receive the **Royal Assent**. It can therefore take a considerable amount of time for a Bill to become law, although statutes can be passed very quickly when there is seen to be an urgent public need.

More recent statutes are often what are termed **enabling Acts**. These statutes provide a broad legislative framework and allow powers for ministers to produce detailed regulations for the operation of the law. These regulations are known as **statutory instruments**. This sort of legislation is flexible in that it allows ministers to make effective changes in the law without the time-consuming need for a new statute. Some 2000 statutory instruments are produced from government departments each year.

When the Veterinary Surgeons Act is eventually redrafted it is likely to become an enabling Act. This will, for example, allow much greater flexibility than does the present Act in regulating the work of para-veterinary professionals such as equine dentists and veterinary nurses.

The UK is part of the European Union and, as such, is also governed by **European law** (European Community Act 1972). The member states have 'pooled' their national sovereignty and, as a result, have formed a superior legal order which has precedence over their individual domestic systems. This is why cases decided in British courts may be overturned in the European Court. In addition, member states of the European Union are subject to EU regulations and directives. Many of these have a major impact on veterinary practice (e.g. COSHH 1988, Manual Handling Regulations 1992).

Legal and ethical accountability of the veterinary nurse

This section deals with the legal accountability of veterinary nurses. **Accountability** means being answerable for one's actions (or omissions). Nurses are accountable in law in four key areas. These cross both civil and criminal law as outlined above. Nurses are also accountable to themselves morally for their actions. In most cases moral and legal accountability are closely linked, but there are some instances where a veterinary nurse may have a moral obligation but no legal liability. An example of this would be a nurse who declines to offer first aid to an injured animal outside of her practice environment. The law does not require that help must be offered and any legal action brought against the nurse would fail.

Accountability: an example

In many instances several different fields of accountability will be involved in a single case.

Mr Brown's pedigree Bengal cat suffered a fractured jaw following dental extractions. The cat was seriously injured as a result of the procedure and its value as a show and/or breeding animal may have been diminished. It transpired that the procedure was carried out by a veterinary nurse. She had qualified in 2004 but had not registered on the RCVS List of Veterinary Nurses.

- Dental extractions are not held to be a minor surgical procedure under the Veterinary Surgeons Act, Schedule 3. Therefore they cannot be legally delegated by a veterinary surgeon to a Listed veterinary nurse.
- The nurse in this illustration had qualified but had not registered on the RCVS List and she was therefore not legally entitled to undertake any delegated veterinary work covered by Schedule 3 (see later).
- Mr Brown could take a civil action against the veterinary surgeon to compensate him for the damage to his valuable cat.
- He could also make a complaint to the RCVS in relation to the delegating veterinary surgeon's professional conduct. (A veterinary surgeon was removed from the RCVS Veterinary Register in 2004 in similar circumstances.)

Accountability to society

All citizens are expected to conduct themselves within the law. Veterinary nurses may be prosecuted for a breach of the law, within the context of either their work (e.g. fraud, drug offences) or their private lives. They may also be called as witnesses in criminal prosecutions brought against animal owners or colleagues, for example cruelty cases.

In the example above, the unlisted veterinary nurse is classed as a lay person. A lay person may not perform any act of veterinary surgery, and she may accordingly be prosecuted in the criminal courts under the provisions of the Veterinary Surgeons Act.

Accountability to the client

A client may bring an action in the civil courts if they have suffered loss or injury as a result of alleged negligence or a breach of contract. This action may be brought against one or more individuals *personally* or against an organization. An organization, such as a veterinary practice, may be directly responsible for damage to an animal because its policies and procedures are at fault. It may also be indirectly (or *vicariously*) liable for the negligent actions of its employees.

In the example given above, the client might bring an action for damages if the harm done to his animal resulted in loss, for example if he could no longer show the cat or breed from it.

A client would be very unlikely to sue a single employee of a veterinary practice (such as the veterinary nurse concerned). The purpose of bringing a civil action in a case like this would be to seek compensation. Litigants will therefore target a business (which carries indemnity insurance) in order to obtain compensation for their loss. In some cases this will amount to many thousands of pounds. However, if the client is successful and is awarded damages for his loss, the practice may take action against its negligent employee to recover the damages.

Duty to the employer

As employees, veterinary nurses have a *duty to obey all reasonable instructions* given by their employers and to carry out their work with due care and diligence. This expectation is an implied term of any contract of employment, meaning that it does not have to be expressly written down.

Employees cannot be required to break the law or to act negligently as part of a 'reasonable instruction'. In the example above, if it were found that the nurse and the veterinary surgeon were acting outside of the normal policy and procedures of the practice, they could be subjected to internal disciplinary procedures. Additionally, the practice may sue employees personally for any loss incurred as a result of their negligent action. However, in practical terms it is rarely cost-effective to pursue such a course of action.

Professional accountability

A veterinary nurse's professional accountability is currently channelled through the veterinary surgeon under whose direction the nurse works. Veterinary surgeons are professionally accountable to the RCVS, which regulates the practice of veterinary surgery, in accordance with the Veterinary Surgeons Act 1966, in the United Kingdom. The professional standards expected of veterinary surgeons are set out in the *RCVS Guide to Professional Conduct*.

The client, in the example given above, may make a complaint to the RCVS against the veterinary surgeon involved in the care of his cat. The RCVS would investigate the conduct of the veterinary surgeon, an issue of which would be his apparent delegation of an act of veterinary surgery to a lay person (the unlisted veterinary nurse). An RCVS disciplinary hearing in 2004 resulted in the removal of a veterinary surgeon from the Register for inappropriately delegating dental extractions to a listed veterinary nurse and other (unqualified) staff.

At present veterinary nurses have no statutory professional accountability for their actions. It is for this reason that Schedule 3 of the Veterinary Surgeons Act permits veterinary nurses to undertake delegated acts of veterinary surgery only under the direction of a veterinary surgeon. The RCVS List of Veterinary Nurses is thus a list only of those who have reached the necessary standard of qualification and continue to pay the required annual retention fee. No nurse may be removed from

the List for misconduct, the primary safeguard against 'unfit' veterinary nurses being through the diligence of their veterinary employers.

In 2007 a new non-statutory Register for veterinary nurses will be introduced. The Register will automatically include all veterinary nurses qualified on (or after) 1 January 2003 and will be open to any other veterinary nurse to join voluntarily. The new Register will stipulate the requirement to adhere to a nurses' Guide to Professional Conduct and to maintain professional competence through continuing professional development (CPD). Nurses on the new Register will be entitled to call themselves **Registered Veterinary Nurses**.

The aim of the new Veterinary Nurses Register is twofold. First, it will, for the first time, make veterinary nurses professionally accountable for their actions. This should increase public and veterinary confidence in veterinary nurses as members of the professional team. Secondly, it will prepare the way for the statutory regulation of veterinary nurses (and possibly other para-veterinary professionals) in future veterinary legislation.

Moral accountability and codes of professional conduct

Codes of professional conduct set out the expected standards of practice within a profession and provide valuable guidance to the courts and professional conduct tribunals of regulatory bodies (such as the RCVS) when they are called to judge the conduct of a defendant. The *RCVS Guide to Professional Conduct* provides guidance on ethical issues, which has been agreed by the veterinary profession. The Guide provides 10 'guiding principles' that are relevant to all those working in veterinary practice, including veterinary nurses. New professional conduct guidance for veterinary nurses, to be published in 2007, reflects this approach.

The *RCVS Guide* represents a broad agreement of the veterinary profession on ethical standards of conduct. It is designed to provide a basis for ethical practice but cannot provide easy answers to the many specific moral dilemmas that may arise in veterinary practice. Those working in veterinary practice must, in addition to heeding the *Guide to Professional Conduct*, also be able to recognize moral problems and arrive at considered solutions that meet the best interests of all concerned.

Negligent practice

Veterinary nurses have a duty in law not to cause harm or loss to clients. Animals count as property and any harm to them must, for an action in negligence to be successful, result in loss to the owner. An example would be damage to a pedigree stud dog that prevented the owner from breeding from him.

In order for negligence to be established, four questions must be addressed:

1. Is there a 'duty of care'? When does the veterinary nurse owe a duty of care and to whom?
2. What is the appropriate standard of care expected and how will the courts decide if that has been breached?
3. Was the injury or loss foreseeable and how must the claimant prove this?
4. What type of harm or loss can be compensated?

The duty of care

Veterinary nurses owe a duty of care to clients of the practice, their employer and colleagues, and certain other individuals. It is important to recognize that, whatever the moral obligations, there is no legal duty of care owed to an animal patient. The duty of care concerning an animal is owed to its owner.

A different situation arises when a nurse acts as a 'Good Samaritan' and causes further injury by administering negligent first aid treatment outside the practice environment (Jones, 1992). However morally obliged a veterinary nurse may feel, there is no legal obligation to provide care and treatment for a stranger. A nurse may walk past an accident with legal impunity (Tingle, 1998). The reason for this is that the law must respect an individual's right to judge whether or not they are competent to deal with a situation and to 'opt out' if they are not. In contrast, professional regulatory bodies often require a different approach in their codes of professional conduct. The RCVS would expect a veterinary surgeon to provide 24-hour emergency cover to all species, to include first aid and pain relief and not to allow any animal to suffer through neglect. The United Kingdom Central Council for Nursing, Midwifery and Health Visiting (UKCC), in its Guidelines for Professional Practice for nurses, makes specific recognition of the difference between legal and professional duty in circumstances such as these. Regulatory bodies thus sometimes place additional moral duties upon their registrants that are over and above the legal definition of a duty of care.

Duty to clients: an example

Sophie, aged 13, took her young dog to the veterinary surgeon for a routine vaccination. The veterinary surgeon allowed her to hold the animal during the procedure but the animal moved suddenly and the needle punctured her hand. Sophie was very upset, had to visit the hospital, and suffered prolonged psychological symptoms following the incident.

- Administering an injection is a professional skill, which involves the safe handling of a syringe and the control of an animal. The likelihood of the animal suddenly moving, or the inexperienced client moving her hand, should have been foreseen by the veterinary surgeon. He could have either warned Sophie or (preferably) asked a veterinary nurse to assist.
- Sophie could therefore take a civil action for negligence against the veterinary surgeon to compensate her for her injury. (A client was awarded £12,000 against a veterinary surgeon in similar circumstances in 2002)

Standards of care and breach of duty

Once it has been established that a duty of care is owed, the injured party (the claimant) must be able to establish negligence. In order to do this, he must be able to show that the veterinary nurse concerned fell below a reasonable standard of practice.

The courts decide what a reasonable standard of practice is by determining what the 'ordinary skilled veterinary nurse' would have done in the circumstances of the case. The **Bolam Test**, which is the starting point in judging all cases of professional negligence, states:

The test is the standard of the ordinary skilled man exercising and professing to have that special skill ... he is not guilty of negligence if he has acted in accordance with a practice accepted as proper by a responsible body of medical men skilled in that particular art.

However, whilst the courts will judge a case according to accepted standards of professional skill, they will not choose between two equally valid courses of practice.

It is important to recognize that a person acting as a veterinary nurse, regardless of experience and whether qualified or not, is expected to demonstrate a level of care and skill in accordance with the Bolam Test. Clients cannot be expected to distinguish between veterinary nurses and students or unqualified staff for themselves. Name badges and uniforms should therefore identify and describe staff clearly and accurately. This is a potential issue in some veterinary practices where unqualified staff are referred to as 'veterinary nurses', or even 'head nurses'. Personnel should not act outside their remit or without adequate supervision, i.e. an unqualified nursing assistant should not perform the work of a listed veterinary nurse.

Foreseeability and remoteness

The consequences of a negligent act must be *foreseeable by a reasonable person in the circumstances*. For instance, if a veterinary nurse fails to dispose of 'sharps' in a bin made for the purpose, it is foreseeable that a colleague may suffer injury as a result. The courts must decide how likely it would be that an action might cause harm.

Res ipsa loquiter

This principle is applied where it is clear that negligence has occurred purely from the effect on the claimant. An example of *res ipsa loquiter* ('the thing speaks for itself') would occur if a swab were inadvertently left inside a patient at operation. It does not matter how this happened; the fact that it should never happen if reasonable care is taken is sufficient.

Establishing loss – causation

A claimant must establish that the harm or loss they have suffered has been caused by the negligence of the defendant. In other words, if a client slips on the surgery floor, they must prove that, but for the negligence of the practice, they would not have suffered injury. However, the courts must take care to establish that the injury is not due to a pre-existing condition. For example, the veterinary surgeon whose car backs into that of a client is only liable for the resulting dent, not the damage caused previously when the client hit a lamp post. Sometimes it can be extremely difficult to establish the cause of an injury. In this case, the courts will decide liability on the balance of probabilities.

Compensation – what can be claimed?

In the UK, the principle that underpins the payment of damages is that the injured party should be put in the position he would have been in had the negligent act not occurred.

The courts will compensate loss of earnings, medical expenses and loss of property and will also allow damages for loss of future earnings and pension (in serious/long-lasting injury), pain, suffering and loss of amenity (reduced ability to lead a normal life). If an animal has been damaged or lost owing to negligence, the owner may sue for the reduction in value or the loss of the animal. As many pets are of limited financial value, it is often not practical to litigate.

Negligence and animals

An individual may be liable for the damage caused by an animal. The most significant legislation in this area is the Animals Act 1971. This area of law is of special importance to veterinary practices.

An individual may be liable in tort (see above) for the actions of an animal that he/she owns or has control of. The range of torts is wide and includes not just negligence (e.g. a dog escapes and causes a road accident) but battery (setting the dog on someone), nuisance (noise or smell from kennels), trespass (allowing animals to enter someone else's land) and even defamation (teaching a parrot to utter slanderous statements).

The Animals Act 1971 provides a framework under which individuals may be liable for damage caused by dangerous species (Section 2(1)) and non-dangerous species (Section 2(2)).

A veterinary surgeon who has temporarily taken responsibility for the care of an animal from its owner becomes its keeper and is accountable in law for any damage it may cause to other people or property.

Where dangerous species are concerned, the Act refers to the species that is dangerous, not to a particular animal. It is therefore no defence to say that a particular animal was tame. With the increasing number of exotic animals that are kept as pets, this is particularly relevant to modern veterinary practice.

The Dangerous Dogs Act (1991) makes specific provision for types of dog that are bred for fighting. The principle of deciding who is the keeper of such a dog (and thus responsible for ensuring that the requirements of this Act are complied with) is similar to that described above. Practices need to take special care when dealing with an animal that is legally construed as a dangerous dog but which the owner may not treat as such.

The Animal Welfare Bill (2006) replaces over 20 current pieces of animal welfare legislation. The Bill, when it becomes the Animal Welfare Act, will impose a duty on everyone to prevent unnecessary animal suffering, whether or not they are the keeper of the animal. This will be based on the 'five freedoms' (see Chapter 12):

- Suitable environment
- Suitable diet
- Freedom to exhibit normal behaviour patterns
- Need to be housed with (or apart from) other animals
- Need to be protected from pain, suffering, injury and disease.

The legislation will apply to all domestic species in England and Wales if they are under human control and not living in a wild state. Amongst the first areas to be brought under the new regulations are riding establishments, livery yards, animal boarding establishments and pet shops. Veterinary surgeons and veterinary practices will have a significant role in educating the public and in identifying animal suffering and those at risk. There is already an Animal Welfare Act in place in Scotland, which is very similar to the proposed England and Wales legislation.

Consent to treatment

Consent to treatment is an area where veterinary nurses must demonstrate an understanding of both legal and ethical issues. In legal terms, written, verbal or tacit consent to treatment constitutes evidence of the contract that exists between the veterinary practice and the client. This one area gives rise to more disputes and complaints than any other single issue. It is thus of paramount importance to ensure that clients, wherever possible, are able to give fully informed consent to treatment.

Informed consent

As a general rule, an individual is legally bound by their signature to a document, whether or not they have read it or fully understood it. A 'consent to treatment' form is often a key document providing evidence of the contract that exists between the veterinary surgeon and the client. Problems can, and do, arise when clients sign such a form without fully appreciating the implications of treatment. Consent forms should therefore be signed by the client only when they understand as fully as possible the implications of treatment. This means that the owner of an animal should be given all the relevant information they need in order to decide on the best course of action. Veterinary nurses are often in a position to support clients during the decision-making process; clients may approach a nurse with their concerns, often expressed obliquely because of embarrassment. It is important to be aware of possible anxieties and always be prepared to explore them. Where a client appears to have serious doubts or misconceptions it is important to report these to the veterinary surgeon.

For further information on consent and confidentiality see Chapter 2.

The Veterinary Surgeons Act 1966

The Veterinary Surgeons Act, in common with other animal protection legislation, sets out to prevent unnecessary suffering to animals. This is achieved through regulating who may provide veterinary care and treatment, i.e. veterinary surgery as defined earlier in this chapter. The Act provides for the regulation of veterinary training, the provision of a register for veterinary surgeons who practise in the UK, and for the regulation of their professional conduct whilst entered on the Register. The title of veterinary surgeon is reserved by law to those whose names appear in the Register of Veterinary Surgeons maintained by the RCVS. Individuals so registered are members or fellows of the RCVS and use the letters MRCVS or FRCVS, respectively. Veterinary surgeons may also be colloquially referred to as veterinarians, a title that is widely recognized in North America and Europe. Only persons who are members or fellows of the RCVS may practise as veterinary surgeons in the UK.

Schedule 3

This schedule of the Veterinary Surgeons Act sets down what non-veterinary surgeons may provide in terms of animal treatment. In June 2002 an amendment to Schedule 3 became law. This widened the scope of veterinary nursing work, previously restricted to the provision of treatment to companion animals (i.e. not farm animals, horses, wild animals or animals kept other than as pets). The provisions of Schedule 3 that apply to veterinary nurses are set out in the box below. Schedule 3 also provides for the owners of pet and farm animals to provide treatment, and for anyone to provide first aid to an animal in an emergency.

Schedule 3 includes 'Treatment and operations which may be given or carried out by unqualified persons'. This is referring to anyone who is not a veterinary surgeon.

There are several important points concerning the provisions of Schedule 3 and the RCVS guidance:

- It does not provide a definitive list of care and treatment, or tasks, that may be carried out by a veterinary nurse. The intention is that a veterinary surgeon may delegate, provided that he/she is satisfied that a nurse is qualified and competent, any procedure or aspect of care that is not excluded (such as surgery entailing entry into a body cavity). Schedule 3 therefore provides for an increasing level of skill, competence and additional qualifications achieved by individual veterinary nurses

- The broad scope of Schedule 3 means that it covers virtually all clinical work undertaken by veterinary nurses, from the administration of medications to minor surgery. The Schedule also permits animal owners or their employees to provide minor medical treatments (otherwise it would be illegal for owners to administer medicines at home)

- The competence of a newly qualified veterinary nurse is defined by the National Occupational Standards for veterinary nursing. However, most veterinary nurses will improve and increase the range of their knowledge and skills after qualification. They may therefore become competent to undertake more complex or specialized care and treatment. The supervising veterinary surgeon must actively ascertain this competence before delegating such work. Conversely, veterinary surgeons must be aware that some nurses do not achieve this progression and must not be expected to undertake work for which they do not possess the necessary expertise.

Veterinary Surgeons Act 1966: Schedule 3 (extracts)

Exemptions from Restrictions on Practice of Veterinary Surgery
Part I
Treatment and Operations which may be Given or Carried Out by Unqualified Persons

1. Any minor medical treatment given to an animal by its owner, by another member of the household of which the owner is a member or by a person in the employment of the owner.

2. Any medical treatment or any minor surgery (not involving entry into a body cavity) given, otherwise than for reward, to an animal used in agriculture, as defined in the Agriculture Act 1947, by the owner of the animal or by a person engaged or employed in caring for animals so used.

3. The rendering in an emergency of first aid for the purpose of saving life or relieving pain or suffering.

…

6. Any medical treatment or any minor surgery (not involving entry into a body cavity) to any animal by a veterinary nurse if the following conditions are complied with, that is to say–
   (a) the animal is, for the time being, under the care of a registered veterinary surgeon or veterinary practitioner and the medical treatment or minor surgery is carried out by the veterinary nurse at his direction;
   (b) the registered veterinary surgeon or veterinary practitioner is the employer or is acting on behalf of the employer of the veterinary nurse; and
   (c) the registered veterinary surgeon or veterinary practitioner directing the medical treatment or minor surgery is satisfied that the veterinary nurse is qualified to carry out the treatment or surgery.

In this paragraph and in paragraph 7 below–
   'veterinary nurse' means a nurse whose name is entered in the list of veterinary nurses maintained by the College.

7. Any medical treatment or any minor surgery (not involving entry into a body cavity) to any animal by a student veterinary nurse if the following conditions are complied with, that is to say–
   (a) the animal is, for the time being, under the care of a registered veterinary surgeon or veterinary practitioner and the medical treatment or minor surgery is carried out by the student veterinary nurse at his direction and in the course of the student veterinary nurse's training;
   (b) the treatment or surgery is supervised by a registered veterinary surgeon, veterinary practitioner or veterinary nurse and, in the case of surgery, the supervision is direct, continuous and personal; and
   (c) the registered veterinary surgeon or veterinary practitioner is the employer or is acting on behalf of the employer of the student veterinary nurse.

In this paragraph–
   'student veterinary nurse' means a person enrolled under bye-laws made by the Council for the purpose of undergoing training as a veterinary nurse at an approved training and assessment centre or a veterinary practice approved by such a centre;
   'approved training and assessment centre' means a centre approved by the Council for the purpose of training and assessing student veterinary nurses.

The provisions of Schedule 3 apply only to veterinary nurses listed by the RCVS, and to enrolled student veterinary nurses (see above). It is therefore important for employing veterinary surgeons to check a nurse's Listed status annually and especially when employing locum staff. Clinical work, which falls within the definitions set out in Schedule 3, undertaken by a qualified but unlisted nurse is outside the law, as is such work undertaken by any unqualified nursing assistant.

Student veterinary nurses may undertake medical treatments or minor surgery only as necessary to further their training. Student nurses must always conduct such work under the supervision of qualified veterinary staff (Listed nurses or veterinary surgeons). In the case of a student undertaking minor surgical procedures, that supervision must be direct, continuous and personal. This means that the supervisor must be present, in control of the situation and able to intervene if necessary throughout the procedure.

Further guidance may be obtained from *RCVS Online*.

RCVS guidance to veterinary nurses on the Veterinary Surgeons Act 1966

Introduction

1. Under the Veterinary Surgeons Act 1966 the general rule is that only a veterinary surgeon may practise veterinary surgery. There are, however, a number of exceptions to this rule, and two of them concern veterinary nurses. This note explains the law as it applies to them.

Definition of veterinary surgery

2. Veterinary surgery as defined in the Act means 'the art and science of veterinary surgery and medicine and, without prejudice to the generality of the foregoing, shall be taken to include–
   (a) the diagnosis of diseases in, and injuries to, animals including tests performed on animals for diagnostic purposes;
   (b) the giving of advice based upon such diagnosis;
   (c) the medical or surgical treatment of animals; and
   (d) the performance of surgical operations on animals.'

What can be done by people other than veterinary surgeons

3. Schedule 3 to the Act allows anyone to give first aid in an emergency for the purpose of saving life and relieving suffering. The owner of an animal, or a member of the owner's household or employee of the owner, may also give it minor medical treatment. There are a number of other exceptions to the general rule, mainly relating to farm animals, in addition to the exceptions that apply to veterinary nurses.

What can be done by veterinary nurses

4. Veterinary nurses, like anyone else, may give first aid and look after animals in ways that do not involve acts of veterinary surgery. In addition, veterinary nurses may do the things specified in paragraphs 6 and 7 of Schedule 3 to the Veterinary Surgeons Act 1966 as amended by the Veterinary Surgeons Act 1966 (Schedule 3 Amendment) Order 2002 (see above).

Listed veterinary nurses

5. Paragraph 6 of Schedule 3 applies to veterinary nurses whose names are entered on the list maintained by the RCVS. They may administer 'any medical treatment or any minor surgery (not involving entry into a body cavity)' under veterinary direction.

6. The animal must be under the care of a veterinary surgeon and the treatment must be carried out at his or her direction. The veterinary surgeon must be the employer of the veterinary nurse or be acting on behalf of the nurse's employer.

7. The directing veterinary surgeon must be satisfied that the veterinary nurse is qualified to carry out the treatment or surgery. The RCVS will advise from time to time on veterinary nursing qualifications that veterinary surgeons should recognize.

8. All listed veterinary nurses (VNs) are qualified to administer medical treatment or minor surgery (not involving entry into a body cavity), under veterinary direction, to all the species that are commonly kept as companion animals, including exotic species so kept. Unless they hold further qualifications, they are not qualified to treat the equine species, wild animals or farm animals. Listed veterinary nurses who hold the RCVS Certificate in Equine Veterinary Nursing (EVNs) are qualified to administer medical treatment or minor surgery (not involving entry into a body cavity), under veterinary direction, to any of the equine species (horses, asses and zebras).

Student veterinary nurses

9. Paragraph 7 of Schedule 3 applies to student veterinary nurses. A student veterinary nurse is someone enrolled for the purpose of training as a veterinary nurse at an approved training and assessment centre (VNAC) or a veterinary practice approved by such a centre (TP). This does not include those who are undertaking the Animal Nursing Assistant course.

10. A student veterinary nurse may administer 'any medical treatment or any minor surgery (not involving entry into a body cavity)' under veterinary direction.

continues ▶

11. The animal must be under the care of a veterinary surgeon and the treatment must be carried out at his or her direction. The veterinary surgeon must be the employer of the veterinary nurse or be acting on behalf of the nurse's employer.
12. The treatment or minor surgery must be carried out in the course of the student veterinary nurse's training. In the view of RCVS, such work should be undertaken only for the purpose of learning and consolidating new skills.
13. The treatment or surgery must be supervised by a veterinary surgeon or a listed veterinary nurse. In the case of surgery the supervision must be direct, continuous and personal.
14. In the view of RCVS, a veterinary surgeon or listed veterinary nurse can only be said to be supervising if they are present on the premises and able to respond to a request for assistance if needed. 'Direct, continuous and personal' supervision requires the supervisor to be present and giving the student nurse his or her undivided personal attention.

Medical treatment and minor surgery

15. The Act does not define 'any medical treatment or any minor surgery (not involving entry into a body cavity)'. Ultimately it would be for the courts to decide what these words mean.
16. The procedures that veterinary nurses are specifically trained to carry out include the following:
    - Administer medication by mouth, topically, by the rectum, by inhalation or by subcutaneous, intramuscular or intravenous injection
    - Administer other treatments, including oral, intravenous and subcutaneous rehydration, other fluid therapy, catheterization, cleaning and dressing of surgical wounds, treatment of abscesses and ulcers, application of external casts, holding and handling of viscera when assisting in operations and cutaneous suturing
    - Prepare animals for anaesthesia and assist in the administration and termination of anaesthesia, including premedication, analgesia and intubation
    - Collect samples of blood, urine, faeces, skin and hair
    - Take X-rays.

Guidance on anaesthesia

17. Particular care is needed over the administration of anaesthesia. A veterinary surgeon alone should:
    - Assess the fitness of the animal to undergo anaesthesia
    - Select and plan a suitable anaesthetic regime
    - Select any premedication
    - Administer anaesthetic if the induction dose is either incremental or to effect.

18. Provided the veterinary surgeon is physically present and immediately available for consultation, a listed veterinary nurse may:
    - Administer selected sedative, analgesic or other agents before and after the operation
    - Administer non-incremental anaesthetic agents on the instruction of the directing veterinary surgeon
    - Monitor clinical signs and maintain an anaesthetic record
    - Maintain anaesthesia by administering supplementary incremental doses of intravenous anaesthetic agents or adjusting the delivered concentration of anaesthetic agents, under the direct instruction of the supervising veterinary surgeon.

Further reading

Dimond B (2005) *Legal Aspects of Nursing, 4th edn.* Pearson Longman, London
Dunstan GRD and Seller MJ (eds) (1983) *Consent in Medicine.* King Edward's Hospital Fund for London
Dyer C (1992) *Doctors, Patients and the Law.* Blackwell, Oxford
Legood G (2000) *Veterinary Ethics.* Continuum, London
Mackay L (1993) *Conflicts in Care: Medicine and Nursing.* Chapman & Hall, London
Mason JK and McCall-Smith RA (1999) *Law and Medical Ethics, 5th edn.* Butterworth, London

McHale J, Tingle J and Peysner J (1998) *Law and Nursing.* Butterworth-Heinemann, London
Royal College of Veterinary Surgeons (2006a) *Guide to Professional Conduct.* RCVS, London (also available online at www.rcvs.org.uk)
Royal College of Veterinary Surgeons (2006b) *The UK Veterinary Profession in 2006.* RCVS, London
Wigens L (ed.) (2004) *Foundations in Nursing and Health Care: Law and Ethics.* Nelson Thornes, London

Websites:
RCVS   www.rcvs.org.uk
Veterinary Medicines Directorate   www.vmd.gov.uk

Chapter 4a

Canine and feline anatomy and physiology

Victoria Aspinall and Melanie Cappello

Learning objectives

After studying this chapter, students should be able to:

- Describe the basic tissues and fluids that make up the mammalian body
- Demonstrate an understanding of the organization of the body cavities and their contents
- Describe the structure of each of the component parts of the body systems
- Describe the role played by each part of a system and how they interrelate to perform a cohesive function
- Understand the anatomical relationship between one body system and another
- Explain the methods by which the body systems contribute to maintaining the balance of the internal environment

This chapter is not intended as a complete source of information on anatomy and physiology and reference should be made to the 'Further reading' list at the end of the chapter.

Introduction

- **Anatomy** – the study of the structure of the body
- **Physiology** – the study of how the body actually 'works'.

Dogs and cats both belong to the Class Mammalia (they suckle their young) and they are both carnivores (they are flesh-eaters). They have a similar anatomical structure and any differences will be highlighted.

Directional terms

It is essential to understand the terms used to describe the position of the parts of the body in relation to each other (Figure 4.1).

Definitions

- **Dorsal** – towards or relatively near the upper surface of the body, the head, neck, tail and the front surface of the paws
- **Ventral** – towards or relatively near the belly and the corresponding surface of the neck and tail
- **Lateral** – on the side or outer surface of the body, i.e. away from the median plane, which divides the body longitudinally into two halves
- **Medial** – towards or relatively near the median plane (i.e. the 'middle' of the body)
- **Cranial / Anterior** – towards or relatively near the head
- **Caudal / Posterior** – towards or relatively near the tail
- **Rostral** – near the nose (structures on the head only)
- **Proximal** – near the main mass of the body or origin (e.g. in the limbs it is the attached end)
- **Distal** – away from the main body mass (e.g. in the limbs it is the free end)
- **Superficial** – relatively near the surface of the body or organ.
- **Deep** – relatively near the centre of the body or organ.

Body fluid compartments

Approximately 60–80% of the body is made of water. The water contains a variety of chemical compounds that are essential for life and it is usually described as 'fluid'. The function of this fluid is to maintain a constant environment in which the normal processes of the body can take place effectively.

Chemical compounds can be divided into two groups:

- **Organic compounds** – those containing carbon (e.g. proteins, carbohydrates and fats)
- **Inorganic compounds** – those that are *not* based on carbon (e.g. sodium, potassium and phosphate).

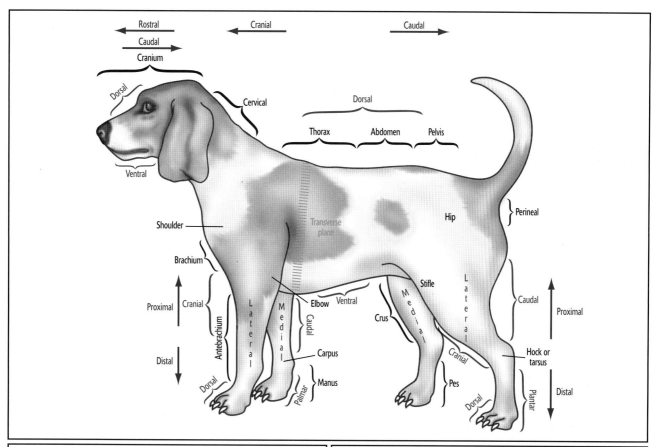

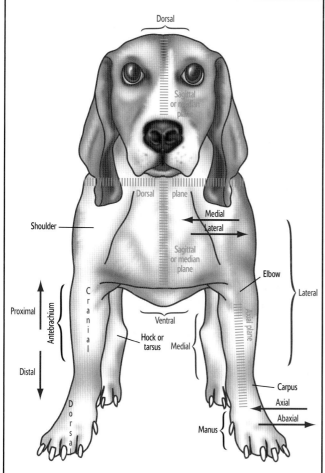

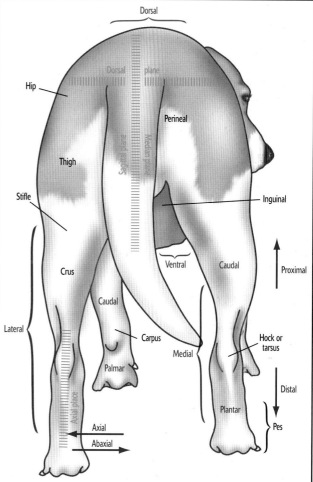

4.1 Anatomical planes and directions.

The most important inorganic compound in the body is **water**. The water content of the body is divided between two main compartments: **intracellular fluid** and **extracellular fluid** (Figure 4.2).

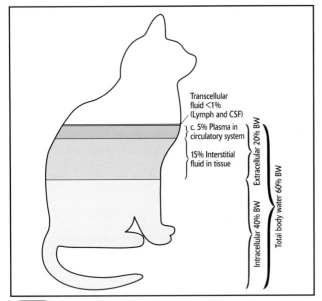

4.2   Water distribution in the body. BW, bodyweight.

- **Intracellular fluid** (ICF) consists of the fluid found within the blood cells and the fluid found within the rest of the cells of the body. It accounts for two thirds of the total body water.
- **Extracellular fluid** (ECF) consists of the fluid part of the blood (**plasma**), the fluid around the cells (**interstitial** or **tissue fluid**) and **transcellular fluid** (lymph, synovial fluid, cerebrospinal fluid). It accounts for one third of the total body water.

The water content of the body may vary. It is slightly *higher* in young and thin animals and slightly *lower* in overweight animals.

A healthy animal takes water into the body in food and drink and loses water from the body in a number of ways, such as in urine and faeces and from the respiratory system. Typical daily water losses from a healthy animal are:

- 20 ml/kg bodyweight in **urine**
- 20 ml/kg bodyweight from the **respiratory system** (i.e. panting, etc.)
- 10–20 ml/kg bodyweight in **faeces**.

Under normal circumstances, an animal requires 50–60 ml of water/kg bodyweight per day to replace the water loss over a 24-hour period.

Within the body fluids and tissues there are a number of other inorganic compounds. These are called **minerals** and they exist in the body in the form of **ions**.

- An **ion** is a charged particle.
- An ion that has one or more *negative* charges is called an **anion**.
- An ion that has one or more *positive* charges is called a **cation**.

The mineral salts (e.g. sodium chloride) present in the body are ionic compounds and when they are dissolved in water they split up into their constituent ions (e.g. sodium and chloride). These free ions allow the passage of electrical currents and are classed as **electrolytes**.

- Within the **ICF** the main cation is **potassium**, though other cations such as sodium and magnesium are present in smaller amounts. The main anion is **phosphate**, with smaller amounts of bicarbonate and chloride. ICF also contains protein.
- Within the **ECF** the main cation is **sodium**, though there are smaller amounts of potassium and calcium and magnesium. The anions present are **chloride**, **bicarbonate** and **phosphate**. ECF does not normally contain protein.

Inside the body there is constant movement of water (by **osmosis**) and electrolytes (by **diffusion**) between the fluid compartments (Figure 4.3). This movement is dependent on the osmotic pressure or tonicity of the ECF – mainly that of plasma and the ICF.

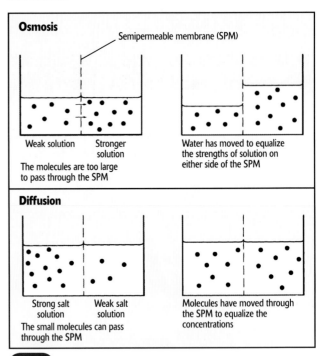

4.3   Osmosis and diffusion.

- The **osmotic pressure** or **tonicity** of a fluid is the pressure needed to prevent osmosis from occurring and is dependent on the number of particles (both ions and undissolved molecules) in a solution.
- A fluid that has the same tonicity as plasma is described as being **isotonic**.
- A fluid that has lower tonicity than plasma is described as being **hypotonic**.
- A fluid that has higher tonicity than plasma is described as being **hypertonic**.

Acid–base balance

- An **acid** is a substance that gives up hydrogen ions when it dissolves or dissociates in water.
- A **base** or **alkali** is a substance that can combine with the hydrogen ions liberated by the dissociation of an acid.

The hydrogen ion concentration of a solution is expressed in its **pH**, which is measured on a scale of 0–14.

- An **acidic** solution has a pH <7.
- An **alkaline (basic)** solution has a pH >7.
- A **neutral** solution has a pH of 7.

If the body is to function effectively it is vital that the pH of the blood and the body fluids remains within the normal range. The normal pH of blood is 7.4. Within the body there are several mechanisms that act to maintain this acid–base balance. They are:

- Respiration, which controls the levels of carbon dioxide dissolved in the blood (excess carbon dioxide makes the blood more acid, i.e. it lowers the pH)
- Sodium and hydrogen ion exchange within the distal convoluted tubules of the renal nephrons (excretion of hydrogen ions will raise the pH)
- The presence of buffers within the blood plasma.

A **buffer** is a substance that can absorb or give up hydrogen ions to keep the pH of a solution within the normal range.

Chapter 19 discusses body fluids in more detail, in the context of fluid therapy.

Cell structure

All living organisms are made of cells and these are arranged into tissues and organs.

In highly organized species such as the dog and cat, different types of cell are specialized to carry out separate functions. However, each cell type has certain features in common (Figure 4.4).

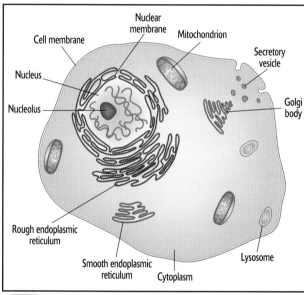

Cell membrane · Nucleus · Nucleolus · Nuclear membrane · Mitochondrion · Secretory vesicle · Golgi body · Lysosome · Cytoplasm · Smooth endoplasmic reticulum · Rough endoplasmic reticulum

4.4 The structure of a cell.

Cell or plasma membrane

This membrane separates the cell from its surrounding environment and controls what enters and leaves the cell. It is said to be selectively permeable, allowing some substances to pass freely through the membrane while others are excluded. The cell membrane is formed by a phospholipid bilayer with protein molecules interspersed within it.

Cells can take in particles by means of two processes:

- **Phagocytosis** ('cell eating') – the process by which extracellular materials are engulfed by a cell into membrane-bound vacuoles within the cytoplasm (see Chapter 6). Some white blood cells are 'phagocytic' and will engulf 'foreign' materials such as bacteria.

- **Pinocytosis** ('cell drinking') – essentially the same as the above process but this is the means by which extracellular fluid is ingested by a cell.

Cytoplasm

This is the aqueous material found within the interior of the cell. The cytoplasm contains the nucleus, organelles and numerous solutes, including glucose, ions and adenosine triphosphate (ATP).

Nucleus

The nucleus controls the cell's activity and contains the hereditary information of the cell within the **chromosomes**. The nucleus is bound by a double membrane that contains a number of pores to allow the entry and exit of molecules. Within the nucleus are one or more **nucleoli**, which manufacture ribosomes (see below).

Organelles

Lying within the cytoplasm are a number of organelles, which carry out the functions of the cell. They are as follows.

Centrioles

These are a pair of structures that act as organizers of the nuclear spindle during cell division (see Figure 4.5).

Mitochondria

These are the sites for cell respiration. They are responsible for the production of **energy** in the form of **ATP** (adenosine triphosphate). Mitochondria have a highly folded inner membrane that increases the surface area on which the processes of respiration take place. They are found in abundance in cells that are very active (e.g. skeletal muscle). When a cell requires energy, a phosphate group is split off the ATP molecule, liberating energy. The resulting molecule has only two phosphate groups and is called **ADP** (adenosine diphosphate). The ADP goes back into the respiratory cycle and is used to make ATP again:

$$ATP \leftrightarrow ADP + energy$$

Ribosomes

These spherical structures float free in the cytoplasm and are responsible for protein synthesis.

Endoplasmic reticulum

This is an elaborate system of membranes and flattened sacs forming a series of sheets. There are two types.

- **Rough endoplasmic reticulum** has numerous ribosomes attached to its surface. Its function is to synthesize protein and transport it within the cell.
- **Smooth endoplasmic reticulum** has no ribosomes on its surface and its function is to synthesize and transport lipids and steroids.

Golgi apparatus or body

This consists of a stack of flattened sacs made of membrane. It modifies a number of cell products and plays a part in the formation of lysosomes.

Lysosomes

These are membrane-bound sacs that contain digestive enzymes. They digest material phagocytosed by the cell, worn-out organelles and the cell itself when it dies.

Cell division

The cells of the body are able to reproduce and make copies of themselves, enabling the body to grow and repair tissues. There are two types of cell division that take place in the body:

- **Meiosis** – occurs in the germ cells of the ovary and testis (see Chapter 5)
- **Mitosis** – occurs in the somatic cells of the body (i.e. all the other cells).

Mitosis

Mitosis (Figure 4.5) involves the replication of the genetic 'information' or DNA that is carried by the chromosomes in every cell. The cell then divides into two new ones by a process known as binary fission. The resulting 'new' cells are called the **daughter cells** and are identical to each other. When the cell is resting between divisions it is said to be in **interphase**, and it is during this stage that the DNA replicates in preparation for mitotic division. The other four stages of mitosis are **prophase, metaphase, anaphase** and **telophase**.

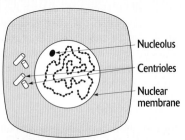

Nucleolus
Centrioles
Nuclear membrane

A Interphase
Cell has normal appearance of non-dividing cell condition: chromosomes too threadlike for clear visibility.

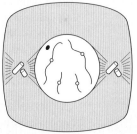

B Early prophase
Chromosomes become visible as they contract, and nucleolus shrinks. Centrioles at opposite sides of the nucleus. Spindle fibres start to form.

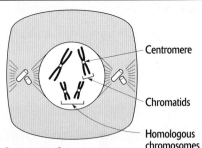

Centromere
Chromatids
Homologous chromosomes

C Late prophase
Chromosomes become shorter and fatter – each seen to consist of a pair of chromatids joined at the centromere. Nucleolus disappears. Prophase ends with breakdown of nuclear membrane.

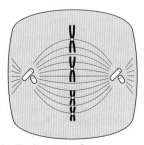

D Early metaphase
Chromosomes arrange themselves on equator of spindle. Note that homologous chromosomes do not associate.

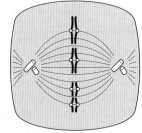

E Late metaphase
Chromatids draw apart at the centromere region. Note that the daughter centromeres are orientated toward opposite poles of the spindle.

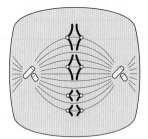

F Early anaphase
Spindle fibres contract and pull the chromatids apart, moving them to the opposite ends of the cell.

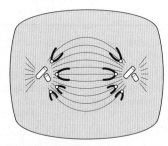

G Late anaphase
Chromosomes reach their destination.

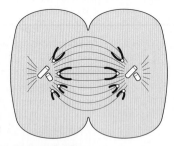

H Early telophase
The cell starts to constrict across the middle.

I Late telophase
Constriction continues. Nuclear membrane and nucleolus reformed in each daughter cell. Spindle apparatus degenerates. Chromosomes eventually regain their threadlike form and the cells return to resting condition (interphase).

Note that the daughter cells have precisely the same chromosome constitution as the original parent cell.

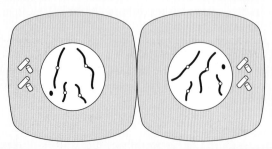

4.5   Cell reproduction: mitosis. (Redrawn after M.B.V. Roberts, *Biology: a Functional Approach*, 4th edn, Nelson, 1986.)

Basic tissue types

- A **tissue** is a collection of cells and their products in which one cell predominates.
- An **organ** is a collection of tissues that performs or is adapted for a specific purpose.
- A **system** is a collection of parts, structures, tissues and organs that are related by function.

The body contains four types of tissue, each of which is highly specialized to carry out a particular function. The types are epithelial, connective, muscular and nervous. Muscular and nervous tissues will be discussed later in this chapter, in the sections on muscles and the nervous system.

Epithelial tissue

Epithelial tissue (Figure 4.6) covers the inner and outer surfaces of the body (e.g. skin, organs, body cavities and blood vessels). It consists of single or layered sheets of cells held together by an intercellular substance. The bottom layer of cells sits on a basement membrane. A single sheet of epithelium is described as **simple**; when it is layered it is described as **stratified**. Epithelial cells may be further described by their cell shape:

- **Cuboidal** – cube shaped
- **Squamous** – flattened
- **Columnar** – tall and column-like.

Epithelial tissue may also contain specialized cells, called **goblet cells**, which produce **mucus** (a proteinaceous secretion that serves to protect the surface of the tissue). It may possess hair-like structures or **cilia** on its surface, which project from the free edge of the epithelial layer and waft the mucus along the surface of the epithelium.

All glandular tissue in the body is derived from epithelial tissue and these tissues may be unicellular (e.g. goblet cells) or multicellular (Figure 4.7).

Types of epithelium		Description/function
Simple squamous epithelium	Cells Basement membrane	Composed of a single sheet of very thin, flat cells. The sheet of cells is thin and delicate, and is found in areas where diffusion occurs (e.g. **alveoli of lungs, lining blood vessels, glomerular capsule**)
Simple cuboidal epithelium		This type of epithelium is found lining many of the **glands** and their **ducts**, and also lining parts of the **kidney tubules**
Simple columnar epithelium		This type of epithelium is found lining the **intestine** allowing the absorption of soluble food material
Ciliated epithelium	Cilia Goblet cells	Usually columnar in shape. It has numerous cilia on the free surface of each cell. This type of epithelium lines tubes and cavities where materials must be moved (e.g. **respiratory tract, oviducts**)
Stratified epithelium		Comprises a series of layers making it tough and it therefore has a protective function. It is found in areas that are subjected to friction (e.g. **oesophagus, mouth, vagina**). In areas where it is subject to considerable abrasion the cells are infiltrated with a tough protein called **keratin**, as seen in the **epidermis** of the skin
Transitional epithelium		A modified form of stratified epithelium. Found in structures that must be able to stretch (e.g. **bladder, urethra**)
Glandular epithelium	Mucus-secreting cells	This type of epithelium has interspersed secretory cells, which secrete materials into the cavity or space they are lining. Folding of glandular epithelium results in the formation of a gland (see Figure 4.7 for examples)

4.6 Types of epithelial tissue.

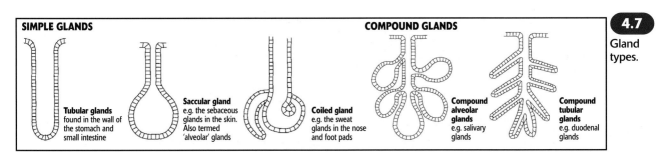

4.7 Gland types.

SIMPLE GLANDS

Tubular glands found in the wall of the stomach and small intestine

Saccular gland e.g. the sebaceous glands in the skin. Also termed 'alveolar' glands

Coiled gland e.g. the sweat glands in the nose and foot pads

COMPOUND GLANDS

Compound alveolar glands e.g. salivary glands

Compound tubular glands e.g. duodenal glands

Connective tissue

Connective tissue is responsible for supporting and binding together all the tissues and organs of the body. It also acts as a transport system, carrying nutrients around the body and removing waste materials.

Connective tissue consists of a **ground substance** or **matrix** that has cells and fibres embedded within it. There are five categories of connective tissue in the body:

- Loose connective tissue – areolar and adipose tissue
- Dense (fibrous) connective tissue – tendons and ligaments
- Cartilage
- Bone
- Blood.

Bone and blood will be discussed later, in the sections on the skeletal and blood vascular systems.

Loose connective tissue

Areolar tissue (Figure 4.8) is found all over the body – beneath the skin, connecting organs and as the 'packing' material in the spaces between tissues. It consists of a ground substance containing cells known as fibroblasts and macrophages, and collagen and elastic fibres.

Adipose (fatty) tissue (Figure 4.8) is similar to areolar tissue but it contains numerous closely packed **fat cells**. Fat is important for the storage of energy and for the insulation of the body.

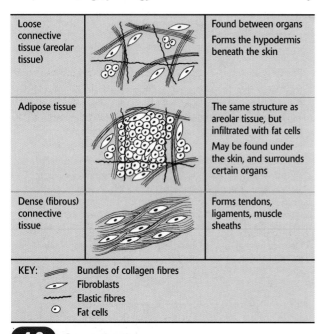

Loose connective tissue (areolar tissue)		Found between organs Forms the hypodermis beneath the skin
Adipose tissue		The same structure as areolar tissue, but infiltrated with fat cells May be found under the skin, and surrounds certain organs
Dense (fibrous) connective tissue		Forms tendons, ligaments, muscle sheaths

KEY:
- Bundles of collagen fibres
- Fibroblasts
- Elastic fibres
- Fat cells

4.8 Connective tissues.

Dense connective tissue

This contains a large number of fibres in proportion to cells in the matrix and may be known as fibrous connective tissue (Figure 4.8). In **tendons** the matrix contains densely packed collagen fibres arranged in parallel, giving great tensile strength. **Ligaments** (yellow elastic tissue) contain a large number of elastic fibres, giving them strength and elasticity.

Cartilage

Cartilage consists of a matrix called **chondrin** with cells or **chondrocytes** and collagen fibres embedded within it. Cartilage is strong but resilient and flexible. It has no blood supply but its nutrition is supplied by the fibrous connective tissue **perichondrium** covering its surface. There are three types of cartilage:

- **Hyaline cartilage** is the simplest and forms the articular surfaces of bones within joints, and the rings of the trachea.
- **Fibrocartilage** has a higher number of collagen fibres within its matrix than hyaline cartilage and is very strong. It occurs where tough support or tensile strength is required. Fibrocartilage contributes to the structure of the intervertebral discs and forms the intra-articular cartilages (e.g. menisci in stifle joint).
- **Elastic cartilage** has a higher number of elastic fibres and is found in areas where support with flexibility is required (e.g. external ear and epiglottis of the larynx).

The body cavities

The body is divided into three separate cavities, which actually are only *potential* spaces, as they are filled with the visceral structures and a little fluid. All the body cavities are lined with a **serous membrane** – an epithelial lining that produces a watery or serous fluid. This lubricates the surfaces of the cavity and the organs within it.

- The serous membrane lining the boundaries of the cavity is described as **parietal** (e.g. parietal pleura).
- The serous membrane covering the organs within the cavity is described as **visceral** (e.g. visceral peritoneum).

The three body cavities are the thoracic cavity, the abdominal cavity and the pelvic cavity.

Thoracic cavity

This is contained within the bony thoracic cage (Figure 4.9). The serous membrane lining the thoracic cavity is called the **pleura**. The different regions of the pleura are named according to their position within the thoracic cavity – the **diaphragmatic pleura** covers the diaphragm, the **costal pleura** covers the inside of the ribs and the visceral **pulmonary pleura** covers the lungs.

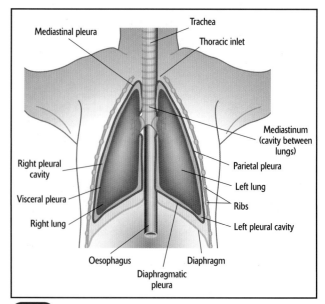

4.9 Horizontal section through the thorax.

The boundaries of the thoracic cavity are:

- *Cranially* – the thoracic inlet
- *Caudally* – the diaphragm
- *Dorsally* – the bodies of the thoracic vertebrae and hypaxial muscle
- *Ventrally* – the sternum
- *Laterally* – the ribs and intercostal muscles.

The thoracic cavity is divided into right and left **pleural cavities** by a double layer of pleura called the **mediastinum**, which contains the pericardial cavity surrounding the heart. Each pleural cavity contains one of the lungs. A small amount of **pleural fluid** (to prevent the organs adhering to each other) facilitates the free movement of the lungs and heart within the thorax.

Abdominal cavity

The abdominal cavity is lined by a serous membrane called the **peritoneum**, which is a continuous sheet forming the closed **peritoneal cavity**. The abdominal cavity is filled with the abdominal viscera or organs. The peritoneal cavity is the potential space between the layers of the peritoneum covering the body wall and the organs in the abdomen. The peritoneal cavity contains no organs: it is filled only with a little serous fluid called **peritoneal fluid**, which acts as a lubricant and prevents adhesions forming between the layers of the peritoneum and the organs. The boundaries of the abdominal cavity are:

- *Cranially* – the diaphragm
- *Caudally* – the pelvic inlet (the abdominal and pelvic cavities are continuous and not separated by a physical barrier)
- *Dorsally* – lumbar vertebrae and hypaxial muscles
- *Ventrally* – muscles of the ventral abdominal wall
- *Laterally* – muscles of the lateral abdominal wall.

The **parietal peritoneum** lines the abdominal cavity while the **visceral peritoneum** covers the surface of the organs within the abdomen. The peritoneum has folds that separate the organs and carry blood vessels and nerves to and from the viscera. There are different names for these folds depending on their position; for example, **mesentery** and **omentum**.

Pelvic cavity

The pelvic cavity is continuous with the abdominal cavity and the cranial part is also lined with **peritoneum**. The boundaries of the pelvic cavity are:

- *Cranially* – the pelvic cavity is continuous with the abdominal cavity but a bony ring referred to as the pelvic inlet forms the entrance to it
- *Caudally* – the pelvic outlet (bony ring that forms the caudal border of the pelvic cavity) and pelvic diaphragm (the set of muscles that closes the caudal end of the pelvic cavity)
- *Dorsally* – the sacrum
- *Ventrally* – floor of the pelvis
- *Laterally* – lateral walls of the pelvis.

The skeletal system

The skeletal system consists of bones, cartilages and joints and is the supportive 'frame' of the body. The functions of the skeletal system are to:

- Provide attachment for the muscles enabling the animal and its parts to move (**locomotion**)
- Provide **protection** for the organs and the soft parts of the body
- Allow formation of blood cells by the bone marrow in the long bones (**haemopoiesis**)
- Provide a **reservoir** of some of the body's essential minerals (e.g. calcium and phosphorus).

Bone tissue

Bone is a specialized type of rigid connective tissue consisting of cells or **osteocytes** in a matrix composed mainly of calcium phosphate, which gives bone its distinctive rigidity and hardness. **Collagen** fibres are also found in bone tissue, contributing to its strength and resilience. These components are arranged in concentric circles, called **lamellae**, around a central channel or **Haversian canal** containing the blood vessels, nerves and lymphatic vessels. There are spaces in the lamellae called **lacunae**, which contain the osteocytes. The whole system is referred to as a **Haversian system**. There are two types of bone tissue: compact and cancellous (or spongy).

- The Haversian systems of **compact bone** are densely packed together. Compact bone is found in the outer edge or **cortex** of all types of bone (Figure 4.10).
- **Cancellous** or **spongy bone** is lighter than compact bone and has a network of interconnected 'bars', called **trabeculae**, providing a 'honeycomb' appearance. Cancellous bone is found at the ends of long bones (Figure 4.11) and in the core of all other types of bone (e.g. flat, irregular).

All bones are covered by a fibrous connective tissue layer: the **periosteum**. Blood reaches the bone via a **nutrient artery**, which enters through a **nutrient foramen**.

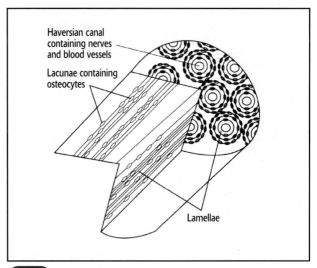

Haversian canal containing nerves and blood vessels

Lacunae containing osteocytes

Lamellae

4.10 Compact bone ultrastructure.

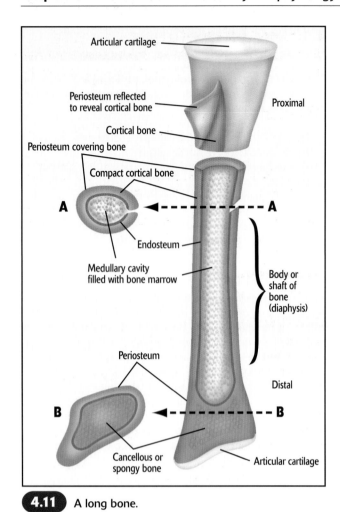

4.11   A long bone.

Classification of bone

Bones can be classified according to their shape:

- **Long bones** – most of the bones of the limbs. They act as levers to facilitate movement and have a long cylindrical shape with a shaft (**diaphysis**) containing a **medullary cavity**. The two ends of a long bone (**epiphyses**) consist of cancellous bone, with a layer of compact bone at the edges (Figure 4.11).
- **Flat bones** – many of the bones of the skull, the ribs and scapulae. These bones have broad flat surfaces. They consist of compact bone at their outer edges, with a core of cancellous bone.
- **Short bones** – found only in the carpus and tarsus. These are small 'cubes' of bone that have a core of cancellous bone covered by a layer of compact bone on the surface.
- **Irregular bones** – including vertebrae and some of the more 'unusual' shapes of bones in the skull. They have an irregular form and consist of a core of cancellous bone surrounded by compact bone on their surface.
- **Sesamoid bones** – small bones that develop in tendons and are shaped like 'sesame-seed'. The function is to reduce the friction and wear on a tendon, by altering the angle at which the tendon passes over a joint (e.g. the **patella**, which contributes to the stifle joint and is found in the tendon of the quadriceps femoris muscle).
- **Pneumatic bones** – bones that contain air (e.g. the frontal and maxillary bones of the skull contain air-filled cavities called **sinuses**). Air-filled cavities enable the bone to maintain its strength while remaining lightweight.

Development of bone

The cells that produce bone are called **osteoblasts**; the cells that reabsorb or remodel bone are called **osteoclasts**. The process by which bone develops is called **ossification**. There are two types: intramembranous and endochondral.

Intramembranous ossification

Many of the bones of the skull develop by this process. The bone develops within a fibrous connective tissue membrane, without a cartilage model.

Endochondral ossification

This type of ossification (Figure 4.12) is the means by which the long bones develop and involves the replacement of a cartilage model within the embryo by bone. The process is not fully completed until the animal has reached maturity.

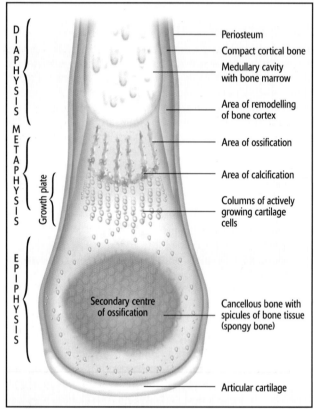

4.12   Endochondral ossification of a long bone.

The process of endochondral ossification in a long bone occurs in the following stages:

1. The cartilage model forms in the fetus.
2. Primary centres of ossification appear in the diaphysis of the bone as the osteoblasts start to replace the cartilage with bone. This progresses towards the ends of the bone.
3. Secondary centres of ossification appear in the epiphyses or ends of the bone. The medullary cavity is formed by the action of osteoclasts reabsorbing the bone tissue in the centre of the diaphysis.
4. Between the developing diaphysis and epiphyses are two bands of cartilage – one at each end of the bone. These are the epiphyseal or growth plates, which allow for elongation of the bone as the animal grows.
5. The epiphyses are replaced by bone and eventually fuse, after which no further growth is possible (i.e. when the animal reaches its adult size).

The skeleton

The skeleton (Figure 4.13) can be divided into three main parts:

- **Axial** – bones of the head, vertebral column and the ribs and sternum
- **Appendicular** – bones of the limbs
- **Splanchnic** – bones that develop within soft tissues.

In order to describe bones it is important to understand the descriptive terminology of the skeletal system and to remember that a **tendon** attaches a muscle to a bone (see Figure 4.24), whereas a **ligament** connects bone to bone.

- **Foramen** (pl. foramina) – a hole in a bone to allow the passage of blood vessels and nerves.
- **Fossa** – a hollow or depressed area on the surface of a bone.
- **Head** – a spherical articular surface on the proximal end of a long bone. The head is joined to the **shaft** of the bone by a narrowed region called the **neck**.
- **Condyle** – a rounded articular surface on a bone.
- **Epicondyle** – a prominence on a bone, lying above a condyle.
- **Trochlea** – a bony structure through or over which tendons pass (e.g. a groove in a bone in which a tendon, acting as a pulley, runs).
- **Tuberosity, trochanter, tubercle** – names given to the various protuberances on bones. They are usually sites for muscle attachment.

The axial skeleton

This forms the axis of the body and runs from the skull to the tip of the tail. It consists of the skull, the vertebral column, the ribs and the sternum.

The skull

The skull consists of a bony **cranium**, which houses and protects the brain, and the **maxilla**, which forms the upper jaw containing the teeth and **nasal chambers**. The skull also houses the sense organs and provides attachment for the lower jaw, or **mandible**, and the **hyoid apparatus**.

The skull consists of a number of bones joined together by immovable fibrous joints called **sutures**. The bones of the skull, some paired and some single, fit very closely together, forming a single rigid structure. In the adult the suture lines are almost invisible.

The shape of an animal's skull varies between species, and, in the case of the dog, even between breeds. There are three morphological forms that are generally recognized, with the difference mainly being expressed in the facial region of the skull.

Skull shapes

- **Mesocephalic** – the 'normal' type of skull, i.e. that which has changed the least from the 'wild type' of skull seen in the ancestor of the dog, the wolf (e.g. Labrador, Beagle)
- **Dolichocephalic** – long and narrow type of skull (e.g. Greyhound, Borzoi, Afghan Hound)
- **Brachycephalic** – short, broad and 'flat' in the facial region (e.g. Boxer, Pug, Pekingese).

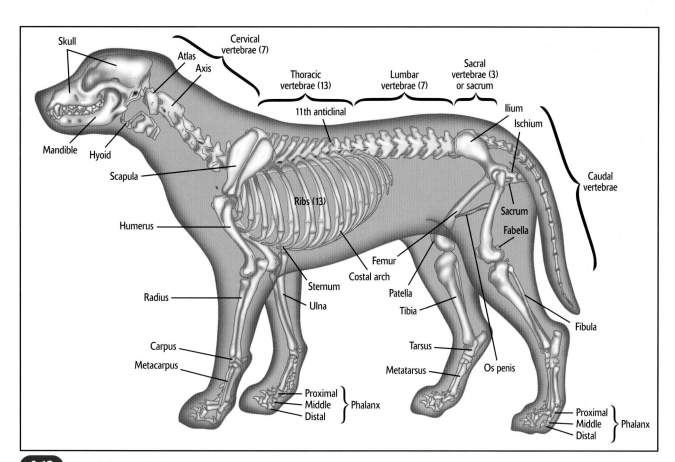

4.13 The skeleton of a dog.

Cranium

Two **parietal** bones form the dorsolateral walls and meet the **occipital** bone, which forms the caudoventral surface of the skull (Figure 4.14). Within the occipital bone is a large hole: the **foramen magnum**, which allows the spinal cord to leave the cranium. On either side of the foramen magnum are the **occipital condyles**, which articulate with the first cervical vertebra (the **atlas**).

The front of the cranium is formed by the **frontal** bones, which contain the air-filled **frontal sinus.** The two **temporal** bones lie ventral to the parietal bones on the lateral surface. On the ventral aspect of the temporal bones are the **tympanic bullae**, which house the middle ear. The **external acoustic meatus** is an opening in the tympanic bulla that is covered by the **tympanic membrane** (ear drum) and is the point where the external ear canal attaches to the skull.

The ventral surface of the cranium is formed by the **sphenoid** bone, with the **ethmoid** bone lying rostral to it.

The **zygomatic** bones form the arches on either side of the skull, which are often called the 'cheekbones'. The **orbit** is the socket in which the eyeball sits. The **lacrimal** bone lies at the base of the orbit and is penetrated by a foramen through which the nasolacrimal duct runs from the eye into the nasal chamber.

Nasal chambers

The nasal bones form the roof of the two chambers, which are divided by the **nasal septum**. Each chamber is filled with fine scrolls of bone covered in ciliated mucous epithelium – the **ethmoturbinates** or **conchae**. The floor of the chambers is formed by the **maxilla**, the **palatine** and the **incisive** bones which also form the roof of the mouth.

The whole structure is penetrated by many foramina to allow for the passage of the numerous nerves and blood vessels that enter and leave the skull.

Mandible

This is the lower jaw, which attaches to the temporal region of the skull at the **temporomandibular joint**. The right and left mandibles are joined together by a cartilaginous joint called the **mandibular symphysis**. Each mandible consists of a horizontal **body** that houses the **alveoli** or **sockets** for the teeth and a vertical **ramus** to which the jaw muscles attach. Caudally an articular surface, the **condylar process**, forms part of the temporomandibular joint.

Hyoid apparatus

This is composed of a number of fine bones joined together in a trapeze-like structure by cartilage. It lies in the neck and is attached to the temporal bone by a cartilaginous joint. The tongue is attached to one side and the larynx to the other side (see Figure 4.50).

The vertebrae

The **vertebral column** or spine consists of a number of **vertebrae** arranged in series in the midline of the body. Its function is to provide a stiff but flexible rod to support the body. It is divided into a number of regions, each of which has a constant number of vertebrae:

- **Cervical or neck** – always 7 vertebrae
- **Thoracic or chest** – 13 vertebrae in the dog and cat
- **Lumbar or lower back** – 7 vertebrae
- **Sacral** – 3 fused vertebrae
- **Coccygeal or caudal** – varies according to length of tail.

All vertebrae share a basic structural plan (Figure 4.15). On the ventral aspect of a typical vertebra is the **body**, which makes up the bulk of the vertebrae. Above it is the **neural arch**. When the arches of all the vertebrae are lined up, they form a 'tunnel' called the spinal or vertebral **canal**, which houses the spinal cord.

Projecting dorsally from the neural arch is a **spinous process**, and projecting laterally are two **transverse processes**. These processes act as sites for muscle attachment and vary in size in the different regions. On the cranial and caudal ends of the neural arch are **articular processes** that form joints with the adjacent vertebrae.

Lying between the bodies of each vertebra are fibrocartilaginous 'shock-absorbers', called **intervertebral discs** (Figure 4.16). The outer part of the disc, the **annulus fibrosus**, is fibrous, while the inner part contains a gelatinous material

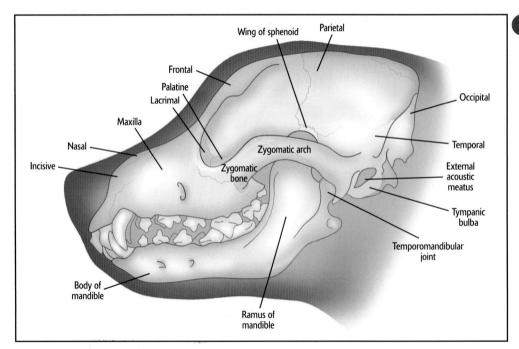

4.14 Lateral view of a dog skull.

Wing of sphenoid
Parietal
Frontal
Palatine
Lacrimal
Maxilla
Nasal
Incisive
Zygomatic arch
Zygomatic bone
Occipital
Temporal
External acoustic meatus
Tympanic bulba
Temporomandibular joint
Body of mandible
Ramus of mandible

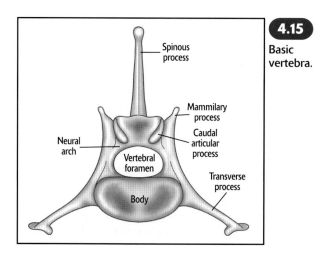

4.15 Basic vertebra.

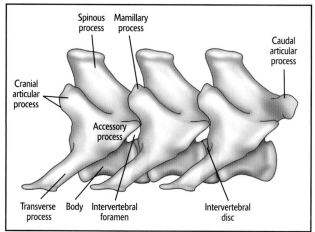

4.16 Part of vertebral column showing two lumbar vertebrae.

called the **nucleus pulposus**. Degeneration of one or more of the intervertebral discs can occur, causing the disc material to 'leak out'. The clinical signs range from pain to complete paralysis due to compression of the spinal cord and nerve roots.

The vertebrae of each region of the vertebral column (Figure 4.17) show the following distinguishing features.

Cervical vertebrae

- The **atlas** or first cervical vertebra consists of two large lateral wing-like processes, joined by ventral and dorsal arches. The atlas articulates with the occipital condyles of the skull in a synovial joint, which allows the head to nod.
- The **axis** or second cervical vertebra has a blade-like spinous process and a cranial projection – the **dens** or **odontoid process**. This articulates with the atlas and allows a rotating movement.

The remaining five cervical vertebrae are similar to each other and follow the basic plan.

A narrowing of the spinal canal in the cervical region may cause compression of the spinal cord and is commonly known as 'wobbler syndrome', as the clinical signs include a 'wobbly' uncoordinated gait. This is most frequently seen in large breeds of dog, such as the Dobermann and Great Dane.

Thoracic vertebrae

Each thoracic vertebra has a short body and a distinctively tall spinous process. Each also has short transverse processes, which have **foveas** (small pits) for articulation with the **tubercles** of the ribs. The bodies of the thoracic vertebrae also have foveas for articulation with the **heads** of ribs (Figure 4.18).

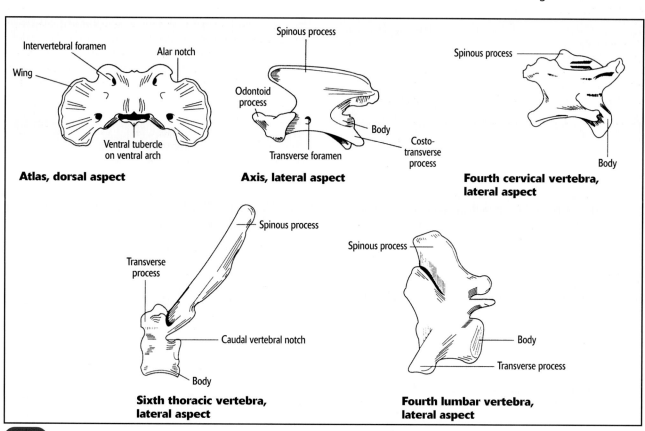

4.17 Regional differences in vertebral structure.

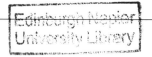

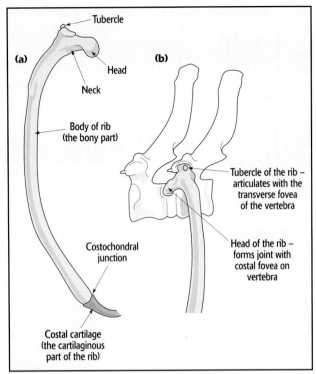

4.18   Structure of a rib and rib articulation.

Lumbar vertebrae
Lumbar vertebrae have longer bodies than thoracic vertebrae and their transverse processes are large and angled cranioventrally.

Sacral vertebrae
The three sacral vertebrae are fused to form the **sacrum**. This articulates with the **ilium** of the pelvis, forming the **sacroiliac joint**.

Coccygeal vertebrae
The first few coccygeal vertebrae have a regular shape but they become progressively smaller and simpler towards the tip of the tail.

The ribs
There are 13 pairs of ribs in the cat and dog, which articulate with the thoracic vertebrae (Figure 4.18). Each rib has a dorsal bony part, which articulates with the appropriate vertebra, and a ventral cartilaginous part – the **costal cartilage**. The costal cartilages of ribs 1–8 articulate with the sternum and are called **sternal ribs**. The costal cartilages of ribs 9–12 touch the cartilage of the rib in front forming the **costal arch** – these are called **asternal ribs**. The last pair of ribs (13) do not articulate with the cartilages of the other ribs and their cartilaginous ends lie free in the muscle wall; these are referred to as the **floating ribs**. This arrangement creates the rib cage.

The sternum
This is composed of eight bones called the **sternebrae**. The most cranial sternebra is called the **manubrium** and lies in the cranial thoracic inlet. The most caudal sternebra is called the **xiphoid process**, which has a flap of cartilage called the **xiphoid cartilage** attached to it.

The appendicular skeleton
This consists of the fore- and hindlimbs (Figures 4.19 and 4.20) and the pectoral and pelvic girdles, which attach the limbs to the axial skeleton.

Canine hip dysplasia is a condition where there is abnormal laxity of the hip joint, which causes the femoral head to move around in the acetabulum, damaging the joint surfaces and leading to osteoarthritis.

Name	Description
Scapula	A flat bone, roughly triangular in shape. Has a prominent **spine** dividing the lateral surface into two fossae (the **supraspinous fossa** and **infraspinous fossa**). At the distal end of the spine is a projection called the acromion. The articular socket at the end of the bone is the **glenoid cavity**
Clavicle	Usually absent in the dog and when present is just a remnant of bone in the muscle cranial to the shoulder. The clavicle is normally present in the cat but does not articulate with any other bones
Humerus	A long bone. Has an articular **head** proximally and a long **body** or shaft. At the proximal end are two prominences, the greater and lesser tubercles, which are sites for muscle attachment. The distal articular surface is the **condyle**, which has a depression, called the **olecranon fossa** and a hole in the centre called the **supratrochlear foramen**
Radius	A long bone that lies alongside the ulna in the forearm. Proximally the depressed articular surface is called the **fovea capitis** (articulates with the humerus). At the distal end there is a rounded projection called the **styloid process** that articulates with the carpus
Ulna	Longer than the radius and has an irregular shape, tapering from its proximal to its distal end. Proximally there is a half-moon-shaped articular surface called the **trochlear notch**, with a hooked projection called the **anconeal process** at its proximal end. At the distal end of the notch are the **medial** and **lateral coronoid processes**). The 'point' of the elbow is formed by the **olecranon**
Carpus	Consists of seven short bones arranged in two rows. The proximal row contains three bones, one of them, the **accessory carpal bone**, projects caudally
Metacarpus	There are five metacarpal bones (I–V), which are small rods of bone. The most medial, metacarpal I, differs from the others as it is shorter and non-weight-bearing (forms part of **dew claw**)
Digits	Digits II–V are composed of three phalangeal bones – a proximal, middle and distal phalanx. Digit I (the dew claw) has only two phalangeal bones. The distal phalanx of each digit bears the **ungual process** that extends into the claw

4.19   The bones of the forelimb.

Name	Description
Pelvis	The pelvis consists of two hipbones joined together ventrally at the **pubic symphysis**. The pelvis articulates with the sacrum dorsally at the **sacroiliac joints**. Each hipbone is composed of three fused bones – the **ilium**, the **ischium** and the **pubis**. The ilium is the largest bone and has a cranial expansion called the **iliac wing**. The ischium is the most caudal pelvic bone and has a prominent caudolateral margin called the **ischiatic tuberosity**. The pubis is the smallest of the bones and forms the cranial portion of the pelvic floor. The three bones unite at the articular socket of the pelvis, called the **acetabulum**, which articulates with the head of the femur via a ball and socket joint. On either side of the pelvic symphysis are two large holes, each being called the **obturator foramen**
Femur	The thigh bone is a typical long bone. Proximally it has an articular **head**, which attaches to the shaft by the **neck**. There is a projection on the proximal femur, lateral to the head, called the **greater trochanter**, and another lies medial to the head, called the **lesser trochanter**. These are sites for muscle attachment. The distal end of the bone has three articular surfaces – the **medial condyle** and **lateral condyle** articulate with the **tibia**, and between them is a smooth groove called the **trochlea**, which articulates with the **patella**
Patella and fabellae	These sesamoid bones are associated with the stifle joint. The **patella** is the largest sesamoid bone in the body and is incorporated into the tendon of the quadriceps femoris muscle, which runs down the front of the thigh. The patella articulates with the trochlea of the distal femur. The **fabellae** are two smaller sesamoid bones, which articulate with the femoral condyles caudally in the stifle joint. The fabellae are located in the tendons of the gastrocnemius muscle
Tibia	The tibia is a long bone and is the main weight-bearing bone of the lower leg. The tibia is expanded proximally providing a wide articular surface for the femur at the stifle joint. Proximally there is a cranially projecting process called the **tibial tuberosity**, which is the point of insertion of the quadriceps femoris muscle. The tibial tuberosity continues distally as a ridge called the **tibial crest**. At the distal end of the tibia is an articular surface and a palpable process called the **medial malleolus**
Fibula	This is a thin long bone, which lies lateral to the tibia. At the distal end there is a prominent bony bulge on the lateral surface of the ankle called the **lateral malleolus**
Tarsus	The tarsus (hock) comprises seven **tarsal bones** arranged in three rows. The proximal row contains the **talus** medially and the **calcaneus** laterally. The calcaneus is extended caudally to form the 'point' of the hock (**tuber calcis**) and serves as a site for the attachment of muscles
Metatarsus	Similar to the metacarpus except that there are only four metarsal bones (although some breeds have a small metatarsal I forming the hind dew claw)
Digits	Similar to the digits in the forepaw but only four digits (II–V) present as the dewclaw is often absent

4.20 The bones of the hindlimb.

The splanchnic skeleton

The only example of a splanchnic bone (i.e. a bone that develops within soft tissue) in the dog and cat is the bone of the penis – the **os penis**. The urethra lies in the **urethral groove** on the ventral surface of the os penis in the dog. In the cat the urethral groove is on the dorsal surface of the os penis, due to the different orientation of the penis (see Figures 4.69 and 4.70).

Joints

A joint or **arthrosis** is the point where two or more bones join together. Joints allow varying degrees of movement and can be classified according to their structure as fibrous, cartilaginous or synovial.

Fibrous joints

The bones forming fibrous joints are united by dense fibrous connective tissue, which allows very little movement. Most fibrous joints are found in the skull, between the flat bones, and are called **sutures**. They are also responsible for attaching the tooth to the bone of its socket.

Cartilaginous joints

The bones forming cartilaginous joints are connected by cartilage and allow little or no movement. They are seen in joints connecting opposite sides of the body and include the **pubic symphysis** between the two hip bones, and the **mandibular symphysis** between the two halves of the mandible.

- **Synarthrosis** – a joint that allows little or no movement (includes fibrous and cartilaginous joints)
- **Amphiarthrosis** – a joint that allows some movement (this type of joint is found between the bodies of the vertebrae).

Synovial joints

Synovial joints (or **diarthroses**) allow a wide range of movement. A fluid-filled space – the **joint cavity**, which is filled with synovial fluid – separates the bones. A **capsule** of dense fibrous connective tissue surrounds the whole joint (Figure 4.21). The outer layer serves as protection while the inner layer or

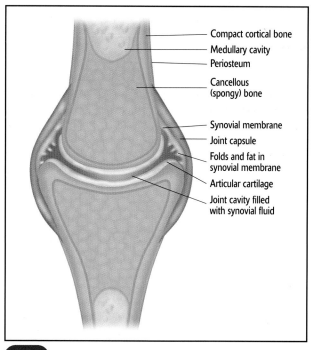

Compact cortical bone
Medullary cavity
Periosteum
Cancellous (spongy) bone
Synovial membrane
Joint capsule
Folds and fat in synovial membrane
Articular cartilage
Joint cavity filled with synovial fluid

4.21 A synovial joint.

synovial membrane lines the joint cavity and secretes synovial fluid, which lubricates the joint. The articular surfaces of the bones are covered by **hyaline cartilage**.

Synovial joints may be stabilized by ligaments. The most common, found on either side of the joint, are **collateral ligaments**. Some synovial joints have stabilizing **intra-capsular ligaments** attached to the articulating bones within the joint (e.g. the cruciate ligament within the stifle joint; Figure 4.22).

Inside a few synovial joints are one or more fibrocartilaginous **menisci** (e.g. the stifle joint has two while the temporomandibular joint has one). These structures help to increase the range of movement of the joint and act as 'shock absorbers'.

Synovial joints allow a wide range of movement between the articulating bones. The motion may be in a single plane or in multiple directions. The types of movement that can occur at synovial joints are:

- **Gliding** – one articular surface slides over the other
- **Flexion** – reduces the angle between the bones (i.e. bends the limb)
- **Extension** – increases the angle between the bones (i.e. straightens the limb)
- **Abduction** – carries the moving part away from the median plane of the body (e.g. when a dog 'cocks' its leg to urinate)
- **Adduction** – brings the body part back towards the median plane of the body
- **Rotation** – the moving bone rotates about a longitudinal axis
- **Circumduction** – allows one end of a bone (e.g. the extremity of a limb) to move in a circular pattern
- **Protraction** – moves a structure away from the body cranially (e.g. moves the foreleg forwards when walking).

- **Retraction** – moves a structure back towards the body (e.g. moves the foreleg back to the original position when walking).

Types of synovial joint

- **Plane or gliding joints** – allow sliding of one bone's surface over the other (e.g. joints between the rows of carpal and tarsal bones)
- **Hinge joints** – allow movement in one plane only (e.g. elbow and stifle joints, which permit just flexion and extension)
- **Pivot joint** – consists of a 'peg' fitted within a 'ring' and allows rotation (e.g. atlantoaxial joint between the first and second cervical vertebrae)
- **Condylar joint** – formed by a convex surface (condyles) that fits into a corresponding concave surface and allows movement in two planes, i.e. flexion, extension and over-extension (e.g. the hock joint)
- **Ball-and-socket joint** – consists of a portion of a sphere or ball received within a corresponding socket. Allows the greatest range of movement (e.g. hip and shoulder joints).

The muscular system

Muscle tissue

There are three types of muscle tissue in the body (Figure 4.23): skeletal (striated/voluntary), smooth (non-striated/involuntary) and cardiac. The muscular system is primarily concerned with skeletal muscle, i.e. those muscles attached to the skeleton.

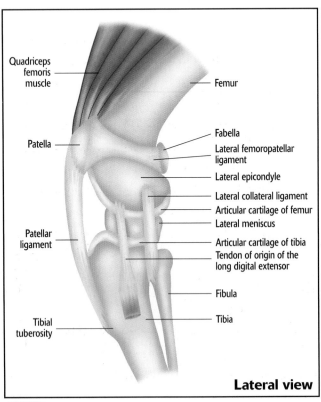

Quadriceps femoris muscle
Femur
Patella
Fabella
Lateral femoropatellar ligament
Lateral epicondyle
Lateral collateral ligament
Articular cartilage of femur
Lateral meniscus
Articular cartilage of tibia
Tendon of origin of the long digital extensor
Patellar ligament
Fibula
Tibial tuberosity
Tibia

Lateral view

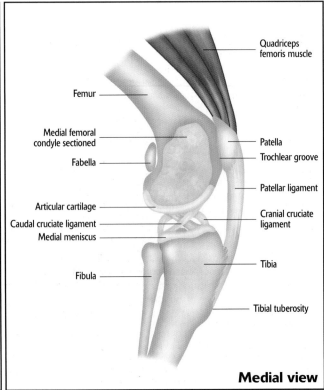

Quadriceps femoris muscle
Femur
Medial femoral condyle sectioned
Fabella
Patella
Trochlear groove
Patellar ligament
Articular cartilage
Caudal cruciate ligament
Medial meniscus
Cranial cruciate ligament
Tibia
Fibula
Tibial tuberosity

Medial view

4.22 A stifle joint.

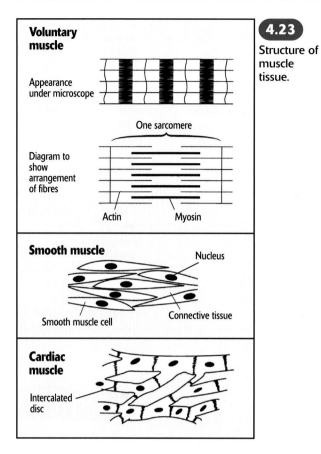

4.23 Structure of muscle tissue.

Voluntary muscle

Appearance under microscope

One sarcomere

Diagram to show arrangement of fibres

Actin   Myosin

Smooth muscle

Nucleus

Smooth muscle cell   Connective tissue

Cardiac muscle

Intercalated disc

Skeletal (striated/voluntary) muscle

This type of muscle is attached to the skeleton and is concerned with locomotion. It is under the conscious or voluntary control of the brain. The cells of skeletal muscle are cylindrical and are called **muscle fibres**. They are arranged in parallel bundles. The muscle fibres are composed of protein filaments called **actin** (thin filaments) and **myosin** (thick filaments), arranged in a way that gives the muscle its striped or **striated** appearance. The skeletal muscles (Figures 4.24–4.29) are responsible for bringing about movement of part of or the whole animal.

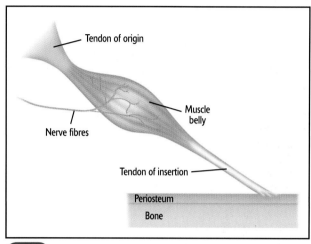

Tendon of origin

Muscle belly

Nerve fibres

Tendon of insertion

Periosteum

Bone

4.24 Muscle and tendon insertion.

Muscle	Origin	Action
Muscles of facial expression	Intrinsic muscles found on the face, around the ears, lips, eyes, mouth and nose. Innervated by cranial nerve VII (facial)	Move the lips, cheeks, nostrils, eyelids and external ears
Muscles of mastication Temporalis Masseter Digastricus	Fills temporal fossa of skull. Coronoid process of mandible Zygomatic arch (lies lateral to mandible). Masseteric fossa of mandible Jugular process of occipital bone. Angle and ventral surface of mandible	Closes the jaw Closes the jaw Opens the jaw
Muscles of the eye Dorsal, ventral, medial and lateral rectus muscles Dorsal and ventral oblique muscles Retractor bulbi	The extra-ocular muscles that move the eye in the socket. They insert on the sclera at the equator of the eye Forms a muscular cone around the optic nerve	Move the eye up, down, inwards and outwards Rotate the eye about the visual axis Pulls the eyeball back into the socket
Muscles of the vertebral column Epaxial group Hypaxial group	Lie in two groups This group of muscles lies dorsal to the transverse processes, i.e. *above* the vertebral column This group lies ventral to the transverse processes, i.e. *below* the vertebral column	Support the spine, extend the vertebral column Flex the head, neck, tail and vertebral column
Muscles of the thorax External intercostals Internal intercostals Diaphragm	The muscles involved in respiration These muscles run from an origin on one rib to a termination on the next, i.e. fill one intercostal space Lie more deeply within the intercostal space, but as with the above they run from one rib to the next The muscle that separates the thoracic cavity from the abdominal cavity Has three openings to allow the passage of structures from the thorax to the abdomen: • **Oesophageal hiatus** transmits the oesophagus and vagal nerves • **Aortic hiatus** transmits the aorta, the azygous vein and thoracic duct • **Caval foramen** transmits the posterior vena cava	Draw the ribs together during inspiration Assist in expiration Inspiration – it contracts to enlarge the thoracic cavity, thus drawing air into the lungs
Muscles of the abdominal wall External abdominal obliques Internal abdominal oblique Transversus abdominis Rectus abdominus	Three muscles make up the lateral wall of the abdomen and one forms the ventral floor of the abdominal wall Form the lateral abdominal wall. All three muscles insert on the **linea alba**, a 'white line' that runs midventrally on the abdomen The deepest of the lateral abdominal muscles Runs in a band either side of the linea alba and inserts on the pubis via the **prepubic tendon**	The fibres run in different directions giving the lateral wall great strength to protect the contents of the abdomen Supports the ventral floor of the abdomen

4.25 Muscles of the axial skeleton.

Muscle	Origin	Insertion	Action
Trapezius	Dorsal midline (level of 2nd cervical to 9th thoracic vertebrae)	Spine of scapula	Protracts the limb (draws the leg forward)
Latissimus dorsi	Broad origin on dorsal midline	Humerus	Retracts the limb (pulls the leg backwards)
Brachiocephalicus	Base of the skull	Cranial aspect of humerus	Bends neck laterally (side to side)
Supraspinatus	Supraspinous fossa of scapula	Greater tubercle of humerus	Extends the shoulder and stabilizes the joint
Infraspinatus	Infraspinous fossa of scapula	Greater tubercle of humerus	Flexes the shoulder and stabilizes the joint
Triceps brachii	Proximal humerus and scapula	Olecranon of ulna	Extends the elbow joint
Biceps brachii	Supraglenoid tubercle of scapula	Radius and ulna	Flexes the elbow joint
Brachialis	Humerus	Radius and ulna	Flexes the elbow joint
Carpal extensor muscles (2)	Humerus (muscle group that runs on the front of carpus)	Carpal bones	Extend the carpus
Carpal flexor muscles (2)	In the group of muscles that run behind the carpus	Carpal bones	Flex the carpus
Digital extensor muscles (2)	Humerus	3rd phalanx	Extend the digits (toes)
Digital flexor muscles (2)	In the group of muscles that run behind the paw	Digits	Flex the digits

4.26 Muscles of the forelimb.

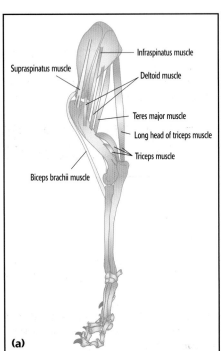

(a)

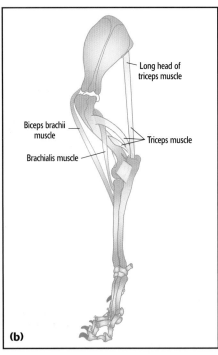

(b)

4.27 Muscles of the forelimb. **(a)** Muscles that move the shoulder joint. **(b)** Muscles that move the elbow joint.

Muscle	Origin	Insertion	Action
Quadriceps femoris	Ilium and femur, runs down the front of the thigh	Consists of four parts, all inserting on the tibial tuberosity	Extends the stifle (tendon contains the **patella**, which articulates with the femur at stifle joint)
Hamstring group Biceps femoris Semitendinosus	Pelvis (ischium) Ischiatic tuberosity (pelvis)	Tibia and calcaneus Tibia and calcaneus	Extends hip, stifle and hock Extends hip and hock; flexes stifle
Semimembranosus	Ischiatic tuberosity	Femur and tibia	Extends hip and stifle
Pectineus Gastrocnemius Cranial (anterior) tibial Digital flexors (2) Digital extensors (3)	Pubis Caudal femur Tibia Run on the caudal surface of the leg Run on the cranial surface of the leg	Distal femur Calcaneus Tarsus Digits (phalanges) Digits	Adducts the limb Extends hock; flexes stifle Flexes hock Flex the toes (digits) Extend the toes (digits)

4.28 Muscles of the hindlimb.

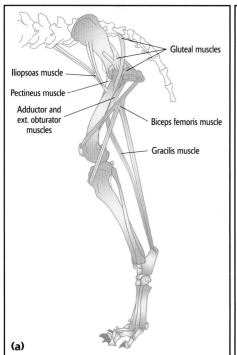

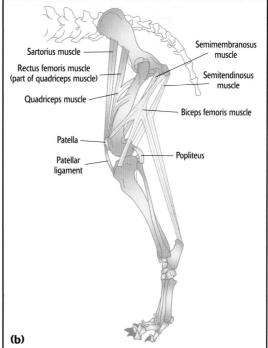

4.29 Muscles of the hindlimb. **(a)** Muscles that protract, retract. adduct and abduct the hindlimb. These muscles also flex and extend the hip joint. **(b)** Muscles that move the hip and stifle joint.

Smooth (non-striated/involuntary) muscle

This type of muscle is found throughout the body (e.g. within the walls of the blood vessels, oesophagus and bladder). Its cells are spindle-shaped (see Figure 4.23) and arranged in sheets or bundles. Contraction of smooth muscle is under the involuntary control of the autonomic nervous system.

Cardiac muscle

This specialized type of involuntary muscle is found only in the heart. It contracts rhythmically and automatically, i.e. the contraction is stimulated from within the muscle tissue itself (**myogenic**). Its fibres are branched and linked by **intercalated discs** and the tissue appears striated (see Figure 4.23).

Muscle contraction

The unit of muscle contraction is called a **sarcomere**. A sarcomere consists of two types of longitudinal protein molecules: **myosin** (thick filaments) and **actin** (thin filaments). Muscle contraction is achieved when the myosin molecules form 'cross-bridges' with the actin molecules. The myosin and actin then slide over one another and the muscle shortens or contracts. This process requires a plentiful supply of energy, in the form of ATP, and free calcium ions.

The cells of skeletal muscle are stimulated to contract by nerve impulses to the muscle fibres. The number of muscle fibres supplied by an individual nerve varies according to the type of movement that the muscle makes. A group of muscle fibres supplied by the one nerve fibre is called a **motor unit**. The size of the motor unit varies; some nerves supply only a few muscle fibres whereas others may supply as many as 200 muscle fibres.

Muscles are always in a slight state of tension, as nerve impulses are constantly being sent to the muscle to keep it prepared for action. This is called **muscle tone**, and it is responsible, for example, for maintaining posture. When an animal is anxious the number of nerve impulses being sent to a muscle

increases. Muscle tone increases and the muscles become 'twitchy' to prepare them for action. The converse is seen when an animal is asleep and fully relaxed. Only a few nerve impulses are sent to the muscle and the animal is more 'floppy'.

The nervous system

The functions of the nervous system are to:

- Receive stimuli from the environment
- Analyse and integrate the stimuli
- Initiate the correct response.

Within the body, the nervous system functions as a well integrated unit, but for descriptive purposes it can be divided into:

- The central nervous system (CNS) – brain and spinal cord
- The peripheral nervous system – all nerves leading away from the central nervous system.

Nervous tissue

The nervous system consists of nervous tissue. The main cell of nervous tissue is the **neuron** (Figure 4.30). Neurons are responsible for the transmission of nerve impulses from one area to another. Each neuron consists of:

- A **cell body** containing the nucleus
- Many fine **dendrites** or thicker **dendrons**, which carry impulses *towards* the cell body
- A single **axon**, which carries impulses *away* from the cell body.

Each neuron is only a few micrometers in diameter, but the length may vary from a few millimetres to a metre. A 'nerve' is made of many neurons held together by connective tissue known as **neuroglia**.

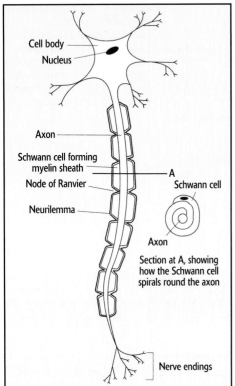

4.30 Structure of a neuron.

Cell body
Nucleus
Axon
Schwann cell forming myelin sheath
Node of Ranvier
Neurilemma
A
Schwann cell
Axon
Section at A, showing how the Schwann cell spirals round the axon
Nerve endings

Nerve type	Definition
Sensory nerve	Carries nerve impulses towards the CNS
Motor nerve	Carries nerve impulses away from the CNS
Intercalated neuron	Lies between a sensory neuron and a motor neuron. May not always be present within a nerve pathway
Mixed nerve	Carries both sensory and motor nerve fibres
Afferent nerve	Carries impulses towards a structure
Efferent nerve	Carries impulses away from a structure
Visceral sensory nerve	Carries information from blood vessels, mucous membranes and visceral body systems, i.e. respiratory, digestive and urogenital systems and the heart to the CNS
Visceral motor nerve	Carries information from the CNS to smooth muscle and glandular tissue within the visceral body systems
Somatic sensory nerve	Carries information from skin, skeletal muscles, tendons, joints and special sense organs to the CNS
Somatic motor nerve	Carries information from the CNS to skeletal muscle
Ganglion	Collection of cell bodies

4.31 Definition of nerve types. NB: The terms efferent/afferent are not restricted to the nervous system and may be applied to blood or lymphatic vessels. Motor nerves are also efferent nerves; sensory nerves are also afferent nerves.

Most axons are covered in a sheath of **myelin**, a white lipoprotein material produced by **Schwann cells** and wrapped like a 'Swiss roll' around the central nerve fibre (Figure 4.30). Between the cells are gaps known as the **nodes of Ranvier** and it is through these that nutrients are able to reach the axon fibre. Myelinated axons conduct nerve impulses faster than nonmyelinated axons. Non-myelinated fibres are rare and may be found in sites such as the retina of the eye and in the grey matter of the central nervous system.

Each neuron terminates in a specialized ending whose function is to conduct nerve impulses:

- From one neuron to another – the ending is called a **synapse** (a single cell body may receive as many as 6000 synaptic endings)
- From a neuron to a muscle fibre – the ending is called a **neuromuscular junction**.

Each nerve pathway consists of neurons and synapses. Nerve impulses travel along the pathway at rates of approximately 100 m/second.

Each synapse consists of a button-like swelling containing vesicles of a **chemical transmitter**. The most common transmitter is acetylcholine, but others include noradrenaline and adrenaline. As the nerve impulse travels towards the synapse, the chemicals are released and stimulate the muscle fibre or cell body with which they are in contact. This process conducts the impulse across the synaptic ending to the next neuron, or brings about contraction of the muscle fibre. The presence of calcium ions is essential for the transmission of a nerve impulse.

A nerve impulse is an 'all or nothing' phenomenon, i.e. each neuron is either stimulated or it is not. A graduated effect is achieved by the relative numbers of neurons in a nerve pathway having an inhibitory effect, compared with the numbers having an excitatory effect.

Figure 4.31 gives definitions of different types of nerve.

Central nervous system (CNS)

The CNS consists of two structures: the brain and the spinal cord. Control by the CNS is voluntary or conscious, i.e. the animal is aware of its actions.

Within the embryo the CNS develops as a hollow **neural tube** from the ectodermal layer of the inner cell mass. It runs along the dorsal surface of the embryo and gives off nerves, which eventually extend to all parts of the body. The anterior part of the tube becomes the brain, while the remainder becomes the spinal cord.

The nervous tissue of the CNS is classified as:

- **White matter** – contains a high proportion of white myelinated fibres
- **Grey matter** – aggregations of cell bodies, with little or no myelin.

In the brain, the white and the grey matter are mixed up, creating an outer grey layer and an inner white layer. Distributed within the white matter are islands of grey matter referred to as **ganglia** or **nuclei**. Each one acts as a relay centre where information, in the form of nerve impulses, is gathered and sent out. In the spinal cord, the grey matter forms a butterfly-shaped core surrounded by white matter.

The brain

The anterior end of the neural tube lying within the cranial cavity swells to form a hollow organ with three distinct regions (Figure 4.32):

- **Forebrain** – cerebrum, thalamus, hypothalamus and associated structures
- **Midbrain** – linking pathway between the fore and hindbrain
- **Hindbrain** – cerebellum, pons and medulla oblongata.

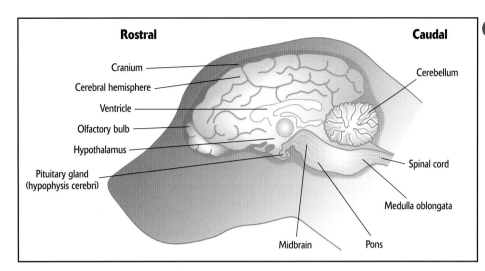

4.32 The dog's brain.

(Diagram labels: Rostral; Caudal; Cranium; Cerebral hemisphere; Ventricle; Olfactory bulb; Hypothalamus; Pituitary gland (hypophysis cerebri); Cerebellum; Spinal cord; Medulla oblongata; Midbrain; Pons)

All the cranial nerves, apart from the olfactory (CN I) and optic (CN II) nerves, arise from the ventral surface of the midbrain and hindbrain.

Forebrain

The **cerebrum** occupies the greater part of the forebrain and consists of the **right and left cerebral hemispheres**. The surface is deeply folded, which enables a large surface area to be fitted into the relatively small cranial cavity (90% of all the neurons in the nervous system are found in the cerebral hemispheres). The folds of the cerebrum are called **gyri** (upfolds) and **sulci** (downfolds).

A central **longitudinal fissure** divides the two cerebral hemispheres. They are linked across the midline by a tract of white matter known as the **corpus callosum**, forming the roof of the third ventricle. Each hemisphere is divided into four lobes: the **frontal, parietal, occipital** and **temporal lobes**, each of which contributes in a different way to conscious thought.

The **thalamus** lies deep in the tissue of the forebrain at the base of the cerebral hemispheres. Its function is to process information from the sense organs and relay it to the cerebral cortex.

The **hypothalamus** lies ventral to the thalamus and dorsal to the pituitary gland and is one of the most vital regions of the brain. Its functions are to:

• Link the nervous and endocrine systems by secreting a series of releasing hormones, which are stored in the pituitary gland (e.g. gonadotrophin-releasing hormone (GRH))
• Help to control the autonomic nervous system affecting activities such as sweating, shivering, vasodilation and vasoconstriction
• Exert a major control on the homeostatic mechanisms of the body (e.g. osmotic balance of fluids, regulation of body temperature, thirst and hunger).

On the ventral surface of the forebrain (Figure 4.32) are:

• A pair of **olfactory bulbs** – responsible for the sense of smell (olfaction); they receive sensory nerve fibres from the mucosa lining the nasal chambers
• **Pituitary gland** – endocrine gland that secretes and stores a wide range of hormones
• The **optic chiasma** – information from both eyes goes to both the right and left sides of the brain via this crossover point.

Midbrain

This short length of brain is difficult to see as it is overhung by the large cerebral hemispheres. Its function is to conduct nerve impulses from the forebrain to the hindbrain and in the opposite direction.

Hindbrain

The **cerebellum is** a globular organ consisting of two hemispheres folded into deep fissures. It lies dorsal to the medulla oblongata and is attached by three pairs of peduncles, through which run tracts of nerves. The function of the cerebellum is to coordinate balance and muscular movement. Nerve impulses initiating voluntary movements begin in the cerebral hemispheres. Fine adjustments are made in the cerebellum and the nerve impulses are sent down the spinal cord to the skeletal muscles and movement results.

The **pons** lies ventral to the cerebellum forming a bridge of fibres from one cerebellar hemisphere to the other. It contains centres involved in the control of respiration.

The **medulla oblongata** extends from the pons to the point where the spinal cord passes through the foramen magnum of the skull. It contains centres responsible for the control of respiration and blood pressure.

Protection of the central nervous system

If an animal is to survive it is vital that the brain is able to function normally. The brain is protected from mechanical damage externally by the bony cranial cavity of the skull and internally by the meninges and the ventricular system.

Meninges

The entire CNS is surrounded by three membranes. From the outside to the inside these are:

• **Dura mater** – a tough fibrous layer. In the cranial cavity this is interwoven with the periosteum of the overlying bones; in the vertebral canal there is a fat-filled **epidural space** between the vertebrae and the dura mater and this is used as a site for local anaesthesia.
• **Arachnoid mater** – a network of collagen fibres and large blood vessels. Between the dura mater and the arachnoid mater is the **subdural space**. Below the arachnoid mater is the **subarachnoid space**, which is filled with **cerebrospinal fluid**.
• **Pia mater** – a fine membrane closely applied to the surface of the brain following the gyri and sulci. It contains many small blood capillaries, which supply the underlying nervous tissue.

Ventricular system

In the embryo, the CNS forms from a hollow neural tube and the central lumen develops into a system of interconnecting cavities, or ventricles, and canals (Figure 4.33).

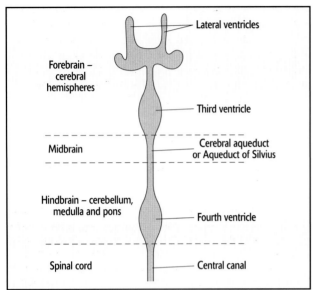

4.33 General plan of the ventricular system and its position within the brain, dorsal view.

A **central canal** runs along the entire length of the spinal cord, surrounded by grey matter. Within the brain, this canal continues as the **fourth ventricle** (in the hindbrain), the **cerebral aqueduct** or aqueduct of Silvius (a narrow canal in the midbrain) and the **third ventricle** (in the forebrain). The latter gives off two **lateral ventricles**, one inside each cerebral hemisphere.

Cerebrospinal fluid

Cerebrospinal fluid (CSF), formed by **choroid plexuses** (capillary networks) in the roof of the ventricles, circulates in the ventricular system and bathes the outer surface of the CNS in the subarachnoid space. It is a clear yellowish fluid resembling plasma but without protein. The function of CSF is to protect the CNS from sudden movement and knocks and to supply the nervous tissue with nutrients.

Spinal cord

The spinal cord is a glistening white structure extending from the medulla oblongata to the lumbar region of the vertebral column. It leaves the cranial cavity via the **foramen magnum** in the occipital bone of the skull and runs in the vertebral canal formed from the interlinked vertebrae. At approximately L6–L7 the cord narrows and breaks up into a group of spinal nerves known as the **cauda equina**. These nerves run towards the hindlimbs and tail. The spinal cord is protected by the surrounding meninges and by the bony vertebral column. Along its length the spinal cord gives off pairs of **spinal nerves**.

In cross-section (Figure 4.34), the tissue of the spinal cord consists of:

- A **central canal** containing CSF
- A butterfly-shaped area of **grey matter** made of non-myelinated neurons (most of the synapses in the spinal cord are in this area)

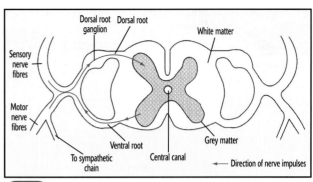

4.34 Cross-section through the spinal cord.

- An outer layer of **white matter** consisting of organized tracts of myelinated nerve fibres running towards (ascending) and away from (descending) the brain. Each tract has a definite origin and destination so that transmission of nerve impulses is fast and efficient.

Peripheral nervous system

The peripheral nervous system consists of:

- **Cranial nerves** (leaving the brain)
- **Spinal nerves** (leaving the spinal cord)
- The **autonomic nervous system** (contains some nerve fibres from the brain, but the majority arise from the spinal cord).

Cranial nerves

There are 12 pairs of cranial nerves, which leave the brain via various foramina in the skull. They are always identified using Roman numerals. Most supply structures on or around the head and so they are short; the longest cranial nerve is the vagus (CN X). Cranial nerves may be sensory, motor or mixed (see Figure 4.35).

Cranial nerve	Type of nerve fibre	Function
I. Olfactory	Sensory	Carries the sense of smell or olfaction from the olfactory bulbs to the brain
II. Optic	Sensory	Carries information about sight from the eyes to both sides of the brain via the optic chiasma
III. Oculomotor	Motor	Supplies the extrinsic muscles of the eye enabling it to make delicate and accurate movements
IV. Trochlear	Motor	Supplies the extrinsic muscles of the eye
V. Trigeminal	Mixed	Carries sensory fibres from the skin around the face and eyes and motor fibres to the muscles of mastication – mainly the temporal and masseter
VI. Abducens	Motor	Supplies the extrinsic muscles of the eye
VII. Facial	Motor	Supplies the muscles of facial expression including those associated with the movement of the lips, ears and skin around the eyes
VIII. Vestibulocochlear (auditory)	Sensory	Vestibular branch carries sensation of balance from the semicircular canals in the inner ear. Cochlear branch carries sensation of hearing from the cochlea of the inner ear

4.35 Cranial nerves.

continues ▶

Cranial nerve	Type of nerve fibre	Function
IX. Glossopharyngeal	Mixed	Carries the sensation of taste or gustation from the taste buds on the tongue and pharynx. Supplies motor fibres to the muscles of the pharynx
X. Vagus	Mixed	Carries sensory fibres from the pharynx and larynx. Supplies motor fibres to the muscles of the larynx. Parasympathetic visceral motor fibres to the heart and various thoracic and abdominal organs including the gastrointestinal tract as far as the descending colon
XI. Accessory (spinal accessory)	Motor	Supplies the muscles of the neck and shoulder
XII. Hypoglossal	Motor	Supplies the muscles of the tongue

4.35 *continued* Cranial nerves.

Spinal nerves

The spinal cord is described as being segmented. Each segment corresponds to a vertebra and gives off a pair of spinal nerves, which leave the vertebral canal by the **intervertebral foramina** – one to the left side of the body and one to the right side. The spinal nerves then travel towards the organs they supply.

Each spinal nerve is divided into the dorsal root and the ventral root (Figure 4.34).

- The **dorsal root** carries sensory fibres from the body towards the spinal cord. A few millimetres from the cord is the **dorsal root ganglion**, a swelling containing all the cell bodies of these neurons.
- The **ventral root** carries motor fibres away from the spinal cord towards the organs. There is no ganglion.

Linking the sensory and motor fibres in the grey matter of the cord there may be one or more **intercalated neurons**.

Once outside the vertebral canal, the sensory nerve fibres entering the dorsal root and the motor nerve fibres leaving the ventral root run together in the same myelin sheath, forming a **mixed nerve**.

Spinal nerves supply the whole musculoskeletal system. In the area of the pectoral and pelvic girdles the spinal nerves are thicker and form a network or **nerve plexus**, which supplies the limbs.

Reflex arcs

A reflex arc may be defined as a fixed involuntary response to certain stimuli. Reflexes are rapid, automatic, always the same and only involve pathways in the spinal cord.

Sensory nerves carry nerve impulses, received from sensory receptors in organs such as the skin, joints and muscles, to the spinal cord. Here they synapse with motor nerves in that segment of the spinal cord and an impulse is sent out to skeletal muscle, which brings about a response. For example: in the pedal reflex, the paw is pinched, pain receptors in the skin send sensory impulses to the spinal cord, a motor impulse is sent to the muscles of the leg and the paw is withdrawn.

Reflex arcs may be described as being:

- **Monosynaptic or simple** – involving only one synapse in the pathway
- **Polysynaptic** – involving at least one intercalated neuron in the pathway.

Reflex arcs may be used in a clinical examination to assess the function of the spinal cord (e.g. after a road traffic accident). The reflex arcs commonly tested include the pedal, panniculus, palpebral, papillary light response, patella and anal reflexes.

The arcs use pathways within a relevant segment of spinal cord, but their presence does not indicate that the spinal cord is intact. However, if the animal cries out or bites when a reflex is tested, it indicates that nerve impulses have also travelled up the spinal cord towards the brain, where they have been consciously perceived; this indicates that the cord is intact.

Reflex arcs are modified by neurons in other segments above (**upper motor neurons**) or below (**lower motor neurons**) that particular segment. If a reflex is extravagant or abnormally suppressed, this could indicate that the cord is severed above or below the area and the modifying effect has been lost.

The brain can override reflex arcs. For example, a person can force themselves to hold their hand on a hot iron even though their reflex would be to pull the hand away. This is a **conditioned reflex**. Conditioned reflexes are made use of in dog training.

Autonomic nervous system

The autonomic nervous system (ANS) (Figures 4.36 and 4.37) can be considered to be a visceral motor system, i.e. it supplies motor nerves to cardiac muscle, smooth muscle and glands within the visceral body systems and the heart. Control of the

	Sympathetic	Parasympathetic
Origin of nerve fibres	Arise from spinal cord from T1 to L4 or L5. Nerve fibres run to ganglia arranged in two chains along the dorsal body wall on either side of the vertebral column – sympathetic chains	Arise from brain in cranial nerves – III, VII, IX and X. Also from spinal cord at S1 and S2
Organs supplied	Eye, salivary glands, heart and lungs. Unpaired ganglia are: • Coeliac – stomach, small intestine, pancreas, large intestine, and adrenal medulla • Cranial mesenteric – large intestine • Caudal mesenteric – bladder and genitals	Eye, salivary glands. Vagus X supplies heart, lungs, stomach, small intestine, pancreas, large intestine. Fibres from S1/S2 supply bladder and genitalia
Length of preganglionic fibres	Short – run to sympathetic chain	Long
Length of postganglionic fibres	Long – ganglia are close to the organ they supply	Short
Transmitter substance at: 1. Synapses within the system 2. Terminal synapses	Acetylcholine Noradrenaline	Acetylcholine Acetylcholine
General effect	Prepares body for 'fear, flight, fight'. Increases respiratory and heart rates, vasodilation, dilates bronchioles, increases levels of stress, reduces gastrointestinal activity, dries salivary secretions, dilates the pupil	Slows the heart and respiratory rates, increases gastrointestinal activity, constricts the pupil, reduces stress levels

4.36 The autonomic nervous system.

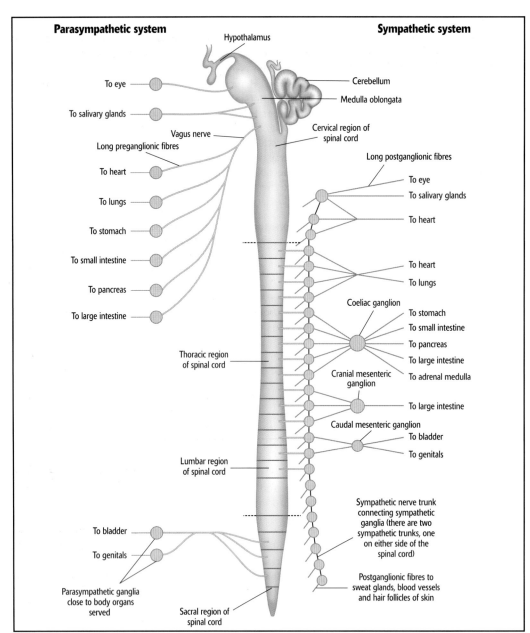

Parasympathetic system

- Hypothalamus
- To eye
- To salivary glands
- Vagus nerve
- Long preganglionic fibres
- To heart
- To lungs
- To stomach
- To small intestine
- To pancreas
- To large intestine
- Thoracic region of spinal cord
- Lumbar region of spinal cord
- To bladder
- To genitals
- Parasympathetic ganglia close to body organs served
- Sacral region of spinal cord

Sympathetic system

- Cerebellum
- Medulla oblongata
- Cervical region of spinal cord
- Long postganglionic fibres
- To eye
- To salivary glands
- To heart
- To heart
- To lungs
- Coeliac ganglion
- To stomach
- To small intestine
- To pancreas
- To large intestine
- To adrenal medulla
- Cranial mesenteric ganglion
- To large intestine
- Caudal mesenteric ganglion
- To bladder
- To genitals
- Sympathetic nerve trunk connecting sympathetic ganglia (there are two sympathetic trunks, one on either side of the spinal cord)
- Postganglionic fibres to sweat glands, blood vessels and hair follicles of skin

4.37
The autonomic nervous system.

autonomic nervous system is involuntary or unconscious. The system can be divided into two parts, the **sympathetic** and the **parasympathetic**, which occupy different areas of the body and have opposite effects. Most organs receive a nerve supply from both systems and control is achieved by balancing the effects.

Special senses

The body has evolved specialized sensory receptor cells, each adapted to respond to particular stimuli in the external environment and housed within organs known as the special sense organs. The special senses are taste (gustation), smell (olfaction), sight, hearing and balance. Gustation is closely allied to olfaction and they often work together. Gustatory and olfactory cells are known as chemoreceptors.

Taste (gustation)

Receptor cells (gustatory cells) lie within discrete organs known as **taste buds**. These are distributed over the dorsal surface of the tongue, the epiglottis and the soft palate.

Chemicals responsible for taste dissolve in mucus covering the oral cavity and stimulate the taste buds. The resulting nerve impulses travel along fine nerve fibres associated with the receptor cells to the facial (CN VII), glossopharyngeal (CN IX) and vagus (CN X) nerves and so to the brain, where the information is interpreted as taste.

Smell (olfaction)

Receptor cells lie within the mucous membrane lining the nasal cavities. Chemicals responsible for smell dissolve in mucus and stimulate the fine nerve fibres of the olfactory nerve (CN I) in close contact with the mucosa. These fibres carry nerve impulses through the cribriform plate of the ethmoid bone at the back of the nasal cavity to the olfactory bulbs of the forebrain, where they are interpreted as smell.

Sight

The eye houses receptor cells (photoreceptors) adapted to respond to light and so bring about sight. Each eye lies within a bony **orbit** in the skull, lateral to the nasal cavities and rostral to the cranium. In the dog and cat the eyes are directed forwards providing a wide field of binocular or three-dimensional (3D) vision. This enables the animal to locate objects accurately, which is important in predatory species.

The eye (Figure 4.38) comprises three main parts: eyeball, extrinsic muscles and eyelids.

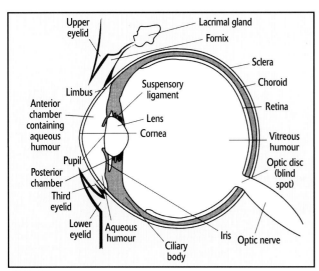

4.38 Longitudinal section through the eye.

The eyeball

This is a globe-shaped structure made of three layers: sclera, uvea and retina.

Sclera

This is a tough fibrous outer coating whose function is to protect the inner structures. The anterior one-sixth of the sclera is the transparent **cornea**, which allows light into the eye and plays a part in focusing light rays on to the retina. The cornea and part of the sclera are covered by a thin protective layer of epithelium called the **conjunctiva**. The junction between the sclera and cornea is known as the **limbus**.

Uvea

This vascular pigmented middle layer consists of the following structures:

- **Choroid** – darkly pigmented and containing blood vessels that supply all the internal structures.
- **Tapetum lucidum** – area of yellow-green iridescent cells lying in the dorsal part of the choroid above the exit of the optic nerve. Its function is to reflect light back to the retina making use of low light levels and improving night vision. Most mammals (except humans) have a tapetum lucidum.
- **Ciliary body** – thickened part of the uvea that projects towards the centre of the eye. It consists of the **ciliary muscle**, which is linked to the lens by the **suspensory ligament**. This arrangement is responsible for controlling the thickness of the lens.
- **Iris** – continues anteriorly from the ciliary body. The iris contains pigment cells and smooth muscle fibres whose function is to constrict and dilate the pupil in response to changes in light intensity.
- **Pupil** – formed by the free edge of the iris and allowing light to reach the lens. The shape of the pupil is characteristic of the species: cats have vertical slits and dogs have round pupils.

Retina

This innermost layer contains the photoreceptor or light-sensitive cells. It consists of the following layers:

- **Ganglion cells** – transmit nerve impulses to the optic nerve (II)
- **Bipolar receptor cells**
- **Photoreceptor cells** – there are two types named according to their shape:
  - **Rods** – black/white vision and night vision
  - **Cones** – colour vision.
- **Pigmented cells** lying close to the choroid.

Light focused on to the retina by the lens travels through the layers of cells and stimulates the photoreceptors. The resulting nerve impulses pass back to the ganglion cells, which transmit them via the fibres of the optic nerve (CN II) to the brain. At the exit of the optic nerve is the **optic disc** (Figure 4.38), an area that contains no photoreceptors and so it is also known as the blind spot.

The central cavity of the eye is divided into three chambers:

- **Anterior chamber** – lies in front of the iris and contains transparent watery fluid called **aqueous humour**, which is secreted by the ciliary body and drains out of the eye back into the circulation at the **limbus**
- **Posterior chamber** – lies between the iris and the lens and also contains aqueous humour
- **Vitreous chamber** – lies at the back of the eye behind the lens and contains vitreous humour.

The function of these humours (fluids) is to maintain the shape of the eye and to provide nutrients to the structures of the eye.

Extrinsic muscles

The eyeball is well supplied with striated extrinsic muscles. These are known as the rectus muscles, which originate on the periosteum and insert on the sclera of the bones of the orbit. They are responsible for the fine movements of the eyeball. These movements are coordinated to provide 3D or binocular vision. These muscles are supplied by the oculomotor (CN III), trochlear (CN IV) and abducens (CN VI) nerves.

Eyelids

The eyes are essential to the survival of an animal and they must be protected from mechanical damage. The posterior two-thirds of the eyeball lies within the bony orbit while the eyelids protect the anterior one-third formed by the cornea and conjunctiva (Figure 4.38).

Each eye has an upper and lower eyelid, which are joined at the **medial canthus**, close to the nose, and the **lateral canthus**. Both eyelids consist of **palpebral muscle** covered in hairy skin. The inner surface is lined with a continuation of the epithelium forming the conjunctiva. On the outer edge of the more mobile upper eyelid is a row of **cilia** or **eyelashes**. Lying within the tissue of the eyelids are the **Meibomian glands**, which secrete fluid to lubricate and protect the eyes.

Deep to the upper and lower eyelids and lying within the medial canthus is the **third eyelid** or **nictitating membrane**. This contains a T-shaped piece of cartilage with associated smooth muscle and glandular and lymphoid tissue. The third eyelid moves across to provide an additional protective layer as the other eyelids close and the eyeball retracts into the orbit. Beneath the third eyelid is the Harderian gland, which sometimes protrudes in a condition known as 'cherry eye'.

The cornea is kept clean, moist and supple by secretions or **tears** from the **lacrimal gland** on the dorsolateral surface of the eye beneath the upper eyelid. Tears flow across the eye, drain into a pair of openings at the medial canthus and then into the **nasolacrimal duct**, which runs through the nasal cavity to open into the nostril.

The eyelids and associated eyelashes of the dog may be affected by several inherited conditions, including **entropion** (inturning eyelids), **ectropion** (drooping of the lower eyelids) and **distichiasis** (ectopic eyelashes). Affected dogs should not be used for breeding.

Formation of an image

1. Light rays from an object pass:
- Through the **cornea** and the **pupil** to hit the **lens**
  - The cornea plays a part in focusing the light on to the retina
  - The iris alters in size and controls the amount of light entering the eye
- Through the lens to be focused on to the **retina**
  - The curvature of the lens is altered by the ciliary muscles and focuses the light rays on to the retina
- Through the layers of the retina to hit the **photoreceptor cells**. Some light is reflected back to the retina by the **tapetum lucidum** to stimulate more receptor cells
2. Resulting nerve impulses, generated by the photoreceptors, travel along the nerve fibres of the **optic nerve (CN II)** to the **brain**
3. On the ventral surface of the brain, a proportion of nerve fibres cross via the **optic chiasma** to opposite sides of the brain so that each cerebral hemisphere receives information from both eyes
4. Information is carried to the **visual cortex** of the cerebral hemispheres, where it is interpreted as an image. The image formed on the retina is smaller than the original and inverted but the brain automatically modifies it.

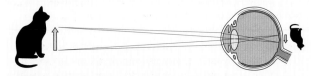

Hearing and balance

The ear (Figure 4.39) contains receptors adapted to respond to sound waves and to the movement of the body. All mammals have two ears, each comprising three parts: external ear, middle ear and inner ear. Inflammation of the ear is common in both dogs and cats. Otitis externa is inflammation of the external ear; otitis media is inflammation of the middle ear; and otitis interna, which may involve loss of balance, is inflammation of the inner ear.

External ear

Pinna
This is also called the ear flap. Each pinna consists of a funnel-shaped flap of elastic cartilage covered in hairy skin. There are fewer hair follicles on the inner surface of the flap.

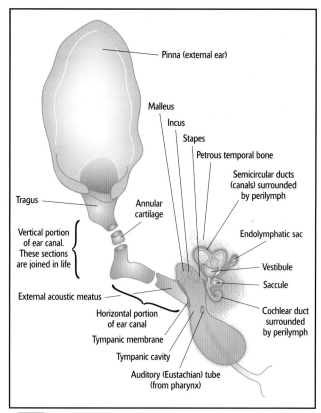

4.39 Cross-section through the ear.

The shape of the pinna is characteristic of the breed. The wolf, from which the domestic dog evolved, has upright ears but years of selective breeding have led to the development of a variety of different ear shapes. Most cats have pointed upright ears.

Both pinnae are very mobile and can move independently, which allows them to pick up sound waves from the environment and to be used as a means of facial expression and communication.

External ear canal
This is also called the external auditory meatus. It is formed by an incomplete tube of cartilage connecting to the pinna and at its distal end to the acoustic process of the **tympanic bulla** of the skull. The canal runs down the side of the head and then turns inwards to run horizontally. It terminates in the **tympanic membrane**.

The canal is lined by modified skin with few hair follicles and many **ceruminous glands,** which secrete wax to protect the ear canal from damage.

Middle ear
This lies mainly within the **tympanic bulla** of the petrous temporal bone of the skull, and is filled with air.

Tympanic membrane
This is also called the eardrum. It is a thin semi-transparent membrane whose function is to convey the vibrations caused by sound waves from the external to the middle ear.

Auditory ossicles
These are three small bones linked by synovial joints to form a flexible chain lying across the dorsal part of the middle ear:

- **Malleus** or **hammer** – in contact with the tympanic membrane
- **Incus** or **anvil**
- **Stapes** or **stirrup** – in contact with the oval window of the inner ear.

Their function is to transmit the vibrations caused by the sound waves from the tympanic membrane to the inner ear.

Eustachian tube

This is also called the auditory tube. It is a short tube connecting the middle ear to the nasopharynx. Its function is to equalize the air pressure on either side of the tympanic membrane, enabling it to vibrate freely and so transmit the sound waves.

Inner ear

This lies within the temporal bone and consists of an inner membranous labyrinth surrounded by an outer bony labyrinth.

Bony labyrinth

This is 'carved out' of the bone and closely follows the shape of the membranous labyrinth. It contains **perilymph**, which flows around the outside of the membranous labyrinth. It is linked to the middle ear by two membranes: the round and oval windows.

Membranous labyrinth

This is a system of interconnecting tubes filled with **endolymph**. Inside the labyrinth are groups of sensory receptor cells adapted to respond to sound and movement. Projecting from each cell is a hair-like structure and touching the base is a nerve fibre from the **vestibulocochlear nerve** (CN VIII). The membranous labyrinth has three parts:

Cochlea

This is responsible for the perception of sound and consists of a tube arranged in a spiral similar to a snail shell. Inside is a group of sensory receptor cells known as the **organ of Corti**. Sound waves are picked up by the **pinna**, travel down the **external auditory meatus** and cause the **tympanic membrane** to vibrate. This starts the **auditory ossicles** vibrating. The third ossicle, the **stapes**, vibrates against the **oval window** of the inner ear, causing first the **perilymph** and then the **endolymph** to move. Movement of the endolymph 'tweaks' the hair cells of the organ of Corti and initiates nerve impulses, which travel along the fibres of the **cochlear branch** of the vestibulocochlear nerve to the brain, where they are interpreted as sound.

Utricle and saccule

These are responsible for maintaining the position of the body when standing still. They are two sac-like structures in the centre of the membranous labyrinth. Each contains a group of receptor cells or **maculae** surrounded by jelly. As the head moves, the jelly responds to the pull of gravity, moving the hairs of the receptor cells and initiating nerve impulses, which travel along the **vestibular branch** of the vestibulocochlear nerve to the brain.

Semicircular canals

These three canals are responsible for maintaining balance when moving. Each canal describes two-thirds of a circle and they lie approximately at right angles to each other. Each canal

is attached to the utricle by a swelling known as an **ampulla**, inside which is a group of receptor cells. As the animal moves, endolymph in the semicircular canals moves, tweaking the hairs of the receptor cells and initiating nerve impulses. These are carried to the brain by the **vestibular branch** of the vestibulocochlear nerve. Within the brain they are interpreted and relayed to the **cerebellum**. Impulses are then sent to the skeletal muscles, bringing about the appropriate muscle movements necessary to maintain balance.

The endocrine system

The endocrine system forms part of the regulatory system of the body. A series of **endocrine glands** secrete chemical messengers known as **hormones**, which are carried by the blood to their **target organs**. These may be some distance away from the gland.

Hormones regulate the activity of the target organ, which responds only to that particular hormone, leaving all other organs unaffected. The response produced by hormones is slower and lasts longer than those of the nervous system, and complements its rapid and relatively short-lived responses.

Endocrine glands

- Pituitary gland
- Thyroid gland
- Parathyroid gland
- Pancreas
- Ovary
- Testes
- Adrenal glands

Endocrine glands are distributed throughout the body (Figure 4.40) and may secrete more than one hormone. Figure 4.41 gives details of the endocrine glands and their associated hormones.

Not all hormones are secreted by endocrine glands. Those that are produced from tissue within other organs include:

- **Gastrin** – produced by the wall of the stomach. As food enters the stomach, gastrin stimulates the release of gastric juices from the gastric glands and digestion begins.

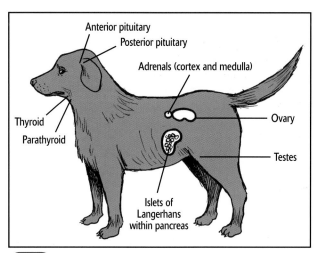

4.40 Components of the endocrine system.

Endocrine gland	Location	Hormone	Function	Control of secretion
Anterior pituitary	Ventral to the forebrain	Thyrotrophic stimulating hormone (TSH)	Stimulates the release of thyroid hormone	Hypothalamus
		Growth hormone or somatotrophin	Controls epiphyseal growth; protein production; regulates the use of energy	Hypothalamus
		Adrenocorticotrophic hormone (ACTH)	Controls the release of adrenocortical hormones	Hypothalamus
		Prolactin	Stimulates the development of mammary glands and secretion of milk	–
		Follicle stimulating hormone (FSH)	Female – stimulates the development of the ovarian follicles. Male – stimulates development of seminiferous tubules and spermatogenesis	Gonadotrophin releasing hormone from the hypothalamus (GRH)
		Luteinizing hormone (LH)	Female – brings about ovulation of the ovarian follicles and development of the corpus luteum	Oestrogen secreted by Graafian follicles
		Interstitial cell stimulating hormone (ICSH)	Stimulates secretion of testosterone from the interstitial cells in the testis	Gonadotrophin releasing hormone from the hypothalamus (GRH)
Posterior pituitary	Ventral to the forebrain	Antidiuretic hormone (ADH) – vasopressin	Acts on the collecting ducts of the renal nephrons – changes the permeability to water	Status of the ECF and blood plasma
		Oxytocin	Stimulates uterine contractions during parturition and milk 'let down'	Suckling by the neonate initiates a reflex arc
Thyroid	Midline on the ventral aspect of the first few rings of the trachea	Thyroxine	Controls metabolic rate. Essential for normal growth	TSH
		Thyrocalcitonin	Decreases the resorption of calcium from bones	Raised blood calcium levels
Parathyroid	On either side of the thyroid gland	Parathormone	Stimulates calcium resorption from bones. Promotes calcium uptake from the intestine	Low blood calcium levels
Pancreas	Within the loop of the duodenum in the peritoneal cavity	Insulin – from the cells in the islets of Langerhans	Increases uptake of glucose into the cells. Stores excess glucose as glycogen in the liver – glycogenesis	Raised blood glucose levels after eating
		Glucagon – from the β cells in the islets of Langerhans	Breaks down glycogen stored in the liver to release glucose into the blood – glycogenolysis	Low blood glucose levels
		Somatostatin – from the cells in the islets of Langerhans	Mild inhibition of insulin and glucagon preventing swings in blood glucose levels. Decreases gut motility and secretion of digestive juices	–
Ovary	One on either side of the midline in the dorsal peritoneal cavity	Oestrogen – from the Graafian follicles	Signs of oestrus; preparation of the reproductive tract and external genitalia for coitus	FSH
		Progesterone – from the corpus luteum	Preparation of the reproductive tract for pregnancy; development of the mammary glands; maintains the pregnancy	LH
Testis	Outside the body cavity within the scrotum	Testosterone from the cells of Leydig	Spermatogenesis. Male secondary sexual characteristics and behaviour	ICSH
Adrenal cortex	Cranial to the kidney in the peritoneal cavity – outer layer	Glucocorticoids, e.g. cortisol	Raise blood glucose levels. Reduce the inflammatory response	ACTH
		Mineralocorticoids, e.g. aldosterone	Acts on the distal convoluted tubules of the renal nephrons – regulate uptake of sodium and acid/base balance	Status of the ECF and blood plasma
		Sex hormones	Very small quantities	–
Adrenal medulla	Cranial to the kidney in the peritoneal cavity – inner layer	Adrenaline and noradrenaline	Fear, flight, fright syndrome	Sympathetic nervous system

4.41 The endocrine glands and their associated hormones.

- **Secretin** – produced by the wall of the small intestine. As food enters the duodenum from the stomach, secretin stimulates the secretion of intestinal and pancreatic juices, which continue the process of digestion.
- **Chorionic gonadotrophin** – produced during pregnancy by the ectodermal layer of the chorion surrounding the conceptus. It helps to maintain the corpus luteum in the ovary throughout gestation.
- **Erythropoietin** or **erythropoietic stimulating factor** – produced by the kidney in response to low levels of blood oxygen. It stimulates the bone marrow to produce erythrocytes (red blood cells).

The blood vascular system

The blood vascular system consists of blood, the heart, the circulatory system and the lymphatic system.

Blood

The functions of the blood include transport, regulation and defence.

Transport
Blood carries:

- Oxygen to and carbon dioxide away from the tissues
- Nutrients to the tissues and waste products of metabolism away from the tissues
- Hormones secreted by endocrine glands to their target organs
- Enzymes to their site of reaction.

Regulation
Blood is responsible for controlling:

- Volume and osmotic balance of the body fluids
- Body temperature (by constriction or dilation of peripheral blood vessels)
- Acid/base balance of fluids (the presence of buffers, e.g. bicarbonate, in the blood regulates levels of hydrogen ions in plasma)
- Blood loss (by the clotting mechanism).

Defence
The white blood cells are responsible for the body's defence against disease and foreign particles such as bacteria and viruses.

Composition of blood
Blood is a specialized type of liquid connective tissue consisting of several types of **blood cell** (Figure 4.42) suspended in a fluid matrix called **plasma**. The pH of blood is 7.4 and it occupies about 7% of the total bodyweight.

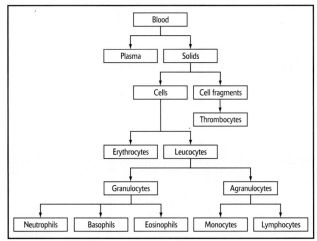

4.42 Components of blood.

Plasma
Plasma is the fluid part of blood and takes up approximately 55–70% of blood. It consists mainly of water containing dissolved substances that are in the process of being transported around the body. Plasma contains:

- **Water** – about 90%
- **Plasma proteins** – albumin, prothrombin, fibrinogen and globulins (these are too large to pass out of the blood and so they help to maintain the osmotic pressure, i.e. they prevent excessive fluid leaving the blood)
- **Gases** – oxygen and carbon dioxide (the majority of oxygen is carried by the red blood cells)
- **Electrolytes** – sodium, potassium, calcium, magnesium, chloride and bicarbonate ions

- **Nutrients** – the products of digestion (amino acids, fatty acids and glucose); these are transported to the cells in the plasma
- **Waste products** of metabolic processes (e.g. urea, creatinine) – transported in the plasma to the kidney and to the liver for excretion
- **Hormones and enzymes** – secreted by endocrine glands directly into the bloodstream and transported in the plasma to their target organs
- **Antibodies and antitoxins** – form part of the body's defence system.

Blood cells
Three types of cells are suspended within the plasma: erythrocytes, leucocytes and thrombocytes.

- **Haemopoiesis** is the formation of blood cells.
- **Erythropoiesis** is specifically the production of red blood cells.

There are two types of haemopoietic tissue in the body:

- **Myeloid tissue** in the red bone marrow produces **erythrocytes** and **granular leucocytes**.
- **Lymphoid tissue** in lymphatic tissues such as the lymph nodes and spleen produces **agranular leucocytes**.

Erythrocytes
These are **red blood cells** (RBCs) and are responsible for transporting oxygen from the lungs to the tissues of the body. Erythrocytes are the most numerous of the blood cells (about 5–8 million/ml). They are small (7 µm diameter) biconcave discs with no nuclei and contain a complex protein pigment containing iron called **haemoglobin**, which gives them their red colour. Haemoglobin combines with oxygen in the lung capillaries which is then transported around the body by the red blood cells.

Erythropoiesis (the formation of erythrocytes) takes place in the bone marrow and is controlled by the hormone **erythropoietin**, secreted by the kidney in response to low blood oxygen levels.

Erythrocytes are formed from nucleated cells known as **erythroblasts**. The nucleus begins to shrink; the cell takes up haemoglobin and is then called a **normoblast**. The nucleus continues to shrink until only fine threads remain; these are known as **Howell–Jolly bodies** and the cells are called **reticulocytes**. A reticulocyte is an immature RBC. Reticulocytes may be seen in the circulation if there is a shortage of mature red blood cells (e.g. in some types of anaemia). As the nucleus completely disappears, the cell becomes a mature erythrocyte and passes into the circulation. Circulating erythrocytes have a lifespan of about 120 days, after which they are destroyed in the spleen or liver.

Erythroblast → normoblast → reticulocyte → erythrocyte

Packed cell volume (PCV or **haematocrit)**, in which the proportion of the erythrocytes in relation to the column of blood as a whole is measured, is used in the diagnosis of anaemia.

Leucocytes
These are **white blood cells** (WBCs) and are nucleated. Leucocytes are far less numerous in the blood than erythrocytes. Each type of leucocyte has a specific function, but they are all involved in the body's defence system. They can be classified as granulocytes or agranulocytes, according to whether they have granulated or clear cytoplasm when stained by Romanowsky stains (Figure 4.43; see also Chapter 17).

Cell type	Numbers present	Appearance	Function
Granulocytes			
Neutrophils	Most abundant WBC 60–75% of leucocytes (5000–9000 per ml)	Cytoplasmic granules do not stain (remain clear). Nuclei have many shapes and are segmented	Phagocytes (i.e. engulf microorganisms and foreign particles). Can move from blood into tissues
Eosinophils	2–10% of leucocytes	Cytoplasmic granules stain with an acidic dye (eosin) and appear red	Inhibit the allergic responses and secrete anti-inflammatory substances. They are also involved in the response to parasitic infections
Basophils	Rare (0.5–1% of leucocytes)	Cytoplasmic granules stain with an alkaline (basic) dye and appear blue	Contain histamine, which is involved in inflammation and allergic reactions. Also contain heparin (anticoagulant)
Agranulocytes			
Lymphocytes	Make up about 30% of circulating leucocytes	Large nucleus surrounded by a narrow rim of cytoplasm	*Immunity* There are two types: **B-lymphocytes** produce antibodies; **T-lymphocytes** are involved in the cellular immune response
Monocytes	5–6% of circulating leucocytes	Largest leucocyte. Clear cytoplasm with a large bean-shaped nucleus	*Phagocytic* Spend a short time in circulation before moving into tissues where they mature into **macrophages**

4.43 Types of granulocytes/agranulocytes.

- **Granulocytes** include neutrophils, eosinophils and basophils. They make up 70% of the leucocytes and have visible granules in the cytoplasm when stained. They have irregularly shaped nuclei and are referred to as polymorphonucleocytes (PMNs) or 'polymorphs'. Granulocytes have a lifespan of about 21 days. They can be further classified according to which type of stain they take up, i.e. neutral, acidic or basic.
- **Agranulocytes** include monocytes and lymphocytes. They do not have visible granules and so have clear cytoplasm. Their nuclei are more uniform in shape.

Leukaemia (literally meaning 'white blood') is a condition caused by an abnormal proliferation of one of the WBC group (e.g. lymphocytic leukaemia). This results in an increase in the numbers of WBCs in the blood and is a form of cancer.

Thrombocytes

These are also called **platelets** and are cell fragments produced from cells in the bone marrow called **megakaryocytes**. They are numerous in the blood (2000–5000/ml) and are involved in the **blood clotting mechanism**.

Blood clotting mechanism

When a blood vessel is damaged, the body is able to 'plug' the wound with a clot of blood to prevent excessive blood loss and the entry of microorganisms. The blood clotting process involves a complicated cascade of events involving several **clotting factors**.

Summary of blood coagulation

1. At the site of a wound the **thrombocytes** release an enzyme called **thromboplastin**.
2. In the presence of **vitamin K** and **calcium ions**, thromboplastin converts the inactive plasma protein **prothrombin** to the active form, **thrombin**.
3. Thrombin converts the soluble plasma protein **fibrinogen** to the insoluble **fibrin**.
4. The fibrin forms a meshwork of fibres across the site, which trap red blood cells to form a clot.

Substances that interfere with the blood clotting mechanism are called **anticoagulants**. Some of these, such as heparin, occur naturally in the body, while others, such as citrate and ethylenediaminetetraacetic acid (EDTA), can be used to prevent blood samples from clotting.

If a blood sample is allowed to clot naturally, the clot will form a compact mass leaving a clear yellow liquid called **serum**. Serum has the same composition as plasma but without the clotting factors (fibrinogen and prothrombin).

The immune system

The immune system is responsible for protecting the animal from disease or damage from foreign materials. It has the ability to recognize anything that is 'foreign' to the body, i.e. 'not self', and it then produces a specific response (see Chapter 6).

Autoimmune diseases occur when the immune system malfunctions and fails to recognize its own cells, treating them as 'foreign'. In autoimmune haemolytic anaemia, the animal produces antibodies against its own erythrocytes.

The heart

The heart is a four-chambered muscular organ that pumps the blood around the body (Figure 4.44). The heart lies in the mediastinum within the thoracic cavity. It is conical in shape and it lies at a slight angle in the thorax, with its base situated craniodorsally above its apex. The heart lies just to the left of the midline with its apex near the sternum.

Heart structure

The heart is completely enclosed by a double-layered membrane called the **pericardium**. The inner layer of this, the **epicardium**, is a serous membrane and directly covers the heart wall. Within the pericardial cavity is a little serous fluid, which lubricates the heart as it beats.

The wall of the heart consists of a layer of cardiac muscle, the **myocardium**, and a thin inner epithelial layer that lines the heart called the **endocardium**. This layer is continuous with the endothelium lining the blood vessels.

The heart is divided into right and left sides by a partition called the **septum**. Each side is divided into two chambers: the thin-walled collecting chamber is called the **atrium** and the thicker-walled pumping chamber is the **ventricle**. The right side of the heart pumps blood into the **pulmonary circulation** (carries blood from the heart to the lungs and back); the left side of the heart pumps blood into the **systemic circulation** (carries blood all around the body).

Heart valves

Within the heart there are two sets of valves whose function is to prevent backflow of blood.

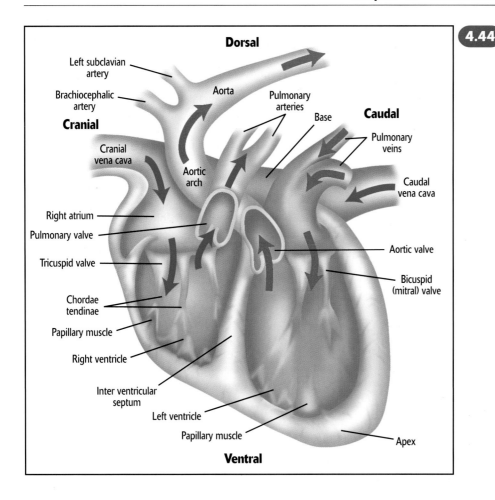

4.44 The structure of the heart and the direction of blood flow.

Atrioventricular valves

These lie between the atria and ventricles and prevent the flow of blood back into the atria when the ventricles contract. They are attached to the **papillary muscles** of the ventricular wall by fibres called the **chordae tendinae**, which prevent the valves being turned inside out by the pressure of the blood flow.

- The **right atrioventricular valve** (also called the **tricuspid valve**) lies between the **right atrium** and **right ventricle** and comprises three fibrous tissue cusps.
- The **left atrioventricular valve** (also called the **bicuspid** or **mitral valve**) lies between the **left atrium** and **left ventricle** and comprises two cusps.

It is the atrioventricular valves closing that can be heard in the **first** heart sound ('**lubb**').

Semilunar valves

These are at the base of the two major vessels leaving the heart.

- The **pulmonary valve** lies at the base of the pulmonary artery and prevents the backflow of blood from the pulmonary artery to the right ventricle.
- The **aortic valve** lies at the base of the aorta and prevents backflow of blood from the aorta to the left ventricle.

It is the semilunar valves closing that can be heard in the **second** heart sound ('**dubb**'). If the valve closure is faulty the flow of blood is disturbed, causing turbulence. This may be heard as a 'whoosh' instead of a 'lubb' or a 'dubb' and is known as **heart murmur**.

Circulation of blood through the heart

Deoxygenated blood is carried back to the heart in the veins. Two major veins collect all the blood and enter the right side of the heart: the **cranial vena cava** and **caudal vena cava** (Figure 4.44). The two atria (left and right) contract in unison, as do the two ventricles:

- The venae cavae empty into the **right atrium**, which contracts when full, sending deoxygenated blood into the **right ventricle** via the right atrioventricular valve.
- The right ventricle contracts, pumping blood into the **pulmonary artery** via the pulmonary valve. The deoxygenated blood is carried in the pulmonary circulation to the **lungs**.
- The blood is oxygenated in the lungs and is then carried back to the left side of the heart in the **pulmonary veins**, which enter the **left atrium**.
- When the left atrium is full it contracts, forcing oxygenated blood into the **left ventricle** via the left atrioventricular valve.
- The left ventricle contracts and pumps blood into the **aorta** (via the aortic valve), which carries the oxygenated blood all around the body in the systemic circulation.

Oxygenated blood is delivered to the tissues and the deoxygenated blood is collected up by the veins and transported back to the heart.

Control of the heartbeat (cardiac cycle)

The heart is made of cardiac muscle, which is a specialized type of muscle tissue that has the ability to initiate a contraction from within the muscle itself (i.e. without a nervous

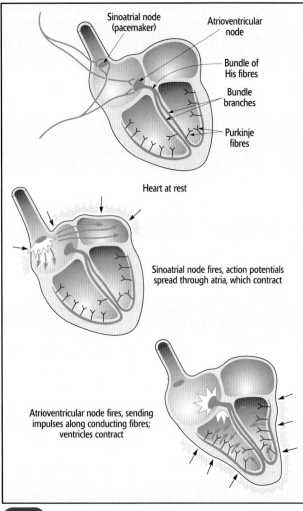

4.45   The conduction mechanism of the heart.

impulse). The mechanism that is responsible for controlling the **rate** of contraction of heart muscle (i.e. the heartbeat) is called the **conduction mechanism** (Figure 4.45).

Within the wall of the right atrium is an area of modified cardiac muscle called the **sinoatrial node** (SA node). This node determines the basic rate of the heartbeat and is referred to as the 'pacemaker'. If the muscles require more oxygen (e.g. during exercise), the SA node will increase the basic rate of contraction so that more oxygenated blood reaches the muscles. During sleep, the SA node will slow the basic heart rate.

1. The SA node initiates a wave of contraction, which passes over the walls of the atria. The myocardium of the atria and of the ventricles, although physically joined, is not in electrical continuity. It is separated, which prevents the wave of contraction in the atria spreading into the ventricles.
2. The impulse is passed to another specialized group of cells called the **atrioventricular node** (AV node) lying at the top of the interventricular septum.
3. The wave of excitation passes down a specialized group of fibres called the **bundle of His**, within the interventricular septum.
4. The impulse is then conducted to the apex of the heart, where it spreads out into the ventricles in specialized nerve cells called **Purkinje fibres**. Thus, the wave of contraction in the myocardium of the ventricles starts at the apex and spreads upwards, forcing blood into the arteries that are situated at the top of the ventricles.

This is called the **cardiac cycle**.

- The period of **contraction** within the heart is called **systole** and is when the blood is being pumped into the ventricles or the pulmonary and systemic circulations.
- The period of **relaxation** in the heart is called diastole and is when the atria are filling with blood.

An **electrocardiogram (ECG)** is the means by which the electrical activity of the heart is assessed.

The circulatory system

This is a branching network of channels that transport the blood from the heart to the tissues, where oxygen and nutrients are delivered, and then transport it back again to the heart. The network consists of arteries, capillaries and veins.

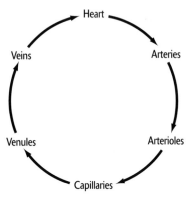

Arteries

An artery is a relatively large vessel that carries blood under pressure *away* from the heart. Most arteries carry oxygenated blood, but the pulmonary artery carries deoxygenated blood from the heart to the lungs. Arteries have thick muscular walls (Figure 4.46) to enable the vessel to dilate or constrict, thus changing the volume of blood flowing through it. Blood travels along the arteries in pulses reflecting the heartbeat and this is felt in the more superficial arteries as the **pulse**.

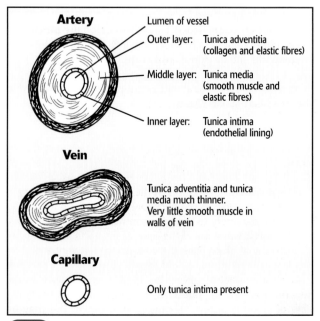

4.46   The structure of an artery, vein and capillary.

As the arteries enter the tissues they branch and get smaller. These are the **arterioles**, which then flow into the capillary networks.

Capillaries

The capillaries form a branching network in all tissues and link the arteries and the veins. They are narrow with thin walls consisting of a single layer of endothelial cells, with no muscle or elastic tissue (Figure 4.46). This means that they are permeable to gases, nutrients and waste products, which diffuse between the blood and tissues and from the tissues back into the blood.

Veins

A vein is a relatively large vessel, which carries blood towards the heart. The walls are thinner than those of arteries and they contain less muscle and elastic tissue (Figure 4.46). Blood flows slowly under low pressure and **valves** may be present in some veins (e.g. the legs) to prevent pooling of blood in the extremities. Most veins carry deoxygenated blood from the tissues, but the pulmonary veins carry oxygenated blood from the lungs back to the heart.

The capillaries collect together to form **venules** or small veins, which eventually drain into the larger veins.

Systemic and pulmonary circulation

The circulation in the mammal is described as being double, as blood passes through the heart twice during one complete circuit (Figure 4.47). There are two parts to the circulatory system:

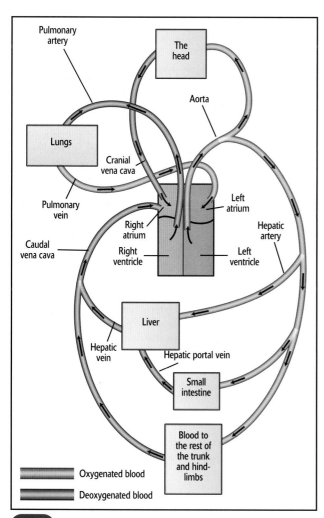

4.47 Circulation of the blood around the body.

- **Systemic circulation** carries oxygenated blood around the body and returns deoxygenated blood to the heart.
- **Pulmonary circulation** carries deoxygenated blood from the heart to the lungs, where it is oxygenated and returned to the heart.

Systemic circulation

Arterial supply

Oxygenated blood leaves the left ventricle of the heart in the major artery known as the **aorta**. This gives off a number of **arteries** that supply the various parts of the body. In the order that they leave the aorta they are as follows.

1. **Coronary arteries** supply the heart muscle.
2. **Brachiocephalic trunk** gives rise to the **common carotid arteries**, which supply the head. The brachiocephalic trunk then supplies the right forelimb as it becomes the **right subclavian artery**, continuing as the **right axillary artery** and then the **right brachial artery** as it passes down the limb.
3. **Left subclavian artery** supplies the left forelimb with blood, becoming the **left axillary artery** and then the **left brachial artery**.
4. The aorta continues through the thorax, passing through the diaphragm into the abdomen and pelvis, giving off branches that supply the bones, muscles and organs of the body. These include:
   - A pair of **renal arteries**, which supply the kidney
   - **Ovarian/testicular arteries**, which supply the gonads
   - **Coeliac artery**, which has branches supplying the stomach, spleen and liver
   - **Cranial mesenteric artery**, which supplies the small intestine
   - **Caudal mesenteric artery**, which supplies the large intestine.
5. The hindlimb is supplied by the **external iliac artery**, which branches into the **femoral artery** in each of the hindlimbs.
6. A branch of the aorta called the **internal iliac artery** supplies the pelvic organs.

Venous return

Deoxygenated blood returns to the heart from the tissues in the **veins**, which follow a similar pattern to those of the arteries and often have the same name (e.g. renal artery and renal vein). The veins of the pelvis, hindlimbs and abdominal viscera all drain into one of the two major veins of the body, the **caudal vena cava**. This empties into the right atrium of the heart.

Venous blood returns:

- From the head in the **jugular veins**
- From the neck and forelimbs in the **cephalic veins**, **brachial veins** and then **subclavian veins** and drains into the **cranial vena cava**, which empties into the right atrium of the heart.

The **azygous vein** carries deoxygenated blood from the thoracic body wall and either joins the cranial vena cava or drains directly into the right atrium.

The deoxygenated blood from the heart muscle drains into the **coronary veins**, which join to form the **coronary sinus**.

The veins that are most commonly used to gain access to the venous system are the **cephalic veins**, found on the cranial surface of the upper part of the forelimb, and the **jugular vein** embedded in the tissue of the ventral surface of the neck.

Hepatic portal system

The hepatic portal system is a modified circulatory system within the systemic circulation. Its function is to carry blood straight from the digestive system to the liver so that the products of digestion can be utilized immediately, rather than having to transport them all round the rest of the body.

Veins draining the small intestine empty into the **hepatic portal vein**, which supplies blood to the liver. The liver thus receives the products of digestion in the hepatic portal vein and oxygenated blood in the **hepatic artery**. Waste products from the liver are drained by the **hepatic vein**, which then flows into the caudal vena cava.

Pulmonary circulation

Deoxygenated blood is pumped from the right ventricle of the heart and is carried to the lungs in the **pulmonary artery**. Within the lung tissue the artery divides into numerous fine capillaries that wrap around the thin-walled alveoli of the lungs. Oxygen in the inspired air diffuses into the blood and carbon dioxide in the blood diffuses into the air in the alveoli.

The newly oxygenated blood is carried to the left atrium of the heart by the **pulmonary veins** and is pumped around the body in the systemic circulation.

The lymphatic system

The lymphatic system is responsible for the circulation of **lymph**, the tissue fluid that leaks out of the blood capillaries and bathes the cells in the interstitial spaces. Lymph is similar to plasma but contains more lymphocytes. The functions of the lymphatic system are to:

- Return excess tissue fluid to the circulation
- Filter out foreign materials (e.g. bacteria) from the lymph by the lymph nodes before being returned to the venous circulation
- Produce lymphocytes as part of the immune system
- Transport digested fats.

The lymphatic system consists of lymphatic capillaries, lymphatic vessels, lymph nodes, lymphatic ducts and lymphatic tissues.

Lymphatic capillaries

The lymphatic capillaries are small thin-walled vessels that are widely distributed throughout all the tissues of the body except the central nervous system. These capillaries are responsible for draining the excess tissue fluid from the interstitial spaces. In the intestinal villi the lymphatic capillaries are called **lacteals** and they collect the majority of the digested fats.

Lymphatic vessels

The lymphatic capillaries in the tissues merge to form larger lymphatic vessels. These are similar in structure to veins and contain valves that prevent backflow of the lymph. The movement of lymph is passive and is dependent upon contraction of the surrounding muscles and the non-return valves.

Lymph nodes

Lymph nodes are bean-shaped structures located at points along the lymph vessels. Each lymph node is enclosed within a connective tissue capsule and is divided into two regions: the cortex and medulla. The cortex contains germinal centres where lymphocytes are produced. There are also phagocytic cells within the lymph node, which remove bacteria and foreign particles as the lymph filters through the node.

- **Afferent** lymphatic vessels carry lymph towards the node and enter it all over its surface.
- A single **efferent** vessel carries lymph away from the node at an indented area called the **hilus.**

Lymph must pass through at least one lymph node before entering the lymphatic ducts that return it to the venous circulation. Some of the lymph nodes (Figure 4.48) are quite superficial and can be palpated. When the body is fighting an infection, the lymph node that lies closest to the source of the infection may become enlarged. If the disease or infection is generalized, all the lymph nodes may become enlarged.

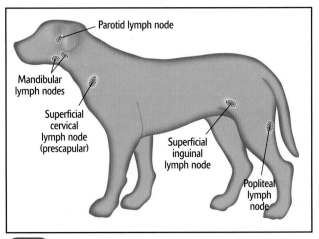

4.48 The lymphatic system: major nodes and ducts.

Superficial lymph nodes include:

- **Submandibular** – located on the caudal edge of the mandible at the angle of the jaw
- **Parotid** – caudal to the temporomandibular joint
- **Superficial cervical** or **prescapular** – just cranial to the scapular
- **Superficial inguinal nodes** – in the groin, between the inner thigh and the abdomen
- **Popliteal** – caudal to the stifle joint within the gastrocnemius muscle.

Lymphatic ducts

After lymph has passed through a lymph node it drains into a larger lymphatic duct. The main lymphatic ducts are:

- **Right lymphatic duct** – collects lymph from the right forelimb and the right side of the head and neck
- **Cisterna chyli** – lies within the dorsal abdomen and collects lymph from the hindlimbs, pelvis and abdomen, including the lacteals
- **Thoracic duct** – collects the lymph from the cisterna chyli, from the left forelimb and from the left side of the upper body.

Both the right lymphatic duct and the thoracic duct empty into either the jugular vein or the cranial vena cava near the heart.

Lymphatic tissues

These are large accumulations of lymphoid tissue, which play an important part in the body's defence system.

Spleen

The spleen is a haemopoietic lymphoid organ found closely attached to the greater curvature of the stomach. The functions of the spleen are:

• Storage of blood
• Removal of old red blood cells
• Production of lymphocytes
• Removal of bacteria and foreign material by the action of the phagocytic cells.

Though the spleen has these important functions, it is not essential to life and can be surgically removed if necessary.

Thymus

This lies in the thorax, cranial to the heart. It is an important site for lymphocyte production in the young animal and plays an essential role in its immune system.

As the animal grows older, the thymus atrophies.

Tonsils

The tonsils form a ring of lymphoid tissue in the subepithelial layer of the pharynx. They provide a defence against the introduction of infection into the digestive and respiratory systems.

The respiratory system

The function of the respiratory system is to extract oxygen from atmospheric air and excrete carbon dioxide, formed by the tissues, out into the air again.

Respiration is the exchange of gases between a living organism and its environment.

It can be considered to occur in two stages:

• **External respiration** is the gaseous exchange between the air and the blood.
• **Internal or tissue respiration** is the gaseous exchange between the blood and the tissues.

The upper respiratory tract is said to consist of the nasal chambers, pharynx, larynx, trachea and primary bronchi while the lower respiratory tract consists of the smaller bronchi, bronchioles and alveoli (i.e. the structures making up the lungs).

Nasal chambers

Air enters the respiratory system through the **external nares** or nostrils to reach the right and left **nasal chambers**. The nostrils are surrounded by the **rhinarium** or nosepad. The nasal chambers are divided by a cartilaginous nasal **septum** and are filled with fine scrolls of bone called **ethmoturbinates** or **conchae** (Figure 4.49). The entire cavity and the ethmoturbinates are covered by **ciliated mucous epithelium**, which is well supplied with capillaries and sensory nerve fibres. These nerve fibres travel the short distance to the olfactory bulbs of the forebrain carrying the sensation of smell or **olfaction.**

Leading from the nasal cavities are small air-filled diverticuli in the surrounding facial bones – the **paranasal sinuses**. They are lined with ciliated mucous epithelium and communicate with the nasal cavity through narrow openings:

• **Maxillary sinus** – not a true sinus in the dog but a recess at the caudal end of the nasal cavities
• **Frontal sinus** – lies within the frontal bone of the skull.

The paranasal sinuses lighten the weight of the skull, allowing the surface area to be used for the attachment of larger muscles. They also act as an area for thermal exchange and for mucus secretion.

The functions of the nasal cavities are:

• To warm and moisten incoming air
• To trap dust and foreign particles in the covering of mucus (the cilia waft them to the back of the nasal cavity, where they pass to the pharynx and are swallowed or coughed out)
• Olfaction.

Pharynx

Inspired air passes into the pharynx. This structure at the back of the oral and nasal cavities is shared by the respiratory and digestive systems. The entrance from the nasal cavity into the pharynx can be sealed off by a musculomembranous partition, the **soft palate** (Figure 4.49), which prevents food from entering the nasal cavities when the animal swallows (see 'Digestive system', below). The soft palate is the caudal extension of the hard palate and divides the pharynx into the **nasopharynx**, which conducts air from the nasal cavity to the

4.49 Midline section through dog's head.

Nasal cavity
Frontal sinus
Ethmoidal conchae with olfactory area
Dorsal concha
Internal nares
Nasopharynx
Ventral concha
Lateral ventricle
Vocal fold
Trachea
External nares
Oesophagus
Hard palate
Tongue
Soft palate
Epiglottis
Oral cavity
Oropharynx
Arytenoid cartilage of larynx

larynx, and the **oropharynx**, which conducts food from the mouth to the oesophagus. During respiratory difficulty or strenuous exercise, 'mouth breathing' may occur and air may enter the pharynx from the mouth as well as the nose, allowing a greater volume of air to reach the lungs.

In addition to these openings there are paired openings into the **Eustachian** or **auditory tubes** that connect the pharynx to the middle ear.

Larynx

The larynx leads from the pharynx and is a complex, mobile structure consisting of a number of cartilages and muscle. It lies in the space between the two mandibles and is suspended from the skull by the bony **hyoid apparatus,** which allows it to swing forwards and backwards like the seat of a swing (Figure 4.50).

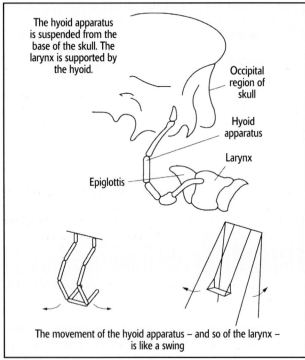

The hyoid apparatus is suspended from the base of the skull. The larynx is supported by the hyoid.

Occipital region of skull

Hyoid apparatus

Larynx

Epiglottis

The movement of the hyoid apparatus – and so of the larynx – is like a swing

4.50 The hyoid apparatus.

The opening to the larynx is the **glottis**, which is closed off by a flap of elastic cartilage, the **epiglottis**, during swallowing (see 'Digestive system', below). When the larynx moves back to its resting position, the epiglottis falls open and air is able to enter the glottis.

Within the lumen of the larynx is a pair of **vocal ligaments** or cords. The mucous membrane covering their inner surface forms the **vocal folds**, which project into the larynx. Sound is produced when air rushes past the vocal folds, causing them to vibrate. Laryngeal paralysis is a condition that may be seen in larger older dogs in which the vocal cords hang within the lumen of the larynx, where they interfere with the free flow of air and cause a roaring noise as the animal breathes. Treatment involves the 'tying back' of the cords to open up the airway.

The functions of the larynx are:

- To prevent entry of anything other than gases into the respiratory tract
- To regulate the flow of gases into the tract
- To produce sounds.

Trachea

The trachea is a permanently open tube attached to the caudal laryngeal cartilages. It lies on the ventral aspect of the neck and extends the full length of the neck. It passes through the thoracic inlet and is carried in the **mediastinum** of the thoracic cavity. It bifurcates into the right and left **primary bronchi** above the heart.

The lumen of the trachea is kept open by a series of C-shaped incomplete rings of hyaline cartilage joined by smooth muscle and connective tissue. The trachea is flexible to allow movement of the head and neck. It is lined with **ciliated mucous epithelium**, which traps and wafts any foreign particles towards the larynx, where they are coughed up and swallowed. Any irritation of the tracheal lining causes coughing, which serves to expel substances from the respiratory tract.

Bronchi and bronchioles

Each of the two primary bronchi leads to the lung on the appropriate side. The bronchus then divides into smaller and smaller branches as it enters the lung tissue. The point at which each bronchus enters the lung is known as the root.

The bronchi are similar in structure to the trachea, but the cartilage rings are complete and gradually reduce as the branches of the bronchi decrease in diameter. The bronchi branch and give off smaller branches – the **bronchioles**. Within the bronchioles the cartilage support reduces and disappears. This arrangement of tubes creates a 'tree-like' pattern referred to as the **bronchial tree**. The whole bronchial tree is lined with ciliated mucous membrane.

The bronchioles continue to branch until they reach their smallest diameter as the **respiratory** or **terminal bronchioles**, at which point each branches into several **alveolar ducts**.

Alveolar sacs

Each alveolar duct ends as an **alveolar sac** consisting of a large number of 'grape-like' **alveoli** (Figure 4.51). The epithelium lining the alveoli is a single-celled non-ciliated **pulmonary membrane** and it is across this that gaseous exchange takes place.

Surrounding the alveoli are thin-walled **capillary networks**, which bring inspired air in the alveoli into close contact with the blood. These networks are branches of the pulmonary arteries and veins.

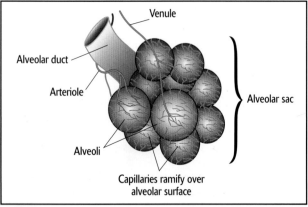

Venule

Alveolar duct

Arteriole

Alveoli

Alveolar sac

Capillaries ramify over alveolar surface

4.51 The terminal air passages.

Gaseous exchange

Oxygen diffuses across the pulmonary membrane into the blood within the capillaries, while carbon dioxide diffuses out of the blood and into the alveoli. There are millions of alveoli in each lung and they provide a large surface area for gaseous exchange. Gaseous exchange takes place *only* in the alveoli. The rest of the respiratory tract conducts the air to the site of gaseous exchange in the alveoli and is called the **conducting system**. Because the component structures of the conducting system have no part in gaseous exchange, they are often collectively referred to as the **dead space**. The volume of the dead space is increased by the attachment of an anaesthetic circuit and it is vital that the size of the animal is considered when selecting the circuit. Small animals such as cats cannot be attached to a large circuit with a large volume, because they do not have the vital capacity to move gas in and out of the tubes (see Chapter 22).

The lungs

The right and left lungs lie within the thoracic cavity, on either side of the mediastinum. Each lung consists of the air passages, blood vessels and surrounding connective tissue, all enclosed within a membrane called the **pulmonary pleura**.

Each lung is divided by deep furrows into lobes. The left lung has three lobes; the right lung has four (Figure 4.52). These lobes are called the **cranial (apical) lobe**, the **middle (cardiac) lobe** and the **caudal (diaphragmatic) lobe**. The fourth lobe of the right lung lies on the medial surface of the caudal lobe and is small and irregularly shaped; this is called the **accessory lobe**.

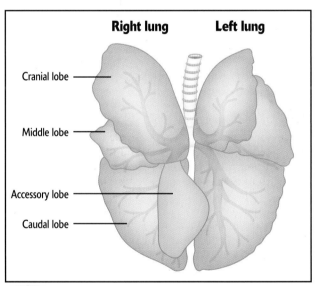

4.52   The lobes of the lung.

Lung volumes

*   **Tidal air** – air passing in and out of the lungs
*   **Tidal volume** – volume of air passing in and out of the lungs during normal respiration
*   **Residual volume** – volume of air left in the lungs after forceful expiration
*   **Total lung capacity** – volume of air breathed in with maximum inspiration or out with maximum expiration
*   **Vital capacity** – total amount of air that can be expired after a minimum respiration
*   **Functional residual capacity** – volume of air let in the lungs after normal respiration
*   **Dead space** – volume of air in the respiratory tract that never reaches the area of gaseous exchange
*   **Respiratory rate** – number of breaths per minute

The mechanism of breathing

Breathing, or pulmonary ventilation, is achieved by the action of muscles that alternately increase and decrease the volume of the thoracic cavity. The muscles that are responsible for breathing are the **diaphragm** and the **external intercostals**.

The pleural membranes divide the thoracic cavity into the right and left pleural cavities. These cavities are closed spaces and there is a vacuum between the lung and the chest wall. Any change in the volume of the thoracic cavity will result in a change in pressure and air will be sucked in or forced out.

*   **Inspiration** occurs when contraction of the external intercostals causes the upward and outward movement of the ribs. The diaphragm contracts, flattens and moves downwards. The volume of the thoracic cavity is increased, creating a negative pressure in the lung tissue, and air is drawn down into the lungs.
*   **Expiration** is mainly passive. The diaphragm and intercostal muscles relax, causing the thoracic cavity to decrease in size. Pressure is put on the lungs and air is pushed out of the lungs.

The internal intercostal muscles are mainly used in **forced expiration** in conjunction with the abdominal muscles, which contract and raise the pressure in the abdominal cavity and force the diaphragm upwards.

Control of respiration

Respiration is an automatic process, which must be constantly adjusted to meet the demands of the body. It is controlled by a system involving receptors, which send information about the status of the body to a central controller in the brain.

Respiratory centres

Respiratory centres in the pons and medulla of the hindbrain affect the basic **rhythm** of respiration:

*   **Apneustic** and **pneumotaxic** centres control expiration.
*   **Inspiratory centre** controls inspiration.

The centres inhibit each other and cannot work simultaneously.

Receptors

Stretch receptors and chemoreceptors within the tissues of the body affect the **rate** and **depth** of respiration.

Stretch receptors

An example of the activity of stretch receptors within the lung tissue is the **Hering Breuer** reflex, which prevents over-inflation of the lungs. As the lung inflates, the stretch receptors send impulses via the **vagus nerve** to the inspiratory centre within the hindbrain and prevent further inspiration. They also stimulate the expiratory centres and the animal breathes out.

Chemoreceptors

These receptors monitor the pH of the blood and the carbon dioxide/oxygen levels in the blood. They are found in the walls of the aorta and carotid arteries. For example, if carbon dioxide builds up in the blood it lowers the pH. This is detected by the chemoreceptors, which send the information to the expiratory centres. The carbon dioxide is exhaled and the pH of the blood returns to normal.

The digestive system

The digestive tract (Figure 4.53) comprises the oral cavity, pharynx, oesophagus, stomach, small intestine (duodenum, jejunum, ileum), large intestine (caecum, colon, rectum) and anus. Associated with the tract are several accessory glands: the salivary glands, pancreas, gall bladder and liver.

The different parts of the system work together to produce energy from the food eaten by the animal (Figure 4.54). The dog and the cat are carnivorous species, i.e. flesh-eaters, and the structure of the digestive tract is adapted to deal with a diet that is relatively easy to digest.

Oral cavity

This is the external opening of the digestive tract and is also called the **buccal cavity** or the mouth. It contains the tongue, teeth and salivary glands and its functions are:

- To pick up food (**prehension**)
- To break up the food and manipulate it into boluses (**mastication**)
- To lubricate the food to aid swallowing.

The oral cavity is supported by the upper jaw (formed by the **maxillary** and **incisive bones**) and the lower jaw (formed by the **left** and **right mandibles**). The **palatine bone** forms the roof of the mouth and is known as the **hard palate**. An outer layer of muscles and skin, which forms the **cheeks**, connects the jaws. Beneath the skin the main muscle of mastication is the **masseter muscle**. The external entrance to the oral cavity is marked by the **lips**, composed of skin and muscle. The upper lip has a central vertical cleft known as the **philtrum**. The entire cavity is lined by mucous membrane, which reflects on to the jawbones forming the **gums** and is pierced by the teeth.

Tongue

This lies on the floor of the oral cavity and is made of striated muscle fibres running in all directions. The tip of the tongue is unattached and very mobile while the root of the tongue is continuous with the larynx and is attached to the hyoid apparatus and to the mandibles.

The tongue is covered in mucous membrane arranged in backward-pointing papillae, giving it a rough surface, which is useful for grooming and for ingestion and manipulation of food. Embedded among the papillae, particularly at the back of the tongue, are the taste buds, which are responsible for gustation

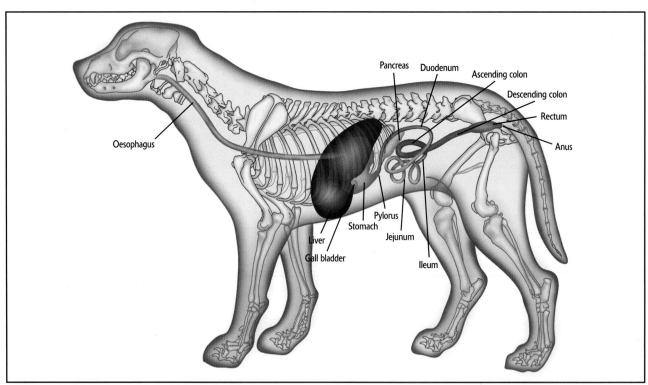

4.53 Position of gastrointestinal tract in the abdomen. Length of intestines has been reduced in order to simplify the diagram.

Process	Definition	Parts of the tract involved
Ingestion	Food is taken into the body	Lips, teeth, tongue
Mastication (chewing)	Food is mixed with saliva and formed into a bolus ready for swallowing	Lips, cheeks, tongue, salivary glands
Digestion	Food is broken down by digestive enzymes into small soluble chemical units	Stomach and small intestine
Absorption	Small units pass through the intestinal wall into the bloodstream	Small intestine
Metabolism	Small units are processed to produce energy and material necessary for normal body functions	Liver and all cells of the body
Excretion	Remaining insoluble material passes out as faeces	Large intestine, anus

4.54 Processes within the gastrointestinal tract.

(see 'Special senses', above). Underneath the tongue is the **lingual vein**, which may be used for venepuncture in an anaesthetized patient.

In the dog the tongue is the main method of thermoregulation. Saliva on the tongue evaporates as the animal pants, causing cooling.

Salivary glands

These are paired glandular structures embedded in the soft tissues of the oral cavity whose secretions enter the cavity by means of ducts. Saliva produced by the dog and cat contains 99% water and 1% mucus. There are no enzymes, as food spends little time in the oral cavity before being swallowed. The main function of the saliva is to aid mastication and swallowing and in thermoregulation. Salivation may be stimulated by the sight or smell of food, irritant smells and tastes, vomiting, pain or poisoning by certain chemicals (e.g. organophosphates).

Teeth

These hard structures are embedded in sockets or **alveoli** in the upper and lower jaw. Each jaw forms a **dental arch**, of which there are four. The mucous membrane covering the gums is called the **periodontal membrane** or the **gingival membrane**.

Structure

All teeth have the same basic structure, as shown in Figure 4.55.

Function

The teeth of the cat and dog are adapted to tearing flesh from the bones of prey. There are four types, each with a different position in the jaw (Figure 4.56) and a different function (Figure 4.57).

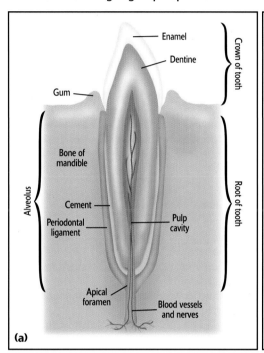

(a)

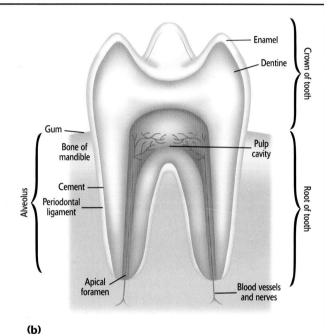

(b)

4.55 Tooth structure. **(a)** Incisor. **(b)** Molar.

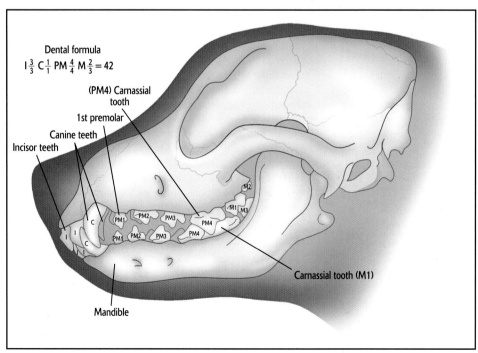

Dental formula

$$I\frac{3}{3}\ C\frac{1}{1}\ PM\frac{4}{4}\ M\frac{2}{3}=42$$

4.56 Skull of a dog to show tooth position.

Type	Shape	Function
Incisor (I)	Lie in the incisive bone of the upper jaw and in the mandible of the lower jaw. Small pointed with a single root	Fine nibbling and cutting flesh. Often used for delicate grooming
Canines (C) – 'eye teeth'	One on each corner of the upper and lower jaws. Pointed with a simple curved shape, single root deeply embedded in the bone	Holding prey firmly in the mouth
Premolars (PM) – 'cheek teeth'	Flatter surface with several points known as cusps or tubercles. Usually have 2 or 3 roots arranged in a triangular position to give stability in the jawbone	Shearing meat off the bone using a scissor-like action. Flattened surface helps to grind up the meat to facilitate swallowing and digestion
Molars (M) – 'cheek teeth'	Similar shape to premolars. Usually larger with at least 3 roots	Shearing and grinding flesh (**NB:** There are no molars in the deciduous dentition)
Carnassials	Largest teeth in the jaw. Similar shape to other cheek teeth **These are the first lower molar and the last upper premolar on each side**	Very powerful teeth sited close to the angle of the lips and used for bone crunching. Only found in carnivores

4.57 Tooth type and function.

Eruption

Dogs and cats have two sets of teeth during their lives:

- **Deciduous, temporary or 'milk' dentition** – present in the jaw at birth and erupt during the first few months of life; smaller and whiter than adult teeth
- **Permanent or adult dentition** – replaces the milk teeth and last for the whole of adult life; larger and show signs of wear as the animal ages.

Eruption times for each type of dentition are shown in Figure 4.58.

Tooth type	Dog	Cat
Deciduous dentition		Entire dentition starts to erupt at 2 weeks and is complete by 4 weeks
Incisors	3–4 weeks	
Canines	5 weeks	
Premolars	4–8 weeks	
Molars	Absent	
Permanent dentition		Variable. Full dentition present by 6 months
Incisors	3.5–4 months	12 weeks
Canines	5–6 months	
Premolars	1st premolars 4–5 months Remainder 5–7 months	
Molars	5–7 months	

4.58 Eruption times for the deciduous and permanent dentitions.

Dental formulae

The number and type of teeth are written as a dental formula, in which I = incisor, C = canine, PM = premolar, M = molar.

Dog

Deciduous teeth:

$$2 \times \frac{\text{I3 \quad C1 \quad PM3}}{\text{I3 \quad C1 \quad PM3}} = 28$$

Permanent teeth:

$$2 \times \frac{\text{I3 \quad C1 \quad PM4 \quad M2}}{\text{I3 \quad C1 \quad PM4 \quad M3}} = 42$$

Cat

Deciduous teeth:

$$2 \times \frac{\text{I3 \quad C1 \quad PM3}}{\text{I3 \quad C1 \quad PM2}} = 26$$

Permanent teeth:

$$2 \times \frac{\text{I3 \quad C1 \quad PM3 \quad M1}}{\text{I3 \quad C1 \quad PM2 \quad M1}} = 30$$

Pharynx

This is a short muscular tube lined with mucous membrane, which acts as a cross-over point between the respiratory and digestive systems. The **soft palate** extends caudally from the hard palate towards the epiglottis of the larynx and divides the pharynx into the **nasopharynx** at the back of the nasal cavity and the **oropharynx** at the back of the oral cavity (see Figure 4.49).

The pharynx conveys food from the oral cavity to the oesophagus by a process known as **swallowing** or **deglutition**.

Swallowing

1. Food is formed into a bolus and pushed to the back of the mouth by the tongue.
2. The walls of the pharynx contract and push the bolus towards the oesophagus.
3. Simultaneously the epiglottis closes to prevent food from entering the larynx.
4. A wave of contraction (peristalsis) pushes the food down the oesophagus.
5. As the food leaves the pharynx the epiglottis falls open, allowing air to pass down the larynx and trachea.

Oesophagus

This simple muscular tube transports food by a series of organized muscular contractions (**peristalsis**) from the pharynx through the thorax and diaphragm to the stomach. In the neck, it lies dorsal to and slightly to the left of the trachea. It is lined with stratified squamous epithelium arranged in longitudinal folds, which allow widthways expansion as food passes down. Beneath this are layers of smooth muscle well supplied with nerves and blood capillaries.

The average time for food to pass down the oesophagus is 15–30 seconds, but this depends on the nature of the food. Food is able to pass back up the oesophagus during vomition and regurgitation.

Stomach

This is a C-shaped sac-like organ lying mainly on the left side of the cranial abdominal cavity (see Figure 4.53). Its functions are:

- To act as a reservoir for food prior to digestion
- To break up the food and mix it with gastric juices
- To begin protein digestion.

Food in the oesophagus enters the stomach via the **cardiac sphincter** and leaves via the **pyloric sphincter**. These muscular structures control the rate of flow of material into and out of the stomach. The outer curve of the stomach is called the **greater curvature** and the inner curve is called the **lesser curvature**. The entire organ is covered in a layer of visceral peritoneum or mesentery – the mesentery attached to the lesser curvature is the **lesser omentum** and that attached to the greater curvature is the **greater omentum**. The **spleen** is closely applied to the greater curvature and lies within the greater omentum.

The walls of the stomach are thick and very distensible. When empty, the stomach lies under the ribs, but when full it may occupy as much as half of the abdomen and can easily be seen from the outside. Sometimes a dog's stomach may become excessively inflated by gas produced during food fermentation or by swallowed air. This results in a condition known as gastric dilatation–volvulus, in which the distended stomach becomes twisted and also presses on other abdominal organs. This is a genuine emergency and treatment must be instigated as soon as possible if the dog is not to die of shock (see Chapter 18).

Structure of the stomach wall

The stomach can be divided into three regions:

- **Cardia** – close to the cardiac sphincter
- **Fundus** – forms the largest region and contains most of the gastric glands
- **Pylorus** – close to the pyloric sphincter.

The walls are lined with mucous membrane, the **gastric mucosa**, which is arranged in deep folds or **rugae** (Figure 4.59) These enable the stomach to stretch when filled with food. Within the mucosa are the **gastric pits**, which consist of three types of cells responsible for the production of gastric juices:

- **Goblet cells** – secrete mucus to aid lubrication of the food and protect the stomach wall from autodigestion
- **Chief cells** – secrete pepsinogen, the precursor of the enzyme pepsin
- **Parietal cells** – secrete hydrochloric acid. This creates an acid pH, which protects against infection and converts pepsinogen to the active pepsin. Pepsin digests protein to form peptides.

The secretion of gastric juices is initiated by the hormone **gastrin**, produced by the stomach walls in response to the distension of the stomach by food.

Beneath the gastric mucosa are three layers of **smooth muscle fibres** lying in all directions. These are responsible for peristaltic contractions, which push the food onwards, and rhythmic segmentation, which mixes the food with the gastric juices.

Within the stomach food is changed into partially digested **chyme** with an acid pH (chyme is defined as food converted by gastric secretion into an acid pulp). This is released in spurts through the pyloric sphincter into the duodenum. The time taken to pass through the stomach depends on food type: liquids may take up to 30 minutes, while more solid or fatty foods may take as long as 3 hours.

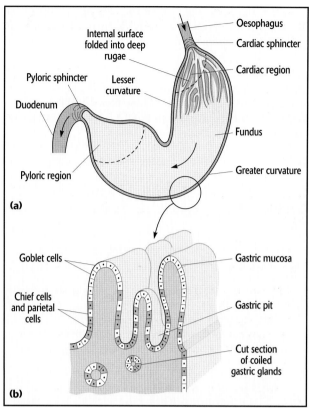

4.59 (a) Cross-section through the stomach wall.
(b) Section showing gastric pits.

Vomiting

Vomiting is the return of ingesta and fluids against the normal direction of swallowing and peristalsis (see Chapter 21).

Vomiting/regurgitation

- **Regurgitation** – overflow of oesophageal contents, no muscle contractions involved
- **True vomiting** – involves active abdominal contractions and expulsion of the vomitus, preceded by a feeling of nausea, and salivation
- **Projectile vomiting** – violent ejection of the stomach contents. This may be seen in cases of pyloric stenosis, which usually occur in neonates and result from the congenital thickening of the muscle of the pyloric sphincter. The sphincter restricts the flow of chyme into the duodenum and affected individuals forcibly vomit within about 30 minutes of eating

Small intestine

This is the main site for the enzymic digestion of food and its subsequent absorption. The small intestine is a long narrow tube divided into three parts (duodenum, jejunum and ileum), each of which has a similar structure but certain functional differences.

Duodenum

This relatively short tube lies in the dorsal abdomen and is held in a U-shaped loop by a short piece of mesentery – the **mesoduodenum**. The **pancreas** lies within the loop. Its secretions enter the duodenum via the **pancreatic duct** near the pyloric sphincter and close to the opening of the **common bile duct** leading from the gall bladder.

Within the walls of the duodenum are **Brunner's glands**. These are digestive glands, which secrete a mixture of enzymes referred to as **succus entericus.**

Jejunum and ileum

These are difficult to distinguish externally and form a long thin tube suspended by the **mesojejunum** and **mesoileum**. This is long and mobile and enables the intestine to fill any free space within the peritoneal cavity.

Within the walls are digestive glands known as the **crypts of Lieberkuhn**. The ileum terminates at the **ileocaecal junction.**

Structure of the intestinal wall

Each part of the intestinal wall has a similar structure (Figure 4.60).

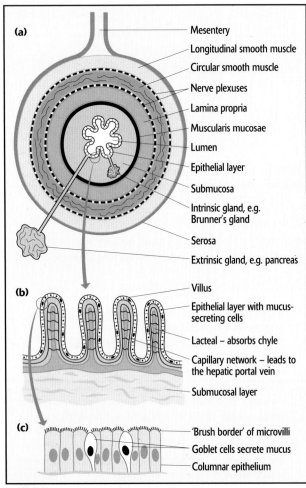

4.60 (a) Cross-section through the intestine wall.
(b) Detail of villus structure. (c) Detail of epithelium.

The epithelium is formed into numerous tiny folds called **villi** (sing. villus). Extending from each epithelial cell is a border of minute microvilli forming a '**brush border**'. Both of these structures increase the surface area for the absorption of digested food.

Inside each villus are:

* A capillary network, which carries digested proteins and carbohydrates to the liver via the **hepatic portal vein**
* A lymphatic capillary known as a **lacteal** which carries **chyle** (a milky liquid containing digested fat) to the **cisterna chyli** in the dorsal abdomen.

Digestion and absorption

Digestion (Figure 4.61) is the process by which proteins (polypeptides), carbohydrates (polysaccharides) and fats (lipids) are broken down into small soluble units, which can then be absorbed by the blood capillaries and the lacteals.

Chemicals known as enzymes are secreted by digestive glands and begin to break down the food as it enters the stomach and small intestine. An **enzyme** is a protein that acts as a catalyst, increasing the speed of a reaction. Enzymes are specifically structured to act on particular materials or substrates and do not affect any other substrates. Some enzymes are produced as precursors, an inactive form that must be activated by another enzyme before it can work.

Absorption is the process by which the small soluble units resulting from digestion are taken into the circulation. The site of absorption is the small intestine and its efficiency is increased by the tube length and by the lining of villi (Figure 4.60), which provide a large surface area with a good supply of blood capillaries and lacteals.

Pancreas and gall bladder

The **pancreas** is a pale pink lobulated gland lying in the loop of the duodenum. It is described as a mixed gland, as it has an endocrine part (see 'Endocrine system', above) and an exocrine part. The exocrine secretions, consisting of several digestive enzymes and bicarbonate, enter the duodenum via the **pancreatic duct**.

The **gall bladder** lies between the lobes of the liver and stores bile formed by the liver. Bile is coloured yellow-green by the pigment bilirubin and contains bile salts needed for the emulsification of fats. It enters the duodenum via the common bile duct.

Large intestine

This is a relatively short tube with a large diameter. The lining is not folded into villi and there are no digestive glands, although there are more goblet cells, which secrete mucus to lubricate the passage of faeces. It consists of the following parts.

Caecum and colon

The **caecum** is a short blind-ended sac, which joins the ileum at the **ileocaecal junction.** It has very little function in the carnivore.

The **colon** is divided into the ascending, transverse and descending colon according to its position in the peritoneal cavity. It is suspended by the short **mesocolon**. Water and electrolytes are absorbed from the remaining indigestible food within the colon.

Rectum and anus

The **rectum** is the part of the colon running through the pelvic cavity. It is held in place by the surrounding connective tissue and muscle.

The **anus** is the external opening of the digestive tract. It forms a muscular sphincter that controls the passage of faeces out of the body. It has two parts:

* Internal anal sphincter – ring of smooth muscle under involuntary control
* External anal sphincter – outer ring of striated muscle under voluntary control.

Digestive juice	Contents	Action	Comments
Stomach secretes gastric juices: The hormone gastrin is produced as food enters the stomach and stimulates the gastric pits to secrete gastric juices			
Goblet cells	Mucus	No enzyme action. Lubricates food. Protects gastric mucosa from autodigestion	
Parietal cells	Hydrochloric acid (HCl)	Denatures protein. Creates a pH of 1.3–5. Converts pepsinogen to active pepsin	Protein digestion is made easier. Acid pH kills most pathogenic bacteria
Chief cells	Pepsinogen	When activated by HCl, pepsin converts protein to peptides	Peptides are smaller molecules
Small intestine:			
Bile from the liver	Bile salts	Emulsifies fats to produce small globules. Activates lipases	As chyme enters the duodenum, the gall bladder contracts forcing bile along the bile duct
Pancreatic juices from exocrine part of the pancreas			Produced in response to gastrin and to the hormone cholecystokinin secreted by duodenal cells as chyme passes through the pyloric sphincter
	Bicarbonate	No enzyme action. Neutralizes the acid pH	Neutral pH stops action of pepsin and enables intestinal digestive enzymes to act
	Trypsinogen	Inactive	Converted to active trypsin by enterokinase present in succus entericus. Spontaneous conversion is prevented by a trypsin inhibitor
	Trypsin	Activates other enzyme precursors. Converts peptides and other proteins to amino acids	Amino acids are absorbed into the bloodstream
	Lipase	Converts fats to fatty acids and glycerol	Activated by bile salts
	Amylase	Converts starches to maltose	Starches are plant carbohydrates
Intestinal juices from Brunner's glands as succus entericus and from the crypts of Lieberkuhn			Produced in response to the hormone secretin, secreted as the chyme passes through the pyloric sphincter
	Maltase	Converts maltose to glucose	Glucose is absorbed by the blood capillaries
	Sucrase	Converts sucrose to glucose and fructose	Glucose and fructose are absorbed by blood capillaries
	Lactase	Converts lactose to glucose and galactose	Glucose and galactose are absorbed by blood capillaries
	Enterokinase	Converts trypsinogen to trypsin	Trypsin is activated
	Aminopeptidase	Converts peptides to amino acids	Amino acids are absorbed into the bloodstream
	Lipase	Converts fats to fatty acids and glycerol	Fatty acids and glycerol are absorbed into the lacteals

4.61 Processes involved in digestion.

The lumen of the anus and the rectum is folded longitudinally, enabling the lining to stretch during the passage of bulky faeces. Between the two anal rings in the '20 to 4' position is a pair of **anal sacs**. These are modified cutaneous glands whose size is approximately that of a pea. They secrete a pungent paste-like material, which coats the faeces as it passes through the sphincter. The characteristic smell is used as a means of territorial marking by the dog and the cat.

Defecation
The faecal mass passes along the colon and rectum by means of peristalsis and by slower, stronger but infrequent contractions known as mass movements. As the faeces enter the pelvic cavity the wall of the rectum is stretched, which stimulates voluntary straining. The anal sphincter, normally held tightly closed, relaxes, the abdominal muscles contract, the animal adopts the correct position and the mass is forced out.

Normal faeces have a smell, colour and shape that is characteristic of the species. Faeces consist of:

- Water and fibre (the relative proportions affect the consistency and shape)
- Dead and living bacteria (these are normal commensals and may contribute to the smell and help to break down any remaining protein)
- Mucus (adds bulk and aids lubrication)
- Stercobilin (derived from bile; gives faeces their colour)
- Sloughed intestinal cells
- Secretion from the anal sacs.

The liver
The liver lies in the cranial abdominal cavity and is the largest gland in the body (see Figure 4.53). The cranial aspect is convex, conforming to the abdominal side of the diaphragm. The caudal aspect is concave and in contact with the stomach, duodenum and right kidney. A normal liver is deep red in colour.

The remnants of the fetal blood vessels from the umbilicus – the **falciform ligament** – is found in the centre of the caudal aspect of the liver and is of no significance in the adult.

Microscopically, the liver consists of millions of cells known as **hepatocytes** arranged in hexagonal **lobules**. Running between the hepatocytes is an interconnecting network of tiny **bile canaliculi** into which bile is secreted. The bile eventually drains into the gall bladder, which lies between the central lobes of the liver on the caudal aspect.

Arterial blood reaches liver tissue via the **hepatic artery**. The products of digestion reach the liver from the small intestine via the **hepatic portal vein** (see Figure 4.47). Blood from these two vessels bathes the hepatocytes, permeating through the liver lobules in minute **sinusoids** and draining into a **central vein** in the middle of each lobule. The central veins flow into the **hepatic vein** and so to the caudal vena cava. There is no contact between the bile canaliculi and the sinusoids.

The liver has many functions and is essential to normal health.

Carbohydrate metabolism

Excess glucose is stored as glycogen in a process known as **glycogenesis** in the presence of **insulin** from the pancreas. When the body requires extra energy, glycogen is broken down to release energy in a process known as **glycogenolysis** in the presence of **glucagon** from the pancreas.

Protein metabolism

This includes:

- Formation of plasma proteins – albumin, prothrombin, fibrinogen
- Conversion of amino acids from the digestion of protein in food into the amino acid of body protein for maintenance and growth – a process known as **transamination**
- Production of urea – surplus amino acids are converted to ammonia and urea in a process known as **deamination**. Urea is excreted in the urine.

Fat metabolism

Fat is the main energy source for the body. Excess fat is deposited around the body. Fatty acids and glycerol resulting from fat digestion are converted into phospholipids for cell membranes and cholesterol for bile salts.

Other functions of the liver

- Formation of bile – stored in the gall bladder and used in digestion
- Destruction of old red blood cells – haemoglobin is excreted as bilirubin in the bile
- Formation of new red blood cells (only in the fetus)
- Storage of vitamins – mainly the fat-soluble vitamins A, D, E and K, but may store some water-soluble ones
- Storage of iron
- Thermoregulation
- Detoxification of certain substances (e.g. alcohol)
- Detoxification and conjugation of steroid hormones.

The urinary system

The urinary system comprises the kidney, ureter, bladder and urethra. It is anatomically linked with the reproductive system, as the urethra (which conducts urine out of the body) runs through the penis of the male and drains into the vagina of the female. Thus the system may be referred to as the urogenital system.

The functions of the urinary system are:

- To excrete nitrogenous waste products from the body in the form of urea
- To regulate the chemical makeup and volume of the body fluids (this process of osmoregulation plays an important role in homeostasis)
- To secrete the hormone erythropoietin or erythropoietic-stimulating factor (see 'Endocrine system', above).

Kidney

Structure

Position

In the normal mammal there is a pair of kidneys (Figure 4.62). One lies on each side of the major blood vessels, the dorsal aorta and caudal vena cava in the cranial dorsal abdomen. They are closely attached to the lumbar hypaxial muscles by the parietal peritoneum and are described as being **retroperitoneal**. The right kidney lies cranial to the left, as the stomach occupies the left side of the cranial abdomen. The kidneys lie cranial to the right and left ovaries and caudal to the right and left adrenal glands.

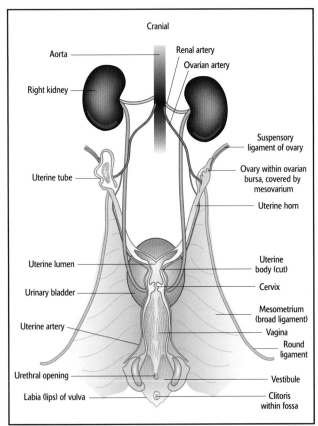

4.62 Ventrodorsal view of the urogenital system of the bitch, showing arterial blood supply.

Shape and size

The kidneys are shaped like a kidney-bean, with a smooth outline, and are normally brownish-red in colour. When examined on a lateral radiograph, the normal kidney measures approximately 2.5 lumbar vertebrae. In acute renal failure the kidneys become swollen, enlarged and very painful; in chronic renal failure they become shrunken and 'knobbly'.

Blood supply

A single **renal artery** from the dorsal aorta carries arterial blood to each kidney, entering via the **hilus**. Blood carried by the renal arteries may be as much as 20% of cardiac output. Within the kidney the renal artery divides into several **interlobar arteries**, which give off capillary networks to supply the tubules and to form the **glomeruli** (sing. glomerulus). The capillaries then recombine to form **interlobar veins**, which enter the single **renal vein**. Venous blood then drains into the caudal vena cava.

Macroscopic appearance

If the kidney is cut longitudinally (Figure 4.63) it is possible to identify the following layers:

- **Fibrous tissue capsule** – tough outer coat closely attached to the cortex (but in a healthy kidney it may be peeled away quite easily). It protects the kidney from mechanical damage and may be surrounded by deposits of fat in obese animals.
- **Cortex** – outer layer of the kidney tissue containing the renal corpuscles and convoluted tubules of the nephrons. Its good blood supply gives it a dark red colour.
- **Medulla** – paler than the cortex. May be possible to see triangular areas called **pyramids**, which contain the collecting ducts of the nephrons. The remainder contains the loops of Henle.
- **Pelvis** – basin-shaped structure made of dense connective tissue. It collects urine formed by the nephrons and is drained by a single **ureter**, which leaves by the **hilus**.

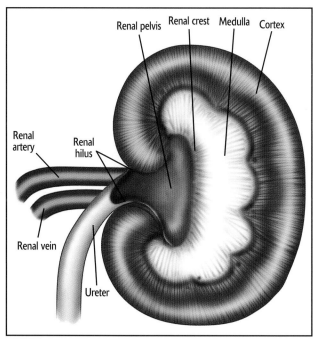

4.63 Longitudinal section through a kidney.

Microscopic appearance

The functional unit of the kidney is the **nephron** (Figure 4.64). Each kidney contains around a million nephrons. Each nephron consists of several parts:

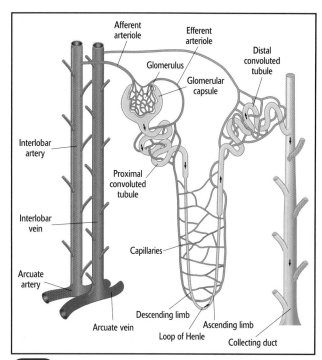

4.64 A kidney nephron. Arrows show direction of urine.

- **Glomerular capsule** – also called Bowman's capsule. A cup-shaped structure enclosing a network of blood capillaries known as the **glomerulus**. A capsule and a glomerulus together form a **renal corpuscle**. The glomerular capsule is hollow and its inner surface forms a **basement membrane** perforated by microscopic pores. This membrane is in close contact with the endothelium of the glomerulus and allows the free flow of fluid from the blood into the lumen of the capsule, but restricts the passage of large molecules (e.g. protein).
- **Proximal convoluted tubule** – long twisted tubule lying within the cortex. Lined with cuboidal epithelium with a brush-border of microvilli, which increases the surface area for reabsorption of water and electrolytes.
- **Loop of Henle** – U-shaped tube extending into the medulla. It has a descending part lined by a thin squamous epithelium and an ascending part lined by a thicker squamous epithelium.
- **Distal convoluted tubule** – lies within the cortex and is lined by cuboidal epithelium without a brush-border.
- **Collecting duct** – each duct collects urine from several nephrons, runs through a pyramid area and empties into the pelvis of the kidney.

Urine formation

The kidneys filter the blood and the filtrate undergoes a series of modifications within the renal tubules to form urine. The urine is very different in composition and volume from the original filtrate; for every 100 litres of fluid removed from the blood, only 1 litre is excreted as urine. The changes to the filtrate reflect the status of the extracellular fluid (ECF) and in particular that of the blood plasma. They are made by different parts of the nephron and make use of different physiological processes (Figure 4.65).

Blood enters the kidneys via the renal artery and reaches the capillaries of the glomerulus.

Process	Description
Osmosis	Passage of water through a semipermeable membrane from a weaker to a stronger solution
Diffusion	Passage of a solute from an area of high concentration to an area of low concentration
Reabsorption	Passage of a substance from the lumen of the renal tubules into the surrounding capillaries and back into the circulation. This is an active process and requires expenditure of energy
Secretion	Passage of a substance from the surrounding capillaries into the lumen of the renal tubules and out of the body in the urine. This is an active process and requires expenditure of energy

4.65   Physiological processes occurring in the renal tubules.

Glomerular capsule

Here the blood is under high pressure because:

- Blood comes straight from the heart via the aorta and the renal artery
- The arteriole leaving the glomerulus is able to constrict under the control of the hormone **renin** (see Figure 4.66), which regulates the pressure in the glomerulus.

This high pressure forces fluid and small molecules out of the glomerulus, through the pores of the basement membrane into the lumen of the capsule. Larger molecules (e.g. red blood cells and protein) are retained in the blood. This process is known as **ultrafiltration** and results in a dilute glomerular filtrate or primitive urine.

Proximal convoluted tubule

This is where 65% of all the resorptive processes take place. These are as follows.

- Sodium ions (Na^+) are reabsorbed.
- By osmosis, 65% of the water is reabsorbed.
- All glucose in the filtrate is reabsorbed. Normal urine does not contain glucose. In cases of diabetes mellitus, urine contains glucose because blood glucose levels are so high that they exceed the renal threshold for glucose and the surplus passes out in the urine. Kidney function in such cases is normal.
- Nitrogenous waste (e.g. urea and creatinine) is concentrated by the reabsorption of water. This is mainly urea from protein metabolism in the liver. Some urea also diffuses back into the blood from the tubules.
- Toxins and certain drugs (e.g. penicillin) are secreted.

Loop of Henle

The **concentration** and **volume** of the urine are regulated here according to the status of the ECF. The filtrate flows into the descending loop and then into the ascending loop, both of which lie in the renal medulla.

- **Descending loop** – the lining cells are *permeable* to water but do not have the mechanism to reabsorb Na^+ ions. Water is drawn out of the filtrate by osmosis, pulled by the high concentration of Na^+ ions in the surrounding medulla. The concentration of the filtrate increases as it travels towards the tip of the loop.
- **Ascending loop** – the lining cells are *impermeable* to water but are able to reabsorb Na^+ ions into the tissue of the medulla and the capillaries. As water cannot leave the filtrate, it becomes less concentrated as it passes upwards.

The result of this mechanism is that the filtrate is the same concentration when it enters the loop as it is when it leaves, but the volume is reduced: water has been conserved in the body. If an animal is dehydrated, more water is reabsorbed; if it is overhydrated, more water is excreted in the urine.

Distal convoluted tubule

The final adjustments are made to the **electrolyte content** of the urine according to the status of the ECF.

- Na^+ is reabsorbed and is replaced in the urine by potassium (K^+) ions.
- Reabsorption of water varies and is controlled by the hormone **aldosterone** (see Figure 4.68).
- **Acid–base balance** is regulated by excretion of hydrogen (H^+) ions. The normal pH of blood is 7.4. If there are excess H^+ ions in the blood, the pH falls (more acidic) and the excess are excreted in the urine, so that the pH returns to normal.

Collecting duct

Final adjustments are made to the **volume of water** in the urine. **Antidiuretic hormone (ADH)** is able to alter the permeability of the walls of the collecting ducts to water to control the volume. If the animal is dehydrated, the walls become more permeable so that water is reabsorbed from the urine into the blood capillaries; and vice versa.

The urine produced by repeated reabsorption and secretion leaves the kidney via the ureter.

Control of kidney function: osmoregulation

Osmoregulation ensures that the volume of the ECF (principally plasma volume) and the concentration of dissolved chemicals in the fluid remain constant so that homeostasis is maintained and the body functions normally. Osmoregulation is controlled by various factors (Figure 4.66) and occurs in two ways: by control of water loss; and by control of salt (Na^+) levels.

Controlling factor	Function
Renin – hormone	Produced by the glomeruli of the kidney in response to low arterial pressure
Angiotensinogen – plasma protein	Converted to angiotensin by the action of renin
Angiotensin – protein	Causes vasoconstriction. Stimulates the release of aldosterone from the adrenal cortex
Aldosterone – hormone – mineralocorticoid	Secreted by the cortex of the adrenal gland. Acts mainly on the distal convoluted tubules but has a lesser effect on the collecting ducts. Regulates the reabsorption of Na^+ ions
Antidiuretic hormone, ADH (vasopressin)	Secreted by the posterior pituitary gland. Mainly affects the collecting ducts by changing their permeability to water. Also has an effect on the distal convoluted tubules
Baroreceptors	Found in the walls of the blood vessels. Monitor arterial blood pressure
Osmoreceptors	Found in the hypothalamus. Monitor the osmotic pressure of the plasma. Affect the thirst centre of the brain and influence the secretion of ADH

4.66   Factors involved in osmoregulation.

Control of water loss

Water is taken into the body in food and drink and is excreted in urine, faeces, sweat and respiration. Small amounts may be lost in vaginal secretions and in tears. If intake is reduced or output is excessive (e.g. vomiting and diarrhoea), the total volume of the ECF falls and the animal becomes dehydrated. This will present as:

- Lowered blood pressure – plasma volume falls and exerts less pressure on the blood vessel walls
- Raised Na^+ ion concentration – a fall in volume concentrates the Na^+ ions, increasing the osmotic pressure of the plasma.

Osmoregulatory mechanisms now begin to work and result in a rise in blood pressure and a fall in urine output. The hormone ADH controls water reabsorption from the collecting ducts (Figure 4.67).

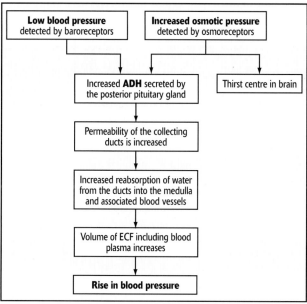

4.67 Mechanism involved in the control of water loss from the kidney.

Raised blood pressure will have the opposite effect and the animal will excrete increased quantities of urine.

- **Blood pressure** is the pressure exerted on the walls of the blood vessels by blood. It depends on the blood volume and is detected by **baroreceptors**.
- **Osmotic pressure** is the pressure needed to prevent osmosis from occurring. It depends on the number of undissolved molecules and ions in the solution and is detected by **osmoreceptors**.

Control of salt levels

Sodium (NaCl) is taken into the body in food and is normally lost in urine, faeces and sweat. It is found in the ionized form Na^+ in all the body fluid compartments and plays an important part in determining blood pressure. High levels of Na^+ in the diet increase osmotic pressure, which draws fluid into the plasma by osmosis, increasing blood volume and thus blood pressure; conversely low Na^+ draws less fluid in and blood volume and pressure fall (Figure 4.68).

Regulation of Na^+ in the plasma occurs mainly in the distal convoluted tubule and is under the control of the hormone **aldosterone** secreted by the adrenal gland.

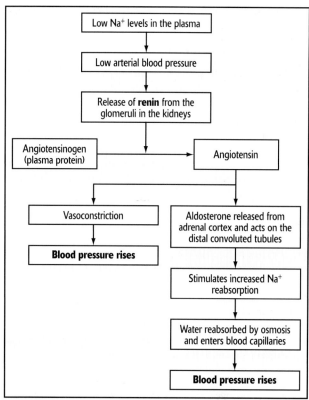

4.68 Mechanism involved in the control of sodium by the kidney.

Excretion

This is the removal of waste products that are produced by the tissues during metabolism. They may be surplus to requirement or may be harmful to the cells and they include nitrogenous waste (e.g. urea and creatinine), water and inorganic ions (e.g. Na^+).

Nitrogenous waste

This results from protein metabolism. Protein taken into the body in food is broken down by digestion into amino acids, which are transported to the liver by the blood. Here they are converted into body protein and used for growth and repair. Surplus amino acids are broken down, or deaminated, and ammonia is formed as a by-product. This is extremely toxic to the nervous system and it must be excreted. It combines with carbon dioxide in a series of biochemical reactions to form urea, which is carried by the blood to the kidneys, from where it is excreted in the urine.

Water

Water forms the bulk of the urine and the volume depends on the status of the ECF and the plasma. It is controlled by osmoregulation (see above).

Inorganic ions

The concentration and type of ions depend on the osmotic pressure of the body fluids and the blood and is controlled by osmoregulation.

The ureter

Urine formed by each kidney is conveyed to the bladder along a single ureter by means of peristaltic waves brought about by contraction of smooth muscle. Each ureter is a narrow muscular tube lined by transitional epithelium, running caudally towards the bladder one on each side of the dorsal abdomen (see Figure 4.62). Each ureter is suspended in a fold of visceral peritoneum – the **mesoureter**.

The bladder

This pear-shaped hollow organ (see Figure 4.69) lies in the midline and is used for the storage of urine. The rounded end points cranially. The size varies according to the volume it contains: when full, the ventral surface may touch the abdominal floor; when empty, the bladder lies entirely within the pelvic cavity.

Each ureter enters the bladder in an area known as the **trigone**, at an oblique angle that helps to prevent backflow of urine up the ureter.

The bladder is lined with transitional epithelium, and the walls contain elastic tissue and layers of smooth muscle. This structure allows expansion as the bladder fills with urine. Flow of urine out of the bladder is controlled by a **sphincter** at the **neck** of the bladder This has an inner layer of smooth muscle under involuntary control and an outer layer of striated muscle under voluntary control.

Formation of bladder stones or calculi is a relatively common condition of dogs and cats and is known as **urolithiasis**. The calculi, whose composition may vary from struvite (triple phosphate), which is the most common, to calcium oxalate, cystine or ammonium urate, may damage the bladder wall, leading to cystitis, or pass down the urethra, leading to an obstruction and consequent inability to pass urine. Blockage is most common in the male animal, as the urethra is longer and narrower. The most common sites for obstruction in the dog are close to the position of the os penis and at the point where the urethra passes over the ischial arch. In the cat, the site of blockage is usually at the tip of the penis close to the os penis.

The urethra

This carries urine caudally from the neck of the bladder to the outside of the body.

In the **female** the urethra is a short tube entering the floor of the reproductive tract at the junction of the vestibule and vagina known as the **external urethral orifice**. A small swelling called the **urethral tubercle** marks the opening.

In the **male** the urethra can be divided into a pelvic and a penile part. There is a difference between the dog and the tomcat:

- In the **dog** – as the urethra leaves the bladder the **prostate gland** and **the deferent ducts** from the testes open into it. The urethra runs caudally through the pelvis and curves over the edge of the ischial arch, where it is surrounded by cavernous erectile tissue to form the **penis**. It continues as the penile urethra and opens to the outside at the tip of the penis.
- In the **tomcat** – there is a short length of urethra cranial to the opening of the prostate gland; this is the **preprostatic urethra**. The urethra runs caudally and opens to the outside ventral to the anus in the perineum. Close to the end of the urethra are the openings from the paired **bulbo-urethral glands**.

From the point at which the deferent ducts join the urethra it conveys both urine and sperm to the outside of the body.

Micturition

Micturition is the act of passing urine. This is normally a reflex activity but can be overridden by voluntary control from the brain. The normal steps are as follows.

1. The bladder is distended by urine formed by the kidneys.
2. Stretch receptors within the smooth muscle of the bladder wall are stimulated and nerve impulses are sent to the spinal cord.
3. Nerve impulses are transmitted back to the smooth muscle by parasympathetic nerves and contraction is initiated.
4. Other nerve impulses trigger relaxation of the internal bladder sphincter and urine is expelled.

If it is inappropriate for the animal to micturate, the brain overrides this reflex pathway and prevents the bladder sphincter from relaxing. At a more appropriate time the brain stimulates the internal and external sphincters and urine is released. Voluntary control develops as the young animal matures and is not fully developed in puppies and kittens until about 10 weeks of age.

Urine is derived from the ultrafiltrate of plasma and reflects the health status of the animal. Normal urine contains only water salts and urea. The clinical parameters used to evaluate a sample of urine (**urinalysis**) are described in Chapter 17.

The reproductive system

The reproductive system shares part of its structure with the urinary system and together they may be referred to as the urogenital system.

Male reproductive system

The reproductive systems of the dog (Figure 4.69) and the tomcat (Figure 4.70) are similar; any differences will be described as appropriate. The parts of the tract are testes, epididymis, deferent duct, urethra, penis, prostate (accessory gland) and bulbo-urethral glands (accessory gland seen only in the tomcat).

Testis

This is the male gonad. Its functions are:

- To produce spermatozoa (sperm) by spermatogenesis
- To secrete the hormone testosterone
- To produce fluids that transport sperm from the testes and aid their survival.

There is a pair of oval testes, which in the adult animal lie in a small almost hairless sac known as the **scrotum**. The scrotum hangs ventral to the pelvis outside the body cavity, where the lower temperature promotes more efficient spermatogenesis. The position of the testis can be altered in response to changes in temperature by smooth muscle within the connective tissue of the scrotum known as the **Dartos muscle** and by smooth muscle in the spermatic cord called the **cremaster muscle**.

The testicular tissue consists of numerous coiled **seminiferous tubules**. These lead into wider **efferent tubules** draining into the **epididymis**, which runs along the dorsolateral border of the testis. The tail or **cauda epididymis** is attached to the caudal extremity and is the site for the storage and final maturation of sperm ready for fertilization.

The epididymis continues as the **deferent duct** (or the vas deferens or ductus deferens), which conveys sperm out of the scrotum into the **urethra** within the pelvic cavity. A spermatic artery and vein and the spermatic nerve accompany the deferent duct; together they form the **spermatic cord**.

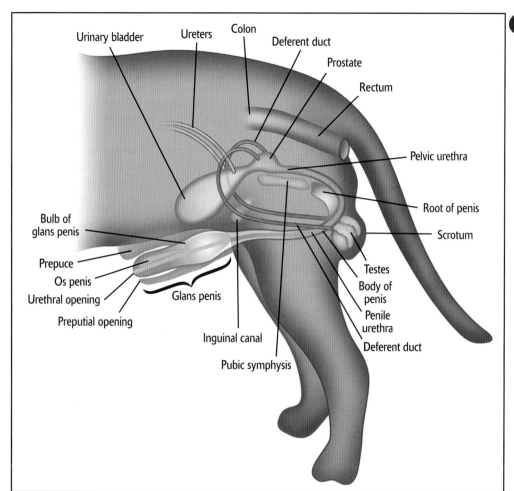

4.69 Reproductive tract of the dog.

Urinary bladder
Ureters
Colon
Deferent duct
Prostate
Rectum
Pelvic urethra
Root of penis
Scrotum
Testes
Body of penis
Penile urethra
Deferent duct
Bulb of glans penis
Prepuce
Os penis
Urethral opening
Preputial opening
Glans penis
Inguinal canal
Pubic symphysis

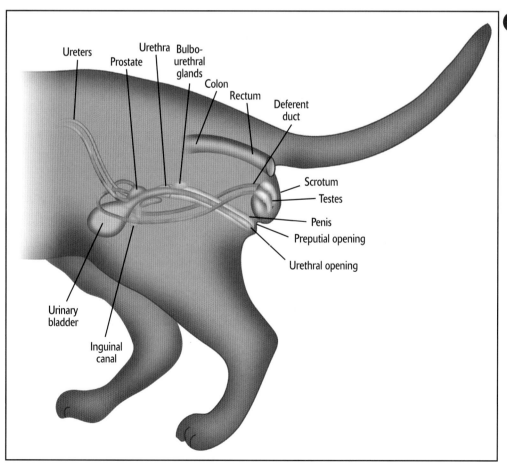

4.70 Reproductive tract of the tomcat.

Ureters
Prostate
Urethra
Bulbo-urethral glands
Colon
Rectum
Deferent duct
Scrotum
Testes
Penis
Preputial opening
Urethral opening
Urinary bladder
Inguinal canal

Microscopically, the seminiferous tubules are lined by two cell types:

- **Spermatogonia** – responsible for producing immature sperm or spermatids by meiosis
- **Sertoli cells** – secrete the hormone **oestrogen** and nutrients to aid the survival of the spermatids as they travel along the seminiferous tubules.

Lying between the tubules are **interstitial cells** or **cells of Leydig**. These are stimulated by **interstitial cell-stimulating hormone** (ICSH) produced by the anterior pituitary gland and secrete the hormone testosterone. **Testosterone** affects:

- Spermatogenesis (the formation of spermatozoa)
- Development of the male reproductive tract, including descent of the testes
- Development of male secondary sexual characteristics (e.g. muscle development, size, male behaviour).

Testicular development

In the embryo, the testes develop within the abdominal cavity close to the kidney. During late fetal and early neonatal life, a band of tissue known as the **gubernaculum**, which is attached at one end to the tail of the testis and at the other to the inside of the scrotal sac, contracts and pulls the testis caudally through the abdomen. It passes out of the abdominal cavity into the scrotum via the **inguinal ring** (a split in the abdominal oblique muscle in the groin of the animal). As it does so, the testis and its associated nerves and blood vessels and deferent duct become wrapped in a fold of peritoneum called the **tunica vaginalis**. During castration the tunica vaginalis is incised to expose the testis and the spermatic cord. The contents of the spermatic cord are then ligated.

The testes should be palpable within the scrotum of the dog and tomcat at about 12 weeks of age. Failure of the testes to descend into the scrotum is known as **cryptorchidism** (see Chapter 25). If one testis is retained in the abdominal cavity this is called **monorchidism**; if both are retained this is called **bilateral cryptorchidism**. The condition may be an inherited characteristic and affected animals should not be used for breeding.

Accessory glands

There are two types of gland:

- **Prostate gland** – bilobed structure surrounding the urethra. In the dog it lies close to the neck of the bladder. In the tomcat there is a short preprostatic urethra cranial to the gland. Secretions of prostatic fluid enter the urethra by short ducts.
- **Bulbo-urethral glands** – found only in the tomcat. The glands lie on either side of the urethra close to the tip of the penis.

The accessory glands produce **seminal fluid**, which:

- Increases the volume of the ejaculate to flush sperm through the penis into the female tract during mating
- Aids sperm survival
- Neutralizes the acidity of the urine within the urethra.

Penis

During ejaculation, spermatozoa produced within the seminiferous tubules are conducted along the **epididymis** and up the **deferent duct** to enter the **urethra** at a point close to the neck of the bladder and to the prostate gland. The urethra runs through the centre of the **penis** and is shared by both the urinary system and reproductive systems (see 'Urinary system', above). The functions of the penis are:

- To conduct sperm and seminal fluid into the female reproductive tract during mating
- To conduct urine from the bladder out of the body
- To direct urine for territorial marking.

The penis of the dog and the tomcat are anatomically different.

Canine penis

In the dog, the penis runs from the ischial arch of the pelvis, passing cranioventrally along the perineum and between the hindlegs. The urethra runs along the centre of the penis and is surrounded by cavernous erectile tissue known as the **corpus cavernosum penis**. During sexual excitement the erectile tissue becomes engorged with blood under pressure. At the proximal end this expands into the **bulb** of the penis and towards the distal end as the **glans penis**. Connective tissue in the form of a pair of **crura** (sing. crus) attaches the penis to the ischial arch, forming the **root** of the penis.

Within the glans penis is a small tunnel-shaped bone, the **os penis**, which aids entry of the penis into the female vagina during mating. The urethra runs *ventral* to the os penis through the 'tunnel', which may restrict its ability to dilate and may be a site for blockage with urethral calculi.

The distal part of the penis is enclosed within and suspended from the ventral body wall by a fur-covered **prepuce**. This is lined with mucous membrane and well supplied with lubricating glands. During mating the prepuce is pushed back to reveal the glans penis.

Feline penis

In the tomcat, the penis is shorter than that of the dog and points caudally; the external opening lies ventral to the anus under the tail. The tip of the **glans penis** is covered in tiny barbs, which elicit a pain response from the female during mating. This stimulates a nerve pathway inducing ovulation within 36 hours of mating (see Chapter 25). The urethra lies *dorsal* to the **os penis** at a point close to the bulbo-urethral glands.

During sexual excitement, the penis engorges and points cranioventrally, allowing the tomcat to mate in a similar position to the dog.

Female reproductive system

The reproductive systems of the bitch (see Figure 4.62) and the queen are similar, varying only in size. The tract is adapted to bear several fetuses in a single pregnancy and is described as **bicornuate**. Species that bear litters of young are said to be **multiparous**. Full details of the oestrous cycle and embryological and fetal development are given in Chapter 25. The processes of the cell cycle and cell division (mitosis and meiosis) are discussed earlier in this chapter and in Chapter 5. The parts of the female reproductive tract are ovaries, uterine tube, uterus (uterine horn and uterine body), cervix, vagina, vestibule and vulva.

Ovary

The ovary is the female gonad. Its functions are:

- To produce ova (eggs) ready for fertilization by the male sperm
- To secrete the hormones oestrogen and progesterone.

There is a pair of ovaries, each one lying on either side of the midline, close to the dorsal abdominal wall. Each ovary lies caudal to the kidney on that side and is held in place by the suspensory **ovarian ligament**, which contains smooth muscle.

The ovary is suspended from the abdominal wall by a fold of the visceral peritoneum, the **mesovarium**, which also carries part of the uterine tube. Part of the mesovarium is folded to form a pouch-like **ovarian bursa**. This completely encloses the ovary and within it is a small opening into the peritoneal cavity.

The ovary consists of a framework of connective tissue, blood capillaries and smooth muscle within which are a large number of germ cells and developing follicles. The process of ovulation is discussed in Chapter 25.

Uterine tube

This is also called the oviduct or the Fallopian tube. Its functions are:

- To collect ova as they are released from the Graafian follicles
- To convey the ova from the ovaries to the uterine horns
- To provide the correct environment for the survival of ova and sperm.

The uterine tube is a narrow convoluted structure lying close to the ovary and suspended in a fold of peritoneum known as the **mesosalpinx**. The proximal end, called the **infundibulum**, is funnel-shaped and the opening is fringed by finger-like processes known as **fimbriae**. The infundibulum is able to move over the surface of the ovary to trap the ova as they ovulate. A lining of ciliated columnar epithelium helps the passage of the ova down the tube.

Uterus

This is a Y-shaped structure lying in the midline of the dorsal abdomen. In the pregnant animal, the weight of the conceptuses pulls the uterus ventrally and at full term it occupies most of the abdominal cavity. Its functions are:

- To contain the fertilized ova until they develop into full term fetuses
- To provide the correct environment for the survival of the developing embryos
- To provide the means by which the developing fetuses are supplied with nutrients (the **placenta**).

The uterus comprises two parts:

- A pair of **uterine horns** – each one leads from a uterine tube and is up to five times longer than the uterine body. During pregnancy the horns contain the developing embryos.
- A short central **body**.

In cross-section, the uterine wall consists of:

- **Endometrium** – inner layer of columnar mucous membrane, blood vessels and glandular tissue (this layer thickens during pregnancy to provide nutrition for the embryo before implantation and to support the placenta)
- **Myometrium** – smooth muscle fibres that contract strongly during parturition
- **Mesometrium** or broad ligament – fold of visceral peritoneum that suspends the uterus and is continuous with the mesosalpinx and the mesovarium.

Blood supply to the tract

The blood vessels that run in the mesometrium, mesosalpinx and mesovarium are:

- **Ovarian artery** – arises from the aorta caudal to the renal artery; supplies the ovary
- **Uterine artery** – anastomoses with the ovarian artery and supplies the caudal part of the tract.

Cervix

This short thick-walled muscular sphincter connects the uterus with the vagina. In the centre of the cervix is a narrow **cervical canal**, which relaxes only to allow the passage of fetuses out during parturition.

Vagina and vestibule

Together these form a highly dilatable channel leading from the cervix to the outside at the vulva. The vagina extends from the cervix to the **external urethral orifice** (the point at which the urethra joins the reproductive tract) while the vestibule runs from the external urethral orifice to the outside at the **vulva** and is shared by both the urinary and reproductive systems. The functions are:

- To convey sperm from the penis of the male into the female tract (sperm is usually deposited at the entrance to the cervix)
- To convey the fetuses from the uterus to the outside
- To convey urine from the bladder to the outside of the body (the vestibule performs this function).

The lumen is lined with stratified squamous epithelium, which shows hormonally induced changes during the oestrous cycle. Study of the epithelial debris is known as **exfoliative vaginal cytology** and can be used to assess the stages of the cycle and to gauge the correct time for mating. The walls are arranged in longitudinal folds, enabling the vagina and vestibule to expand widthways during parturition.

Vulva

This is the external opening of the female tract. It consists of two parts:

- **Labiae** – two vertical lips joined ventrally and dorsally and made of fibrous and elastic connective tissue, smooth muscle and fat. The **vulval cleft** lies between them. The vulva may be enlarged during pro-oestrus and oestrus in the bitch.
- **Clitoris** – small knob of cavernous erectile tissue lying in the **clitoral fossa** just inside the ventral part of the vulval cleft.

Mammary glands

Although these are not strictly part of the reproductive tract, the mammary glands are the defining feature of the Class Mammalia. All mammals feed their young on milk from the mammary glands produced by a process known as **lactation** (see Chapter 25).

Mammary glands are modified cutaneous glands, which lie on either side of the midline on the external ventral wall of the abdomen and the thorax. The bitch has five pairs and the queen has four pairs. The glands are present in both sexes.

Each gland (Figure 4.71) consists of glandular tissue lined with secretory epithelium. The secreted milk drains through a network of sinuses into **teat canals**, which open on to the surface of the teat as **teat orifices**. Each gland has one teat, but each teat has several orifices.

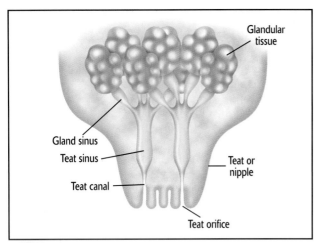

4.71 Section through a mammary gland.

The integument

The integument is said to be the largest organ of the body and includes the skin, hair, footpads and claws.

The skin

The skin completely covers the external surface of the body and blends with the mucous membranes at the various natural openings.

Functions of the skin

Protection
The skin protects the underlying structures of the body from:

- Physical damage
- Invasion by microorganisms (by creating an intact barrier and by the secretion of sebum from the sebaceous glands, which has antibacterial properties)
- Drying out or becoming waterlogged (by creating a waterproof barrier)
- Damage by ultraviolet radiation (by the presence of pigments in the skin and hair).

Sense organ
The skin contains numerous nerve endings to detect temperature, pain and touch. These provide sensory information to assist the body in monitoring its external environment.

Secretory organ
Secretions are produced by various skin or cutaneous glands. These include:

- **Sebaceous glands** – associated with the hair follicles; they secrete sebum, which waterproofs the coat, has an antibacterial action and contains the precursor to vitamin D that is activated by the action of ultraviolet light
- **Sweat glands** (also called sudoriferous glands) – only found on the nose and the footpads of the dog and cat; secrete sweat, which cools the body by evaporation
- **Ceruminous glands** – modified sebaceous glands that secrete protective wax (cerumen) on to the skin lining the ear canal
- **Mammary glands** – modified sweat glands that secrete milk
- **Glands of the anal sacs** – produce a secretion with a characteristic smell used for territorial marking.

Storage
Fat is stored under the skin as adipose tissue and acts as an energy store and as a thermal insulating layer.

Thermoregulation
Heat loss is prevented by:

- Constriction of surface blood capillaries, which diverts blood away from the skin's surface
- Erecting the hairs and trapping a layer of insulating air between the body and the outer surface
- Layer of adipose tissue insulates the body.

Communication
Specialized glands produce **pheromones**, which are natural scents used for intraspecific communication. Other scents used for communication include those secreted by the **circum-anal glands** and glands of the **anal sacs**. The integument also provides **visual communication** (e.g. a dog raises its hackles when threatened).

Structure of skin
The skin is composed of three layers: epidermis, dermis and hypodermis (Figure 4.72).

Epidermis
The epidermis is composed of **stratified squamous epithelium** arranged in multiple layers (or strata) of cells. Cells are constantly being produced to replace the cells that are lost or damaged by injury and wear. The epidermis is avascular and receives nutrients from the underlying dermis. The layers of the epidermis are, from deep to superficial:

- **Stratum basale (germinativum)** – a single layer of cells that divide by **mitosis**. As the new cells are produced they push those above into the next layer of the epidermis. **Melanocytes** containing granules of the pigment melanin are also present. This pigment gives skin and hair its characteristic colour.
- **Stratum granulosum** – the cells are flattened and the process of **keratinization** (infiltration of the cells by the structural protein **keratin**) begins.
- **Stratum lucidum** – the cells lose their nuclei.
- **Stratum corneum** – the most superficial layer. The cells have no nuclei (they are dead), are fully keratinized and are flattened in shape. They are known as **squames** and flake off from the skin surface.

Dermis
The dermis is composed of dense connective tissue with collagen and elastic fibres. It has a generous supply of blood vessels and nerves. Also found in the dermis are the **hair follicles**, **sebaceous glands** and **sweat glands**, which are only active in the hairless skin of the nose and footpads of the dog and cat.

Hypodermis
The hypodermis, or subcuticular layer is not actually part of the skin, but is a layer of loose connective tissue and fat, which lies beneath the dermis. It also contains elastic fibres, which gives the skin of the dog and cat its ability to move and return to its original position.

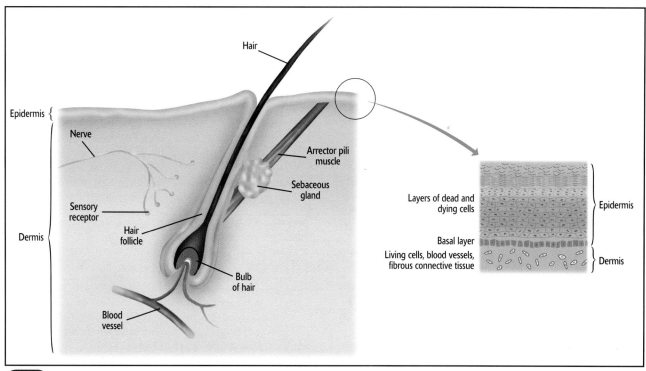

4.72   Cross-section through skin to show the structure.

The nose pad

The **rhinarium**, or nose pad, is covered by thickened, hairless pigmented skin and surrounds the nares or nostrils. The epidermis on a dog's nose has a unique patterning that is much like a human 'fingerprint'. The nose also has active sweat glands.

Hair

Hair is a keratinized structure and is a distinctive characteristic of mammals. It covers the entire body of the dog and cat with the exception of a few areas such as the nose and footpads.

The visible part of the hair above the skin's surface is called the **hair shaft** and the part that lies within the skin is called the **hair root**. Each hair grows from a **hair follicle**, which develops from epidermal cells. These grow down into the underlying dermis and form a 'hair cone' over a section of dermis called the **dermal papilla**. From the hair cone, the cells keratinize and form a hair (Figure 4.73). As the hair grows up through the epidermis to the skin's surface the cells at the point of the cone die, forming a channel – the hair follicle. The hair continues to grow until it eventually dies and becomes detached from the follicle. Hair growth is cyclical; once the hair is shed a new hair will start to grow from a new follicle.

Moulting

Moulting (the shedding of hair) is influenced by seasonal factors, such as temperature and day length. Most dogs moult more heavily in the spring and autumn. Cats moult most heavily in spring and this is followed by a less heavy hair loss throughout the summer and autumn. However, pet cats and dogs are usually kept inside centrally heated houses with electric lighting; this disrupts the natural seasonal triggers and they may moult all year round.

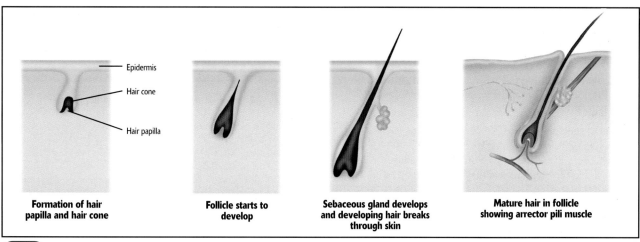

Formation of hair papilla and hair cone

Follicle starts to develop

Sebaceous gland develops and developing hair breaks through skin

Mature hair in follicle showing arrector pili muscle

4.73   The formation of hair.

Hair types

There are three main types of hair: guard hairs, wool hairs and tactile hairs (vibrissae).

Guard hairs

These are the thicker and longer hairs that form the outer protective coat of the animal. The nature of the guard hairs gives the coat its waterproof quality so that water 'runs off', preventing it from penetrating the coat. One guard hair grows from each follicle and is associated with an involuntary muscle called the **arrector pili muscle** (Figure 4.72). This raises the hair from its resting position, trapping a layer of warm air close to the body. The muscle contracts in response to cold, but can also be stimulated by fear or threat, such as the 'bottlebrush effect' of the hairs of the tail in the cat as a response to threat.

Wool hairs

These form the soft undercoat. They are thinner, softer and shorter than guard hairs and are more numerous. Their number fluctuates with the seasons: in winter they serve to keep the body warm by providing an insulating layer. The thickness of the wool hairs also varies between breeds; for example, Huskies have a very thick undercoat and are well adapted to extreme cold, whereas Dobermanns have a very short outer coat and no undercoat and so they do not tolerate cold weather. There may be a number of wool hairs growing from one follicle with one guard hair.

Tactile hairs

These are the **vibrissae**, also called 'whiskers' or sinus hairs. They are much thicker than guard hairs and protrude outwards beyond the rest of the coat. They are specialized hairs that grow from follicles found deep in the hypodermis. Each follicle is surrounded by nerve endings that are responsive to mechanical stimuli and provide sensory information from the environment. Tactile hairs are mostly found on the face, principally on the upper lip and near the eyes. They are also found in other areas, such as the cluster of tactile hairs on the palmar surface of a cat's carpus and the tuft of whiskers on a dog's cheek. In the fetus they are the first hairs to be formed.

Footpads

The footpads are covered by thick, keratinized, hairless epidermis. The surface is roughened by conical **papillae**, which provide traction when the dog walks. The surface of the cat's pads is smoother.

The dermis is also thickened, contains fatty tissue and is very vascular. This forms the **digital cushion**, which acts as a shock absorber as the animal walks and runs. Active sweat glands are found in the footpads of dogs and cats. There are seven pads on each forepaw and five on each hindpaw.

There are three types of pad (Figure 4.74):

- **Digital pads** protect the distal interphalangeal joints – one pad per digit (including the 'dew' claw)
- **Metacarpal/metatarsal pads** protect the phalangeal/metacarpal or metatarsal joint – heart-shaped in the dog, rounder in the cat
- **Carpal pad** (also called the **stop pad**) – found only on the forepaw and lies just distal to the carpus.

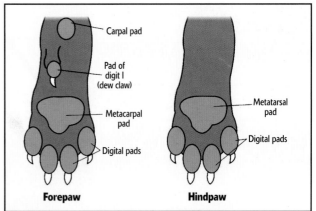

4.74 Ventral view of dog's forepaw and hindpaw, showing footpads.

Claws

The claws (Figure 4.75) are modified epidermal structures and form the outer layer of the distal or third phalanx, where they cover the **ungual process**. The epidermal cells contain a high proportion of keratin, which makes them hard and protective, and the tissue is referred to as **horn**.

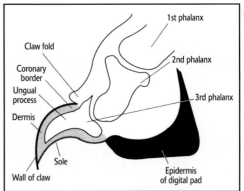

4.75 Longitudinal section of dog's toe, showing claw.

Each claw grows from a specialized region of epidermis, the **coronary border**, which lies underneath a fold of skin called the **claw fold**. The claw consists of two hard, laterally compressed **walls**. In a groove between the walls on the ventral surface is the softer horn of the **sole**. The **dermis** or 'quick' lies at the base of the claw and contains blood capillaries and nerve fibres.

Dog claws are non-retractable. Cat claws are held retracted by means of elastic ligaments that run from the second and third phalanges. When the cat unsheathes its claws, the digital flexor muscle overcomes the tension in the elastic ligaments.

Further reading

Aspinall V (2005) *Essentials of Veterinary Anatomy and Physiology*. Elsevier, Oxford

Aspinall V (ed) (2006) *The Complete Textbook of Veterinary Nursing*. Elsevier, Oxford

Aspinall V and O'Reilly M (2004) *Introduction to Veterinary Anatomy and Physiology*. Butterworth Heinemann, Oxford

Boyd JS (2001) *Colour Atlas of Clinical Anatomy of the Dog and Cat*, 2nd edn. Mosby, London

Tartaglia L and Waugh A (2005) *Veterinary Physiology and Applied Anatomy* (revised reprint). Elsevier, Oxford

Chapter 4b

Anatomy and physiology of exotic pets

Simon Girling

Learning objective

After studying this chapter, students should be able to:

- **Describe the significant anatomical and physiological differences between commonly seen exotic pets and cats and dogs**

Small mammals

Principally, the species within the rodent, lagomorph (primarily rabbit) and mustelid (primarily the domestic ferret) groups will be considered here. Biological parameters for small mammals are given in Figure 4.76.

Species	Average life expectancy (years)	Adult weight	Body temperature (°C)
Rabbit	5–8	1–10 kg (breed-dependent)	38.5–40
Ferret	8–10	600 g (jill) 1.2 kg (hob)	37.8–40
Mouse	1–2.5	20–40 g	37–38
Rat	3	400–800 g	37.6–38.6
Gerbil	1.5–2.5	70–130 g	37–38.5
Syrian hamster	1.5–2	100–200 g	36.2–37.5 [a]
Chinese/ Russian hamster	1.5–2	20–40 g	36–38
Guinea pig	4–7	750–1000 g	37.2–39.5
Chinchilla	10–15	400–500 g	37–38
Chipmunk	3–5	80–150 g	37.8–39.6 [a]

4.76 Biological parameters of small mammals. [a] Hibernates in the wild.

Musculoskeletal system

The basic quadruped form is found in all of the common species of small pet mammals seen. There is some variation in limb lengths: rabbits and chinchillas in particular have elongated rear limbs that allow jumping and rapid turns of speed. Rabbits and chinchillas also have a lightweight skeleton. The rabbit's skeleton on average comprises 7% of its bodyweight, as compared with a cat's, which is nearly double this at 13%. This means that the bones are often more brittle and so comminuted fractures are common.

The number of digits apparent on each limb also varies from species to species. The majority considered here have four digits on their forelimbs and five digits in their hindlimbs. The exceptions are: the guinea pig, which has three digits on the hindlimb; the rabbit, which has four digits on the hindlimb and five on the forelimb; and the ferret, which has five digits on the forelimb.

Some species, such as the rat, mouse, gerbil and chinchilla, have a prominent tail. Others, such as the hamster and guinea pig, have a vestigial tail.

Rats may have open growth plates, particularly in the males, well into the second year of their lives.

The pubic symphysis in many female rodents, particularly the mouse and the guinea pig, separates shortly before parturition to allow widening of the pelvic canal. If the female guinea pig is not bred before she reaches 12 months of age, there is a risk that the pubic symphysis will fuse in its narrow maiden state and so any attempts to farrow may result in dystocia.

Respiratory system

In general, the lungs and trachea are similar in small mammals to those seen in cats and dogs. The main difference is that the proportion of their body given over to the thoracic cavity in relation to the abdominal cavity is smaller than that seen in cats and dogs. Respiratory disease therefore tends to cause problems sooner in small mammals. In addition, many of the rodents and lagomorphs are obligate nasal breathers, with the epiglottis above the soft palate.

Digestive system

This is perhaps where some of the greater differences occur between small mammals and cats and dogs.

Rabbits

Rabbits have the dental formula I 1/1, C 0/0, PM 3/2, M 3/3. Therefore, like the other small herbivores considered here, there is a gap or **diastema** between the incisors and the premolars.

The rabbit stomach and small intestine are similar to those of the cat and dog. Like horses, rabbits are hindgut fermenters; therefore they have developed a capacious large intestine and caecum to provide chambers in which the bacteria and protozoa that help them to digest hemicellulose and cellulose can live. At the junction of the ileum and caecum lies the sacculus rotundus, which is rich in lymphoid tissue and is a common site for foreign body impactions. The caecum itself is large and sacculated and spiral-shaped, ending in a blind-ended vermiform appendix, again rich in lymphoid tissue.

The start of the large intestine is the ampulla coli, which is smooth-walled. The rest of the large intestine has bands of fibrous tissue (**taeniae**), which create sacculations (**haustra**). At the end of the proximal colon the taeniae and haustra cease; the gut wall thickens and becomes the fusus coli, a section containing large amounts of nerve ganglia that act as pacemakers for the complicated bowel contractions. The final distal descending colon then connects to the rectum.

The physiology of the rabbit gut is such that partially digested food material is moved into the caecum for further microbial breakdown. Any remaining partially digested material is then pushed out of the bowel and covered in mucus to be re-eaten directly from the anus. This forms the **caecotroph**, the mucus being necessary to protect much of the bacteria within the caecotroph from the acid pH of the stomach. Caecotrophs are dark green and produced generally overnight in domesticated rabbits. The waste indigestible fibre that the microbes cannot breakdown is excreted as a dry faecal pellet, which is generally a light brown colour.

Chinchillas, guinea pigs and degus

All three species have the dental formula I 1/1, C 0/0, PM 1/1, M 3/3. As with the rabbit, these species are hindgut fermenters. The small intestine is relatively long. At the junction of the ileum and large intestine lies the caecum, which can be 20 cm long and contain up to 70% of all the gut contents in the guinea pig. The caecum is slightly smaller in the chinchilla and degu, but in all species has taeniae along its length and is sacculated. In the chinchilla, the proximal portion of the colon is also sacculated, whereas in the guinea pig it is smooth surfaced along its entire length. The large bowel of the guinea pig is coiled into a complicated spiral.

Other rodents

Rats, mice, hamsters and gerbils have the dental formula I 1/1, C 0/0, PM 0/0, M 3/3. Rodents such as the hamster and the chipmunk possess cheek pouches for carrying food. The hamster, gerbil and rat also have two sections to their stomach: a non-glandular portion and a more traditional glandular section. In the hamster in particular, the non-glandular portion of the stomach allows a moderate amount of microbial fermentation of food.

Ferrets

The digestive tract of the ferret is very similar to that of the cat, except that ferrets do not possess a caecum.

Cardiovascular system

This is broadly similar to that of cats and dogs. The exception is the ferret, which has one vessel arising from the aorta (the innominate artery 1) where the cat and dog would have separate vessels for the right and left carotid artery. The innominate artery 1 then divides cranially at the thoracic inlet into the left and right carotid arteries.

Urogenital system

Urinary tract

The urinary system of rodents, lagomorphs and mustelids is broadly similar to that of dogs and cats. Important differences include the separate external orifices for the urinary system and reproductive tract in rodents. In addition, species such as the desert rodents (gerbils and jerboas) have longer loops of Henle, which means that they can produce more concentrated urine and so conserve water.

Most of the herbivorous mammals considered here produce urine that is slightly cloudy because of the presence of calcium carbonate or calcium oxalate crystals. The colour variation may be great, particularly when the animal is fed high beta carotene-containing foods such as leafy greens and beetroot, when the urine may be almost blood red in colour due to the excretion of porphyrin pigments. Generally, apart from the mustelids, the normal urine pH should be alkaline.

Reproductive tract

The variations in oestrous periods and gestation are wide in rodents, lagomorphs and mustelids (see Chapter 25). In rodents, the reproductive tract of the female has a separate opening from the urinary tract. Many of the species considered here have subtly different uterine structures. The rabbit, for example, has no common uterine body, rather two separate uterine horns, each of which has a cervix and joins separately to the vagina. Ferrets are much the same in uterine structure as the cat.

In males, in all of the species here except the ferret, the testes may be retracted into the abdomen voluntarily.

Sexual dimorphism is apparent in all small mammals (see Chapter 25). In many rodents the sex is determined by examining the ano-genital distance, which is greater in the male. Careful examination of the female rodent may also show the presence of the separate reproductive tract opening (see Chapter 25).

Skin

In general, the skin structure of rodents, lagomorphs and mustelids is similar to that of cats and dogs. Certain differences exist, such as the presence of cutaneous scent glands in many species (generally more prominent in the male of the species), including the ventral scent gland in gerbils, the flank scent glands in hamsters and the perianal scent glands in rabbits.

Other differences include dewlaps and the absence of foot pads in rabbits, fragile fracture planes in the tail of gerbils (these allow degloving of the skin should a predator attack) and the absence of sweat glands in the skin of nearly all of the species considered here. This makes pet rodents and lagomorphs in particular prone to heat stress.

Nervous system

This is generally similar to that of dogs and cats. The main differences lie in some of the small herbivores that have larger collections of myenteric nerves supplying the capacious large intestine and caecum.

Lymphatic system

Thymus
In most of the rodents and lagomorphs, the thymus survives largely intact in the adult animal and may be seen on radiographs cranial to the heart.

Spleen
The spleen is similar to that found in cats and dogs. There is some size variation between the species, but it is located adjacent to the stomach on the left side.

Birds

Musculoskeletal system
The majority of birds have the ability to fly. This requires a number of adaptations of the basic terrestrial mammalian skeleton in order to lighten and strengthen the avian skeleton. For example, many of the bones have no bone marrow, instead being filled with a light trabecular structure. Some of the bones (such as the humerus and often the femur) are pneumatic, i.e. they are air-filled and communicate with the respiratory system, further decreasing their weight.

Skull
The beak is a defining feature of avian species, and is also one of the most varied structures seen. It may be short and thickened, as is seen with many seed eaters such as the finch family, or long and slender as in many wading birds, ideal for probing the mud for food. It may be curved and powerful ideal for ripping food apart, as in many birds of prey, or it may be thickened with a powerful hinge joint ideal for nut and seed cracking, as in many parrots. In all cases, a lower (mandibular) and upper (maxillary) beak are present. These are covered in a layer of keratin, known collectively as the **rhamphotheca**. The keratin covering the maxillary beak is referred to as the **rhinotheca**, and that covering the mandibular beak is referred to as the **gnatotheca**.

The eyes and therefore orbits of birds are relatively large. The eye shape is maintained by cartilage and a ring of small bones, known as **scleral ossicles**, which are situated within the sclera at the scleral corneal junction. The connection between the skull and the first cervical vertebra is different in birds from that seen in mammals as there is only one occipital condyle in birds. This makes the head extremely mobile.

The infraorbital sinus is a cavity situated below the eye. It connects with the nasal passages and is unusual in that it has no bony lateral wall, being only covered by skin and soft tissues. Infection of this sinus is commonly associated with respiratory disease, as it has very poor drainage and easily fills with exudates. The main nasal passages communicate with the oropharynx via a midline slit in the hard palate, known as the **choana**.

Axial skeleton, pelvis and ribcage
The cervical vertebrae are small and box-like in form and freely articulate with each other. Their number varies from species to species and may be anywhere from 11 to 25. The thoracic vertebrae are fused together in many species to form a single bone, the **notarium**. This overlies and protects the semi-rigid lungs beneath. There is one free thoracic vertebra caudal to the notarium, allowing some limited movement. Caudal to this are the fused vertebrae of the sacral area, which merge into the pelvic bones to form the **synsacrum**. This bone protects the kidneys, which lie close to its ventral surface. Caudal to the synsacrum are a limited number of mobile coccygeal vertebrae. These are followed by a single bone comprising fused coccygeal vertebrae known as the **pygostyle**, which forms the base for the attachment of the tail feathers.

The pelvic structure is largely fused into the sacral vertebrae. The pubic bones are elongated in comparison with mammals and are not fused. They support the musculature of the abdominal wall. The acetabulum is not fully ossified in birds, and there is a ridge on the pelvis, dorsal to the hip joint, known as the **antitrochanter**. This articulates with the trochanter of the femur and allows the pelvic limb to lock in place and prevent adduction when perching.

There are eight pairs of ribs in most parrots. Each rib has a dorsal or 'vertebral' and a ventral or sternal segment. At the junction of the two is a caudally projecting process. The ribs can move laterally and allow the sternum to move ventrally so that inspiration can occur. The sternum has a ventral midline ridge on to which the pectoral muscles attach. This ridge may be well developed in some species, such as parrots (Figure 4.77) and birds of prey, or almost absent in species such as ducks, where the sternum is a more boat-like structure to improve flotation.

Appendicular skeleton
The shoulder joint is complicated and is formed by the humerus, scapula and coracoids. The scapula is much reduced in birds and lies along the lateral ribcage. The coracoid is an additional bone in birds which forms a strut from the keel up to the shoulder and is there to counteract the immense downward forces imparted by the beating of the wings. The humerus articulates with the radius and ulna. In birds the ulna is the larger bone of the two. It also forms the attachment for the secondary flight feathers. The radius and ulna then articulate with a reduced number of carpal bones, one radial and one ulnar carpal bone. These then articulate with three metacarpal bones. The first is the equivalent of the avian thumb, and is referred to as the **alula** or bastard wing. The remaining two are referred to as the major and minor metacarpal bones as they are each made up of a fused carpal bone and metacarpal bone. These articulate with the first phalanx and the minor digit. The first phalanx then articulates with the second phalanx at the distal extremity of the wing.

The wing is drawn ventrally by the action of the superficial pectoral muscle, which attaches to the sternum. It is brought dorsally again by the **supracoracoid** muscle, which also attaches to the sternum but then attaches to the dorsal aspect of the humerus after passing through the triosseal canal formed by the meeting of the humerus, coracoid and scapula bones. The elastic recoil of the wing itself is enhanced by the wing web, or **propatagium**, a sheet of fine muscle and elastic tissues connecting the humerus to the carpal joint.

The hip joint is a ball and socket joint. The femur may be pneumatic. It articulates with the **tibiotarsus** distally at the stifle joint. The stifle joint has a patella, meniscal cartilages and cruciate ligaments. The tibiotarsus is formed from the fusion of the tibia and the proximal row of tarsal bones. The tibiotarsus

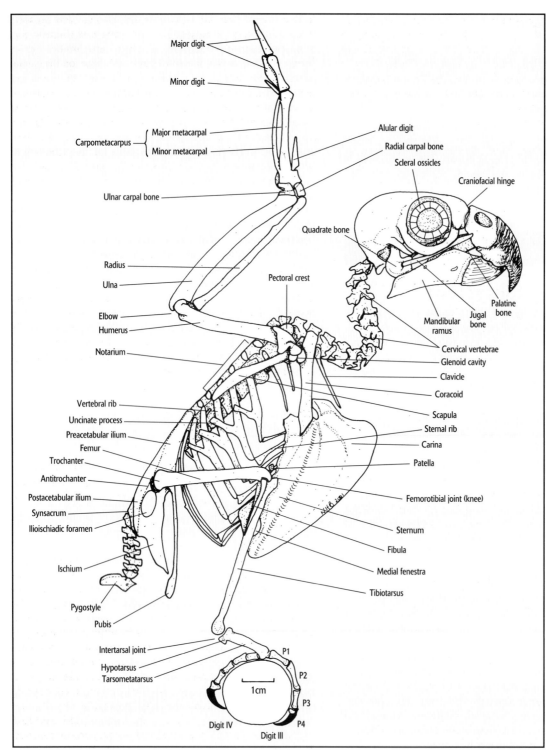

4.77

Right lateral view of the skeleton of a blue-headed parrot (*Pionus menstruus*) in a normal perching position. The wing is elevated. (Reproduced from *BSAVA Manual of Exotic Pets, 4th edition.* © Nigel Harcourt-Brown)

then articulates distally with the **tarsometatarsus**, formed from the fusion of the distal row of tarsal bones with the proximal metatarsal bones. The joint between the tibiotarsus and the tarsometatarsus is the **intertarsal joint**, although it may be referred to colloquially as the hock or suffrage joint. The tarsometatarsus then articulates with the phalanges. In parrots, two digits point forwards (the second and third) and two backwards (the first and fourth) creating a **zygodactyl** limb. In perching birds and many birds of prey, three toes point forwards (the second, third and fourth) and one backwards (the first), creating an **anisodactyl** limb. In some species, such as the osprey, the fourth digit may move forwards or backwards (to enhance the capture of slippery fish) and this is referred to as a semi-zygodactyl limb.

Respiratory system

Upper respiratory system

The nares are generally situated at the base of the beak, though this is variable between species. The nasal passages have a main nasal turbinate or concha, and then communicate with the sinuses of the head (the main one being the infraorbital sinus), which are blind ending. They also communicate with the oropharynx via the choana in the hard palate. At rest, the **glottis** (the rudimentary larynx) is positioned immediately ventral to the choana. The glottis of birds, unlike the larynx of mammals, lacks an epiglottis, thyroid cartilage and vocal folds, and guards the entrance to the trachea. The glottis is held closed at rest.

The trachea of avian species has complete signet-ring-shaped cartilages to support its structure. It is often relatively long in birds (it may be coiled inside the sternum in some swans) and finishes at the bifurcation into the two main bronchi. There is considerable species variation in the shape of the trachea; some penguins have a midline septum dividing the trachea into two as far cranially as the glottis. Male ducks have a diverticulum, or bulla, of the trachea just inside the body cavity.

At the caudal end of the trachea may be found the **syrinx**, or avian voice box. This comprises a series of muscles and two membranes which can be vibrated, independently of inspiration or expiration, to produce the bird's 'voice'. It is also often the site for fungal infection growth, such as is seen in aspergillosis.

Lower respiratory system

There are two lungs, which are semi-rigid in birds and so do not inflate or deflate significantly during inspiration and expiration. They are attached to the underside of the dorsal body wall and protected by the notarium. There is no diaphragm in birds, and the common body cavity so formed is a **coelom**, although the terms thoracic and abdominal may still be used.

The two primary bronchi enter the lungs and rapidly divide into secondary and tertiary (or parabronchi) bronchi. The tertiary bronchi are arranged into two areas: the paleopulmonic portion of the lung, where they are arranged in a regular pattern and only allow air to flow from caudal to cranial; and the neopulmonic portion, where they are arranged more haphazardly and allow air to flow both from cranial to caudal and vice versa. Only at the level of the tertiary bronchi does gas exchange start to occur. Their walls have a series of pits, or **atria**, from which small tubes or air capillaries branch, where further gaseous exchange can take place.

In birds, as there is no diaphragm and the lungs are semi-rigid, air is moved through the lungs by moving the sternum downwards and the ribcage outwards. This allows inspiration, and air is sucked in through the lungs into a series of **air sacs** (Figure 4.78), which act as passive bellows. There are nine air sacs in most species. These include the minor sacs: a single

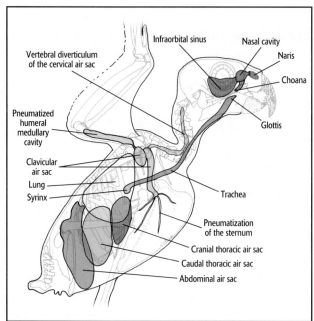

4.78 Right lateral view of the respiratory system of a parrot. (Reproduced from *BSAVA Manual of Exotic Pets, 4th edition.* © Nigel Harcourt-Brown)

cervicocephalic sac, which communicates only with the nasal sinuses; and a single cervical sac, which lies between the lungs and dorsal oesophagus. The main air sacs involved in respiration include the so-called cranial air sacs: the single clavicular air sac, which has two diverticula, one around the heart and one around the bones and muscles of the pectoral girdle and crop (and communicates with the pneumatic humeral bones); and the paired cranial thoracic air sacs, which lie laterally, ventral to the lung field and caudal to the heart. In addition there are the so-called caudal air sacs: the paired caudal thoracic air sacs lie immediately caudal to the cranial thoracic air sacs, and the paired abdominal air sacs caudal to these. The abdominal air sacs connect with the lungs at their most caudal aspect and extend around the gastrointestinal tract. They also communicate with other pneumatic bones, such as the femora, and the notarium and synsacrum.

The respiratory cycle in birds is complex and involves two cycles of inspiration and expiration. On inspiration, air moves into the lungs and into the caudal air sacs; air expelled from the caudal air sacs then moves back into the lungs where gaseous exchange takes place; the air then moves into the cranial air sacs and is exhaled via the bronchi. Birds can therefore extract oxygen from air on both inspiration and expiration, making them much more efficient at gaseous exchange than mammals.

Digestive system

Oral cavity

The beak has already been mentioned. The tongue may be strap-like and rudimentary, as in many perching birds (Passeriformes), or highly muscular and mobile, as in parrots (Psittaciformes).

Oesophagus and crop

Several species of bird, including many seabirds and owls, do not possess a crop and instead make use of a highly distensible oesophagus. In those species that do possess a crop, the oesophagus is split into a proximal segment (that cranial to the crop) and a distal segment (that between the crop and the true stomach). The crop itself also varies in structure according to species. In many, such as the parrots, it acts purely as a storage chamber and takes no part in digestion. It is situated at the base of the neck, predominantly on the right side. In species such as the pigeon and dove family (Columbiformes), the crop can produce a secretion (known as 'crop milk') which is used to feed and raise their young. It is composed of exfoliated lipid-containing cells from the lining of the crop, produced under the control of the hormone prolactin during the breeding season. Both male and female pigeons can produce this 'milk'.

The 'stomachs'

Birds possess two stomachs. The first is the 'true' or acid-secreting stomach, referred to as the **proventriculus** (Figure 4.79), which is where digestion starts. Here there are compound acid- and pepsinogen-secreting glands, as well as separate mucus-secreting glands. The proventriculus then empties immediately into the second stomach, referred to as the **ventriculus** (also known as the 'grinding' or '**gizzard**' stomach). This may be well developed in seed-eating species that are required to grind their food, or merge into the proventriculus in species such as birds of prey where little or no grinding action is needed.

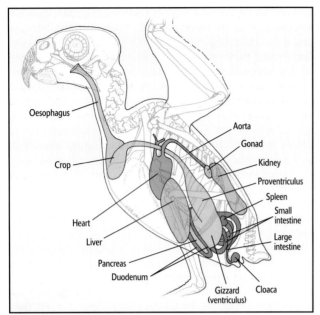

4.79 Left lateral view of the viscera of a parrot. (Reproduced from *BSAVA Manual of Exotic Pets, 4th edition.* © Nigel Harcourt-Brown)

Small intestine

This is short in comparison to an equivalent sized mammal species. It is composed predominantly of (from cranial to caudal) a large duodenum (divided into a descending and an ascending limb), followed by a smaller jejunum and ileum.

Large intestine

This is frequently referred to as the 'rectum' in birds, owing to its small size. It is responsible for the resorption of water and electrolytes. At the junction of the ileum and rectum are situated the **caeca**. These may be large and paired, seen in ratites such as the emu and ostrich, or may be totally absent, as in many parrots. They aid in the digestion of hemicellulose and cellulose present in the diet by providing a site for microbial fermentation. The rectum empties into the coprodeum portion of the cloaca.

Cloaca

This is the communal chamber into which the digestive, urinary and reproductive tracts empty. It is divided into three main sections. The **coprodeum** receives faeces from the gastrointestinal tract. This is separated from the next section of the cloaca, the **urodeum**, by a mucosal fold. The urodeum receives urinary waste via the ureters from the kidneys as well as the opening of the oviduct (females) or vas deferens (males). The next section is the **proctodeum**, where faeces and urinary waste are combined before exiting through the vent. The proctodeum also communicates with the **bursa of Fabricius**, which is the site for B-cell lymphocyte production in juvenile birds.

Liver

The liver is bilobed and situated caudal to the heart, ventral to the proventriculus and cranial to the ventriculus (Figure 4.79). Some species possess a gall bladder, but many parrots do not. The main bile pigment in birds is **biliverdin**, and not bilirubin as is the case in mammals. As its name suggests, the pigment biliverdin is green, and evidence of liver inflammation or damage may be indicated by the presence of this green pigment in the droppings: the white urates turn mustard yellow to lime green.

Pancreas

This gland is tubuloacinar in structure and has three lobes in most species. It produces the same digestive enzymes and bicarbonate ions as in mammals.

Cardiovascular system

Heart

The avian heart is four chambered, as with mammals, but proportionally larger with respect to body size, averaging 1–1.5% of bodyweight as opposed to the mammalian average of 0.5%.

The sinus venosus is a separate chamber in birds and receives blood from the caudal vena cava and right cranial vena cava. The left vena cava empties nearby but is separated from the sinus venosus by a septum.

There are two coronary arteries, as in mammals, but four coronary veins as opposed to one in mammals.

Blood vessels

The major artery, the aorta, curves to the right side as it leaves the heart in birds, rather than the left as in mammals. The other major difference in avian vasculature is the supply to the kidneys. In birds there are three blood vessels supplying each kidney, one for each lobe (cranial middle and caudal). The gonads are supplied by an offshoot of the cranial renal artery.

The pelvic limbs are supplied by a femoral artery arising from the external iliac artery, but this is not the main supply. This arises from the ischiadic artery, which arises from a common vessel offshoot of the aorta that also creates the middle and caudal renal arteries and so passes through and over the kidney structure.

The venous system has some differences from the mammalian model. The right jugular vein is significantly larger than the left. This vessel is often used for blood sampling.

There is an enterohepatic portal system as in mammals, except that there are two hepatic portal veins instead of one. There is also a renal portal system. Here the main vein from the leg (the femoral vein) runs into the external iliac vein and so either into the renal portal vein, which surrounds the renal tubules, or directly into the common iliac vein and so bypasses the kidney.

Blood cells

The bird erythrocyte is nucleated. The main leucocyte is the **heterophil**, which is broadly similar to the mammalian neutrophil. The other main difference is that the platelet (referred to as the thrombocyte) is also nucleated.

Urogenital system

Urinary tract

The avian kidney is different in shape from the mammalian one, being trilobed, and relatively large. It is located on the dorsal body wall, immediately ventral to the synsacrum over the pelvis. There is no urinary bladder in birds; instead the ureters empty directly into the urodeum portion of the cloaca.

The avian kidney also differs from the mammalian one in its microscopic structure. It possesses two different types of nephron, one of which is similar to the mammalian model and has a loop of Henle and produces mildly hypertonic urine. The other is a reptilian form of nephron that does not have a loop of Henle and so can only produce isotonic urine. In addition, the biggest physiological difference in birds is that their main waste product of protein metabolism is not urea, as in mammals, but the compound **uric acid**. This is removed from the body by active proximal tubule excretion. Uric acid has a low solubility and so appears in a semi-solid state as the 'whites' or urates present in the normal bird dropping. Damage to the kidneys or severe dehydration can lead to a precipitation of uric acid inside the body, which can lead to a deposition of urates on internal organs (visceral gout) or in joints (articular gout).

Reproductive tract

In the male the two testes are located internally, cranial to the kidneys. The testes often increase in size during the reproductive season, sometimes by as much as 20 times their non-breeding size. Each testis empties into a vas deferens, which in turn runs down to the urodeum portion of the cloaca.

There is no phallus in many avian species, transmission of sperm from male to female occurring purely by the apposition of the vents. The exceptions include many of the duck family (Anseriformes). In these species the phallus lies on the ventral floor of the cloaca at rest. When erect, it develops a corkscrew shape and projects out of the vent. It has no urethra, but there is a groove along its surface into which the sperm runs and so is guided into the female cloaca. The phallus therefore plays no part in urination.

In the female, in many species, there is only one ovary (the left) and one oviduct. The oviduct is divided from cranial to caudal into the following divisions functionally: the **infundibulum**, which is responsible for catching the oocyte (composed of the ovum plus yolk) from the ovary and is the part of the tract where combination of sperm and oocyte occurs and where the initial supporting membranes (**chalazon**) are laid down; the **magnum**, which is responsible for laying down the bulk of the egg white (**albumen**); the **isthmus**, which is responsible for laying down the shell membranes; the **shell gland**, which is responsible for laying down the egg shell, and where '**plumping**' (the addition of fluids to the albumen) occurs. At the caudal aspect of the shell gland is a muscular sphincter, followed by the vagina, which is responsible for the outer layer or cuticle of the shell and which then opens into the urodeum portion of the cloaca.

The sex of birds, as with mammals, is determined by chromosomes, but the female is the heterozygous individual, nominated 'ZY', and the male is homozygous, 'ZZ'. Many species show no obvious sexual dimorphism, but others do; for example, in the canary the male sings and female does not.

Skin

Avian skin is relatively thin in comparison with mammalian skin. The major difference is the presence of feathers. These are arranged in tracts, known as **pterylae**. This leaves areas of skin without feathers, known as **apterylae**. Avian skin is relatively inelastic and loosely attached to the underlying subcutis over most of the body, except over the head and the lower legs. Over the lower legs, the skin is thrown up into a series of thick scales in many species.

The feathers are adapted into a number of different forms. The flight feathers are arranged into **remiges** (comprising the primaries and secondaries on the wings) and the **rectrices** or tail feathers. The primary feathers are attached to the carpus and distal wing; the secondaries are attached only to the ulna. These flight feathers have a central shaft or **calumus**, and from this arise a series of barbs. These are linked to their neighbour by **barbules**, and these are further interlinked by small hooklets or **hamuli**, creating an effective solid surface.

Insulation is provided by a series of short undercoat feathers that lack interlocking barbules. These are referred to as **down feathers**. Further short feathers that possess some interlocking barbs and barbules overlie these and are referred to as the **contour feathers**.

There are highly specialized feathers, particularly around the face, which possess a very thin short bare shaft. They are responsible for touch sensation and are referred to as **bristle feathers**. Longer versions of these, known as **filoplumes**, lie alongside each of the flight feathers, and allow the bird to appreciate the position of each individual flight feather.

Finally, there are also short blunt **powder feathers**, responsible for secreting **powder down**, which aids water proofing and the integrity of the plumage.

Moulting

Moulting is the shedding of old feathers and replacement with new plumage. Moulting occurs in many temperate species once a year, usually just after the breeding season in the late spring and early summer. Some species moult more frequently, having a winter and summer plumage. Most species do not lose their feathers all in one go; rather, they lose the flight feathers in a set pattern, one or two at a time, and so can still fly. The exceptions are some of the duck family, which lose all of their flight feathers at once and so become flightless during the moult.

Nervous system

Birds have 12 cranial nerves, as with mammals. The brain lacks **gyri** (the folds on its surface) and has proportionally larger optic lobes, reflecting the importance of sight as the main sense in birds.

Another important feature of the avian nervous system is the nervous supply to the legs. The main supply passes through the kidneys, therefore any swelling of the kidneys, such as a tumour or nephritis, may lead to pressure on the ischiadic nerve and so lead to limb paresis or paralysis.

Finally, the sensory nervous system in birds is geared towards monitoring the position of the flight feathers, allowing the bird to make fine adjustments continuously to prevent stalling. This is performed by the supply of sensory nerves to the roots of filoplume feathers; each flight feather can be associated with up to six filoplumes.

Lymphatic system

Spleen

The spleen is spherical in shape in many species and sits adjacent to the proventriculus. It is particularly important in systemic infectious diseases, as there are no peripheral lymph nodes in many species.

Thymus

This is generally not one discrete organ, but a series of islands of tissue scattered along the neck and thoracic inlet. As with mammals, it is responsible for the production and maturation of T-lymphocytes.

Bursa of Fabricius

This structure is unique to birds. It is located in the dorsal wall of the proctodeum segment of the cloaca. It is responsible for producing B-lymphocytes and decreases in size as the bird matures.

Lymph nodes

These are not found in most species of bird, though rudimentary structures do exist in some waterfowl. Instead, lymphatic tissue is scattered throughout the internal body organs, such as the liver, kidneys, lungs and digestive tract.

Reptiles

Reptiles are **ectothermic**, i.e. they rely on an external heat supply to achieve their preferred body temperature (**PBT**), which they need to reach for optimum bodily functions to occur. This means that the reptile must be kept within a temperature gradient so that it can position itself to either raise or lower its body temperature as required. This ideal temperature gradient is often referred to as the preferred optimum temperature zone (**POTZ**).

Musculoskeletal system

Chelonians

The most obvious feature of the chelonian musculoskeletal system is the presence of the shell. This is divided into an upper domed portion (the **carapace**) and a lower flattened portion (the **plastron**). These are connected to each other between the fore- and hindlimbs by the **pillars** of the shell. The shell is composed of coalesced islands of bone within the dermis, covered by a hard keratin. The ribcage is fused to the ventral surface of the carapace, and the shoulder blades are found inside the ribcage (a feature unique to chelonians). The cervical vertebrae are mobile, but they fuse with the ventral surface of the carapace at the cervicothoracic junction. The vertebral column then remains fused with the carapacial bone as far as the coccygeal vertebrae caudally, which are again mobile.

Lizards

There are one or two limbless lizards, such as the slow worm; otherwise the basic body form is similar to other quadruped animals.

Snakes

The skeletal system of snakes is defined by the absence of limbs. However, the evolutionary older species of snake, such as the boa and python families, still possess remnants of a pelvis.

The skull of a snake is extremely flexible. The mandible can separate at the rostral symphysis as well as there being a kinetic joint at the junction of the maxilla and calvarium. This, combined with laxity in the joint between the mandible and skull itself, allows the gape of the snake to be enlarged quite dramatically, enabling consumption of prey much larger than the snake's head.

The vertebral column is long and highly mobile, with large epaxial muscles running the length of the body. There are paired ribs rising from each vertebral body. Only the coccygeal vertebrae caudal to the vent do not have ribs. These support the body wall and allow attachment of the ventral muscles, which allow movement.

Body systems

Figures 4.80 to 4.82 illustrate the main body organs of a tortoise, lizard and snake.

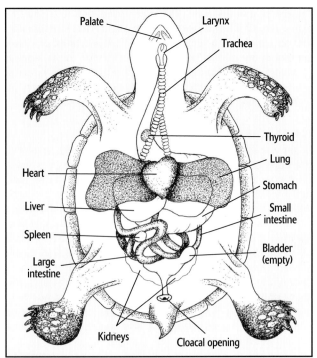

4.80 Ventral view of the main organs in the body cavity of a tortoise (plastron removed). (Reproduced from *BSAVA Manual of Reptiles, 2nd edition*)

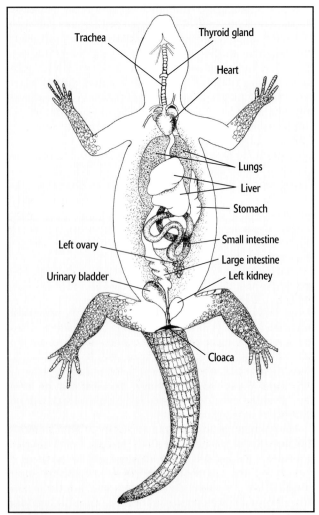

4.81 Ventral view of the main organs in the body cavity of a lizard. (Reproduced from *BSAVA Manual of Reptiles, 2nd edition*)

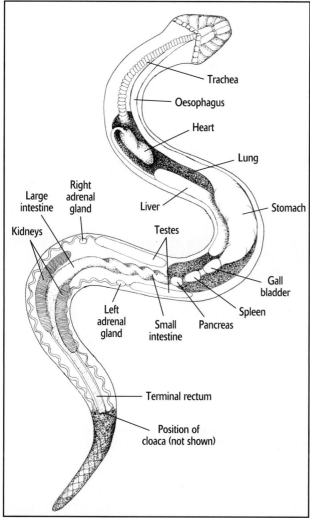

4.82 Ventral view of the main organs in the body cavity of a snake. (Reproduced from *BSAVA Manual of Reptiles, 2nd edition*)

Labels on figure: Trachea; Oesophagus; Heart; Lung; Large intestine; Right adrenal gland; Liver; Testes; Stomach; Kidneys; Gall bladder; Left adrenal gland; Small intestine; Pancreas; Spleen; Terminal rectum; Position of cloaca (not shown)

Respiratory system

Chelonians
There is no hard palate in chelonians. The trachea has complete rings of cartilage and in many land-based chelonians it bifurcates into the primary bronchi high in the neck (see Figure 4.80). The two lungs are elastic in nature and situated in the dorsal part of the carapace. There is no true diaphragm, although a pseudodiaphragm is present.

Lizards
There is no hard palate present. The trachea has C-shaped rings of cartilage, as with mammals, and this divides into two primary bronchi, which supply the paired lungs. There is no diaphragm. The lungs are alveolar and elastic in nature.

Snakes
There is no hard palate in snakes. The long trachea is similar to that in lizards, but some species have a tracheal lung – an outpouching of the lining of the trachea. In the majority of snakes there is only one major lung: the right; the left lung becomes vestigial. This is the case in many species such as Colubridae (e.g. kingsnakes and cornsnakes) and Viperidae. In boas and pythons two lungs are present, though the left is smaller. Air sacs are often present at the ends of the lungs, and these may be well developed in aquatic species. There is no diaphragm.

Digestive system
The lack of a diaphragm means that there is no division between 'abdominal' organs (such as the liver and gut) and 'thoracic' organs (such as the heart and lungs). Instead there is a single body cavity known as the **coelomic cavity**. The liver therefore tends to be situated beneath and in contact with the lungs.

The digestive system of reptiles is generally similar to that seen in mammals, but the tongue may have considerable variation. It is fleshy and immobile in chelonians, strap-like and forked in snakes, and fleshy and mobile in many lizards. Only the snakes and lizards have teeth; the chelonians have a keratin beak. Snakes have six rows of teeth (four in the maxilla and two in the mandible) and they are replaced continually as they are shed. Lizards have four rows of teeth: some species replacing the teeth continually, as in snakes, and are referred to as having a **pleurodont** dentition (e.g. iguana family); others have the same teeth for the whole of their life and are referred to as having an **acrodont** dentition (e.g. chameleon and agamid families). Some lizards (e.g. water dragons) have mixed dentitions.

The oesophagus is similar to its mammalian counterpart except in some marine species, such as turtles, which may have caudally pointing barbs to enable consumption of slippery prey such as jellyfish.

The stomach is simple, with compound tubuloacinar pepsinogen- and acid-secreting glands. The small intestine has few obvious differentiations into duodenum, jejunum and ileum visible to the naked eye. The greatest variations exist in the large intestine, which may become multi-chambered in herbivores such as the green iguana, where the increased folding of the bowel provides a greater surface area for microbial fermentation to occur to help in the digestion of hemicellulose and cellulose. The large intestine empties into the coprodeum portion of the cloaca, as with birds.

The cloaca is split into three main chambers, as in birds: the **coprodeum**; the **urodeum**, which receives the ureters and the vas deferens (males) or oviducts (females); and the **proctodeum**, which is the last chamber before the vent.

The commonly seen lizards, snakes and chelonians all possess a liver similar to that found in mammals. The majority possess a gallbladder, but as with birds the main bile pigment is biliverdin and not bilirubin. A pancreas is also present and may be fused with the spleen as a **splenopancreas**.

Cardiovascular system
The heart is generally considered to be three chambered in lizards, snakes and chelonians, as there is no physical division between the right and left ventricle. They function, though, as a four-chambered heart, with deoxygenated blood being preferentially directed towards the lungs and oxygenated blood to the rest of the body. There is an additional chamber, the sinus venosus, which receives blood from the caudal vena cava and right cranial vena cava.

Lizards, snakes and chelonians have paired aortae leaving the heart, one going to the right and one to the left. These then fuse to form a single abdominal aorta, dorsally. Reptiles possess a renal portal system, as is seen in birds. This means that blood returning from the caudal part of the body of the reptile can either pass through the parenchyma of the kidney before emptying into the caudal vena cava, or it can bypass the kidneys altogether. This has a theoretical importance when administering drugs to reptiles: if the drugs are given in the caudal part of the body, they may go to the kidneys before the rest of the body and so either be removed from the body before having a chance to work, or, if the drug is nephrotoxic (such as the aminoglycoside antibiotics), they may cause higher levels of kidney damage than if administered in the cranial part of the reptile.

Major blood vessels used for blood sampling include the ventral tail vein in lizards and snakes, the dorsal tail vein in chelonians, the jugular veins in chelonians and the palatine veins in anaesthetized snakes. Cardiac puncture to collect a blood sample may sometimes be performed in snakes and lizards consciously, but sedation or anaesthesia may be required.

The erythrocyte is nucleated in reptiles. The main leucocyte is the **heterophil**, which is broadly similar to the mammalian neutrophil. The other main difference is that the platelet (referred to as the thrombocyte) is also nucleated.

Lymphatic system

There are no lymph nodes in reptiles. The lymphoid tissue is scattered in nodules throughout the internal organs such as the liver and gut.

Urinary tract

Reptiles possesses a form of nephron that does not have a loop of Henle. In addition, the biggest physiological difference in reptiles is that, as with birds, the main waste product of protein metabolism is not urea (as in mammals) but the compound uric acid. This is removed from the body by active proximal tubule excretion. Uric acid has a low solubility and so appears in a semi-solid state as the 'whites' or urates present in the normal reptile dropping. Damage to the kidneys or severe dehydration can lead to precipitation of uric acid inside the body, leading to deposition of urates on internal organs (visceral gout) or in joints (articular gout).

Chelonians

The kidneys are bean shaped and situated on the ventral aspect of the carapace, caudally. As with lizards, they have a single ureter each, which drains into the urodeum portion of the cloaca. A separate urinary bladder is present, also attached to the cloaca as with lizards. This is often large and bilobed in terrestrial chelonians.

Lizards

The kidneys are generally bean-shaped. They are often situated in the pelvic region. As with snakes, each kidney is drained by one ureter, which enters the urodeum portion of the cloaca. Some lizards do possess a urinary bladder, but it has a separate connection to the cloaca. Therefore the urine passes from the kidneys to the cloaca and then refluxes into the urinary bladder. Lizard urine is therefore not sterile. It is possible that some fluid reabsorption may occur across the urinary bladder epithelium, and it is known that isotonic urine produced by the kidneys and excreted into the cloaca can be refluxed into the caudal rectum, where electrolyte and water reabsorption may also occur.

Snakes

The snake has paired elongated kidneys, situated in the caudal third of the body cavity. Each kidney has a single ureter draining it. This travels caudally to the urodeum portion of the cloaca. There is no urinary bladder in snakes.

Reproductive tract

The reproductive tract of female reptiles is similar to that seen in birds, except that the single oviduct of birds is paired into a right and left oviduct in reptiles. The oviducts are separated into the same sections as seen in birds: an infundibulum that has the fimbrial portion adjacent to the ovary and the tubular portion; the magnum; the isthmus; the shell gland/uterus; and then the muscular vagina. The vagina opens into the urodeum portion of the cloaca. Each oviduct empties independently into the cloaca.

In males, the testes are internally situated, cranial to the respective kidneys. The vas deferens empties into the urodeum portion of the cloaca. Males do possess a rudimentary penile structure. In snakes and lizards, there are two such structures, known as **hemipenes**. These are situated as invaginations in the base of the tail, opening adjacent to the vent either side of midline ventrally. When blood engorges the hemipenis, it inflates and projects out from its invagination to lie beneath the vent. Sperm then drips into the cloaca, out of the vent and into a groove on the surface of the hemipenis. The hemipenis is inserted into the female cloaca to allow insemination. The hemipenes therefore have no urethra and play no part in urination. In chelonians, there is a single hemipenis or phallus, which lies on the ventral floor of the cloaca. It too has no urethra, only a groove on its surface, and so only functions as a reproductive organ.

Nervous system

There are 12 cranial nerves in reptiles, as with mammals. The olfactory lobe of the brain is relatively well developed in species such as snakes that use scent to track prey. In snakes, paired nerves arise at each intervertebral joint and supply the ventral musculature. By firing alternately, these cause waves of contraction in the ventral body muscles, propelling the snake along the ground. In chelonians, the spinal column becomes encased in the carapace in the thoracic and lumbar regions.

Snakes do not have an external ear. Instead they use the vibrations of animals moving over the ground, which are transferred to the jaw bones and so to the internal ear. Lizards and chelonians do have an external ear drum/tympanum, and a single auditory ossicle to transmit vibrations from this to the internal ear.

Some snakes also possess infra-red heat-sensing pits. In the case of older evolutionary species such as the boas and pythons these are labial pits, a series of depressions around the upper jaw line. In the more recent evolutionary species, such as the pit vipers, there is a single pit between the nostril and the eye on either side. These are extremely sensitive to heat variations and can act together in a binocular fashion to pinpoint prey even in the dark.

Skin

The epidermis is relatively thin yet is heavily keratinized. The underlying dermis is thrown into folds, covered by the epidermis, to create the scales. In snakes these are obvious and large, and tend to overlap each other, the caudal edge of a proximal scale overlying the cranial edge of the next. This is less obvious in lizards, where the scales are often smaller. Chelonians possess small scales over the head, neck, limbs and tail, but over the shell large **scutes** of keratinized material are found.

Chromatophores are found in the dermis, and in species such as chelonians the dermis also forms bone to create the shell. Many special adaptations of the skin can be found in reptiles, including heat-sensitive skin pits (see 'Nervous system', below) as well as vestigial so-called **parietal eyes** in some species. This rudimentary structure is found on the dorsum of the head, between the two conventional eyes, and is obvious in many iguanids. It is very well developed in the unique reptile, the tuatara, where the structure actually possesses a lens. The function of the parietal eye is thought to be in transmitting information regarding diurnal light patterns to the pineal gland in the brain, which in turn controls seasonal behaviour such as breeding.

Shedding

Reptiles regularly shed their skin, a process known as **ecdysis**. This may occur as a complete shed of the whole skin, as seen in snakes, or it may occur in small pieces, as more commonly seen in lizards and chelonians. The process starts with the formation of a new layer of epidermal skin cells beneath the old skin. Lymphatic fluid and proteases are then secreted in between the new and old layer of skin, so cleaving them apart from each other. This is often seen as a dulling in the colour of snakes, and a blueing of the eyes (snakes eyelids are fused over the surface of the cornea and have become transparent – the so-called 'spectacles'). Once this has occurred, the fluid is reabsorbed, the snake returns to its normal coloration, and a few days later the snake starts to rub its mouth on an abrasive surface to start peeling the old skin away.

The frequency of shedding is dependent on: the age of the reptile (more frequent when young and growing rapidly); time of year; health status of the reptile; environmental temperature and humidity. An incomplete or abnormal sloughing of the skin is referred to as **dysecdysis**.

Fish

Fish are **poikilothermic**, i.e. their body functions at temperatures found in their environment (sometimes referred to as being 'cold-blooded'). They have no internal source of heat production and function at body temperatures generally lower than those found in the ectothermic reptiles or homeothermic birds and mammals.

The fish that are commonly seen in veterinary practice are referred to as **teleost** or bony fish. There is no clear division of the body cavity into a thorax and abdomen as in mammals and so the common internal cavity is referred to as a coelomic cavity, as with birds and reptiles.

Musculoskeletal system

The skeleton is simple. There is a complex skull shape with mobile maxilla and mandible. The former is particularly loosely attached to the skull itself. In addition, there are bones in the operculum to cover the gills. Immediately caudal to the ventral skull lies the pectoral girdle, which articulates with a vestigal scapula and coracoid bone. These then articulate with the bones of the pectoral fin.

The spine is composed of 60 or more bony vertebrae. The trunk vertebrae (except the first two) have short paired processes projecting ventrally, which then articulate with slender pleural ribs. In the tail region the ventral paired processes join to make a haemal arch. The most caudal vertebrae are flattened and have broadened processes, which fuse together to form a strong support for the caudal fin (where present). The rest of the fins possess dermal fin rays, paired slender bones that support the integument. There are pectoral fins, pelvic fins, dorsal fins and anal fins (Figure 4.83). Salmonids possess an adipose fin between the dorsal fin and the tail, dorsally.

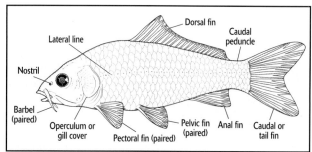

4.83 External anatomy of a carp. (Reproduced from *BSAVA Manual of Ornamental Fish, 2nd edition*)

Respiratory system

Fish use gills to extract oxygen from the water. Each gill contains a gill arch. This supports a series of paired, leaf-like structures that project at right angles from the arch and are referred to as primary **lamellae**. The primary lamellae are divided into secondary lamellae, all of which are highly vascularized. The water flows through the gills to create a countercurrent system (blood and water flow are in opposite directions) to ensure maximum oxygen extraction from the water. Water is forced through the gills by the closing of the mouth and the raising of the floor of the buccal cavity.

The frequency of gill movements is governed by alterations in blood chemistry of the partial pressure of oxygen and carbon dioxide, as well as its pH. The gill movements are then monitored by mechanoreceptors and proprioceptors located in the pseudobranch, a rudimentary gill arch found under the operculum.

Digestive system

Teeth are often present on the maxilla and sometimes on the mandible, depending on the species. These are peg-like in general. Some species, such as the carp family, have teeth in the pharyngeal region only, which bite upwards on to a horny pad attached to the dorsal surface of the pharynx.

Food is prevented from passing over the gills by gill rakers. Food then passes into the distensible gullet, which can secrete mucus from its lining, and on into the stomach. In some species, such as the carp family, there is no true stomach. The intestine may have small blind-ended tubes projecting from its lumen, known as **pyloric caecae**; these can enhance enzymatic digestion of food. In herbivorous fish, the gut is generally longer than carnivorous ones.

The liver is found around the stomach. It is often dark but varies between species and depending on diet. The gallbladder is a separate organ found further caudally. The pancreas is present in most fish and is often scattered throughout the mesenteric fat, or it can be incorporated within the liner as the hepatopancreas.

The **swimbladder** (Figure 4.84) is a structure unique to fish. It originates as a diverticulum of the oesophagus and has a thin wall. In some species its connection to the gut remains (**physostomous** fish) and in others it is now completely separate (**physoclistous** fish). In many cases the swimbladder has an area that actively secretes gas (the so-called **gas gland**) and another which absorbs it (the **oval gland**). Homeostasis between the two allows the swimbladder to maintain neutral buoyancy. Physostomous fish can augment the gas in the swimbladder by rising to the surface and gulping in air, which can then pass through the gut and into the swimbladder.

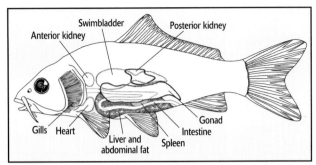

4.84 Internal anatomy of a carp. (Reproduced from *BSAVA Manual of Ornamental Fish, 2nd edition*)

Cardiovascular system

The heart has only one atrium and one ventricle. Blood returns to the heart via two blood vessels: the common cardinal vein, which receives blood from both the head and the body, and the hepatic vein(s). These empty into a small antechamber, the sinus venosus, which then empties into the atrium. Valves separate the atrium from the ventricle. The ventricle empties into the conus arteriosus, a muscular precursor to the ventral aorta. The ventral aorta moves cranially and divides into the branchial arteries, which supply the gills with blood. These move on to coalesce into the dorsal aorta, which then moves caudally to supply the rest of the body with oxygenated blood.

There is a renal portal system in fish, similar to that seen in birds and reptiles, and a hepatoportal system.

Fish erythrocytes are nucleated.

Urogenital system

Urinary tract

The kidneys are found just ventral to the spinal column, above the swimbladder. They are paired and are often fused together. The cranial portion of the kidney is responsible for producing erythrocytes, whilst the caudal part is excretory. The structure of the kidney itself differs depending upon whether the fish in question is a marine, freshwater or brackish (slightly salty) water dweller. In general they cannot produce hyperosmotic urine. It is important to note that the gills, not the kidneys, are the most important organ for the excretion of ammonia, the main waste product of protein metabolism.

The ureters lead to the urinary papillae and may fuse and deliate to form a bladder in some species.

Osmoregulation and excretion

Marine fish are hyposmotic in relation to their environment and so lose water across the gills continuously. This is counteracted by the fish drinking sea water, but this results in a build-up of salts. As the kidneys cannot produce hyperosmotic urine, the excess salt is excreted in marine fish via salt glands in the gills, which actively excrete sodium and chloride ions. The kidneys remove the divalent ions such as magnesium and calcium.

In freshwater fish the opposite situation occurs, as the fish tissues are now hyperosmotic in relation to the environment. They therefore need to excrete water and this causes loss of salts as well. Any deficiencies in individual elements such as sodium or chloride is made up by active absorption across the gills.

Reproductive system

In males and females, the gonads are paired and internal and tend to lie alongside and slightly ventral to the swimbladder. In the males, a vas deferens connects the testis to the vent. In females, the gonads may be extremely large, producing hundreds of eggs and filling most of the coelomic cavity. Fertilization of the oocytes in most fish takes place externally, once they are shed from the vent. The male passes over the top of the shed oocytes and in turn sheds sperm from his vent.

Sex is determined by chromosomes in many teleosts (females being XX and males XY). In many species there is sexual variation between the sexes, with the males being more colourful than females, but some species show no sexual dimorphism.

Skin

The outer layer of the skin (the epidermis) is thrown into a series of folds, covering the underlying scale structure, which projects from within the dermis. The epidermis has a basement membrane and then a series of fibrous Malpighian cells, which become progressively flattened as they mature towards the surface. Other cells in the epidermis include goblet cells and club cells, as well as immune system cells such as lymphocytes and macrophages. The secretions of the mucus cells allow a build-up of a mucopolysaccharide layer of cellular material and mucus often referred to as the **glycocalyx**. It provides a protective function from pathogens, reduces friction with the water when swimming and reduces osmotic loss/gain of water across the skin.

The scales are small dermal bony plates that overlap one another. They derive from scale pockets, with growth occurring around the attached edge producing a series of concentric rings. Scales are only replaced when lost, there being no 'moulting' of scales. Some species have evolved or been bred without scales. Coloration of the skin arises from chromatophores present in the skin.

Nervous system

Fish have only 10 cranial nerves. The spinal column gives off segmental nerves supplying the muscles of the trunk. There is an internal ear, and fish use a system of pressure sensors running along the midline of each flank, known as the **lateral line** system. The efficiency of sight varies between species. Focusing is achieved by the movement of the lens, rather than its contraction or relaxation. Some use **electrolocation** (the emission of weak electrical signals) to locate obstacles and prey.

Further reading

Girling SJ (2003) *Veterinary Nursing of Exotic Pets*. Blackwell Publishing, Oxford

Girling SJ and Raiti P (2004) *BSAVA Manual of Reptiles, 2nd edn*. BSAVA Publications, Gloucester

Harcourt-Brown N and Chitty J (2005) *BSAVA Manual of Psittacine Birds, 2nd edn*. BSAVA Publications, Gloucester

Harcourt-Brown N and Forbes N (1996) *BSAVA Manual of Raptors, Pigeons and Waterfowl*. BSAVA Publications, Gloucester

Meredith A and Redrobe S (2000) *BSAVA Manual of Exotic Pets, 4th edn*. BSAVA Publications, Gloucester

Wildgoose W (2001) *BSAVA Manual of Ornamental Fish, 2nd edn*. BSAVA Publications, Gloucester

Chapter 5

Genetics

Susan E. Long

Learning objectives

After studying this chapter, students should be able to:

- **Describe the structure of DNA**
- **Define the terms:**
  - **autosome, sex chromosome**
  - **gene, gene locus, allele**
  - **dominant, recessive, epistasis**
  - **homozygous, heterozygous**
- **Describe mitosis and meiosis and explain the difference**
- **Define Mendel's first and second laws and describe the modern interpretation**
- **Describe methods for identifying animals carrying a recessive gene**
- **Describe X inactivation and show how this is demonstrated in tortoiseshell cats**
- **Define inbreeding, line breeding, outcrossing and heterosis**
- **Describe the eradication schemes for:**
  - **hip dysplasia and elbow dysplasia in dogs**
  - **inherited eye disease in dogs**
  - **polycystic kidney disease in cats**
- **Describe the principles of DNA testing**

Introduction

Genetics is the science of inheritance, i.e. how characteristics are passed from one generation to the next. For ease of description the field is often divided into molecular genetics, cytogenetics, Mendelian genetics and population genetics.

- **Molecular genetics** deals with the molecular structure and manipulation of deoxyribonucleic acid (DNA), the genetic material found in the nucleus of a cell.
- **Cytogenetics** deals with chromosomes, which are molecules of DNA linked to protein.

- **Mendelian genetics** deals with inheritance in individuals of characteristics that are governed by a single gene or just a few genes. Genes are blocks of DNA and form the units of genetic inheritance. The field is named after Gregor Mendel, an Augustinian monk who lived in what is now the Czech Republic. He first described the principles of heredity in the middle of the 19th century.
- **Population genetics** deals with characteristics or traits that are governed by a large number of genes. Each gene obeys the principles of Mendelian genetics but because there are so many interacting genes the effect of each individual gene is difficult to predict. Such characteristics are best studied within a group or population of animals.

Genetic material

DNA

DNA has a unique structure (Figure 5.1). It consists of two chains of sugar and phosphate molecules (the 'backbone') joined together by other molecules, rather like the rungs of a ladder. The 'steps' of the ladder are formed by pairs of nucleotide bases: either adenine (A) and thymine (T), or guanine (G) and cytosine (C). A always links with T, and G always links with C. For example, if on one side of the ladder there is a sequence of AGTAACGGC, then on the other side of the ladder the sequence *must be* TCATTGCCG. Thus, the steps of the ladder are a sequence of **base pairs**. The structure of the base pairs is such that they cause the sides of the ladder to twist, forming a double spiral, or **double helix**.

In between the genes the base pairs have a random or non-coding sequence and this is often called **junk DNA**. Over millions of years individual variation in the non-coding part of DNA has developed because changes in this part of the DNA do not affect the viability of the animal. It is possible to detect this individual variation and so produce **genetic fingerprints**. DNA can be broken into small pieces by attacking certain base pair sequences. These particular sequences occur at different sites along the DNA molecule in different individuals. If these broken pieces are separated by electrophoresis, the differently

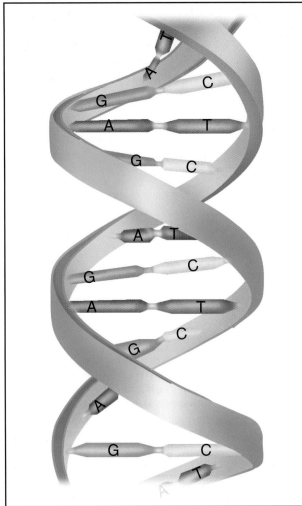

5.1 The structure of DNA. The 'steps' of the 'ladder' are a sequence of *base pairs* and their structure is such that they cause the sides of the ladder to twist, forming a double spiral, or double helix.

- **Sex-linked genes:** the orange coat colour gene in cats and the gene for haemophilia A in dogs are both found on the X chromosome and are therefore examples of sex-linked (or X-linked) genes.
- **Sex-limited genes:** the genes associated with milk quality are carried by both males and females but can only be expressed in the females; therefore these genes are said to be sex-limited.
- **Lethal genes:** the gene that causes lack of a tail in the cat is the manx gene. When two copies of this gene are present, this is lethal and the embryo dies *in utero*.

Mutations

Mutations are permanent changes in the structure of DNA. If they occur in a somatic cell (i.e. a body cell other than sperm or eggs), when that cell divides the new cell will have the mutation but it will not be passed to any offspring. If they occur in the cells that produce either sperm or eggs, that mutation can be passed on to offspring. A mutation is not necessarily bad. Most mutations do not occur in a part of the DNA where a gene is located, but if they do, one of two things may happen:

Either:

The change is so great that the gene can no longer produce an instruction for its protein. In this case the gene is destroyed and lost. If this occurs in an embryo, it may result in an abnormality or even death of the animal.

Or:

The change allows coding but a slightly different instruction is produced. The gene still exists but there has been a small change. A gene that has been changed is said to be an **allele** of the original gene. Not all mutations are 'bad'. Most have a neutral effect, i.e. they are neither advantageous nor disadvantageous as regards the survival of the individual. A few are advantageous and convey a competitive advantage to the individuals that carry them.

Alleles

Alleles are alternative forms of a gene. A gene can have any number of alleles, depending on how often mutations have occurred at that place in the DNA. However, there can only be a maximum of two different alleles in a cell, because alleles are found at the same locus and there are only two loci in a cell (one on each homologous chromosome).

- If there are two different alleles in the cell, the animal is said to be **heterozygous** for that gene.
- If there are two copies of the same allele, the animal is said to be **homozygous** for the gene.

The gene **locus** is the 'gene address' on the chromosome. Each gene has a different address and cannot 'live' at another address on the chromosome (which can be thought of as a block of flats with a series of different addresses). Since chromosomes come in homologous pairs, there will be two 'blocks of flats' with the same addresses in each. **Alleles** are members of the same family that live at the same address (i.e. locus), but only one allele can be 'at home' at the same time. Thus, even though a gene may have many alleles, only two alleles can be present in a cell – one on each homologous chromosome at the appropriate locus.

sized pieces move at different rates. This results in a pattern like a barcode that is different for different animals and this is the genetic fingerprint.

A **microsatellite** is a short DNA sequence that is repeated many times within the animal or organism. The number of repeats at a particular site is highly variable between individuals of the same species and therefore characteristic of that individual.

Genes

Genes are specific sequences of the base pairs. They act to instruct the production of proteins. Each gene has a specific location on a specific chromosome which is called the **gene locus**. Since chromosomes are in pairs it follows that genes come in pairs.

If a gene locus is on the sex chromosome, the gene is said to be **sex-linked**. Genes are usually expressed in the same way in either sex but some genes control characteristics that are only expressed in one sex. Such genes are said to be **sex-limited**.

Some genes or gene combinations are not compatible with life and these are said to be **lethal genes** or **lethal factors**. If an individual receives such a gene or genes, that individual dies.

Chromosomes

Within the cell nucleus the DNA molecule is very tightly folded and coiled and is surrounded by protein to form the chromatin fibres of the **chromosomes**. The chromosomes are usually considered in pairs. One of each pair is inherited from each parent. The chromosomes in a pair are alike in morphology and the types of genes that they carry, and are therefore said to be **homologous** (meaning 'same').

Each species has a characteristic number of chromosomes. For example, the number of chromosomes in the cell of a cat is 38 (Figure 5.2), in a dog is 78, and in a horse is 64. If all the chromosomes from a cell in each of these species were weighed, the total weight of the genetic material would be more or less the same; in other words, they have roughly the same amount of genetic material but it is cut into a different number of pieces.

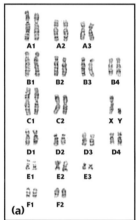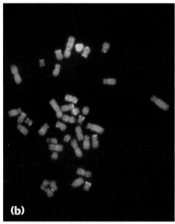

(a)

(b)

5.2 Cat chromosomes. **(a)** Karyotype showing 2n = 38,XY. Stained by Giemsa-banding. **(b)** Fluorescence microscopy image of metaphase, following hybridization with chromosome-specific DNA paint probes, showing the X chromosome (red) and Y chromosome (bright green). (Courtesy of Professor MA Ferguson-Smith and Dr Fengtang Yang, Cambridge University Centre for Veterinary Science)

Sex chromosomes and autosomes

Two of the chromosomes are called the **sex chromosomes** and are designated X and Y. In mammals, females have two X chromosomes (XX), and males have one of each of the sex chromosomes (XY). In males the Y chromosome is inherited from the father and the X chromosome is inherited from the mother. In females one X chromosome is inherited from the mother and the other X chromosome is inherited from the father. Thus females are said to have a maternal and paternal X chromosome.

The chromosomes that are not the sex chromosomes are called **autosomes**.

Chromosomal abnormalities

It is possible to use the ordinary light microscope to examine chromosomes and therefore assess the number and morphology of any abnormalities. Chromosomal abnormalities often mean that the affected chromosomes have difficulties pairing during cell division. This is most apparent during meiosis (see later) and so chromosome anomalies often result in reduced fertility or even sterility.

The cell cycle and cell division

When a cell is carrying out its normal day-to-day functions, it is said to be in **interphase (G1)**. In order to replicate itself, it first has to synthesize new genetic material – the **synthesis (S)** stage. This is followed by a **resting** stage, called **G2** (G stands for 'gap'). Then there is separation of the new genetic material into the two new cells; this is the **nuclear division** or **M** phase. The two new cells can then get on with their jobs, so they are again said to be in interphase. Thus, there is a **cell cycle** (Figure 5.3).

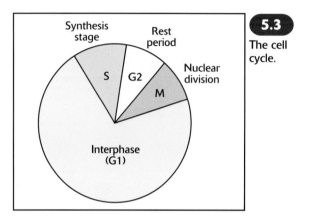

5.3 The cell cycle.

When a cell divides, the chromosomes must replicate exactly; otherwise the new cells would not be coding for the same characteristics. Many cells in the body are continually replicating (e.g. cells from the lining of the intestine) and it is important that the new cells can carry on the functions of the old. In these circumstances the nuclear division is by a process called **mitosis**. Mitotic division results in two new cells with nuclei (and hence genetic material) that are exactly the same as in the original cell.

The cells forming sperm and eggs divide in a different way, called **meiosis**. This results in the new cells having only half the amount of the original DNA ('haploid'), and the genes are mixed up a little. Thus, when a sperm fertilizes an egg, the new embryo has the right amount of genetic material ('diploid') and a mixture of DNA from the mother and father.

Mitosis

Mitosis occurs after the S phase and so each chromosome already has an exact replica of itself (see Chapter 4). The original and replica chromosomes are joined together at the **centromere**. In the S phase, the two copies of the same chromosomes that are held together at the centromere are called **chromatids** (Figure 5.4).

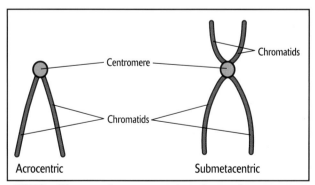

5.4 Diagramatic representation of metaphase chromosomes.

The final separation of the chromosomes and creation of two new cells is a dynamic process, but for the purposes of description it is divided into four stages:

1. **Prophase** – this is when all the chromosomes condense and become shorter and thicker.
2. **Metaphase** – the nuclear membrane breaks down and during this stage the chromosomes line up in the middle of the cell and become attached to fibres that are called the cell **spindle**.
3. **Anaphase** – at this stage the old and new chromosomes separate by moving to different sides of the cell. This is possible because the centromere divides.
4. **Telophase** – the nuclear membrane forms around each group of chromosomes to create two new nuclei and the cytoplasm divides to form two new cells.

Meiosis

A different type of cell division is necessary for those cells that are going to develop into **gametes** (eggs and sperm). This is called meiotic division. It is made up of two cell divisions (**meiosis I** and **meiosis II**), during which the number of chromosomes in the daughter cells are halved. The stages are similar to those of mitotic division, i.e. prophase, metaphase, anaphase and telophase, but the first meiotic division is a longer and more complicated process (Figure 5.5).

The chromosomes have to be separated into different gametes in such a way that the total number is reduced by half and yet there is still one copy of each pair of alleles that was present in the parent cell. In this way, when the two gametes fuse to form a zygote, the new individual has the right number of chromosomes for the species and the right combination of

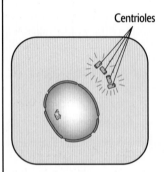

Interphase I

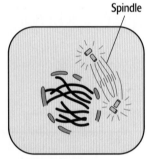

Prophase I

This is divided into five stages: leptotene, zygotene, pachytene, diplotene and diakinesis. During this time the chromosomes contract and crossing over takes place.

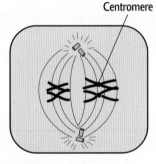

Metaphase I

Homologous pairs of chromosomes lie side by side on the cell spindle so that there are two rows of chromosomes (unlike in mitosis when there is a single row).

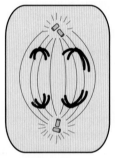

Anaphase I

The spindle fibres contract and homologous chromosomes separate to opposite ends of the cell. The centromeres do not divide as in mitosis.

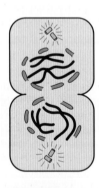

Telophase I

This is the stage of cytoplasmic division. In the female two separate cells are produced (the ovum and first polar body) but in the male cytoplasmic division is often incomplete and the cell has a dumb-bell shape with two sets of chromosomes.

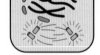

Prophase II

The chromosomes remain contracted.

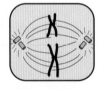
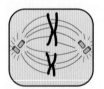

Metaphase II

This is like mitotic metaphase. The chromosomes line up one below the other on the equator of the spindle.

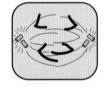
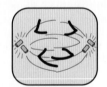

Anaphase II

Like mitotic anaphase. The spindle fibres contract, the centromere divides and the chromatids are pulled apart and move to opposite ends of the cell.

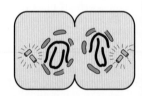
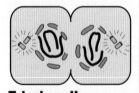

Telophase II

The cytoplasm divides. In the female this forms the ovum and second polar body and in the male the spermatids.

 Meiosis.

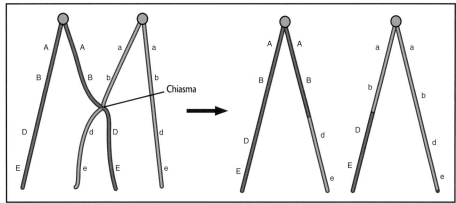

5.6 Crossing over. During prophase I of meiosis, homologous chromosomes, each comprising two chromatids, come to lie next to each other. At random points the chromatids break and reunite with their homologous partners. Thus, alleles that were on one chromosome cross over to the homologous chromosome.

genes in order that each cell can perform its function. Thus, each individual receives half its chromosomes (and so half the genes) from one parent and half from the other.

Before meiosis I, new DNA is synthesized in the S phase of the cell cycle, as with mitosis, and the new chromosomes are held together at the centromeres.

In meiosis I, prophase is much longer than in a mitotic division and so it is described as having five stages: leptotene; zygotene; pachytene; diplotene; diakinesis. During the latter stages of meiotic prophase, crossing-over takes place (Figure 5.6).

During metaphase I the chromosomes line up in the centre of the cell with homologous chromosomes lying side by side. The homologous chromosomes then move to opposite ends of the cell so that half the chromosomes are on one side and half on the other. This is anaphase of the first meiotic division. Telophase is the division of the cytoplasm but the second cell division begins immediately and this is just like a mitotic division. Thus, from one original cell, four new cells are formed, each of which contains half the original number of chromosomes. The new individual inherits the genetic material from each parent but with some variation because of the crossing-over.

Differences between mitosis and meiosis

- In meiotic prophase I, the homologous chromosomes lie side by side. In mitotic prophase they do not
- In meiotic metaphase I, the homologous chromosomes line up on the metaphase plate side by side. In mitosis they line up one below the other
- In meiotic telophase I, the nuclear membrane does not reform and a second division begins immediately.

Inheritance

Mendel's laws

Gregor Mendel (1822–1884) was the first to propose 'laws' governing inheritance. The laws were formulated so that people could calculate the expected outcome of crossing animals or plants even though at that time the mechanism of inheritance was not understood.

Mendel's first law

Mendel's first law states that **alleles separate** to different gametes. It is now known that this is because alleles are on different homologous chromosomes and these separate to different gametes at meiosis.

Mendel's second law

Mendel's second law states that there is **independent assortment** of pairs of alleles, i.e. alleles of different genes separate at random. For the most part this is true. However, it is now known that gene loci that are close together on a chromosome are more likely to be inherited together and so it is not entirely a random process. This is because gene loci can be separated during crossing-over. If two genes lie far apart on a chromosome, there is a greater chance of a cross-over event than if they are lying close together. Genes lying close together on a chromosome are said to be **linked** or to show **linkage**. This is an advantage if both genes are desirable but a disadvantage if a breeder is trying to retain one gene and eradicate the other.

Dominant and recessive genes

If there are two different alleles in a cell, it might be expected that both alleles would be 'expressed', i.e. their effects would be apparent in the animal's appearance. In fact this does happen in many circumstances when the genes are **co-dominant** (e.g. the genes coding for blood groups). However, some alleles are only expressed if there are two copies of the same allele in the cell. These are said to be **recessive** genes. Genes that can be expressed when only one copy is present and which can suppress the other allele are said to be **dominant** genes. The different types of gene are symbolized by a capital letter for a dominant gene and a lower case letter for a recessive gene.

Example

The black coat-colour gene in the Labrador is dominant to the brown gene that codes for chocolate. Therefore, the black gene is designated *B* and the brown gene is designated *b*.

A black Labrador can have either *BB* or *Bb* genes, because black is dominant to brown and the *B* gene will suppress the expression of the *b* gene. Thus *BB* and *Bb* animals have the same **phenotype** (i.e. the same appearance) but a different **genotype** (i.e. different genetic make-up).

Chocolate Labradors must all be *bb*, because brown is recessive and can only be expressed if two copies of the allele are present.

Identification of animals carrying a recessive gene

Animals homozygous for a particular gene will always breed true when bred together, but heterozygous animals will sometimes produce offspring that are homozygous for the recessive gene. Usually (but not always), the recessive gene is unwanted and so breeders would like to be able to identify those animals that are heterozygous for a recessive gene and avoid breeding from them.

Identification of the recessive carrier can be done by test mating to a homozygous recessive animal. This test mating is known as the 'back cross to the recessive'. Such a mating is useful if the recessive gene involves something like coat colour but it is not possible if the homozygous animal has an abnormality or demonstrates a disease. In that case the mating has to be with a known heterozygous carrier.

The animals that are mated are the **parent generation** and the offspring are the **filial** or **F_1 generation**. If the offspring were to be mated they would produce the **F_2 generation** and so on.

Test mating with a homozygous recessive animal

If you have a black Labrador and you want to know whether its genotype is *BB* (i.e. homozygous for the dominant *B* black allele) or *Bb* (i.e. heterozygous for the recessive *b* brown allele) then you can cross it with a chocolate (*bb*) Labrador.

- If the black Labrador is *BB* then all the offspring will be black puppies (although with the genotype of *Bb*).
- If the black Labrador is *Bb*, it will still produce black puppies, but it will also produce chocolate (*bb*) puppies.

How this arises is demonstrated below.

Checkerboard for determining the genotype of offspring:

Bb (father) × *bb* (mother)

Sperm of father	*B*	*b*
Eggs of mother		
b	*Bb*	*bb*
		offspring
b	*Bb*	*bb*

It can be calculated mathematically that if the black Labrador produces seven black puppies when mated to the chocolate Labrador then you can be 99% sure that its genotype is *BB*. The more black puppies that are produced, the more certain you can be that the genotype is *BB*. If just one chocolate puppy is produced, irrespective of the number of black, then you know that the black Labrador must be *Bb*. You do not have to mate the black Labrador to the same chocolate Labrador to get the offspring: it is the number of offspring that is important.

Test mating with a known heterozygous carrier

If a black Labrador has previously produced a chocolate puppy, then that black Labrador *must* be *Bb*, i.e. a known heterozygote. You can therefore mate your unknown black Labrador with this known heterozygote. If the unknown Labrador is really *Bb* , the checkerboard will be:

Sperm of father	*B*	*b*
Eggs of mother		
B	*BB*	*Bb*
		offspring
b	*Bb*	*bb*

This time 16 black puppies would have to be produced before you could be 99% sure that the animal was *BB* and not *Bb*. Again, these puppies do not have to be produced from a single mating and the birth of just one chocolate puppy will prove the dog to have been *Bb*.

Epistasis

The terms dominant and recessive apply to the interaction of alleles. Some genes can interact with other genes that are not their alleles, i.e. they suppress the effect of genes at a different locus. These genes are said to have epistatic effects on the other genes, or to show epistasis. An example is the albino gene blocking the expression of all the coat-colour genes.

Sex chromosomes and X inactivation

The Y chromosome is usually quite small and carries the genes that code for maleness. Very few other genes are carried on the Y chromosome. In contrast, the X chromosome is often one of the largest chromosomes and carries a number of genes that are important in the day-to-day metabolism of the cell. Since females have two X chromosomes (XX) and males have one X chromosome and one Y chromosome (XY), it follows that females must receive twice the number of genes that are carried on the X chromosome compared with males. In order to compensate for this, only one X chromosome in each cell of a female is activated and the genes on this chromosome are functional. The other X chromosome becomes highly contracted and most of the genes are inactivated and non-functional. This is called the **Lyon hypothesis of X inactivation and gene compensation** (after the person who first put forward the hypothesis). The decision as to which X chromosome is to become inactive in a cell (i.e. the paternal or maternal X chromosome) is a random process and is settled very early on during embryogenesis. Thereafter, all the daughter cells have the same X chromosome inactivated. Thus a female has some cells where the paternal X chromosome has activated genes and other cells where it is the maternal X chromosome that has activated genes.

The tortoiseshell coat colour and male tortoiseshell cats

The tortoiseshell coat colour in cats is a mixture of ginger and black/tabby etc., and is usually only seen in females. It is produced as the result of the epistatic effects of the sex-linked orange (*O*) gene on the autosomal black/tabby etc. genes. In cells with an *O* gene on the X chromosome, the hair colour will be ginger even if there are other coat-colour genes on the autosomes. Therefore, male cats may have an X chromosome that carries the orange gene and be $X^O Y$. This produces the ginger coat colour. Alternatively, their X chromosome may not have the orange gene and therefore they are $X^- Y$ and their autosomal coat colour genes will be expressed.

Females, with two X chromosomes, have three possibilities: $X^- X^-$ cats will be black or tabby etc. depending upon which autosomal genes they have; $X^O X^O$ cats will be ginger (yes, it *is* possible to have ginger female cats); and $X^- X^O$ cats will be tortoiseshell, i.e. patches of ginger and patches of black/tabby etc. There are patches of colour because in a female cell only one X chromosome is functional and the other is inactivated (Lyon hypothesis, see above). Since the inactivation takes place at random at about day 12 of gestation in the cat, there are groups of cells with a different active X chromosome and therefore groups of cells in the skin that produce the ginger coat colour or black or tabby.

In theory, male tortoiseshell cats should not occur. However, a few do appear and they are chromosomally abnormal in that they either have an extra X chromosome in each cell (e.g. XXY, called the **Klinefelter syndrome**) or have more than one cell line (i.e. they are **chimaeric**, e.g. XX/XY or XX/XXY or XY/XXY etc.). The XXY Klinefelter cats have always been infertile. Some of the chimaeric cats with a normal XY cell line are fertile but an XY cell line does not guarantee fertility.

Multifactorial inheritance and the influence of environment

Some characteristics are governed by single genes but many characteristics are controlled by the cumulative effect of many genes. Such characteristics are said to be **polygenic**.

Sometimes, when a characteristic is controlled by many genes the expression of the characteristic can vary in degree. That is, the characteristic is said to show **variable expressivity**. All the animals carrying the main gene for the trait express the trait but the expression is modified by other genes to create the variation in expression.

Some other polygenic characteristics show **incomplete penetrance**. That is, not all the animals that carry the major genes express them, because of modification by minor genes. However, all the animals that *do* express the trait do so to the same extent.

Some characteristics will be affected by the environment. For example, the size of a dog will depend on many genes but also on the amount of food available. When the environment can influence a characteristic, as well as genes, that characteristic is said to be **multifactorial**. It is obvious that these characteristics will have great variation and be very difficult to control by selection.

The proportion of the variation of a characteristic within a population that is due to different genes (i.e. not the variation in environment) is called the **heritability** of the characteristic. For example, if only half the variation is due to variation in genes, the heritability is 50% (also written as 0.5).

Parentage analysis

The ability to identify the parentage of an individual depends upon two basic facts:

- There is genetic variation. That is, no two individuals are *exactly* alike genetically, because regions of DNA show **polymorphism**
- An individual inherits its genes from its parents. That is, the genotype can be traced back to the parents.

In general the dam is known and it is the sire that is in doubt. If neither parent is known the process is more complicated but the principles are the same. Parentage analysis can be carried out in two ways:

- **By looking at the expression of genes and alleles** in the individual and possible parents. This is what is done when parents are identified using **blood typing**. Red cell surface antigens, white cell surface antigens and serum proteins can be examined and those of the individual and putative sires can be compared. If the offspring has something that is not found in the dam, it is assumed to have been inherited from the sire. All sires without that characteristic can therefore be excluded. The more

characteristics that are examined, the more sires there are that can be excluded, until only one possible candidate remains
- **By looking at the DNA itself.** This is usually described as **DNA profiling**.

DNA profiling

In practice, what is done is to look at a specific type of DNA called **microsatellites**, which are tandem repeats of base pairs found at the same site along the genome in different animals of the same species. They are highly polymorphic, i.e. there can be a different number of repeats, but related individuals inherit the same number of repeats. For the purposes of international comparability the microsatellites are tested to ensure that there is sufficient variation in a population before it is used. The more microsatellites used, the easier it is to exclude possible parents. A trial by the American Kennel Club showed that the use of between 10 and 15 microsatellites could provide a universal canine panel.

Microsatellites that are associated with a trait are called **markers**, because they mark the presence of the gene responsible for the trait and are inherited along with that gene.

DNA profiling can be carried out using any cells that contain DNA. In practice, the most convenient source of cells is from a **blood sample**. Alternatively, cells from the **buccal mucosa** can be collected on a swab, but this does not generally provide as many cells from which to extract the DNA for analysis.

As a result of parentage analysis, possible parents can be *excluded* with 100% certainty on the basis that they could not have been able to contribute to the genome of the individual.

Those that are not excluded *could* be a parent. The aim is to use sufficient tests such that the probability of two *possible* parents having the same combination would be so small as to be negligible.

Breeding strategies

When breeders wish to ensure that their animals breed true, they try to make them homozygous for the genes governing the desirable characteristics. The quickest way to increase homozygosity is to inbreed.

Inbreeding

Inbreeding is the breeding of two individuals more closely related than the population as a whole. Related individuals are more likely to have the same alleles and so more likely to produce offspring that will be homozygous for the genes. The more closely related the individuals, the more likely it is that the offspring will be homozygous at any particular gene locus. This is called the **coefficient of inbreeding**, which is the probability that two alleles at any locus will be alike by descent, i.e. the alleles will be alike because they have been inherited down the maternal and paternal line through a common ancestor (Figure 5.7).

Unfortunately, inbreeding will create homozygosity, i.e. it will fix the 'bad' alleles as well as the 'good' alleles. This is why inbreeding is generally considered as dangerous. The chances of good or bad alleles being fixed are the same.

One way to reduce the intensity of inbreeding (and hence the likelihood of producing homozygosity for a bad gene – or a good gene) is to carry out line breeding.

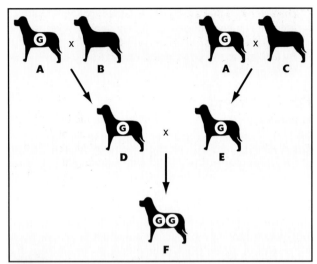

5.7 How an individual can be homozygous for a gene, by descent. The individual F will inherit genes from individual A through the paternal and maternal lines. Thus it is possible for two copies of the same allele to be inherited by F (one via the maternal line and one via the paternal line), who will therefore be homozygous by descent.

Line breeding

Line breeding is a form of inbreeding that involves mating within a certain family or line and which aims to maintain a relationship with a particular popular ancestor (e.g. show champion). Whilst the animals to be mated are related, they are not as closely related as, for example, father and daughter or brother and sister. They are more likely to be grandparents and grandchildren or cousins. The rationale is that whilst the relatives are chosen because they have the same 'good' alleles for the required trait, it is hoped that they will have different 'bad' alleles for the other characteristics. The hope is that the offspring will be homozygous for the chosen trait but remain heterozygous for all the possible bad alleles.

Outcrossing

The best way to reduce the chances of the offspring being homozygous for any given allele is to outcross. Outcrossing (or outbreeding) is the mating of two individuals less closely related than the population as a whole. Outcrossing masks the effect of recessive alleles, because unrelated individuals are unlikely to have the same unwanted recessive alleles. The offspring of an outcross show **hybrid vigour**, or **heterosis**, i.e. they are often 'bigger and better' than their parents. The major disadvantage of outcrossing is that the F_1 generation will not breed true, because they are heterozygous and not homozygous for their alleles.

Breed variation

Cats and dogs have been kept as pets for hundreds of years and during this time humans have selected certain characteristics that were deemed either useful or attractive. This has resulted in considerable breed variation. There are over 170 different breeds of dog, divided into 7 groups: Hound; Gundog; Terrier; Utility; Working; Pastoral; and Toy. Each breed has characteristics defined by the Kennel Club.

In cats, there are 37 different breeds recognized by the Cat Fanciers' Association.

In both dogs and cats, these breed characteristics are artificial in that they are defined by humans and are not necessarily those characteristics that make the animal best adapted to its environment.

Hereditary diseases and eradication schemes

Hereditary diseases or abnormalities are those caused by genes and which can be passed from one generation to another. Diseases or abnormalities that are present at birth are said to be **congenital**. Not all congenital diseases or abnormalities are hereditary. For example, a virus infection during gestation may result in the birth of abnormal offspring. This would be congenital but not genetic.

Conversely, not all genetic diseases will be manifested at birth. It may take a number of months or years for the defect to become apparent. This is true for a number of genetic eye defects.

Eradication schemes are based upon the identification of animals carrying the unwanted genes. This is easy for the problems caused by dominant genes, because every animal carrying even one copy of a dominant gene will express that gene and so they can be eliminated from the breeding population. Eradication is more difficult when the defect is caused by recessive genes. In these cases only homozygous individuals will express the defect and whilst these can be removed from the breeding population the heterozygous carriers will remain. Unfortunately, the majority of genetic abnormalities in dogs show a recessive mode of inheritance.

Traditionally, heterozygous carriers have been identified by test matings (backcross to the recessive) but increasingly it is possible to identify carriers using molecular genetic techniques.

Polygenic conditions, such as hip and elbow dysplasia, are also difficult to control because it is the combination of genes that causes the problem and many animals may have some of the genes but appear completely normal.

British Veterinary Association (BVA)/Kennel Club/International Sheep Dog Society Eye Scheme

This was the first eradication scheme to be set up in Britain. It currently covers 11 hereditary eye conditions in 47 different breeds. The causal gene and mode of inheritance of an anomaly can be different in different breeds, but many are recessive.

Interpretation of the morphology of the eye and its structures is very complex and so all the examinations are carried out by veterinary specialists in ophthalmology. These specialists comprise the Eye Panel Working Party. Dogs are best first examined before they are 1 year old and thereafter an annual examination will reveal any later developing anomalies.

The breeds and conditions are divided into Schedule 1 and Schedule 3. **Schedule 1** lists the *known* inherited eye diseases in the breeds where there is enough scientific information to show that the condition is inherited in that breed and often what is the mode of inheritance. For breeds in Schedule 1, a certificate is issued with results of 'affected' or 'unaffected' and these results are recorded and published by the Kennel Club. **Schedule 3** lists those breeds in which the conditions are only *suspected* as hereditary and therefore are 'under investigation'. With further work, breeds and conditions in Schedule 3 may be confirmed as inherited and therefore moved to Schedule 1.

BVA/Kennel Club Hip Dysplasia Scheme

Hip dysplasia is a polygenic multifactorial condition of the hips. Clinically there is a malformation of both the femoral head and acetabulum of the hip, which results in lameness, pain and degenerative joint changes. It is a particular problem in certain breeds of dog where the genes responsible for the condition have been concentrated, presumably during the inbreeding that produced the breed. The condition is exacerbated by increased exercise and rapid growth in the young prepubescent animal.

The basis of the scheme is radiographic examination of young adult animals in order to identify signs of malformation. For most breeds the examination takes place after the animal is 12 months old but for giant breeds it is delayed until they are 18 months old.

The radiographs are taken by the client's own veterinary surgeon and are then interpreted by a panel of experts. It is very important for accurate interpretation that the radiographs are taken with the animal in the correct position. A number of parameters are assessed on each hip by a member of the panel of experts and each parameter is given a score. The total for each examined point is the hip score. The lowest score, 0, indicates normality; the highest score, 106, indicates the worst possible expression of hip dysplasia.

The names and scores of dogs scored under the scheme are sent to the Kennel Club for publication and inclusion on the animals' documents.

Over the years a number of dogs have been examined from each breed and so it is possible to calculate a 'breed mean score' (BMS) for hip dysplasia. The recommendation is that only animals with a score well below the BMS should be used for breeding purposes. The BVA informs the Kennel Club of registered dogs with a score of 8 or less and no more than 6 on either hip. By following these recommendations the aim is slowly to reduce the BMS. The genes responsible for the condition will then be eliminated from the breed.

BVA/Kennel Club Elbow Dysplasia Scheme

Elbow dysplasia is the abnormal development of the cartilage of the elbow joint, with resultant wear leading to secondary osteoarthritic changes and eventually lameness. Like hip dysplasia, it is polygenic and multifactorial. In the dog there are three primary lesions: osteochondritis dissecans (OCD); fragmented or ununited coronoid process (FCP); and ununited anconeal process (UAP).

The eradication scheme is run in a similar manner to the hip dysplasia scheme. Two radiographic views of the elbow joint are required: extended lateral and flexed lateral. The client's own veterinary surgeon takes the radiographs when the animal is one or more years old and these are examined by a panel of experts. Each elbow is graded on a 0–3 scale, with 0 indicating normality and 3 indicating severe elbow dysplasia.

The names and scores of dogs graded under the scheme, together with the results, are sent to the Kennel Club for publication and inclusion on the relevant documents. It is recommended that only animals with a grade of 0 or 1 are used for breeding.

Feline Advisory Bureau (FAB) Polycystic Kidney Disease Screening Scheme

Polycystic kidney disease (PKD) is caused by a single autosomal dominant gene and so every animal carrying even a single copy of the gene will show clinical signs. Homozygosity for the gene causes such gross abnormal development of the kidneys that there is prenatal death. The condition is particularly common in Persian cats and related breeds.

The screening programme is based upon ultrasonographic examination of the kidney by a veterinary specialist. The cats should be over 10 months old in order that, when no cysts are found, there is confidence that small cysts have not been missed. A copy of the result of the scan is sent to the FAB.

Recently a genetic test has been developed to identify cats that carry the gene for PKD. This gene test is being validated and is likely to replace the ultrasound screening scheme.

Molecular genetic screening

Molecular genetic screening (also known as **DNA testing**) examines DNA and can differentiate between affected and carrier animals as well as normal animals. In the UK, the Animal Health Trust offers molecular genetic screening for a number of diseases in the dog, as follows.

Canine leucocyte adhesion deficiency (CLAD)

This is an immune deficiency disease found in Irish Setters. The test probes directly for the gene in DNA from a blood sample.

Congenital stationary night blindness in Briards

Again, the test probes directly for the gene and distinguishes affected, carrier and normal individuals. The test can be carried out on material from buccal mucosa.

Copper toxicosis in Bedlington Terriers

This test is based upon the fact that a microsatellite acts as marker DNA, which is inherited along with the gene causing the disease. For each dog tested, three to five generation pedigrees with disease status indicated are also requested. By this means, the test can be refined as more data are collected. Submitted samples can be either buccal mucosa or peripheral blood. Results are made available to the Bedlington Terrier Association.

Fucosidosis in English Springer Spaniels

Fucosidase is an enzyme necessary for the normal activity and function of nerves. The disease is caused by a deletion in the normal gene. It is identified using the polymerase chain reaction (PCR) to amplify the region of the gene that spans the deletion and then separating the DNA fragments on the basis of their size. The DNA fragment from the disease gene can be recognized because it is smaller than that from the normal gene. The test is carried out on DNA from a blood sample.

Phosphofructokinase deficiency in English Springer Spaniels

Deficiency of this enzyme leads to haemolytic anaemia and jaundice after exercise. The genetic defect is a small mutation in the phosphofructokinase gene. The DNA test involves determining the structure of the gene in the critical region, using DNA from a blood sample.

Progressive retinal atrophy (PRA) in Miniature Long-haired Dachshunds

Many forms of PRA exist, each form being confined to one or a few breeds only. The disease in Miniature Long-haired Dachshunds is caused by a mutation in one of many genes involved in sight. The test can be carried out on DNA from either blood or buccal mucosa.

PRA in Irish Setters

The test probes directly for the gene and can be done using a blood sample. DNA testing for PRA in Irish setters is carried out under a screening scheme run with the Kennel Club. Results are made publicly available through the Kennel Club website.

Pyruvate kinase deficiency in West Highland White Terriers

This disease results in a deficiency of the enzyme in red blood cells, resulting in haemolytic anaemia and disorders of the bone marrow and the liver. The test probes for the gene itself and can be carried out on DNA from a blood sample.

Further reading

Long SE (2006) *Veterinary Genetics and Reproductive Physiology: A Textbook for Veterinary Nurses and Technicians.* Elsevier (2006)

Nicholas FW (1996) *Introduction to Veterinary Genetics, 2nd edn.* Blackwell Publishing, Oxford

Robinson R (1991) *Genetics for Dog Breeders, 2nd edn.* Pergamon, Oxford

Vella CM, Shelton LM, McGonagle JJ and Stanglein TW (1999) *Robinson's Genetics for Cat Breeders and Veterinarians, 4th edn.* Butterworth-Heinemann, Oxford

Chapter 6

Infection and immunity

John Helps

Learning objectives

After studying this chapter, students should be able to:

- **Understand and define the common terms listed in bold type**
- **Describe relationships between microorganisms and host in health and disease**
- **List factors that may influence the occurrence, onset and severity of disease**
- **List possible routes of entry of infectious agents into the host, with examples**
- **Describe how pathogens establish, spread and multiply within the host, triggering disease**
- **List ways in which infections may be shed and transmitted**
- **Understand the principles involved in the control of infectious disease**
- **Describe the functional components of the immune system**
- **Understand the underlying principles of vaccines and vaccination**
- **Understand the principles of hypersensitivity and other immune disorders**

Principles of infection and infectious disease

Definitions

- **Infection** is the colonization of an individual (host) by a foreign microorganism. Infective agents that cause harm are termed **pathogens**, living within or on the host and disrupting physiological function. ▶

- **Disease** occurs when normal body function is sufficiently impaired to reduce performance, leading to recognizable clinical signs. Though infection is a common cause of disease, there are many other potential causes.
- Infectious diseases may be **contagious**, i.e. spread directly or indirectly from one individual to another. Important examples of contagious diseases are given in Chapter 21. The capacity of a pathogen to spread varies and depends on:
    - **Transmissibility** – the ability to pass from one host to another, typically determined by the capacity of the pathogen to survive outside the body
    - **Infectivity** – the ability to penetrate host defences.
- **Pathogenicity**, the ability of a pathogen to cause disease, depends on both its capacity to spread and its ability to harm the host, or **virulence** (Figure 6.1).
- **Epidemiology** is the study of the occurrence, spread and distribution of disease and is of vital importance in the design and monitoring of effective control policies.
- **Endemic** refers to a disease present at a normal level in a country or region. For example, myxomatosis is now an endemic disease in wild rabbits in the UK.
- **Epidemic** refers to a disease where a pronounced increase in incidence has been observed within a country or geographical region. The foot-and-mouth epidemic in the UK in 2001 led to controls on movement and widespread slaughter of infected and at-risk livestock.
- **Pandemic** refers to epidemic disease that spreads across many countries or continents. Avian influenza is a potential threat to the human population if mutation and recombination with the human influenza virus allows person-to-person infection and spread. This could potentially lead to a global pandemic similar to that seen in 1918–1919.
- **Epizootic** is sometimes used to refer to an animal disease epidemic. The outbreak of canine parvovirus in the 1970s was an epizootic. Widespread vaccination has ensured that this disease is now only encountered sporadically in the UK.

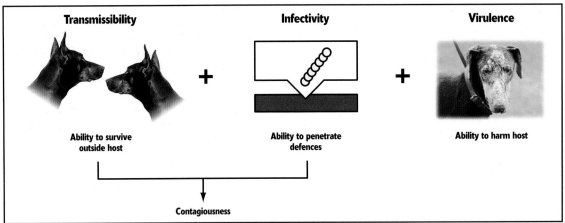

Transmissibility   **Infectivity**   **Virulence**

Ability to survive   Ability to penetrate   Ability to harm host
outside host   defences

Contagiousness

6.1
Factors influencing pathogenicity.

The resident microflora

Most microorganisms, or **microbes** (see Chapter 7), are useful to humans or even vital for life; relatively few are associated with ill health. The skin, oral cavity, conjunctiva, gastrointestinal tract and distal urogenital tracts all house a varied resident **microflora,** consisting of billions of microbes – principally bacteria. These organisms are described as **commensal,** because they share the body and usually do no harm; however, their presence may help to prevent the colonization of more harmful organisms.

Non-contagious disease

Microbes that normally live benignly on or within the host or environment can cause disease. Such infections, most commonly bacterial, are less likely to lead to disease in other in-contact individuals, but gain advantage in the affected host because normal innate immunity (see below) is weakened or bypassed, or abnormal local conditions favour infection.

Common examples include:

- Cat-bite abscesses
- Wound infections
- Bacterial skin infection (pyoderma)
- Bladder infection (bacterial cystitis).

Factors influencing occurrence and severity of disease

In order to trigger disease, pathogens need to:

- Penetrate host defences and establish themselves
- Multiply on or within host tissues
- Overcome the initial natural defence mechanisms inside the host
- Harm the host in some way.

The expression of disease in an individual depends on a balance between the nature of the infectious challenge and the resistance of the host.

The capacity of an infection to cause disease is determined by:

- The **infective dose,** i.e. the number of agents, such as bacteria or viral particles
- The **virulence** of the agent; this may vary between different **strains.**

Host susceptibility may be increased by:

- Immaturity
- Stress (e.g. transport, novel environment)
- Concurrent disease
- Genetic factors (e.g. inbreeding, breed predispositions)
- Lack of or reduction in immunity
- Medication (e.g. immunosuppressive drugs such as corticosteroids)
- Malnutrition.

Based on the balance between the infectivity of an agent and host susceptibility, a number of outcomes are possible:

- The pathogen may be eliminated by the immune system without consequence to the host
- **Subclinical infection** may occur, i.e. *without* disease but with the possible risk of transmission to other animals
- Disease may occur, associated with infection or risk of transmission to others.

The **incubation period** for an infectious disease is the time interval elapsing between exposure to the causative pathogen and the first clinical signs appearing. For many diseases this period is a few days but it may be weeks, months or even years. Dose and virulence of the infecting pathogen, as well as host susceptibility, can impact on both incubation period and severity of disease, so that within a group of infected individuals both the severity and onset of clinical signs can vary markedly.

Routes of entry

Pathogens infect new hosts via a variety of routes:

- **Ingestion** (taken in via the mouth): in contaminated food or water; during hunting or mutual grooming; through **coprophagia** (ingestion of faeces); through contact with infected items (fomites, see below)
- **Inhalation** (breathing in) of infected particles (droplet infection) (e.g. kennel cough)
- **Through the skin:** through bite or surgical wounds; via vectors such as fleas, ticks or mosquitoes
- **Via skin contact** (e.g. ectoparasites, ringworm)
- **Across mucous membranes:** gastrointestinal and respiratory epithelia are frequent entry routes; *Leptospira* bacteria may penetrate intact mucosae as well as damaged skin
- **Across the placenta or during birth** (e.g. *Toxocara canis,* feline panleucopenia, feline leukaemia virus).

Spread within the host

Pathogens commonly establish and multiply at the point of entry. For many viral pathogens, this is in the epithelial cells of the gastrointestinal or respiratory tracts. From these initial entry points spread to local lymph nodes may then occur. Infection may remain localized in response to a rapid immune response and/or because of a preference (**predilection, tropism**) for certain cell types. Alternatively the agent may spread into the blood circulation. The occurrence of virus within the blood is called **viraemia**. Bacterial infection may also remain localized, but serious infections can seed systemically via the bloodstream (**bacteraemia**). **Septicaemia** occurs if bacteria actively multiply in the bloodstream.

How pathogens trigger disease

Harm may be caused in a variety of ways:

- The cells within tissues may be destroyed by the pathogen itself. For example, in order to reproduce and propagate, viruses 'hijack' the normal metabolic processes of the host cell, finally rupturing and destroying the cell as new virus particles leave to infect other cells
- Biological poisons (**toxins**) may disrupt normal physiological function. The presence of toxins in the circulation is called **toxaemia**. In severe sepsis, circulatory collapse caused by endotoxic shock is a potentially life-threatening consequence. (See Chapter 7 for more discussion on microbial toxins)
- The response of the immune system to infection may cause damage. For example, in feline infections peritonitis (FIP), damage occurs as a result of the body's immune response to attempt to eliminate the coronavirus that triggers the disease. This may damage organs, commonly including the kidneys, eyes and central nervous system ('dry' form of FIP), or may lead to exudation of large quantities of fluid into the chest or abdominal cavity ('wet' form of FIP). See also 'Allergy and hypersensitivity reactions', below.

Transmission

For pathogens to succeed and propagate they need both to infect a host and to have the capacity to spread to other susceptible individuals.

Direct transmission

Spread by direct contact, direct transmission is particularly important for fragile pathogens such as feline leukaemia virus (FeLV) and feline immunodeficiency virus (FIV), because they are unable to survive for long outside the host.

Indirect transmission

This occurs if infection is acquired from a contaminated environment, or via a vector.

Mechanical vectors

Also known as **fomites**, these may be inanimate objects such as bedding, grooming kit, bowls and litter trays. People may also act as vectors by transporting infection on skin, clothing or shoes. For example, canine parvovirus persists for many months or years in the environment and is susceptible to few disinfectants. Virus is excreted by infected puppies for only a few days. Because of the virus's survival ability, indirect spread via ingestion from an environment contaminated by the faeces of infected dogs is the most significant route. Of course, direct ingestion of the faeces of an infected dog (coprophagia) would also be a possible route of transmission.

Biological vectors

These are organisms that may not cause disease in their own right but may convey infectious agents from one host to another. A number of significant canine diseases, for which dogs travelling to Europe and beyond may be at risk, are transmitted by biological vectors. Important examples of such vectors are: sandflies, which transmit leishmaniasis; ticks, which may transmit a number of serious infections including Lyme disease (borreliosis), babesiosis and ehrlichiosis; and mosquitoes, which may carry the *Dirofilaria immitis* heartworm.

Horizontal transmission

This term is sometimes applied to direct or indirect spread of infections between individuals of the same generation.

Vertical transmission

In some infections, transmission occurs from dam to offspring, either before or during birth. Possible effects of fetal infection include:

- Fetal death, resorption, mummification, abortion or stillbirth
- Birth of individuals showing clinical signs of disease
- Poor viability (e.g. fading kittens or puppies)
- Birth of infected carriers showing no disease signs.

Different infective agents may be excreted or 'shed' by a variety of routes. Careful consideration of likely routes of transmission enables appropriate disease control measures to be implemented.

Routes of transmission

- In saliva, via bites (e.g. rabies, FIV)
- In nasal or ocular discharges (e.g. feline upper respiratory tract disease, *Chlamydophila felis* conjunctivitis in cats)
- In urine (e.g. leptospirosis, infectious canine hepatitis)
- In faeces or vomitus (e.g. canine parvovirus, bacterial enteritis, panleucopenia
- In blood, via a biological vector (e.g. feline infectious anaemia caused by *Mycoplasma haemofelis* is transmitted by fleas)
- In milk (e.g. feline leukaemia virus, FIV, *Toxocara*)
- Across the placenta (transplacentally) to the fetus *in utero* (e.g. *Toxocara canis*, panleucopenia)
- By aerosol (i.e. airborne) (e.g. 'kennel cough', canine distemper)
- By skin contact (e.g. ectoparasites, ringworm)
- During coitus or parturition (e.g. panleucopenia, FIV).

Carriers

In some diseases infected animals, known as **carriers**, may continue to shed infective agents despite showing minimal or no signs of disease. For example, cats infected with feline herpesvirus (FHV) carry infection throughout their lives and may 'shed' virus *intermittently*, throughout life, with or without signs of disease, following episodes of stress. Between periods of shedding, the infection remains **latent** (dormant) and the virus cannot be isolated on swabs. In contrast, cats infected with feline calicivirus (FCV), shed virus *continuously* following apparent recovery from disease. Unlike FHV infection, most FCV-infected individuals eliminate the infection completely within weeks or months.

Controlling infection and disease

A range of measures needs to be taken in order to contain the potential spread of infection between animals and to humans (see 'Zoonoses', below) and to reduce the risk of disease occurring. Hygiene measures include:

• Efficient cleaning and appropriate use of disinfection of accommodation, paying attention to potential fomites (see Chapter 12)
• Careful cleaning and disposal of faeces, urine, body fluids and discharges; appropriate disposal of contaminated waste (see Chapter 12)
• Good hygiene in all stages of storage, handling and preparation of pet food. High quality tinned and dry diets are available and avoid the potential hazards of offering raw meat, which can potentially present a source of food-poisoning bacteria and parasites.

Animal management risks should be considered:

• Wear suitable protective clothing whenever handling animals and change once this becomes soiled
• Wash/disinfect hands between patients (Figure 6.2) and before touching any potential fomites – consider pens, clinical notes, cigarettes, door handles, food, cups, etc.
• Quarantine animals with suspected contagion and newly introduced animals of unknown health status (see below)
• 'Barrier nurse' cases of suspected infectious disease (see below).

To manage disease risk factors, consider the following.

• Ensure good draught-free ventilation and low stocking rates in multi-animal facilities such as kennels and catteries. Avoid mixing animals in large groups and in the same airspace.
• Rest accommodation following occupation for as long as practicable, depending on the likely persistence of the infectious agent(s) of concern, to reduce the risk of residual environmental contamination.
• Minimize stress through good husbandry. Ensure optimum nutrition and prompt attention to any ancillary health issues.

• Control disease vectors, such as external parasites. Where appropriate reduce populations of stray animals, via rescue centres and neutering programmes.
• Use appropriate vaccines in animals, both routinely and targeted where specific disease risks are identified.

Owners should be educated regarding disease risks, hygiene and good husbandry, including parasite control and vaccination.

Zoonoses

Zoonoses (singular: **zoonosis**) are diseases transmissible from animals to humans. Some are potentially life-threatening (e.g. rabies, leptospirosis), while others may pass unnoticed unless an individual is particularly susceptible. Toxoplasmosis is mainly a risk in pregnancy and immune-suppressed individuals. Figure 6.3 lists some important examples of zoonotic infections.

Apparently healthy animals may harbour infection and it may be unclear that an animal carries a zoonosis, so care should always be exercised. In addition to general risk-reduction measures listed above, some special precautions should be taken.

Precautions against the spread of zoonotic infections

• Do not allow animals to lick humans (particularly on the face and mouth) and especially children, as they have higher susceptibility and lower awareness of basic hygiene.
• Facilities and utensils for animal food preparation and washing up should be separate from those for human use.
• Avoid unnecessary exposure to infections: reduce unnecessary animal handling and ensure that handling technique minimizes risk (e.g. from bites/scratches).
• Pregnant women should be especially vigilant about personal hygiene after animal contact, since infection risks to the unborn are greater.
• Always seek medical advice if human infection is suspected.
• Tetanus immunization is advisable for all veterinary nurses. If working with zoo animals or captive primates, rabies and hepatitis vaccinations should also be considered.

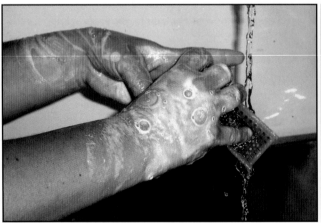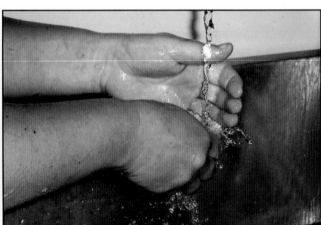

6.2 Hands should be washed thoroughly between handling each patient.

Disease/infection	Risk sources
Major enteric infections	
Campylobacter spp.	Contaminated food (esp. poultry meat); faeces of livestock, poultry, dogs, cats, wild birds
Salmonella spp.	Contaminated food; faeces of carrier mammals including livestock and pets, and of birds, reptiles and fish
Escherichia coli (Strain VTEC O157)	Contaminated food; faeces of healthy carrier livestock and birds
Cryptosporidiosis	Contaminated water; livestock (esp. calves, lambs)
Notifiable animal diseases in the UK	
Anthrax	Cutaneous form from contact with imported infected hide (very unlikely)
Avian influenza (fowl plague)	Airborne from infected poultry
Bovine spongiform encephalopathy (causes variant Creutzfeld-Jakob disease in humans)	Ingestion of contaminated beef
Bovine tuberculosis (TB)	Unpasteurized milk (now unlikely in the UK). Most cases due to human TB
Brucellosis	Contact with infected aborting cattle
Rabies[a]/European bat lyssavirus (EBL-2)	Mammalian hosts (esp. dogs) via bites. Risk in UK of EBL from bites from infected bats.
West Nile virus (WNV)[a]	Mosquito transmission – wild birds, horses
Other important zoonoses	
Hydatid disease[b]	Dog faeces
Leptospirosis	Water-borne; urine of infected rats, dogs, cattle
Orf	Viral skin infection of sheep
Pasteurellosis	Animal bites – cats and dogs
Psittacosis	Infected birds (esp. psittacines)
Ringworm	Contact with infected dogs, cats, livestock and wildlife (e.g. hedgehogs)
Toxocariasis	Dogs, cats (roundworms)
Toxoplasmosis	Cat faeces; uncooked meat

6.3 Some important examples of zoonoses. [a] Disease currently absent from UK; [b] *Echinococcus granulosus* tapeworm in UK, *E. multilocularis* currently absent from UK but present in mainland Europe.

Nosocomial infections

Infections acquired by patients in hospital are termed **nosocomial** infections and are of particular concern because the patient's immunity may be compromised by underlying disease, drugs, surgery, invasive supportive care (e.g. intravenous or urinary catheters), malnutrition or stress. Poor hygiene and transfer of pathogens between patients, combined with the potential for build-up of antimicrobial resistance, lead to increased risk of exposure and of more severe consequences if infection occurs.

Examples of nosocomial infections include:

- Urinary tract infection following repeated catheterization
- Wound infection following surgery
- Diarrhoea due to overgrowth of antibiotic-tolerant microbes.

Nosocomial infections may be minimized by:

- Adequate cleaning and disinfection of kennels between patients
- Good barrier nursing technique
- Reducing infection risk through:
  - Good wound management, e.g. changing soiled bandages
  - Correct management and hygiene of indwelling catheters and drains.

Antibacterial agents, although helpful in treating susceptible infections, may select for resistant microorganisms. An increase of antimicrobial resistance has reduced the ability to treat some formerly treatable infections in humans and animals. To reduce the build-up of resistance, antibiotics should be used only when strictly necessary and never as a substitute for good patient care and practical infection control measures.

MRSA: methicillin-resistant *Staphylococcus aureus*

MRSA is one notable example of a bacterium that can be acquired as a nosocomial infection. Harmless to most healthy individuals, it may be carried on the skin and mucous membranes of the nose, from where it may spread to susceptible hospital patients. Although not necessarily more pathogenic than other *Staphylococcus aureus* strains, it may cause serious disease in both human and animal hospital patients. MRSA is resistant to methicillin (a penicillin antibiotic), making it more difficult to treat than other staphylococci. Unfortunately, in some cases MRSA acquires multiple drug resistance against a wide range of antimicrobials.

Sterilization and disinfection

In microbiology, **sterilization** is the complete elimination of microorganisms from equipment and surfaces. To achieve this, surgical equipment is typically subjected to high temperatures and pressure within an **autoclave**.

Disinfection is the physical or chemical destruction of micro-organisms. A range of chemical disinfectants is available in order to achieve this. Because pathogens vary in their structure and properties, their susceptibility to different disinfectants varies too; true sterilization may be difficult to achieve by chemical means. For optimum effect an appropriate disinfectant needs to be selected, instructions for the correct dilution should be carefully followed and the product should be used in a physically clean environment. The use of disinfectants is described in Chapter 12.

Good wound management

All wounds, whether clean or contaminated (see Chapter 24), need proper care to reduce the risk of complications:

- Always wear sterile gloves
- All swabs, cotton buds or instruments entering the wound should be sterile
- Irrigation fluids used for flushing should be sterile
- Bandaging materials should also be sterile
- Dressings should always be changed regularly and if they become soiled or wet
- Self-trauma should be prevented if necessary by using an Elizabethan collar and by providing adequate pain relief.

Isolation and quarantine

Isolation

This is the physical segregation of an animal or group of animals suspected of having, or proven to have, a contagious disease, so as to eliminate the potential for transmission to other susceptible individuals. Isolation is also required for the exclusion of infections from 'high health status' animals, such as specific pathogen-free (SPF) animals used in research.

A self-contained isolation ward should be established with its own facilities for washing and disposal. It should hold a range of stock solely for use within the unit, including:

- Gloves, gowns, masks, overshoes for protection of personnel and clothing from contamination
- Bedding, food bowls, litter trays
- Disinfectants
- Medications, syringes, needles
- Appropriate diagnostic/monitoring equipment.

Ideally, the ward's entrance and its ventilation should be separate from those of the main hospital. A footbath at the entrance for disinfecting footwear and the allocation of different personnel to the isolation unit are useful precautions.

Potential routes of transmission (see above) should be carefully considered in designing procedures to avoid the spread of infection. The risk of spread of airborne pathogens can be minimized by reducing the number of animals in the same airspace and ensuring a good rate of air exchange. Within buildings, positive pressure ventilation may be used to encourage airflow from cleaner to potentially contaminated zones.

Barrier nursing

This is the term describing the precautions used in nursing an animal kept in isolation. This subject is covered in Chapter 12.

Quarantine

This is the segregation of individuals of unknown disease status for a period prior to entry to a new premises or country, to limit the risk of disease introduction. The UK has been free of terrestrial rabies since 1922, though endemic European bat lyssavirus has been identified in Daubenton's bats and has been responsible for causing 'bat rabies' in humans. Prior to the PETS travel scheme, 6 months of compulsory quarantine for all pet dogs and cats entering the UK successfully prevented reintroduction of the disease.

Pet Travel Scheme (PETS)

The **Pet Travel Scheme** has replaced the 6-month quarantine rule for dogs and cats entering the UK from designated countries, including EU member states, the USA, Japan, Australia, New Zealand and many rabies-free islands. The scheme operates via certain carriers and designated entry points within the UK, including Eurotunnel, major ports and airports. For countries outside these areas and for animals that fail to comply with PETS rules, the 6-month quarantine rule still applies.

'Pet Passports', recognized throughout the EU, hold all the relevant certification in booklet form and double as entry documents for many EU countries, simplifying export procedures.

To qualify to enter or return to the UK, a number of criteria have to be met. For an animal new to the Scheme, these are (in chronological order):

1. Identichip implantation.
2. Rabies vaccination.
3. Blood sample (2–4 weeks after vaccination).
4. Passing a serological test carried out on this sample to show adequate rabies immunity.
5. A correctly completed Pet Passport with the relevant identification, vaccination and blood testing details.
6. Waiting 6 months from the date of the blood test before animals can be considered for entry to the UK (note: the pet may qualify immediately to travel abroad).
7. A visit to a veterinary surgeon 24–48 hours prior to the return to the UK for tick and tapeworm treatment and certification to that effect.

In order to keep 'Passports' valid, rabies boosters need to be repeated *within* the duration of immunity of the particular vaccine used. Animals that lapse, even by one day, have to be revaccinated, blood tested again and observe a 6-month wait before they can enter the UK.

The up-to-date requirements of the Department for Environment, Food and Rural Affairs should always be checked: see www.defra.gov.uk .

The immune system

This is the defence system by which the body resists microbial or parasitic invasion. The immune system functions on three basic levels: physical barriers, innate immunity and acquired immunity. Throughout life, individuals are continuously exposed to a range of foreign antigens. These are delivered to the immune system, such that over time the individual becomes resistant to a wide range of pathogens.

Physical barriers

Physical barriers to invasion (the skin and the surfaces of the gastrointestinal, respiratory and urogenital tracts) provide an initial obstacle. The movement of mucus secretions up the respiratory tract, coughing, sneezing, urine flow, vomiting and diarrhoea all aid in clearing pathogens.

Innate immunity

Innate immunity constitutes the next layer of defence. Components of innate immunity are either pre-existing or rapidly activated:

- **Pre-existing**: e.g. enzymes such as lysozyme in tears and saliva, and various proteins that can bind to bacteria and hasten their destruction
- **Rapidly activated**: cells such as macrophages and neutrophils can recognize molecules on the outside of invading microbes before engulfing (by phagocytosis) and destroying them (Figure 6.4). Inflammation allows blood flow to increase to areas of damaged tissue, allowing such cells to be directed to the site of injury.

Innate immunity is a vital and effective layer of defence, but many pathogens successfully overcome it and more sophisticated and specific approaches are therefore required.

Acquired immunity

Acquired immunity recognizes and responds to specific foreign pathogens. Following infection, the immune system learns to produce specific cells and antibodies directed precisely against the particular pathogen involved. In contrast to the rapid response of innate immunity, this active immunity takes several days to begin to act against infections not previously encountered. However, because specific **memory cells** are formed following initial exposure, a much more rapid response may be expected if challenged by the same pathogen again.

Active immunity is initiated when components of foreign substances and microbes that trigger immune recognition (**antigens**) are collected by **antigen-presenting cells** (e.g. dendritic cells and macrophages) and delivered to lymph nodes, where they are presented to lymphocytes. Some lymphocytes specifically recognize the antigen and become activated.

There are two major divisions of acquired immunity: humoral and cellular.

Humoral immunity

Humoral immunity (Figure 6.5) is associated with B lymphocytes (B cells), which mature within bone marrow. Activated B lymphocytes develop into plasma cells, which manufacture proteins called **antibodies** (composed of immunoglobulins). Antibodies lock on to specific foreign antigens and neutralize them, or facilitate the binding of other components of the immune system. Humoral immunity can be measured by assessing the level of specific antibodies in the blood. Such tests are commonly used as diagnostic tests for specific infections (see Chapter 17).

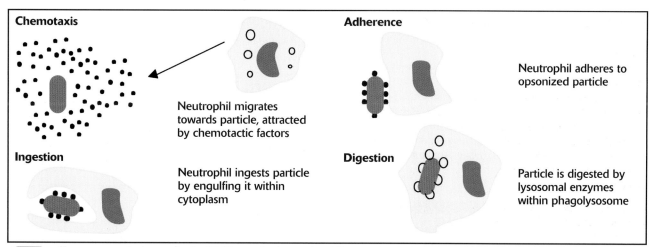

Chemotaxis

Neutrophil migrates towards particle, attracted by chemotactic factors

Ingestion

Neutrophil ingests particle by engulfing it within cytoplasm

Adherence

Neutrophil adheres to opsonized particle

Digestion

Particle is digested by lysosomal enzymes within phagolysosome

6.4 The process of phagocytosis. (1) **Chemotaxis**: neutrophils are attracted to areas of infection by chemical factors from bacteria or damaged cells. (2) **Adherence** of the neutrophil is facilitated by presence of **opsonins** such as antibodies or protein components known as **complement**. (3) **Ingestion**: the neutrophil engulfs the particle within its cytoplasm. (4) **Digestion**: the particle is digested within a phagolysosome by lysosomal enzymes.

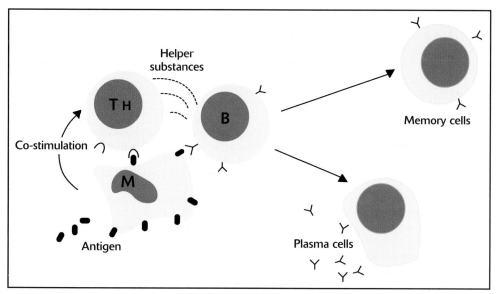

Helper substances

T H

B

Co-stimulation

M

Antigen

Memory cells

Plasma cells

6.5 B cells differentiate into antibody-producing plasma cells and memory cells. Interaction with and stimulation by antigen-presenting cells such as macrophages (M) and helper T cells (TH) is needed for this to occur.

Humoral immunity can be acquired via **passive transfer** of antibodies. In nature, this is by passage of **maternally derived antibodies (MDA)** across the placenta and in the first milk (colostrum) from a dam to her offspring. Whereas in humans the vast majority of MDA pass across the placenta before birth, in dogs and cats few MDA are received in this way and the vast majority are present in the colostrum. The intestine of neonatal animals is initially permeable to the passage of these antibodies, allowing an efficient transfer into their circulation. However, the efficiency of this transfer declines rapidly within hours of birth and this means that significant delays to colostral intake by young animals may lead to poor passive immunity and increased risk of infection. Whereas active immunity invokes immunological memory, passive immunity confers only *temporary* protection. Within a few weeks of birth, MDA decline to non-protective levels, whereupon young animals become more susceptible to disease.

Cellular immunity

This is associated with the activity of T lymphocytes (T cells), which mature within the thymus. Activated T lymphocytes manufacture chemical messengers called **cytokines**, which help to direct immune cell functions and responses. There are a number of different types of T lymphocyte:

- **Helper T cells** recognize processed antigen and coordinate macrophages and B cells in the immune response, promoting immune function (see Figure 6.5)
- **Cytotoxic T cells** destroy cells infected with intracellular pathogens such as viruses
- **Suppressor T cells** keep the immune system in check by suppressing immune reactions within tolerable limits. Decreased activity of these cells is one mechanism by which the immune system may begin to damage the body's own tissues and organs (see 'Autoimmune disease', below).

Principles of vaccination

The purpose of a vaccine is to stimulate an active immune response in the recipient against one or more specific pathogens, such that an improvement in clinical outcome is seen following infection. Resulting immunity varies, depending on the pathogen and vaccine, from full protection of the host against clinical disease, infection and shedding (**sterilizing immunity**) to simply a reduction of clinical signs following infection. The contribution made by vaccination towards preventing and reducing the incidence of major infectious diseases in humans and animals is, without doubt, enormous. Many serious contagious diseases are seldom seen today, but continued widespread vaccination is essential if this is to remain so.

Immunization may be passive or active:

- **Passive immunization** involves administration of **antisera** or **antitoxins**, containing concentrated antibodies against either a pathogen or a toxin, respectively. Used in the treatment of disease or at the time of possible exposure, passive immunization cannot give long-term protection, because the levels of antibody decline over several weeks. An important example is the preventive use of tetanus antitoxin (TAT) in horses with wounds and for therapy of animals with clinical tetanus

- **Active immunization**: most vaccines stimulate immunity by exposing the immune system to foreign antigens associated with specific infections. **Immunological memory** stimulated by such exposure means that, if challenged by the same infections, acquired immunity quickly neutralizes or minimizes the threat.

Types of vaccine

There are three broad categories of vaccine product designed for active immunization (see also Chapter 9): attenuated (live) vaccines; inactivated (killed) vaccines; and subunit, recombinant and vector vaccines.

Attenuated (live) vaccines

Live vaccines usually contain weakened (**attenuated**) strains of the pathogen, i.e. strains that cannot cause disease in the host. The immune response following vaccination with such products mimics what occurs following natural infection. Good cellular and humoral immunity is usually stimulated, and a protective immune response can often be expected rapidly after one dose. A potential concern of using live vaccines is reversion of the vaccine strain to virulence, but stringent trials required for licensing make this an unlikely scenario.

Inactivated (killed) vaccines

Inactivated vaccines remove the potential for reversion to virulence by containing pathogens that have been inactivated or killed. Many inactivated vaccines contain an **adjuvant** – a chemical substance that helps to stimulate a satisfactory immune response. Killed vaccines often also require two or more doses to stimulate an effective response (Figure 6.6) and are usually better at stimulating humoral than cell-mediated responses. In some cases, the immunity to a killed vaccine may not be as durable or complete as with a live equivalent.

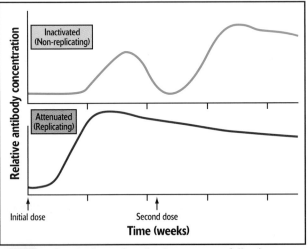

6.6 Comparison of antibody responses following inoculation with an inactivated vaccine (top) and a live attenuated vaccine (bottom). In this example, one dose of live vaccine is adequate to stimulate active immunity whereas a second dose of the inactivated product is required to stimulate a protective 'anamnestic' response.

Inactivated toxins used as vaccines are known as **toxoids**. Most commonly used in horses, tetanus toxoid stimulates active immunity to give longer-term protection in contrast to antitoxins, which are for short-term treatment and prophylaxis only.

Subunit, recombinant and vector vaccines

Subunit vaccines contain a small fragment or fragments of pathogen that contain the necessary antigens. Some are termed **recombinant** vaccines because they are manufactured using genetic engineering techniques. These products have the potential advantage of reducing unnecessary material in the vaccine.

Vector vaccines try to combine the potential advantages of live vaccines with some of the advantages of using an inactivated subunit vaccine. In vector vaccines the useful subunits are incorporated into a different non-pathogenic live virus. One feline leukaemia vaccine currently available in the UK uses a canarypox virus, genetically modified to contain important feline leukaemia virus (FeLV) antigens, to stimulate immunity.

Administering vaccines

Some vaccines contain single components (e.g. parvovirus alone) but, for convenience, a number of different components are often packaged together as a **multivalent** vaccine, conferring activity against more than one pathogen. Recommendations for use of different vaccines vary and are detailed within product data sheets. Live vaccines are often freeze-dried, requiring reconstitution with a diluent prior to use (Figure 6.7). Vaccine antigens available for use in dogs, cats and rabbits in the UK at the time of writing are listed in Figure 6.8.

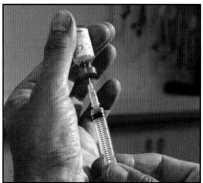

6.7 Preparing a vaccine for use.

For dogs
Canine distemper
Infectious canine hepatitis
Canine parvovirus
Leptospirosis (*L. canicola* and *L. icterohaemorrhagiae*)
Rabies
Kennel cough:
Canine parainfluenza virus [a]
Bordetella bronchiseptica [b]
Canine herpesvirus
Tetanus toxoid

For cats
Feline panleucopenia
Cat flu:
Feline calicivirus
Feline herpesvirus
Bordetella bronchiseptica [b]
Chlamydophila felis
Feline leukaemia virus
Tetanus toxoid

For rabbits
Myxomatosis
Viral haemorrhagic disease

6.8 Disease antigens currently available as vaccines for small animals in the UK. [a] Parenteral or intranasal combined vaccines available. [b] Intranasal vaccine available.

Not all vaccines are administered by injection. Figure 6.9 shows a *Bordetella* vaccine being administered intranasally to a cat. Intranasal administration stimulates the rapid formation of specific antibodies on the lining of the respiratory tract, which neutralize infection at the point of entry. Intranasal vaccines typically work within a few days and can be effective in the face of MDA, allowing some such products to be used to protect even very young animals.

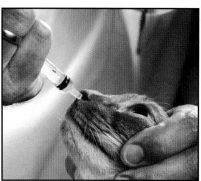

6.9 Intranasal vaccination in a cat.

Primary vaccination

Primary vaccination describes the initial administration or course of administrations that establishes immunity. Significant levels of passive antibodies (e.g. MDA) can interfere with the immune response to the vaccine. The recommendations for timing of primary vaccine course doses are based on an understanding of when MDA will decline to levels that will not interfere with the immune response (Figure 6.10). Canine vaccines currently in use in the UK have recommendations for the final dose of the primary course to be given at 10 or 12 weeks of age; for cats, 12 weeks is most commonly the age at which the final dose of the primary course is given.

A **turnout** period (often around 7–14 days) should be carefully observed following final vaccination before protective immunity is established and individuals can be exposed to risk.

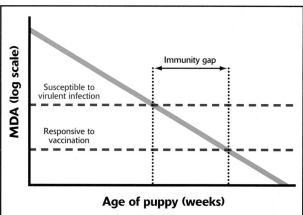

6.10 The fall in maternally derived antibody (MDA) is depicted by the solid line. As MDA interferes with response to vaccination, the final vaccination is timed to coincide with the expected decline in MDA to a point where a response is possible. The period between the decline in MDA to non-protective levels and vaccinal immunity developing is known as the **immunity gap**. Animals exposed to infection during this period will not be protected.

Booster vaccinations

Booster vaccinations (Figure 6.11) are required in those individuals where immunity may decline to non-protective levels. For some UK canine vaccines against distemper, hepatitis and

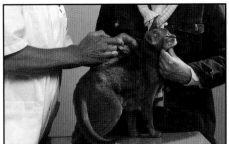

Administering a booster vaccination to a cat.

parvovirus, the recommended licensed intervals have changed to every 3 years (though recommendations vary with manufacturer). Available evidence shows that annual boosters against other diseases, such as leptospirosis, are still essential to maintain optimal immunity.

Immune-mediated disorders

Allergy and hypersensitivity reactions

Allergy is a state of exaggerated immune sensitivity induced by exposure to a particular, usually harmless, antigen (or **allergen**), resulting in harmful immunological reactions on subsequent exposures. Allergies may be localized problems in one organ (e.g. skin, intestinal tract, respiratory tract) or can result in systemic and potentially life-threatening reactions.

Hypersensitivity reactions are the inappropriate immune responses that result from exposure to a foreign antigen and are the underlying mechanisms for allergies as well as a number of other important autoimmune diseases (see below) and rare drug and vaccine reactions. Different forms occur. A **type I** (or **immediate-type**) hypersensitivity reaction is perhaps the most familiar and is the classical underlying mechanism for allergic reactions such as hay fever in humans, urticaria (wheals) and atopic dermatitis. Clinical signs vary from mild and localized (hay fever) through to systemic and life-threatening (anaphylactic shock).

Other hypersensitivity reactions are underlying mechanisms for a number of diseases, including autoimmune disease. Figure 6.12 summarizes the different types of hypersensitivity reactions seen in animals and gives examples of diseases where such reactions are noted.

Autoimmune disease

Autoimmunity occurs if the immune system reacts to one or more of the body's own tissues as foreign. Although rare, such conditions can prove life-threatening and difficult to manage. Examples include: pemphigus complex, where the immune system specifically attacks the skin and/or mucocutaneous junctions; rheumatoid arthritis; and immune-mediated haemolytic anaemia (IMHA), which is characterized by the breakdown of red blood cells, resulting in anaemia. Some types of endocrine disease, such as diabetes and hypothyroidism in dogs, may also arise as a result of an immune-mediated destruction of glandular tissues.

Graft rejection

Transplanting organs and tissues is a regular occurrence in human surgery and there is now some interest in the veterinary field. A potential problem is rejection of the graft or implant because the recipient's immune system may recognize transplanted tissue as foreign and attack it. Careful tissue matching reduces such risks; nevertheless, lifelong use of immunosuppressive drugs by the recipient is usually necessary.

Hypersensitivity reaction	Type	Components	Disease examples
I	Immediate-type (anaphylaxis)	Antigen binds to IgE antibodies on mast cells, which release histamine and other inflammatory mediators	Atopy; hay fever; urticaria; anaphylactic shock
II	Antibody-dependent or cytotoxic	Antibodies attach to antigens on the body's own cells (e.g. red blood cells), triggering their destruction	Immune-mediated haemolytic anaemia; transfusion reactions; pemphigus complex; babesiosis
III	Immune complex	Immune complexes of antibody and antigen form in tissues (e.g. joints, kidneys, blood vessels), precipitating damage	Immune-mediated polyarthritis; glomerulonephritis; vasculitis
IV	Delayed-type	A cell-mediated reaction involving cytotoxic T cells, helper T cells and macrophages	Tuberculosis; allergic contact dermatitis; feline infectious peritonitis (FIP)

6.12 Hypersensitivity reaction types.

Acknowledgement

The author would like to thank Intervet International for their assistance with preparation of the charts and images used in this chapter.

Further reading

Day MJ (1999) *Clinical Immunology of the Dog and Cat.* Manson Publishing, London
NOAH *Compendium of Data Sheets for Veterinary Products*
Thrusfield N (1997) *Veterinary Epidemiology, 2nd edn.* Blackwell Science, Oxford
Tizard IR (2004) *Veterinary Immunology – an Introduction, 7th edn.* Elsevier, Philadelphia

MRSA BSAVA Guidelines
http://www.bsava.com/resources/mrsa (18/08/06)

Pet Travel Scheme
http://www.defra.gov.uk/animalh/quarantine/index.htm (18/08/06)
http://www.bsava.com/resources/petpassport (18/08/06)

Vaccination issues
www.future-of-vaccination.com (18/09/05)

Chapter 7

Elementary microbiology

Maggie Fisher and Helen Moreton

Learning objectives

After studying this chapter, students should be able to:

- **Describe the important bacterial, viral and fungal infections of cats and dogs and be aware of some examples from other companion animals**
- **Describe the theoretical and practical skills necessary to identify microbial infection in animals**
- **Describe the measures used to control and treat infectious diseases**

Introduction

The microorganisms that will be described in this chapter vary in size from the relatively large ringworm fungi to viruses that can only be seen with an electron microscope (Figure 7.1). These microorganisms represent only a very small proportion of all microorganisms, and are those that interrelate with animal hosts in some way. Figure 7.2 shows the major similarities and differences between the different types of microorganism.

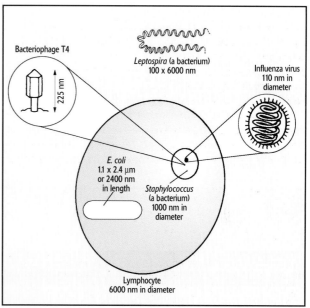

7.1 Relative sizes of various microorganisms, plus a white blood cell for comparison.

Characteristic	Bacteria	Viruses	Fungi	Protozoa	Algae
Size	0.5–5 μm	20–300 nm	3.8 μm (yeasts)	10–200 μm	0.5–20 μm
Cell arrangement	Unicellular	Non-cellular	Unicellular or multicellular multicellular	Unicellular	Unicellular or multicellular
Cell wall	Present; mainly peptidoglycan	Absent	Present; mainly chitin	Absent	Present; mainly cellulose
Nucleus	No true membrane-bound nucleus	Absent	Membrane-bound nucleus	Membrane-bound nucleus	Membrane-bound nucleus
Nuclei acids	DNA and RNA	DNA or RNA	DNA and RNA	DNA and RNA	DNA and RNA
Reproduction	Asexual by binary fission	Replicate only within another living cell	Asexual and sexual by spores, budding in yeast	Asexual and sexual	Asexual and sexual

7.2 Major similarities and differences between different types of microorganism.

continues ▶

Characteristic	Bacteria	Viruses	Fungi	Protozoa	Algae
Nutrition	Mainly heterotrophic – can be saprophytic or parasitic; a few are autotrophic	Obligate parasites	Heterotrophic – can be saprophytic or parasitic	Heterotrophic – can be saprophytic or parasitic	Autotrophic
Motility	Some are motile	Non-motile	Non-motile except for certain spore forms	Motile	Some are motile
Toxin production	Some form toxins	None	Some form toxins	Some form toxins	Some form toxins

7.2 *continued* Major similarities and differences between different types of microorganism.

There are several ways in which microorganisms can relate to hosts (Figure 7.3), some of which may be beneficial or neutral in effect. The focus in this chapter will be upon those that cause infection or disease in dogs, cats and other companion animals. A few important organisms that are carried by cats and dogs without clinical signs but are capable of causing disease in humans (i.e. are zoonotic) are included.

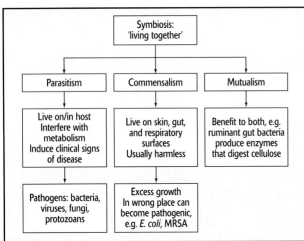

7.3 Relationships between microorganisms and animal hosts.

Viruses

Structure and naming

Viruses are extremely small and are sometimes not classified as living organisms, as they are incapable of reproduction without a host cell. A virus particle, or **virion**, is little more than a package containing instructions for the recreation of further virus particles. Each virus particle is composed of two parts (Figure 7.4):

- *Nucleic acid* – RNA or DNA (never both) forming a central core
- *A protein coat* – the **capsid**.

Together, these two parts form the **nucleocapsid**. For some viruses, this is all that an individual virus particle will comprise. Various shapes of virus nucleocapsid have been identified (Figure 7.5):

- Helical
- Icosahedral
- Complex (poxvirus)
- Composite (some bacteriophages).

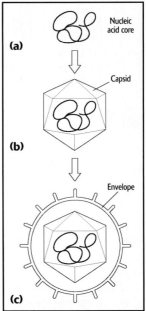

7.4 General virus components: **(a)** central core of nucleic acid; **(b)** capsid surrounding the nucleic acid to form a nucleocapsid (with icosahedral symmetry); **(c)** in addition, some viruses possess an outer envelope.

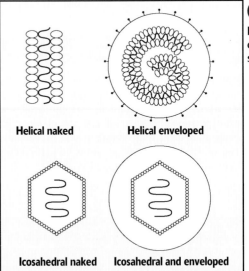

7.5 Four types of viral structure.

Some viruses have an additional envelope around the outside, often formed of the host cell membrane (Figure 7.4c). Each of the helical or icosahedral shapes of the nucleocapsid can be enveloped or non-enveloped (Figure 7.5), giving four possible basic shapes for viruses. In fact, there are no animal viruses (only plant viruses) that are helical and non-enveloped, so viruses of dogs and cats can be grouped by and large into the other three types. Viruses have been classified together on the basis of structural similarities. For example, the group of viruses causing true flu are the influenza viruses but the disease called cat flu is caused by two viruses, neither of which is an influenza virus.

Viral replication

A virus is only able to attach to cells that carry a compatible receptor. For example, influenza viruses can only attach to ciliated epithelial cells in the respiratory tract. This specificity of viruses for specific tissues is known as **tissue tropism**. Viruses normally have only one or two host species that they are able to infect; e.g. parvovirus in dogs does not infect cats, and measles virus will only infect humans and apes. Once attached, virus particles are taken into the host cell (Figure 7.6) by fusing the virus envelope with the host cell membrane or, in the case of non-enveloped viruses, by causing the host cell to engulf the virus particle into the cell. Once inside the cell, the virus is able to switch the cell's normal metabolism to obey the instructions of the virus. The virus may cause this to happen immediately, so that the cell begins to produce the constituents of new virus particles within hours of infection. Alternatively, as in the case of AIDS, the virus may join with the host cell's own nucleic acid for an extended period before making any changes to cell metabolism (see Chapter 21). New virus particles are then assembled and released from the cell. Depending on the virus, this may leave the host cell intact or may cause its rupture and destruction.

Transmission

Viruses are transmitted from host to host either directly (e.g. by a cat licking feline calicivirus in nasal secretions off the face of another cat) or indirectly (e.g. a dog licking the floor of a kennel that had been occupied by a dog with parvovirus

infection and had not been adequately cleaned). Different viruses have adapted their means of transmission according to their structure (which affects their ability to survive in the environment) and their location in the host. For example, a respiratory tract virus is often transmitted by virus particles being sneezed from one host into the air breathed in by another host. This is ideal for influenza virus, as these enveloped viruses are not very robust and do not survive for extended periods in the environment. An ability to survive in the environment for longer periods is beneficial for canine parvovirus. The virus must be licked up and ingested by another dog for infection of the gastrointestinal tract to occur.

Incubation

Once a host animal has been infected with a small number of virus particles, there is a time lag before the symptoms that are associated with the infection are seen; this is the **incubation period**. During this time, the virus reaches the cells that it can invade and initially infects a small number of cells in order to increase the number of virus particles. Symptoms (or signs) are seen once large numbers of virus particles infect a large number of cells.

Viral diseases

Some infections in dogs and cats that are caused by viruses are shown in Figures 7.7 and 7.8. Some viral infections of other companion species are shown in Table 7.9. More details of viral diseases can be found in Chapter 21.

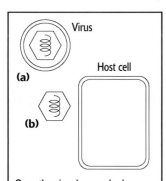

Once the virus has reached a suitable host cell, it attaches to receptor sites on the host cell membrane.

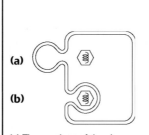

(a) The envelope of the virus may fuse with the cell wall and release the nucleocapsid into the cell or (b) the virus may be taken into the cell by endocytosis.

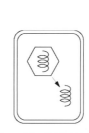

The virus enters the host cell and the protein coat (capsid) breaks down to release the viral nucleic acid.

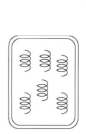

The viral nucleic acid replicates (either in the host cell cytoplasm or nucleus) and directs the host cell metabolism to make new virus material.

7.6 Replication of animal viruses.

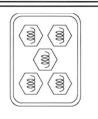

The new viruses are assembled.

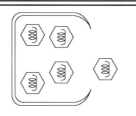

They leave the host cell either by rupture of the cell membrane; or

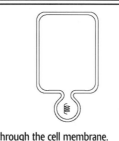

through the cell membrane.

Name of virus	Disease caused	Nucleic acid type	Shape of nucleocapsid	Enveloped?
Parvovirus	Parvovirus	DNA	Icosahedral	No
Canine adenovirus 1 (CAV-1)	Infectious canine hepatitis	DNA	Icosahedral	No
Canine adenovirus 2 (CAV-2)	Infectious canine tracheobronchitis	DNA	Icosahedral	No

7.7 Some viral diseases of dogs.

continues ▶

Name of virus	Disease caused	Nucleic acid type	Shape of nucleocapsid	Enveloped?
Canine distemper virus	Distemper	RNA	Helical	Yes
Canine parainfluenza virus	Part of kennel cough syndrome	RNA	Helical	Yes
Rabies virus	Rabies	RNA	Helical	Yes
Canine herpesvirus	Disease and death in very young pups	DNA	Icosahedral	Yes
Canine coronavirus	Vomiting and diarrhoea	RNA	Helical	Yes

7.7 *continued* Some viral diseases of dogs.

Name of virus	Disease caused	Nucleic acid type	Shape of nucleocapsid	Enveloped?
Feline parvovirus (panleucopenia)	Feline infectious enteritis	DNA	Icosahedral	No
Feline herpesvirus	Feline rhinotracheitis; cat flu	DNA	Icosahedral	Yes
Feline calicivirus	Cat flu	RNA	Icosahedral	No
Feline coronavirus	Feline infectious peritonitis (FIP)	RNA	Helical	Yes
Feline leukaemia virus	Feline leukaemia	RNA	Icosahedral	Yes
Feline immunodeficiency virus	FIV infection	RNA	Icosahedral	Yes
Rabies virus	Rabies, although cats are less susceptible to infection than dogs	RNA	Helical	Yes

7.8 Some viral diseases of cats.

Name of virus	Disease caused	Nucleic acid type	Shape of nucleocapsid	Enveloped?	Host species
EIAV (a lentivirus)	Equine infectious anaemia ('swamp fever')	RNA	Icosahedral	Yes	Horses
West Nile virus (a flavivirus)	West Nile	RNA	Polyhedral/spherical	Yes	Birds, horses, zoonosis
Equine influenza virus	Influenza	RNA	Segmented	Yes	Horses
Equine herpesvirus 1–4	Depends on type (e.g. type 1 sub-strains cause rhinopneumonitis, abortion and myoencephalopathy)	DNA	Icosahedral	Yes	Horses
RHV calicivirus	Haemorrhagic fever	RNA	Icosahedral	No	Rabbits
Myxoma (a poxvirus)	Myxomatosis	DNA	Brick-shaped, slightly pleomorphic	Yes	Rabbits
Influenza A H5N1 virus	Bird flu	RNA	Helical	Yes	Birds, zoonosis if close contact

7.9 Some viral diseases of other species.

Diagnosis of viral infections

Viral infections may be diagnosed on the basis of their symptoms and the animal's history. Often there are several infections that may cause similar signs and it may be important to be able to confirm the particular virus present. This may be carried out in a number of ways, including the following:

- Virus particles are too small to be seen with the light microscope but they may be seen with an electron microscope
- Large numbers of virus particles may clump together in cells; the clump may then be seen with the light microscope. Large groups of rabies virus are seen in cells of animals infected with rabies; these are known as Negri bodies. An animal can only be examined for these and a number of other virus-related changes at postmortem
- Serology may be carried out to detect virus antigen or the antibody produced by the host in response to infection.

Treatment of viral infections

Viral infections can be combated in a number of ways. Treatment of animal virus infections normally involves supportive nursing, including:

- Fluids to prevent dehydration in the case of canine parvovirus infection
- Tempting foods for cats with cat flu
- Antibacterials to limit secondary bacterial infection.

Animals may also be vaccinated in order to stimulate an immune response (see Chapter 6).

There are now some specialized treatments for a few viral infections in humans, such as AIDS, the shingles form of chickenpox and herpes simplex (the cause of cold sores). Some antiviral treatments are also used in companion animals, though this is mainly confined to ophthalmic treatment and to treatment of cats infected with feline leukaemia or feline immunodeficiency virus (e.g. zidovudine for FIV).

Prevention of viral infection

As viral infections are difficult to treat once the animal is infected, control has been aimed at preventing infection, particularly of severe viral diseases. This can be done at a number of levels:

- A country can have a border policy to prevent entry of diseases that are not present in a country (e.g. countries seek to prevent entry of rabies by quarantine or vaccine policies) (see Chapter 6)

- Catteries may be designed so that airborne viruses are not readily transmitted from cat to cat (see Chapter 12).
- Suitable disinfectants can be used to kill viruses that may be present in animal cages between occupants (see Chapter 12)
- Individual animals may be protected by vaccination (e.g. canine distemper, canine parvovirus, feline leukaemia). More details about vaccination may be found in Chapters 6 and 9.

Prions

Prions are very small protein particles that cause infections within the central nervous system, leading eventually to the death of the animal. The incubation period is usually long; it takes from 2 months to 20 years before signs of disease become apparent. Until relatively recently, the study of prion diseases was highly specialized work carried out by a few people. Researchers had investigated scrapie, a prion infection of sheep that has been recorded in Europe for the last 200 years. Interest and research in prion infections increased greatly following

the outbreak of bovine spongiform encephalopathy (BSE), which was first identified in the UK in the mid 1980s. It appears that BSE may be transmissible to humans as a result of eating infected beef. There have been over 100 deaths attributed to a new variant (vCJD) of a human encephalopathy, Creutzfeldt–Jacob disease. Around 20 cases of a similar disease, feline spongiform encephalopathy (FSE), in cats and other felids have been recorded since 1990. Affected cats exhibit nervous signs and incoordination. It is thought that these spongiform encephalopathies may originally have derived from scrapie. Much research effort is now aimed at being able to confirm disease in the live animal. At present, diagnosis is normally based on the appearance of brain tissue at postmortem examination.

Bacteria

Size and shape

Bacteria (singular: **bacterium**) are single-celled organisms (Figure 7.10) and most range in size from 0.5 μm (micrometres or microns; 10^{-6} m) to 5 μm in length, though there are some

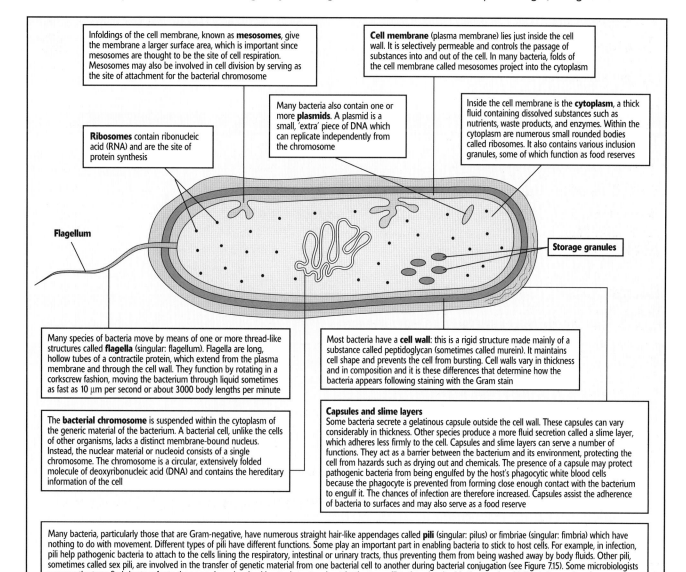

Infoldings of the cell membrane, known as **mesosomes**, give the membrane a larger surface area, which is important since mesosomes are thought to be the site of cell respiration. Mesosomes may also be involved in cell division by serving as the site of attachment for the bacterial chromosome

Cell membrane (plasma membrane) lies just inside the cell wall. It is selectively permeable and controls the passage of substances into and out of the cell. In many bacteria, folds of the cell membrane called mesosomes project into the cytoplasm

Many bacteria also contain one or more **plasmids**. A plasmid is a small, 'extra' piece of DNA which can replicate independently from the chromosome

Inside the cell membrane is the **cytoplasm**, a thick fluid containing dissolved substances such as nutrients, waste products, and enzymes. Within the cytoplasm are numerous small rounded bodies called ribosomes. It also contains various inclusion granules, some of which function as food reserves

Ribosomes contain ribonucleic acid (RNA) and are the site of protein synthesis

Flagellum

Storage granules

Many species of bacteria move by means of one or more thread-like structures called **flagella** (singular: flagellum). Flagella are long, hollow tubes of a contractile protein, which extend from the plasma membrane and through the cell wall. They function by rotating in a corkscrew fashion, moving the bacterium through liquid sometimes as fast as 10 μm per second or about 3000 body lengths per minute

Most bacteria have a **cell wall**: this is a rigid structure made mainly of a substance called peptidoglycan (sometimes called murein). It maintains cell shape and prevents the cell from bursting. Cell walls vary in thickness and in composition and it is these differences that determine how the bacteria appears following staining with the Gram stain

The **bacterial chromosome** is suspended within the cytoplasm of the generic material of the bacterium. A bacterial cell, unlike the cells of other organisms, lacks a distinct membrane-bound nucleus. Instead, the nuclear material or nucleoid consists of a single chromosome. The chromosome is a circular, extensively folded molecule of deoxyribonucleic acid (DNA) and contains the hereditary information of the cell

Capsules and slime layers
Some bacteria secrete a gelatinous capsule outside the cell wall. These capsules can vary considerably in thickness. Other species produce a more fluid secretion called a slime layer, which adheres less firmly to the cell. Capsules and slime layers can serve a number of functions. They act as a barrier between the bacterium and its environment, protecting the cell from hazards such as drying out and chemicals. The presence of a capsule may protect pathogenic bacteria from being engulfed by the host's phagocytic white blood cells because the phagocyte is prevented from forming close enough contact with the bacterium to engulf it. The chances of infection are therefore increased. Capsules assist the adherence of bacteria to surfaces and may also serve as a food reserve

Many bacteria, particularly those that are Gram-negative, have numerous straight hair-like appendages called **pili** (singular: pilus) or fimbriae (singular: fimbria) which have nothing to do with movement. Different types of pili have different functions. Some play an important part in enabling bacteria to stick to host cells. For example, in infection, pili help pathogenic bacteria to attach to the cells lining the respiratory, intestinal or urinary tracts, thus preventing them from being washed away by body fluids. Other pili, sometimes called sex pili, are involved in the transfer of genetic material from one bacterial cell to another during bacterial conjugation (see Figure 7.15). Some microbiologists now use the term fimbriae to refer to the appendages involved in attachment and restrict the term pili to those involved in the transfer of DNA during conjugation

7.10 Components of a generalized bacterial cell and their functions.

exceptions. The morphology of bacteria can affect their physiology and pathogenicity. The shape and physiology of bacteria present in infections are used to identify their species and thus assess prognosis and suitable treatments. Three basic shapes are generally recognized and these are sometimes used as a means of classification and naming of bacteria (Figure 7.11):

- Cylindrical or rod-shaped cells are called **bacilli** (singular: bacillus). Some bacilli are curved and these are known as **vibrios**

- Spherical cells are called **cocci** (singular: coccus). Some cocci exist singly while others remain together in pairs after cell division and are called **diplococci**. Those that remain attached to form chains are called streptococci and if they divide randomly and form irregular grape-like clusters they are called **staphylococci**
- Spiral or helical cells are called **spirilla** (singular: spirillum) if they have a rigid cell wall or **spirochaetes** if the cell wall is flexible.

Structure

Some of the structures shown in the generalized bacterial cell depicted in Figure 7.10 are common to all cells; others are only present in certain species or under certain environmental conditions. Figures 7.12 and 7.13 give details of some bacteria that cause disease in dogs and other species.

Naming bacteria

All bacteria, in common with plants and animals, are named according to the binomial system. The first word starts with a capital letter and indicates the genus to which they belong (e.g. *Escherichia*). This is followed by the species name (e.g. *coli*). Thus *Escherichia coli* is one of the species of the genus *Escherichia*, and *Homo sapiens* (modern humans) is one of the species of the genus *Homo*. The generic name is frequently shortened to an initial letter, e.g. *Escherichia coli* becomes *E. coli*; *Staphylococcus aureus* may be seen written as *Staph. aureus*. Both generic and specific names are written *in italics*.

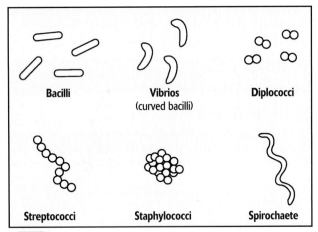

7.11 Classification of bacteria by shape.

Name of bacterium	Disease caused	Gram stain	Shape	Aerobic?
Salmonella spp.	Diarrhoea	–ve	Rod/bacillus	Yes
Campylobacter spp.	Diarrhoea	–ve	Curved rods	Yes (but prefer less oxygen than in air)
Bordetella bronchiseptica	Kennel cough	–ve	Short rods/bacilli	Yes
Leptospira spp.	Leptospirosis	–ve	Helically coiled (spirochaete)	Yes
Borrelia burgdorferi	Lyme disease	–ve	Helically coiled (spirochaete)	Yes
Streptococcus spp.	Infection, particularly in puppies, occasionally otitis externa, metritis	+ve	Cocci (arranged in chains)	Yes
Staphylococcus spp.	Pyoderma or wound infection	+ve	Cocci (arranged as bunches of grapes)	Yes
Clostridium tetani	Tetanus (rare)	+ve	Long rods (bacilli)	No

7.12 Some bacterial diseases of dogs. See Chapter 21 for more details.

Name of bacterium	Disease caused	Susceptible species	Gram stain	Shape
Mycoplasma felis	Mycoplasmal conjunctivitis	Cat	–ve (but stain poorly)	Pleomorphic as there is no rigid cell wall
Pasteurella spp. and other organisms	Cat-bite abscess	Cat	–ve (*Pasteurella*)	Rod or cocco-bacilli
Bacillus anthracis	Anthrax	Most mammals, often farm stock, a zoonosis	+ve	Rod
Streptococcus equi equi	Strangles	Equine species	+ve	Coccus
Rhodococcus equi	Summer pneumonia	Foals	+ve	Coccus
Pasteurella multocida	Pasteurellosis (many types, such as respiratory diseases)	Rabbits ('snuffles', conjunctivitis etc.) and many other livestock	–ve	Rods or cocco-bacilli
Mycobacterium avium	Avian tuberculosis	Birds – many species	+ve (but stain very poorly so alternative 'acid-fast' stain is used)	Rods
Chlamydophila psittaci	Psittacosis	Birds, and is zoonotic	–ve (but stain poorly so require specialized stain)	Cocci

7.13 Some bacterial diseases of other species.

Endospores

Some species of bacteria produce dormant forms called endospores (or simply **spores**), which can survive unfavourable conditions. They are formed when the vegetative (growing) cells are deprived of some factor, e.g. when the supply of nutrients is inadequate. It is important to note that endospore formation (or **sporulation**) is not a method of reproduction: one vegetative cell produces a single spore which, after germination, is again just one vegetative cell. Spore formation is most common in the genera *Bacillus* and *Clostridium*. These genera contain the causative agents of tetanus, anthrax and botulism. These diseases are zoonoses, commonly affecting domestic and farm animals. Species susceptibility to each disease varies; for example, dogs only infrequently suffer from tetanus, whilst horses are very susceptible and require routine vaccination, as do humans.

Many endospore-forming bacteria are inhabitants of the soil but spores can exist almost everywhere, including in dust. They are extremely resistant structures that can remain viable for many years. They can survive extremes of heat, pH, desiccation, ultraviolet radiation and exposure to toxic chemicals such as some disinfectants. The reason why endospores are so resistant is not completely understood, but heat resistance is thought to be due to the fact that a dehydration process occurs during spore formation which expels most of the water from the spore. The spore develops within the bacterial cell and under the microscope it appears as a bright, round or oval structure.

The fact that spores are so hard to destroy is the principal reason for the various sterilization procedures that are carried out in veterinary practice. Common techniques employed to kill spores include:

- Autoclaving (moist heat, 121°C under pressure 6.9 kPa for more than 15 minutes)
- Tyndallization (repeated steaming)
- Dry heat (160°C for at least 2 hours).

Conditions necessary for bacterial growth

Bacteria can grow and reproduce only when environmental conditions are suitable. The essential requirements for growth include:

- A supply of suitable nutrients
- The correct temperature (the temperature at which a species of bacterium grows most rapidly is the optimum growth temperature; most mammalian pathogens grow best at normal body temperature)
- The correct pH (the majority of mammalian pathogens grow best at pH 7–7.4)
- Water
- The correct gaseous environment (many species of bacterium can grow only when oxygen is present).

Bacteria that must have oxygen for growth are called strict or **obligate aerobes**. Some, known as **obligate anaerobes**, can only grow in the absence of oxygen, while others, the **facultative anaerobes**, grow aerobically when oxygen is present but can also function in the absence of oxygen. A few species, the **microaerophiles**, grow best when the concentration of oxygen is lower than in atmospheric air.

Reproduction of bacteria

If their environment is suitable, bacteria can grow and reproduce rapidly. The time interval between successive divisions is called the **generation time**. In some bacteria the generation time is very short; for others it is quite long. For example, under optimum conditions the generation time of *E. coli* is 20 minutes, whereas for the tuberculosis bacterium *Mycobacterium tuberculosis* it is approximately 18 hours. Given appropriate conditions, growth is exponential, i.e. one bacterium produces two, then two produce four and so on.

Bacteria reproduce asexually by simply dividing into two identical daughter cells, a process called **binary fission** (Figure 7.14). Prior to cell division, the cell grows; once it has reached a certain size, the circular chromosome or nucleoid replicates to form two identical chromosomes. As the parent cell enlarges, the chromosomes are separated and the cell membrane grows inwards at the centre of the cell. At the same time, new cell wall material grows inwards to form the septum and this divides the cell into two daughter cells. These may separate completely, but in some species (e.g. streptococci, staphylococci) they remain attached to form the characteristic chains or clusters. Replication of pathogenic bacteria usually takes place outside the host's cells – unlike pathogenic viruses, where reproduction is intracellular.

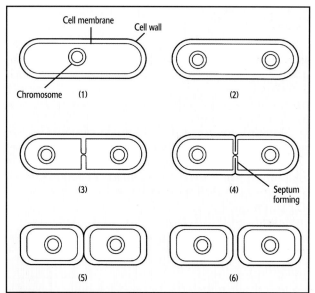

7.14 Replication of bacteria by binary fission. (1, 2) The cell grows and the chromosome replicates to form two identical chromosomes. (3) As the cell enlarges, the chromosomes are separated and the cell membrane grows inwards at the centre of the cell. (4) At the same time, new cell wall material grows inwards to form the septum. (5, 6) The cell divides into two daughter cells.

Conjugation

The process of conjugation (Figure 7.15) involves the passage of DNA from one bacterial cell (the donor) to another (the recipient) while the two cells are in physical contact. The cells are pulled together by an appendage called the **sex pilus**, which is formed by the donor cell. Once contact has been made, the pilus retracts so that the surfaces of the donor and recipient are very close to each other. The cell membranes fuse, forming a channel between the two cells, and DNA then passes from the donor to the recipient.

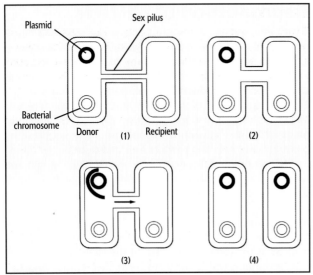

7.15 Sequence of events in conjugation. (1) Donor and recipient cells are pulled together by the sex pilus, which is formed by the donor cell. (2) The pilus retracts, bringing the two cells very close to each other, and the cell membranes fuse to form a channel between the two cells. (3) The plasmid replicates and one strand passes through the channel to the recipient. (4) The two cells separate. The recipient becomes a donor, because it now has the plasmid.

Frequently, a plasmid is transferred from the donor to the recipient but sometimes part of the donor cell chromosome, or even the whole chromosome, is transferred. Conjugation is important because the recipient acquires new characteristics. For example, one plasmid, the R plasmid, carries genes for resistance to antibiotics.

Conjugation is rare among Gram-positive bacteria but common among those that are Gram-negative. It is sometimes regarded as a primitive type of sexual reproduction but this is misleading because, unlike sexual reproduction in other organisms, it does not involve the fusion of two gametes to form a single cell.

Identification of bacteria

It can be important to identify the bacteria causing an infection, perhaps so that appropriate antibacterials can be selected for treatment. The simplest and quickest way to identify bacteria is to make a smear and stain with a mixture of stains that turns bacteria either blue (Gram-positive) or red (Gram-negative) (see Chapter 17). This also allows the structure of the bacterial cell to be observed.

There are often several bacteria that look alike at this stage and so it may be necessary to culture the bacterium so that the identity can be determined more precisely. Figure 7.16 shows how this process might occur for the investigation of an infection causing otitis externa in a dog's ear.

Practically, samples are often cultured initially in order to obtain quantities of a pure growth of the bacterium responsible for the infection. The characteristics of the colony can then be observed and there is enough bacterial material to carry out any further tests that are necessary. Culture also allows an experienced microbiologist to differentiate important colonies from those of bacteria that are normally present or otherwise insignificant in the infection.

Bacterial cultivation in the laboratory

The cultivation of bacteria in the laboratory requires an appropriate nutrient material or culture medium (see Chapter 17). The culture medium must contain a balanced mixture of the essential growth requirements – carbon, nitrogen and water. Culture can also be used as a method of bacterial identification as many bacteria have specific individual requirements for optimal growth.

Respiratory requirements

The different respiratory requirements of bacteria, described above, can be used in helping to identify bacterial pathogens, as can the detailed biochemical pathways that they use to provide energy. Bacteria that will grow in the amount of oxygen in the air may be cultured in an incubator. For anaerobes and microaerophiles (including most *Campylobacter* species), Petri dishes containing appropriate culture medium can be placed in an anaerobic jar to minimize atmospheric oxygen and

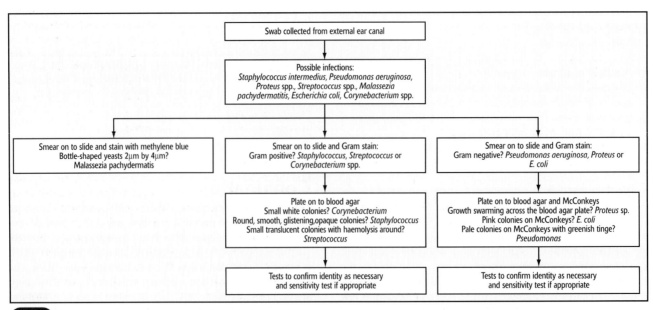

7.16 Flow chart for the identification of bacteria or *Malassezia pachydermatis* from a dog with chronic otitis externa.

encourage the growth of the bacteria. If the appropriate conditions for a particular organism are not provided, its presence may not be recognized as it fails to grow in the laboratory. Respiratory mechanisms of any particular bacterium can be identified by testing for the presence of enzymes that are involved in oxidative processes, such as catalase and cytochrome oxidase.

Diseases caused by bacteria

A variety of bacteria are capable of infecting dogs and cats; some can cause signs of infection in the dog or cat. Important disease-causing bacteria are shown in Figures 7.12 (for dogs) and 7.13 (for some other species of animal). Sometimes the same bacterium is responsible for causing disease in a number of species; other infections are more species-specific.

The signs of infection may be directly associated with the presence of the bacteria; they may be related to damage caused to local tissue by the presence of the infection, the inflammatory reaction stimulated by the infection or due to toxins produced by bacteria.

Rickettsias and chlamydias

Both rickettsias and chlamydias possess a cell wall like other Gram-negative bacteria but both need to live inside other cells, i.e. they are obligate intracellular organisms. These bacteria are responsible for a number of diseases in animals.

Rickettsias

These are transmitted by vectors such as the tick, louse, flea and mite. A particularly pathogenic species is the tick-transmitted infection *Ehrlichia canis*, which is endemic in France and the Mediterranean basin.

Chlamydias

Various strains of *Chlamydophila* (formerly *Chlamydia*) *psittaci* are the cause of psittacosis in psittacine birds (parrots, parakeets) and mammals. Psittacosis is a zoonotic infection that humans can acquire by inhaling the organism in the airborne dust or cage contents of infected birds. Feline pneumonitis is caused by *Chlamydophila felis,* which may also cause conjunctivitis in the cat. The bacteria are transmitted by inhalation of infectious dust and droplets and by ingestion. There is also evidence to suggest that vector-borne infection may occur.

Identification

Generally, the identification of rickettsias and chlamydias is more difficult and thus more specialized than that of most bacteria. Diagnosis of infection may be based on demonstration of the organisms themselves or on the demonstration of increased titres in paired serum samples. Rickettsias are smaller than most bacteria and are barely visible using a light microscope. They can only be cultivated in tissue culture or in the yolk sac of embryonated eggs. Typically, they are rod-shaped and measure about 0.8–2.0 μm.

Mycoplasmas

Mycoplasmas are tiny bacteria-like organisms but they do not possess a cell wall. They include *Mycoplasma felis*, a cause of chronic conjunctivitis in cats. *Mycoplasma* spp. have been implicated in complicating respiratory tract infections in a number of animal species, notably calves.

Mycoplasmas will grow on agar-based media but, as they are so fragile, isolation and identification are specialized skills. More information about the diseases caused by these small bacteria may be found in Chapter 21.

Toxins

Toxins are poisonous substances that have a damaging effect on the cells of the host. The effects of the toxin are felt not only in the affected cells and tissues but also elsewhere in the body as the toxin is transported through the tissues. Two types of toxin are recognized:

- Exotoxins, which are manufactured by living microorganisms and released into the surrounding medium
- Endotoxins, which are part of the microorganism and only liberated when it dies.

Exotoxins

Exotoxins are proteins produced mainly by Gram-positive bacteria during their metabolism. They are released into the surrounding environment as they are produced. This can be into the circulatory system and tissues of the host or, as in food poisoning, into food that is then ingested. Microbial toxins include many of the most potent poisons known and may prove lethal even in small quantities. The body responds to the presence of exotoxins by producing antibodies called **antitoxins**, which neutralize the toxins, rendering them harmless.

Exotoxins, as they are proteins, are destroyed by heat and some chemicals. Chemicals such as formaldehyde are used to treat toxins so that they lose their toxicity but not their ability to elicit an immune response. These treated toxins are called **toxoids** and will stimulate the production of antitoxins if injected into the body. For example, tetanus toxoid is used to provide immunity to tetanus.

Effects of toxins

The effects of toxins are usually very specific. For example, when spores of the anaerobic tetanus bacillus *Clostridium tetani* get into a wound that provides favourable conditions, they may germinate and grow in the tissues. The bacteria do not spread through the tissues but secrete an exotoxin that travels along peripheral nerves to the central nervous system, where it interferes with the regulation of neurotransmitters that control the relaxation of muscle. This leads to uncontrollable muscle spasms and paralysis. Tetanus toxin is called a **neurotoxin** because of its activity in the nervous system. Unlike tetanus, which is caused by exotoxins produced while the organism is growing within the host, botulism, caused by the saprophytic bacterium *Clostridium botulinum*, is the result of ingestion of food containing the toxins. In botulism, the exotoxin affects the nervous system, leading to paralysis; it too is therefore a neurotoxin. Other exotoxins formed outside the body include those produced by *Staphylococcus aureus*, the bacterium that causes staphylococcal food poisoning. This is an **enterotoxin** because it functions in the gastrointestinal tract, causing vomiting and diarrhoea.

Endotoxins

Endotoxins are part of the cell wall of certain Gram-negative bacteria and are released only when the cells die and disintegrate. Compared with exotoxins, they are less toxic, cannot be used to form toxoids and are able to withstand heat. Blood-borne endotoxins are responsible for a range of non-specific reactions in the body, such as fever. They also make the walls of blood capillaries more permeable, causing blood to leak into the intercellular spaces, sometimes resulting in a serious drop in blood pressure (a condition commonly called endotoxic shock). They are also responsible for the change in capillary blood flow in equine hooves that leads to laminitis.

Aflatoxin

Toxins are not made exclusively by bacteria. The saprophytic fungus *Aspergillus flavus* produces a toxin called aflatoxin. The fungus grows in warm, humid conditions and contaminates a variety of agricultural products such as peanuts, cereals, rice and beans. Aflatoxin has been implicated in the deaths of many farm animals that have been fed on mouldy hay, corn or on peanut meal.

Bacteria carried by cats and dogs

There are a number of bacteria that are normally carried by cats and dogs without causing any clinical signs. However, in certain circumstances, disease can result from infection.

- *Bartonella henselae* is a small Gram-negative bacterium present in a proportion of the cat population and is not normally pathogenic to cats. It may be transmitted to a human in the course of a cat scratch and may result in a local or more general infection in the person, so-called cat-scratch disease.
- CDC group M5 is a Gram-negative bacterium that normally lives in the mouth of dogs without causing any disease. It may be transmitted to humans in a dog bite, where it can cause a local infection.
- Some *Staphylococcus aureus* developed resistance to methicillin (methicillin-resistant *Staphlococcus aureus*, or **MRSA**) in the 1960s. Since then some strains have developed resistance to many antibacterials. These resistant bacteria can live on the skin or in the nasal passages of dogs, cats or humans without clinical signs. However, if infection establishes in a wound or other organ, severe damage can be caused. As the organism is resistant not only to methicillin but also to other antibacterials, the infection can be very difficult to treat. The presence of infection in a veterinary hospital ward may necessitate the closure of the ward and thorough cleaning until the infection is eliminated.

Treatment of bacterial infections

Bacterial infections can occur in many different locations within an animal and so the treatment will depend on the location and the type of bacteria present.

Choice of antibacterial agent

- A surface infection or a cat bite abscess might be treated with local cleaning with an antibacterial wash (e.g. chlorhexidine).
- Other infections can be treated with systemic antibacterials or antibiotics. Depending on the infection, treatment might be administered by mouth or by injection. Some antibacterials can be administered intravenously when speed of activity is essential. Some antibacterials are broad-spectrum and so are effective against a range of Gram-positive and Gram-negative organisms; others are effective against a more narrow range of organisms and so it is necessary to have an idea of the infection present in order to choose an appropriate antibacterial.
- Choice of an antibacterial also requires an understanding of where that antibacterial will get to in the body. For example, if treatment of cystitis is required, an antibacterial that is not broken down before it reaches the urinary tract should be selected. ▶

- Some antibacterials can destroy the microflora necessary for normal functioning. This is a particularly important consideration when choosing a treatment for small mammals such as rabbits, gerbils and hamsters.

Bacterial sensitivity testing

Sometimes it is important to identify the antibacterials to which the bacteria causing an infection will respond. A bacterial sensitivity test can be conducted where, for example, the bacteria are spread on an agar plate and discs containing different antibacterials are placed on top. After incubation the patterns of growth around the discs are examined:

- If the growth occurs right up to a disc, that antibacterial will not be effective.
- If there is a wide zone of inhibition of bacterial growth around a disc, the antibacterial contained in that disc is likely to be effective (see Chapter 17).

Fungi

There are many different fungi (as can be seen by looking at a mouldy slice of bread) but only a few are able to infect animals. Fungi grow aerobically (using oxygen) and gain their energy from the organic substances on which they grow. They can be divided into two categories and the fungal pathogens seen in small animal veterinary practice include both types.

- **Moulds** (Figure 7.17) are multicellular. Example: the 'ringworm' dermatophytes ('skin eaters')
- **Yeasts** (Figure 7.17) are unicellular. Examples: *Malassezia pachydermatis* and *Candida albicans*.

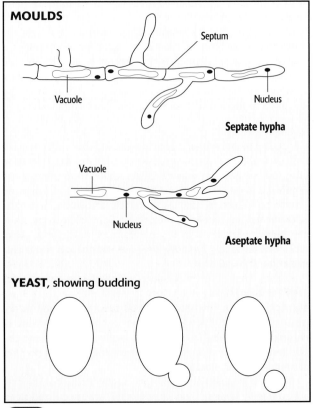

MOULDS

Septum

Vacuole

Nucleus

Septate hypha

Vacuole

Nucleus

Aseptate hypha

YEAST, showing budding

7.17 Different forms of fungi.

Dermatophytes

Fungal infections of **keratin** (the horny tissue that forms nail, hair and skin) can affect cats, dogs, rabbits and guinea pigs. The condition broadly known as **ringworm** is caused by dermatophytes such as the species *Trichophyton mentagrophytes* (in dog, cat, rabbit and guinea pig) and *Microsporum canis* (in dog and cat), amongst others.

In its most obvious form, ringworm appears as circular areas of hair loss with active fungal infection around the edge of the lesion. The lesions may be small and discrete or large and co-alescing, with an irregular outline. Some are not very inflamed and cause little irritation, whilst others may show severe inflammation. A more marked reaction is common in dogs.

Transmission may be directly from affected animal to animal, or to humans (many dermatophytes are zoonotic). Long-haired cats, in particular, may appear normal but may be carriers of infection. There may also be indirect transmission via bedding, cages etc. Ringworm spores can remain viable in the environment for prolonged periods.

Diagnosis

This can be done by staining hair pluck or skin scrape samples, by examining for fluorescence with a Wood's lamp or by culture on specialist media (see Chapter 17).

Treatment

Topical

Treatments include a fungicidal wash (such as enilconazole) or painting the affected area with povidone–iodine. Topical treatment is usually repeated after an interval to effect a full cure. It may be possible to treat the area of a discrete lesion only or it may be necessary to wash the whole animal. In severe or non-responsive cases, e.g. some long-haired cats, it will be necessary to clip the affected part or even the entire animal to facilitate treatment.

Systemic

Itraconazole or ketoconazole can be administered orally for the treatment of dermatophytes in dogs and cats. Griseofulvin is administered in tablet form and has to be given for a prolonged period as the levels build up gradually in the skin. Care, including the wearing of gloves, should be taken when handling griseofulvin as it is **teratogenic** (i.e. it can cause malformation of a fetus in a pregnant woman).

Candida albicans

Candida albicans is often present in the intestinal tract of animals without causing disease but it can become pathogenic in certain circumstances. *Candida* infections are usually opportunistic, i.e. they take advantage of a young, debilitated or immunocompromised animal and cause disease. Infection may also be seen after prolonged antibacterial treatment or following skin damage such as that incurred in a burn. The infection is known as 'thrush' and is commonly seen on mucous membranes, e.g. in the mouths of puppies or kittens. Rarely, it can occur on skin, particularly mucocutaneous junctions. Humans can acquire the infection but transfer of infection would be highly unlikely unless the person were immunocompromised in some way (for example, a person with AIDS).

- Infection of the skin of a dog may appear as an ulcer that does not respond to antibacterial therapy.
- Infection of the mouth may appear as a white growth and ulceration of the affected area in a puppy or kitten and may be associated with unwillingness to suck.
- In birds, *C. albicans* can infect the crop, particularly after prolonged antibacterial treatment.

Treatments for candidiasis include amphotericin B and injectable flucytosine.

Malassezia pachydermatis

Malassezia pachydermatis is a yeast that may be found on normal skin. In some situations, particularly seborrhoeic conditions, overgrowth may cause pruritic dermatitis (localized or generalized) or otitis externa, usually in dogs, but cats are sometimes infected. Infection occurs most commonly in warm summer months. Lesions may appear greasy and may have a distinct odour.

Suspected lesions can be sampled by pressing adhesive tape to the area (see Chapter 17). The strip is stained with methylene blue, attached to a microscope slide and examined microscopically. *Malassezia* appear as small, blue, bottle-shaped yeasts (see Chapter 17). As they are present on normal skin in low numbers, significant infection is indicated by an increase in numbers, perhaps when multiple organisms are seen in each high-power field of view under the microscope. Infection can be treated with a shampoo containing chlorhexidine and miconazole.

Other fungal infections

Occasionally, dogs, cats and other companion animals develop internal fungal infections. A number of different fungi can be responsible. For example, *Aspergillus fumigatus* can infect the nasal passages of the dog, the guttural pouches of horses and the respiratory system of birds. Fungi such as *Saprolegnia* spp. can infect fish and may cause severe disease and death of affected fish.

Further reading

Gillespie S and Bamford K (2000) *Medical Microbiology and Infection at a Glance*. Blackwell Science, Oxford

Heritage J, Evans EGV and Killington RA (1996) *Introductory Microbiology*. Cambridge University Press, Cambridge

Quinn PJ, Carter ME, Markey BK and Carter GR (1994) *Clinical Veterinary Microbiology*. Wolfe Publishing, London

Trees A and Shaw S (1999) Imported diseases in small animals. *In Practice* **21**, 482–491

Chapter 8

Elementary parasitology

Maggie Fisher and Vicky Walsh

Learning objectives

After studying this chapter, students should be able to:

- **Describe the ectoparasites and endoparasites that affect dogs and cats**
- **Describe the geographical distribution and zoonotic potential of parasites**
- **Discuss how the life cycle of a parasite determines the possible routes of infection**
- **Identify parasites on the basis of their location on or in the host and their morphology**
- **Discuss treatment options for parasite control**
- **Describe options for prophylaxis to prevent parasite infection**

Definitions

- **Parasite**: one eukaryotic organism living off another (the host) to the advantage of the parasite
  - **Ectoparasites** live on the outside of the host
  - **Endoparasites** live inside the host
- **Eukaryote**: organism in which the chromosomes are enclosed in a nucleus (e.g. animals, plants, fungi).

Ectoparasites

Ectoparasites belong to the animal kingdom and have a hard chitinous outer shell or exoskeleton. They include:

- **Insects**, where the adult has three pairs of legs and the body is divided into head, thorax and abdomen (e.g. lice, fleas)
- **Arachnids**, where the adult has four pairs of legs and the body is divided into two parts only: cephalothorax and abdomen (e.g. mites, ticks).

Usually it is the adult stage, often together with the immature stages, that is parasitic. There are two cases where it is only an immature form that is parasitic: the first is a mite, *Trombicula autumnalis*, and the other is the larva of the blowfly.

Ectoparasite morphology is illustrated below and diagnostic features are listed in Chapter 17.

Insects

The diagnosis and control of insect ectoparasites are described in Figure 8.1.

Lice

Infection with lice is also known as **pediculosis**. Lice are subdivided into biting lice (Figures 8.2 and 8.3) and sucking lice (Figure 8.4), reflecting their manner of feeding.

Infection is transmitted by close contact, as the louse spends its entire life cycle on the host. Infection may also be transferred by eggs collected on grooming equipment. However, individual louse species are highly host-specific and will not survive if transferred to another host. Cats, dogs, rabbits, rodents and birds may be affected with lice. Often young or debilitated animals are the worst affected. Large numbers of lice cause intense irritation and concomitant self-inflicted injury. In addition, the sucking lice may cause anaemia if they are present in large enough numbers.

Life cycle

Adult female lice lay their eggs individually and cement them to hairs. The eggs ('nits') are just visible to the naked eye (Figure 8.5). When these hatch, immature lice that are identical to the adult emerge and, after several moults, become adults. The whole life cycle takes about 2–3 weeks.

Fleas

Adult fleas bite the host in order to take a blood meal. The area that has been bitten shows something of an inflammatory reaction and causes some irritation. A heavy flea infestation may cause anaemia. Fleas can transmit disease as they feed and fleas appear important in the spread from cat to cat of *Bartonella henselae*, the agent responsible for cat scratch disease

	Diagnosis	**Control**
Lice	Demonstration of the eggs attached to hairs. Visualization of the adult louse. The adult lice may be seen with the naked eye on close examination of an animal's haircoat or may be seen in a skin scrape/brush	Thorough cleaning Topical surface treatment with an insecticidal wash, spray or spot-on.
Fleas	Demonstration of an adult flea or their faeces in the coat of a dog or cat by combing the coat thoroughly, preferably with a very fine toothcomb (ideally a human louse comb). The animal may be brushed over a sheet of damp white paper. Flea faeces will be seen on the paper as small black dots. Since they contain a large amount of undigested blood, a ring of red is seen around the black spot when moistened. There is also a skin test for allergy to fleas	Control of the environment at stages: – Hoovering, particularly around where the pet sleeps – Applying an environmental insecticide and/or an insect growth regulator such as methoprene or pyriproxyfen, for example, to kill the immature stages. Depending on the formulation these products may be applied to the animal or directly to the environment. The chitin synthesis inhibitor (lufenuron) is given orally to the dog or cat or by injection to the cat. It prevents eggs hatching and/or larval development
		Control of adult fleas on the animal: – Thorough grooming, e.g. using a human louse comb – Applying an insecticide in the form of, for example, a spray, impregnated collar, powder, shampoo or spot-on. The active ingredient in insecticides is now less often an organophosphate or a carbamate as these have been replaced by synthetic pyrethroids, phenylpyrazole (fipronil), chloronicotinyl nitroguanidine (imidacloprid) or avermectin (selamectin)
Dipteran fly larvae	An affected animal will often stop eating and appear restless and later depressed. The animal should be thoroughly examined to find the larvae and thus diagnose the problem	In order to treat the infestation, the first step is to remove the larvae: – Wash the affected area with a mild antiseptic solution, ensuring that the larvae are removed in the process – Lightly towel-dry the area. Apply antiseptic ointment Any underlying problem (e.g. diarrhoea) that may have predisposed the animal to becoming 'fly blown' should be investigated and treated and apply an antiparasitic agent such as cyromazine

8.1 Diagnosis and control of insect ectoparasites.

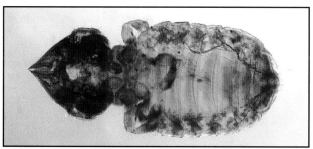

8.2 Dorsal view of the biting louse *Felicola subrostratus*. Found on cats, it is approximately 2 mm long. If viewed from the side, the louse would appear dorsoventrally flattened.

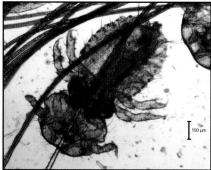

8.3 The species of biting louse found in dogs is *Trichodectes canis*. Biting lice tend to have shorter, broader heads than sucking lice.

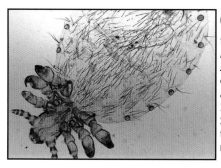

8.4 Ventral view of the sucking louse *Linognathus setosus*. Found on dogs, it is approximately 2 mm long. Sucking lice tend to have elongated, narrow heads.

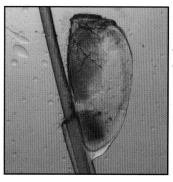

8.5 Louse egg ('nit') attached with 'cement' to the shaft of hair.

in humans. It is believed that a cat's claws may be coated in the bacteria, probably derived from the cat grooming infected flea faeces out of its coat.

Some animals become sensitized to **allergens** (particles that an individual may become sensitized to on repeat exposure) in flea saliva and develop severe lesions after just a few bites. This is known as flea allergic dermatitis. The species of flea may be identified by the appearance of the head. Most fleas on cats and dogs are the 'cat flea' *Ctenocephalides felis felis* (Figure 8.6) (often abbreviated to *C. felis*) but dogs in a dog-only situation (e.g. greyhound kennels) may be infected with

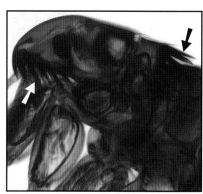

8.6 Lateral view of the head of the cat flea, showing the characteristic combs.

the dog flea *Ctenocephalides canis*. Infrequently other fleas, e.g. hedgehog fleas, are found on cats or dogs. Birds have their own species of flea, the immature stages of which live in the bird's nest.

Life cycle of the cat flea

The life cycle of the cat flea is shown in Figure 8.7. The adult is laterally compressed, which allows the flea to move readily between the host's hairs. The female flea feeds, then mates on the host and lays eggs. These are smooth and fall off into the environment, particularly around where the animal usually lies. After 2–14 days the eggs hatch out into larvae that look like small maggots. These feed on skin debris, the faeces of adult fleas and other organic matter in the environment. After about a week, each mature larva spins a cocoon and pupates. The outside of the cocoon is sticky and so bits of debris from the environment stick to it. After a further 10 days (though this can be considerably longer in cold or dry conditions) the adult flea is fully developed inside the pupa. Before it emerges, it waits for signs of a host being available, e.g. pressure (this is one explanation for the stories that occur of occupants going into an empty house and being bitten by fleas within hours). Once emerged from the pupal case the flea will locate a host and jump on to it.

Dipteran flies

Myiasis ('fly strike') is parasitism by larvae of dipteran flies (green-, blue- and black-bottles). The life cycle is shown in Figure 8.8. The flies lay their eggs on a suitable site, which might be, though is not necessarily, on an animal, such as in the fleece of a sheep or around the anus of a rabbit. Flies are particularly attracted to a smelly animal, e.g. one that is soiled by diarrhoea. Attraction can be minimized by ensuring that animals are kept clean. The larvae (maggots) hatch after as little as 12 hours and begin to traumatize the skin surface and feed off the damaged tissue. Larval development can be prevented by treating the animal with a larval growth inhibitor such as cyromazine. After several moults the larvae drop to the ground. Here they may overwinter as larvae before pupating or they may pupate immediately. Eventually the adult fly emerges from the pupal case.

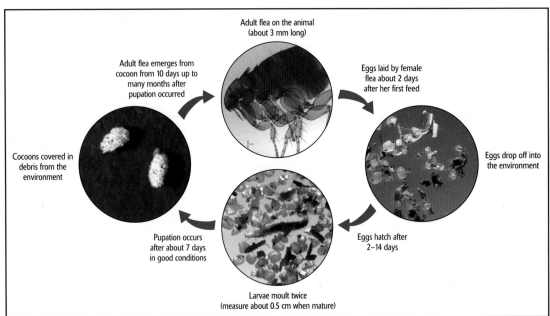

8.7

Life cycle of the cat flea.

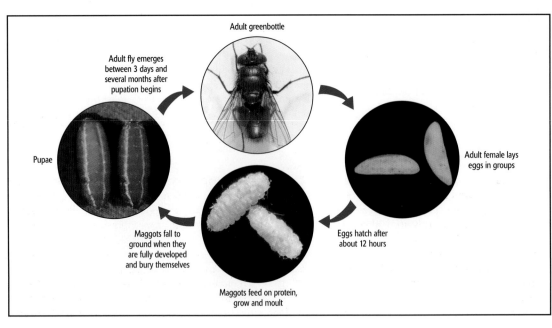

8.8

Life cycle of the blowfly. (Images courtesy of J McGarry)

Arachnids

The arachnids of veterinary importance are the ticks and the mites. The immature larvae that emerge from the eggs appear like a smaller version of the adult, except that they have only three pairs of legs, whereas the nymph and adult stages each have four pairs of legs.

Mites

The mites are all permanent ectoparasites (they spend their entire life cycle on the host) except for *Trombicula autumnalis*, where it is only the larva that is sometimes parasitic. Mites may be subdivided into the burrowing and the surface mites. Both types cause dermatitis, which may or may not be itchy, depending on the species of mite present. Diagnosis is usually by inspection of coat brushings, skin scrapes or hair plucks. Surface brushings are most readily examined in a Petri dish under a low-power dissecting microscope. Specific guidance on diagnosis and treatment of each mite is given in Figure 8.9 (see also Chapter 17).

Diagnosis	Presence of mite in:	Treatment
Sarcoptes scabiei	Skin scrapes or blood test	Mite infections may be treated with a suitable acaricide such as amitraz, selamectin or imidacloprid and moxidectin. Where no authorized product is available, treat with, e.g. fipronil. Where no prolonged activity, repeat treatments after 10–14 days to ensure all immature stages killed. Also treat the environment in *Cheyletiella* infection.
Notoedres	Skin scrapes	
Cnemidocoptes	Skin scrapes	
Demodex	Skin scrapes or hair plucks	
Cheyletiella	Coat brushings or sellotape strips (adult mite and/or eggs)	
Otodectes cynotis	Ear wax	Clean the ear canal; instil ointment containing suitable acaricide, often in combination with antibiotic. Also treat in-contact animals to clear reservoir of infection. Alternatively, selamectin or moxidectin spot-on may be used

8.9   Diagnosis and treatment of mites.

Burrowing mites

Burrowing mites live in small tunnels within the surface layers of the skin. They lay their eggs within small nests within these tunnels. There are three genera of burrowing mite typically seen in domestic pets: *Sarcoptes scabiei* var. *canis*; *Notoedres* spp.; and *Cnemidocoptes* spp. (The burrowing mite found in the guinea pig is *Trixacarus caviae*.)

Sarcoptes scabiei var. *canis*

This mite (Figure 8.10) affects dogs and, very rarely, cats. (Different *Sarcoptes* species may cause mange in rodents and one species is responsible for causing scabies in humans.) Animals become infected by close contact with infected animals or by acquiring mites or eggs that are present in bedding or the environment. The mite normally lives on a host throughout its life cycle, but mites may be shed by heavily infected individuals and can survive for several days in good conditions. Often the tips of the ears, elbows and then the face are the first areas affected but large areas of the body may be infected in severe cases. Affected areas become hairless, thickened and inflamed. This is partly due to the effect of the mites themselves and

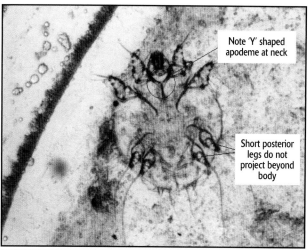

Note 'Y' shaped apodeme at neck

Short posterior legs do not project beyond body

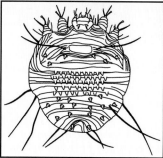

8.10   Adult *Sarcoptes* mite (0.4 mm long). The drawing (dorsal view) shows the short, stubby legs that barely project beyond the body, spines and pegs, terminal anus, and pedicles with suckers at the ends of the legs. Photo courtesy of Donald Mactaggart

partly due to the trauma that the animal causes by rubbing and scratching the affected area – the condition is very itchy. Sarcoptic infection in dogs will infect humans but normally the lesions are small and self-limiting.

Notoedres

This burrowing mite of the cat (Figure 8.11) is seen very rarely in the UK but it causes similar signs to *Sarcoptes scabiei* in the dog. *Notoedres* infestation also occurs in rats.

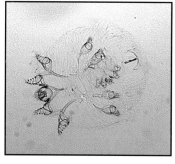

8.11   Dorsal view of adult female *Notoedres* mite (0.36 mm long) showing concentric circles on body and the dorsal anus.

Cnemidocoptes spp.

These mites are the cause of 'scaly leg' and 'scaly face' in birds, particularly budgerigars.

Demodex

This small cigar-shaped mite (Figure 8.12) may be found in normal hair follicles without necessarily causing any problem. In young dogs with an apparent genetic predisposition and in older dogs with immunosuppression, the number of *Demodex* mites can increase dramatically to cause a dermatitis that is characteristically an area of non-itchy alopecia. In localized demodicosis, where lesions are small, the face is often affected, particularly around the eyes or mouth. Generalized demodicosis can affect any area, with involvement of the feet being especially painful and problematic. *Demodex*

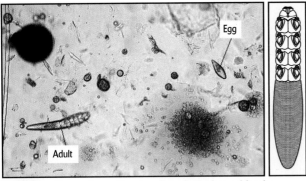

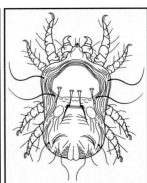

8.12   *Demodex* mite, showing cigar-shaped body (0.2 mm long) plus an egg. Photo courtesy of Donald Mactaggart

can be trickier to find than the other burrowing mites as it is smaller and dwells deep within the hair follicle. Hair plucks are often useful to find this mite. *Demodex* may also cause mange in hamsters and gerbils.

Surface mites

Otodectes cynotis

These are the small ear mites in dogs and cats (Figure 8.13). They live within the ear canal, often stimulating a dark brown waxy discharge. Mites may be seen on the surface as small white moving dots. Secondary bacterial infection may result in a pus-like discharge. Many cats are infected, often without showing clinical signs. Some cats and most dogs show clinical signs of head shaking and ear rubbing when infection is present. This may result in trauma to the ears and haematoma formation in the ear flap. Ferrets can also be infected with *Otodectes cynotis*. (Ear 'canker' in rabbits is caused by *Psoroptes cuniculi*.)

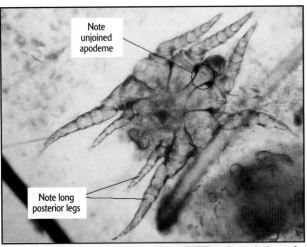

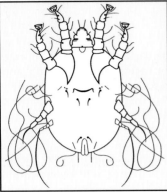

8.13   Dorsal view of *Otodectes* mite (0.4 mm long). Note the longer legs protruding from the body and unjoined pedicles (stalks) with suckers on the ends. Photo courtesy of Donald Mactaggart

Cheyletiella

Animals affected with this fur mite are often described as having 'walking dandruff', since infection often leads to the production of excess scale and since the mites are just visible with the naked eye (they are almost 0.5 mm long; Figure 8.14). Infection does not usually cause any marked loss of hair. Often the mites will move on to humans handling the animals and will often bite, though they will not survive for long periods. Small raised red spots appear in the affected areas of the human body and the condition is itchy.

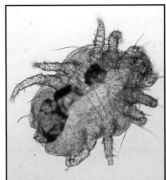

8.14   Dorsal view of *Cheyletiella* mite (0.4 mm). Note the 'comb' on the end of each leg and the large palps on either side of the head, each with a large claw.

Trombicula autumnalis

This mite (also known as *Neotrombicula autumnalis*) normally becomes a problem in late summer and autumn, particularly in chalky areas of southern England. The larval mites (Figure 8.15) attach themselves to the legs of passing animals, including dogs or cats, and feed, causing intense irritation to the host.

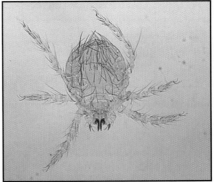

8.15

Trombicula autumnalis (harvest mite) larva (1 mm long, orange-brown in colour). Note that there are only three pairs of legs.

Dermanyssus

This is the 'red mite' that sucks blood of chickens and occasionally other animals. All stages live off the host, e.g. in the eaves of poultry houses. The mites visit chickens to feed, particularly at night. Infection causes irritation and debility, with anaemia in heavy infections. Control is by cleaning the hen-house and treatment with an acaricide.

Ticks

Ticks on livestock are important in many parts of the world as carriers or 'vectors' of disease (see Chapter 6). A heavy tick burden may cause anaemia. In small animal practice it is more usual to encounter just one or two ticks on a cat or dog, with an owner who is concerned about how to get rid of them. Even in these low numbers, ticks can transmit infections such as the Lyme disease agent *Borrelia burgdorferi*.

Since the advent of the Pet Travel Scheme, there has been an increased opportunity for some of the tick-transmitted diseases present in mainland Europe to be introduced into the UK. In order to prevent infected ticks entering the UK, it is mandatory for dogs or cats to be treated with an approved **acaricide** (a substance that is toxic to ticks and mites) before their return to the UK. Details of the latest requirements may be found on the DEFRA website (www.defra.gov.uk).

Several species of tick may affect dogs in the UK and one of these (*Ixodes canisuga*) is host-specific to the dog. However, by far the most common ticks seen on small animals are the sheep tick (*Ixodes ricinus*) (Figure 8.16), particularly in country dwellers, and the hedgehog tick (*Ixodes hexagonus*), especially in urban areas. These ticks are remarkably cosmopolitan and will attach to many different hosts. Initially all that is visible is a small greyish swelling, firmly attached to the animal. Inspection reveals pairs of legs close to the attachment with the host; the mouth parts (Figure 8.17) are buried into the animal's flesh. Once the tick has fed fully it will drop off its host. Diagnosis is based on finding the ticks. The identification of the species of tick is a specialized skill.

The life cycle of the sheep tick is shown in Figure 8.18. It should be noted that some other ticks, such as the dog tick, remain on the host from larva to adult and only drop off once they are fully fed adults.

Individual ticks may be removed by dabbing with a cotton-wool bud that has been treated with an acaricide. Once dead, the tick can be gently removed. A number of tick removal devices are also available. At times of tick challenge it may be worthwhile carrying out prophylactic treatment to ensure that any ticks are repelled from the dog or cat and that any that do attach are killed soon afterwards. There are a number of products available to achieve this, some of which will protect against flea infestation at the same time.

⚠ WARNINGS

- Never try to pull off a live tick unless using an effective 'tick remover', as its mouthparts may be left embedded in the animal and may become a focus for infection.
- Avoid local application of a spot-on acaricide to remove a tick close to an animal's mouth.

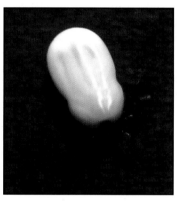

8.16 Engorged adult female sheep tick *Ixodes ricinus*, measuring approximately 7 mm. Note the small dark brown scutum or plate near to the head.

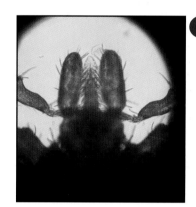

8.17 Mouth parts of a tick.

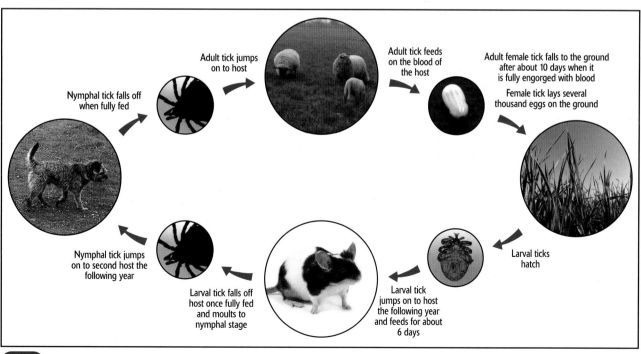

Adult tick jumps on to host

Adult tick feeds on the blood of the host

Adult female tick falls to the ground after about 10 days when it is fully engorged with blood

Female tick lays several thousand eggs on the ground

Nymphal tick falls off when fully fed

Larval ticks hatch

Nymphal tick jumps on to second host the following year

Larval tick falls off host once fully fed and moults to nymphal stage

Larval tick jumps on to host the following year and feeds for about 6 days

8.18 Life cycle of the sheep tick.

Endoparasites

Endoparasites may be divided into helminths and Protozoa.

- **Helminths** are the worms and are subdivided into three types:
  - **Flukes** (which are found in the liver of sheep and cattle but do not normally affect dogs or cats in the UK)
  - **Tapeworms** (cestodes)
  - **Roundworms** (nematodes)
- **Protozoal** parasites are small unicellular organisms.

Figure 8.19 lists the species in each category seen in small animal veterinary practice.

Group	Species	Affects
Helminths		
Flukes		
Cestodes (tapeworms)	*Echinococcus granulosus granulosus*	Dogs
	Echinococcus granulosus equinus	Dogs
	Echinococcus multilocularis [a]	Dogs, cats
	Dipylidium caninum	Dogs, cats
	Taenia spp.	Dogs, cats
Nematodes (roundworms):		
Ascarids	*Toxocara canis*	Dogs
	Toxascaris leonina	Dogs, cats
	Toxocara cati	Cats
Hookworms	*Uncinaria stenocephala*	Dogs
	Ancylostoma tubaeforme	Cats [b]
	Ancylostoma caninum	Dogs
Whipworm	*Trichuris vulpis*	Dogs
Heartworm	*Dirofilaria immitis* [c]	Dogs, cats
Capillaria	*C. plica*	Dogs
	C. hepatica	
Lungworms	*Aelurostrongylus abstrusus*	Cats
	Angiostrongylus vasorum	Dogs
	Oslerus osleri, formerly *Filaroides osleri*	Dogs
Protozoa		
Coccidia	*Eimeria intestinalis*	Rabbits
	E. flavescens	Rabbits
	E. stiedae	Rabbits
	Isospora sp.	Dogs, cats
	Cryptosporidium parvum	Dogs, cats
	Sarcocystis spp.	Dogs, cats
	Toxoplasma gondii	Cats
	Neospora caninum	Dogs
	Hammondia sp.	Cats
Flagellate	*Giardia* sp.	Dogs
Piroplasma	*Babesia* sp.	Dogs [d]

8.19 Species of endoparasite. [a] Mainland Europe only; [b] Hookworm infection occurs rarely in cats in the UK; [c] Not UK – endemic in the Mediterranean area; [d] Not in the UK, though infected dogs may be imported from the southern part of mainland Europe.

Helminths

Cestodes (tapeworms)

A cestode is tape-like and has no alimentary tract. It is composed of three parts: the head or scolex; an area behind this where segments or proglottids form; and finally the maturing segments (Figure 8.20). Tapeworms are hermaphrodites, with a set of male and female reproductive organs in each segment. As the segment matures, reproduction takes place and then eggs develop within the segment, so that when fully mature it is simply an egg-containing structure. Each tapeworm has an immature stage that develops in a separate or intermediate host; the exact structure varies according to the species of tapeworm.

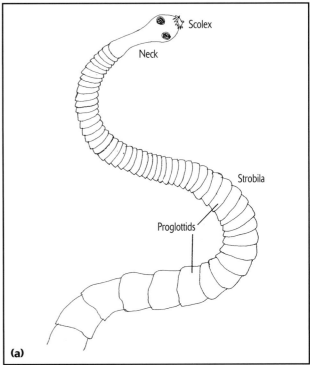

(a)

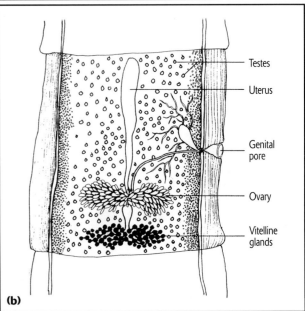

(b)

8.20 (a) A typical adult cestode. (b) A mature proglottid. (Reproduced from Urquhart *et al.*, 1996, with the permission of Blackwell Publishing)

Tapeworms found in cats and dogs in the UK are *Echino-coccus granulosus* (dogs), *Dipylidium caninum* (dogs and cats) and the *Taenia* species (one species in cats and several species in dogs). Their presence is not normally any problem to the final host, though the sight of tapeworm segments is repugnant to owners. There is more often a problem with infection of the intermediate host, either because the presence of the tapeworm cysts causes disease or because affected meat is condemned as unfit for human consumption.

Tapeworm definitions

Adult tapeworm:

- **Scolex**: head of a tapeworm – used for attachment to the host's intestine using suckers and the rostellum (where present) for attachment
- **Rostellum**: the anterior part of the scolex, present in most tapeworms; it is a protrusible cone and is armed with hooks in some species
- **Strobila**: the chain of individual segments
- **Proglottid**: name for each individual segment that makes up the strobila.

Immature tapeworms (**metacestodes**):

- **Cysticercus**: fluid-filled cyst containing a single invaginated scolex attached to the cyst wall
- **Cysticercoid**: single evaginated scolex (this is the form found in invertebrate intermediate hosts)
- **Hydatid cyst**: large cyst containing many scolices, some loose in the fluid inside and some contained within 'brood capsules'
- **Coenurus**: a cyst with many invaginated scolices attached to the cyst wall.

Dipylidium caninum

This is probably the most common tapeworm of cats and dogs in the UK. The intermediate host is the flea, and the biting louse in the case of the dog. It is normally diagnosed by the presence of motile segments (shaped like rice grains) around the anus or in the faeces of a cat or dog (Figure 8.21). The life cycle is shown in Figure 8.22. Control depends on treating the existing infection then eliminating any flea or louse problem to break the transmission cycle. *Dipylidium caninum* occasionally infects humans.

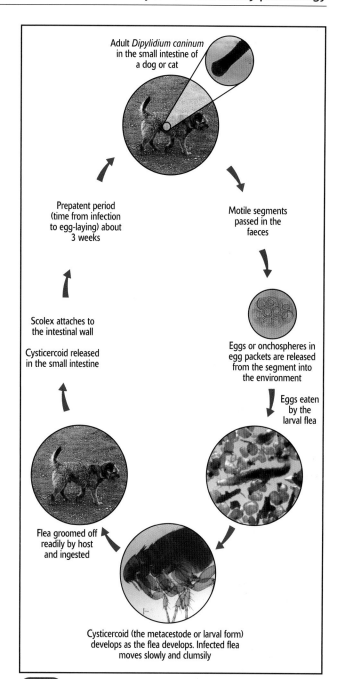

Adult *Dipylidium caninum* in the small intestine of a dog or cat

Prepatent period (time from infection to egg-laying) about 3 weeks

Motile segments passed in the faeces

Scolex attaches to the intestinal wall

Cysticercoid released in the small intestine

Eggs or onchospheres in egg packets are released from the segment into the environment

Eggs eaten by the larval flea

Flea groomed off readily by host and ingested

Cysticercoid (the metacestode or larval form) develops as the flea develops. Infected flea moves slowly and clumsily

8.22 Life cycle of *Dipylidium caninum*.

Taenia spp.

Dogs and cats may be affected with taeniid tapeworms when they eat raw meat, either in the form of uncooked meat or offal or through catching and eating prey containing the intermediate stages. The life cycle of *Taenia hydatigena* is shown in Figure 8.23 and the names of the specific tapeworms with their final and intermediate hosts are shown in Figure 8.24. Diagnosis is based on seeing segments passed by the animal. More rarely, eggs liberated from the segments are seen during microscopic examination of a faecal sample. *Taenia* eggs (Figure 8.25) are smaller than those of *Toxocara* (see Figure 8.29), measuring about 40 µm in diameter. Control is based on treating the current infection and then preventing the animal having access to uncooked flesh, which is something that is easy to do where the animal is fed by the owner but more difficult if the infection is derived from wild prey.

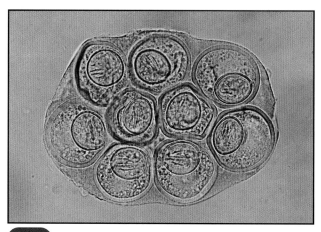

8.21 A *Dipylidium caninum* 'egg packet'.

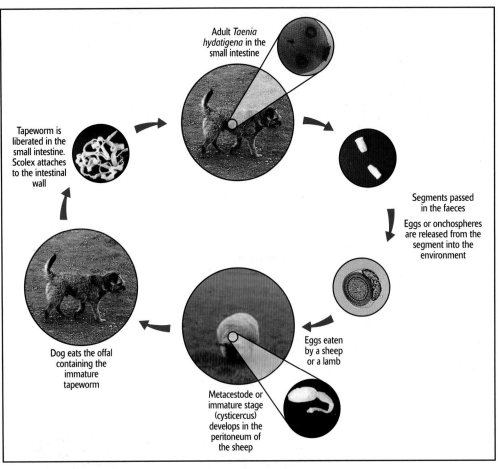

8.23 Life cycle of *Taenia hydatigena*. (Cysticercus courtesy of J McGarry)

Adult *Taenia hydatigena* in the small intestine

Tapeworm is liberated in the small intestine. Scolex attaches to the intestinal wall

Segments passed in the faeces

Eggs or onchospheres are released from the segment into the environment

Dog eats the offal containing the immature tapeworm

Eggs eaten by a sheep or a lamb

Metacestode or immature stage (cysticercus) develops in the peritoneum of the sheep

Taenia species	Final host	Intermediate host
T. taeniaeformis	Cat	Rat or mouse (*Cysticercus fasciolaris* in the liver)
T. serialis	Dog	Rabbit (*Coenurus serialis* in connective tissue)
T. pisiformis	Dog	Rabbit (*Cysticercus pisiformis* in the peritoneum)
T. ovis	Dog	Sheep (*Cysticercus ovis* in muscle)
T. hydatigena	Dog	Sheep/cattle/pig (*Cysticercus tenuicollis* in the peritoneum)
T. multiceps	Dog	Sheep/cattle (*Coenurus cerebralis* in the central nervous system)

8.24 Hosts of *Taenia* tapeworms.

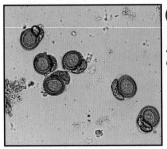

8.25 *Taenia* spp. eggs, each approximately 40 μm in diameter.

Echinococcus granulosus granulosus

This organism has a dog-to-sheep life cycle (Figure 8.26). It is an important zoonotic pathogen that occurs in the UK but is fortunately fairly rare. It is endemic in two areas of the UK –

Wales and the Hebrides – where dogs have the opportunity to feed on sheep carcasses on the hills. Following accidental ingestion of eggs, hydatid cysts can develop in humans, particularly in the liver or lungs.

The adult parasite is very small, only about 6 mm long, and several thousand may be present in the intestine of a single dog. Dogs in affected areas should be regularly treated with an effective anthelmintic and denied access to sheep carcasses. If a human ingests a proglottid or individual eggs, then a hydatid cyst may develop in the liver or lungs in the same way as it will develop in the sheep. This forms a space-occupying lesion that may grow to some considerable size. Treatment of affected people is based on anthelmintics followed by draining the cyst and then surgically removing the wall of the cyst. This is quite a hazardous procedure for the patient.

Echinococcus granulosus equinus is a separate tapeworm that has a dog-to-horse life cycle. It occurs particularly where hounds are fed on horse offal. It is not believed to pose a zoonotic risk.

Echinococcus multilocularis

This is a related tapeworm found in continental Europe, where it was particularly recognized in Switzerland but has now spread to include a wide area of central Europe, including Germany and eastern France. The intermediate stage, a multilocular invasive cyst, is normally found in rodents but humans can also be infected. Dogs, foxes and cats can act as final hosts, though cats are considered to be a poorer host. This parasite is the reason for the necessity to treat animals returning to the UK with praziquantel. Up-to-date information about this and other requirements of the pet travel scheme may be found at www.defra.gov.uk/animalh/quarantine/index.htm.

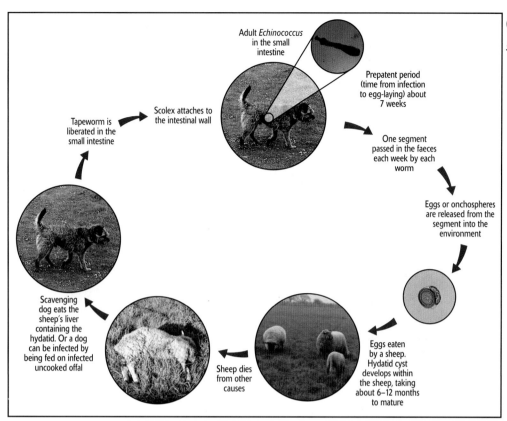

8.26 Life cycle of *Echinococcus granulosus granulosus*.

Adult *Echinococcus* in the small intestine

Scolex attaches to the intestinal wall

Tapeworm is liberated in the small intestine

Prepatent period (time from infection to egg-laying) about 7 weeks

One segment passed in the faeces each week by each worm

Eggs or onchospheres are released from the segment into the environment

Scavenging dog eats the sheep's liver containing the hydatid. Or a dog can be infected by being fed on infected uncooked offal

Sheep dies from other causes

Eggs eaten by a sheep. Hydatid cyst develops within the sheep, taking about 6–12 months to mature

Cestode infections in other animals

Birds and other animals, such as rabbits, mice, rats and hamsters, may all be infected with adult tapeworms specific to the host species. In most cases infection has no effect on the host. Occasionally a heavy tapeworm burden in hamsters may be associated with weight loss and perhaps intestinal blockage. In each case the intermediate host is an invertebrate such as a beetle or mite.

Treatment of cestode infections

Adult tapeworms can be killed by a number of anthelmintics. These may be products that only have activity against tapeworms, in which case they are known as **cestocides**. Alternatively, the preparation may have activity against other helminths, particularly nematodes, as well as tapeworms; these are known as **broad-spectrum anthelmintics** (see Chapter 9). It is much more difficult to kill the immature tapeworm infections in the intermediate hosts and this is not usually carried out.

Nematodes

Nematode worms are round in cross-section and have a digestive tract. Most have a direct life cycle, but some (e.g. lungworms) have a slug or snail as intermediate host. Others may be carried by a **paratenic host** (one that acts as carrier only; no development of the parasite occurs in a paratenic host).

Important nematode groups seen in small animal veterinary practice include **ascarids** (especially *Toxocara canis, Toxascaris leonina* and *Toxocara cati* in dogs and cats). These large fleshy worms (Figure 8.27) are most numerous and frequent in young animals. Ascarids occur commonly in other animals, including reptiles (e.g. tortoises) and birds (especially parakeets); in each case the ascarid species is host specific. Heavy burdens may be associated with poor growth or intestinal impactions.

Other nematode groups are shown in Figure 8.19.

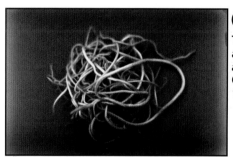

8.27 Typical appearance of adult ascarids (approximately 10 cm long).

Toxocara canis

This is a very important worm, since it is a zoonotic pathogen and can also cause disease in young puppies. Its life cycle is shown in Figure 8.28.

Puppies are first infected before birth by larvae that pass from the bitch's muscles to her uterus after about the 42nd day of pregnancy. These larvae migrate through the liver and lungs of the young puppies and are then coughed up and swallowed. They remain in the small intestine, where they develop to adult worms by the time that the puppies are 3 weeks old. Puppies can receive further infection from infective eggs in the environment and by infective larvae that pass in the mother's milk, but usually the majority of the infection will have occurred across the placenta. Puppies that have a heavy *Toxocara* burden will typically be stunted, with distended bellies; they may vomit and/or have diarrhoea, and severe infections may lead to a total blockage of the intestine. As immunity develops following exposure, and possibly related to an increase in age, puppies begin to expel their *Toxocara* infection spontaneously from about 7 weeks of age. Most have expelled all of their adult worms by 6–7 months of age. Normally further larvae that are ingested pass from the intestine to muscle, where they enter a resting state.

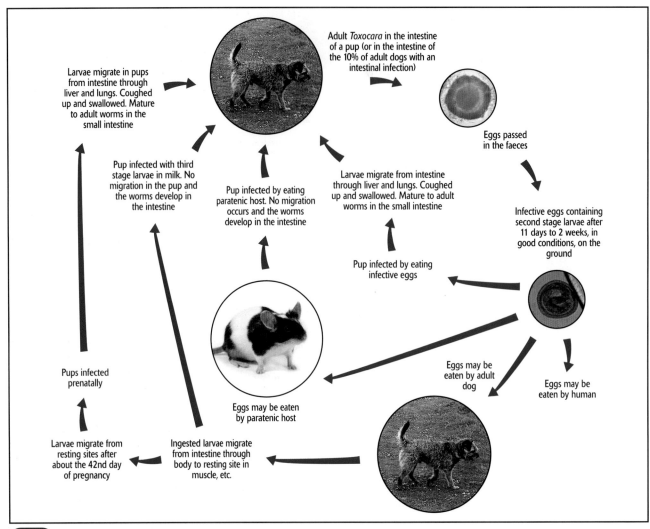

Larvae migrate in pups from intestine through liver and lungs. Coughed up and swallowed. Mature to adult worms in the small intestine

Adult *Toxocara* in the intestine of a pup (or in the intestine of the 10% of adult dogs with an intestinal infection)

Eggs passed in the faeces

Pup infected with third stage larvae in milk. No migration in the pup and the worms develop in the intestine

Pup infected by eating paratenic host. No migration occurs and the worms develop in the intestine

Larvae migrate from intestine through liver and lungs. Coughed up and swallowed. Mature to adult worms in the small intestine

Infective eggs containing second stage larvae after 11 days to 2 weeks, in good conditions, on the ground

Pup infected by eating infective eggs

Pups infected prenatally

Eggs may be eaten by paratenic host

Eggs may be eaten by adult dog

Eggs may be eaten by human

Larvae migrate from resting sites after about the 42nd day of pregnancy

Ingested larvae migrate from intestine through body to resting site in muscle, etc.

8.28   Life cycle of *Toxocara canis*. (Embryonated egg courtesy of J McGarry)

Adult worms pass large numbers of eggs (as many as several thousand eggs per gram of faeces in a 3-week-old puppy). Each egg is surrounded by a thick wall (Figure 8.29), which is very resistant to either physical or chemical damage. The eggs are not immediately infective but require time for a larva to develop inside. In ideal conditions this will take about 14 days, but it may take much longer in low temperatures. Since the larva remains in the shell until eaten by an animal, the eggs may remain infective in the environment for at least 2 years. If the animal that ingests the eggs happens to be a bitch, the larvae remain in this resting state until she becomes pregnant; some of the larvae will migrate to infect her pups; and others will remain to infect her subsequent litters.

Larvae that are accidentally eaten by other animals (including humans) migrate from the intestine and enter a resting state in other tissues. If a human ingests a large number of infective eggs and these all migrate together through the body, a condition known as visceral larva migrans may develop, associated with signs of damage to the organs through which the larvae are migrating. If only a few larvae are ingested, they will usually migrate through the human body without any signs of illness, except in the rare case where they come to rest in the eye, when sight dysfunction or even blindness may result. Infection is usually seen in children, as they are the most likely to have unhygienic habits.

To perpetuate their life cycle, dormant larvae in the tissues of birds or animals other than dogs depend upon their paratenic host being eaten by a dog.

In some adult dogs, for one reason or another, including a low level of challenge, adult worms will develop in the small intestine. Lactating bitches are particularly likely to have a patent infection, probably due to the change in their hormonal status. Their infection may come from a number of sources, including young worms passed by the pups that the bitch ingests as she cleans up around the nest. Usually the bitch expels her remaining infection shortly after the pups are weaned. Single-sample surveys showed 5–10% of dogs infected. In a recent Swiss survey with monthly sampling over 12 months, 30% of dogs were infected at least once during the year.

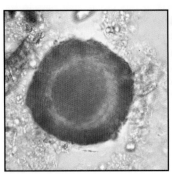

8.29

Toxocara canis egg (approximately 80 μm diameter). Note the dark contents and dark shell with pitted edge.

Control of *Toxocara canis*

The aims are:

- Control of infection in the dog, to prevent disease in puppies and to prevent eggs being put into the environment
- Prevention of infection in children.

Control in dogs is based on the following.

- Prenatal infection in puppies may be controlled by treating the bitch, prior to whelping, with a product that will kill the migrating larvae, e.g. fenbendazole from the 40th day of pregnancy to 2 days post whelping.
- Alternatively, puppies may be treated at regular intervals with a suitable anthelmintic, starting from 2 weeks of age. The bitch should be treated at the same time.
- Reducing the number of eggs in the environment is very difficult once the eggs are present. Scorching with a flame-thrower has been found to be the most effective method, but education of the dog-owning public is the best way to reduce egg output in the future.

The most important methods of preventing children from becoming infected are to ensure that:

- Dogs defecate in specified areas in parks
- 'Pooper scoopers' or other means of appropriate faeces disposal are used
- Children wash their hands before eating
- Children are discouraged from handling young puppies unless the animals have been thoroughly wormed.

Toxascaris leonina

This ascarid will infect both cats and dogs. Its life cycle is shown in Figure 8.30. It has rarely been implicated as a zoonosis. There is no prenatal infection; therefore infection is usually first seen in adolescent animals. The worm is not normally associated with clinical signs, since large burdens are reasonably well tolerated. The egg (Figure 8.31) can be distinguished by the smooth outer wall to its shell.

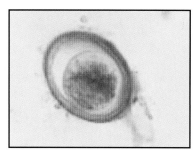

8.31 *Toxascaris leonina* egg (approximately 85 μm long). Note the smooth outer wall. Contents are paler than those of *Toxocara* species.

Toxocara cati

This organism is responsible for ascarid infection in cats, particularly kittens. It is transmitted to kittens by their mothers' milk; infection also occurs through infective eggs in the environment and ingestion of paratenic hosts (Figure 8.32). A heavy infection may cause stunting of kittens and a pot-bellied appearance. The adult worm can be distinguished by the appearance of the alae or 'wings' either side of the head end (Figure 8.33). The egg is grossly indistinguishable from that of *Toxocara canis*. Control is by regular treatment of kittens from about 3 weeks of age until they are several months of age. Kittens are infected via the milk and so will be about 6 weeks of age before the first infection becomes patent.

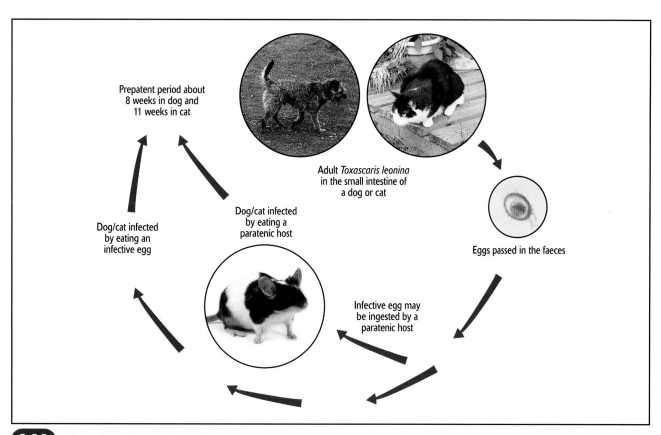

Prepatent period about 8 weeks in dog and 11 weeks in cat

Adult *Toxascaris leonina* in the small intestine of a dog or cat

Dog/cat infected by eating a paratenic host

Dog/cat infected by eating an infective egg

Eggs passed in the faeces

Infective egg may be ingested by a paratenic host

8.30 Life cycle of *Toxascaris leonina*.

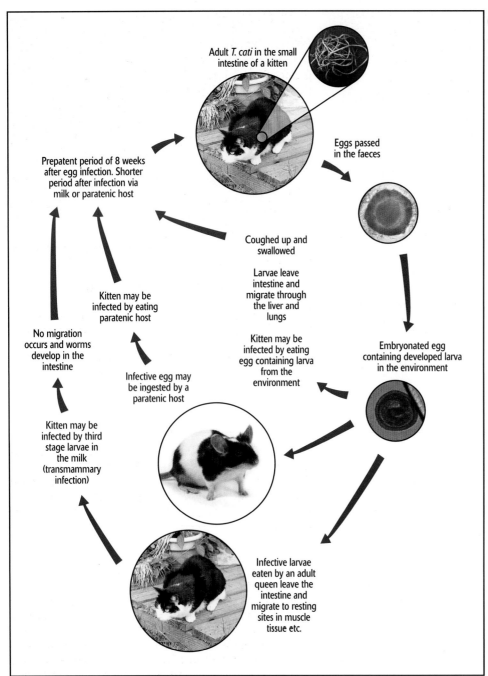

Adult *T. cati* in the small intestine of a kitten

Eggs passed in the faeces

Prepatent period of 8 weeks after egg infection. Shorter period after infection via milk or paratenic host

Coughed up and swallowed

Larvae leave intestine and migrate through the liver and lungs

Kitten may be infected by eating paratenic host

Kitten may be infected by eating egg containing larva from the environment

Embryonated egg containing developed larva in the environment

No migration occurs and worms develop in the intestine

Infective egg may be ingested by a paratenic host

Kitten may be infected by third stage larvae in the milk (transmammary infection)

Infective larvae eaten by an adult queen leave the intestine and migrate to resting sites in muscle tissue etc.

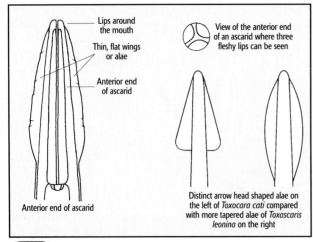

Lips around the mouth

Thin, flat wings or alae

Anterior end of ascarid

View of the anterior end of an ascarid where three fleshy lips can be seen

Anterior end of ascarid

Distinct arrow head shaped alae on the left of *Toxocara cati* compared with more tapered alae of *Toxascaris leonina* on the right

8.33 Anterior end and alae of adult ascarid.

Hookworms

Hookworms are short stout worms with hooked heads (Figure 8.34). *Uncinaria stenocephala* and *Ancylostoma caninum* occur in the small intestine of the dog. Of the two species, *U. stenocephala* is the more common in the UK and is known as the northern hookworm; it is particularly seen in Greyhounds or hunt kennels. The species may be distinguished by the appearance of the head: *A. caninum* has three pairs of large teeth; *A. braziliensis* (Figure 8.35) has two pairs of similar teeth; and *U. stenocephala* has plates in the mouth cavity.

The life cycle is shown in Figure 8.36. The worms attach to the intestinal mucosa by their mouthparts. They use their teeth to damage the surface and then feed off the tissue fluids, particularly blood in the case of *A. caninum*. A heavy burden of *Uncinaria* spp. may cause a dog to be thin and *Ancylostoma* spp. may cause anaemia. Eggs produced by the adult female worms are passed in the faeces. The infective larvae of both worms may penetrate the skin. Larvae of *Uncinaria* spp. simply

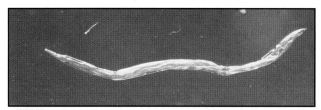

8.34 Adult female hookworm measuring just over 1 cm in length.

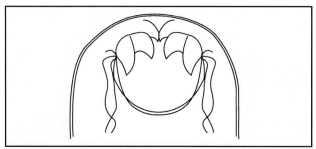

8.35 Head of *Ancylostoma braziliensis*, showing two pairs of teeth at the entrance to the buccal capsule. *Uncinaria stenocephala* has a similarly sized buccal capsule but with cutting plates instead of teeth. *A. caninum* has three pairs of teeth.

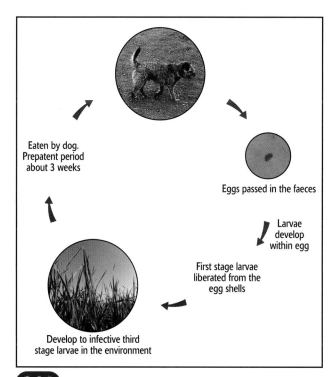

Eaten by dog. Prepatent period about 3 weeks

Eggs passed in the faeces

Larvae develop within egg

First stage larvae liberated from the egg shells

Develop to infective third stage larvae in the environment

8.36 Life cycle of *Uncinaria stenocephala*.

cause a dermatitis, as they are incapable of travelling further, whereas those of *Ancylostoma* spp. may travel to the intestine and develop into adults. Bitches may infect their pups with *Ancylostoma* spp. larvae via their milk. Cats can be infected with hookworm but infection appears to be rare in the UK.

Whipworm

Trichuris vulpis, the whipworm of the dog, has a whip-like appearance (Figure 8.37). The worms burrow into the mucosa of the large intestine, leaving the thicker caudal end in the intestinal lumen. A low burden is well tolerated but a heavy infection may be associated with a bloody mucus-filled diarrhoea. The eggs in which the larvae develop are characteristic (Figure 8.38)

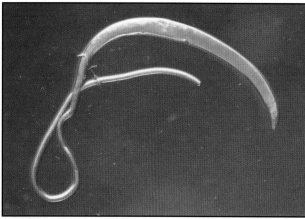

8.37 Whipworm (*Trichuris vulpis*). Note the wide posterior end and the narrow anterior end normally buried in the mucosa of the largest intestine (1–3 cm).

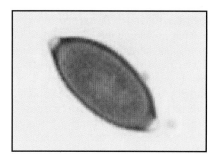

8.38 *Trichuris vulpis* egg (approximately 70 μm long). Note plugs at both ends.

and are covered in a thick shell, which makes them resistant to damage in the environment. Eggs containing infective first-stage larvae may survive for several years in the ground. *T. vulpis* therefore tends to cause problems when dogs have access to permanent grass runs but clinical signs are rarely seen in the UK.

Heartworm

Dirofilaria immitis does not occur in the UK but may be seen in dogs that have been imported from warmer countries. The adult worms live in the heart; immature larvae are known as **microfilariae**. These are dispersed in the host's blood and transmission occurs when a mosquito transfers the larvae from one host to another. A light infection in a dog may be well tolerated but a larger burden can lead to right-sided heart failure. Infection in cats is somewhat less common but clinical effects of just a single worm can be severe in cats.

This is another parasite to consider when owners are planning to take their pet to mainland Europe, as heartworm is endemic from the Mediterranean area of France southwards. Prophylactic treatment should be carried out by owners, using one of the treatments now licensed in the UK and following data sheet instructions.

Bladder and liver worms (*Capillaria* spp.)

Adult worms of *Capillaria plica* live in the bladder and so the eggs are passed in the urine of affected dogs. The eggs appear very like *Trichuris* eggs, but are smaller with less distinct plugs. Infection is rarely seen in the UK.

Capillaria hepatica is a parasite of rats, particularly wild rats. The adult worm lives in the liver of the host, where it lays its eggs. These are only released when the rat dies or is eaten by another animal. Cats, dogs and humans may be infected, but this occurs very rarely. Other *Capillaria* species specific to birds may cause diarrhoea in pigeons.

Lungworms

Cats become infected with *Aelurostrongylus abstrusus* (cat lungworm) by eating a slug or snail containing the infective larvae. The adult worm lives within the lung tissue of the cat. Infection with many worms may cause coughing, but a few worms often go unnoticed. Adult females produce larvae (rather than eggs) that are coughed up and swallowed. Diagnosis is confirmed by finding larvae in the faeces using the Baermann technique (see Chapter 17).

Dogs acquire *Angiostrongylus vasorum* infection through eating a snail containing the infective larvae. Transmission of this infection in England was confined to Cornwall and South Wales, but it is now being seen in most of England.

The slender adult worms live in the pulmonary artery of the dog. The adult females produce eggs that travel to the alveoli and hatch; the larvae then penetrate the alveolar walls. The larvae are coughed up, swallowed and passed in the faeces. Clinical signs include coughing and dyspnoea.

Oslerus osleri (formerly *Filaroides osleri*)

The adult worms live in small nodules at the bifurcation of the trachea (in dogs, particularly Greyhounds). The nodules can be seen on endoscopy and they may cause coughing in some dogs, but others tolerate their presence without showing symptoms.

The adult female worms produce larvae that are coughed up and swallowed. The life cycle is direct (i.e. the parasite passes directly from one host to the next without having to infect an alternative or intermediate host) and the bitch may infect her puppies as she grooms them.

Diagnosis of nematode infections

It is important that faecal samples are fresh and are quickly picked up from the ground, otherwise the sample can become contaminated with free-living nematodes and their eggs from the environment. The main diagnostic methods are modified McMaster techniques to detect nematode eggs in faeces and the Baermann technique (see Chapter 17) to detect larvae.

Treatment of nematode infections

Treatment of nematode infections is carried out in three main situations.

Regular treatment

A broad-spectrum anthelmintic with additional cestocidal activity is often used to remove any infections that may have accumulated since the animal was last wormed. Adult dogs and cats will usually be treated at intervals of 3–6 months depending on the likelihood of infection. There is now an option to control nematodes and fleas at the same time by using either selamectin (Stronghold) or imidacloprid and moxidectin (Advocate) in cats and dogs, or lufenuron and milbemycin (Program Plus) in dogs; all treatments are administered at monthly intervals. Control of tapeworms, where necessary, has to be carried out separately.

Toxocara infections in puppies and kittens

Since these infections occur in the vast majority of litters, it is normal to control them by treating all puppies and kittens regularly.

Diagnosed nematode infection

Where the presence of a nematode infection has been diagnosed as the cause of a clinical problem, the product with the best activity against that infection will usually be chosen for treatment of the animal.

Protozoal parasites

Coccidia

Coccidia may cause marked diarrhoea in young animals, particularly lambs, birds and rabbits. Rabbits may be infected with any of three *Eimeria* spp., all of which have the typical coccidian life cycle (Figure 8.39):

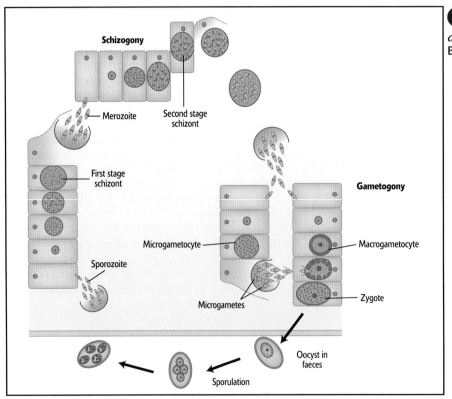

8.39 Life cycle of *Eimeria* spp. (Redrawn from Urquhart *et al.*, 1996, with the permission of Blackwell Publishing)

- *Eimeria intestinalis* and *E. flavescens* infect the caecum, causing diarrhoea and emaciation.
- *E. stiedae* infects the bile ducts in the liver, causing wasting, diarrhoea and excess urine production.

Diagnosis is based on finding oocysts present in the faeces (Figure 8.40). The small rod-like organisms found in the faeces of sick rabbits are not coccidia and are not believed to be significant. Treatment such as sulphonamide may be given in rabbits' drinking water, or to pet rabbits on an individual basis. Control is based on making sure that the rabbits have clean bedding and that droppings or diarrhoea are not allowed to build up in the feeding area.

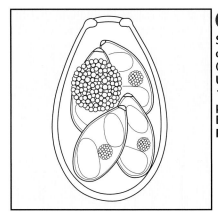

8.40
Sporulated oocyst of *Eimeria* spp. (Reproduced from Urquhart *et al.*, 1996, with the permission of Blackwell Publishing)

Isospora

This protozoan is also known as *Levineia*. Two species infect cats and another two infect dogs. The animals are infected when they ingest either sporulated oocysts (oocysts are not sporulated until a few days after they have been passed in the faeces) or infected intermediate hosts. Reproduction occurs in the cells lining the small intestine. Infection is usually associated with few clinical signs, but there may be transient diarrhoea. Heavy infection may cause severe diarrhoea in puppies and kittens.

Cryptosporidium parvum

This small protozoan parasitizes epithelial cells in the small intestine. Both asexual and sexual reproduction occur in the intestine; and small oocysts, the result of sexual reproduction, are passed in the faeces. Infection occurs by ingesting sporulated oocysts; this has been associated with diarrhoea in young puppies and kittens and the young of other domestic animals. Humans may be infected, usually only causing a transient diarrhoea, though severe diarrhoea may be associated with infection in immunocompromised individuals.

Diagnosis is based on finding the oocysts (4.5–5 μm diameter) in the faeces. Identification may be assisted by staining with Ziehl–Neelsen, as the oocysts are acid fast, or by immunofluorescence techniques. There is currently no licensed treatment for the infection in small animals.

Sarcocystis

This organism has a more complex life cycle than the coccidia and is therefore classified separately. The intermediate hosts are ruminants, pigs or horses. Large unsightly cysts are formed in muscle and so infected meat is condemned. In addition, infection may result in marked illness in the infected animal. The final host for each species is the dog or the cat. For example, *Sarcocystis tenella* (also known as *Sarcocystis ovicanis*) is a parasite of sheep and dogs. Reproduction occurs in the small intestine without clinical signs. The oocysts, measuring approximately 10–15 μm, are already sporulated when passed.

Toxoplasma gondii

The final host for *T. gondii* is the cat (Figure 8.41). Sexual reproduction occurs in the epithelial cells of the small intestine. Oocysts are produced that are passed in the faeces. The

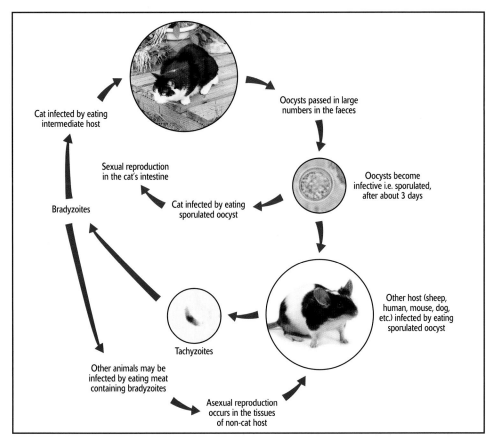

8.41 Life cycle of *Toxoplasma gondii*. (Tachyzoites and oocyst courtesy of J McGarry)

Cat infected by eating intermediate host

Oocysts passed in large numbers in the faeces

Sexual reproduction in the cat's intestine

Oocysts become infective i.e. sporulated, after about 3 days

Bradyzoites

Cat infected by eating sporulated oocyst

Other host (sheep, human, mouse, dog, etc.) infected by eating sporulated oocyst

Tachyzoites

Other animals may be infected by eating meat containing bradyzoites

Asexual reproduction occurs in the tissues of non-cat host

cat usually shows no sign of infection and normally, after excreting oocysts for about 10 days, becomes immune and stops production.

Asexual reproduction occurs in the extra-intestinal (outside the intestine) tissue of almost any animal. Following ingestion of oocysts or asexual stages, the sporozoites leave the intestine and travel to tissue, particularly muscle or brain. Here they divide to form **tachyzoites**. Once an immune response is started by the host, these undergo slower division; they are then known as **bradyzoites**, which remain in the tissue in the hope that they will one day be eaten by a cat.

These cysts in tissue are minute and cause little problem except in certain circumstances:

- A ewe is infected for the first time during pregnancy. Some cysts may occur in the placenta and may cause abortion.
- A woman is infected for the first time during pregnancy, perhaps by eating meat containing bradyzoites or accidentally swallowing sporulated oocysts. Infection of the fetus may result and, depending on the stage of pregnancy, this may result in abortion, severe abnormalities or no clinical signs at all. Fortunately, infections during human pregnancy are not common. Further information and leaflets can be obtained from Tommy's, The Baby Charity (www.tommys.org), who have taken over the work of the Toxoplasmosis Trust in the UK.
- Infection in humans may be associated with malaise and flu-like symptoms that vary in severity from individual to individual.
- Cysts in immunosuppressed individuals may begin to undergo rapid division and cause severe tissue lesions.

In order to try to prevent these infections occurring:

- Farmers are advised to prevent cats, particularly young cats, from getting into food stores intended for sheep.
- There is now a vaccine against *Toxoplasma* for sheep.
- Pregnant women are advised to take precautionary measures. For example, they should not clean out cat litter trays, they should wear gloves when gardening and they should ensure that all meat is thoroughly cooked before eating it.

There is no effective treatment to prevent oocyst shedding in the cat. Children who have been infected prenatally are treated with antiprotozoals to prevent any long-term effects.

Neospora caninum

This parasite causes incoordination in young dogs and abortion in cattle. In the past, infection was normally ascribed to *Toxoplasma gondii*. It is believed that the dog is the final host for this parasite. Treatment of affected puppies may be necessary. Breeding bitches can be screened serologically for signs of infection.

Hammondia

This is another protozoan parasite where the cat is the final host. Infection is not normally associated with clinical signs. Sexual reproduction occurs in the intestine of the cat and oocysts are produced that appear similar to those of *Toxoplasma*. The intermediate hosts for *Hammondia* are rodents and so the presence of these oocysts does not present a human health risk.

Giardia spp.

This flagellate protozoan may parasitize the small intestine of humans and domestic animals. It is still unknown how important *Giardia* infection in pet animals is as a source of human infection, but it may cause death in cage birds such as cockatiels and budgerigars.

Infection may be asymptomatic or may be associated with transient or chronic diarrhoea. Puppies are at greatest risk. Diagnosis is based on demonstration of the cysts (Figure 8.42), which are small (approximately 10 μm) and may be passed intermittently in the faeces. Even when a sample is positive, cysts may be present in low numbers, so a sensitive detection technique is used, such as centrifugal flotation using saturated zinc sulphate solution. The cysts can then be stained with Lugol's iodine to increase visibility. It is suggested that collecting samples for 3 days and pooling the sample may help to overcome intermittent excretion.

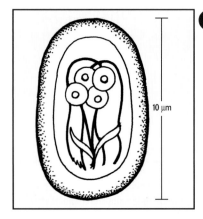

8.42 Cyst of *Giardia* spp.

Other protozoal infections

Some protozoal infections are not endemic in the UK, but clinical disease may be seen in animals that are imported from, for example, parts of Europe, where the disease is endemic. These include *Babesia*, a parasite that infects the red blood cells of dogs, thereby causing anaemia. This is a tick-transmitted infection endemic in southern Europe. Leishmaniosis is caused by a flagellate protozoan and is transmitted by sandflies. It occurs in many warmer parts of the world, including the Mediterranean area. Incubation can be particularly long and it is often extremely difficult to clear the infection completely with treatment. More information about these diseases may be found in the review by Trees and Shaw (1999).

Further reading

Bishop Y (2005) *The Veterinary Formulary, 6th edn.* Pharmaceutical Press, London

Bowman DD (2000) *Georgi's Parasitology for Veterinarians, 7th edn.* WB Saunders, Philadelphia

Fisher M: BSAVA review of worm control in dogs. www.bsava.com

Fisher M: BSAVA review of worm control in cats. www.bsava.com

Overgaauw PAM (1997) Aspects of *Toxocara* epidemiology: toxocarosis in dogs and cats. *Critical Reviews in Microbiology,* **23**, 233–251

Trees A and Shaw S (1999) Imported diseases in small animals. *In Practice,* **21**, 482–489

Urquhart GM, Armour JA, Duncan JL and Jennings FW (1996) *Veterinary Parasitology, 2nd edn.* Blackwell Science, Oxford

Chapter 9

Medicines: pharmacology, therapeutics and dispensing

Jonathan Elliott and Amanda Rock

Learning objectives

After studying this chapter, students should be able to:

- Categorize drugs used in routine veterinary practice into their therapeutic groups
- List the routes by which drugs can be administered and explain the effect that drug formulation and route of administration have on the rate of absorption of a drug into the body
- Calculate drug dosages accurately, regardless of the units of drug concentration used in describing a particular formulation
- List the legislation that governs the storage, handling, use and supply of medicines used in veterinary practice
- Discuss the implications that the legislation has for the working of a veterinary practice
- Recognize significant adverse drug reactions and state to whom they should be reported

---

Introduction

Definitions

- **Pharmacology** – the science of drugs.
- **Pharmacokinetics** – how the body acts on the drug. This involves the following processes: absorption, distribution, metabolism (usually in the liver) and excretion, either of the drug itself or its metabolites into the bile, urine or via the respiratory tract.
- **Pharmacodynamics** – how the drug acts on the body. Most drugs interact with a receptor in the body. They may stimulate the receptor and produce a full effect (**agonists**), or stimulate it and produce a partial effect (**partial agonists**), or block the receptor by binding to it without producing an effect (**antagonists**). Some drugs inhibit enzymes or block ion channels ▶

that serve physiological functions in the body or the infective organisms.

- **Clinical pharmacology** – the study of how drugs affect diseased patients.
- **Therapeutics** – the rational and optimal use of drugs in the management of disease states or in the manipulation of physiological functions. In order to use drugs in a rational and optimal way, an understanding of the nature of the disease process and of the pharmacology of the drugs to be used is required.
- **Pharmacy** – the preparation and dispensing of drugs.
- The **preparation** of drugs, and their formulation into medicines, is usually done by a pharmaceutical company.
- **Dispensing** (giving out) the drug can be done direct from the veterinary practice, as veterinary surgeons have a *privilege* to dispense medicines. Only pharmacists have the *right* to dispense by law, when presented with a **prescription** (written instruction) from the veterinary surgeon responsible for the care of the animal. Under exceptional circumstances veterinary surgeons can dispense drugs against a prescription from another veterinary practice. Practices are also obliged to inform their clients that they can request prescriptions from their veterinary surgeons but obtain the medications from a pharmacist rather than directly from the veterinary practice.

Drug classification

Drugs can be classified according to the way in which they bring about their effect on the body and which body system (or infective agent) they affect. This is the most useful form of classification for the practice pharmacy as it determines what the drugs are used for in clinical situations and gives an indication of likely **side effects**. When these effects compromise the health of an animal they are termed **undesirable** or **adverse drug reactions** and should be reported to the Veterinary Medicines Directorate (VMD) on special (yellow) SARSS (Suspected Adverse Reaction Surveillance Scheme) reporting forms (Figure 9.1).

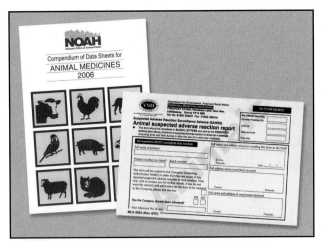

9.1 Special yellow Veterinary Medicines Directorate forms for reporting adverse drug reactions.

Recognition of significant adverse drug reactions

Nurses are often consulted by owners for advice about adverse drug effects and, if in doubt, should consult the veterinary surgeon about specific cases. Examples of significant potential adverse drug effects where immediate veterinary attention should be sought are given below (this list is by no means exhaustive):

- Vomiting, anorexia and lethargy with non-steroidal anti-inflammatory drugs and with digoxin
- Skin lesions, lameness and lethargy with potentiated sulphonamide preparations
- Mucoid ocular discharge in dogs taking preparations containing sulphonamides
- Weakness and incoordination in animals taking vasodilator and other cardiac medications
- Lethargy, anorexia and depression in cats taking antithyroid drugs (e.g. carbimazole, methimazole), griseofulvin or diazepam
- Any vague signs of illness in animals taking cancer chemotherapy agents (these should be taken seriously)
- Haematuria in dogs taking cyclophosphamide
- Loss of balance, nystagmus and circling in animals prescribed ear medications.

Therapeutic index

Any drug that is administered at dosages above those recommended for therapeutic use (accidentally or deliberately) may cause **toxic effects** in the animal. The **therapeutic index** of a drug is the ratio between the dose that causes toxic effects and the dose required to produce the desired therapeutic effect:

$$\text{Therapeutic index (TI)} = LD_{50}/ED_{50}$$

where LD_{50} is the lethal dose in 50% of experimental animals, and ED_{50} is the dose that was effective in 50% of animals.

The higher the TI, the safer is the drug. Low ratios mean that a particular drug may be more dangerous to use and the margin of error that can be allowed when determining the dose for a particular animal is smaller. Examples of drugs with low therapeutic indices include digoxin, the cancer chemotherapeutic agents and the anticoagulant drugs.

A statement of LD_{50} is no longer required as part of the safety package for drug registration. Hence the TI as traditionally defined is not possible to calculate precisely; however, the underlying principle still applies.

Drug names

Wherever possible the **generic** (approved or official) name rather than a **proprietary** (brand or trade) name should be used when referring to drugs. Throughout this chapter examples have been given where a product exists that has been approved (**authorized**) for use in small animals.

Drugs used in the treatment of microorganisms

Definitions

- **Antimicrobial agents** are drugs used to treat infections by bacteria, fungi, viruses or protozoans.
- **Antibiotics** are drugs that are natural products of another microorganism or semi-synthetic products that inhibit the growth of microorganisms (**bacteriostatic**) or kill them (**bactericidal**).

These drugs show **selective toxicity**: they target and damage processes that are essential to the microorganism but which do not take place in animal cells.

Antibacterial drugs

- **Narrow-spectrum** antibacterials are active against only a narrow range of organisms, usually only Gram-negative or only Gram-positive bacteria.
- **Broad-spectrum** antibacterials are active against a wide variety of bacteria (both Gram-positive and Gram-negative) and other microorganisms such as protozoans.
- **Potentiated** antibacterials are formed when two agents are used in combination to produce an effect greater than the additive effects of the two drugs when each is used alone. An example is the potentiated sulphonamides, which are a combination of a sulphonamide plus trimethoprim.

Antibacterials are classified into families of drugs that are chemically related. For example, the penicillins all have the same mode of action (preventing the cross-linking of bacterial cell walls) and so are all bactericidal and share common side effects. If one agent induces allergic reactions in a sensitive animal or person, the whole family should be avoided. Small changes in their structure, however, can change their spectrum of activity. Figure 9.2 summarizes the main antibacterial drug families and gives examples of each.

Good prescribing practice involves selecting an agent on the basis of several factors, including the organism involved, the site of infection and the immunocompetence of the patient. To avoid the development of resistance, prophylactic use should be reserved for specific situations, such as orthopaedic surgery, and some drug groups (e.g. the fluoroquinolones) should be reserved for treatment of serious bacterial infections.

Family	Example	Spectrum of activity	Bactericidal or bacteriostatic
Penicillins [a]	Benzyl penicillin Amoxicillin	Narrow (Gram-positive) Broad	Bactericidal Bactericidal
Tetracyclines	Oxytetracycline	Broad	Bacteriostatic
Aminoglycosides	Neomycin	Narrow (Gram-negative)	Bactericidal
Lincosamides	Clindamycin	Narrow (Gram-positives and anaerobes)	Bacteriostatic
Sulphonamides	Sulfadiazine	Broad	Bacteriostatic
Potentiated sulphonamides	Sulfadiazine plus trimethoprim	Broad	Bactericidal
Nitroimidazoles	Metronidazole	Narrow (anaerobes)	Bactericidal
Chloramphenicol	Chloramphenicol	Broad	Bacteriostatic
Fluoroquinolones	Enrofloxacin	Broad	Bactericidal

9.2   Antibacterial drug families. [a] Penicillins and cephalosporins (e.g. cefalexin) are related chemically and collectively called β-lactams.

Antifungal drugs

Antifungal drugs can be used topically to treat skin, mucous membrane or corneal infections. The hair should be clipped from affected areas and the nails clipped to expose lesions fully before application of the antifungal agent. Perseverance is often an essential element of therapy. Some topical antifungal agents that have been used with success include:

- Iodine preparations: tincture of iodine, potassium iodide
- Copper preparations: copper sulphate
- Dyes: crystal (gentian) violet
- Imidazoles: miconazole, clotrimazole, econazole
- Polyene antibiotics: amphotericin B, nystatin.

Griseofulvin

Griseofulvin is a systemic antifungal agent that is effective against the common dermatophytes that cause ringworm in the dog and cat. It works by distorting the hyphae of the fungus and hence is **fungistatic** (stopping the growth of the fungus) rather than **fungicidal** (killing the fungus). Its absorption from the gut is variable and is enhanced by high-fat meals. The new growth of hair, nail and horn is free from fungal infection, but the infection persists in old hair until it is naturally shed, which means that long courses of up to 6 weeks are recommended unless the patient is shaved at the start of therapy. Griseofulvin is contraindicated in pregnant animals because it is teratogenic (i.e. can harm a developing fetus), but it has good selective toxicity otherwise, as it is preferentially taken up by susceptible fungi rather than by mammalian cells.

Lufenuron

The anti-flea product lufenuron may have some efficacy against feline dermatophytosis, but no well controlled clinical trials have been undertaken to prove this. Hence, this is not an authorized indication for this product.

Antiviral drugs

There are not many antiviral agents as it is not easy to find drugs that can impair the virus without damaging the host, because viruses are obligate intracellular parasites and they use the host's genetic machinery to produce new virus. This is known as poor selective toxicity. Other complications include the infrequency with which definitive diagnosis is made attributing a disease to a virus.

Aciclovir

The only antiviral agent commonly used in veterinary medicine is aciclovir, which is used topically in the eye to treat feline herpesvirus infection.

Antiprotozoal drugs

These are used to treat infections by protozoal organisms such as *Toxoplasma gondii*. An example is pyrimethamine.

Leishmaniasis

Therapy for leishmaniasis involves treatment for several months with one or more of amphotericin B, meglumine antimonate and allopurinol.

Drugs used in the treatment of parasitic infections

Endoparasiticides

Endoparasiticides (**anthelmintics**) are drugs used to treat helminth infestations, mainly nematode (roundworm) and cestode (tapeworm) infections. Each drug has its own indications and side effects. Some of the products currently available are listed in Figure 9.3.

Drug	Tapeworms		
	Echinococcus	*Taenia*	*Dipylidium*
Febantel	0	2	0
Fenbendazole	0	2	0
Mebendazole	1	2	0
Milbemycin	0	0	0
Nitroscanate	1	2	2
Piperazine	0	0	0
Praziquantel	2	2	2
Pyrantel	0	0	0
Selamectin	0	0	0

9.3a   Anthelmintic activity against tapeworms. 2, excellent activity; 1, very good activity; 0, poor or ineffective.

Drug	Roundworms		
	Toxocara/ Toxascaris	Whipworms (Trichuris)	Hookworms (Uncinaria)
Febantel	2	2	2
Fenbendazole	2	2	2
Mebendazole	2	2	2
Milbemycin	2	1	2
Nitroscanate	2	2	0
Piperazine	1	1 [a]	0
Praziquantel	0	0	0
Pyrantel	2	2	2
Selamectin	2	2	2

9.3b Anthelmintic activity against roundworms. [a] Effective at 1.5 times the normal dose. 2, excellent activity; 1, very good activity; 0, poor or ineffective.

Anthelmintics must be selectively toxic to the parasite. Parasitic helminths must maintain an appropriate feeding site, and nematodes and trematodes must actively ingest and move food through their digestive tracts to maintain an appropriate energy state, which requires appropriate neuromuscular coordination. The pharmacological basis of the treatment for helminths generally involves interference with one or both of these energy processes, causing starvation of the parasite, or paralysis and subsequent expulsion of the parasite.

Ectoparasiticides

Use of ectoparasiticides has moved away from the organophosphate compounds (e.g. dichlorvos) to treat fleas, mites, ticks and lice, because of increasing resistance and growing fears about the health risks involved.

Commonly used ectoparasiticides

- **Fipronil** is an effective adulticide against fleas. Treatment with 10% fipronil solution has been shown to be effective not only in controlling fleas on animals, but also in significantly reducing the environmental burden. In one study, three monthly applications of fipronil resulted in a reduction in flea burden by 96.5% and the flea numbers in the environment were reduced by 98.6% without the use of an adulticide or insect growth regulator in the environment.
- **Selamectin** also kills adult *Sarcoptes*, the mite responsible for fox mange.
- **Lufenuron**, **methoprene** and **pyriproxyfen** are insect growth regulators. Lufenuron inhibits chitin development and so prevents the adult flea from producing viable eggs and larvae, contributing to environmental control of fleas within a household. Methoprene and pyriproxyfen mimic juvenile hormones and prevent metamorphosis to the adult stage.

- **Imidacloprid** is used in the management of flea infestations in cats, dogs and rabbits. It causes salivation if it is licked off the coat as the authorized product tastes bitter.
- **Permethrin**, a widely used pyrethroid, is an active ingredient in collars, sprays, shampoos, dips and topical concentrations for control of fleas and ticks in dogs and cats. **CATS ARE PARTICULARLY SENSITIVE TO PYRETHROIDS AND OVER-THE-COUNTER PRODUCTS FORMULATED FOR DOGS CAN KILL CATS.** Some forms of synthetic pyrethroids are formulated for application to carpets to provide persistence of the drug in the environment and are not for application to the animal.

Systemic oral preparations

Advantages of systemic oral preparations over topical applications:

- Reduce the exposure of pet owners and the environment to the insecticides
- Efficacy is not influenced by external factors such as rain, sunlight or animal behaviour
- Make it easy to avoid overdosing or underdosing, incomplete coverage or contamination of sensitive body parts such as the eyes.

Disadvantage of systemic oral preparations:

- Rely on the parasites ingesting the drug with a blood meal, which can result in the activation of allergy or the introduction of infections.

Ivermectin

Although not authorized, ivermectin is occasionally used. Dog breeds sensitive to ivermectin include:

- Collies
- Australian Shepherd Dog
- Old English Sheepdog
- Shetland Sheepdog.

This sensitivity occurs in about half of these animals, due to a mutation in the *MDR-1* gene (which normally prevents ivermectin crossing the blood–brain barrier). Homozygotes lack the *p*-glycoprotein pump for which this gene encodes.

Ivermectin must not be used in chelonians, as it is highly toxic.

Drugs acting on the gastrointestinal system

These drugs are shown in Figure 9.4.

Main drug class	Class	Mode of action	Examples
Antidiarrhoeal agents		Suppress diarrhoea non-specifically [a]	
	Adsorbents	Coat the gut wall, adsorb toxins	Charcoal, kaolin, bismuth
	Modulators of intestinal motility	Reduce gastrointestinal motility	Loperamide, diphenoxylate
	Chronic antidiarrhoeals	Anti-inflammatory agents	Sulfasalazine, prednisolone
Anti-emetic drugs		Prevent or suppress vomiting (emesis)	Metoclopramide (vomiting due to gastritis) Aceatis) Acepromazine (motion sickness)

9.4 Drugs acting on the gastrointestinal system. [a] Specific treatment relies on identifying the underlying cause. In some cases, for example, antibacterial drugs or anthelmintics may be indicated. *continues* ▶

Main drug class	Class	Mode of action	Examples
Emetic drugs		Stimulate vomiting	Washing soda (orally) Xylazine (by injection)
Laxatives	Lubricant laxatives Bulk-forming laxatives Osmotic laxatives Stimulant laxatives	Increase defecation Lubricate faecal mass Increase volume of faeces Hypertonic solutions, poorly absorbed Stimulate local reflex gut motility	Liquid paraffin *Isphagula* husk Phosphate (enemas) Dantron
Antacids		Neutralize acid secreted in stomach	Aluminium hydroxide
Ulcer-healing drugs		Inhibit acid secretion in the stomach and allow ulcers to heal Stimulation of mucosal defences and repair mechanisms	Cimetidine Ranitidine Sucralfate
Pancreatin supplements		Contain protease, lipase and amylase activity to aid digestion in exocrine pancreatic insufficiency	

9.4 *continued* Drugs acting on the gastrointestinal system. ᵃ Specific treatment relies on identifying the underlying cause. In some cases, for example, antibacterial drugs or anthelmintics may be indicated.

Drugs used in the treatment of disorders of the cardiovascular system

These can be grouped into agents acting on the heart, blood vessels, blood coagulation system and kidney, respectively.

Drugs acting on the heart

- **Myocardial stimulants** (positive inotropes) stimulate the heart muscle to beat more forcefully. Examples: digoxin and the drug pimobendan, a calcium-sensitizing agent.
- **Sympathomimetics** mimic the action of the sympathetic nervous system and hence increase the heart rate. These can be used in an emergency to treat heart block. Example: isoprenaline.
- **Antidysrhythmic drugs** suppress dysrhythmias (abnormal rhythms). Examples: lidocaine (without adrenaline) for the treatment of ventricular dysrhythmias; and diltiazem to treat atrial dysrhythmias.

When the heart muscle fails to relax properly to allow adequate filling during diastole (e.g. hypertrophic cardiomyopathy in cats), drugs that reduce the force of contraction and/or slow the heart rate are used, e.g. diltiazam and the beta-blocker atenolol.

Drugs acting on the blood vessels

Vasodilators relax the smooth muscle of blood vessels and lower resistance to blood flow, so reducing the work the heart has to do.

- **Arterial dilators** (e.g. hydralazine) act primarily on the arterial smooth muscle.
- **Venodilators** (e.g. glyceryl trinitrate) act primarily on the venous smooth muscle.
- **Mixed dilators** (e.g. enalapril) act on both sides of the circulation.

Hypotension (lowering of the blood pressure) is a potential side effect of these agents and so they are called **antihypertensive drugs** when they are used to treat hypertension. Amlodipine (a calcium-channel blocker with selectivity for vascular smooth muscle) is used in cats with hypertension arising secondary to diseases such as chronic renal failure.

Drugs acting on the blood-clotting system

- **Anticoagulants** prevent blood clotting (e.g. heparin, warfarin)
- **Fibrinolytic agents** break down clots once they have formed (e.g. streptokinase)
- **Haemostatics** arrest haemorrhage and are usually applied topically to local bleeding areas (e.g. calcium alginate).

Drugs acting on the kidney

Diuretics are drugs that act on the kidneys to increase the production of urine. By preventing the reabsorption of sodium, an increased volume of urine is produced, reducing the circulating blood volume and lowering the blood pressure. The diuretics all work on different parts of the nephrons making up the kidney, as shown in Figure 9.5 and vary in their ability to induce diuresis. Some of the available drugs are listed below.

- **Loop diuretics** (e.g. furosemide)
- **Thiazide diuretics** (e.g. hydrochlorothiazide)
- **Potassium-sparing diuretics** (e.g. spironolactone) (can be used with the above two agents to counteract the potassium loss they cause).

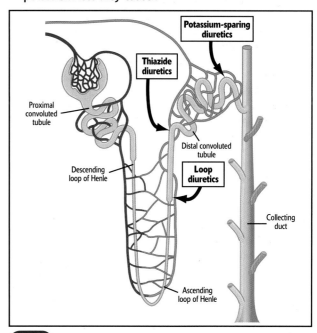

9.5 Sites of action of diuretics on the kidney nephron.

ACE inhibitors

Angiotensin-converting enzyme (ACE) inhibitors can be regarded as potassium-sparing diuretics as they block the formation of angiotensin II and thus the secretion of aldosterone, but they also have balanced vasodilator activity. Examples include benazepril, enalapril, imidapril and ramipril. The ability of ACE inhibitors to lower glomerular capillary pressure is thought to be one way in which they may slow the progression of chronic renal failure.

Drugs used in the treatment of disorders of the respiratory system

Inhalation of infective agents or allergens (e.g. pollen) stimulates inflammation and tissue damage, leading to reflex stimulation of coughing and bronchoconstriction. The sites at which drugs may counteract some of these disease processes are shown in Figure 9.6.

Drugs acting on the nervous system

Sedatives

Sedatives (e.g. acepromazine and medetomidine) are agents that cause calmness, drowsiness and indifference of the animal to its surroundings. They are often used as premedicants for animals that are to be anaesthetized, to promote smoother induction and recovery and to allow a reduction in the dose of general anaesthetic. **Sedative antagonists** (e.g. atipamezole) are available for some sedatives to reverse the effects.

Tranquillizers (e.g. diazepam) cause calmness without drowsiness. **Narcotics** produce deep sedation (narcosis).

Opioid analgesics relieve pain by acting on opioid receptor sites in the brain and spinal cord (e.g. morphine and buprenorphine). **Neuroleptanalgesics** are combinations of sedatives and opioids that produce deeper sedation than sedatives alone. **Opioid antagonists** (e.g. naloxone) reverse the sedation.

General anaesthetics

General anaesthetics produce unconsciousness so that painful procedures can be performed.

- **Injectable general anaesthetics** may be used for induction of anaesthesia (e.g. thiopentone).
- **Inhalational anaesthetics** may be used for maintenance of anaesthesia (e.g. isoflurane).

Antimuscarinic drugs (e.g. atropine, hyoscine) may be given before anaesthesia to counteract the salivation and increased bronchial secretions that can obstruct the airway, and to prevent the **bradycardia** (reduced heart rate) seen as a result of increased vagal nerve stimulation during some surgical procedures.

Muscle relaxants

Muscle relaxants prevent the message from the nerve reaching the muscle. The skeletal muscle paralysis that ensues is not associated with depression of the central nervous system; the animal is fully conscious throughout the period of immobility. Indications for the use of muscle relaxants include:

- Muscle relaxation for surgery
- To facilitate endotracheal intubation in the cat
- Fracture reduction and replacing dislocated joints
- Mechanical ventilation
- Tetanus.

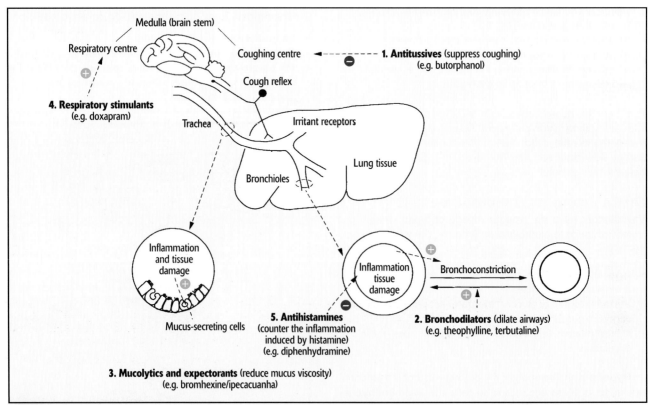

9.6   A schematic representation of the respiratory system showing the sites at which drugs act in the treatment of respiratory disorders (⊕ = stimulation; ⊖ = inhibition of the processes indicated). Inhalation of allergens or infective agents initiates inflammation, bronchoconstriction, increased mucus secretion and coughing (via the cough reflex, which stimulates the coughing centre in the medulla).

Examples of competitive (non-depolarizing) agents include gallamine and pancuronium. Suxamethonium is an example of a depolarizing agent. Neostigmine is a **muscle relaxant antagonist** that can reverse the paralysis caused by competitive (non-depolarizing) agents and will potentiate and prolong the effects of depolarizing agents.

Local anaesthetics

Local anaesthetics temporarily prevent conduction of an impulse along a nerve fibre. Sensory nerves are affected first, causing loss of sensation, followed by loss of function when motor nerves are paralysed. Vasoconstrictors (e.g. adrenaline) are sometimes added to prolong the action of the drug by reducing the blood flow to the area.

- **Lidocaine** (formerly known as lignocaine) is the prototypical local anaesthetic agent used in veterinary practice, being rapid in onset of action and having minimal tissue irritant effects, effective tissue penetration and a relatively short duration of effect (1–1.5 h).
- **Mepivacaine**, is used in equine practice and causes even less tissue irritation than lidocaine but is more expensive.
- **Bupivacaine**, has no tissue irritant effects but has different properties to lidocaine that dictate its clinical use. It has a prolonged duration of effect (4–6 hours) but is slow in its onset of action (15 minutes).

Some local anaesthetics are formulated for topical (surface) applications, e.g. **proxymetacaine**, for ophthalmic use. **EMLA cream** is a eutectic mixture of lidocaine and prilocaine and can be applied to skin 45 minutes before cannulation.

Anti-epileptics

Anti-epileptics are used to control convulsions or seizures. Control of canine epilepsy can be achieved in up to 80% of cases with one drug only (e.g. phenobarbital). The drug is metabolized in the liver, and it increases the rate of hepatic clearance of other drugs, including itself, resulting in more drug being required to produce a given effect over time. Other examples of anti-epileptics include potassium bromide, phenytoin and diazepam.

Drugs used in the treatment of disorders of the endocrine system

Treatment of endocrine disorders involves replacing deficient hormone or prevention of overproduction. Some of the available drugs are listed in Figure 9.7. Anterior pituitary hormones (or their analogues) are used in diagnostic tests for endocrine disorders; for example, tetracosactrin is used in the ACTH stimulation test to diagnose hyperadrenocorticism and hypoadrenocorticism.

- **Steroid hormones** share a common chemical structure and are produced by the adrenal cortex (**adrenal corticosteroids**) or by the ovary and testes (**sex steroids**). Figure 9.8 compares the effects of some of the steroids.
- **Anabolic steroids** (e.g. nandrolone) are derivatives of testosterone and are used to increase muscle mass and to promote tissue repair in convalescing animals.

Gland	Disease state	Drug class	Example
Adrenal gland	*Deficiency:* Hypoadrenocorticism (Addison's disease)	Adrenal corticosteroids Mineralocorticoids (sodium conserving) Glucocorticoids	Fludrocortisone Prednisolone, dexamethasone
	Excess: Hyperadrenocorticism (Cushing's disease)	Adrenolytic agent Glucocorticoid synthesis inhibitor	Trilostane, mitotane, ketoconazole
Thyroid gland	*Deficiency:* Hypothyroidism	Thyroid hormone replacement	Levothyroxine
	Excess: Hyperthyroidism	Antithyroid agent	Methimazole, carbimazole
Endocrine pancreas	*Deficiency:* Diabetes mellitus (hyperglycaemia)	Insulin Oral hypoglycaemic agent	Protamine zinc insulin Glipizide
	Excess: Hypoglycaemia (low blood glucose)	Glucose (intravenous) Anti-insulin agents	Dextrose solution Dexamethasone (glucocorticoids)
Posterior pituitary gland	Diabetes insipidus (deficiency of ADH)	Posterior pituitary hormone (ADH analogue)	Desmopressin

9.7 Drugs used in the treatment of endocrine disorders.

Corticosteroid	Glucocorticoid potency (anti-inflammatory)	Mineralocorticoid potency (electrolyte disturbance)	Alternate-day therapy
Hydrocortisone	1	1	No: anti-inflammatory effect short-lived
Prednisolone	4	0.8	Yes: adrenal gland function not suppressed after 36 h
Methylprednisolone	5	0	Yes
Dexamethasone	30	0	No: results in complete adrenal gland suppression
Betamethasone	30	0	No: results in complete adrenal gland suppression

9.8 Comparison of activity of corticosteroids.

Drugs acting on the urogenital tract

Figure 9.9 describes sex hormones (sex steroids), luteolytic agents (prostaglandins), myometrial stimulants (ecbolics) and drugs used to treat urinary tract disorders. Drugs used in the management of disorders of urination are shown in Figure 9.10.

Drugs used to treat malignant disease

Cancer is the unrestrained growth of cells that, by either local invasion or metastatic spread, can destroy normal tissues. **Cancer chemotherapy** is the medical treatment of cancer using **cytotoxic drugs** (e.g. cyclophosphamide, vincristine) and its success depends on the ability to balance the killing of tumour cells against the toxicity of many of these drugs to host cells.

Agents	Examples	Uses
Oestrogens	Diethylstilbestrol Oestradiol benzoate	Prevent implantation following accidental mating (misalliance) Treat urinary incontinence [a] Reduce the size of an enlarged prostate gland and anal adenomas
Progestogens Steroids which mimic the actions of progesterone	Megestrol acetate Delmadinone Proligestone	Postpone or suppress oestrus in the bitch and queen Management of some behavioural problems (aggression in male dogs)
Androgens Esters or analogues of the male sex hormone, testosterone	Methyltestosterone	Hormone alopecia in dogs and cats Deficient libido in males
Luteolytic agents (prostaglandins)	Dinoprost	(unauthorized use) Synchronization of oestrus in cattle and sheep Induction of parturition in pigs
Myometrial stimulants (ecbolics)	Oxytocin (extract of posterior pituitary gland)	Stimulate the uterus to contract. Dystocia due to weakness of the uterine muscle (uterine inertia)
Urinary acidifers Lower the pH of the urine	Ethylenediamine	In the management of urolithiasis (struvite calculi) Cystitis (aid action of antibacterials and urinary antiseptics)
Urinary alkalinizers Raise the pH of the urine	Sodium bicarbonate	In the management of urate uroliths
Urinary antiseptics Hydrolyse in acidic urine to release formaldehyde	Hexamine	Prophylaxis and long-term treatment of recurrent urinary tract infection

9.9 Drugs used in the treatment of reproductive and lower urinary tracts. [a] First line drug for the medical management of urinary incontinence secondary to urethral sphincter mechanism incompetence would be phenylpropanolamine (see Figure 9.10).

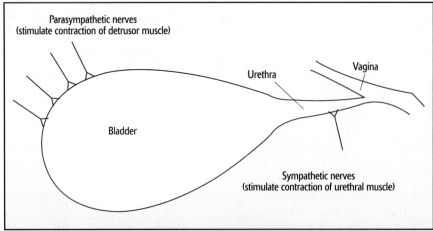

9.10 The bladder, and drugs that affect urination. The process of urination is brought about by parasympathetic stimulation of the detrusor muscle and inhibition of sympathetic tone to the urethral smooth muscle, allowing the bladder to contract and empty through the relaxed urethra. When the bladder fills, the sympathetic nervous system is active, maintaining continence by closing the urethra; the parasympathetic system is inactive, allowing the detrusor muscle to relax and the bladder to fill.

Clinical problem	Signs	Drug class and action	Example
Atonic bladder	Bladder overfills and may leak (overflow incontinence)	Parasympathomimetic (stimulates detrusor muscle to contract)	Bethanechol
Weak bladder neck (intra-pelvic bladder)	Dribbles urine particularly at rest	Sympathomimetic (increases urethral tone)	Phenylpropanolamine
Urethral spasm	Unable to pass stream of urine	Sympathetic antagonist (lowers urethral tone)	Phenoxybenzamine (α-adrenoceptor antagonist)

- The narrow therapeutic indices of these agents means that **dosages** are calculated on body surface area rather than body mass.
- Antineoplastic agents are commonly administered in various combinations referred to as treatment **protocols**.
- The main **indication** for cancer chemotherapy as a first-line treatment is systemic disease such as lymphoma, myeloma and forms of leukaemia.
- Cytotoxic drugs are also used as an **adjunct** to surgery or radiotherapy, or to help prevent metastasis of solid tumours.
- Cytotoxic drugs and the urine and faeces of treated animals are a **hazard** to those handling them and should be avoided by women of childbearing age, particularly if they are, or are liable to become, pregnant. (See also COSHH regulations and risk assessments later in this chapter.)

Drugs used to treat disorders of the musculoskeletal system and joints

Anti-inflammatory drugs

Anti-inflammatory drugs are used to relieve pain, swelling and fever caused by acute inflammation anywhere in the body.

- **Corticosteroids** of the glucocorticoid group will suppress inflammation and at high doses produce immunosuppression. This is required in the treatment of immune-mediated diseases that sometimes cause polyarthritis in the dog.
- **Non-steroidal anti-inflammatory drugs (NSAIDs)** mostly work by inhibiting the formation of prostaglandins (PGs) and related compounds which are important mediators of acute inflammation. Those that selectively inhibit the formation of PG made by the COX-2 enzyme are termed COX-2 selective drugs.

Lack of COX-1 inhibition will improve safety by reducing gastric ulceration as a side effect. Potential toxicity on the kidney will be probably similar. Figure 9.11 lists some examples.

Chondroprotective agents

Chondroprotective agents (e.g. pentosan polysulphate sodium) prevent further breakdown of cartilage and stimulate the synthesis of new articular cartilage.

Drugs acting on the eye

Antimicrobial and anti-inflammatory agents can be applied topically in drop form or as an ointment. Local anaesthetic (e.g. proxymetacaine) is available for topical application.

- **Mydriatics** and **cycloplegics** dilate the pupil (mydriasis) and reduce spasm in the ciliary muscle (e.g. **antimuscarinic agents** atropine, homatropine).
- Glaucoma (raised intraocular pressure) can be treated with **mitotics** to constrict the pupil and thus open up the drainage angle for ocular fluid (e.g. the **parasympathomimetic** pilocarpine, which mimics parasympathetic nerve stimulation to the eye).
- **Carbonic anhydrase inhibitors** also reduce the formation of aqueous humour and so treat glaucoma. Examples: e.g. dorzolamide (given topically), acetazolamide (given orally).

To replace the tear film when treating keratoconjunctivitis sicca (dry eye), hypromellose drops are the most commonly used drug. Acetylcysteine, a **mucolytic**, may be beneficial when the tears are mucoid and viscous. Pilocarpine may stimulate lacrimal secretion.

Drugs acting on the ear

Topical treatments combining several drugs are popular. Figure 9.12 lists some available therapies.

Drug	Authorized for veterinary use	Comments
Aspirin	No	Also used to prevent arterial thromboembolization
Carprofen	Cats, dogs and horses	COX-2 selective (particularly in dogs, though this selectivity is not great) Cats do not seem to benefit from same level of safety as dogs: should only be used in short term for cats
Flunixin meglumine	Dogs and horses	Very potent Helps with endotoxaemia as it has anti-endotoxin effects at doses below those that produce anti-inflammatory effects
Ketoprofen	Dogs, cats and horses	Powerful anti-inflammatory, analgesic and antipyretic properties
Meloxicam	Dogs and cats	PG sparing as COX-2 selective, though relatively poorly selective
Paracetamol	No	*Do not use in cats, as they lack glucuronyl transferase enzymes required to metabolize this drug* Mainly used for antipyretic and analgesic properties Considered a poor anti-inflammatory
Phenylbutazone	Dogs and horses	
Piroxicam	No	Used to reduce size of bladder carcinomas
Ibuprofen	No	GI erosions occur consistently in dogs
Firocoxib	Dogs	One of the new generation of coxib NSAIDs that show greater selectivity for the COX-2 enzyme

9.11 Non-steroidal anti-inflammatory drugs (NSAIDs).

Use	Comments	Examples
Cleaning	Avoid use if tympanic membrane ruptured	Ceruminolytics and detergents Solvents used are usually squalene or propylene glycol
Acidification	Useful against Gram-negative bacteria	Acetic acid (vinegar), benzoic acid, salicylic acid
Anti-inflammatory	Relief of pain as well as reducing swelling and redness	Topical glucocorticoids very useful
Antibacterial	Most common isolates are Gram-positive *Pseudomonas* (Gram-negative) can also be problem in ears	Fusidic acid against Gram-positive Aminoglycosides (e.g. gentamicin) effective against Gram-negatives
Antifungal	Most common isolates are *Malassezia pachydermatis* and *Candida albicans*	Nystatin commonly used
Antiparasitic	Must treat all animals in household	

9.12 Drugs acting on the ear.

Drugs acting on the skin

The skin can be treated with drugs given orally, parenterally or topically.

Topical therapy

Advantages of topical therapy include:

- Target organ easily accessible
- Less systemic absorption, therefore fewer side effects (but it should not be assumed that absorption is negligible – absorption of steroids, for example, can be sufficient to cause suppression of the hypothalamus–pituitary–adrenal axis)
- Maximum drug concentration at desired site of action.

Disadvantages of topical therapy include:

- Potential ingestion
- Human exposure
- Messy and laborious nature
- Perceived simplicity by the owner of this approach.

Topical preparations contain 'active ingredients' and additives such as stabilizers, emulsifiers, preservatives, colour and fragrance and a vehicle to carry the agent. Figure 9.13 lists the traditional and modern methods of drug delivery

Traditional methods	Modern methods
Solids	Wipes
Greases	Liposomes
Aqueous or alcoholic solutions	Multi-lamellar micro- or nano-capsules Microparticles Spherulites Microemulsions for slow release of drugs Chitosanide (agent often added to preparations to help topical spreading)

9.13 Methods of drug delivery to the skin.

Topical medicines are classed as:

- Shampoos (short duration)
- Cream rinses (medium duration)
- Leave-on sprays or conditioners (prolonged action).

Therapies include antibacterial, antifungal, ectoparasiticides or treatment to restore and maintain skin barrier function in cornification disorders and atopic dermatitis. Other therapies might be:

- **Topical antimicrobials**, including iodine and chlorhexidine, the latter available at the following concentrations: 7.5% solution; 2% shampoo (Malaseb, also containing Miconazole); 4% surgical scrub (Hibiscrub); 0.05% aqueous solution for ophthalmic use; or several oral cleansing solutions
- **Antiseborrhoeics (keratolytics and keratoplastics)**, including sulphur, salicyclic acid, coal tar, benzoyl peroxide and selenium sulphide
- **Essential fatty acids**, which have potential anti-inflammatory properties, e.g. gamma linolenic acid (GLA), eicosapentaenoic acid (EPA)
- **Antihistamines**, used to reduce pruritus associated with atopy.

Drugs affecting nutrition and body fluids

Electrolyte and water replacement solutions (crystalloid fluids)

These solutions are used to treat animals suffering from dehydration.

Oral rehydration solutions

These consist of mixtures of sodium, potassium, chloride ions and an anion that is metabolized by the liver to form bicarbonate (e.g. citrate). In addition, glucose and amino acids such as glycine are included, not for nutritional purposes but because they help the transport of sodium and water across the gut wall and into the bloodstream.

Parenteral solutions

These are used to replace fluid losses in cases where the oral route is unsuitable and a parenteral (usually intravenous) route is chosen. The composition of the fluid used depends on the type of losses sustained. For example, replacement of extracellular fluid volume requires a fluid with plasma concentration of sodium (about 140 mmol/l). When parenteral fluids are given to maintain hydration in an animal that is unable to drink, fluids that are much lower in sodium are more appropriate. Isotonicity of such fluids is maintained by the addition of glucose (e.g. 4% glucose and 0.18% sodium chloride). Concentrated additives such as potassium chloride, glucose (dextrose monohydrate) and sodium bicarbonate are available for addition to commercially available fluids so that the composition of the fluid can be adjusted to suit the requirements of the animal being treated.

Nutrient solutions

These are available to provide nutrition by the intravenous route (parenteral nutrition). They consist of concentrated solutions of glucose or emulsions of lipid to provide calories and amino acids. They should only be administered through the jugular vein as the risk of phlebitis and infection when given through a small peripheral vein is high.

Hypertonic saline

This special type of crystalloid fluid (e.g. 7.0% sodium chloride) is used in the treatment of hypovolaemic and endotoxaemic shock. Small volumes are given for the pharmacological effect this has on cardiac output and arterial blood pressure. Volume replacement with conventional isotonic crystalloid fluids or colloids (see below) should still form part of the treatment of such patients.

Plasma substitutes

Plasma substitutes (e.g. gelatin) are large-molecular-weight colloids in solution which are retained in the circulation rather than leaving capillaries and distributing into the whole extracellular fluid volume (as is the case with crystalloid fluids). Thus, a smaller volume of such colloid preparations will restore the circulating fluid volume in an animal suffering from haemorrhagic shock when compared with the volume of replacement crystalloid solutions required.

Blood substitutes

Haemoglobin glutamer-200 (bovine) is a recent addition to the parenteral fluids available for use in veterinary practice and it has oxygen-carrying capacity as well as being a colloid. This cross-linked bovine haemoglobin solution is called Oxyglobin (Biopure Corp.) and can be used for animals requiring oxygen-carrying capacity. Indications for its use include acute blood loss or haemolytic crises where a source of cross-matched blood is not available.

Vitamins and minerals

These can be used as supplements for sick and debilitated animals, and, as such, would be regarded as medicines. Nutritional deficiencies may occur but are uncommon in the dog and cat nowadays with the use of commercial pet foods. Specific indications for a mineral would include eclampsia in the bitch, where calcium gluconate would be given intravenously. Phytomenadione (vitamin K1) is the specific antidote to warfarin poisoning.

Vaccines and immunological preparations

Immunity results from natural infection or from being given protection through some form of vaccination.

Active immunity

This is when the body produces immunity in response to an antigen (see Chapter 6).

Agents inducing active immunity

- **Live vaccines** – consisting of living organisms of a slightly different strain from that which causes the natural disease. The organisms in live vaccines multiply inside the host and stimulate a rapid, long-lasting response.

- **Live attenuated vaccines** – the antigen is sufficient to stimulate the immune response but the organisms have been heat treated or cultured at an unfavourable temperature. There is always the potential to revert to virulence, but because they are similar to the actual organism, they elicit a strong immunity.
- Killed vaccines (**inactivated organisms**) – the organisms are unable to reproduce and are therefore incapable of causing disease. They provide a weak immune response of shorter duration and often require large doses to yield protection.
- Extracts of organisms or exotoxins produced by organisms (**toxoids**) – these subunit vaccines present a low risk for adverse reactions, but they do not elicit strong immunity and cost more to produce.
- **Autogenous vaccines** – these are prepared from material collected from an animal and administered back to that same animal.
- **Multivalent vaccines** – those protecting against several infectious diseases as all-in-one vaccines. Concerns have been raised about whether this causes immunosuppression through antigen overload, though this has yet to be substantiated.

In addition to the antigen, vaccines contain **adjuvants**, i.e. materials added to enhance their immunogenicity. Examples include other antigens, protein from tissue culture of egg yolk, preservatives such as antibiotics, and carrier substances such as aluminium. Animals may react to these substances.

Shedding of live virus can occur and care must be taken not to administer a vaccine by an alternative route than intended – for example, an in-contact cat grooming the coat of a vaccinated animal and ingesting some vaccine, or an aerosol being created from a syringe.

Passive immunization

Agents inducing passive immunity

- Maternally derived humoral antibodies (**colostrum**)
- Passive transfer of **immune cells** (lymphocytes are taken from an infected animal and transferred to an uninfected animal; the ability to respond to an infection is also transferred)
- Passive transfer of **hyperimmune serum** (by inoculating a species not usually susceptible to a disease); for example, inoculating a horse with foot-and-mouth, a disease that only affects cloven-hoofed animals, and then harvesting the serum after the animal's immune system has produced antibodies (immunoglobulins) to the organism. The serum will contain antibodies to protect the recipient without them having to mount an immune response of their own, but the immunity only persists for a few weeks.

A multivalent anti-endotoxin immunoglobulin is authorized for use in dogs to protect them against Gram-negative septicaemia. This form of passive immunity can be useful in protecting animals at risk of developing septic shock, e.g. puppies with parvovirus or bitches with pyometra.

Formulation and administration of drugs

Systemically administered drugs

If a drug cannot be applied locally (topically) to the site at which its action is desired, it must be **absorbed** into the blood circulation (systemically), from which it **distributes** around the body. The efficiency of absorption and distribution is affected by the route of administration and the physical and chemical form in which the drug is given.

Oral preparations

Advantages:

- The oral route is the most convenient route for owners
- Some drugs are not absorbed from the gut and act as local therapy without having systemic effects (e.g. neomycin used for enteric infections).

Disadvantages:

- Absorption is slower and less complete than when drugs are injected (given by a parenteral route) (Figure 9.14). The drug must dissolve and some drugs rely on the stomach emptying before they are absorbed in the small intestine
- Vomiting makes oral administration unreliable
- Some drugs are unstable in gastric acid or are destroyed by the enzymes of the gut (e.g. penicillin G, insulin)
- The liver may break down the drug and prevent it reaching the circulation (e.g. lidocaine, glyceryl trinitrate) or a higher dose is required when given orally (e.g. propranolol)
- Food may delay the entry of a drug into the bloodstream (e.g. digoxin) or reduce the amount of drug absorbed (e.g. ampicillin). Fatty foods help the absorption of some drugs (e.g. griseofulvin, lufenuron, mitotane).

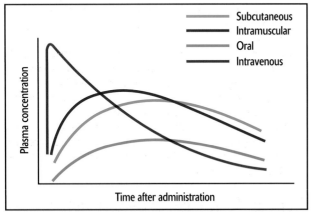

9.14 Plasma concentration versus time curve for a 'typical' drug following its administration by: intramuscular, intravenous or subcutaneous injection, or oral administration.

Tablets

These contain the active drug and some inert ingredients (binders and excipients). They may be coated for several reasons, including:

- Protection from the atmosphere and moisture
- To delay disintegration and protect the active drug until through the acidic environment of the stomach

- To protect the stomach from irritant effects of the drug (e.g. aspirin)
- To hide a bitter taste (e.g. erythromycin).

Breaking or grinding up tablets that are enteric coated may render the drug inactive and it is important to check with the manufacturer before undertaking such actions.

Capsules

These contain either powder or granules. The outer case, made up of hard gelatin in two halves that slot together, prevents the drug (which may taste bitter) from contacting the oral mucosa.

Slow or sustained release of drugs is achieved by using granules of differing sizes and compositions which dissolve at different rates (e.g. slow-release theophylline or diltiazem). The rate of passage through and the conditions inside the gastro-intestinal tract vary from species to species and so 'off-label' use may lead to poor absorption (and therefore lack of effect) or too rapid absorption (and toxicity).

Mixtures

- **Solutions** are liquid medications containing a freely soluble drug.
- **Suspensions** are liquids containing insoluble drugs (e.g. kaolin in water). They require mixing and should be labelled 'Shake well before use'.
- **Syrups/linctus** are drugs contained in a concentrated sugar solution.
- **Emulsions** are a mixture of two immiscible liquids.

Parenteral preparations

Any route other than oral is considered parenteral, but it is generally taken to mean injectable routes and therefore all preparations should be sterile and pyrogen free. Routes include:

- **Intravenous** – directly into venous blood
- **Intramuscular** – into muscular tissue, usually the hamstrings, gluteals or back
- **Subcutaneous** – into the tissue beneath the skin.

Intravenous route

Useful sites in the cat and dog include the jugular, cephalic and saphenous veins (see Chapter 15).

Advantages:

- Fastest distribution of the drug to its site of action
- Peak plasma concentrations achieved are higher
- Drugs that are irritant to the tissues can be given by this route (e.g. vincristine, thiopentone).

Disadvantages:

- Drug concentrations often decrease rapidly, as absorption from the site of injection is instantaneous and does not continue over a period of time (see Figure 9.14)
- Preparations must be either aqueous solutions, where the drug is dissolved in sterile water, or another type of solvent
- Injections must be given slowly to prevent a bolus of drug or solvent reaching the brain or heart with detrimental effects
- Suspensions cannot be given intravenously as the particles may block lung capillaries and cause death
- Accidental injection of irritant drugs outside the vein (extravascular injection) can cause severe tissue damage.

Intramuscular route
Advantages:

- More convienient for less cooperative patients
- Drugs in suspension can be given by this route.

Disadvantages:

- Accidental intravenous injection can occur unless the needle is drawn back on after insertion to ensure that its tip is not in a blood vessel within the muscle
- Injections may be painful; the severity depends on the volume, viscosity and chemical nature (e.g. pH) of the compound.

The drug diffuses from the injection site by dissolving in the tissue fluid surrounding the muscle cells and is then absorbed into the blood capillaries and lymphatics supplying the muscle.

Subcutaneous route
Advantages:

- Can be made anywhere there is loose skin, usually over the neck or back. To improve uptake, injections can be made behind the elbow so that movement of the limb will encourage absorption of the drug. This is especially useful for insulin injections in cats
- Larger volumes can be administered than by the intramuscular route.

Disadvantages:

- Formulations should be of blood pH and blood fluid tonicity and should not be irritant or cause vasoconstriction as this will impede absorption of the drug.

Absorption rates

- Drugs are generally absorbed faster from intramuscular sites, due to the larger blood supply.
- Combinations of different salts of a drug can be produced. The sodium salt of penicillin G is highly soluble and so rapidly absorbed. The procaine salt is more slowly absorbed and the benzathine salt, which is poorly soluble, is slowly absorbed. These long-acting injections are called **depot injections**.
- Insulin preparations have different times to onset of action and duration of effect. Protamine zinc insulin may only need injecting once a day, whereas isophane insulin has a shorter duration of activity and requires two injections a day.
- Implants of a small disc or cylinder of relatively insoluble drug (often a hormone) can be inserted under the skin in a sterile manner to release drugs over an extended period of time.

Other injection sites
These are all forms of local therapy, as the injection site is the site at which the drug is desired to produce its effect.

- **Intradermal** – into the dermis (e.g. allergy testing in dogs)
- **Intraperitoneal** – delivery of drugs into the abdominal cavity. Potential disadvantages include the variable onset and duration of action of drugs given by this route, the potential for puncture of abdominal organs and the formation of adhesions
- **Intra-articular** – into a joint cavity (e.g. corticosteroids)

▶

- **Intrathecal** – into the cerebrospinal fluid (e.g. contrast media for myelography). Therapeutic agents are not given this way in veterinary medicine
- **Epidural** – into the vertebral canal outside the dura matter (e.g. spinal analgesia when local anaesthetics are injected)
- **Subconjunctival** – under the conjunctival membranes of the eye
- **Intracardiac** – injection through the chest wall, directly into the heart chambers. It allows the drug to access the bloodstream quickly. Euthanasia and cardiac resuscitation drugs are occasionally administered this way
- **Intra-osseous** – injection of a substance directly into the bone marrow in the medulla of a suitable long bone (e.g. femur or humerus). It is most often used to provide fluids to very small patients, those with damaged veins or those with very low blood pressure.

Disposal of administration equipment
Care should be taken that all used needles and other 'sharps' are placed into 'sharps' bins, which will then be collected for incineration. It is advisable that 'sharps' are disposed of immediately after use. The 'sharps' bin must be an approved container (see Chapter 1), which can be sealed and which has a handle. Unofficial containers, such as used tablet pots, are not acceptable.

Syringes containing medicines should be disposed of in appropriate containers (see Chapter 1).

Other ways of administering drugs to produce systemic effects

- **Inhalation** supplies drugs to the respiratory tract and allows drugs such as gaseous anaesthetics to be absorbed into the bloodstream.
- **Nebulization** requires drugs in solution to be produced in a very fine mist of droplets that are then inhaled by the animal (e.g. bronchodilators). There are obvious safety implications for the operators.
- Administration may be **across mucous membranes** such as the conjunctiva, nasal mucosa or buccal membranes (e.g. desmopressin drops, which cannot be administered orally as the agent is a small peptide and is broken down by enzymes in the gastrointestinal tract).
- **Penetration of the skin** and absorption into the bloodstream is posssible (e.g. the nitrovasodilator, glyceryl trinitrate, which cannot be given orally as it is removed so effectively by the liver).

Topically administered drugs
Topically administered drugs are applied directly to the site of action, usually the skin, eyes and ears.

- **Enemas** involve the administration of fluids into the rectum to soften the faecal mass.
- **Intramammary** preparations and **vaginal** suppositories or pessaries are used in large animal medicine.

Drugs can be absorbed across mucous membranes and even intact skin (e.g. the organophosphate insecticide, fenthion, and lipid-soluble drugs such as corticosteroids) and so these drugs should not be assumed to be without systemic effects.

Examples of topical preparations

- **Creams** – semi-solid emulsions of oil or fat and water (which usually contain the drug). They spread out easily without friction and penetrate the outer layers of the skin, particularly if the fat used is lanolin. Water-soluble drugs are more active in creams than in ointments.
- **Ointments** – semi-solid greasy, insoluble in water and the drugs are present in a base of wax or fat (usually petroleum jelly). They are non-penetrating and more occlusive than creams and are most suitable for dry chronic lesions.
- **Dusting powders** – finely divided powders for application to the skin containing usually ectoparasiticides or antibacterials. Powders can act as foreign bodies in ears and wounds.
- **Wettable powders** – applied to the skin as a suspension after mixing with a large quantity of water. The animal is air dried, leaving the powder in the coat (i.e. it is not rinsed off).
- **Lotions** – liquid preparations consisting of solutions of the drugs in water (e.g. calamine lotion).
- **Medicated shampoos** – aqueous solutions or suspensions of drugs that have a detergent base, which gives good penetration of the coat. Contact time should be adhered to and the product thoroughly rinsed off.
- **Aerosol sprays** – a way of applying liquid solutions or suspensions of drugs in fine droplet form. The liquid is packaged under pressure.
- **Eye medications** – ointments or drops. Both forms should be sterile and once opened they should be discarded after the recommended length of time.
  - Ophthalmic ointments are more liquid than standard ointments having a soft paraffin base. When applied to the cornea they melt to form a thin film that covers the whole surface of the eye.
  - Eye drops are aqueous solutions of drugs and are generally shorter acting, requiring more frequent application.

Prescribing and dispensing for exotic species

Drug therapy in avian and exotic veterinary medicine presents some interesting and challenging problems:

- The range of species dealt with is enormous
- Very few drugs are authorized for use in exotic species
- Treatment is, sadly, often initiated without a diagnosis
- Small size may make accurate dosing difficult
- Differences in metabolic rate may need to be taken into consideration
- Targeted drug delivery to specific tissues may require specialist techniques and preparations
- Important differences may exist between species in the areas of:
  - Drug pharmacokinetics
  - Animal handling
  - Route of administration
  - Water consumption
  - Drug side effects.

In many cases drugs will have to be specially prepared to take these differences into consideration. Specialist advice should be sought in such situations and informed consent should be obtained from the client for such off-label use.

Calculations of drug dosages

Veterinary nurses may be asked to calculate the dosages of medications. Although at present the responsibility lies with the veterinary surgeon whose care that animal is under, nurses should understand how to calculate dosages of drugs.

Weights, volumes and concentration

The minimal level of attainment should include the ability to convert units such as micrograms into milligrams and grams and having an understanding of percentage solutions and proportions.

1 kilogram (kg) = 1000 grams (g)
1 g = 1000 milligrams (mg)
1 mg = 1000 micrograms (μg)
1 μg = 1000 nanograms (ng)

1 litre = 1000 millilitres (ml)
1 ml = 1000 microlitres (μl)

Percentage concentrations

The strength of a drug may be expressed as a **percentage**, meaning parts per 100 parts. This can be expressed in four ways, as shown in Figure 9.15.

Term	Abbreviation	Example
Percentage weight in volume	% w/v	5% w/v would contain 5 g of drug in 100 ml of product
Percentage weight in weight	% w/w	5% w/w would contain 5 g of drug in 100 g of product
Percentage volume in volume	% v/v	5% v/v would contain 5 ml of drug in 100 ml of product
Percentage volume in weight	% v/w	5% v/w would contain 5 ml of drug in 100 g of product

9.15   Percentage strengths.

If the weight relates to a tablet or capsule, each tablet or capsule contains the stated weight of active drug. A quick method of converting percentage solution into mg/ml is to multiply by 10 (e.g. a 2.5% solution contains 25 mg/ml). Conversely, to convert mg/ml into percentage solution, divide by 10 (e.g. a solution containing 10 mg/ml is a 1% solution).

Some drugs are unstable in solution and so are supplied as a solid in a vial, with the solvent (often water) supplied separately. The drug is reconstituted by adding the solvent to the vial and the percentage solution (or mg/ml) and the date should be written on the vial. The reconstituted drug may be stable for several days but storage conditions must be adhered to.

Exceptions to standard weights and volumes

Drugs such as insulin, oxytocin and heparin are extracted from animal tissues and are not produced in a pure form.

The concentration of the drug in the product is determined by its effect in a laboratory test system (bioassay) against international standard. The concentration is usually given in terms of international units (IU) per standard volume (usually per millilitre).

For example, insulin for human use is produced at 100 units/ml and there is an insulin authorized for veterinary use containing insulin at a concentration of 40 IU/ml. Syringes for insulin administration are graduated in units rather than in millilitres and the correct syringe must be selected, i.e. a 40 IU syringe for insulin concentration 40 IU/ml.

Dosages

Drug dosage rates are usually expressed in terms of weight of drug per weight of the animal (e.g. 2 mg/kg). Some drugs, especially chemotherapeutics, are dosed on a weight of drug per body surface area (e.g. mg/m² body surface area). Conversion charts are available that give the body surface area from the animal's weight in kilograms.

EXAMPLE 1

You are asked to dispense enrofloxacin tablets for a dog weighing 20 kg at a dose rate of 2.5 mg/kg twice daily for 7 days. The drug comes in tablet sizes of 15, 50 and 150 mg. Which tablet sizes would be most appropriate, how many tablets would you dispense and what instructions for dosing would you give to the owner?

Amount of drug required (mg)
= dose (mg/kg) x bodyweight (kg)
= 2.5 mg/kg x 20 kg
= 50 mg

Thus, the most appropriate tablet size to use would be 50 mg and the owners should be instructed to give one tablet twice a day for 7 days. The number of tablets required will be 14.

EXAMPLE 2

A 6 kg miniature poodle requires digoxin for treatment of congestive heart failure. The dose rate required is 0.01 mg/kg each day, which should be divided into two equal doses (0.01 mg/kg divided twice daily). The tablet sizes available are 62.5, 125 and 250 µg. What tablet size would you use, what would your dosing instructions to the owners be and how many tablets would you dispense for a 30-day course?

Daily dose required (mg)
= dose (mg/kg) x bodyweight (kg)
= 0.01 mg/kg x 6 kg = 0.06 mg

To convert milligrams to micrograms (µg), multiply by 1000. Thus:
0.06 mg = 0.06 x 1000 µg
= 60 µg

This dose should be divided into two equal daily doses, so each dose should contain:
60/2 µg = 30 µg

Thus, the most appropriate size to use would be the 62.5 µg tablets, and the owners should be instructed to give half a tablet every 12 hours before food. For a course of 30 days the owners would require 30 tablets.

EXAMPLE 3

For injection, you are given a drug in solution which is 7.5% w/v. The dose required for the dog you are treating is 10 mg/kg and the dog weighs 18 kg. What volume of the drug should be given to this dog by injection?

Concentration of drug in solution
= 7.5 g in 100 ml (7.5% w/v)
= (7.5/100) g in 1 ml
= 0.075 g in 1 ml
= (0.075 x 1000) mg in 1 ml
= 75 mg/ml

Amount of drug required
= dose (mg/kg) x bodyweight in kg
= 10 mg/kg x 18 kg = 180 mg

Volume of drug required (ml)
= Amount of drug (mg)/concentration (mg/ml)
= 180 mg/75 (mg/ml)
= 2.4 ml

Tips for calculations

- It is important to be sure of the position of the decimal point in all drug calculations, so always write 0.01 rather than simply .01.
- The dose required in Example 2 is slightly lower than the convenient tablet size. Digoxin is a drug with a lower therapeutic index and care should be taken not to overdose an animal. In this case, the inaccuracy was deemed so small as to be of no consequence but judgement should always be made by the veterinary surgeon in charge of the case.
- In dosing with digoxin, food can interfere with the rate of absorption of the drug from the gut, so an instruction to give the medication before meals is important.
- In Example 2 the total daily dose rate was given and had to be divided into two equal doses. An alternative way of expressing this would be to say the dose required is 0.005 mg/kg to be given twice daily, which was the way the dose rate in Example 1 was expressed.
- To convert the concentration of a solution expressed in percentages into mg/ml, multiply the percentage figure by 10.

Legal aspects of medicines and prescribing

The legislation that governs the storage, handling, use and supply of medicines in veterinary practice includes:

- Veterinary Medicines Regulations (VMR) 2005
- Misuse of Drugs Act 1971
- Health and Safety at Work etc. Act 1974
- Control of Substances Hazardous to Health Regulations 1999

Aspects of these are also considered in Chapters 1, 2 and 3.

The Government ensures the quality, safety and efficacy of medicines for human and animal use by a system of licences approved by the Department of Health and the Department for Environment, Food and Rural Affairs (DEFRA), respectively. Before a product can be manufactured, imported and distributed widely, the company or person who devises it has to gain a marketing authorization by showing that the drug is safe, efficacious (produces the effects that the data sheet claims) and that the manufacturing process ensures a consistent quality of the product. Manufacturers and wholesale dealers of medicinal products require a manufacturer's and wholesale dealer's marketing authority, respectively. As part of the licensing procedure, the company may need to perform a clinical trial of the drug in question and for this purpose they apply for an animal test certificate.

An exemption to this law is that veterinary surgeons do not require a product licence to prepare a medicinal product themselves (or to request another veterinary surgeon to prepare such a product for them) for a particular animal or herd under their care. The veterinary surgeon is only allowed to stock a very limited supply of a medicine prepared in this way (2.5 kg of solid and 5 litres of liquid). It is not permissible for vaccines (other than autogenous vaccines) to be prepared in this way.

Use of unauthorized products in veterinary medicine

For non-food-producing animals, the regulations state that a product that has a veterinary marketing authorization for the species and the condition to be treated, or is authorized for another condition or another veterinary species, should, if possible, be chosen before a product that is authorized only for human use. Products authorized only for human use may be used if no veterinary authorized alternative exists. Special products made by the veterinary surgeon or by a pharmacist for the veterinary surgeon that have no marketing authorization at all should be used only if a veterinary or human authorized product does not already exist. These regulations (commonly referred to as the medicines **cascade**) have been produced to protect the consumer of animal products from drug residues. Their application to small animal veterinary practice has been clarified by guidance notes issued by the Veterinary Medicines Directorate (VMD) (AMELIA 8). Using unauthorized drugs requires informed consent (see Chapter 2) and the appropriate form should be signed.

Prescribing and dispensing for exotic species

The lack of suitable authorized products for exotic pet species means that the prescribing cascade will frequently be referred to and presents the veterinary surgeon with some interesting choices. A good understanding of exotic animal medicine is required for appropriate choices to be made. Specialist advice should therefore be sought wherever possible, in order to ensure that clients are informed about the full range of options available to them and given the most up-to-date advice.

Selection of an appropriate medication will follow the prescribing cascade for non-food-producing animals. Certain companion animals may, however, also be food-producing animals and this fact should be ascertained from the client.

If there is no medicine authorized in the UK for a condition affecting a non-food-producing species, the veterinary surgeon responsible for treating the animal may, in order to mitigate unacceptable suffering, treat the animal in accordance with the following sequence:

1. A veterinary medicine authorized in the UK for use in another animal species, or for a different condition in the same species (e.g. the use of fenbendazole to worm tortoises).
2. A medicine authorized in the UK for human use (e.g. haloperidol for the management of feather plucking in parrots).
3. A veterinary medicine authorized for veterinary use in accordance with Directive 2001/82 (as amended) in another EU Member State can be imported in accordance with an import certificate (e.g. importation of an injectable doxycycline preparation for the treatment of chlamydophilosis in parrots)
4. A medicine prepared extemporaneously, by a veterinary surgeon, a pharmacist or a person holding an appropriate manufacturer's authorization, as prescribed by the veterinary surgeon responsible for treating the animal (e.g. dilution of ivermectin (1%) in propylene glycol to make a 0.1% solution, which can be more accurately dosed in small mammals).

If there are no such products, advice should be sought from the VMD as to whether a product authorized for veterinary or human use can be imported from the rest of the world.

Legal categories of medicines

The VMR 2005 apply the relevant provisions of European law and set out UK provisions in areas such as fees, distribution, appeals, advertising, inspection and enforcement of any veterinary medicinal product (VMP). VMPs are defined as:

'a. any substance or combination of substances presented as having properties for treating or preventing disease in animals; or
b. any substance or combination of substances which may be used in, or administered to, animals with a view either to restoring, correcting or modifying physiological functions by exerting a pharmacological, immunological or metabolic action, or to making a medical diagnosis.'

The VMR 2005 sets out the distribution categories for UK drugs as follows:

- Prescription Only Medicine – Veterinarian (**POM–V**)
- Prescription Only Medicine – Veterinarian, Pharmacist, Suitably Qualified Person (**POM–VPS**)
- Non-Food Animal – Veterinarian, Pharmacist, Suitably Qualified Person (**NFA–VPS**)
- Authorized Veterinary Medicine – General Sales List (**AVM–GSL**)

POM-V

A VMP that has been classified as POM–V may only be dispensed by a veterinary surgeon or pharmacist and a clinical assessment must be made by the veterinary surgeon first. A product is included in this category when it:

- Contains a new active ingredient not previously used in a veterinary medicine in the EU
- Requires a strict limitation on its use for specific safety reasons
- Requires the specialized knowledge of a veterinary surgeon for use/application

- Has a narrow safety margin requiring above average care in its use
- Is Government policy to demand professional control at a high level
- Requires specific use, linked to a prior clinical assessment of the animals.

POM–VPS

A POM–VPS drug can be supplied by a Responsible Qualified Person (RQP), which is defined as:

- A registered veterinary surgeon
- A registered pharmacist
- A registered suitably qualified person (SQP).

SQPs will be registered with a body that has provided training to them and they will have had to pass an examination and be present at each sale of the VMP. Although a clinical assessment of the animal is not a prerequisite, the prescribing RQP must be satisfied that the person administering the product has the competence to do so safely.

NFA–VPS

These drugs may be supplied by an RQP without a clinical assessment but with advice relating to any warnings or contraindications of use.

AVM–GSL

This may be supplied by any retailer, as there are no restrictions on its supply.

Prescriptions and recording of medicines

The *Veterinary Medicines Guidance Notes* outline how a prescription should be written. The following information should be included (Figure 9.16):

- The name and address of the prescriber
- The particulars substantiating that the prescriber is a veterinary surgeon (e.g. MRCVS)
- The name and address of the person to whom the product is supplied

Mr A. Vet MRCVS
50 High Street, Anytown, Anyshire
Tel: 01234 56789

25th September 2002
Mr J. Smith's dog 'Smarty'
23 The Green,
Anytown

Rx
Tablets Pethidine 50 mg
Send 10 (ten)

Label: Given half a tablet twice a day for 5 days

For Animal Treatment Only

This animal is under my care

No repeats

9.16 Example of prescription form for a controlled drug.

- A description of the animal(s) it is prescribed for
- The date
- The name(s) and strength(s) of drugs to be dispensed. The proprietary or generic name may be provided (in the latter case the pharmacist may dispense any suitable product)
- The directions that the prescriber wishes to appear on the label
- A declaration that the prescription is issued in respect of an animal under the care of the prescriber
- Any instructions for repeating the prescription
- The prescriber's usual signature

It is good practice to include:

- The species of animal and its name/number
- The total amount of the medicine to be supplied and the dose
- 'For animal treatment only'.

The prescription should be written in ink or another indelible format, and it should be signed or otherwise authenticated by the prescriber.

The practice of issuing repeat prescriptions is one that should be done at the discretion of the veterinary surgeon in charge of the case, taking note of the stability of the animal's condition and the need for re-examination.

Veterinary surgeons should keep a full record of all incoming and outgoing medicinal products and at least once a year should carry out a detailed audit reconciling these with stock, recording any discrepancies. Records must be kept by keepers of food-producing animals outlining the purchase of all medicines and the identification of the animals treated. The act of dispensing, including quantity and batch numbers, should be recorded in the animal's or farm's clinical records. All retailers of POM–V and POM–VPS must also record the following information in respect of each incoming or outgoing transaction, and keep the records for 5 years:

- Date
- Precise identity of the VMP
- Manufacturer's batch number
- Quantity received or supplied
- Name and address of the supplier or recipient
- If there is a written prescription, the name and address of the person writing the prescription and a copy of the prescription.

All prescriptions should be detailed and a copy kept for 5 years. Wholesalers should keep their records for at least 3 years.

All withdrawal periods for meat, milk and eggs in food-producing animals should be recorded both on the medicine dispensed and in the farm client's Medicines Record Book.

Ordering/requisitioning procedures

Automated ordering systems, similar to ESCOS, are commonly used that have a built-in stock level specific to the practice and that transfer the order directly to the supplier.

The Misuse of Drugs Regulations 2001 was amended in 2003 to allow computer-generated requisitions for controlled drugs but all Schedule 2 medicines require an original order with a veterinary surgeon's signature before they can be processed. Schedule 3 drugs under the Misuse of Drugs Act (MDA) 1971 require an MDA form.

Pharmacy stock management

There must be an efficient stock control system to ensure a continuous supply of all products and removal of out-of-date medicines (see Chapter 2). Depending on the workload of the practice, some agents may be used infrequently, which results in some drugs exceeding their shelf-life. Many of the common injectable and oral agents require refrigeration; these agents should be kept away from animal or human food sources.

Although cytotoxic drugs are not controlled by law, they can be abused (with serious results) and locked refrigeration is recommended. Drug residues have been found on the outside of manufacturer's packaging and on surfaces adjacent to stored unused cytotoxic products. Thus from the time the drug arrives in the practice, the agent should be handled with gloves and should only be dispensed by trained personnel. It is also wise to store agents in clear plastic ziplock type bags.

Storage of medicines

There are many specific storage requirements for drugs (see also Chapter 2) and it is always wise to consult the data sheets for any unfamiliar drugs on unpacking. For example, some carprofen preparations should be stored in the refrigerator until the vial is opened and then kept at room temperature.

Guidelines on storage of medicines

- Maximum/minimum thermometers should be used both in drug refrigerators and in the dispensary to ensure that environmental conditions do not fluctuate outside the recommended ranges.
- Light-sensitive drugs, such as injectable oxytetracycline, should not be dispensed in clear syringes. The syringe should be placed in a brown envelope or bag until used.
- All environmental variables should be considered, including humidity. It is unwise to store drugs near to the autoclave.
- Health and safety considerations include storing large containers on the ground and any potentially hazardous chemicals away from the general public.
- Affix a practice label to each item before it is placed in stock and write the date of first use on broached multi-dose vials to ensure that the recommended period of use is not exceeded.
- Once stock has been dispensed it should not be accepted back into the dispensary, because there may have been storage problems whilst the product was not under your care.
- To avoid storing surplus stock, some practices may charge the client for the entire amount of drug in a pack. If small amounts of medicines are only required for occasional use, the provision of a prescription is often more suitable.

Disposal of unwanted medicines

Pharmaceutical products, veterinary compounds and prescription only medicines (POMs) constitute clinical waste and therefore must be disposed of in accordance with the Hazardous Waste Regulations 2005 (see Chapter 1).

Disposal of Schedule 2 drugs

Schedule 2 drugs (see 'The Misuse of Drugs Act' below) that are no longer required should be stored and destroyed in the presence of a police officer from the Drugs Squad or a member of the Home Office, who will countersign the Controlled Drugs book. Schedule 2 drugs should be destroyed in a manner that renders them unavailable for further use.

Packaging of medicines

The Royal Pharmaceutical Society of Great Britain recommends that when repackaging medicines from bulk containers, they must be dispensed in appropriate containers, both for the product and the user (Figure 9.17). The dispenser has a duty to ensure that the owner understands any instructions on the label and knows how to use the product safely.

Container	Contents
Coloured flute bottles	Medicines for external application Examples: shampoos, soaps, lotions Enemas and eye and ear medications should be similarly dispensed if not already packaged in a suitable plastic container
Plain glass bottles	Oral liquid medicines
Wide-mouthed jars	Creams, dusting powders, granules
Paper board cartons/wallets	Sachets, manufacturer's strip or blister-packed medicines
Airtight glass, plastic or metal containers (preferably childproof)[a]	All solid oral medicines (tablets and capsules)

9.17 Recommended containers for different medicines. [a] Discretion can be exercised with childproof containers. Some aged and infirm clients may request screwtop containers.

Under *The Medicines (Fluted Bottles) Regulations 1978*, certain medicinal products for external use should be dispensed in fluted bottles so that they are recognizable by touch. This requirement does not apply to volumes in excess of 1.14 litres or to eye or ear drops supplied in plastic containers.

Labelling medicines

The Medicines (Labelling) Regulations 1976 recommend the following;

- The label must be mechanically printed or indelibly and legibly printed or written in accordance with statutory requirements. Biro, felt tip or ballpoint pen are acceptable; ink and pencil are not.
- The words 'for external use only' or 'not to be taken internally' should be included for medicines that are for topical use (e.g. eye or ear formulations, lotions, liquid antiseptics).
- Ideally the label should not obscure the expiry date of the preparation or important printed information on the manufacturer's label or pack. Small tubes may be dispensed in an appropriately labelled envelope.
- Product information leaflets should be dispensed with the product where possible.
- If the drug is to be used in food-producing animals, the label must also include the withdrawal period (the time between the last dose of the drug and the use of meat, milk or eggs from the animal for human consumption).

Figure 9.18 indicates essential information that has to be provided by law and also the optional (but desirable) information.

Essential

Owner's name
Owner's address
Veterinary practice name
Veterinary practice address
For Animal Treatment Only
Date
Keep Out of Reach of Children

Optional

Precautions relating to the use of the product
Quantity and strength of drug
Instructions for dosing
Total quantity of drug dispensed
Initials of person dispensing

9.18 Label details, including information required by law and additional desirable details.

RCVS Guide to Professional Conduct

The changes made to the *RCVS Guide* that took effect on 3 November 2005 are detailed below. The RCVS enforces these recommendations, made by the Competition Commission. Any complaints are investigated by the Preliminary Investigation Committee and may be referred to the Disciplinary Committee. Key changes relate to providing information to clients about the availability of prescriptions and the prices of most of the commonly prescribed medicines.

- Clients must be able to obtain prescriptions as appropriate.
- Clients must be informed of the price of any medicine to be prescribed or dispensed and the price must be made available to other parties who make reasonable requests.
- Itemized invoices must be made available to distinguish between fees charged for services and medicines, and where possible itemized for individual products.
- Clients must be informed of the frequency of and charges for further examinations and repeat prescriptions.
- New and existing clients must be provided with this information in writing.
- There must be a sign in the waiting room detailing the current prices of the ten veterinary medicinal products most commonly prescribed during a recent and typical 3-month period (Figure 9.19).
- The exceptions to these requirements are when a delay in supply or administration would be unreasonable or where the medication is to be administered by injection and is only available in packs containing multiple doses.

The RCVS also gives advice about communication with clients via the internet about animals that are under their care. The VMR do not define the phrase 'under his care' and the RCVS has interpreted it as meaning that:

- The veterinary surgeon must have been given the responsibility for the health of the animal or herd by the owner or the owner's agent
- That responsibility must be real and not nominal
- The animal or herd must have been seen immediately before prescription; or
- Recently enough or often enough for the veterinary surgeon to have personal knowledge of the condition of the animal or current health status of the herd or flock to make a diagnosis and prescribe
- The veterinary surgeon must maintain clinical records of that herd/flock/individual.

Prescriptions are available from this practice.

You may obtain relevant medicinal products from your veterinary surgeon OR ask for a prescription and obtain these medicines from another veterinary surgery or a pharmacy.

Your veterinary surgeon may prescribe relevant veterinary medicinal products only following a clinical assessment of an animal under his or her care.

A prescription may not be appropriate if your animal is an inpatient or if immediate treatment is necessary.

You will be informed, on request, of the price of any medicine that may be prescribed for your animal.

The general policy of this practice is to reassess an animal requiring repeat prescriptions for, or supplies of, relevant veterinary medicinal produces every *XX* months, but this may vary with individual circumstances. The standard charge for a re-examination is £*XX*.

The current prices for the ten relevant medicinal products most commonly prescribed during *XX* [a typical 3-month period] were:
[*List the ten most commonly prescribed medicines and their prices.*]

Further information on the prices of medicines is available on request.

9.19 Client advice that must be displayed prominently on a large sign in the waiting room.

What amounts to 'recent enough' must be a matter for the professional judgement of the veterinary surgeon according to the circumstances of each case.

The RCVS Guide to Professional Conduct provides the following advice on retail supplies:

'A veterinary surgeon who supplies POM–V, POM–VPS or NFA–VPS veterinary medicinal products must:
(a) Always advise on the safe administration of the VMP
(b) Advise as necessary on any warnings or contraindications on the label or package leaflet; and
(c) Be satisfied that the person who will use the product is competent to use it safely, and intends to use it for a use for which it is authorized.

A veterinary surgeon who makes retail supplies of POM–V veterinary medicinal products on the prescription of another veterinary surgeon (i.e. for animals that are not under his or her care) should ensure that those to whom the medicines are supplied, or may be supplied, are informed that such supplies are made without a clinical assessment of the animal and that the animal is not under his or her care.

A veterinary surgeon who is associated with retail supplies of POM–VPS, NFA–VPS or AVM–GSL VMP (or makes such supplies) should ensure that those to whom the medicines are supplied, or may be supplied, are informed of:
(a) The name and qualification (veterinary surgeon, pharmacist or SQP) of any prescriber
(b) The name and qualification (veterinary surgeon, pharmacist or SQP) of the supplier; and
(c) The nature of the duty of care for the animals.

Veterinary surgeons may prescribe POM–VPS VMP in circumstances where there has been no prior clinical assessment of the animals and the animals are not under his or her care. In these circumstances veterinary surgeons should prescribe responsibly and with due regard to the health and welfare of the animals.'

AMTRA has been given the authority to run training courses in conjunction with some colleges to allow qualified and listed veterinary nurses to upgrade to become SQPs. The modules will be designed to allow SQPs to supply for all animals or for all food-producing animals, horses, companion animals or particular species. Listed veterinary nurses will be able to supply POM–VPS and NFA–VPS products in their own right if they become SQPs.

Legislation is constantly updated and takes into account reviews of and changes in both UK and European legislation. Up-to-date information can be obtained from reliable sources such as the RCVS and the VMD.

Misuse of Drugs Act 1971 and Misuse of Drugs Regulations 2001

This legislation controls the production, supply, possession, storage and dispensing of drugs where the potential exists for abuse by humans. These are the **controlled drugs (CDs)**, a special category of POM-V products, and there are five schedules:

Controlled drugs: schedules

- Schedule 1 (S1) – addictive drugs such as cannabis and the hallucinogens mescaline and LSD
- Schedule 2 (S2) – the opiate analgesics morphine, etorphine, fentanyl and pethidine, plus cocaine and amphetamine
- Schedule 3 (S3) – the barbiturates pentobarbital and phenobarbital, plus the opiate analgesics buprenorphine and pentazocine
- Schedule 4 (S4) – benzodiazepines such as diazepam and chlordiazepoxide
- Schedule 5 (S5) – certain preparations of cocaine, codeine and morphine that contain less than a specified amount of the drug (e.g. codeine cough linctus, kaolin-and-morphine antidiarrhoeal suspension).

A veterinary surgeon does not have any general authority to possess or supply drugs from Schedule 1. Some of the other controlled drugs are subject to more stringent regulations than general POM–V medications.

Management of controlled drugs

Purchase

Purchase of a CD requires a handwritten (in indelible ink) requisition from the veterinary surgeon to a wholesaler, manufacturer or pharmacist that includes:

- The veterinary surgeon's signature
- Their name and address and profession
- The purpose for which the drug is required
- The total quantity of the drug required.

If a messenger is sent to collect the drug, written authority has to be given by the veterinary surgeon. Schedule 3 drugs also require a written requisition for their purchase. This does not have to be handwritten but must be signed by the veterinary surgeon making the request.

Storage

S2 drugs and buprenorphine (S3) and temazepam (S3) must be kept in a locked cupboard that is attached to a wall. The veterinary surgeon is responsible for the key and it should only be opened with their authority. Ketamine may be the subject of misuse and so should be stored in the controlled drugs cabinet and its use recorded in an informal register.

Records

A bound register of all transactions involving S2 drugs must be kept. Details of incomings (purchases) of S2 drugs and their outgoings (drugs used on the premises or dispensed) should be recorded in separate parts of the register, e.g. pethidine should be recorded separately from morphine. Commercial registers are available and they should be kept for 2 years from the last entry.

Prescriptions

Prescriptions require the following information to be handwritten:

- Name and address of the client
- The date and the quantity (in words and numbers)
- The strength of the prescription.

The prescription should not be dispensed later than 13 weeks from the date of issue, whereas other prescriptions can be dispensed for up to 6 months from the date of issue. In addition, no repeats are allowed (unlike other prescriptions, which can stipulate the number of repeats).

Health and Safety at Work etc. Act 1974 and Control of Substances Hazardous to Health (COSHH) Regulations 2002

When common sense is used and a few general ground rules are followed, the medicines used in most veterinary practices present a relatively small hazard to the health of employees. All data sheets of authorized medicines will discuss any hazards the medicine might pose to the operator (the person dispensing and administering the drug). The practice should also have produced a COSHH Assessment for the substances (including drugs) which staff come into contact with during the working day (see Chapters 1 to 3). It is important that these documents are read and the safety measures followed to keep any risk to the absolute minimum.

Drugs can get into the body by accident and have systemic effects in the operator in a number of ways, such as the following.

Absorption across the skin

This can occur with certain drugs, including:

- Prostaglandins (luteolytic agents)
- Insecticides
- Nitrovasodilators
- Compounds containing the solvent DMSO (dimethyl sulphoxide), which aids penetration of substances dissolved in it across the skin.

The following safety precautions should be taken:

- Wear gloves when handling the above or when handling any medications with cuts or abrasions.
- Wash hands after handling any medication.
- Wash splashes or spills off skin immediately.

Absorption across mucous membranes

The membranes of the eye (conjunctiva), nose and oral cavities may be contaminated by drugs in aerosol form from liquid formulations or dust from powders containing the drug. Aerosols are most often formed when reconstituting (dissolving) drugs for injection in the diluent supplied and when expelling air bubbles from a syringe. To reduce the risks:

- Do not pressurize the contents of vials when reconstituting drugs.
- Keep the needle cover on when expelling air bubbles from the syringe.
- Cytotoxic (potentially dangerous) drugs should only be reconstituted by trained personnel in designated areas.
- Should accidental contamination occur, washing or flushing with copious amounts of water should be the initial first aid treatment and further medical help should be sought depending on the drug involved.

Accidental ingestion of drugs

This can occur through aerosols or dust, as described above, or through eating contaminated food. Food and drink must not be consumed or stored in areas where drugs are being handled, including areas where topical sprays (e.g. flea sprays) are applied to animals. Smoking should also be prohibited from these areas.

Inhalation

Inhalation of volatile agents such as gaseous anaesthetics (e.g. isoflurane), dust from powders and droplets from aerosols may cause irritation of the respiratory tract or the drugs may be absorbed and cause systemic effects.

- Hazards from inhalational anaesthetics can be minimized by the use of adequate scavenging circuits attached to the anaesthetic circuit and by providing good ventilation.
- Dust masks and eye protection should be worn when dispensing powders from bulk packs, where a large amount of dust is inevitable.
- Insecticidal sprays should be used in well ventilated areas.

Accidental injection

This is the final way in which drugs may get into the body. The risk may be minimized by keeping all needles covered until the injection is made and disposing of the used needle in a safe way immediately after use. The quantity of drug that enters the body following penetration of the skin with a needle is very small, but oil-based vaccines can produce very severe reactions. Some drugs, such as etorphine, are extremely toxic to humans, such that even these minute quantities are hazardous.

Hazardous drugs used in veterinary practice

The groups of drugs mentioned below carry special risks and so are worthy of note. It is important to realize that whilst some drugs may produce acute effects on the operator that are obvious shortly after exposure, other drugs can have cumulative effects, when exposure to small quantities occurs over a long period of time, which can be just as detrimental. For this reason it is good practice to keep exposure to all drugs handled to an absolute minimum by following the ground rules mentioned above.

- **Etorphine** – highly toxic following accidental injection or exposure of skin or mucous membranes to the drug.
- **Halothane** – repeated inhalation may damage the liver and has been incriminated in increasing the risk of miscarriages.
- **Cytotoxic** drugs – many are **mutagenic** (damaging genetic material), **carcinogenic** (causing cancer) and **teratogenic** (damaging the unborn fetus).
- **Prostaglandins** – may cause asthma attacks, have serious effects on the cardiovascular system and cause uterine contraction. Should not be handled by asthmatics or women of childbearing age. The British Veterinary Association has drawn up a code of practice for using prostaglandins in cattle and pigs.

Antimicrobial agents

- **Griseofulvin**, the antifungal drug, is teratogenic and should not be handled by women of childbearing age. Protective clothing, impervious gloves and a dust mask should be worn when handling the powdered form and when adding this to feed.
- **Penicillins** and **cephalosporins** may cause hypersensitivity on exposure in operators who are allergic to these drugs. The reaction can range from mild skin rash to swelling of the eyes, lips and face with difficulty in breathing – symptoms that require immediate medical attention. Drugs in these two families should not be handled by those have a history of allergy to them.
- **Chloramphenicol** can cause a fatal aplastic anaemia in humans, a reaction that is not related to the dose received and occurs in a very small number of people exposed to the drug when prescribed for them by doctors. Nevertheless, it is wise to avoid unnecessary exposure to this drug by taking the precautions mentioned above, including avoiding direct contact of the drug with the skin.

Handling hazardous drugs

It can be seen from the above discussion that hazards are greatest from drugs that are formulated in a liquid or powder form, where aerosols, accidental injection or dust can lead to significant exposure of the operator. Many capsules and tablets can be safely handled with minimal or no contact with the drug, provided that they are not broken or ground up to release the contents in a powdered form. For all tablets it is good practice to wear gloves when handling them (e.g. cyclophosphamide, mitotane and griseofulvin). The use of a triangular metal or plastic tablet counter facilitates the counting of tablets and reduces any contact between the operator and the tablets to a minimum.

Dispensing drugs to owners

Practical tips

- Make sure the owner is aware of any special storage conditions that apply to the drug product (e.g. store in the fridge or out of direct sunlight). Label the product accordingly.

continues ▶

continued

- If dispensing a suspension, make sure the owner is aware that the product should be shaken well before use. Label accordingly.
- Go through the dosing instructions with the owner and make sure they understand them.
- If dispensing products containing penicillins (any members of the penicillin family), ask whether the owner has a penicillin allergy and alert the veterinary surgeon to this fact.
- If dispensing products that are potentially harmful to owners (e.g. cytotoxic drugs, mitotane, griseofulvin, chloramphenicol ointments) make sure the veterinary surgeon has discussed the safe handling of these products with the owner and ask whether protective gloves are to be given out with the drug products.
- Encourage the owner to administer the full course of medication prescribed and make sure they are aware of when the animal needs to be seen again.
- If dispensing tablets, ask the owner how they will give the tablets.
  - If they propose to give them with food, check with the veterinary surgeon that this will be acceptable.
  - If they propose to crush the tablets, check whether this will be acceptable. Drugs with film coatings or capsules generally should not be crushed.
- When dispensing childproof bottles, check that the owner is able to open these containers.
- Always advise owners to bring back the containers (with any unused drugs) to their next consultation.
- Do not reuse empty containers that clients have returned unless you are sure these have not been washed out. Residual moisture will damage most products.

Common prescribing abbreviations

Directions should preferably be in English without abbreviation. It is acceptable, however, to use some Latin abbreviations when dispensing and prescribing. These should be limited to those in Figure 9.20.

a.c.	before meals (*ante cibum*)
ad lib.	at pleasure (*ad libitum*)
amp.	ampoule
b.i.d.	twice a day (*bis in die*)
cap.	capsule
e.o.d.	every other day
g	gram
h, hr	hour
i.m.	intramuscular
i.p.	intraperitoneal
i.t.	intratracheal
i.v.	intravenous
l, L	litre
m^2	square metre
mg	milligram
ml	millilitre
o.m.	in the morning
o.n.	at night
p.c.	after meals (*post cibum*)
p.r.n.	as required (*pro re nata*)
q	every (e.g. 'q12h' means 'every 12 hours')
q.i.d., q.d.s.	four times a day (*quater in die*)
q.s.	a sufficient quantity
s.i.d.	once a day (*semel in die*)
Sig:	directions/label
stat	immediately (*statim*)
susp.	suspension
tab	tablet
t.i.d., t.d.s.	three times a day (*ter in die*)
µl	microlitre

9.20 Common abbreviations used in veterinary medicine.

Further reading

Bishop Y (2000) *BVA Code of Practice on Medicines*. BVA Publications, London

Bishop Y (2004) *The Veterinary Formulary, 6th edn*. The Pharmaceutical Press, London

Brander GC, Pugh DM, Bywater RJ and Jenkins WL (1991) *Veterinary Applied Pharmacology and Therapeutics, 5th edn*. Baillière Tindall, London

Tennant B (2005) (ed) *BSAVA Small Animal Formulary, 5th edition*. BSAVA Publications, Gloucester

Veterinary Medicines Directorate (Executive Agency of the Department for Environment, Food and Rural Affairs):
Veterinary Medicines Regulations 2005
Veterinary Medicines Guidance Notes 2005
Veterinary Medicines Directorate's Clarification Note on record keeping

Wilkins S (1991) Hazards of handling veterinary medicines. *Veterinary Nursing Journal*, **6**, 15–17, 53–55

Chapter 10

Handling and control of small and exotic animals

Trudi Atkinson and Simon J. Girling

Learning objectives

After studying this chapter, students should be able to:

- **Describe how the veterinary nurse should handle and restrain animals for examination or treatment**
- **Describe basic canine and feline 'body language', including signals indicating fear and potential aggression**
- **Explain how to minimize fear and stress in veterinary patients during approach, handling and restraint**
- **Identify the techniques used when handling aggressive or potentially aggressive animals, and list the equipment that may be required**
- **Apply the principles of handling and restraint to everyday veterinary practice**

Introduction

A frequent task for the veterinary nurse in practice is the handling and restraint of animals requiring treatment or examination. How an animal is handled can greatly affect the ease and efficiency with which procedures may be carried out. Inefficient or inappropriate handling can subject the patient to unnecessary stress and discomfort, which is not only damaging to patient welfare but may also result in the development of, or an increase in, defensive aggression towards veterinary staff. Proficiency in handling and control is one of the most essential and valuable skills for a veterinary nurse to acquire.

The aims of the nurse when restraining an animal should be as follows:

- To enable an examination or procedure such as the application of dressings or the administration of medication to be carried out as efficiently as possible

- To avoid injury or further injury to the patient. (For example, if sharp instruments such as scissors are used to cut the animal's hair or a scalpel blade is used to take a skin scrape for examination, injury may result if the animal moves excessively; or injury may be caused if a patient moves unexpectedly whilst attempts are made to examine or treat a fracture or open wound.)
- To prevent injury by the animal to themselves or other persons
- To achieve all of the above without causing additional or unnecessary pain or distress to the animal.

Canine and feline communication

Pain and fear may cause an animal to behave very differently in the veterinary surgery from how it might do under other circumstances. An elementary knowledge of canine and feline communication can help the veterinary nurse assess the possible reactions of an individual animal in its current situation and adapt the means of handling and restraint accordingly.

Canine 'body language' and facial expressions

Figure 10.1 illustrates the typical range of canine body postures (changes in body posture will also occur depending on the dog's current activity). Figure 10.2 shows the typical range of facial expressions in dogs.

Tail wagging

A wagging tail can have several meanings, including a willingness to interact (possibly aggressively) by an assertive dog, or a sign of appeasement by a nervous and potentially defensively aggressive dog. A handler should always consider other aspects of the dog's body language and never assume that a dog with a wagging tail is friendly and will not bite.

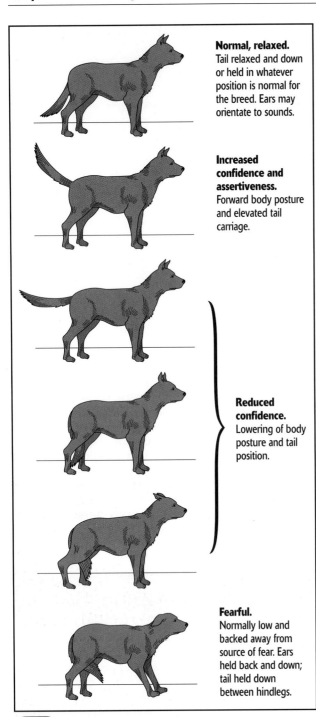

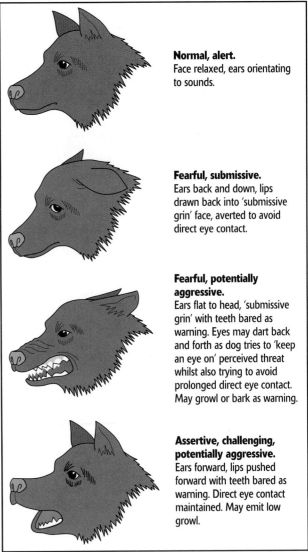

Normal, relaxed.
Tail relaxed and down or held in whatever position is normal for the breed. Ears may orientate to sounds.

Increased confidence and assertiveness.
Forward body posture and elevated tail carriage.

Reduced confidence.
Lowering of body posture and tail position.

Fearful.
Normally low and backed away from source of fear. Ears held back and down; tail held down between hindlegs.

10.1   Canine body language.

Normal, alert.
Face relaxed, ears orientating to sounds.

Fearful, submissive.
Ears back and down, lips drawn back into 'submissive grin' face, averted to avoid direct eye contact.

Fearful, potentially aggressive.
Ears flat to head, 'submissive grin' with teeth bared as warning. Eyes may dart back and forth as dog tries to 'keep an eye on' perceived threat whilst also trying to avoid prolonged direct eye contact. May growl or bark as warning.

Assertive, challenging, potentially aggressive.
Ears forward, lips pushed forward with teeth bared as warning. Direct eye contact maintained. May emit low growl.

10.2   Canine facial expressions.

Dominance, aggression and fear

'**Dominance**' should not be equated with aggression. Not only are the 'rules' of a canine hierarchy designed to reduce the risk of physical confrontation, but also conflicts or misunderstandings over hierarchy are more likely to occur with members of the dog's social group, i.e. the people or other animals that it lives with. Episodes of **aggression** towards people outside that social group are more commonly due to **fear**, especially in a veterinary situation. However, a fearful dog may appear confident and assertive if it has previously had the opportunity to learn that aggression can be effective in making a potential threat 'back off' or keep its distance, even if only momentarily. It is important to realize that attempts to reprimand such a dog physically will only result in an increase in fear and consequently an increase in aggression. (See also Chapter 11.)

Feline communication

Figure 10.3 shows typical body language for a cat.

Relaxed

- *Body*: if resting, may be on back with belly exposed, or curled up. Feet may not be in contact with the ground.
- *Eyes*: may be half closed if cat is relaxed, pupil size dependent on available light. A 'slow eye blink' may be directed towards other animals, including people, as a signal of 'non-confrontation'.
- *Ears*: normal 'relaxed'.
- *Tail*: extended or loosely wrapped if cat is resting. If standing or if in motion, tail may be held down in 'U' shape away from body, or upright, sometimes with curl at the end as friendly greeting.
- *Vocalization*: may purr while relaxed, or chirrup or meow as friendly greeting.

Tense

- *Body:* may explore area looking for ways of escape or rest in 'ready' position with feet in contact with the ground so cat can move quickly if necessary.

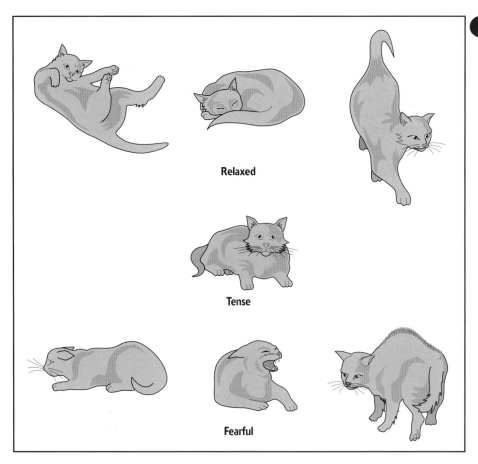

Relaxed

Tense

Fearful

- *Tail*: usually wrapped around body.
- *Ears*: slightly flattened sideways.
- *Eyes*: open, pupils dilated.

Fearful

- *Body*: may be held low and away from source of fear with all four feet on the ground, or may attempt to hide.
- *Tail*: very tight to body.
- *Ears*: flattened sideways.
- *Eyes*: wide, with dilated pupils.

Fearful/defensively aggressive

- *Body*: flattened and backed away from source of fear. If approached, may 'lash out' with front feet, but with body held back.
- *Tail*: tightly wrapped or 'lashing'.
- *Ears*: fear and submission signalled by holding ears down and to the side; however, to protect them from injury, ears are held back and down if an aggressive encounter becomes more likely.
- *Eyes*: wide, pupils fully dilated, and focused on the source of fear.
- *Vocalization*: may growl, hiss or spit.

A cat confronted by a sudden, unexpected danger, such as an unknown or unfriendly dog, may arch its back and fluff out the hairs along the back and tail in an attempt to appear much larger than it really is.

Purring

Cats often purr when relaxed or as a way of soliciting food or attention, but they may also purr when in extreme pain or distress. This may be one way that the cat tries to reduce its level of stress, in the same way that people may whistle or hum if anxious or frightened. It should not always be assumed that a cat is not stressed or in pain because it is purring.

Initial approach and handling

Dogs

Whenever possible, a dog should be encouraged to approach the handler rather than their directly approaching the dog. Cornering a dog, leaning over it or prolonged direct eye contact, which the dog may consider threatening, should be avoided. Crouching down to the dog's level can help with nervous individuals, but not so close that the face could be within 'biting' distance. Grabbing a dog by the collar or scruff should be avoided, as this could frighten the dog and cause it to turn and bite.

Nervous animals that are normally obedient may be reassured by giving them a few easy commands to help them relax, especially if the owner has previously associated these responses with rewards.

Occasionally, dogs are reluctant to leave the safety of a hospital kennel and may become defensively aggressive if confronted or if attempts are made to enter the kennel in order to remove them. If a lightweight lead is left on the dog, the end can be extracted using a broom handle or cat catcher, allowing the handler to take hold of the lead safely without needing to confront the dog. In most instances, once the handler has hold of the lead the dog will leave the kennel and walk willingly with the handler.

⚠ **WARNING**
A lead must *never* be attached to a check chain or slip lead and the dog must be regularly supervised whilst in a kennel with a lead attached.

Handling with the owner present

It should always be remembered that, to the owner of a beloved pet, how they witness their animal being handled may reflect on the type and standard of care that they expect from the practice in general. If the pet is handled roughly or inefficiently they may choose to take their pet and their custom elsewhere.

- Spend a little time 'chatting' with the owner before attempting to handle or approach a dog. This time can be spent watching the dog and making a general assessment of its temperament.
- The dog will take cues from its owner as to whether or not something or someone is a potential threat. A minute or so interacting with the owner in a 'friendly' manner can often help to convey the message to the dog that you are not a threat. However, it is not a good idea to attempt to shake the owner's hand, as the dog may regard this as a threatening gesture and may become aggressive.

It may be tempting to ask an owner to help in handling or restraining their pet, particularly if it is nervous; however, if the client should be injured during this process the practice may be liable, even if the owner volunteered their services (see Chapter 2). Owners might usefully administer treats or distractions to their pet to ease examinations etc. but generally should be dissuaded from putting themselves in any position of potential risk.

Some owners may unintentionally reinforce their pet's fear and aggression, and if a dog is difficult to handle it may be easier to deal with away from the owner. When separating dog and owner it is often more successful to ask the owner to leave the room first and then lead the dog away.

Cats

Examination or procedures should be carried out on cats as soon as possible. Cats often have a limited 'tolerance period', i.e. they will put up with so much for so long and then suddenly decide that they have had enough and try to escape or become defensively aggressive. Cats often feel very vulnerable in hospital kennels. Providing them with a box in which they can hide will often help them to feel more secure and therefore easier to approach and handle.

Extracting a cat from a carrier

Top-opening carriers

1. Lift the lid slowly. Most cats will prefer to stay in the carrier but some may try to jump out as soon as the lid is lifted, so be prepared.
2. Stroke the cat to settle it and assess its temperament.
3. Make sure the cat is well supported underneath (see later on lifting and carrying) and lift it out and on to the examination table.

▶

Front-opening carriers

1. Open the front and try to encourage the cat out without putting a hand inside the carrier, which the cat may find threatening, making it less willing to leave the safety of the carrier.
2. If the carrier can be separated into two halves, remove the top half and lift the cat out as you would with a top-opening carrier. Some front-opening carriers have a tray in the base in which the cat sits. If so, this can be gently pulled out, bringing the cat out with it.
3. If none of the above is possible, gently tilt the carrier, which may help to encourage the cat out.

A cat should only be physically extracted from its carrier as a last resort; try to do so gently and be aware that the cat may become defensive. *Do not scruff the cat and pull it out unless it is absolutely necessary to do so and all other methods have been tried.*

Once the cat is out of its carrier, place the carrier on the ground away from the cat. If the carrier is left in its sight, the cat may repeatedly try to get back in and may become fractious when prevented from doing so.

Moving, transporting and lifting animals

Dogs must be on a lead attached to a well fitting collar if they are to be walked from one area of the surgery to another.

- Always check that the collar is not too tight, or so loose that the dog could slip out of it.
- For added security, use a lightweight slip lead as well.

If cats or other small animals are to be transported from one area to another they must be securely contained in an appropriate carrier.

Lifting and carrying

Handlers should be aware of any possible medical condition or injury that may be causing an animal pain or discomfort before attempting to lift or carry it. Points of pain should be kept away from the handler's body as the animal is carried, to reduce the risk of causing further discomfort.

It is important to ensure that the animal is aware of the handler's approach and intent before an attempt to lift it is made.

- Small to medium-sized dogs may be lifted by one person (Figure 10.4). Assistance may be required to carry drips or open doors, etc.
- Large, heavy (>20 kg) or injured dogs should be lifted and carried by two people (Figure 10.5).
- Large, immobile or severely injured dogs are best carried by two or more people in a blanket (Figure 10.6) or on a stretcher (Figure 10.7).
- Cats should be tucked in under the arm with the forearm supporting the underneath of the cat and with the hand gently holding its front legs (Figure 10.8). The other hand can be used to stroke the cat over the head and neck, ready to take hold of its scruff if necessary.

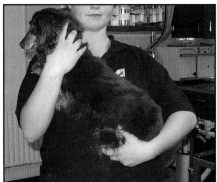

10.4

Lifting a small dog. (Courtesy of J Niehoegen)

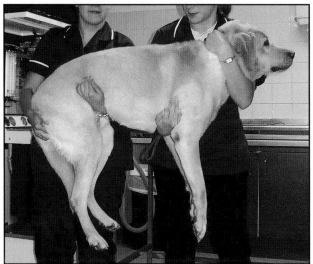

10.5 Lifting a large dog requires two people. (Courtesy of J Niehoegen)

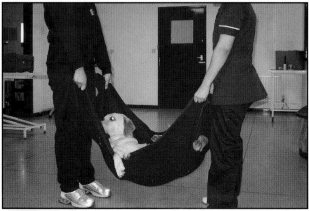

10.6 Lifting a dog with a blanket. (Courtesy of J Niehoegen)

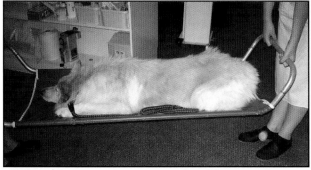

10.7 Carrying a dog on a stretcher. (Courtesy of E Mullineaux)

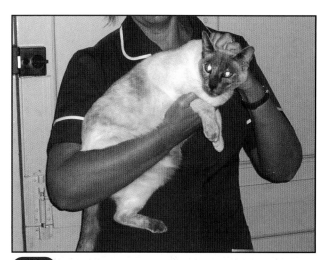

10.8 Lifting a cat.

Manual handling
Always follow the health and safety rules when lifting:

- Keep the back straight, legs slightly apart and bend at the knees
- Always get assistance before attempting to lift a heavy or awkward weight
- Keep the load close to the body.

Transport of anaesthetized or unconscious animals
Anaesthetized or unconscious animals should be transported on a wheeled trolley, or similar, and monitored at all times. To maintain the animal's airway the neck should be pulled slightly forward and the tongue extended. Placing the tongue under the patient's lower jaw will prevent the tongue falling back into the mouth and blocking the airway if the animal is not intubated.

Restraint for examination or treatment

Restraint of pet animals should be firm but gentle, using no more than the minimum amount of restraint necessary. Care must be taken not to cause undue pain or discomfort by applying any more pressure than is required. It may be necessary to adjust the firmness of your hold momentarily, depending on the animal's reactions to the procedure being performed.

The means of restraint used is dependent on both the procedure to be performed and the reactions of the individual animal.

Restraint of dogs
Figure 10.9 shows two methods of steadying a dog's head. The rolled-up towel method is particularly useful with small brachycephalic breeds and can be used to prevent a dog from turning round to bite when it is not possible to use a muzzle.

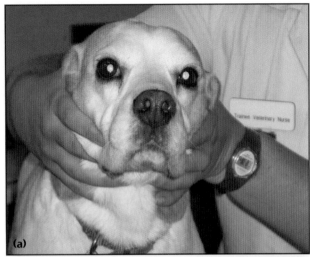

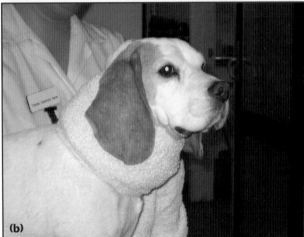

10.9 Restraining a dog's head. **(a)** The hands are placed either side of the neck and the head is gently pushed forwards with the fingers. **(b)** A rolled-up towel is held firmly but gently around the dog's neck. (Courtesy of E Mullineaux)

Figure 10.10 shows a dog being held for cephalic venepuncture. It is often useful to have an additional person available to steady the back end of the dog if it starts to struggle.

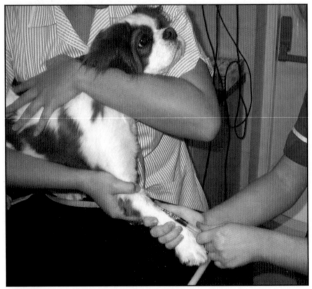

10.10 Holding a dog for cephalic venepuncture. (Courtesy of D Mactaggart)

Figure 10.11 shows a dog being restrained on its side. It may be possible to manoeuvre a dog into this position by first getting the dog to lie down, on command if possible or by drawing the dog's legs forward whilst it is in a sitting position, and then gently rolling the dog over using the forearm to push the dog's head down whilst also holding on to the dog's legs. If the position cannot be achieved by the above method, the dog's legs that are closest to the handler are grasped and pulled away, causing the dog to fall towards the handler. The dog is then gently lowered down against the handler's chest and on to the surface. However, it is necessary to be aware that this manoeuvre and being held in this position can be frightening and may cause the dog to panic and attempt to bite. Gentle reassurance is essential and muzzling the dog beforehand may be advisable.

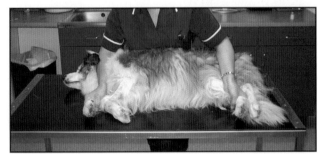

10.11 Restraining a dog on its side. (Courtesy of J Niehoegen)

Restraint of cats

Figure 10.12 shows general restraint for examination or treatment of the head area. The cat's body should be held close to the handler to prevent the cat from backing away. A firm but gentle hold around the front legs prevents the cat using its front claws.

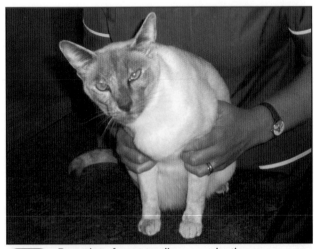

10.12 Restraint of a cat to allow examination or treatment of the head.

Figure 10.13 shows raising of the cephalic vein or restraint for examination or treatment of the foreleg. Figure 10.14 shows two methods of restraint for jugular venepuncture.

It is sometimes necessary to hold a cat by the scruff of the neck if firmer restraint is required. Other methods should always be tried first as many otherwise calm and tolerant cats can become fractious and difficult to handle as soon as attempts are made to handle them by the scruff.

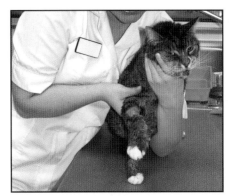

10.13
Raising a cat's cephalic vein or restraint for examination of the foreleg. (Courtesy of C Clarke)

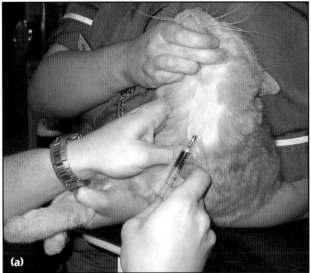

(a)

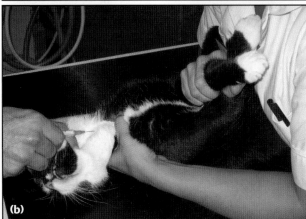

(b)

10.14 Alternative methods of holding a cat for jugular venepuncture. (a, Courtesy of D Mactaggart; b, Courtesy of E Mullineaux)

Distraction

Gentle distractions can often help to calm an animal and allow procedures to be carried out more efficiently.

- Talking to the animal in a calm and friendly manner, especially if the animal's name is used, can often help to distract and calm a patient.
- Use the fingers gently to stroke, scratch or massage the animal.
- A short whistle can often 'still' a struggling dog, allowing a few moments to get a needle into a vein, take a radiograph or perform any other procedure that requires the animal to be still and distracted for a second or two.

Handling difficult or aggressive dogs and cats

Most animals are scared by the veterinary clinic and what happens there. It is a strange place where potentially unpleasant things can happen. Good sensitive handling will obviously help to minimize this problem. The use of dog and cat pheromone diffusers (e.g DAP or Feliway, Ceva Animal Health) in the clinic may also help to reduce the anxiety of the animal. Remember that a frightened animal may use aggression as a defence. Therefore any unnecessary actions that may cause an animal to be fearful or that may increase its fear should be avoided.

Dogs

Raising of the paw, lip-smacking, yawning and looking away are all signs shown by dogs in the clinic that suggest they may be anxious. The handler should look for these signs and intervene before the animal shows more overt signs. Giving the animal something to do, which it knows how to do and for which it is normally rewarded (such as a sit), can be a good way of switching the animal into a more positive mood. However, it is important that such actions are taken before the animal gets too worked up.

Growling

If a dog growls:

- Do *not* attempt to punish the dog: a confrontation will only teach the dog that it has good reason to be defensive.
- Do *not* attempt to comfort or reassure the dog: this may actually reward and so reinforce the unwanted behaviour.
- *Do* muzzle the dog: a growl may not cause you to back off but a set of sharp teeth heading in your direction will. If this happens the dog will learn that direct aggression is effective even if a warning growl is not. Dogs that have already learnt this can be some of the most dangerous and unpredictable to handle.
- *Do* try to appear unconcerned by the growl: backing away or appearing fearful or angry may reinforce the growling and potential aggression.
- *Do* try to understand why the dog may be growling. Is the dog in pain? Is it the way in which it is being handled? Is it the procedure that is being carried out? Unless the procedure is almost finished, or is one that will only take a few seconds, it is best to stop and then continue once the dog is muzzled.

Muzzles

Whenever possible, a dog should be muzzled *before* it tries to bite. It can be far more difficult to get a muzzle on a dog that has already decided that you are a threat and has discovered that trying to bite is effective in making you back off.

A variety of cloth, plastic and leather muzzles are available (Figure 10.15). A good selection of different types and sizes should always be at hand. Note that open-ended muzzles may still allow a dog to 'nip' with its front teeth.

If a dog is to be muzzled for longer than a few minutes, it is important always to use a basket-type muzzle that allows the dog to open its mouth, enabling it to pant or vomit. A dog must never be left unattended for any length of time whilst muzzled.

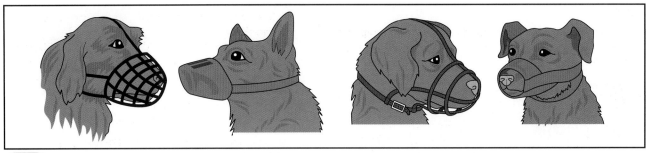

10.15   Variety of muzzles.

If a dog is a regular patient and frequently needs to be muzzled, a good idea is to provide the owner with a suitable muzzle to take home. The owner should be advised to put the muzzle on the dog frequently for short periods and reward the dog with food treats, play, affection, and even walks whilst wearing the muzzle. The dog will then make pleasant associations with wearing the muzzle, making it easier for the owner to put the muzzle on the dog before bringing it into the surgery.

Applying a tape muzzle

Figure 10.16 shows the steps in applying a tape muzzle. The tape must be pulled tight in order for the muzzle to be effective, but this can be uncomfortable for the dog and may even cause some slight injury. Therefore this muzzle should only be used in an emergency or if it is not possible to get close enough to the dog to use any other type of muzzle.

Using a 'dog-catcher'

The noose of the dog-catcher (Figure 10.17) is dropped over the animal's head and then tightened, thereby reducing the risk of injury to the handler when taking hold of a severely aggressive dog. The use of a dog-catcher can be highly traumatic for a dog, so it should only ever be used as a last resort.

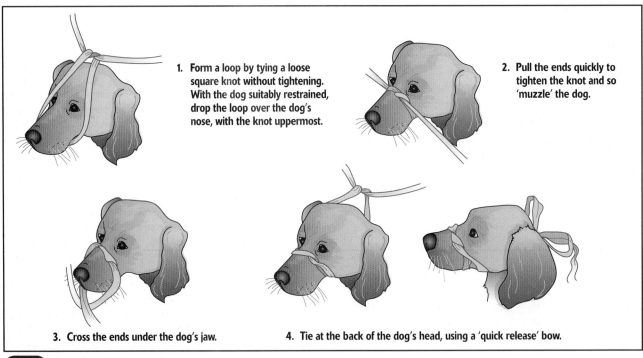

1. Form a loop by tying a loose square knot without tightening. With the dog suitably restrained, drop the loop over the dog's nose, with the knot uppermost.

2. Pull the ends quickly to tighten the knot and so 'muzzle' the dog.

3. Cross the ends under the dog's jaw.

4. Tie at the back of the dog's head, using a 'quick release' bow.

10.16   Applying a tape muzzle. Use a length of tape or non-stretch bandage at least 100 cm long for a medium-sized dog.

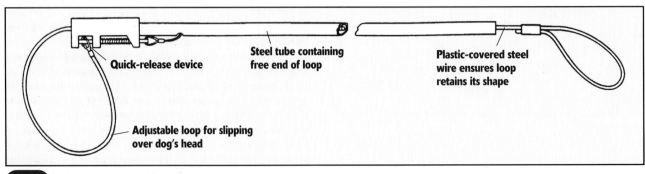

Quick-release device

Steel tube containing free end of loop

Plastic-covered steel wire ensures loop retains its shape

Adjustable loop for slipping over dog's head

10.17   A dog-catcher.

Cats

Fractious cats can often be adequately restrained by wrapping them in a large towel (Figure 10.18). An alternative is a 'cat restraining bag'.

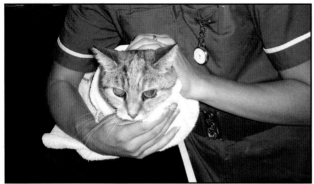

10.18 A fractious cat can be wrapped in a towel. (Courtesy of E Mullineaux)

Use of a 'crush cage' may be necessary with cats that cannot be handled. This is similar to a wire cat carrier but with a movable partition that is used to press the cat against one side of the cage, allowing an injection to be given through the mesh of the cage. If a crush cage is not available, or if the cat cannot be moved from its carrier, the lid or door of the carrier can be opened just enough to allow thick towels to be pushed into the carrier but not enough to allow the cat to escape. The towels are then used to press the cat against the side of the cage, allowing an injection to be given.

Handling and restraint of small mammals

Pet mammals come in many different shapes and sizes, and from many different backgrounds. They range from those more adapted to human cohabitation, such as mice and rats, through to the more recently adopted pets such as chipmunks, which are still semi-wild in nature.

Initial assessment

In order to safeguard the small mammal patient's welfare, there are several points to consider before restraint is attempted.

- **Is the patient severely debilitated and in respiratory distress?**
  Examples include the pneumonic rabbit, with obvious oculonasal discharge and dyspnoea, or the chronic lung disease seen so often in older rats. Excessive or rough handling of these patients is contraindicated.

- **Is the species a tame one?**
  Examples of the more unusual small mammals that may be kept include chipmunks, marmosets and other small primates, opossums and raccoons. All of these are potentially hazardous to handlers and themselves, as they will often bolt for freedom when frightened, or turn and fight. Even the more routinely kept small mammals, such as hamsters, may be aggressive.

- **Is the patient suffering from a metabolic bone disease?**
  This is often seen in small primates, young rabbits and guinea pigs. The diet may have been inadequate with regard to calcium and vitamin D3 and exposure to natural sunlight may be absent, hence long-bone mineralization during growth will be poor, leading to spontaneous or easily fractured bones.

- **Does the patient require medication or physical examination?**
  If so, restraint may be essential.

Handling techniques for small mammals

There are many common handling errors made with small mammals. For example, most species find an approach from above very threatening: to them it may seem like a predator swooping down and it is not surprising that they try to escape, biting if necessary. In general, allowing an animal to approach first or trying to entice it with a treat rather than reaching in and grabbing it is preferable. Taking extra time at this stage can save time in the long run.

Because of the wide range of species grouped under the heading 'small mammal', this section is easier if considered under specific groups and orders.

Rabbits

The majority of domestic rabbits are docile, but the odd aggressive doe or buck, usually those not used to being handled, does exist. The potential dangers to the veterinary nurse arise from the claws, which can inflict deep scratches rivalling those inflicted by cats, and the incisors, which can produce deep bites. Aggression is frequently worse at the start of the breeding season in March/April. In addition to the damage they may cause the handler, a struggling rabbit may lash out with its powerful hindlimbs and fracture or dislocate its own spine. Severe stress can even induce cardiac arrest in some individuals. Rapid and safe restraint is therefore essential.

To this end, an aggressive rabbit may be grasped by the scruff with one hand whilst the other hand supports underneath the rear legs. If the rabbit is not aggressive, one hand may be placed under the thorax with the thumb and first two fingers encircling the front limbs, whilst the other is placed under the rear legs to support the back.

When transferring the rabbit within a room it must be held close to the handler's chest. Non-fractious individuals may also be supported with their heads pushed into the crook of one arm, with that forearm supporting the length of the rabbit's body; the other hand is then used to place pressure on or grasp the scruff region (Figure 10.19). When transporting rabbits in a pet carrier or basket it is sensible to place a towel over a top-opening carrier before opening it, to prevent a frightened rabbit from jumping out.

Once caught, a rabbit may be calmed further by wrapping it in a towel so that just the head protrudes (Figure 10.20) (similar to the method used for restraining cats). There are also available specific rabbit 'papooses' that zip up along the rabbit's dorsum, leaving the head and ears free for blood sampling but confining the limbs to prevent escape or self-harm. It is important not to allow rabbits to overheat in this position, as they, like a lot of small mammals, do not have significant sweat glands and do not actively pant. They can therefore quickly overheat if their environmental temperature exceeds 23–25°C, with fatal results.

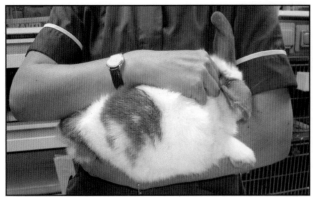

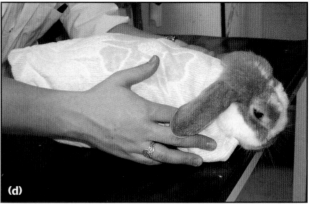

10.19 Carrying a docile rabbit, with its head in the crook of the elbow. Most rabbits find this method of restraint settling. (Reproduced from the *BSAVA Manual of Rabbit Medicine and Surgery, 2nd edition*)

10.20 *continued* The 'bunny burrito': restraining a rabbit by wrapping it in a towel. **(d)** The remaining side of the towel is wrapped across the dorsum and tucked in ventrally on the opposing side to complete the wrap. (Reproduced from the *BSAVA Manual of Rabbit Medicine and Surgery, 2nd edition*)

Covering a rabbit's eyes will often help to calm it (Figure 10.21).

⚠ WARNING

Care should be taken if there is a need to restrain a rabbit on its back for examination or minor treatment of the ventral area. This should be avoided if possible, as the rabbit may injure its back if it suddenly attempts to escape or turn itself upright. The rabbit may go into a state known as tonic immobility when turned on its back, and the transition from a passive animal to one engaged in very active escape can be instantaneous and unpredictable.

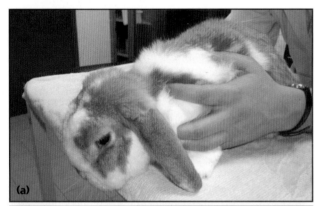

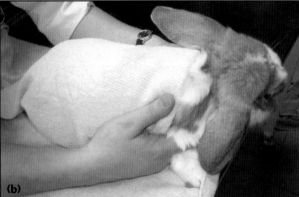

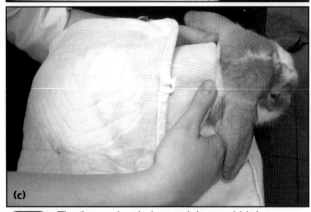

10.20 The 'bunny burrito': restraining a rabbit by wrapping it in a towel. **(a)** The rabbit is placed on a towel, facing away from the handler. **(b)** One side of the towel is wrapped firmly across the dorsum, covering the forefeet but leaving the head exposed. **(c)** The back of the towel is folded up over the lumbar region. *continues ▶*

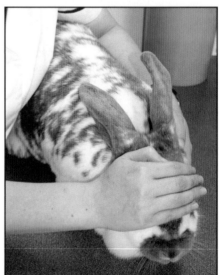

10.21

A hand over the rabbit's eyes helps to keep the animal calm. (Courtesy of C Clarke)

Rodents

The Order Rodentia contains the following groups:

- Myomorpha, which contains the families Muridae and Cricetidae
  - Muridae contains mice and rats
  - Cricetidae contains hamsters and gerbils
- Caviomorpha (hystricomorph rodents), which contains the families Caviidae (guinea pigs) and Chinchillidae (chinchillas)
- Sciuromorpha contains the family Sciuridae (chipmunks).

Mice and rats

Mice will frequently bite an unfamiliar handler, especially in strange surroundings. It is useful first to grasp the tail near to the base and then position the mouse by this means on a non-slip surface. Whilst still grasping the tail, the scruff may now be grasped firmly between thumb and forefinger of the other hand (Figure 10.22).

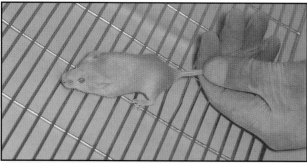
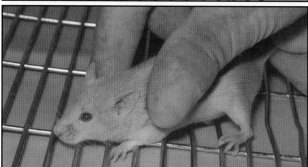
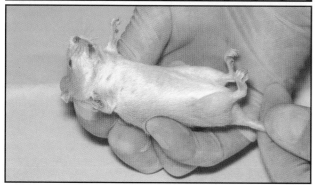

10.22 Handling techniques for mice. (Reproduced from *BSAVA Manual of Exotic Pets, 4th edition*)

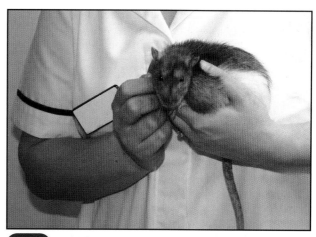

10.23 Holding a tame rat. (Courtesy of C Clarke)

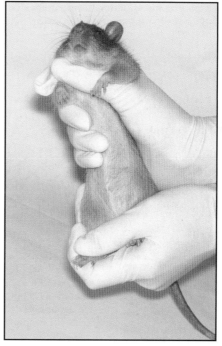

10.24 Restraining a rat. (Reproduced from *BSAVA Manual of Exotic Pets, 4th edition*)

Rats will rarely bite unless roughly handled (Figure 10.23). They are best picked up by encircling the pectoral girdle (immediately behind the front limbs) with the thumb and fingers of one hand whilst bringing the other hand underneath the rear limbs to support the rat's weight (Figure 10.24). The more fractious rat may be temporarily restrained by grasping the base of the tail before scruffing it with thumb and forefinger.

Under no circumstances should mice or rats be restrained by the tips of their tails, as degloving injuries to the skin covering them will occur.

Hamsters and gerbils

Hamsters can be relatively difficult to handle as, being nocturnal, they are never pleased at being awoken and picked up during daylight hours. If the hamster is relatively tame and used to being handled, simply cupping the hands underneath the animal is sufficient to transfer them from one cage to another.

Some breeds of hamster are more aggressive than others and the Russian, Djungarian or hairy-footed hamsters are notorious for their short temper. In these cases, the hamster should be placed on a firm flat surface and gentle but firm pressure should be placed on the scruff region with finger and thumb of one hand. Then as much of the scruff should be grasped as possible, with the direction of pull in a cranial manner to ensure that the skin is not drawn tight around the eyes (hamsters have a tendency to proptose their eyes if roughly scruffed). If a very aggressive animal is encountered, the use of a small glass or perspex container with a lid for examination and transport purposes is useful.

Gerbils are relatively docile, but can jump extremely well when frightened and may bite if roughly handled. For simple transport they may be moved from one place to another by cupping the hands underneath the gerbil. Like all small mammals, they should always be approached from the sides and low levels, so that the handler's hands do not startle the animal by mimicking the swooping action of a bird of prey.

For more rigorous restraint the gerbil may be grasped by the scruff between thumb and forefinger of one hand after placing the animal on a flat level surface. It is vitally important not to grasp a gerbil by the tail as this will lead to stripping of the tail's skin, leaving denuded coccygeal vertebrae. This will never regrow and the denuded vertebrae will undergo avascular necrosis and drop off later.

Jerds and **jerboas** are related species and handling techniques are the same.

Guinea pigs, chinchillas and degus

Guinea pigs are rarely aggressive, but they become highly stressed when separated from their companions and normal surroundings. This makes them difficult to catch, as they will move at high speed in their cage. To aid restraint, dimmed lighting can be used and environmental noise should be restricted to reduce stress levels. Restraint is also easier if the guinea pig is already in a small box or cage, as there is less room for it to escape.

To restrain a guinea pig it should be grasped behind the front limbs from the dorsal aspect with one hand, whilst the other is placed beneath the rear limbs to support the weight (Figure 10.25). This is particularly important as the guinea pig has a large abdomen but slender bones and spine, which may be easily damaged.

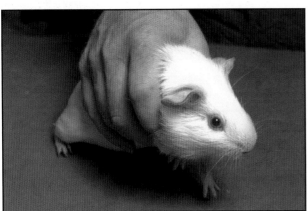

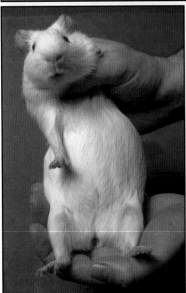

10.25 Restraining a guinea pig. The animal is first grasped around its shoulders. It can then be lifted, with the hindquarters supported.

Chinchillas are equally timorous and rarely if ever bite. They too can be easily stressed and so dimming the room lighting and reducing noise can be useful during capture. When restrained they must not be scruffed under any circumstances, as this will result in the loss of fur at the site held. Even if no physical gripping of the skin occurs, chinchillas may lose some fur due to the stress of the restraint. This 'fur slip', as it is known, will leave a bare patch that will take many weeks to regrow.

Some chinchillas, when particularly stressed, will rear up on their hind legs and urinate at the handler with surprising accuracy. It is therefore essential to pick up the chinchilla calmly and quickly, with minimal restraint, placing one hand around the pectoral girdle from the dorsal aspect just behind the front legs, and the other hand cupping the hind legs and supporting the chinchilla's weight.

Degus may be handled in a similar way to chinchillas.

Chipmunks

There are at least 24 species of chipmunk, with the commonest seen in the UK currently being the Siberian species, though smaller North American species are also kept. As a species they are extremely highly strung and the avoidance of stress and fear aggression is essential to avoid fatalities. Generally they are very difficult to handle without being bitten unless they have been hand reared, in which case they may be scruffed quickly or cupped in both hands. To catch them in their aviary-style enclosures the easiest method is to use a fine-meshed aviary net or butterfly net, preferably made of a dark material. The chipmunk may be safely netted and quickly transferred to a towel for manual restraint, examination, injection or chemical restraint.

Ferrets

The Mustelidae family contains ferrets, polecats, martens, weasels and stoats. In practice the commonest seen is the domestic ferret. Ferrets can make excellent house pets and many are friendly and hand tame. However, in the UK the most frequent use for which ferrets are kept is for rabbit hunting, hence many ferrets are not regularly handled and so may be aggressive.

For excitable or aggressive animals, a firm grasp of the scruff, high up at the back of the neck, should be made. The ferret may be suspended from this whilst stabilizing the lower body with the other hand around the pelvis (Figure 10.26). Animals that are more tame may be suspended with one hand behind the front legs, cupping between thumb and fingers from the dorsal aspect, with the other hand supporting the rear limbs (Figure 10.27a). This may be varied somewhat in the more lively individuals by placing the thumb of one hand underneath the chin, so pushing the jaw upwards, and the rest of the fingers grasping the other side of the neck (Figure 10.27b). The other hand is then brought under the rear limbs as support.

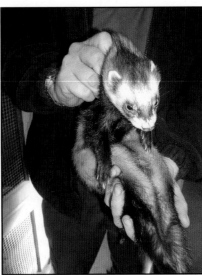

10.26 Holding a potentially aggressive ferret, using the scruff. (Courtesy of S Redrobe)

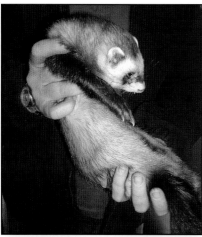

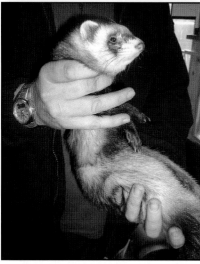

10.27

Holding a less aggressive ferret. (Courtesy of S Redrobe)

Handling and restraint of birds

As with small mammals, a decision needs to be made on whether the bird in question is safe to restrain. This is not only because of the danger to the handler (in the case of an aggressive or potentially dangerous bird of prey) but also because of the medical aspects of the patient's health.

Initial assessment

- Is the bird in respiratory distress, and is the stress of handling going to exacerbate this?
- Is the bird easily accessible, allowing quick, stress-free and safe capture?
- Does the bird require medication via the oral or injectable route, or can it be medicated via nebulization or food or drinking water?
- Does the bird require an in-depth physical examination at close quarters or is cage observation enough?

It is not always necessary for a bird to be restrained. It is important to remember that many avian patients are highly stressed individuals, so any restraint that is performed should involve minimal periods of handling and capture.

Initial techniques useful in handling avian patients

It is helpful to remember that the majority of birds seen in practice (with the obvious exception of owls) are **diurnal** (active during the day) and so reduced or dimmed lighting in general has an immediate calming effect. This can be used to advantage when catching a flighty or stressed bird. In the case of the Passeriformes ('perching birds' such as canaries and finches) and Psittaciformes (members of the parrot family, including budgerigars and cockatiels), turning down the room lights or drawing the curtains or blinds is enough. For raptors (birds of prey) there may well be access to the practice's or the bird's own 'hoods' (see below).

It is advisable to keep noise levels to a minimum when handling birds, as the acuity of their hearing is second only to the acuity of their vision. With these two initial approaches, stress and time for capture can be greatly reduced.

Prior to the capture of the avian patient, all obstructing items should be removed from their cage or box (e.g. toys, water bowl, food bowl). This helps to avoid self-induced trauma by the bird and reduces the time needed to capture the patient. Once these initial arrangements have been made, the avian patient can be approached.

Equipment used in avian handling

Birds of prey

There are two main categories of birds of prey commonly seen in practice:

- **Falconiformes** is the Order that contains falcons, hawks, vultures and eagles. These birds are mainly diurnal and make up the most commonly seen group
- **Strigiformes** is the Order that contains owls. These are generally relatively docile. They differ from falcons in two main areas:
  - They rely more heavily on silent flight and excellent hearing to capture their prey
  - They are generally nocturnal and so use of hoods and darkening the room will not quieten these birds.

Hoods (Figure 10.28) are leather caps that slot over the head, leaving the beak free but completely covering the eyes. They are used to calm falcons and hawks when on the wrist or during handling or transporting. Many of these birds will also have **jesses** on their legs. These are the leather straps attached to their 'ankles' (lower tarsometatarsal area) and they allow the falcon to be restrained whilst on the owner's fist.

Leather gauntlets (Figure 10.28) should be worn by all handlers for all birds of prey, as their talons and the power of grasp of each foot can be extremely strong. The feet of birds of prey represent the major danger to the handler and not the beak. When the bird of prey is positioned on the gauntleted hand it is important to note that the wrist of this hand (traditionally the left hand in European falconers) is kept *above the height of the elbow*. If not, the bird has a tendency to walk up the arm of the handler, with potentially serious and painful results. The type of gauntlet should either be a specific falconer's gauntlet or one of the heavier-duty leather pruning gauntlets available from garden centres.

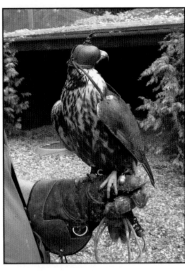

10.28
A hood keeps a raptor calm. (Courtesy of J Chitty)

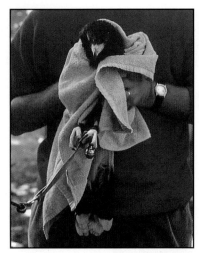

10.29
Casting a Harris' hawk. (Reproduced from *BSAVA Manual of Exotic Pets, 4th edition*)

1. Place the gauntleted hand into the cage or box or beside the bird's perch.
2. Grasp the jesses with the thumb and forefinger of the gauntleted hand and encourage the bird to step up on to the glove.
3. Once the bird is on the hand, retain hold of the jesses and slip the hood over the bird's head.

The bird may then be safely examined 'on the hand' and frequently is docile enough to allow manipulation of wings and beak and for small injections to be administered or for oral dosing to occur.

If the bird does not have jesses on but is trained to perch on the hand, it may well step up on to the gauntlet of its own accord. If not, the room lighting needs to be darkened for Falconiformes (a blue or red light source could also be used, allowing the handler to see the bird but preventing the bird of prey seeing normally). There are then two possible approaches.

1. The bird may be grasped from behind in a thick towel, ensuring that the handler is aware of where the bird's head is (this is known as **casting** the bird; Figure 10.29). The bird is restrained across the shoulder area with the thumbs pushing forward underneath the beak to extend the head away from the hands. The hood can then be placed over the bird's head and the bird placed on a gauntleted hand. The majority of birds are happier and struggle less when their feet are actually grasping something, rather than being held in a towel with their feet freely hanging.
2. Alternatively the hooded bird may be held from behind with the middle and fourth finger of each hand grasping the leg on the same side and directing the feet away from the handler. This method of holding the legs prevents the raptor from grasping one foot with the other, which would cause severe puncturing of the skin leading to secondary infections known as bumblefoot.

If the raptor is loose in its aviary, for the majority of raptors catching them at night is advised. Owls should be caught during the day. The use of nets and towels is often required.

Finally, it is important to remember that the majority of birds of prey are regularly flown and so it is vital to preserve the integrity of their flight or tail feathers. Unfortunately, not many falconers will thank the veterinary surgeon for saving their bird's life if they then cannot fly that bird until after the feathers have been replaced at the next moult (moulting usually occurs in the autumn).

Parrots and other cagebirds

Parrots are often trained to step up on to the hand. If the owner does not have the bird already trained to do this, they should be encouraged to do so. A tasty treat can be held in front of the bird, with the other hand just in front and above the internal perch. The treat should be at such a distance that the bird must step on to the hand to get to the treat. It is important to be aware that nervous birds especially may reach down to the hand, as it is normal for many parrot species to use the beak as a third limb to help balance. The novice handler may mistake this for an attempt to bite and pull the hand away, making matters worse as the bird is now even less sure about stepping on to the hand and may grab at the hand in a desperate attempt to pull itself on to the hand, biting in the process.

With all this group, the use of subdued or blue or red light will calm the bird and allow restraint with minimal fuss.

- With **psittacine birds**, the main weapon is the beak and a powerful bite is possible. (The hyacinth macaw, the largest in the family, can produce 330 pounds per square inch of pressure with its beak. This means that it can easily crack the largest Brazil nuts and badly damage or even sever a finger.)
- With **passerine birds**, the main weapon may again be the beak, though this is less damaging as a biting weapon. It may still be a sharp stabbing weapon in the case of starlings and mynah birds.

Heavy gauntlets are not recommended for either family group for restraint, as they do not allow easy judgement of the strength of the handler's grip on the patient. Instead it is better to use dish or bath towels for the larger species and paper towels for the smaller ones, as these provide some protection from being bitten without masking the true strength of the grip.

Important note: birds do not have a diaphragm and so rely solely on the outward movement of their ribcage and keel bone for inspiration. Restriction of this movement with too tight a grip can be fatal.

1. The bird's cage should first be cleared of all obstacles that might hinder capture or result in injury of the patient.
2. The towel and hand are then introduced into the cage and the bird is firmly but gently grasped from the back (Figure 10.30). It must be ensured that the head is located first, to allow the thumb and forefingers to be positioned underneath the lower beak, in order that it can be pushed upwards thus preventing the bird from biting.

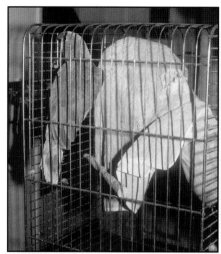
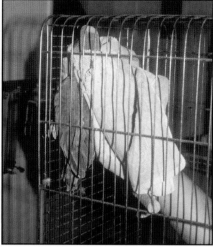
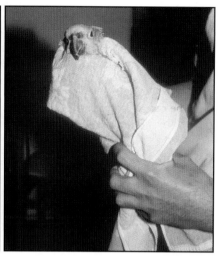

10.30 Removing a parrot from its cage. (Reproduced from *BSAVA Manual of Psittacine Birds, 2nd edition*)

3. The rest of the towel is then used to wrap around the bird to gently restrain its wing movement. This will avoid excessive struggling and wing trauma.
4. The patient may then be cocooned in the towel with the head still held extended from behind through the towel and the rest loosely wrapped around the bird's body.
5. The limbs may then be removed from the towelling one at a time for examination or medication.

The towel technique is also more beneficial than gloves alone because it presents a larger surface area for the bird to try to evade. The bird is then less likely to make a bolt for freedom, whereas a single hand can be a much smaller target and encourages escape attempts.

For smaller cagebirds:

1. A piece of paper towel may be used and the bird then transferred to the hand. Latex gloves may be worn.
2. The neck of the bird should be held between the index and middle fingers (Figure 10.31).
3. The thumb and forefinger can be used to manipulate legs or wings.
4. The rest of the hand should gently cup the bird's body to resist struggling.
5. Care should be taken not to overconstrain as this could cause physical harm.

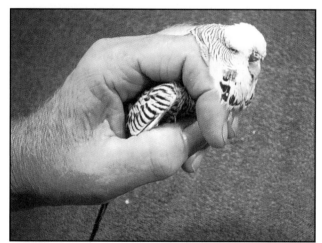

10.31 Holding a budgerigar for examination. (Reproduced from *BSAVA Manual of Psittacine Birds, 2nd edition*)

In the case of particularly aggressive parrots that are very difficult to handle, leather gauntlets may be employed, but remember that too strong a grasp around the bird's body can prove fatal.

Less commonly seen avian species

Toucans and hornbills
A group of birds increasingly kept in private collections includes the toucans and hornbills. These have impressive beaks with a serrated edge to the upper bill. Provided that the head is initially controlled using the towel technique described previously for parrots, an elastic band or tape may be applied around the bill to prevent biting. The handler still needs to be wary of stabbing manoeuvres and it may be sensible to work with a second handler. Otherwise restraint is the same as for passerine birds.

Waterfowl
Ducks, geese and swans are often kept in farm situations, but are also kept by smallholders and so may well be brought in for treatment. Restraint of these species is relatively straightforward but may become hazardous with the larger birds. With swans and geese the following approach may be necessary:

1. The first priority is to concentrate on capturing the head. This can be done manually, by grasping the bird around the upper neck from behind.
2. Make sure that the fingers curl around the neck and under the bill whilst the thumb supports the back of the neck and the potentially weak area of the atlanto-occipital joint. Failing this, a swan or shepherd's crook or other such adapted smooth metal or wooden pole-attached hook can be used to catch the neck – again high up under the bill.
3. Next, it is essential that the often powerful wings are rapidly controlled before the bird has a chance to damage itself or the handler. This can be most easily achieved by using a towel, thrown or draped over the bird's back and loosely wrapped under the sternum. Some practices may have access to more specialized goose or swan cradle-bags, which wrap around the body, containing the wings but allowing the feet, head and neck to remain free.
4. The bird may now be safely carried or restrained by tucking its body (contained within the towel or restraint bag) under one arm and holding this close to the torso. With the other hand, the neck can be loosely held from behind just below the bill.

Escaped avian patients

Where a bird is loose in a room or in an aviary flight cage, a number of capture methods can be applied. Darkening the room and reducing its area if possible are both very helpful to calm and confine the bird.

- In the case of larger parrots, throwing a heavy bath towel over the bird can confine them for long enough to allow the handler to restrain the head from behind and then wrap the patient into the towel.
- For very small birds, a fine aviary net or butterfly net (preferably made of very fine dark mesh) is extremely useful for catching the bird safely either in mid-flight or against the side of the cage or room. Larger nets are available from specialist retailers for catching the larger species of birds.

Handling and restraint of reptiles

Reptiles tend to be less easily stressed patients than birds and so restraint of the debilitated animal may be performed according to the degree of risk. The need for restraint should be considered carefully before physical attempts are made.

Initial assessment

It is worth considering one or two aspects that may make restraint dangerous to animal and handler alike:

- **Is the patient in respiratory distress?**
  Examples include pneumonic cases, where mouth breathing and excessive oral mucus may be present and where excessive manual manipulation can exacerbate the condition.

- **Is the species a fragile one?**
  The small day geckos (*Phelsuma* spp.) are extremely delicate and very prone to shedding their tails when handled. Similarly some species such as green iguanas (*Iguana iguana*) are prone to conditions such as metabolic bone disease, whereby their skeleton becomes fragile and spontaneous fractures are common.

- **Is the species an aggressive one?**
  Some are naturally so, e.g. alligator snapping turtles (*Macroclemys temminckii*), Tokay geckos (*Gekko gecko*) and rock pythons (*Python sebae*).

- **Does the reptile patient require medication/ physical examination?**
  In these cases, restraint is essential.

Techniques and equipment

Because of the variety of reptile species and their diversity, this section is best considered under specific groups.

⚠ WARNING

It should be borne in mind that many species of reptile have a bacterial flora in their digestive systems which frequently includes *Salmonella* species. To prevent zoonotic diseases, therefore, personal hygiene is very important when handling these patients.

Chelonians (tortoises, turtles and terrapins)

This group includes all land tortoises, terrapins and aquatic turtles. Size differences in this order are not as great as for the other two reptilian families, but it is still possible to see chelonians varying from the small Egyptian tortoises (*Testudo kleinmanni*), weighing a few hundred grams, all the way up to adult leopard tortoises (*Geochelone pardalis*) at 40 kg, and the Galapagean tortoise (*Geochelone nigra*) family, which can weigh several hundred kilograms. The majority of chelonians are harmless (though surprisingly strong). The exceptions include the snapping turtle (*Chelydra serpentina*) and the alligator snapping turtle, both of which can give a serious bite. Most of the soft-shelled terrapins have mobile necks and can also bite. Even red-eared terrapins (*Trachemys scripta elegans*) may give a nasty nip.

- For mild-tempered chelonians such as the Mediterranean *Testudo* species, the animal may be held with both hands, one on either side of the main part of the shell behind the front legs (Figure 10.32a). To keep it still for examination, a tortoise may be placed on a cylinder or stack of tins. This ensures that the legs are raised clear of the table and the tortoise is balancing on the centre of the underside of the shell (plastron).
- For aggressive species it is essential that the shell is held on both sides behind and above the rear legs to avoid being bitten (Figure 10.32b). In order to examine the head region in these species it is necessary to restrain them chemically.
- For the soft shelled and aquatic species, soft cloths and latex gloves (non-powdered) should be used in order not to mark the shell.

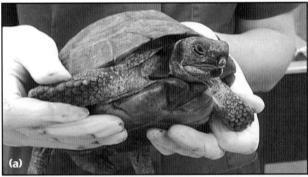

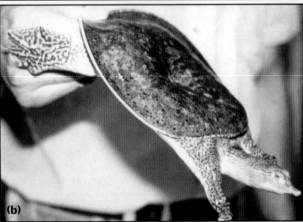

10.32 Handling chelonians. **(a)** Lifting a docile species. **(b)** Handling an aggressive species by grasping the caudal part of the carapace. (Reproduced from *BSAVA Manual of Reptiles, 2nd edition*)

Lizards

Lizards come in many different shapes and sizes, from the adult green iguana at 1.2 m long down to the green anole (*Anolis carolinensis*), which is only a tenth of that length. They all have roughly the same structural format, with four limbs (though these may become vestigial in the case of the slow worm, for example) and a tail. The potential dangers to handlers include claws and teeth, and in some species (e.g. iguanas) their tails, which can lash out in a whip-like fashion.

Geckos other than Tokay geckos are generally docile, as are lizards such as bearded dragons (*Pogona* spp.). Others, such as green iguanas, may be extremely aggressive, particularly sexually mature males. They may also be more aggressive towards female owners and handlers, as they are able to detect pheromones secreted during the menstrual cycle.

Restraint

Restraint is best performed by grasping the pectoral girdle with one hand from the dorsal aspect, so controlling one forelimb with forefinger and thumb and controlling the other forelimb between middle and fourth finger (Figure 10.33). The other hand is used to grasp the pelvic girdle from the dorsal aspect, controlling one limb with the thumb and forefinger, and the other limb between middle and fourth finger. The lizard may then be held in a vertical manner with the head uppermost and the tail out of harm's way underneath the handler's arm. When holding a lizard in this manner, the handler should allow some flexibility as the lizard may wriggle, and if the restraint is overly rigid the spine can be damaged. It is then possible to present the head and feet of the lizard away from the handler to avoid injury.

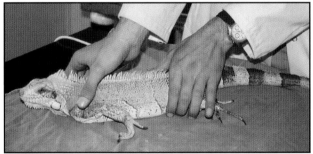

10.33 Holding the forelimbs and hindlimbs against the thorax and tailbase, respectively, restrains medium to large lizards such as this iguana. (Courtesy of S Redrobe)

Some of the more aggressive iguanas may need to be restrained prior to this method of handling. Here, as with avian patients, the use of a thick towel to control the tail and claws is often very useful. In some instances gauntlets are necessary for particularly aggressive large lizards, and for those that may have a poisonous bite, such as the Gila monster (*Heloderma suspectum*) and the beaded lizard (*Heloderma horribilis*). It is important to ensure that not too much force is used when restraining lizards, as those with skeletal problems (e.g. metabolic bone disease) may be seriously injured. In addition, lizards do not have a diaphragm and so overzealous restraint will lead to the digestive system pushing against the lungs and compromising respiration.

Geckos can be very fragile and the day geckos, for example, are best examined in a clear plastic container rather than being physically restrained. Other geckos have easily damaged skin and so latex gloves and soft cloths should be used and the gecko cupped in the hand rather than restrained physically.

Small lizards may have their heads controlled between the index finger and thumb to prevent biting.

It is important that lizards are never restrained by their tails. Many will shed their tails at this time, but not all of them will regrow. Green iguanas, for example, will only regrow their tails as juveniles (less than $2^{1}/_{2}$–3 years of age); once they are older than this, they will be left tailless.

Vago-vagal reflex

There is a procedure that may be used to place members of the lizard family into a trance-like state. It involves closing the lizard's eyelids and placing firm but gentle digital pressure on both eyeballs. This stimulates the parasympathetic autonomic nervous system, resulting in a reduction in heart rate, blood pressure and respiration rate (the vago-vagal reflex). Provided that there are no loud noises or environmental stimuli, after 1–2 minutes the lizard may be placed on its side, front or back, allowing radiography to be performed without using physical or chemical restraint. To maintain pressure on the eyeballs, a cotton-wool ball may be placed over each closed eye and a bandage wrapped around the head holding these in place. Loud noises or physical stimulation will immediately revert the lizard to its normal wakeful state.

Snakes

There is a wide range of sizes among snakes, from the enormous anacondas (*Eunectes murinus*) and Burmese pythons (*Python molurus bivittatus*), which may achieve lengths of up to 10 m or more, down to the thread snake family (*Leptotyphlid*), which may be a few tens of centimetres long. All snakes are characterized by their elongated form with an absence of limbs. The potential danger to the handler is from the teeth (and in the case of the more poisonous species, such as the viper family, the fang teeth) or, in the case of the constrictor and python family, the ability to asphyxiate the 'prey' by winding themselves around the victim's chest or neck. With this in mind, the following restraint techniques may be employed.

Non-venomous snakes

These can be restrained by initially controlling the head. This is done by placing the thumb over the occiput and curling the fingers under the chin. Reptiles, like birds, have only the one occipital condyle and so the importance of stabilizing the occipital/atlantal joint cannot be underestimated. It is also important to support the rest of the snake's body, so that not all of the weight of the snake is suspended from the head. With smaller species, this is best achieved by allowing the snake to coil around the handler's arm, so that the snake is supporting itself.

In the larger species (those longer than 3 m) it is necessary to support the body length at regular intervals (Figure 10.34). Indeed, it is vital to adopt a safe operating practice with the larger constricting species of snake. For this reason a 'buddy system', as with scuba diving, should be operated whereby any snake longer than 2.5–3 m should only be handled by two or more people. This is to ensure that if the snake were to enwrap the handler, the 'buddy' could disentangle them by unwinding from the tail end first. Above all, it is important not to grip the snake too hard as this will cause bruising and the release of myoglobin from muscle cells that will lodge in the kidneys, causing damage to the filtration membranes.

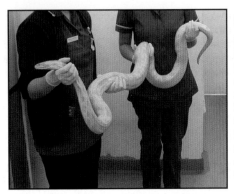

10.34
Carrying a large snake requires support from more than one handler. (Reproduced from *BSAVA Manual of Reptiles, 2nd edition*)

Venomous and aggressive snakes

Venomous snakes, such as vipers and rattlesnakes, and very aggressive species, such as anacondas and pythons, may be restrained initially using snake tongs (Figure 10.35) or hooks – 0.5–0.75 m steel rods with a blunt shepherd's hook at one end. They are used to loop under the body of a snake to move it at arm's length into a container. The hook may also be used to trap the head flat to the floor before grasping it with the hand. Once the head is controlled safely the snake is rendered harmless – unless it is a member of the *spitting cobra* family. Fortunately it is rare to come across these in general practice, but those who do handle them must wear plastic goggles, or a plastic face visor, as they spit poison into the prey/assailant's eyes and mucous membranes, causing blindness and paralysis.

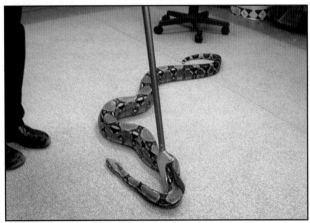

10.35 Grasping a non-venomous snake with a pair of snake tongs. The tongs exert pressure over a wide area and are spring-loaded to prevent excessive force on the snake, which can then be seized behind the head. (Reproduced from *BSAVA Manual of Reptiles, 2nd edition*)

Examination and restraint of amphibians

Examination of the amphibian patient should be performed at the species' preferred optimum body temperature (this is also the case for reptile patients). A rough guide is between 21 and 24°C, which is lower than the more usual 22–32°C reptile housing conditions.

The examination table should be covered with unbleached paper towels soaked in dechlorinized water, preferably purified. More purified water should be on standby to be applied to the patient to prevent dehydration during the examination.

Initially it is useful not to restrain the patient until the extent of any problem is assessed, as many have severe skin lesions that are extremely fragile.

- Newts and salamanders should be examined only in water, as removal from the water results in skin damage. Some of the larger species, such as the hellbender species (*Cryptobranchus* spp.), can also inflict unpleasant bite wounds on handlers.
- Smaller species and aquatic species may be best examined in small plastic or glass jars.

Gloves and goggles

Once an initial assessment has been made, the patient may be restrained manually. It is advisable to use a pair of non-powdered hypoallergenic latex gloves. This minimizes irritation to the amphibian's skin caused by the normally acidic human skin, and prevents irritation caused by the powder in many prepacked latex gloves. The wearing of gloves is also essential in handling members of the toad family or the arrow tree frogs, which can secrete irritant or even potentially deadly toxins from their skin. These toxins can be absorbed through unprotected human skin. It may also be necessary to wear goggles when handling some species of toad; for example, the giant toad *Bufo marinus* can squirt a toxin from its parotid glands over a distance of several feet.

Method of restraint

The method of restraint will depend on the animal's body shape.

- The elongated forms of salamanders and newts require similar restraint to that of a lizard, with one hand grasping the pectoral girdle from the dorsal aspect, index finger and thumb encircling one forelimb, second and third fingers the other, and the opposite hand grasping the pelvic girdle, again from the dorsal aspect in a similar manner. Some salamanders will shed their tails if roughly handled and so care should be taken with these species.
- Large frogs and toads can be restrained by cupping one hand around the pectoral girdle immediately behind the front limbs, and placing the other hand beneath the hindlimbs. Care should be taken with some species that have poison glands in their skin, as mentioned above. Care should also be taken with species such as the Argentinian horned frog, as amphibians can bite.

Handling and restraint of fish

Physical restraint of fish should be performed carefully, and generally avoided unless essential. Even light handling can damage the protective outer layer of mucus present on the body surface of most fish and so increase the risk of opportunistic infection. Where handling is required, powder-free latex gloves should be worn and the fish kept moistened with water from its own tank during the procedure. Fine-meshed nets may be used with caution to restrain the fish in a tank initially, but these may again result in abrasions that can lead to secondary infections. An attempt should be made to cover the eyes of the fish during handling to minimize sensory stimulation.

Handling and restraint of invertebrates

The species involved will naturally determine the methods by which the patient can be restrained safely (for handler and invertebrate alike). Many invertebrates present no direct threat to the handler. Examples include giant land snails, stick insects and cockroaches. These may be gently picked up and cupped in the hand, or allowed to walk on to a towel or similar non-slip surface to assess for movement. Aquatic invertebrates should be examined and moved in water, either within their own tank or in a clean plastic, perspex or glass container.

Hazardous species

Other species, such as the mygalomorph spider family, may present multiple hazards. These may flick setae (the small hairs that cover their abdomens) at the handler if stressed or if they feel threatened. The setae are highly irritant on the skin and particularly dangerous if they come into contact with the conjunctiva. In addition, many of these spiders have a nasty bite. The bites are rarely fatal but still cause similar pain and potential harm as a bee or wasp sting. These species should be transferred into a perspex, glass or plastic container (Figure 10.36) and only ever handled with latex gloves. If it is necessary to pick up such a spider, it may either be cupped in paired hands or grasped with either fingers or atraumatic forceps immediately behind the cephalothorax, around the 'waist' of the spider. Protective goggles should be worn if the spider is to be removed from its container.

Scorpions present a similar problem, with the tail sting being the most obvious danger. The majority of scorpions kept in captivity, such as the imperial scorpion, are not seriously dangerous, though the sting may be likened to a wasp or bee sting. To restrain these species safely, they may be transferred into a perspex, plastic or glass container, or alternatively a sheet of clear plastic may be laid gently but firmly over the top of the scorpion to confine it for examination or to allow a better grasp. They may also be lifted gently by the tip of the tail using atraumatic forceps, with a sheet of card or plastic supporting the body from underneath.

Acknowledgement

Trudi Atkinson would like to thank Daniel Mills for comments and contributions made during an earlier draft.

Further reading

Bessant C (1992) *How to Talk to Your Cat.* Smith Gryphon, London

Bradshaw JWS (1992) *The Behaviour of the Domestic Cat.* CAB International, Wallingford, Oxon

Bradshaw JWS and Nott HMR (1995) Social and communication behaviour of companion dogs. In: *The Domestic Dog: Its Evolution, Behaviour and Interactions with People*, ed. J Serpell. Cambridge University Press, Cambridge

Dunbar I (1979) *Dog Behavior: Why Dogs Do What They Do.* TFH Publications, New Jersey

Fowler ME and Ames L (1995) *Restraint and Handling of Wild and Domestic Animals, 2nd edn.* Iowa State Press, Ames, Iowa

Fox MW (1971) The comparative ethology of the domestic dog. In: *Behaviour of Wolves, Dogs and Related Canids*, pp. 183–214. Jonathan Cape, London

Girling SJ (2003) *Veterinary Nursing of Exotic Pets.* Blackwell Publishing, Oxford

Heath S (2001) Understanding dominance in dogs. *Veterinary Nursing*, **16**(4), 124–126

McBride A (1995) The human–dog relationship. In: *The Waltham Book of Human–Animal Interaction: Benefits and responsibilities of pet ownership*, ed. I Robinson. Pergamon, Oxford

McCune S (1992) Temperament and Welfare of Caged Cats. PhD Thesis, University of Cambridge (unpublished)

Meredith A and Redrobe S (2002) *Manual of Exotic Pets, 4th edn.* BSAVA Publications, Cheltenham

Overall KL (1997) Canine aggression. In: *Clinical Behavioral Medicine for Small Animals*, pp. 88–137. Mosby, St Louis

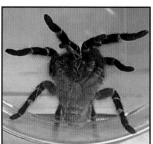

10.36 Placing a spider in a transparent container allows it to be examined easily. (Courtesy of E Morgan)

Chapter 11

Animal training and behaviour

Kendal Shepherd and Daniel Mills

Learning objectives

After studying this chapter, students should be able to:

- **Describe the factors that influence the behaviour of animals in general and in a given situation**
- **Describe the principles of learning and how they operate in real-world situations both intentionally and unintentionally**
- **Identify high-risk situations for problem behaviour in the clinic and propose strategies to prevent and manage such situations in the veterinary practice setting**
- **Address a range of common misconceptions relating to companion animal behaviour and training**
- **Provide behavioural first aid advice for a range of common client behaviour queries**
- **Identify the most appropriate course of action for more challenging problems**

Introduction

In a relatively recent survey of UK veterinary nurses, more than 80% reported involvement in educating and advising clients on issues of pet behaviour. Unfortunately, 91% felt that their training did not provide them with sufficient knowledge of companion animal behaviour. Unwanted behaviour also remains a common reason for euthanasia, especially in the dog. It is therefore essential that the compulsory element of education required for success in professional qualifications is supplemented with further reading and education. It is also important that, whatever the circumstances, individuals do not attempt to handle an animal beyond their competence or offer advice beyond their own knowledge as this can have disastrous consequences for the individual and the patient, as well as the client and the practice as a whole.

All animals are behaving all the time, in that they are responding to the environment around them in a manner that seems to them to be likely to achieve the most advantageous results. Their decision as to how to behave is based upon an amalgam of genetic factors and what life's experiences have taught them. The principles guiding the learning process are exactly the same whether an animal is being naturally trained by random environmental events or by a human 'trainer'. Cats are almost entirely trained by uncontrolled environmental events whereas dogs generally spend some time being deliberately 'trained'. However, this training for the vast majority of dogs tends to be very specific in nature, namely: when they are young; for a tiny proportion of the dog's life; and in specific contexts only, such as training class. Deliberate training of dogs rarely extends into every area of real life and, most pertinently for the purpose of this book, into the veterinary surgery. The surgery can become another context, in which an individual animal may be left entirely without human guidance and therefore behaves appropriately or not entirely by accident, depending upon what history and experience have taught it.

There are several areas in which the veterinary nurse can and should be involved in dealing with behavioural issues. Answering direct questions from clients, mainly regarding what to do about perceived behaviour problems, is an area that has recently increased in importance owing to public awareness and demand and the delegation of responsibility by veterinary surgeons. Running puppy parties and classes is advocated as the way forward to educating dogs for their future lives, not least in how to behave in a convenient way (to all-round benefit) at the surgery. What is less immediately obvious is the need to recognize the impact of what veterinary staff do on an animal's behaviour, whether or not an owner is present. It is impossible to treat physical ailments thoroughly without considering an animal's environment and its behavioural responses to it. It is also essential that the same message is delivered to the patient by all veterinary staff, from reception through to the consulting room, kennels and operating theatre. Whether treating behaviour problems or trying to prevent them, the impact of any environment upon behaviour and the principles underlying how an animal learns must inform everything we do.

Assessment of animal behaviour

In order to assess the behaviour of an animal, a broad history is necessary. An animal's behaviour at any given moment is a response to certain immediate influences. These can be divided into external and internal factors.

- External factors include the management of the animal and the specific environment at the time the behaviour is shown.
- Internal factors include its physiological and psychological state.

The two are linked: the external environment brings about changes in both internal physiology and behaviour. Psychology simply reflects the ongoing physiology of the brain. So an understanding of physiological processes and how they affect behaviour and the mind is essential.

Normal physiology can not only bring about changes in the immediate behaviour of an individual but also shape future development and behavioural predispositions in a much more permanent way. For example, some forms of aggression seen during false pregnancy are intimately associated with the hormonal changes in the bitch at that time, which bring about perceptual changes that encourage protective aggression. Learning at this time may mean that the animal is more aggressive in future, even though the hormones involved are no longer present.

To understand behaviour, it is necessary to be aware of how these factors interact with other features such as the genetics and early history of the animal. The knowledge base for dealing with behaviour therefore draws on very disparate fields, including just about every branch of zoology as well as various branches of psychology, veterinary medicine, animal management and nutrition. Disease may result in an apparent behaviour problem, e.g. aggression in the hyperthyroid cat, or in an animal with chronic low-grade pain.

To assess behaviour fully requires consideration of not only what is happening but where, when, with whom and why. Some owners will hold back information either because they think it is not important or because they feel guilty about some aspect of it. It is essential to establish a bond of trust with the client when trying to extract information about their pet's behaviour.

There can be a tendency to consider behaviour as being either largely influenced by the animal's genes (nature influences) or shaped by the environment (nurture influences). However, it must be recognized that both come together in a given animal to make it an individual. These two elements are considered below:

Genetics – the influence of nature

Genetics provides the blueprint for the behaviour of the individual. Genetic factors not only determine what is normal but may also set certain limits. This can be seen at three levels: species-typical behaviour; breed characteristics; and individual characteristics.

Species-typical behaviour

This describes those behaviours that define a dog as a dog and a cat as a cat, or an African Grey parrot as an African Grey parrot. Many popular texts make analogies to wild relatives, such as the wolf in the case of the dog, but dogs are not wolves and their behaviour is quite different, as they have evolved to survive in very different environments. This means that the value of such analogies is limited and can lead to inaccurate advice. On the other hand, it is essential to be well versed in the normal behaviours of a species in order to appreciate if something is genuinely abnormal and therefore to be able to advise an owner correctly. For example, an owner may think that the behaviour of their female cat in oestrus, i.e. rolling on the floor and 'calling', is abnormal or indicative that the animal is in pain. In the case of pet birds, there are enormous differences in the natural biology of the different species and generalizations are rarely valid.

Breed characteristics

Just as the dog is not a wolf, neither are all breeds of dog or cat alike. Thus breed characteristics also determine what is normal (e.g. vocalization in the Siamese cat, or fixed eye in the Border Collie). Likewise breed behaviour may indicate what problems may be likely in a given breed (e.g. nipping by Border Collies, or attachment in Siamese cats). An understanding of the breed is also important when trying to advise a potential owner about a new pet.

Individual characteristics

In any population there is variation and some of this has a genetic basis. Even within a breed, some animals are predisposed to being more fearful than others and nervousness, for example, has been reported to have a relatively high heritability for a behaviour trait. This information is particularly important when considering the prevention of behaviour problems through selective breeding as well as appreciating the limits of behavioural modification for a given individual.

Many differences between the sexes, whilst obviously having a genetic basis, actually reflect differences in physiology that can be changed, rather than differences that are genetically controlled. For example, urine spraying in cats is more common in males, but neutering usually helps in the prevention and treatment of the problem in both sexes by altering their physiological state. The effect of physiology on behaviour is usually complex. For example, aggression is neither a male-typical nor steroid-dependent behaviour, but is influenced by numerous physiological factors. Therefore it should be recognized that castration may make matters worse in some cases, and simple generalizations about the management of behaviour should be avoided.

Sexual maturity is a good example of a time when changes may be seen in an animal's behaviour owing to a change in sensitivity to certain stimuli. The interaction between internal and external factors is very clear at this time but exists for all behaviour. At maturity, the opposite sex suddenly becomes more interesting and attention may become biased in entire animals.

Such internal physiological changes also underpin other phases when certain types of change may be more or less likely. These include sensitive phases in early development (see next section), but also changes associated with ageing. As an animal gets older, not only are there pathological changes, such as the loss of sight, hearing or pain related to arthritis, which can influence behaviour, but also specific age-related changes in the brain. This can result in a condition known as cognitive dysfunction, which has presenting signs, such as house-soiling and increased vocalization, that can resemble those caused by a range of other diseases and certain more exclusively behavioural problems (such as separation anxiety). In order to differentiate these conditions and protect the welfare of the dog or cat, any problem with a late age of onset must be particularly carefully evaluated by a veterinary surgeon to determine possible medical causes, before a behavioural plan is implemented.

By the same measure, even if a problem is largely medical in origin, behavioural management will be important. The distinction between behavioural and medical management is therefore a false one, if a clinic is really focused on patient welfare. Nonetheless, the next section considers ways in which the environment can have a particularly marked effect.

The environment – the influence of nurture

In early life, dogs and cats have 'sensitive phases' when they learn more rapidly or form impressions that can affect their behaviour and temperament. Animals reared in impoverished environments often do not develop well intellectually and may have difficulty in regulating their emotions. This not only predisposes an individual to a variety of problems, but also reduces the prognosis for treatment.

One particularly important sensitive phase is the socialization phase, as it has a large impact on the way the animal will tend to respond to both the physical and social elements of its environment. This period appears to be between the 4th and 10th week of age in the puppy and between the 2nd and 7th week in the kitten. It is vital that pets receive pleasant experiences at this time associated with all things that are to be accepted later. For example, they should be handled gently by a range of handlers, old and young, so that they do not shy away from people later in life. It seems that controlled exposure to an urban environment, with all the sights, sounds and smells of traffic and various people, may be one of the most important factors in building confidence at this age, which prevents fearful avoidance later in life.

Over-stressing the animal (for example, by excessive exposure or early weaning) should be avoided as this interferes with the animal's learning ability. Early weaning has also been implicated in fundamental emotional changes and a reduced ability to cope with stress in a range of species. Around this life stage, temperament is shaped and any damage done is much harder to undo later. Many problems arise because the animal has not been properly socialized or trained when young. It is far easier to teach appropriate behaviour from the outset than it is to correct problems later on.

Environmental influences can also include external additives such as drugs and diet, which act internally. Drug therapy affects an animal's physiological state, since it alters the balance of nerve transmitters in the brain. Whilst there are some drugs, such as antidepressants and anxiolytics, that are specifically designed for the purpose, other drugs may produce behaviour changes as a secondary effect. For example, phenylpropanolamine, used to control urinary incontinence in dogs, may also cause aggression in some cases.

Diet can influence behaviour through its physiological effects. These range from the ingestion of stimulants that result in over-activity and hence associated problems, to the manipulation of diet to maximize the availability of precursors of neurotransmitters. It is being increasingly recognized that dietary reactions may also play quite an important role in some behaviour problems. These are not the same as allergies, but may respond to similar dietary changes.

Behaviour does not just happen. It is in part a response to the situation in which an animal finds itself. This is why so much about the management of behaviour, whether it is the manner of restraining the nervous dog or treating its fear in the longer term, focuses on environmental changes – including those that are designed to bring about learned changes (training) and those that might simply aim to change the immediate response (e.g. environmental enrichment).

Principles of animal learning

There is a common assumption that behavioural modification and training are in some way different. In practice, a **modified behaviour** tends to imply a reduction in the expression of something undesirable, such as trying to bite passers-by or urinating in the wrong place, whereas a **trained behaviour** assumes an increase in a more desirable performance, such as sitting rather than lunging at a passer-by, or urinating in the garden rather than in the sitting room. Both processes, in fact, are dependent upon the alteration of an animal's conditioned response to environmental information and both are therefore practical manifestations of the behavioural effects of an animal's learning.

Conditioned or **learned responses** involve memories, associated emotions and their behavioural expression, and are evoked by changes in the environment. The manner in which environmental information is presented can change (or modify) behaviour immediately, sometimes giving a false impression that a particular task has been learned. Only by consistent presentation of information in all contexts in which an animal 'behaves' will resultant behaviour be sufficiently rehearsed and learned to be able to say that 'training' has occurred.

Associative learning (or **conditioning**) often occurs in one of two main ways (see the section below on habituation for information on non-associative learning):

- **Pavlovian** (or **classical**) **conditioning** occurs when physiological and behavioural responses change as a response to environmental events.
- **Operant** (or **instrumental**) **conditioning** occurs when an individual uses its behaviour to alter the response of the environment.

Classical conditioning

Classical conditioning is named after Pavlov's classical finding that once a stimulus (the ringing of a bell) that previously had no significance to dogs was closely associated with the presentation of food, salivation (an unconditioned response that did not need to be learned) occurred equally to the sound of the bell alone as to the presentation of food. The sound of the bell thus became a conditioned (or learned) stimulus predicting the arrival of food and subsequently elicited similar physiological, emotional and behavioural responses as the unconditioned (unlearned) stimulus of food.

Examples of classical conditioning abound in the average dog's life and vary from the sight of a lead predicting the excitement of a walk, or the sound of a particular car engine predicting an owner's imminent arrival home, or the sound of a tin-opener or rustle of a crisp packet predicting food, to the sight of a syringe in a veterinary surgeon's hand predicting pain. All these stimuli have no intrinsic meaning to a dog until they are paired with an emotionally significant outcome.

Operant conditioning

Operant conditioning is the learned effect that consequences of behaviour have upon whether the same behaviour is performed again (**operated**) or not. All trained behaviour is led by its consequences, i.e. what happens *after* a particular behaviour is performed. A common misconception is that a dog will sit, for example, on hearing the command word 'sit' because it has 'been told what to do'. In reality, the dog sits because the word and the action of sitting have become usefully paired with a desirable consequence from the dog's perspective. This consequence is predicted to the dog by environmental information of all kinds, verbal information being only one category upon which a dog will depend. Visual cues are often more powerful and may override verbal ones, even if they are unintentional. The simple reason why words fail in so many situations, frustrating both clients and their pets alike, is that in certain circumstances the environment of the dog, which comprises an amalgam of visual, auditory and olfactory information, predicts rewarding consequences for entirely different behaviours, e.g. it looks like it will be a better idea to run away rather than sit at this particular time. The behaviour required by the owner therefore becomes redundant as far as the dog is concerned.

In all real life situations, classical and operant conditioning are inextricably linked. The sound of a crisp packet may herald food (classical conditioning) but unless a dog runs towards the source of food and uses a previously successful behaviour, such as sitting and begging in an appealing manner (operant learning), the food reward will not materialize. Some dogs may be usefully taught that staying in one's bed is a more likely way of getting the food to arrive, whereas others learn to steal when no one is looking. Likewise, the sight of a syringe and needle may signify the association of pain, but it is the behaviour that seems to make such unpleasantness go away that will be operantly conditioned. Some dogs learn that sitting calmly does indeed eventually work in getting a veterinary surgeon to retreat, whereas others rely upon wriggling, growling and attempting to bite.

Reward and punishment

Whether a behaviour is repeated or not depends upon the reliability or predictability of consequence and this phenomenon is used in both training and behaviour modification. It is important to realize that although there may be a human assumption that rewards are 'nice' and punishments are 'nasty', the terms are defined only by their results upon an animal's behaviour, not by the human view of desirability or unpleasantness. Attempted punishments by pet owners, such as shouting or smacking, frequently merely exacerbate problem behaviours and therefore should not be called punishments at all. In the same vein, a 'reward' in the form of a titbit of food offered for sitting is not reinforcing if, at that particular moment, a dog's preferred option is to chase ducks or escape the veterinary surgeon's clutches.

- **Reinforcement** is defined as an environmental event that *increases* the likelihood of a behaviour being performed.
- **Punishment** is defined as an environmental event that *decreases* the likelihood of a behaviour being performed.

Both reinforcement and punishment can be positive or negative.

Arrival and removal

The **arrival** of both reinforcing and punishing events induces behavioural change as follows:

- **Positive reinforcement** is the arrival of an event, as a direct consequence of a behaviour, that *increases* the likelihood of that behaviour being performed: for example, the presentation of food as a result of sitting. Only if the arrival of food increases the likelihood of a dog sitting can food be termed a **positive reinforcer**.
- **Positive punishment** is the arrival of an event, as a direct consequence of a behaviour, that *decreases* the likelihood of that behaviour being performed: for example, jerking on a check chain as a result of a dog pulling ahead. Only if the arrival of a tight check chain reduces the likelihood of a dog pulling in future can it be called a **positive punishment**.

The effects of the **removal** of both reinforcing and punishing events are defined as follows:

- **Negative reinforcement** is the removal of an event, as a direct consequence of a behaviour, that *increases* the likelihood of that behaviour being performed: for example, the slackening (i.e. removal of tightness) of a check chain as a result of walking to heel. Only if a slack check chain increases the likelihood of a dog walking to heel can it be called a **negative reinforcer**.
- **Negative punishment** is the removal of an event, as a direct consequence of a behaviour, that *decreases* the likelihood of that behaviour being performed: for example, denying a dog a food reward if he jumps up. Only if the removal of the food reward decreases the likelihood of a dog jumping up can it be called a **negative punishment.**

These consequences of behaviour are shown in Figure 11.1 and can be practically applied and usefully harnessed, during training and behaviour modification, to channel behaviour in directions convenient to us.

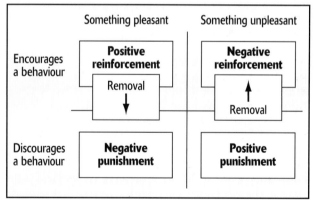

11.1 The effects of reinforcement and punishment, both positive and negative, from the animal's perspective.

Other examples of potential positive reinforcers are toys, human attention and play. Withdrawal or denial of any of these will constitute negative punishment of the behaviour that produced it. Therefore a dog that jumps up wanting attention will be punished by absolute denial of attention, but intended reprimand in the form of a telling off may have the opposite effect as it gives social attention. Further examples of potential positive punishments include a water spray, rattle can, shouting and smacking. Withdrawal of any of these punishments will constitute negative reinforcement of the behaviour that produced it, and so a dog that avoids being shouted at by going to his bed will be rewarded by cessation, or lack of, shouting.

Balancing reinforcement and punishment

Intrinsic to the use of these principles is the understanding that negative punishment (e.g. absence of food) cannot operate without the contrast of positive reinforcement (presence of food), just as negative reinforcement (e.g. absence of choking) cannot operate without the contrast of experienced positive punishment (presence of choking). Equally important is the knowledge that, despite spurious claims and distinctions among trainers that 'only reward-based methods are used in class', *all* training methods have a rewarding consequence, whether it be the gaining of a positive reward or the avoidance of a positive punishment. The emotion of relief is an extremely potent one. It may be more relevant in certain circumstances (and therefore more reinforcing) for a dog to use behaviours that successfully avoid or reduce human threat and anger, whether applied in training or real, than those that gain a tasty piece of food.

Humans appear to have a natural tendency to resort by default to attempted punishment when their dogs misbehave, implying that, for anyone involved in improving the relationship between people and their pets, a through grounding in the nature of punishments and how they do, or don't, work is essential.

A useful exercise to develop awareness of the relationship between behaviour and events is simply to observe dogs wherever they may be, while asking the questions, 'What is that dog doing and why?' Everyday observations will include a dog sitting at the kerbside, a dog pulling on lead, a dog not pulling on lead, a dog chasing a ball, a dog not coming when called, a dog jumping up in greeting, a dog trying to jump off a consulting room table and a dog sitting still. All too often in considering behaviour, we notice only behaviours that are obviously happening rather than what is *not* happening. How much more often do we ask the question, 'Why did this particular dog bite?' rather than asking why that particular dog *didn't* bite? But both questions and their answers are equally valid and are crucial to fully understanding and improving an animal's behaviour. Understanding motivation to behave 'well', and using this knowledge to create more of the same behaviour, treats behaviour problems just as effectively as preventing them.

Practical applications of animal learning theory

Processes

Habituation

Habituation is a form of non-associative learning and is the process whereby an animal becomes used to and learns to ignore environmental events that have no consequence. In effect, environmental stimuli have neither positive nor negative significance but become emotionally neutral. Habituation is part of the socialization process in young puppies and prevents the development of adverse fearful responses that might otherwise be expressed in the face of novelty. The more real-life experiences a puppy has, the less novel the world and its contents will seem later in life and the less likely fearful responses become (see 'The environment' above).

Latent inhibition

Latent inhibition is the process whereby previous experiences and associations made with certain contexts serve to block future associations. Thus previous positive experiences may protect an animal against subsequent less favourable experiences in the same situations. In effect, once such learning is in place, an animal is less likely to react fearfully or aggressively. Awareness of the protective effect of latent inhibition is of particular importance during an animal's first contact with the veterinary surgery – for example, at puppy vaccination. However, by the same measure, a bad initial experience can be much harder to put right. It is therefore important always to start well in a new context. Puppy socialization largely depends on developing latent inhibition to help protect the animal from the consequences of future bad experiences as well as habituating it to otherwise arousing stimuli.

Desensitization

Desensitization is a similar process to habituation but tends to be used in behavioural management to describe the loss of existing negative emotions and their behavioural results, which have become associated with environmental information and events. It is therefore used in treating problem behaviour rather than preventing it. Once an animal is already afraid of a particular stimulus (for example, the sight and sound of fireworks), the stimulus must initially be presented at a low enough intensity to induce no emotional and behavioural reaction. The intensity of the stimulus is increased very gradually to ensure continued lack of response. Proof of success in desensitization, as in habituation, is seeing nothing, i.e. no undesirable behavioural response.

Counter-conditioning

Counter-conditioning involves the creation of new more positive emotional associations linked to a particular event. This may be achieved by presenting the animal with something that it enjoys, such as food or a game, in the presence of something it would normally avoid, such as a sound recording of an unpleasant noise. However, unless the animal is in a largely neutral emotional state, such rewards may be immaterial and so such recordings should be played quietly initially. The ability of a dog to eat or play can also therefore be practically used as a rough gauge of positive emotional state, as a warning of going 'too far, too fast' in training, and as a measure of success of a desensitization programme. In practical terms, it is not possible to create new associations with an event without operant conditioning (*how* an animal gains an emotionally significant reward) coming into play. Counter-conditioning may therefore encompass creating positive associations with a specifically trained response (**operant counter-conditioning** or **response substitution** – see below) as well as more reflexive physiological and emotional change (**classical counter-conditioning**).

Response substitution

In behaviour management, **response substitution** usually refers to the specific *replacement* of one behaviour (something inconvenient to humans) with another more appropriate behaviour. For example, a dog who habitually lunges and barks at other dogs when on lead can be taught to look to his owner instead for an expected game with a tennis ball. Jumping up in greeting can be replaced with 'sit to greet'. It is essential that an accurate assessment is made of *why* a dog lunges at other dogs or jumps up – in other words, its motivation – before attempting to compete with this during training. There is no point in attempting to entice a dog with food if his overriding desire is to play or fight. It may be necessary to combine reinforcers (e.g. tasty food + tennis ball + owner's attention) to create more behavioural leverage, as well as present a stimulus at very low intensity (e.g. the sight of a dog 100 yards away) before an alternative behaviour can begin to be learned and trained.

Extinction

The process of **extinction** refers to a behaviour becoming gradually redundant, owing to a lack of reinforcement (negative punishment), and therefore its elimination from an animal's behavioural repertoire. This is only achieved if an expected reward is no longer forthcoming. It is essential that this lack of reward and reinforcement is absolute and consistent. For example, a dog that jumps up in greeting may be used to being petted and cuddled in certain convenient situations but being reprimanded in others. In both cases, attention given continues to reinforce the behaviour and maintains it as a result. The sudden withdrawal of attention, by folding arms and turning away as a result of the same behaviour, is the dog's first signal that jumping up is not working as it used to. Clients must be warned of the **extinction burst**, whereby a dog may initially try harder to gain his accustomed reward. Giving in to a dog's increased demands at this time, as the behaviour may seem to get worse before it gets better, is a very common reason for failure of otherwise sound advice.

Combining the processes

Although habituation, desensitization, counter-conditioning (including response substitution) and extinction are all described as separate processes, in practical terms they often happen at the same time when treating behaviour problems. There is no point in attempting to provide motivation for alternative, more convenient, behaviours (*response substitution*) if accidental or deliberate reinforcement is still continuing for what is not wanted (failure of *extinction*). However much a family may want to say hello to their dog on their return to the house, they will not be doing their visitors, or passers-by on the street, any favours by continuing to reward jumping up. The most humane way to alter emotions (*desensitization* and *counter-conditioning*) is to train alternative behaviours (*response substitution*) using positive reward-based training methods, by which a dog will look forward (*positive emotional change*) to doing exactly as humans require, with implied loss (*extinction*) of undesirable behaviour. In this way, both emotions and behaviour are changed for the better at the same time.

Conditioned reinforcers and punishments

All potential reinforcers and punishments can be divided into:

- **Primary** – those events that are inherently rewarding (e.g. food, water, rest and play) or punishing (e.g. pain and danger) to an animal
- **Secondary** – those events whose significance has to be learned, such as the sound of a whistle, the sound of a word, the sight of a raised hand or the sound of training discs or a clicker (see below). Such stimuli, once associated with primary rewards or punishments, are termed **secondary** (or **conditioned**) **reinforcers** and **punishments**. Secondary reinforcers and punishments are used deliberately in dog training and also occur inadvertently in every aspect of day-to-day life.

Although assumed to be intrinsically rewarding – in other words, a primary reinforcer – human praise or pleasure works most efficiently when contrasted with human displeasure or sternness. Rather than being a true positive reinforcer, therefore, it may be that praise is effective via negative reinforcement, i.e. a dog learns to perform behaviours that stop humans being angry. Praise is also frequently linked to, and therefore

predicts, more tangible rewards in the form of food and cuddles, and, as such, is a secondary reinforcer. A sternly issued command or pointed finger, both threatening in themselves, may be predictors of worse to come if disobedience continues. In predicting punishment, but not actually administering it, such human gestures are secondary punishers. Both secondary reinforcers and secondary punishments, as long as they are consistently followed by a primary reinforcer or punishment, come to induce the same emotional and behavioural change as the primary reinforcer or punishment they predict.

Clicker training

Clicker training makes use of the sound of a click as a secondary reinforcer. Once paired with the reliable and imminent arrival of a food reward (associative learning), the click becomes a 'good news' sound, inducing the same emotional change as the primary reinforcer. It therefore becomes a sound that a dog (or other animal) wants to hear. Behaviours are subsequently performed ('offered') by the dog in order to make the click happen and thereby operantly conditioned. No verbal cue (later to become a 'command') is given until a behaviour is consistently being performed. The choice of what behaviour to perform is entirely up to the dog. The consequences of a dog's choice of behaviour are marked either with a 'click and treat', signifying success, or no click, indicating not only failure but 'try again' in a different way.

Clicker training allows for **successive approximations** – in other words, stages in progress towards a completed task, to be marked and rewarded. For example, in training a retrieve or picking up a set of keys by an assistance dog, the first step to be 'clicked and treated' is a dog sniffing at the object on the ground. Once this is consistently being performed, the anticipated click is withheld in order to frustrate the dog into trying harder to gain a click ('raising the criteria'). Among the behaviours that a dog will reliably try next is to begin to mouth or pick up the object, which then earns the expected 'click and treat' for progress in the desired direction.

Failure of clicker training results from:

- Insufficient preparation in creating the close association between the sound and a food reward so that the click sound does not develop the significance that it should
- The use of the clicker as a distraction or form of 'remote control' in order to alter a dog's behaviour (if so used, the click will mark 'wrong' behaviours rather than 'right' ones)
- Lack of patience in waiting for a dog to make the 'right' choice without speaking to it.

Good clicker-training candidates are those dogs considered to be the most inquisitive and mischievous and who are always 'getting themselves into trouble'. Clicker training does not create behaviours; it merely selects, from a dog's existing repertoire, those behaviours that humans approve of. The more extensive the repertoire is to start with (the definition of a 'mischievous' dog for some people!), the more there is to select from.

Training discs

Training discs are a set of brass discs making a distinctive sound if knocked together. Used correctly, they should signify the exact opposite of the sound of the clicker. They indicate failure or 'non-reward' and the sound of them becomes therefore a *secondary punishment*. Rather than the click predicting the arrival of a food reward, the sound of the discs is deliberately associated with removal or loss of food (*negative punishment*). Once trained to the significance of the sound, an animal should therefore decide for itself to desist from whichever behaviour seems to induce the 'bad news' sound.

As with the clicker, training discs are frequently misused as distractions or a means of startling a dog into behaving differently rather than truly communicating a specific message.

Vocal communication

An owner should not consider themselves bereft of means of communication with their dog if they do not happen to have such gadgets in their pocket. The word 'Yes!', if used consistently, can replace the sound of a click to mark a successful behaviour, just as by contrast the word 'No!' can, and should, signify simple failure and 'Try again!' Almost universally, however, 'No!' is used in a 'Stop it or I'll kill you!' fashion in conjunction with threatening human body gestures and, as such, becomes a predictor of positive, rather than negative, punishment. The practical consequence is the considerable number of dogs presented for behaviour therapy that growl and bite when reprimanded, or in situations when historically a physical reprimand has been proved very likely. All too often, a dog has no idea how to pre-empt the threat of punishment; in other words, a human-approved or 'correct' behaviour has never been reinforced in the first place and punishment has been applied inconsistently. If this is the case, anxiety and subsequent aggression are a common consequence.

If the correct behaviour has already become established, an animal knows exactly how to avoid a threatened punishment and can remain in control of a situation, without the generation of uncertainty and anxiety.

Advice on dog training and communication pitfalls

Ultimate behavioural goals

One of the reasons for the success of an experienced trainer over a typical pet-dog owner, whether using positive or negative reinforcement to direct behaviour, is the ability to recognize an ultimate behavioural goal. Experienced trainers have a specific end in sight for which they not only select the most suitable dog, but also have the ability to train the dog they have already selected. A dog that shows inappropriate behaviours and traits for a given task is not selected in the first place. Successful trainers will also work towards a specific goal and appreciate that they are training their dog whenever and wherever they are with it, rather than exist in an inconsistent or ill-defined behavioural relationship. These goals are clearly communicated to the dog through consistent and unambiguous signals, which persist across all real-life contexts.

Pet-dog owners, on the other hand, frequently 'fall in love' with the most unpromising material while at the same time having no idea of what they need or how to educate a dog to perform to requirements. By this means, the least suitable dogs fall into the least experienced and least able hands. This must be taken into account in any advice given to pet-dog clients but without implying fault for any ill-informed choices. However, for the majority of the time, the dog–human relationship is successful on this basis without any deliberate professional intervention. Any advice given must take the emotional needs of each party into consideration while at the same time giving practical and educational advice.

Positive training for real life

Just as a client's primary concern regarding physical illness and injury is that the clinical sign (e.g. limping, vomiting, scratching) goes away, the ubiquitous requirement when help is needed for behaviour problems is that the dog should stop doing whatever behaviour it is that has become irritating, dangerous or expensive, or a combination of all three. In order to try to stop a dog biting, chewing the contents of the house or urinating in the kitchen at night, for example, various means of punishment will usually have been tried already with little or no success.

Merely trying to stop behaviour using punishment, with or without forethought and planning, implies a belief that a dog must have 'misbehaved' to justify the action. Unfortunately the minds of most companion animals are not adapted to deal with such concepts. The punishment will give the animal no clue as to what it should be doing instead, because no specific behavioural goal has been set. The means whereby punishment is avoided, i.e. which behaviour is negatively reinforced, is largely left to chance and may or may not result in behavioural improvement. Indeed, human anger is frequently instrumental in triggering potentially dangerous aggression.

Rarely is enough time spent even deciding how a dog should behave in all real-life contexts, let alone training it to perform as required. The assumption is made that early training lasts for life and that a dog will continue to sit 'because we said so', rather than for anything more tangible. In addition, in situations for which a dog has not been trained and where it may find the 'right' decision impossible to make, it will often be viewed as disobedient and stubborn and not deserving of reward.

In practical terms, the greatest reward must be on offer at the very times when a dog may be about to be the worst behaved, to encourage it to make the right choice. For example, the most desirable food or toy may need to be used to pre-empt, rather than distract in response to, snapping on veterinary handling.

Using positive reward-based training methods not only ensures that behaviour is channelled consistently in the right direction but also reduces the number of decisions that a dog has to make on a 'threat/no threat' (i.e. punishment versus negative reinforcement) basis. Any communication with dogs that does not involve threatening them will also significantly reduce, if not actually eliminate, the need for an aggressive response.

Obedience and good behaviour

Owners are generally unaware of the difference between an obedient dog and a well behaved one. It is perfectly possible for a dog to be obedient and not at all well behaved and, vice versa, to be exceptionally well behaved without knowing the meaning of a single obedience command. Well trained obedient dogs appear to be presented as frequently for counselling owing to their unacceptable behaviour as are completely uneducated ones.

Often, dogs are only well behaved by chance: they are making their own choice as to what to do but their behaviour happens to be convenient and pleasurable to their owners. In effect, information from the environment is sufficient for the dog to make an appropriate decision; for example, the television is turned on and the dog lies down at his owner's feet. Such ideal dogs may be the result of evolutionary selection for an ability to read human behaviour rather than the training skill of the owner. Commands therefore appear to be unnecessary, as the dog is already doing as his owner wishes for the vast majority of the time.

The result is that the very words that are needed to give a dog successful guidance when life gets difficult, distracting or threatening are never thoroughly rehearsed when the dog is calm and amenable enough to teaching and learning. In real life, as opposed to training class, owners often try to change a dog's mind only when he has already made an inconvenient, dangerous, damaging or painful decision. They do not practise achieving a truly obedient dog, i.e one whose choice of behaviour can be altered to coincide with theirs by means of a cue word, until the situation is so distracting, exciting or threatening that the dog will find it impossible to comply.

Canine appeasement behaviour and body language

The appearance of canine appeasing (or calming) and threat-averting behaviour is, for the most part, enormously appealing to humans and is likely to have formed at least part of the basis upon which selection and rejection have been made since the domestication process began. In other words, people love dogs who look like they love them. Recognizing what appeasement behaviour looks like, understanding its purpose and responding appropriately to it are therefore all of crucial importance in preventing dogs from needing to bite. On the other hand, misunderstanding and misinterpreting the nature and purpose of appeasement behaviour frequently results in inappropriate human responses that ultimately damage a dog's trust in people, with consequent behavioural deterioration.

The Ladder of Aggression (Figure 11.2) is a sequence of calming and threat-averting gestures that dogs give, regardless of their status relative to another, with the intention of achieving an immediate reduction in the threat perceived. If responded to appropriately, escalation to overt and potentially damaging aggression is pre-empted and avoided. The more

intense the gesture (higher up the ladder), the more important it is that an animal's expression of unease and discomfort is understood. If it is not, the risk of being injured or being forced to injure as a response increases significantly.

The apparently guilty dog (see middle rungs of ladder and Figure 11.3) who 'knows he's done wrong' is in reality giving threat-averting gestures designed to calm and appease. Such body language has a genetic basis and will be displayed the instant that uncertainty and threat are perceived. Once an association has been made by the dog between specific environmental information (such as urine in the kitchen, a chewed sofa or raided rubbish) and an unpleasant and threatening event (such as human anger and punishment) (Figure 11.4), a learned attempt to pre-empt and avert a predicted threat will be made. The dog does not know that such behaviours are inherently 'wrong', nor can it make such a retrospective connection between its own previous behaviour and punishment; nonetheless an almost universal human assumption is made that such body language indicates an acknowledgement of guilt and apology. This in turn seems to justify the use of punishment on the premise that the dog knew he shouldn't do it and will thereby 'learn not to do it again'.

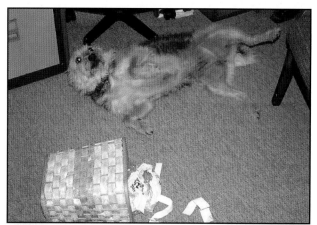

11.3 The 'lying down, leg up' gesture (see 'Ladder of Aggression') signifying 'You're threatening me – please stop it now' is almost universally misinterpreted as an expression of guilt. Continuing to reprimand and punish risks inducing aggression. © Kendal Shepherd.

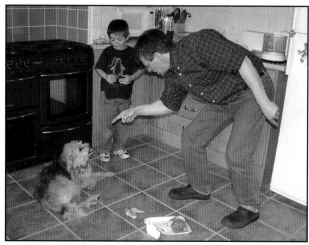

11.4 This dog has already growled in response to reprimand and is also at risk of associating the presence of a child with punishment and its own need for an aggressive response. So-called unpredictable aggression towards children may therefore emerge in the future. © Kendal Shepherd.

The Ladder of Aggression:

- Bite
- Snap
- Growl
- Stiffening up, stare
- Lying down, leg up
- Standing crouched, tail tucked under
- Creeping, ears back
- Walking away
- Turning body away, sitting, pawing
- Turning head away
- Yawning, blinking, nose licking

11.2 The Ladder of Aggression. (Reproduced from *BSAVA Manual of Canine and Feline Behavioural Medicine*)

Such a human response merely increases the threat to an already threatened dog and is perceived as unjustified aggression, thereby warranting an aggressive response. If a dog learns that the more subtle calming and 'negotiating' stages of the Ladder of Aggression (such as turning the head away, walking away or even growling) are ineffective, they may be dispensed with and a bite selected immediately as the only strategy that humans seem to understand. By punishing the 'guilty' look, the very behaviours for which dogs have been selected are devalued. Many so-called 'unpredictably' aggressive dogs result from the very predictable misinterpretation by humans of the Ladder of Aggression. From a dog's perspective, much of what humans do, particularly when coercive and threatening training methods are used, is simply intrusive, unpredictable and incomprehensible.

Dominance

Another common area of misunderstanding for owners, widely perpetuated by popular literature and culture, is the concept of dominance. Dominance describes a relationship, not an individual. One is not a 'dominant' dog or person in oneself, but is relatively more dominant or subordinate in specific relationships or situations. Moreover, a dominance relationship is established by the actions of the subordinate, who decides to yield to avoid further conflict – not by the dominant partner. Where real and stable dominance–subordinance relationships exist, the subordinate individual reliably defers to the dominant through avoidance or some of the signs indicated on the Ladder of Aggression. The decision whether or not to defer, however, will depend on circumstances and may be altered by the apparent value or scarcity of resources. The purpose of a dominance relationship is to avoid completely the need for aggression through the establishment of predictable outcomes and expectations.

'Dominance aggression' is therefore a contradiction of terms. Aggression is a sign of an uncertain relationship, not a dominant one, since aggression is always a potentially risky strategy and means that the two individuals have not established who takes precedence in a less risky way. There is also no direct evidence that dogs use the concept of social dominance (i.e. a desire to be in overall control) to motivate their behaviour. In fact it is doubtful that they are capable of such a concept. They will compete in individual circumstances, if they have a need for a resource, and also learn that they usually get their own way, but this is not the same as trying to be dominant. Dominance is created by outcomes and becomes the expectation, but is not the intention.

In the human–dog relationship, accidental deference to a dog occurs in many day-to-day circumstances. For example, a dog scratches at the back door and is let out to relieve himself. He presents a ball at his owner's feet or lap and is obediently played with. These are not seen as significant events by humans, and indeed may be convenient and pleasurable, but they have a continual and cumulative effect upon the dog's perception of the consequences of their interactions with their human companions. This may not cause a problem until the owner tries to take control in a situation that is unexpected by the dog. Threatening behaviour on the part of an owner may, if convincing enough, elicit threat-averting behaviour, which can be wrongly interpreted as 'submission' or even 'obedience', but in some cases, it may be seen by the dog as a reason to escalate overt aggression in response.

Commonly recommended exercises, such as rolling a dog on its back to assert dominance are a test of control in a given context only and probably do nothing to create a perception of a human's superiority. If a dog is fearful of human handling, these exercises are extremely ill-advised as they can be very dangerous. Supposed attempts at asserting dominance by humans may be seen as unjustified aggression and are particularly risky if attempted by individuals who do not normally take control. Such exercises should not be recommended as part of treatment or even a preventive behaviour management programme, when there are much less risky ways of altering a dog's choice of how to behave.

Prevention of behaviour problems

Pet selection

With a breeder, problem prevention begins in choosing which animals to breed from and how their offspring are reared before they are sold. For most pet owners, the issue begins when trying to select the correct pet.

It is important for owners to appreciate the behaviour and needs of the species and breed of pet they are choosing. Some time should also be spent preparing their home for the new arrival to check that the environment provided is set up to encourage the right behaviours from the outset. An animal in the wrong environment will be stressed and much more likely to develop problems (and in the case of small mammals, reptiles and birds, standard housing is often not the same as appropriate housing). Owners may need advice on suitable toys for their animal. They should also be advised about reputable sources, as a poor early environment will predispose an animal to behaviour problems later in life.

Early development

Owners need to appreciate the optimal age to purchase a given animal and what they should expect of an animal of a certain age. For example, youngsters may not be physically mature enough to be dry through the night. Whilst castration may help to prevent certain problems, there is also growing evidence that neutering can increase certain forms of reactivity and so the decision to neuter on behavioural grounds is perhaps not as straightforward as is often claimed.

If veterinary staff are working with breeders, it is important to emphasize the importance of their role in problem prevention. The breeder of any puppy or kitten, pure or cross-bred, has a responsibility to ensure that from the start a puppy is gently but routinely exposed to the range of environmental stimuli that it will be expected to cope with in later life, including, most importantly, human handling. Owners of 'rescued' dogs will often interpret fear and aggression as the result of previous 'deliberate cruelty and abuse', but it is far more likely to be the result of a lack of appropriate environmental experience in the first 3 months of life.

The age at which caution begins to override the desire to explore, and therefore the age at which the ability to learn good things about one's environment begins to be inhibited by fear, is for most breeds of dog quite early at between 7 and 8 weeks. Certain breeds, especially guard breeds like the German Shepherd Dog, may become fearful as early as 5 weeks of age.

However much breeder clients may give the impression that they already 'know it all', it is a duty of the veterinary practice team to inform them of the essential nature of the socialization process and how routine exposure to real life should not be left to chance. This process should be deliberately arranged by the breeder and continued in the puppy's or kitten's new home.

It is essential to explain to owners that their new acquisition is much more advanced in developmental terms than they may realize. A 10-week-old puppy (Figure 11.5) is the equivalent of a 5-year-old child and is equally capable of learning to say 'please' nicely. Treating puppies as babies whose demands must be met leads the puppy to believe that demanding behaviour is what owners want. Inappropriate, inconvenient or sometimes dangerous behaviours are thus maintained into adolescence and adulthood.

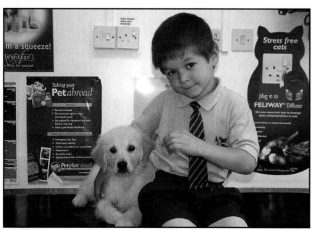

11.5 This 10-week-old puppy and 5-year-old schoolchild are developmental equivalents but will be treated very differently by average parents and dog owners.
© Kendal Shepherd.

All too often owners are still being told that a puppy must be kept indoors until at least a week after the second vaccination, resulting in a puppy's first contact with the world being as late as 14 weeks of age. An appropriate balance must be struck between the small risk of infection and the big risk of under-socialization and habituation, with consequent development of equally life-threatening antisocial and fear-related problems. Carrying a dog out into a town where it can see and experience the sights, sounds and smells of the city is a simple way to habituate a dog to many stimuli at minimal risk.

Puppy parties and classes

The assumed aim of puppy parties and classes is to create a sociable animal that will be able to cope with all life events without becoming fearful or aggressive. Although the terms 'party' and 'class' are frequently used interchangeably, **puppy parties** refer to pleasantly habituating the puppy to the surgery, the consulting room table, other puppies and human handling, whereas **puppy classes** imply specific obedience training content as well.

However they are conducted, for classes or parties to contribute to success, owners must be realistic as to what will be achieved by attendance. Over-optimistic expectations on the part of both dog and owner may be more damaging than not attending at all. Most owners have the frequently unrealistic requirement that their dogs should ignore all other dogs when out walking or 'play nicely' with them, should the opportunity arise and it is convenient for the owner. An animal cannot learn to 'play nicely' unless it has the chance to practise, nor will a dog ignore other dogs upon request unless its owner makes deliberate, concerted and continual efforts to remain the most important feature in the dog's life, whatever else is happening. If great care is not taken, ignoring the owner completely in favour of the highly self-rewarding behaviour of play may be all that is learned instead.

The essential lessons of puppy classes are that the dog's owner must be instructed in how to retain mental control of their dogs at all times and in all situations, and that practising such control must continue throughout a dog's life. A common finding in treating behaviour problems later is the false assumption that puppy class lessons last for life without rehearsal and also without considering it necessary to continue to reward a dog for a job well done. Puppies are given food rewards, but adults are expected to obey and tolerate anything life presents to them for human pleasure alone.

Veterinary practices should consider running their own puppy classes if the expertise exists to manage them appropriately. Alternatively, one of a growing number of professional puppy trainers may be used to deliver a structured programme. It is obviously important to check the qualifications and experience of anyone invited to deliver classes in the name of the practice, as the standard of service can vary enormously.

These classes may combine basic obedience training with socialization, plenty of handling and lots of novel stimuli provided in a controlled and pleasant environment. Puppies are taught what is acceptable, and what is not (e.g. biting). All vaccinated puppies can be invited to the classes and given the opportunity to mix with puppies of their own age and new people. A recommended 4-week programme is given below. The classes are not only an important service but also excellent public relations for the practice, as well as a lot of fun for all involved. (See also Chapter 2.)

Four-week puppy class programme

The whole family should be encouraged to attend the classes and take part in the exercises. The principles of training should be described as part of the course, so that owners understand not only what they should do but also why.

Each week new skills are taught and established ones are reinforced. It is important to explain the principles behind the tasks and to provide handouts, since the owners will inevitably be distracted by their puppies some of the time.

If classes are to be run outside normal surgery hours or at a different venue to the normal site of the veterinary practice, it is important to check that the practice insurance still applies.

Examples of exercises to be demonstrated to clients

Week 1
- **Sit**: With the puppy standing, move a small food treat back over its head and then slightly lower it. The nose should follow the treat and the back legs naturally fold underneath as the treat is lowered. Try to avoid putting pressure on the hindquarters.
- **Stand**: Move the food lure slightly up and forward in front of the sitting puppy.
- **Down**: Move the food to the floor just in front of the puppy and keep it there.
- **Watch me**: Hold a treat to the side of your face next to your eyes.
- **Recalls**: Take the puppy away from the owners and get them to encourage it towards them. Make sure that there are no distractions for the puppy when you do this for the first time and tell the owners always to be pleased to see the puppy, to crouch down to greet it and have ample food rewards at the ready. Instruct them to take hold of the puppy's collar before giving a food reward.

continues ▶

continued
- **Chew control**: Select a range of toys for the puppy and either smear an edible reward (like peanut butter) on them or load hollow toys with treats that fall out as the puppy chews on them.
- **Bite control**: Whilst playing calmly with the puppy, slip your hand into his mouth, as the teeth make contact with your skin and well before it hurts, say "Ouch! (but try not to frighten the pup or others nearby), withdraw your hand and walk away. After a short time repeat the exercise. Soon the puppy will learn to inhibit its bite towards people. This is one of the most important lessons a dog can learn.
- **Handling exercises**: Ask someone to reward the puppy with gentle praise and small treats as the dog is handled all over. Make sure you include an examination of the ears, under the tail, between the toes and in the mouth. This will need to be done in stages initially.

Week 2
- **Off and Take it**: Show the puppy some food in your hand, say 'Off', and then close your hand over the treat. Ignore all efforts to investigate your hand until the puppy pulls its nose away from your hand. Immediately open your hand to present the reward and add a 'Take it' request as you reveal the treat.
- **Stay**: Steadily increase the time the puppy has to wait for a reward once the command word has been given. Then gradually move further away. The reward should be given when you return to the pup, not if the pup runs to you.
- **Recall from play**: Ask all the owners in the class, other than the one who will be giving the recall command, to grab their puppies when the owner doing the training calls their puppy. The puppy should be given lots of praise as it approaches the owner.
- **Off lead heel**: Hold a treat (toy or favourite food) by your side approximately level with the puppy's head. Encourage the puppy to walk beside you as you move forward just a few steps. As you stop, ask the puppy to sit. When you turn for the first time, turn towards the puppy so your leg will guide him round if necessary.

Week 3
- **Relax**: Quietly and gently reassure the puppy as a suitable command word like 'time out' is softly repeated. Keep going until the puppy is totally relaxed.
- **Heeling on lead**: Allow a lead attached to the puppy's collar to trail on the ground, while encouraging the puppy to stay with you as in Week 2 exercises. When the end of the lead is picked up, the puppy should not notice the difference between a trailing lead and a held one.
- **Greeting people**: Whilst walking the puppies on lead, stop as you meet other owners. Each owner then gives the other person's puppy a 'sit' command, bends down, and gives the puppy a treat. Children must also learn how to behave around dogs. They should not encourage mouthing, chasing or clothes chewing, but should give treats when the puppy is well behaved.
- **Socialization**: Encourage owners to get out and about with their puppies. The idea is to expose the puppy to every situation it might need to accept in its adult life in the next few weeks, without getting it overexcited, frightened or overtired. So do not let owners do too much in one go.

▶

Week 4
- **Tricks**: The principles of learning are explained earlier in the course and all owners are asked to teach their dog a trick in preparation for this week. This helps them demonstrate their understanding of training. Certificates can be given to all making it this far. These might include a picture of the puppy taken earlier in the course and make a great souvenir.

Top tips for puppy classes
- Make sure that the puppy can perform a behaviour reliably before labelling it with a command.
- Say a command word ('sit', 'stand', 'watch me' etc.) only *after* a puppy sits, stands or watches.
- Praise the behaviour (e.g. 'Good sit'), not the dog – praise should maintain behaviour, not end it.
- Reward difficulty of task, not quality – the puppy finding it the hardest deserves the most reward.
- Keep body gestures consistent in all contexts, with or without food in hand.
- Practise the 'Whose idea is it?' rule (Figure 11.6) – an obedience command is simply a means of changing a dog's mind.

The 'Whose idea is it?' rule
To remind you to routinely practise changing your dog's mind in calm, emotionally neutral situations, you must ask yourselves, whatever he is doing and wherever he is: 'Whose idea was it?' The more ideas that are yours, the better control of him you will be developing. Successfully changing the dog's mind throughout the day will imply that you are:

- Routinely considering the choices available to your dog
- Making positive requests for 'good' behaviour rather than merely trying to stop the 'bad'
- Using all routine 'life resources', including your attention, to improve your bargaining power
- Rehearsing obedience commands before you need them to work
- Teaching your dog when he is in 'emotional neutral' and finds it easiest to learn
- Not giving in to attention-seeking.

11.6 The 'Whose idea is it?' rule.

Minimizing behavioural damage during veterinary intervention
Reading the signs
It should be remembered that:

- The purpose of appeasement behaviour is to deflect threat and restore harmony
- Devaluing appeasement behaviour forces a dog towards aggressive behaviour.

Unfortunately, appeasement behaviour is consistently ignored, misunderstood and devalued in the veterinary consulting room and surgery, to the detriment of staff, owners and of course the pet.

An animal's preferred option when faced with a threat is to retreat from it. The minute such retreat is unavailable, the conversion of 'flight' to 'fight' becomes more likely, if not inevitable. The simple raising of a paw, tucking tail under or putting ears back are all evidence of a dog's desire for a perceived threat to diminish; similarly the hunching or laying back of the ears of a cat are a sign of avoidance. Whenever veterinary attention and interference continue in spite of such signalling, the animal is slightly less likely to use such signals next time and more likely to opt for overt aggression. Every effort must therefore be made to understand what the animal in the clinic is indicating and to avoid forcing it to learn that aggression is necessary in this situation.

Vaccination

A pet's vaccination may be its first experience of the surgery and must be viewed as an opportunity to predict the same message as is conveyed in puppy or kitten parties or classes. If an animal has already attended a class, there is a chance to reinforce overtly what has already been learned. If a concerted effort is not made to make the surgery appear 'nice' and things are left to chance, there is the very real possibility that the perception will be converted to one of 'nasty', with the risk of consequently fearful and aggressive responses. It is a sad indictment of a consistent lack of veterinary attention to the nurturing of a positive attitude among their patients that so many clients assume that their pets 'hate coming to the vet's'.

In addition, what is demonstrated at this time should not only create animals that are convenient and safe for veterinary staff to handle in the future, but should also provide a role model for humane and educational owner interaction with their pet for the rest of its life.

Whatever time is available for a vaccination consultation, the majority of it should be spent feeding or playing with the puppy or kitten and using ample and tasty food rewards to demonstrate the principles of both associative and operant conditioning. At this stage in their lives, there are very few puppies that will not want to eat – but only if nothing nasty is done to them first. There is little point in trying to 'make friends' *after* the event.

Asking the owner to feed a puppy or kitten while its ears, teeth, skin and nails are examined creates pleasant associations with handling. Waiting until a puppy or kitten sits on the table before food is given, rather than pestering at the hand containing food, demonstrates *operant conditioning*. If these very simple lessons are taken into every aspect of a pet's life, fewer behaviour problems will occur later.

These exercises can all be dealt with in a special consulting room by a nurse, before the veterinary surgeon arrives to deliver the injection. However, it is important that the veterinary surgeon, too, takes the small amount of time required to make friends with the pet before delivering the injection. At the point of giving the injection, the owner should be asked to release the animal and tease it instead with a particularly tasty treat or toy. The owner should be instructed to present the food at the exact time of the injection itself. Such an approach produces animals who very rarely even notice the procedure – and who may indeed look forward positively to the next one – and prevents the apparent need to grab the animal suddenly and restrain it to prevent escape. The stimulus of restraint itself, once associated with pain, is at great risk of triggering a fearful and aggressive response during subsequent visits.

Using negative reinforcement

Although nearly all puppies are happy to eat in the consulting room, unfortunately a proportion of adult dogs simply turn and back away as a result of previous bad experiences. A typical owner response is, 'He won't take food from strangers' (which should be interpreted as 'He's worried by strangers') or, 'He remembers what happened last time' (and is therefore worried by specific strangers, such as veterinary surgeons and nurses). For these dogs, use can still be made of desirable events in order to try to maintain behaviour that allows a veterinary surgeon or nurse to do their job (Figure 11.7).

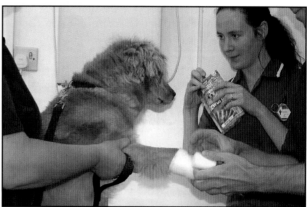

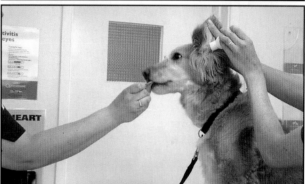

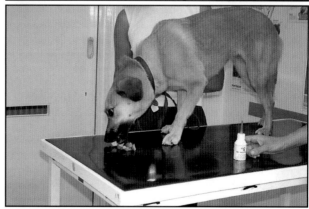

11.7 Food should be used to make pleasant associations with common veterinary procedures, regardless of whether a dog appears to need it. 'Good dogs' are frequently taken for granted. For example, fearful dogs may need the time to make pleasant associations with the sight of a bottle of ear drops before approach and application are possible. © Kendal Shepherd.

Most clinical tasks can be performed with a dog that reliably sits and stays sitting for a prerequisite time. The reward, which can be offered to a dog in order to maintain a 'sit' as a useful behaviour in the consulting room, is the opportunity to leave the room, which can be trained using the following procedure:

1. With the dog in the clinic on a lead restraint, ask the dog to sit.
2. Open the door only if the dog obeys the request straight away.
3. If the dog does not comply immediately, in addition to not opening the door, ask the owner to turn away from their dog, keeping the lead slack, thereby demonstrating how to effectively deliver punishment by withdrawal of attention (negative punishment) and without the need for threat.

Most dogs will quickly learn to sit and wait to regain their owner's attention and to leave the room (Figure 11.8). Sitting thus becomes a valuable behaviour in the clinic as well as elsewhere and can then be used to take control of a dog's behaviour in the clinic. A little patience is all that is required.

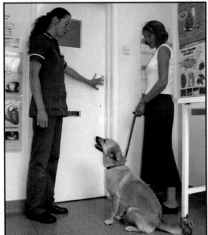

11.8

Leaving the consulting room is a rewarding event for most dogs. Learning to sit to achieve this reinforces sitting as a useful behaviour for all concerned inside the consulting room as well as elsewhere. © Kendal Shepherd.

Using conditioned emotional responses
Although a dog may not take food if offered from the hand of a veterinary surgeon or nurse, the same food item may be readily accepted from the hand of the owner, the explanation simply being that one hand is less threatening than the other. For a certain number of dogs, however, their emotional state is such as to prevent food from being taken even from the hand of the owner. If the same dog is asked to sit by the owner, at the same time ensuring that the owner's body language is relaxed and happy rather than stressed by being in the surgery, a considerable proportion of dogs will not only comply with the command, but will then also accept the food item. In this situation, the previous experience of the 'sit' word and body language of the owner are being used to produce a conditioned emotional response.

Such emotional change for the better, induced when the word is heard and gestures seen, allows the dog to relax sufficiently to feel like eating. In other words, the 'sit' command results in eating, rather than a dog sitting in order to gain food. It is then highly likely that a 'sit' command issued by the veterinary surgeon or nurse will also be obeyed and food eaten as a result. Once this breakthrough in communication is made, a window of opportunity is created whereby a dog's view of the surgery and consulting room can be improved.

Behaviours and commands for the clinic
An essential part of training is the clarity of the message given. How often are owners heard to give meaningless instructions such as 'Come on, behave yourself!' or 'Now, it's only going to take a little while so just settle down, will you?', which the dog has never heard before? If owners can simply be persuaded to give a clear 'sit' and 'stay' command to their dog, preceded

only by the dog's name, many will achieve remarkably instant results.

Nonetheless, owners should be advised about behaviours to be rehearsed at home in preparation for the visit to the surgery. Veterinary staff should also decide upon and train specific behaviour that will be of use, if not essential, for the future. Conditioning positive emotional expectations and associated behaviour to commands will ensure that both behaviour and underlying emotions will remain stable, if not actually improve, with subsequent visits.

Commands of particular use include:

- 'Sit' (all four feet and bottom on floor)
- 'Stand' (all four feet on floor)
- 'Stay' (remain in previous position)
- 'Watch me' (watch owner rather than anything else)
- 'This way' (follow as handler turns away).

However well such commands and behaviours are rehearsed at home or in training class, a consistent result will not be produced if the verbal and visual signals given by the owner vary from one situation to another, or depending on whether they have food rewards in their hand or not. Similarly, a dog that has been trained to sit via the threat of a jerk on the lead or check chain will not perform if the predictive lead or check chain is not present. A very common reason for dogs to become 'disobedient' in certain contexts is that environmental information predicting what they should do, and why, is changed or missing altogether (**context-specific learning**). Training classes are very rarely conducted with a handbag in one hand and a baby buggy in the other, but owners must pretend and act as if they are in training class or in their kitchen at home if dogs are to be expected to behave in the same way.

Minimizing stress on admission
There are now pheromone products (Feliway and DAP, Ceva Animal Health) that appear to have a calming effect on dogs and cats in the clinic, by helping to reduce the perceived novelty of the environment, but there are also many other simple measures that can help to shift the balance away from fearful or anxious expectations. The more that the same commands the dog is familiar with at home can be used in the clinic, the less novel the environment will seem. Conditioned emotional responses to standard obedience commands are invaluable in buffering the dog against potentially fear-provoking novelty. In order to minimize the impact of the hospital, it is therefore worth asking a few basic questions as part of the admission procedure. The following questions are equally relevant to day patients and to hospitalized ones, the only difference being that dogs staying overnight or longer have more opportunity for learning.

- How has the dog been trained? (*What emotional responses have been conditioned and why?*)
- What words does the dog know? (*Use the same ones!*)
- Any concerns regarding reactivity to noises? (*Protect dog in hospital, or early intervention for treatment*)
- Where does dog usually eliminate? On command, or 'asks' to go out? (*Gravel, grass, earth, concrete*)
- What is the dog's reaction to other dogs? (*May govern kennelling choice*)
- What is the usual lead restraint? How does the dog behave on lead? (*Pre-prepare with Halti or Gentle leader*)
- How does the dog react to grooming, both at home and at groomer's? (*If better at groomer's, possibly consider owner-absent examination/basket muzzle training*)

'First aid' for common behaviour problems

Many problems are amenable to retraining using the general principles discussed above, but common problems such as aggression, house-soiling and house destruction are complaints for which there are many causes. The specific cause for a given case needs to be identified if it is to be treated effectively and this will require specialist evaluation. The veterinary nurse should explain this clearly to the client and also give behavioural first aid advice to contain the problem in the mean time.

Aggression

Aggression is a serious concern for all involved and should only be tackled by skilled handlers. Aggression that is associated with perceived threat, defence and control of resources must be distinguished from that associated with medical disorders, play and predation, which are functionally very different behaviours. Medical assessment by a veterinary surgeon is essential, as pain will often present as increased irritability and risk of aggression. Animals often assume an aggressive stance when there is uncertainty or frustration in the environment, and previous or anticipated punishment is likely to exacerbate the situation.

Prior to specialist evaluation, the risks to others from an aggressive animal should be minimized. This involves the following:

- Owners must be informed of their responsibility to prevent injury to others.
- Owners should aim to avoid situations that are likely to exacerbate the condition. This may include identifiable trigger stimuli, such as: other pets and children; opportunities for competition; uncertain, frustrating or fear-provoking situations.
- The animal should not be approached when it has no opportunity to retreat.
- If it is safe to do so, the owner should be encouraged to muzzle-train an aggressive dog away from arousing or dangerous environments (Figures 11.9 and 11.10). The most common problem with muzzles is that they are only used when the dog is already showing aggression and will resent restraint. This is why training should begin away from distractions and the trained dog should be muzzled before a problem arises.
- A special appointment should be made to discuss the problem further.

IF YOUR DOG IS AGGRESSIVE ... FIRST AID ADVICE

The following advice is designed to do no more than prevent incidents and to help you manage your dog's aggression in the short term. Specific advice aimed at resolving the problem cannot be given until we understand *why* your dog is acting aggressively. This can only be achieved through a combination of both behavioural and veterinary investigation. Therefore if your dog is aggressive it is advisable to seek help from a qualified behaviourist but only *after* your dog has first undergone a physical examination by your veterinary surgeon.

If your dog is aggressive to you or other family members:

- **Avoid confrontations and actions that the dog may regard as challenging or threatening.** Do not fight your dog for possessions. Avoid prolonged direct eye contact, leaning over or handling the dog in any way that may provoke aggression.
- **Keep your distance and avoid unintentional provocation.** Sudden movements or flapping of the hands can provoke aggression, as can moving into the dog's personal space (typically within about 2 metres of the dog).
- **Defuse any threat of aggression by the dog** by looking away, slumping your shoulders and *slowly* walking away.
- **Do not attempt punishment** as this is likely to increase a fearful dog's need to be defensive and aggressive, and an assertive dog may be more willing to rise to the challenge of a confrontation and react with increased aggression.
- **Anticipate and avoid any potential situations that may result in your dog becoming aggressive.** For example, if your dog is aggressive around food, do not give him bones or long-lasting chews and ensure that he is not disturbed whilst eating his dinner.
- **Keep in mind that a growl is a warning and a normal part of canine 'language'.** If you are doing, or about to do, something to a dog that causes him to growl, by continuing with that action the dog may feel the need to get the message across with a bite.
- **Attach a long lightweight lead to your dog's collar** if he attempts to bite you whenever you try to move him, so that you can lead him away without needing to handle or confront him. *However, it is important that your dog is supervised at all times while the lead is attached.*
- **Never leave your dog alone unsupervised with children.** This is advice that is applicable to *any* dog, not just dogs that are known to be aggressive.

If your dog is aggressive to other dogs or people:

On walks

- **Avoid exercising your dog in public places until professional help is obtained.** Every time your dog uses aggression he is likely to learn that it is a successful way to make other people or dogs 'go away' or keep their distance. In other words, he will learn that 'aggression works' and therefore the behaviour will increase.
- **Do not attempt to punish your dog.** This includes pulling back roughly on the lead. Doing so will cause discomfort, even pain, that your dog is likely to associate with the main focus of his attention at the time, i.e. the other dog or person, which will have the effect of increasing aggression in the long run.
- **Do not attempt to reassure your dog or use food treats as a distraction** whilst he is acting aggressively, as doing so may actually reward and so reinforce the aggressive behaviour.
- **Never leave your dog tied up in public places.**
- **Ensure that your dog is under your control**, on the lead and/or muzzled **at all times**.

11.9 Aggression First Aid Client Handout. (Courtesy of Trudi Atkinson and Francesca Riccomini)

continues ▶

In or around the home

- **Do not allow your dog to encounter people at the boundary of his territory,** for example at the front door or garden gate.
- **Ensure that all perimeter fences etc. are secure.**
- **Avoid visitors to the house until professional help is obtained.** If this is not possible ensure that the dog is securely shut away for the duration of the visit. If the dog cannot be shut away, he should be kept on a lead and/or muzzled whilst the visitor is in the house. Also instruct the visitor to ignore the dog, as any attempts to approach the dog or direct eye contact could provoke an aggressive response. For visits of long duration (a day or more) it may be better to board your dog at kennels while the visitor is in the house. It is essential to explain to the kennel owner why you need to board your dog and explain that he may be aggressive.

IT IS IMPORTANT THAT YOU ARE AWARE THAT A DOG'S OWNER IS RESPONSIBLE IN LAW FOR THE SAFETY OF OTHERS

SHOULD YOUR DOG CAUSE INJURY YOU COULD BE AT RISK OF PROSECUTION, WITH AN ORDER THAT YOUR DOG IS DESTROYED

DO NOT TAKE ANY UNNECESSARY RISKS

11.9 *continued* Aggression First Aid Client Handout. (Courtesy of Trudi Atkinson and Francesca Riccomini)

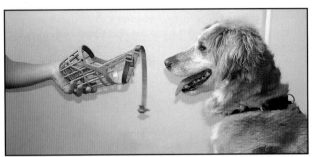

11.10 Food is used to make pleasant associations with a muzzle and encourage voluntary rather than forceful application. This must be thoroughly rehearsed before a dog is deemed to need muzzling. © Kendal Shepherd.

House-soiling

When asked about a house-soiling problem it is important to establish what form of elimination is involved and, if it involves urine, whether the animal is scent marking (spraying in the cat or spot marking in the dog), as these represent fundamentally different behaviours to urinary and faecal elimination. In all cases of inappropriate urination, possible medical causes should first be investigated and ruled out by a veterinary surgeon. The next step is to establish that the animal has been properly housetrained.

Cats

Feline urine spraying, where it is not due to cystitis, may be treated with a commercial preparation of feline facial pheromone and may not require any additional retraining advice. Marked areas should be cleaned with a solution of biological washing powder followed by surgical spirit. The area should then be rinsed with water and wiped dry with paper towels.

Cats that have been urine marking for some time may also stop using the litter box. Other reasons for indiscriminate elimination include lower urinary tract disease, litter box and litter aversions, an emotional problem or substrate preferences. It should be checked that the litter box is positioned away from the cat's food and bed in a quiet, secluded area where the cat cannot be disturbed, that the box is cleaned regularly and completely and that there have been no changes to the normal routine (e.g. change of litter type). Bleach, ammonia-based disinfectants or strong-smelling cleaners are not recommended, as the smell may be aversive to the cat. If the cause is not readily identifiable and the animal is healthy, expert advice should be sought.

Dogs

In the dog, house-soiling is most commonly a result of lack of sufficient housetraining, loss of housetraining, scent marking, disease, fear or separation distress. First, any disease must be investigated and treated promptly, but in all cases the pet will need retraining. This is most effectively achieved by ensuring that the dog is taken out regularly to a particular toilet area and returned without comment if it does not eliminate. If it does eliminate, it should be given lots of praise and a treat. This might be a game, a longer walk or a titbit. Neutering (surgical or chemical) can often be an effective treatment for scent marking.

Dogs may urinate when they feel threatened, as this is a normal appeasement gesture. Owners often get upset and angry at this reaction and so may make matters worse by telling their dog off. Eye contact alone may be sufficient to trigger this appeasement behaviour in some dogs. Owners should be encouraged not to appear threatening in any way towards their pet, especially on their return to the house, and in particular should avoid eye contact.

Dogs also eliminate when they are frightened (e.g. during thunderstorms) or are distressed in some other way such as by the departure of the owner.

Owner-absence behaviour

The term 'separation anxiety' is often wrongly used to describe any problem that arises in the owner's absence. Such complaints are more accurately described as 'separation-related behaviour' and are purely descriptive of what happens, rather than assigning or identifying any specific cause.

There are many reasons why an animal may not be able to cope with the absence of its owner. These may include over-attachment to the owner, in which case treatment must focus on reducing this attachment, or developing an owner substitute. Alternatively, the animal may be fearful of the isolation experienced when left alone or, more specifically, of fear-provoking events, such as a thunderstorm that happens to have occurred when the owner was out of the house. In this case a companion might help and the animal may be trained gradually to cope, with steadily increasing periods of isolation as well as desensitization and counter-conditioning. A third factor may relate to the stress of confinement or barrier frustration and results in primary attempts at escape. These cases often carry a poorer prognosis. In some cases, the owner may simply be expecting too much from a young or ageing animal.

Whatever the cause, behaviour modification advice is generally essential for the long-term resolution of the problem, but for maximum success this should be tailored to address the factors underlying the behaviour. Drugs such as clomipramine or commercial preparations of dog pheromones may help to speed up the rate of response in certain cases.

These problems may also occur in cats, with soiling usually being associated with the owner's bed or some other personal area.

Modifying separation-related behaviour

- Although the correct use of indoor crates can be useful (Figure 11.11), animals should not be simply caged when left alone. Shutting the door may alleviate owner distress by restricting damage and soiling, but will do nothing for the animal's emotional state. It is important to train the animal to the cage first so that going into it becomes a positively desirable experience.
- All dogs should be provided with stimulating toys when left alone for long periods of time. These can be made attractive at the time of leaving by smearing them with food paste or filling them with food. The toy can be taken up when the owner returns so that access is limited and its value to the dog increased.
- Dogs should be trained to chew on appropriate items at all times, not just when left alone, and it should not be assumed that they will naturally stop chewing on things when they stop teething.

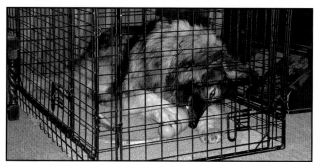

11.11 Making the indoor kennel or crate a rewarding place to be must be carried out as part of a dog's daily routine, not just reserved for potential problem situations. Ideally, whether the door is open or shut should be immaterial as far as the dog is concerned. © Kendal Shepherd.

Noise fears

The following hints may be given to owners when managing an animal for its fear of noises.

- Drugs may be useful in some cases, but should only be used under veterinary supervision. If using any such remedies, they should be given so they take effect *before* any noise starts or panic sets in. Sedation is not the object of such treatment.
- Do not punish the animal when it is scared – it will only confirm that there was something to be afraid of.
- Do not fuss or try to reassure the scared animal, as this rewards the behaviour. If you are cheerful, your behaviour will help to counteract the fear.
- Ignore any fearful behaviour that occurs for no good reason.
- Make sure that the pet is kept in a safe and secure environment at all times so that it does not bolt and escape if a sudden noise occurs. The use of pheromone treatments will help to provide an emotionally secure environment.

- Provide a safe and secure retreat for the frightened animal as this will help it cope and so reduce the intensity of the fear response. When the noise 'season' begins it may help to black out one of the quietest rooms in the house and place toys for the animal to play with, and preferably things for the owner to do as well, so that the room is associated with positive experiences. Some animals appreciate the opportunity to withdraw and the provision of a retreat such as a cupboard under the stairs may help them to cope. Duvets and blankets not only make the area comfortable but can also help to soundproof the area. Blacking out the room removes the potentially additional problems of flashing lights in the case of firework or thunderstorm fears.
- Ignore the noises and try to engage the animal in some form of active game.
- Put some music on. Calming music can help.
- Feeding a dog a good protein-rich meal with added vitamin B6 mid to late afternoon, with plenty of carbohydrate a little later, can help to calm a nervous animal, but do not try this if the dog is prone to diarrhoea when scared or at other times. If necessary, do not feed the dog at any other time in the day, to ensure a good appetite.
- If there is a dog that is not scared by the noises and which gets on with the noise-phobic dog, keeping the two together during the noise period may help. Playing with the non-fearful dog may help to persuade the other dog that the noise is not so bad after all.
- Ear plugs can be made by taking a piece of cotton wool, dampening it, squeezing out any excess water, rolling it into a long thin cylinder and twisting into the animal's ear so as to pack the canal. Care must be taken that the cylinder is not so thin that it goes too deep into the ear canal nor so wide that it cannot be secured. The plug should be secure and firm but not so tight that it irritates the animal. Remember to remove it later that day and do not reuse ear plugs from one day to the next. A support stocking over the ears may help to hold the plugs in place.
- Do not just ignore the problem because it only happens once or twice a year. Instigate a desensitization programme once the 'season' is over and you have control over the environment again. There are many good commercial products available which owners can use in their home. It is important to read the specific instructions associated with a given programme. Desensitization training works better if sessions are frequent rather than longer.
- Do not be afraid to seek professional advice, as this is a serious welfare problem for any pet.

Acknowledgement

The authors would like to thank Trudi Atkinson for her useful comments on early drafts of the chapter.

Further reading

The APBC/CABTSG Manual of Behavioural First Aid, available from http://www.apbc.org.uk/books1.htm
Heath S and Mills D (2005) *Client Information Handouts, Behaviour*. Lifelearn Ltd, Newmarket
Horwitz D, Heath SE and Mills DS (2002) *BSAVA Manual of Canine and Feline Behavioural Medicine*. BSAVA Publications, Gloucester

Useful website:
Companion Animal Behaviour Therapy Study Group: www.cabtsg.org

Chapter 12

Maintaining animal accommodation

Louise Monsey

Learning objectives

After studying this chapter, students should be able to:

- **Outline optimal environmental conditions for animal accommodation**
- **State the advantages and disadvantages of different construction and bedding materials in relation to animal accommodation**
- **Explain the general principles and considerations of kennel and cattery management in relation to an animal's needs**
- **Describe different types of specialized animal housing, including housing for exotic species**
- **Outline the principles of cleaning and disinfection of kennel and hospital environments**

Animal housing

Anyone responsible for animal care should be aware of and always bear in mind the animal's basic needs. The RSPCA terms these 'The Five Freedoms for Animals'.

The Five Freedoms

- **Freedom from Hunger and Thirst**
  By ready access to fresh water and a diet to maintain full health and vigour
- **Freedom from Discomfort**
  By providing an appropriate environment including shelter and a comfortable resting area
- **Freedom from Pain, Injury or Disease**
  By prevention and/or rapid diagnosis and treatment
- **Freedom to Express Normal Behaviour**
  By providing sufficient space, proper facilities and company of the animal's own kind
- **Freedom from Fear and Distress**
  By ensuring conditions and treatment that avoid mental suffering

Environmental requirements

All animal accommodation must be soundly constructed to provide conditions that will ensure suitable temperature, humidity and ventilation. All animals should be clean, dry and comfortable at all times. (See also specific requirements for kennels and catteries later in the chapter.)

Temperature

Animals must be protected from extremes of temperature. Very old and very young animals, which are more sensitive to changes in temperature, may require provision of heating or cooling. The temperature of accommodation for dogs and cats should not be allowed to drop below 7°C and the temperature in the sleeping area should not be allowed to drop below 10°C. It is often excess temperatures that are more difficult to control, but the temperature of the accommodation should not exceed 26°C unless there is access to a shaded area where the animal can seek cooler temperatures (Figure 12.1).

Adult dogs	7–26°C Should not drop below 7°C Sleeping area should be at least 10°C
Adult cats	10–26°C
Hospital and isolation kennels	18–23°C
Whelping/kittening and neonate accommodation	Parturition area: 18–21°C Neonates: • First week 26–29°C • Second week 21–26°C • Until weaning 20°C

12.1 Environmental temperatures for housing cats and dogs.

Lighting

Lighting should be as similar to the duration and intensity of natural conditions as possible. Sunlight is the preferred means of lighting for birds and mammals, provided that shaded areas are available. Artificial lighting is necessary to allow the animal housing to be thoroughly cleaned and animals to be checked.

Ventilation

Ventilation should be adequate to keep animal housing areas free from dampness, noxious odours and draughts. Fans should not be placed near windows because air would just travel in a small circle and would not reach the rest of the room. Under normal conditions four to eight air changes should take place per hour but the rate can be increased depending on weather conditions, occupancy, presence of disease, being in isolation units or other considerations.

Bedding

Beds and bedding offer warmth, comfort, security, protection and absorbency and represent the animal's own territory whilst in the kennel or hospital environment. The bedding area should be large enough to enable the animal to stretch out but small enough to ensure that it feels secure. Properties of a good bedding material include:

- Good insulator
- Soft and comfortable
- Absorbs body fluids to keep the animal dry
- Non-irritant and presenting no harm to the animal
- Easy to launder and disinfect
- Easy to store
- Does not damage or soil the animal's coat
- Economical – durable, long-lasting, reusable, inexpensive and difficult to chew or tear.

The advantages and disadvantages of different bedding materials are considered in Figure 12.2.

Type of bed/bedding	Use	Advantages	Disadvantages
Acrylic veterinary bedding	Veterinary surgeries, kennels, domestic	Easy to launder
Absorbs body fluids into bottom layer leaving top layer dry for the animal to lie on
Supportive
Does not harbour parasites
Long-lasting/durable	Expensive
May be chewed
Blankets	Domestic, kennels	Warm	Expensive
Difficult to launder and dry
May be chewed
May harbour dust mites
Expensive unless donated
Several layers needed for comfort
Easily saturated with urine
Bean bags, acrylic-filled beds	Domestic	Comfortable
Supportive
Good insulators	Easy to chew
Expensive
Difficult to launder
Easily saturated with urine
Covered foam pads	Veterinary surgeries for recumbent animals	Comfortable
Warm
Supportive – excellent for recumbent animals	May be chewed
Difficult to clean
Shredded paper	Small mammals	Comfortable
Allows nesting behaviour
Absorbent
Does not harbour parasites
Cheap	Not very warm
Straw, hay	Small mammals	Comfortable
Warm
Allows nesting behaviour	Not very absorbent
May harbour parasites and *Aspergillus* spores (may cause respiratory problems)
Expensive
Acrylic/nylon wadding	Small mammals	Comfortable
Warm
Does not harbour parasites	Not very absorbent
Expensive
May constrict around limbs
Newspaper	Lining of kennels/cages	Very absorbent
Usually free of charge	Not comfortable unless shredded
Urine may be drawn across paper
Animals may eat/rip
May dirty pale coats
Sawdust	Base of small mammal cages
Not for hospitalized animals – impractical to change and observe animal and may stick to wounds	Comfortable
Allows tunnelling and nesting
Warm
Absorbent	Expensive
May harbour parasites
May emit turpens, which irritate mucous membranes
Pre-sterilized peat	Base of small mammal cages
Not for hospitalized animals – impractical to change and observe animal and may stick to wounds	Comfortable
Warm
Allows tunnelling and nesting
Does not harbour parasites
Very absorbent
Reduces odours	Expensive

12.2 Types of bedding.

General principles of kennel and cattery management

Managers of animal boarding establishments are responsible for:

- Providing accommodation and facilities to suit the physical and behavioural requirements of the animals held
- Providing protection for the animals in their care from adverse natural or artificial environmental conditions, other animals and interference from the general public
- Providing sufficient space for animals to stand, move around freely, stretch fully and rest
- Providing sufficient and appropriate exercise for the requirements of the animal
- Providing sufficient quantities of appropriate feed and water to maintain good health
- Protecting animals as far as possible from disease, distress or injury
- Providing prompt veterinary or other appropriate treatment in cases of disease or injury
- Maintaining the hygienic status of the premises and the health of the animals
- Directly or indirectly supervising daily feeding and watering, and inspecting the animals to ensure their welfare
- Providing adequate training and supervision of staff
- Collating and maintaining relevant records.

Licensing

The location and construction of animal boarding establishments must comply with local government requirements. Boarding kennels are licensed by local councils on an annual basis as required by The Animal Boarding Establishments Act 1963. A licence will be granted at the discretion of the local authority and will only be granted if:

- Animals will, at all times, be kept in accommodation suitable in respect of construction, size of quarters, number of occupants, exercising facilities, temperature, lighting, ventilation and cleanliness
- Animals will be adequately supplied with suitable food, water and bedding material, adequately exercised, and (so far as necessary) visited at suitable intervals
- All available precautions will be taken to prevent and control the spread of infectious or contagious diseases among animals, including the provision of adequate isolation facilities
- Appropriate steps will be taken for the protection of the animals in case of fire or other emergency
- A register will be kept containing a description of any animals received into the establishment, date of arrival and departure, and the name and address of the owner. The register must be available for inspection at all times by an officer of the local authority or veterinary surgeon.

A licence does not have to be sought if accommodation is provided for other people's animals in connection with a business of which the accommodation is not the main activity (though this will change with the new Animal Welfare Bill; see Chapter 3). Therefore, there may be premises that are run without proper concern and there is currently no power under the law to inspect premises where owners have not applied for a licence. Veterinary staff are advised not to recommend boarding establishments to clients without having knowledge of or having visited the premises themselves. Clients should be advised to inspect a premises and ask questions of the owner or manager of the kennels or cattery to ensure that they feel confident about the establishment before leaving their pet in its care.

Location

Animal boarding establishments should be located in an area that is not subject to flooding and where they are accessible to members of the public but away from sources of noise and pollution that are likely to cause injury or stress to the animals and far enough away from residential areas to minimize complaints regarding the noise from barking dogs.

Sharing of facilities

Generally there should be no sharing of facilities, except where written agreement is obtained from the keeper of animals from the same household. No more than three cats from the same household should be housed together.

Strays should only be boarded following licensing approval and then kept separately from other boarded animals.

Animal identification

All animals must be clearly identified. Records that must be kept for each animal admitted for boarding include:

- The animal's name
- The owner's name, address and telephone number
- The emergency/contact telephone number of the owner or the owner's nominee
- A description of the animal, including:
  - Sex
  - Breed or type
  - Colour
  - Age
  - Distinguishing features
  - Date of admission
  - Expected date of collection
  - Details of medical, dietary, bathing and grooming requirements
  - The animal's condition and, when possible, its weight on arrival
  - Any collar, leads or belongings brought in with the animal
  - Vaccination status
  - Name and contact number of the veterinary surgeon who normally attends to the animal.

Hygiene and safety

Disease control

Disease control involves the consideration of many issues in kennel design and operation, including:

- Construction
- Disinfection
- Vaccination
- Communal exercise area
- Isolation facilities
- Efficient ventilation

- Rodent control
- Veterinary surgeon (call at first signs of disease)
- First aid kits
- Emergency medications
- Muzzles
- Protective barriers between units.

Cleaning and disinfection

Animal housing and exercise areas must be cleaned and disinfected so that the comfort of animals can be maintained and disease controlled. Excreta must be removed as necessary. Kennels should be cleaned out and disinfected at least once daily. Cleaning and disinfecting agents should be chosen on the basis of their suitability, safety and effectiveness. Manufacturer's instructions for the use of these agents should be followed. After cleaning, animal housing areas should not be allowed to remain wet. Poor ventilation and humidity increases the spread of kennel cough.

Pest control

Efforts must be made to control pests, including flies and wild rodents, effectively. Some pesticides and rodenticides are toxic to dogs and cats and should be used with extreme care. If chemicals are used, they must only be used according to the manufacturer's instructions. All animals must be completely excluded from that part of the facility until the poison programme is complete.

Waste disposal

Waste disposal must be in accordance with the requirements of the local authority. Solid waste must be collected from all parts of the facility and be disposed of in a suitable fashion (see Chapter 1).

Emergencies/fire

An adequate plan must be provided to cover emergency measures. All staff should be aware of the plan. A sign should be displayed referring anyone to an emergency contact if nobody is present at the facility. Fire extinguishers should be placed at easily accessible places, and fire exits should be clearly marked.

Welfare

Vaccination

Dogs and cats must be vaccinated before admission. A current vaccination certificate (i.e. certifying that the vaccination was done within the preceding 12 months) must be produced. Dogs and cats under 4 months old should not be admitted for boarding other than in exceptional circumstances, and then preferably held in isolation. All risks must be explained to the owner prior to admittance. Dogs and cats should be treated for internal and external parasites before admission.

Observation of animals

Each animal should be checked at least once daily to monitor its health and comfort. Any change in health status should be reported promptly to the animal boarding establishment manager.

Veterinary services

The boarding establishment manager should establish liaison with a veterinary surgeon to attend the premises whenever required. Veterinary attention must be sought for any animal showing signs of disease. The animal's insurance cover should be known.

Isolation

Animals known or suspected to be suffering from a contagious disease should not be admitted for boarding, other than in exceptional circumstances. They must be held in isolation facilities.

An infected animal should never be admitted into a kennels where no separate, specific isolation facilities exist. The usual reason for providing these facilities in kennels and catteries is to enable the isolation of animals that have developed suspicious symptoms after they have been admitted, since by then this will be the only course of action to protect the other animals housed.

The recommended rate for isolation is at least one isolation kennel per 50 dogs and one isolation kennel per 30 cats. Isolation kennels must be separate from the main kennels and are usually physically separated by at least 5 m (this distance is based upon the distance that a dog sneeze travels). In existing catteries there must be a minimum of 3 m physical separation from the main cat accommodation units. Cat isolation cages should have solid rather than wire mesh doors to act as sneeze-barriers. Where new kennels and catteries are being built it is recommended that isolation facilities are built 10 m from the main accommodation units.

Animals that have been in contact with a contagious case should be isolated from both the contagious case and the healthy animals. Veterinary advice should be sought in the management of specific outbreaks of disease. Facilities should be designed in such a way to prevent cross-infection and to be easily cleaned and disinfected, i.e. non-porous kennel surfaces, minimal equipment kept within the facility, washing facilities available at the entrance to the facility, protective clothing available etc.

Further practical details are given in 'Isolation procedure' later in this chapter.

Animals receiving medication

The boarding establishment must follow all written medication protocols they are given, unless they receive advice from a veterinary surgeon to change them. The type of drug (name, amount and description) should be noted on the animal's reception card along with details of the veterinary surgeon who prescribed the medication. The staff member administering the medication must record that each treatment has been administered (what and when) and a permanent record of this must be kept for reference purposes.

Nutrition

Sufficient food of adequate nutritional value must be supplied daily to every animal. Fresh water should always be available.

The manufacturer's instructions should be adhered to for the feeding of commercial food. Details of any special feeding requirements should be obtained from owners on admission of the animal. Owners can be encouraged to bring the pet's usual food if the kennel/cattery does not stock it.

Food should be prepared hygienically in a separate kitchen area (Figure 12.3a). It should be stored appropriately, e.g. dry food should be kept in a rodent-free place and fresh meat kept refrigerated (Figure 12.3b).

Food and water bowls should preferably be solid, heavy containers that are chew-proof and not prone to spillage. They must be readily accessible and cleaned at least daily.

Where dogs leave food uneaten, the food should be removed and disposed of promptly so that it does not spoil or attract vermin or flies.

Ideally, cats should be offered their daily food requirements (divided into small portions) several times a day.

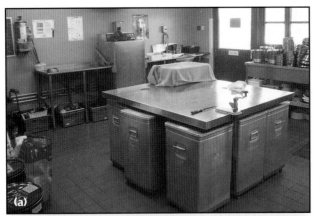

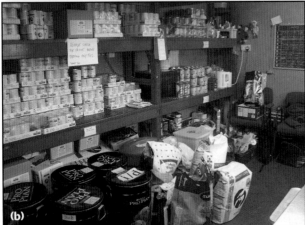

12.3   **(a)** Separate kitchen area. **(b)** Food storage area.

Exercise

Dogs must have the opportunity for exercise to:

- Allow them to urinate and defecate
- Give them contact with humans and, if appropriate, with other dogs
- Allow muscular activity
- Allow staff to monitor the dog's gait and behaviour.

Exercise can be provided by:

- Allowing dogs access to an exercise area for at least 15 minutes twice daily (Figure 12.4); and/or
- Walking dogs on a lead for at least 15 minutes twice daily.

Very active dogs may require more and old dogs less exercise than specified above.

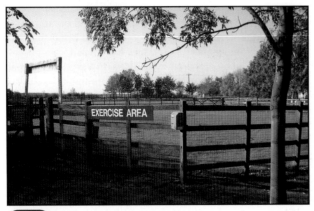

12.4   Dog-exercising area.

Cats must have sufficient room to enable them to stretch and to move about freely. Cats should be monitored for gait and mobility.

Unclaimed animals

Animal boarding establishments should have a policy for dealing with unclaimed animals, giving owners a reasonable opportunity to collect boarded animals.

Staff

All staff should respect the animals and have experience in their handling. They should be aware of their responsibilities and competent to carry them out. Cats and dogs require frequent human contact and time should be spent with each animal.

Kennel and cattery unit design

Construction materials

The advantages and disadvantages of the many different materials used for the construction of kennel and cattery units are considered in Figure 12.5.

Material	Advantages	Disadvantages
Concrete	Indestructible Easily cleaned if sealed and good drainage system Cool in summer Easily laid Relatively inexpensive	Uncomfortable Planning permission required Cold in winter Takes a long time to dry after cleaning Porous if unsealed
Wood	Inexpensive Warm Easy construction Movable	Not long-lasting or durable Requires maintenance Destructible Difficult to clean and disinfect (cross-infection risk) Not escape-proof
Fibreglass	Easy to clean Warm Indestructible Durable Minimal maintenance required	Expensive Installation difficult Some disinfectants may cause damage
Stainless steel	Easy to clean Durable Indestructible Minimal maintenance required	Expensive Cold Noisy Installation difficult
Tiles	Indestructible	Cold Difficult to clean Tiles may crack Slippery when wet Expensive to install
Glass	Easy to clean Allows natural light in	Expensive (glass should be toughened and double glazed) Breakable
Brick	Insulating Strong Easily built Can paint to seal	Porous (harbours bacteria) Difficult to clean Not chew-proof
Breeze blocks	Inexpensive Durable Good sound-proofing Insulating	Porous (harbours bacteria) Difficult to clean Rough Unattractive
Plastic	Warm Inexpensive Easy to clean	Not very strong Dogs may chew Some disinfectants may damage

12.5   Types of construction material.

Flooring

Floors of the animal housing areas of kennels and catteries should be made of an impervious material to facilitate cleaning and drainage. Sealed concrete is ideal.

Drainage

Proper drainage is vital. Solid easy-to-clean channels without covers are recommended. Covered drains gather dirt and are difficult to clean. Kennel and cattery floors should be sloped to enable waste and water to run off.

Size of animal units

Animal housing areas must provide at least enough space for each animal to feed, sleep, sit, lie with limbs extended, stretch and move around. The recommended kennel sizes for short-term housing of dogs are shown in Figure 12.6 and those for cats in Figure 12.7.

Size of dog	Height of unit	Exercise area (floor area)	Sleeping area (floor area)
Up to 60 cm at shoulder	1.85 m	2.46 m²	1.9 m²
Over 60 cm at shoulder	1.85 m	3.35 m²	1.9 m²

12.6   Recommended sizes of kennel units for short-term housing.

Number of cats	Height of unit	Exercise area (floor area)	Sleeping area (floor area)
One cat	1.85 m	1.7 m²	0.85 m²
Up to three cats	1.85 m	3.0 m²	1.5 m²

12.7   Recommended sizes of cattery units for short-term housing.

Kennels

Kennels must be separated by either solid partitions or chain-wire dividers. The partitions must not allow the animals to have physical contact with each other, where injury or cross-infection may occur. Any mesh or chain-wire must be of sufficient strength to contain the animals. Mesh size should not exceed 50 mm square and wire should be of at least 2 mm in diameter.

Kennels should be designed for ease of cleaning and control of disease and the internal surfaces with which animals have contact must be constructed of impervious, solid, washable materials. Joints and corners should be properly sealed (Figure 12.8).

All kennels should be provided with a raised sleeping area covered with a dry, soft bedding material (Figure 12.9).

Catteries

Cats should have access to an exercise area twice daily for a period of no less than 1 hour (Figure 12.10). Each cat unit should include a night box, to allow the cat to withdraw (Figure 12.11a). Cats often feel safer if allowed to retreat to higher ground; they may be housed in an area where the bedding is off the ground and accessed via a ladder, which is more economical of space and encourages climbing, which forms part of a cat's natural behaviour (Figure 12.11b). Scratching posts, toys etc. provide exercise and prevent boredom.

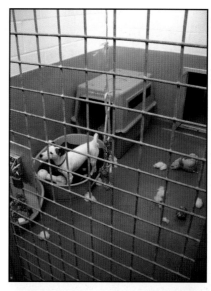

12.8   Kennel designed for easy cleaning, with sealed joints and corners.

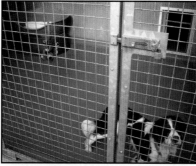

12.9   Kennel with a raised sleeping area.

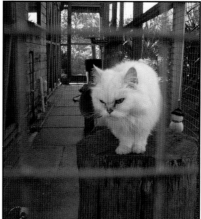

12.10   View of cat exercise area.

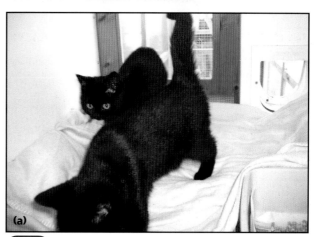

(a)

12.11   (a) Night box for cats.

continues ▶

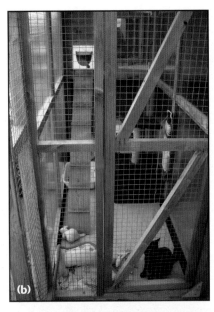

12.11

continued
(b) Cat's ladder access to off-the-ground bedding area.

Cats must be provided with litter trays. Sufficient suitable litter material, such as commercial cat litter, untreated sawdust or shredded paper, should be provided. Litter should be changed and litter trays cleaned and disinfected at least daily.

Heating

Heating and insulation are required in kennel buildings to:

- Provide warmth and comfort to the animals
- Allow rapid drying following cleaning and disinfection
- Lower the risk of respiratory diseases by reducing condensation
- Provide comfortable working conditions for staff
- Prevent damage caused by frost or damp.

The use of a maximum/minimum thermometer helps in assessing the variations in temperature throughout the day.

There are many methods of heating that can be used to heat whole kennel or cattery blocks or individual units. The types of heating and their advantages and disadvantages are considered in Figure 12.12.

Type	Advantages	Disadvantages
Central heating	Easily controlled Safe Use of thermostats ensure minimum temperature kept constant Economical	Expensive to install Requires regular maintenance Additional heat in individual kennels may be necessary Requires suitable wall space for fitting Difficult to clean and disinfect
Electric fan-assisted heating/fan heaters	Convenient Rapid-heating effect	Heater should not be placed too close to animal as overheating may occur Noisy Expensive to run Spread of airborne diseases risk increased Move dust around
Total air-conditioning/heating	Temperature easily controlled Animals have no potential contact with heating source Wall space not an issue	Expensive to install Expensive to run
Underfloor heating	Floors dry quickly Very comfortable for animals to lie on	If insulation is poor floors can become very hot Faecal material difficult to remove Expensive to install and repair
Portable radiators	Mobile Cheap to purchase	Take a long time to heat an area Supervision required May be knocked over in a busy area Surface temperature may injure staff or animals if they come into contact Cables must be protected from animals Switches and sockets should be waterproof Sockets in kennels must be covered when not in use
Portable electric fan heaters	Good for boosting the temperature rapidly Emergency back-up if heating system fails Can be controlled individually Heat can be directed towards animals	Heater should not be placed too close to an animal's kennel (overheating) Noisy Expensive to run Spread of airborne diseases risk increased Move dust around Fire risk
Infra-red heating lamp	Easy to install Correct heat can be directed on to animal's sleeping area Produces heat without light Height of lamp can be adjusted to regulate heat reaching the animal Can be controlled by using thermostats	Requires a socket in each kennel – needs to be waterproof and covered when not in use Animals may interfere with cables – risk of electric shock Fire risk Animal may be either too hot or too cold if incorrectly positioned (use a thermostat)
Heated beds/pads	Enjoyed by animals Low constant heat Cheap to buy and run	Damaged by chewing Risk of electric shock (use circuit breaker) Difficult to clean/disinfect Only used for supplementary heat Overheating Burns
Hot-water bottles	Cheap Rapid, direct warmth	Risk of burns/scalds Water cools rapidly Used only as supplementary heat source

12.12 Types of heating.

Lighting

Dogs and cats require light to keep them active during the hours of daylight, providing mental stimulation and avoiding boredom. It is preferable to use natural sources of light wherever possible and to supplement with artificial lighting when needed. Artificial lighting is usually used in addition to natural lighting to facilitate procedures and observation, but it should be noted that artificial lighting produces heat and may cause overheating during hot summer months.

The most common type of lighting is fluorescent strip lights with diffusers to avoid shadows. Hanging light bulbs are not recommended. All electricity cables should be encased to keep them waterproof and they should be made inaccessible to animals. Waterproof switches and sockets should be used.

During the night, lighting should be dimmed to allow the animals to rest. Most prefer to sleep in a darkened area and cats often prefer to eat when it is dark. The use of screens or blinds may need to be considered for animal housing areas that receive a lot of natural light or direct sunlight, as animals may find it difficult to rest or may become restless very early in the morning. Direct sunlight can cause overheating in summer months.

Ventilation

Good ventilation is vital in kennels and catteries for four reasons:

- To provide clean air for staff and animals by removing odours, fumes (ammonia) and gases (expired carbon dioxide)
- To reduce the risk of cross-contamination of airborne infections
- To control humidity
- To assist in temperature regulation.

There are two types of ventilation: passive and active.

Passive ventilation

Fresh air is provided by opening windows, doors and vents. This is an ineffective method of ventilation when used alone within a kennel or cattery environment: there is no control over the number of air changes per hour, draughts are caused, heat will be lost (which is not economical) and there is the risk of animals escaping.

Active ventilation

Active ventilation actively 'pulls in' fresh air and forces out stale air. This dramatically reduces the risk of cross-infection of airborne disease but does not rule it out, so an animal suspected of having an infection that can be passed via the airborne or aerosol route should always be isolated. Active ventilation can be achieved by extractor fans or air-conditioning systems.

Extractor fans can be set to draw air out of or into the unit. Alternatively passive vents can be used in conjunction with extractor fans: if extractor fans are set to draw air in, passive vents will let air escape because a positive air pressure within the building or area will be caused. If extractor fans are set to suck air out of the building or area, passive vents will allow air in because a negative air pressure will be caused. The movement of air within the facility and individual areas should be carefully considered and ideally be designed to pass fresh air over individual animals and then extract the air from the building before it can be inhaled by other animals.

With **air-conditioning systems**, induction vents actively push air into each individual kennel unit from an external 'clean' source. The air is then actively extracted by another vent immediately outside the unit (for example, in a corridor). The efficacy of air-conditioning units is reduced by the opening of windows and doors. Air-conditioning units can be incorporated into a heating system so that the exact temperature required can be set. The humidity level can also be controlled. These units are very useful when considering optimum housing conditions for different species, though they are expensive to install and run.

Noise

Design, construction and management of kennels should be such as to minimize noise levels. Dogs should be separated visually to discourage barking at each other (Figure 12.13).

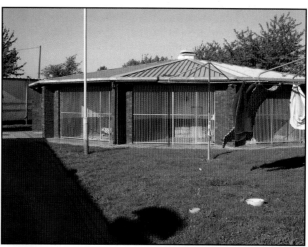

12.13 Parasol kennel. As the dogs cannot see each other, they are less likely to bark.

Cats should be housed away from dogs as they may be disturbed by the barking. Noise barriers such as earth banks and tree belts may be helpful and the site should be large enough to limit any noise disturbance. Double doors and double-glazed windows will also limit noise; acoustic tiles may also be used.

Security

Kennel and cattery buildings must be kept locked when nobody is in attendance. Each individual kennel, cat cage, module or colony must be fitted with a secure closing device that cannot be opened by the animals held. Where dogs are boarded, a security barrier at least 3 m high should be constructed to prevent the escape of animals or unauthorized entry.

The kennel compound wall may form part of the security barrier. In the case of cats, all buildings in which animals are housed should be fitted with double doors to prevent the loss of any animals that may escape from cages or other facilities.

Other facilities

Each boarding establishment must provide:

- An area for reception
- An area for records storage
- Washing and toilet facilities for staff
- Hygienically maintained facilities for bathing, drying and grooming animals
- An area suitable for cleaning and disinfecting food and water bowls and any other equipment used in the preparation of food
- A hygienic food storage area where there is no risk of contamination of the food by vermin or spoilage by other organisms, and refrigerator space for foods that are likely to spoil at ambient temperatures.

Specialized animal housing

Hospital kennelling

Hospital kennels are specifically designed for short-stay patients that are undergoing surgery or treatment. It is for this purpose that the kennels are restrictive to ensure strict rest and allow good observation. Separate accommodation for hospital patients from any animals being groomed or boarded is recommended.

The RCVS Practice Standards Scheme states that in-patient facilities must be of a suitable size, securable, sturdy, escape-proof, without potentially injurious faults and easily cleanable. Ideally kennels or cages, and their fittings, should be made of non-permeable materials so as to be easily cleaned and disinfected.

There must be adequate heating, lighting and ventilation of the hospitalization area. A range of bedding, feedstuffs and clean fresh water must be available. There should be facilities for hospitalization of the full range of species and size of animals routinely admitted. Walk-in kennels should be available for the hospitalization of large-breed dogs.

Informed consent should be sought for all procedures for which an animal is admitted into a veterinary hospital. The veterinary hospital should also provide accommodation and have a written policy for the isolation of contagious cases.

Figure 12.14 shows the minimum recommended sizes for hospital kennels.

Animal	Height (cm)	Width (cm)	Depth (cm)
Cat	45.72	45.72	72.39
Small dog	45.72	60.96	72.39
Medium dog	76.20	76.20	72.39
Large dog	76.20	121.92	72.39
Giant dog	91.44	152.40	72.39
Walk-in kennel	180	140	110

12.14 Minimum recommended sizes of hospital kennel units.

Whelping accommodation

People owning two or more bitches that are actively breeding at any one time and who are making financial gain need a dog breeding licence. The kennels must be inspected and licensed by the local council. The kennels must have a suitable whelping area included in the design.

Special considerations for whelping

- Small enough for the bitch to feel secure in, yet not too small
- Quiet and away from ringing telephones and other barking dogs
- Warm and comfortable, with bedding in which the bitch can make a nest
- Additional heating provided for the puppies (e.g. an infra-red lamp), which the bitch can move away from should she become too warm
- Gives privacy for the bitch allows observation

- Ideally a 'cut-out' of one side of the box to prevent the puppies escaping but allowing the bitch to leave the box to urinate and feed
- The bitch and puppies to be under protective isolation, away from other dogs, and hygiene should be of utmost importance
- The whelping area should be escape-proof.

Puppy accommodation

Puppies should be under protective isolation away from other dogs. The accommodation should be escape-proof, with the ability to regulate the temperature of the environment. A stable-type door is ideal, with the bottom half being low enough to allow staff to step over whilst not allowing the puppies to escape.

Dangerous and stray dogs

Accommodation for aggressive animals should be labelled as such to ensure staff safety. Any animal of an unknown disposition should be isolated and observed initially to assess its behaviour. A full history is useful in identifying any specific behaviour traits. Any procedure or behaviour likely to cause aggressive behaviour in an animal should be well communicated to all staff. Staff should ensure their own safety at all times.

It should be remembered that dogs which are extremely friendly and non-aggressive under normal conditions may become aggressive when stressed, in pain or when kennelled. 'Kennel-guarding' may occur; dogs become territorially aggressive when placed into the confines of a kennel. In a veterinary hospital it is recommended that all kennelled dogs are fitted with a collar before being put into a kennel. This makes it easier for staff to remove the animal from the kennel should kennel-guarding occur. In some practices, dogs will be attached to their kennel door via the use of a long length of indestructible metal chain to ensure that the dog can be removed from the kennel.

Security is very important when housing aggressive animals and access to the kennels and runs should ideally be from separate service passages with double doors to ensure that the animal does not escape (Figure 12.15). Staff should be provided with a means of personal communication, such as walkie-talkies or mobile-phones, so that they can obtain assistance if necessary.

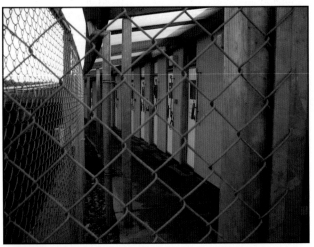

12.15 Double-doored separate service passage for access to kennels and runs.

Exotic pets

Rabbits

Rabbit accommodation should be large enough to enable the rabbit to stand on its hindlimbs without its ears touching the top and of a good size to enable the rabbit to exercise and display normal behaviour. A hutch with access to a grass run is often used. The accommodation should ideally incorporate access to grazing for a period every day. Some owners keep their rabbits inside but the pets should only be allowed to run loose in the house when supervised, as they may chew electrical cables. At other times they can be housed in a secure hutch or pen indoors. The accommodation should provide protection from predation and extremes of heat; temperatures should be kept below 26°C. A darkened area or sleeping box allows the rabbit to retreat and feel secure. Nesting material should be provided for females. There should be a litter tray; rabbits easily learn to use one and it makes the accommodation much more hygienic and easier to clean. The housing area should be well ventilated. Rabbits can be provided with toys, tubes, tunnels and apple wood to gnaw on to enrich their environment and prevent boredom (Figure 12.16; note the channel drain for ease of cleaning).

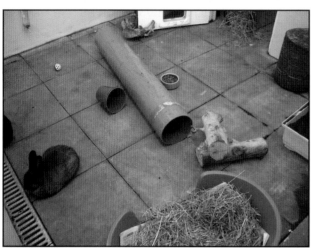

12.16 Enriched environment in accommodation for a rabbit.

Guinea pigs

Guinea pigs should have separate summer and winter accommodation. They are particularly sensitive to damp conditions and it is best to house them indoors in winter. Indoor cages should allow at least 0.2 m² of floor space per animal. In summer a mobile run, provided that they have access to a dry covered area, is ideal. Pens should be at least 30 cm high to avoid escape and should be covered to prevent predation. A sleeping/nest area with bedding material should always be provided, as well as lots of places for the guinea pigs to hide and retreat to. Temperatures between 12°C and 20°C are ideal, and extremes of temperature should be avoided.

Chinchillas

Accommodation should allow for plenty of exercising. Tall multi-level cages with plenty of branches work well. The cages should be made from wire mesh, as chinchillas love to chew. At least half of the cage's mesh floor should be covered with wood or toughened glass to lessen the pressure on their feet. Newspaper or wood shavings can be placed over the wire mesh.

A wooden nest box should be provided and the enclosure placed somewhere that is quiet during the day, as chinchillas are nocturnal, and this is when they will rest. Chinchillas have a unique grooming habit and should be provided with access to a dust bath containing chinchilla sand deep enough for the animal to roll around in every day (Figure 12.17). Removing the bath after use keeps it clean of urine and faeces. Branches should be provided for chewing, which helps to keep teeth filed down. A pumice stone is also useful for chewing.

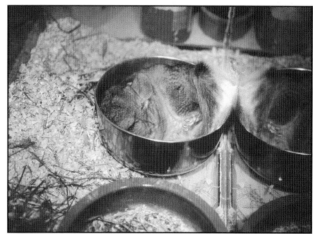

12.17 Shallow bowls of dust give chinchillas an opportunity for a spinning dust bath. (Reproduced from *BSAVA Manual of Exotic Pets, 4th edition*)

Rats, mice, hamsters and gerbils

Rats and mice enjoy climbing and so the accommodation should be tall and provide plenty of opportunity for this. A large aquarium with a wire lid to provide adequate ventilation may be used. Branches may be provided for them to chew as well as climb.

Hamsters can also be built an interesting environment in a large aquarium (Figure 12.18). Commercial hamster accommodation is available but it should be ensured that this is large enough, chew-proof and adequately ventilated.

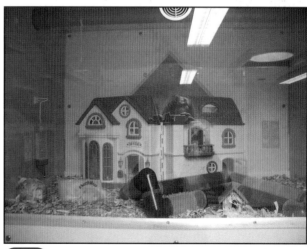

12.18 Aquarium-style hamster accommodation.

Gerbils are ideally housed in an aquarium half-filled with a mixture of peat and straw and furnished with branches, allowing them to dig, chew and explore. Alternatively, the aquarium may be deep littered with shavings, which has the advantage of making soiled bedding easier to see.

Cages should be escape-proof and gnaw-resistant, and should always be well ventilated. Suitable substrates to line the cage include dust-free commercial pet bedding or paper-based cat litter.

All of the small mammals should be provided with a sturdy nest box containing nesting material (shredded paper is preferable to acrylic bedding). Small mammals also appreciate lots of places to hide and retreat to and so their environment should be enriched in this way (Figure 12.19; note also the ventilation considerations of this accommodation).

If exercise wheels are used only solid-bottomed wheels should be provided, to prevent fractured limbs.

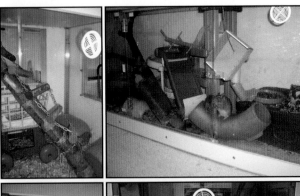
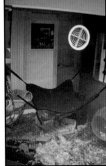
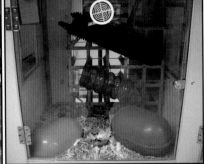

12.19 Accommodation suitable for small mammals. Note the ventilation system in each unit.

Chipmunks

Chipmunks do not really do very well in captivity and they develop stereotypical behaviours in anything but the largest enclosures. The best accommodation is a large, secure outdoor enclosure that they can't dig or chew their way out of. Due to their origin, they cope easily with cold temperatures, but they need shelter from hot days and should be provided with a nest box to retreat to. They should be kept in dry and draught-free conditions with plenty of branches to climb and opportunity to dig burrows. Their enclosures should be escape-proof. Enclosures for chipmunks should be sited well away from televisions, strip lighting or computer terminals that may emit 50 Hz wavelength radiation, as this frequency can induce manic neurological behavioural problems in this species.

Ferrets

Ferrets may be housed indoors or outdoors but should be protected from temperatures above 26°C. They need protection from the rain and draughts, somewhere dry to sleep and plenty of things to prevent boredom, such as tunnels, toys, branches, things to hide in (e.g. tubes and boxes). They are not good climbers but are very good at burrowing and escaping through small holes. Ferrets quickly learn to use a litter-tray. The construction of the cage should ensure an impervious surface, as urine and faeces are strong-smelling.

Birds

Birds should be ideally housed in cages that allow free movement and, in the case of smaller birds, flight. The minimum legal requirement is that the bird should be able to stretch its wings in all three dimensions.

Natural wood perches are best (Figure 12.20) but should be replaced regularly. Sandpaper perch coverings should be avoided, as these can abrade the feet and lead to secondary foot infections.

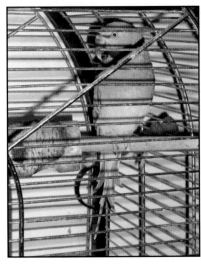

12.20 Birdcage with wooden perches.

Bathing facilities should be supplied or the bird should be sprayed regularly.

Caged birds benefit from exposure to either natural ultraviolet (UV) or artificial UV light on a daily basis; specific UV lights are available for indoor birds.

A nest box is often appreciated and cages should be covered at night to allow rest.

Birds should not be kept in the same room as gas fires or in the kitchen, where fumes can cause respiratory problems. These include fumes from Teflon-coated pots and pans, released when the utensils are allowed to become overheated; although these cannot be detected by humans they are rapidly lethal to birds. It is also not recommended that birds be kept by people who smoke.

The cage should ideally be placed high up or at least to the side of the room. The cage should not be so filled with toys that the bird cannot move, but birds often appreciate a few toys and these can be rotated so that the bird does not become bored with them. Parrots are very destructive and their toys should be the tough acrylic type available.

Food and water containers should be placed where the bird can reach them easily and cannot defecate in them. Whether the species normally feeds on or off the ground should be taken into consideration.

Aviaries

Birds may be kept in aviaries. Aviaries should have deep foundations or a solid concrete base and wire covering the bottom of the aviary to protect against rats and mice. A frost-free shelter should be provided, with provision for heating and lighting the shelter during the winter months. Solid roofing material will reduce the possibility of disease spread from wild birds and a safety (double) door will reduce the possibility of escapes. The environmental conditions required by each species should be researched before attempting to provide housing, so that these conditions can be accommodated. These will depend upon where the birds come from, their natural habitat and the climate.

Reptiles

Reptiles are housed in a controlled environment known as a vivarium (Figure 12.21). The important points to consider when setting up a vivarium are heating, lighting, humidity, ventilation, structure and furnishing.

Heating

A temperature gradient should be provided across the vivarium. The range should be maintained within the inhabitant's preferred optimum temperature zone (POTZ) to enable the reptile to maintain its preferred body temperature (PBT).

12.21 Reptile environments: **(a)** clinical; **(b)** arboreal; **(c)** semi-aquatic.

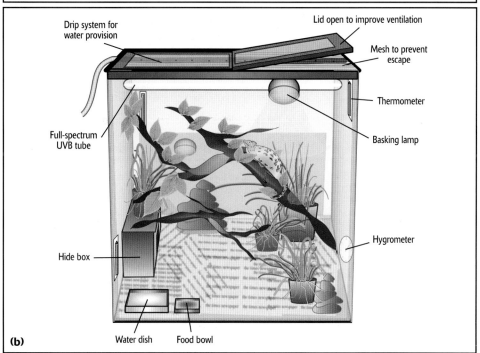

(a)

Solid back and sides are best

Ventilation grille

Thermometer

Hide box for privacy

Full-spectrum fluorescent tube accessible from hot and cool ends of tank

Sliding glass doors with locking device

Food bowl

Water dish

Ceramic heat bulb protected by wire cage

OR

Infrared heat pad placed along back of vivarium connected to thermostat

Thermometer

Hygrometer

Substrate of newspaper

(b)

Drip system for water provision

Full-spectrum UVB tube

Hide box

Water dish

Food bowl

Lid open to improve ventilation

Mesh to prevent escape

Thermometer

Basking lamp

Hygrometer

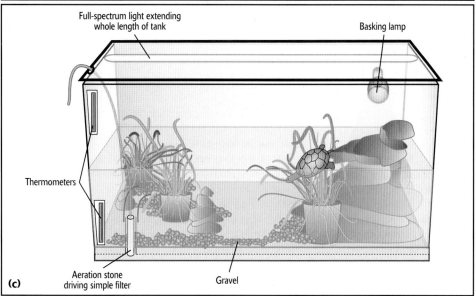

(c)

Full-spectrum light extending whole length of tank

Thermometers

Aeration stone driving simple filter

Gravel

Basking lamp

The heating element should be attached to a thermostat and monitored using a separate maximum–minimum thermometer. Overhead heating is a more natural way of supplying heat than heat-mats but must be shielded from the reptile: thermal burns are common as reptiles often will not move away from a heat source that is actually burning them.

Lighting

Lighting should be of daylight quality for lizards and chelonians, for activity and foraging. Fluorescent tubes that provide a good daylight spectrum, including ultraviolet (UV-B is specifically required to allow synthesis of vitamin D3 in many reptiles and UV-A is required to stimulate some forms of behaviour, such as breeding and in some cases appetite), should be selected and these should be changed every 6 months, as the UV portion of their spectrum has a limited life.

Reptiles from desert habitats will require a higher light intensity than those from forests.

Humidity and water

Powerful heaters tend to dry the atmosphere, and regular spraying with water is required to maintain a reasonable degree of humidity. This should be done regularly, even for desert species, and very often for rainforest species.

A source of water for drinking and bathing should also be provided. It should be noted that many species of reptile (e.g. chameleons and many iguanas) will not drink from bowls, but only from water droplets in the vivarium. This means regular misting of the cage with water, or setting up a drip system to supply continually dripping water, is necessary.

Ventilation

Adequate air vents are essential to ensure good air circulation. If ventilation is poor, an airline powered by a small aquarium pump will encourage the circulation of fresh air.

Structure

Glass or Perspex aquariums are easy to clean but are often extremely heavy. Custom-built vivaria are made out of melamine-covered chipboard (with the corners sealed with aquarium sealant) or fibreglass and generally have front-opening sliding doors to make access easier. They are generally easier to clean.

Furnishing

Arboreal species will require branches for climbing and burrowing species will require sufficient depth of substrate to hide in. Substrates used to line the bottom of the vivarium include bark chippings, peat, aquarium gravel and sand. Sand tends to be used only for desert species of lizard and burrowing species of snake. Sand can cause scale abrasions in snakes.

All species should have hide areas or hide boxes – if possible at least one more hide area than there are reptiles in the tank.

Aquatic or semi-aquatic reptiles and amphibians

The natural history of the species should be researched. It is important when considering housing to know the animal's natural habitat, climate and whether it lives on land, in water or makes use of both.

The requirements for amphibians are similar to those for many aquatic species of reptile. Some amphibians are totally aquatic (e.g. many newts, the axolotl and amphisbaenids); others prefer to have an aquatic and a terrarium area (e.g. many frogs) or just a very moist terrarium (e.g. many members of the toad family).

Aquatic and semi-aquatic species need glass or Perspex aquarium tanks, because of the relatively high level of humidity required. Totally aquatic species need a tank equipped as a fish tank, with good water filtration. Terrestrial species need a vivarium similar to that for a reptile but with increased humidity.

Species that need both land and water need an aqua-terrarium (Figure 12.22). A glass tank may be used and the land area may be provided by using a piece of glass to separate it from the water, sealed with aquarium sealant. The land area is then filled with soil, moss or gravel or by building up rocks within the terrarium to provide a land area. In this case it is difficult to provide live plants and there is no area for egg-laying. The rocks should be set securely and ideally glued so that they do not become dislodged.

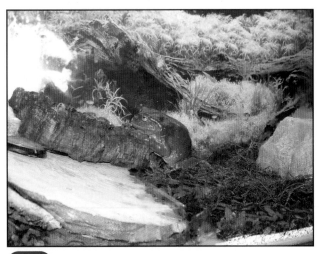

12.22   Frogs will need an aqua-terrarium.

Filtration

Where free water is provided it must be changed regularly, or (preferably) an effective aquarium filtration system should be installed, to minimize the build-up of environmental bacteria. If reptiles require to be fed in the water, it is better to move them into a separate tank for feeding as the volume of detritus produced often exceeds the capacity of most filtration devices.

Heating

Some species require heated water, in which case an aquarium heater should be used. The water area must be deep enough to submerge the heater completely and the heater should be protected from the reptile to prevent injuries.

Some species need to bask out of water and in this case a basking heat source and a UV-emitting fluorescent lamp should be provided over the land area. Supplemental heating is generally not required for most species of amphibian that originate in temperate climes, but a UV light source is still recommended for anurans (frogs and toads) to prevent metabolic bone disease.

If condensation becomes a problem, an air pump with an air line can be installed to keep the glass clear.

Fish

Fish need to be kept in a carefully controlled environment (see *BSAVA Manual of Ornamental Fish, 2nd edition*) and the following aspects are particularly important to consider.

The water for most species of fish should be kept at pH values between 7.0 and 7.5. Water hardness should be over 10 mg/ml for most freshwater fish.

Fish require oxygen either from live plants, diffusion from the surface or by artificial aeration of the water using air pumps. Carbon dioxide is removed from the tank by live plants or the aeration system.

Fish produce ammonia as a waste product of protein metabolism and this needs to be removed from the tank. Ammonia is used by live plants to build protein but if there are no live plants within the aquarium it must be removed by an under-gravel filter. Bacteria break down nitrogenous waste by converting ammonia to nitrite and then to nitrate; these products need to be kept under control by efficient filtration and should be monitored regularly using a water-testing kit. In general, ammonia is most toxic to fish and its toxicity is exacerbated by higher water temperatures. Nitrites are the next most toxic and nitrates are the least toxic of the three waste products.

Wildlife

When housing wildlife, for treatment or rehabilitation, the natural habitat and behaviour of the species should be considered in order to fulfil their basic needs (see *BSAVA Manual of Wildlife Casualties*). The following points should be considered:

* Does the animal nest?
* Is the animal nocturnal or diurnal?
* What temperature does the animal prefer?
* Is the animal arboreal?
* Does the animal perch?
* Can the animal gnaw through bars?

Caging wild animals will cause stress to the animal and steps should be taken to minimize stress wherever possible. They should be housed in a quiet area. Lighting may be subdued and the front of the cage covered to calm them. Wild animals should be handled and disturbed as little as possible whilst still maintaining adequate care. They will appreciate a box or area or plenty of hay or straw to hide in. Birds should be provided with perches and water birds should be provided with a water bowl to bathe in. Bats and swifts will appreciate a towel within the accommodation to hang from. Deer should not be kennelled, as they will panic, but should be housed in a barn away from any noise.

Cleaning and disinfection

Methods of preventing the spread of infection

* Cleaning and disinfection
* Isolation
* Barrier nursing
* Protective clothing
* Quarantine
* Treatment
* Sterilization
* Vaccination
* Prevention
* Improved diet
* Owner compliance
* Hygiene
* Ventilation

Definitions

* **Disinfection** is the removal of microorganisms, but not necessarily all pathogens and their spores (reduction in the number of microbes).
* **Sterilization** is the removal of all microorganisms, including bacterial spores.
* **Disinfectant** is a chemical agent that kills, or prevents the multiplication of, microorganisms on inanimate objects. May be known as an 'environmental disinfectant'.
* **Antiseptic** is a disinfectant safe to use on living tissue. May be known as a 'skin disinfectant'.
* **Antisepsis** is the prevention of sepsis, achieved by disinfection. Usually refers to the prevention of infection in living tissues by the use of an antiseptic.
* **Asepsis** is the exclusion of all microorganisms and spores; a sterile state. Achieved by sterilization.
* **-cide** is a suffix meaning kills (e.g. a bactericide kills bacteria).
* **-stat** is a suffix meaning preventing growth or multiplication (e.g. a bacteriostat prevents further multiplication of bacteria).

Disinfection is a process by which pathogenic microorganisms are destroyed or removed from inanimate objects. It is an important method of controlling the spread of disease within the veterinary practice and is achieved by both physical and chemical actions.

The physical action of scrubbing and cleaning is just as important as the chemical actions of the disinfectants themselves. This is because foreign materials, such as blood and faecal matter, are ideal breeding grounds for pathogens but the efficacy of disinfectants is greatly reduced when used in the presence of organic material. The disinfectants must have direct contact with the microorganisms to destroy them and so the organic materials must first be removed. Only when all the debris has been removed will the actions of the disinfectant be effective. The most efficient method of disinfection is to use **chemical disinfection** following **mechanical cleaning**.

Heating is another method of disinfection and way of achieving antisepsis. Microorganisms are destroyed by high temperatures, e.g. during steam cleaning and machine washing of bedding. The efficacy of chemical disinfectants is also increased by mixing them with warm rather than cold water.

Cleaning a clinical environment

Each area of the practice should be assessed for risk according to the potential for cross-infection. Standard Operating Procedures should then be established for the cleaning and disinfecting of each area according to its risk (Figure 12.23). All staff should be aware of the procedures and potential risks.

* **Low-risk** areas include offices and corridors. They require an easy-to-use product that combines cleaning and disinfection.
* **High-risk** areas include any that may become contaminated by body fluids (e.g. theatres, kennels and consulting rooms).

Standard Operating Procedure for cleaning a kennel
1. Remove animal from kennel to a safe, secure holding area (not another dog's kennel).
2. Remove all items from the kennel (feeding bowls, bedding, toys etc.).
3. Remove any gross contamination.
4. Sweep or hose out any hair or debris.
5. Scrub all surfaces of the kennel (including the door) with a detergent[a].
6. Rinse with water[a].
7. Apply disinfectant at the correct dilution rate[a].
8. Allow for contact time of disinfectant.
9. Rinse thoroughly if applicable.
10. Dry.
11. Leave to air dry.
12. Return/replace bedding etc. as necessary.
13. Return animal to kennel.
14. All feeding bowls, litter trays etc. should be washed in detergent (e.g. washing-up liquid) rinsed, sprayed with or soaked in disinfectant, rinsed and then dried (alternatively, feed bowls may be sterilized using an autoclave or ethylene oxide).
15. Bedding should be machine washed at 60°C (most microorganisms will be destroyed).
16. Mop-heads and cleaning equipment should also be regularly washed and disinfected.

12.23 Example of an SOP for cleaning a kennel.
[a] Many of the more recently developed kennel disinfectants are a combination of specialist detergents and disinfectant agents, mixed by manufacturers as part of the active ingredient formulation. This principle potentiates the activity of the disinfectant and accelerates the microbicidal process. When using these products, follow actions 1–5, using the combined detergent/disinfectant instead of a detergent, and cut out steps 6 and 7.

Certain areas may seem low-risk but the potential for cross-infection is high. An example is the reception area/waiting room – every animal that enters the practice will enter the reception area. Control measures should be put into place: for example, any animal suspected of having a contagious disease should be isolated immediately into a separate area whilst waiting for the veterinary surgeon to attend; and owners of puppies arriving for first vaccinations should be advised not to let them on the floor of the reception area or allow them to mix with the other animals waiting.

High-risk areas should be thoroughly cleaned and disinfected daily using a fast-acting, broad-spectrum disinfectant:

- Areas (surfaces and floors) should first be cleaned using a detergent to ensure the removal of all organic material.
- Walls should be cleaned regularly to a height of 1.5 m with both detergent and disinfectant.
- Mop-heads should be machine washed daily and replaced regularly.
- Surfaces in theatres and consulting room tables should also be cleaned *between* patients; any potential contaminants (hair, body fluids, tissue, contaminated instruments and equipment) should be removed and cleaned or disposed of as appropriate.
- Clipper blades should also be cleaned between patients.
- Throughout the day surfaces and floors should be spot-cleaned if they become soiled.

The use of daily and weekly cleaning checklists is an effective way of ensuring that all tasks are completed in each area and therefore minimizing the risk of cross-infection within the veterinary practice. Figure 12.24 shows an example of such a cleaning checklist.

Consulting room daily cleaning checklist	Date:
Task	Initial when completed
Dispose of clinical and household waste accordingly	
Empty clinical and household waste bins, disinfect bins and replace bin bags	
Clean and disinfect/sterilize any used equipment accordingly	
Wipe all surfaces (including walls to a height of 1.5 m) with detergent	
Wipe all surfaces (including walls as before) with disinfectant	
Clean clippers	
Change hand towel	
Change disinfectant and cotton wool in thermometer pot	
Refill disinfectant spray, surgical spirit and antiseptic bottles	
Restock all consumables	
Vacuum floor	
Mop floor with detergent	
Mop floor with disinfectant	

12.24 Example of a cleaning checklist.

Many practices will use one particular agent for main use. The dilution rate may depend upon the intended use, and the manufacturer's data sheet or instructions for use should always be checked before using any chemical within the veterinary practice. For example, the dilution rate of many disinfectants is halved for high-risk areas (i.e. twice the concentration of disinfectant is used). Too weak a solution will be ineffective, but too strong a solution would be wasteful and may be harmful to animals and personnel.

Types of antiseptic and disinfectant

Disinfectants, by their very nature, are toxic. They are designed to kill organisms. There is no such thing as a completely non-toxic disinfectant. Before choosing any disinfectant, it is important to know what organisms are to be killed. Typically, these organisms are viruses, bacteria, fungi or spores.

Several factors will influence the selection of a particular type of disinfectant or antiseptic:

- Intended use of the product (environment or living tissue, high- or low-risk area)
- Range of activity against microorganisms
- Contact time
- Safety of staff and animals (i.e. how toxic is it?)
- Corrosive/staining effects
- Ease of use
- Cost and economy of the product
- Ability to be mixed with other products without causing unexpected toxicity
- Stability of the product
- Odour.

There are different classes of disinfectants, based on the types of agent they contain. Figure 12.25 gives examples of the different types of disinfectants and antiseptics.

Disinfectant class	Examples
Alcohol	70% Isopropyl alcohol
Biguanides Chlorhexidine	Nolvasan, Savlon, Dinex, Hibiscrub
Cationic surfactants Quaternary ammonium compounds	Vetaclean
Halogens and halogen-containing compounds Chlorine-based Iodine-based Halogenated tertiary amines	Sodium hypochlorite (chlorine bleach), Domestos Iodine, iodophors, povidone–iodine, Betadine Trigene
Oxidizing agents Peroxides Peroxygen compounds	Hydrogen peroxide Virkon, Vetcide
Phenols and related compounds Phenolics Synthetic phenol	Phenol (carbolic acid), Cresol (cresylic acid), Lysol, pine tar, pine oil, Izol, Jeyes Fluid Chloroxylenols; Dettol
Reducing agents Aldehydes	Glutaraldehyde, formaldehyde, Cidex, Parvocide, Formula H

12.25 Types of disinfectant.

Types of agents

Alcohol

Alcohol is very effective against bacteria, fungi and some viruses but is not sporicidal. It is non-penetrating and so the skin needs to be cleaned first. It is often used as the final step in the surgical scrub routine of the patient. It is more expensive but mixes well with other antiseptics. It is flammable and can be irritant as it tends to dry skin.

Chlorhexidine

This has a good action against Gram-positive bacteria but is less effective against Gram-negative bacteria and mycobacteria. It has a variable viral activity with antifungal action. It is inactivated by organic matter, soaps and plastics but is unaffected by body fluids. It is an excellent skin and wound disinfectant and has a residual effect in the tissues.

Quaternary ammonium compounds

These have a good action against Gram-positive bacteria but are less effective against Gram-negative bacteria and have no sporicidal action. They have good fungicidal activity but very limited activity against viruses. They are only really suitable for disinfecting low-risk areas and tend to be inactivated by hard water and organic matter.

Chlorine-based halogens

Hypochlorites (bleach) are very effective against viruses, bacteria, fungi and spores. They are cheap but very corrosive and bleaching may occur. They produce strong vapours that can cause airway irritation. Organic matter reduces their efficacy and they deteriorate with storage and exposure to sunlight. They should not be used in the presence of urine as they can produce a noxious gas when mixed together.

Iodine-based halogens

Iodine and iodophors have a broad spectrum of activity against bacteria, viruses and fungi and some action against bacterial spores. They are inactivated by organic matter and may corrode metal and cause staining. Some people may be allergic to iodine. They are used as skin antiseptics and for open wound cleansing.

Halogenated tertiary amines

These contain a quarternary ammonium compound and have a wide range of action against bacteria, fungi, viruses and bacterial spores. They are not inactivated by organic matter and usually contain a detergent. They are irritant at concentrate level but they are generally of low toxicity and have low corrosion effects.

Peroxygen compounds

Peroxygen compounds have a good range of activity against bacteria (except mycobacteria), viruses and fungi and a variable action against bacterial spores. Their efficacy is reduced in the presence of organic material and they are irritant in powder form. They are corrosive to some metals.

Phenols

Phenolics may be described as black, white or clear. They have good bacterial and fungal activity but a variable efficacy against viruses. They have a poor action against bacterial spores. They are not easily inactivated by organic material. They are toxic and irritant and should not come into contact with skin.

Phenols are irritant, strong smelling and *highly toxic to cats*. They are absorbed by rubber and plastics and may stain. They are cheap to purchase.

Synthetic phenols have a poor action against Gram-negative bacteria and their efficacy is reduced in the presence of organic matter. They are less irritant and can be inactivated by hard water.

Aldehydes

Glutaraldehyde has a wide range of bacterial, fungal and viral activity and is sporicidal but is slow acting. It is not inactivated by organic material. It is highly irritant and highly toxic to skin, eyes and respiratory mucosa. This chemical can also cause sensitization, leading to further health problems with continued exposure. Due to its toxic nature, it is not recommended that this product be used as a wash-down disinfectant and should only be used where the necessary precautions to ensure safety of personnel can be taken.

Susceptibility of microbes to disinfection

Some bacteria are naturally more resistant to certain disinfectants than other bacteria. This is known as **intrinsic resistance**. Other, normally sensitive, bacteria can become resistant after exposure to a disinfectant; this is **acquired resistance**. Some viruses also demonstrate intrinsic resistance to disinfectants, but it is unlikely that viruses would develop acquired resistance under natural conditions. Non-enveloped viruses, such as canine parvovirusand feline calicivirus, are more resistant than enveloped viruses such as feline leukaemia virus and feline herpesvirus.

- Bacterial spores are bacterial 'embryos' surrounded by several different layers that make spores extremely resistant to chemical attack.

- Gram-negative bacteria (e.g. *Salmonella*) have a different type of cell wall which acts as a barrier to some disinfectants and so they tend to be more resistant to some disinfectants than Gram-positive bacteria (e.g. *Staphylococcus*).
- Mycobacteria are even more resistant to disinfectants, because of additional waxy layers in the cell wall.
- Plasmids are bacteria that acquire resistance by mutation or acquisition of extra genetic material.

Figure 12.26 shows the susceptibility of microbes to different types of disinfectant and antiseptic.

Precautions and the safe use of disinfectants

- Read manufacturer's instructions and use as directed.
- Wear protective gloves/clothing and avoid direct contact with skin.
- Only use disinfectants for the purpose recommended by the manufacturer.
- Use the correct dilution according to manufacturer's instructions.
- Add the disinfectant to the container after filling with the correct amount of water (to reduce inhalation of vapours or possibility of direct contact with concentrated disinfectant).
- Use only freshly made solutions.
- Mix with water at the recommended temperature.
- Leave the disinfectant for the recommended contact time.
- Concentrated solutions and powders may be harmful so care must be taken when handling them.
- Keep chemicals in their original containers.
- Ensure that all lids are secured.
- Store away from children and animals.
- Do not mix chemicals.
- Minimize skin splashes.
- When spraying disinfectants use the 'squirt' setting or apply the product with a cloth or sponge to avoid atomizing the disinfectant.
- Only mix enough product as is necessary, to avoid introducing excess material into the sewage system.
- Wash hands thoroughly after use.

Isolation and barrier nursing

Cleaning and disinfection are obviously of utmost importance when nursing a contagious or potentially contagious case and strict procedures should be followed for the nursing and care of these patients and the cleaning and disinfection of the isolation facility to ensure the safety of all the animals within the veterinary practice. The first rule should always be: *if there is any doubt as to whether or not an animal has a contagious disease, it should be isolated immediately, assumed as contagious and treated as such*. If this rule is not followed, then by the time it is established that the patient is potentially contagious, that patient has probably entered and contaminated several areas of the practice, contaminated several personnel and been in contact with other animals within the practice. It follows that all reception staff require adequate training to be able to recognize the signs and symptoms of different contagious diseases. It might be set within practice policy, for example, that any animal presenting for an appointment with vomiting and/or diarrhoea should be isolated until seen by the veterinary surgeon, as these are common symptoms of many contagious diseases.

Definitions

- **Isolation** is the physical separation of the animal suspected of or proved to have a contagious infectious disease, thus eliminating the possibility for contact, direct or indirect, to be made with other susceptible animals, or people if the disease is zoonotic.
- **Quarantine** is the compulsory isolation (with associated strict protocols) of animals with, or potentially exposed to, notifiable diseases.
- **Barrier nursing** describes the methods used when nursing a potentially contagious or infectious animal that create a 'barrier' between the contagious animal and the nursing staff and other animals, thus reducing indirect contact (e.g. wearing protective clothing, using separate equipment for that animal). This is usually carried out in conjunction with isolating the animal but can be employed alone if no isolation facilities exist.

▶

Disinfectant	Bactericidal activity	Effect on bacterial spores	Effect on viruses	Effect on fungi
Alcohol	Good	No	Variable	Good
Chlorhexidine	Gram-positive: yes Gram-negative: less so Poor against mycobacteria	No	Variable	Fair
QACs	Gram-positive: Yes Gram-negative: less so None against *Mycobacterium tuberculosis*	No	Very limited	Yes
Chlorine-based halogens (bleach)	Good	Good	Good	Good
Iodine/iodophors	Good	Some	Good	Good
Halogenated tertiary amines	Good	Good	Good	Good
Peroxygen compounds	Good, but poor against mycobacteria	Variable	Good	Good
Phenols	Good	No	Poor	Good
Aldehydes	Good	Good but slow	Good	Good

12.26 Susceptibility of bacterial, viral and fungal organisms to disinfectant.

- **Protective isolation** is the isolation of very susceptible animals (e.g. very young, very old, after surgery, or with compromised immunity) in an attempt to protect them from potential sources of infection.

Isolation procedure

When an animal is admitted to the hospital suspected of having a contagious disease, it should be isolated immediately, without entering any other rooms within the practice. The isolation facilities should be labelled as being in use, thus preventing the admittance of any other animals into the ward and ensuring that access by staff and the public is restricted.

Visitors should not be allowed into the isolation unit. A method of colour coding might be appropriate so that all staff are immediately aware on glancing at the facility that a contagious case has been admitted. The isolated case should have no contact with other animals.

Equipment for the isolation facility (Figure 12.27) should be collected together so that it is only used within the isolation ward and also to limit the number of times staff have to enter and leave the ward when nursing the patient.

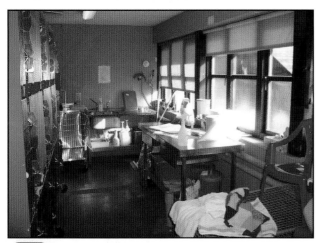

12.27 A self-contained fully-equipped isolation facility.

Necessary equipment within the isolation facility might include the following (this list is not exhaustive):

- Protective clothing, e.g. coveralls, aprons, hoods, clogs, shoe covers, hats, facemasks (for nursing animals with airborne zoonoses, such as psittacosis), gloves etc.
- Food and water bowls and feeding equipment (e.g. cutlery, jug, scales)
- Litter trays and cat litter
- Thermometer
- Cleaning equipment
- Bucket
- Detergent and disinfectant
- Incontinence pads
- Newspaper
- Clinical waste bags.

Ideally, one or two members of the nursing staff should be assigned to nursing the isolation case and, if at all possible, should nurse only that patient, to minimize the potential for indirectly passing the infection to other patients. If it is not possible for those members of staff to nurse only that patient, it must be ensured that the infectious case is nursed and treated last, before the other patients are attended to. Under no circumstances should the same staff nurse both the isolated cases and the very susceptible (i.e. the very young, very old or immunosuppressed).

- A footbath containing a disinfectant effective against the disease being treated should be placed at the entrance to the isolation facility and shoes should be dipped on entering and leaving the isolation ward. The value of this may be minimal, because most disinfectants require a contact-time period to allow the disinfectant to work, and so a change of footwear might be more appropriate.
- Protective clothing should be donned when entering the ward and should ideally be discarded after use.
- Hands should be thoroughly washed with an appropriate antiseptic on leaving the ward and disposable hand towels should be used to dry hands.

Ventilation within the facility must be considered. The unit should be under mild negative pressure (meaning that air will move into the unit when the door is opened, rather than air rushing out into another ward or area of the practice). This can be achieved by the use of extractor fans, with the fan in the isolation ward set to expel air out of the building and the fan in the room adjoining the facility set to draw air inwards. If active ventilation has been installed, the number of air changes per hour should be increased to 12.

After the contagious case has been discharged, a strict cleaning and disinfection regime must be followed. An example of such a routine is as follows:

- Separate cleaning equipment must be used for the isolation facility (e.g. mop and bucket, cloths) and ideally disposed of after use.
- All consumable equipment (newspaper, aprons, gloves, gowns, shoe covers, hats, masks, etc.) should be disposed of as clinical waste and incinerated.
- Ideally all equipment used within the ward should be disposed of, so the use of disposable feeding bowls, gowns/coveralls, bedding (newspaper) etc. is recommended.
- Any equipment that is intended to be re-used should ideally be sterilized or, if this is not possible, soaked for 12 hours in a disinfectant known to be effective against the particular contagious disease and then rinsed.
- Bedding, gowns etc. should then be boil-washed after soaking.
- All surfaces within the ward should be cleaned with disinfectant (including windows, walls, door handles, all kennels, cupboards, sinks, floors etc.) and left to soak for 12 hours.
- All surfaces should then be rinsed and disinfection repeated and left for a further contact time of 12 hours.
- All surfaces should then be rinsed again and allowed to dry.

Further reading

Animal Boarding Establishments Act 1963. Available from the RSPCA

Girling S (2002) *Veterinary Nursing of Exotic Pets.* Blackwell Publishing, Oxford

Meredith A and Redrobe S (2002) *BSAVA Manual of Exotic Pets, 4th edn.* BSAVA Publications, Gloucester

Mullineaux E, Best R and Cooper JE (2003) *BSAVA Manual of Wildlife Casualties.* BSAVA Publications, Gloucester

Stocker L (2004) *Practical Wildlife Care.* Blackwell Science, Oxford

Wildgoose W (2001) *BSAVA Manual of Ornamental Fish, 2nd edn.* BSAVA Publications, Gloucester

Williams D (1998) *Ask The Vet – Exotic Pets.* Lifelearn, Newmarket

Chapter 13

Observation and assessment of the patient

Jennifer Seymour

Learning objectives

After studying this chapter, students should be able to:

- **Describe the procedure for performing a general health check on a hospitalized patient**
- **Recognize the possible causes of abnormalities observed in hospitalized patients**
- **Apply the knowledge of normal and abnormal appearance of animals to evaluate the condition of patients in the surgery**
- **Recognize signs of pain in the hospitalized patient and demonstrate methods of pain relief**

Observation

During the course of a working day veterinary nurses will come into contact with patients that range from healthy animals of many species and temperaments to those that require intensive treatment and nursing procedures. They must recognize the normal and abnormal appearance and behaviour patterns of those in their care, and report all relevant information to the veterinary surgeon. The nurse's observations can give valuable input to the case history of the patient and may assist the veterinary surgeon's diagnosis and subsequent treatment. All observations should be noted and any abnormalities reported immediately.

Dogs and cats in the hospital environment

It should be remembered that each patient is an individual. Signs considered normal for one patient may be abnormal for another. It is necessary, therefore, to become familiar with each animal and to recognize their normal appearance and behaviour patterns.

The veterinary practice is not usually a relaxed environment for dogs, cats or small animals. Patients will be surrounded by faces, smells and sounds unfamiliar to them, and therefore may be expected to behave in an abnormal fashion. Normally placid animals may become nervous and exhibit signs of aggression or submission. Furthermore, these patients are often required to be secured in a small enclosed space from which there is no visible means of escape. When approached by an unfamiliar person the animal may feel threatened and react to the 'flight or fight' instinct by growling or snapping at the perceived threat. Cats, being solitary animals, are particularly inclined to feel stressed away from their home territory and will often resort to attack as their only means of defence.

Fear and anxiety are not conducive to a smooth and speedy recovery. By considering the natural environment and routine of patients, many simple measures may be implemented to reduce stress and provide a calm non-threatening atmosphere.

Guidelines for reducing stress

- Wherever possible, avoid placing cats in cages where they can see and be seen by other patients. If necessary, cover the cage with a blanket, but ensure that regular observation of the patient is maintained.
- Provide cats with the security of somewhere to hide. This is easily achieved by the inclusion of an igloo or cardboard box in the pen.
- Dogs may enjoy the stimulation of everday activity around them, but try to avoid potentially confrontational situations.
- Direct eye contact may be perceived by a dog as a challenging gesture and one that demands an aggressive response. This should be avoided.
- Noise levels should be kept to a minimum and any sudden loud noises should be avoided. Barking dogs should be isolated if practical and returned home as soon as possible.
- Ample provision should be made for urination and defecation. Animals easily become agitated if this is not allowed and are often distressed if they soil their kennel. Cats should always be provided with a litter tray, unless the veterinary surgeon has specifically given other instructions.

- Male dogs can become extremely agitated if kennelled in close proximity to a bitch in season. It is advisable not to admit bitches in oestrus to the veterinary practice unless absolutely necessary.
- A stressed nurse will increase the anxiety of a nervous animal. Providing a calm environment and using a quiet, gentle voice can do much to soothe a frightened patient.
- Ideally, each patient should be monitored and cared for by a specific nurse. This will provide continuity and allow mutual trust to develop.
- The provision of 'TLC' to all patients should be a major priority of the veterinary nurse.

Assessment of the patient

A routine health check of the patient should be performed on admission and regularly throughout its stay in the hospital. The general demeanour, temperament and overall condition of the animal can be assessed before performing a physical examination. Factors such as posture, gait, orientation and respiration may be considered before approaching the patient and this may yield valuable information. Furthermore, these may be evaluated without causing undue stress to the patient.

By looking at the patient 'head on', factors such as ataxia, head tilt or lameness may be observed and breathing abnormalities such as tachypnoea or dyspnoea may be identified. Also the stance of the patient may be viewed to ascertain pain or respiratory distress. Animals with abdominal pain will often assume a 'praying' position in order to relieve their suffering, whereas those with respiratory embarrassment may attempt to increase their lung capacity by abduction of the elbows.

A basic assessment of visual and auditory function may also be considered at this time. The ability of the patient to respond to its environment and external stimuli may be monitored by establishing the response to people, objects and sounds in the vicinity. Patients with visual or auditory impairment may feel especially vulnerable in the hospital environment; therefore particular care should be taken to ensure that any distress or anxiety is minimized.

Normal clinical signs of the healthy animal

- Clean, patent nares and nasal passages
- Stable teeth with absence of tartar
- Pink, moist mucous membranes
- Capillary refill time of 1–2 seconds
- No obstruction of oral cavity
- Clear, bright eyes with absence of discharge
- Regular pupil size with normal pupillary responses
- Clean ears with absence of discharge or odour
- Good general skin and coat condition with no evidence of wounds, parasites, swelling, irritation or 'tenting'
- Free mobility of limbs with no evidence of fracture, dislocation, stiffness or pain
- Normal parameters of temperature, pulse and respiration   ▶

- Clear pale yellow urine passed without pain or difficulty
- Firm, brown faeces passed without undue straining or pain
- Interest shown in food if offered, with an ability to eat and drink comfortably
- Keen reflexes with sharp reaction to stimuli
- Suitable weight for breed and size with no signs of obesity or wasting.

Physical examination

Physical examination of the patient should be carried out starting at the external nares and progressing methodically caudally to the tail. All findings should be recorded and reported.

Head area

The nares should be moist and provide a patent airway into the nasal passages. Any nasal discharge, serous or mucopurulent, should be noted. Nasal discharge is most commonly caused by infection (viral, bacterial or fungal). Other causes include foreign bodies and tumours.

Nasal haemorrhage is referred to as **epistaxis**; this may be caused by trauma, foreign body, neoplasia or clotting abnormalities. Sneezing or dyspnoea may accompany nasal discharge.

The mouth should be checked to assess the state of the teeth, tongue and mucous membranes. The bones of the jaws should be examined for evidence of fractures or misalignment. Neonates should be checked for the congenital abnormalities of cleft palate and harelip. Teeth should be tartar free with no bleeding around the gum line. The breath should be odourless: abnormal-smelling breath can be an indicator of ill health; uraemia associated with kidney disease may be evidenced by a smell of ammonia, acetone (pear drops) may be indicative of diabetes mellitus and rotten decaying teeth have an unmistakable fetid odour.

Mucous membranes

The colour and hydration status of mucous membranes are a good indicator of the general health of an animal and will sometimes signal the need for emergency action; they should be moist and pink in colour, indicating adequate blood flow and oxygenation of tissues. Tacky or dry membranes are indicative of dehydration.

- Pallor of mucous membranes is indicative of inadequate blood volume or low haemoglobin concentration and may be seen in shocked patients or those with haemorrhage, anaemia or circulatory collapse.
- Blue-tinged (**cyanotic**) membranes indicate insufficient transport of oxygen to the body tissues and may be caused by respiratory obstruction, dyspnoea and some poisons (such as paracetamol in cats). This is a critical situation that requires immediate attention.
- Yellow (**icteric/jaundiced**) membranes may be due to an increased concentration of circulating bilirubin, indicative of liver disease
- Brick red membranes are seen in cases of septic shock, caused by the release of bacterial endotoxins into the blood.
- Cherry red coloration is observed in patients with a carbon monoxide build-up in the blood. This may be caused by overexposure to car exhaust, coal, gas or wood fire fumes.

Petechiae are small pinpoint red haemorrhages on the mucosa. These may be seen in patients suffering from clotting disorders such as von Willebrand's disease. It is particularly indicative of animals poisoned with anticoagulant rodenticides.

While noting the colour of the mucosa, the capillary refill time (CRT) may be assessed (Figure 13.1). This should be carried out by application of pressure on the gum with a clean thumb or finger. This will cause a blanching of the area, which should return to its normal colour within 1–2 seconds. An increased CRT may indicate shock, dehydration, hypovolaemia or hypotension. Patients in pain or with septic shock or fever may demonstrate a decreased CRT.

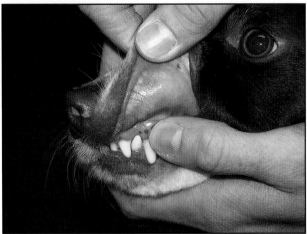

13.1   Assessing capillary refill time (CRT). The animal's lip is curled back and pressure is applied on the gingival mucosa until it blanches. The CRT is the time taken for full colour to return. (Courtesy of A Boag)

Eyes

The eyes should be examined carefully without touching the surface of the cornea. Any abnormal bulging of the eyeball should be noted; this may indicate increased intraocular pressure seen in **glaucoma**, or oedema of the conjunctiva described as **chemosis**. Prolapsed eyeball is referred to as **proptosis**; this should be considered an emergency requiring immediate veterinary attention (see Chapter 18). The protective coverings of the eye should be observed for evidence of **entropion** (inward-turning lashes) or **ectropion** (outward-turning lashes).

The position of the nictitating membrane or third eyelid should be assessed. This is situated in the medial canthus of each eye. In normal healthy animals this membrane is not visible, but in emaciated or dehydrated animals the eye sinks back into the socket, causing the membrane to protrude from the canthus.

The cornea should be glossy and clear with no evidence of opacity, scratching or ulceration. The colour of the sclera should be noted: it should be white with no evidence of vascularity or jaundice.

Any secretion should be noted; discharge may be present in patients with infectious disease or abnormal eyelid or eyelash structure. Foreign bodies such as grass seeds and any allergic response may also produce an ocular discharge.

Irritation of the eye can cause considerable distress to a patient and signs such as pawing at the face and rubbing the head against the floor may be seen.

Further information may be gained by examination of pupil size and reflex. Pupil sizes should be symmetrical and there should be a pupillary light reflex. This may be assessed by shining a bright light directly into the eye. In a normal animal, the pupils will react to the light by constricting, thus restricting the amount of light entering the eye. Once the stimulus is removed, the pupils should rapidly return to their normal diameter. Unequal pupil size is referred to as **anisocoria** and may be indicative of brain damage.

Ears, lymph nodes and skull

The ear pinnae should be checked for inflammation and wounds such as haematoma, and the ear canal examined for signs of redness, foreign bodies, ear mites and excess wax production.

Whilst examining the head area, the parotid and submandibular lymph nodes may be palpated. Lymph nodes are small accumulations of lymphoid tissue located throughout the body. They play a major role in the defence mechanism of the body. They most commonly become enlarged in cases of infection or neoplasia.

The examination should now progress to the skull, checking for evidence of fractures or wounds.

Skin and coat

The loose skin of the neck should be lifted to check for suppleness. The skin of an adequately hydrated animal will rapidly return to its normal position once released. Slow return or 'tenting' indicates dehydration and this should be addressed.

The overall condition of the coat and skin should be assessed. Macroscopic ectoparasites such as fleas, lice and ticks may be identified and redness or irritation may indicate infestation with microscopic parasites such as demodectic or sarcoptic mange mites. Open or closed wounds may be observed, which may confirm involvement in a fight, road incident or physical abuse. Eczema, allergic reaction and hair loss may also be apparent.

Forelimbs

The forelimbs should now be examined for lameness, wounds, crepitus, fractures, heat or swelling. The prescapular lymph node is located cranial to the scapula and this may be palpated. The state of the claws should be assessed: split or scuffed nails often provide evidence of involvement in a road traffic incident. Toes should be checked for foreign bodies, irritation or discharge and pads examined for dryness, cracking, lesions or tenderness.

Thorax and abdomen

The examination should now progress to the thorax, where the ribs and thoracic vertebrae should be gently felt to identify fractures, and the overlying skin checked for wounds irritation or swelling. The apex beat of the heart may be located on the left side of the ventral chest between ribs three and six and the intensity, rate and character of the heartbeat should be noted. The normally functioning heart has a characteristic 'lub dub' sound. Auscultation of the chest using a stethoscope may be carried out to detect crackles or rales, which may be indicative of pulmonary oedema, pneumonia or haemothorax.

The abdomen should be palpated with care by applying light pressure of the flattened finger ends (not the fingertips) to identify tenderness, pain or abnormal swelling. Deeper structures may be palpated if required; the kidneys, bladder, spleen, small and large intestines can be located, although these may prove difficult to locate in a tense or obese animal.

Pelvis, hindlimbs and anus

The pelvis and hindlimbs should be examined in the same manner as the forelimbs. The femoral pulse may be monitored on the medial aspect of the proximal femur and the popliteal lymph node palpated within the gastrocnemius muscle caudal to the stifle.

The anus should be examined for evidence of soiling, trauma or discharge. Anal glands situated on either side of the anus should be inspected for signs of impaction or infection.

Reproductive organs, tail and weight

The penis and testicles of the male animal should be examined. Entire dogs should have two descended testes within the scrotum.

The vulva of the female animal should be examined for swelling or discharge. Vaginal discharge is associated with the reproductive cycle of the bitch and may be normal or abnormal. In pro-oestrus, vulval swelling and blood-red discharge are to be expected followed by a straw-coloured discharge in oestrus. A dark green/brown discharge signals imminent parturition and is caused by the breakdown of the marginal haematoma from the zonary placenta (in the queen, this discharge is brown). A brown/black discharge is seen as a sign of metritis, while a foul-smelling black flow may indicate the death and decomposition of an unborn fetus or fetuses. A purulent green or pale coffee-coloured secretion is a consequence of an open pyometra commonly seen in middle-aged entire bitches.

The final action of the examination is to run the hands along the tail to check for wounds or damage to the coccygeal vertebrae. The patient should then be weighed and the weight recorded.

Physiological assessment

In addition to the physical examination of the patient, the following factors should be considered.

Appetite changes

Alterations in feeding patterns may occur in the practice situation as a result of disease processes or the change in environment or diet.

- **Loss of appetite** is often the first sign that an animal is unwell. There may be a number of contributory factors, such as mouth trauma, ulceration or pain, **dysphagia** (difficulty with eating), infectious and metabolic diseases or pyrexia. Nasal congestion may cause impaired olfactory function and therefore a reluctance to eat. This is particularly significant in cats, as their sense of smell is an important factor in their willingness to eat.
- **Voracious appetite** with subsequent loss of weight and condition may be a symptom of exocrine pancreatic insufficiency (EPI), or hyperthyroidism in cats.
- **Pica** is craving for unnatural foodstuffs and may occur as a result of dietary imbalance, but is often merely an undesirable habit. **Coprophagia** (ingestion of faeces) is an example of this condition.
- An animal with a **capricious** appetite is a picky or fickle eater. Cats are notoriously capricious, particularly when they are ill or stressed.

Urination patterns

Urine output can provide valuable information regarding kidney and circulatory function. The average quantity of urine produced in the dog is 1–2 ml/kg/hour.

- Increased urine production is described as **polyuria** and may be indicative of a number of conditions, such as diabetes mellitus, diabetes insipidus, nephritis, hyperadrenocorticism (Cushing's disease) and pyometra. Polyuria is typically accompanied by an increased thirst described as **polydipsia**.
- Bitches in pro-oestrus will demonstrate increased frequency of urination to maximize the attraction of male suitors by the secretion of pheromones in the urine.
- Reduced urine production may be the outcome of dehydration, shock, acute renal failure, feline lower urinary tract disease (FLUTD) or urinary tract trauma, restriction or obstruction. A urine output of <0.5 ml/kg per hour is described as **oliguria** and this may signify a requirement for fluid replacement.
- **Anuria** is the absence of urine production; this may be caused by acute kidney failure or urinary tract obstruction. It should be considered a potentially urgent situation that requires immediate veterinary attention.

All changes in urination patterns should be monitored and water intake and urine output should be measured accurately. This is best carried out by the use of an indwelling catheter attached to a collection bag. The colour, smell and turbidity of the urine passed should be assessed and any abnormalities reported.

It is important for an animal to be able to pass urine freely without pain or discomfort. Conditions such as cystic calculi, feline lower urinary tract disease, prostatic enlargement, obstruction of the urinary tract and trauma to the pelvis or urinary tract may produce difficult or painful urination, a state known as **dysuria**.

Haematuria indicates the presence of blood in the urine, which may be caused by trauma, neoplasia, infection or inflammation of the urinary tract. Iatrogenic trauma and urinary calculi may also lead to this condition.

Changes in defecation patterns

The volume and frequency of faecal material passed should be monitored and recorded. The faeces should be assessed for colour, smell and texture and examined for the presence of blood, mucus or parasitic worms. Microscopic examination may also be carried out.

- **Constipation** (the failure to evacuate faeces, which may lead to straining) may be caused by a number of factors, including ingestion of foreign material, tumours in the rectum or colon, environmental factors such as soiled litter trays or confinement, enlargement of the prostate gland or feline dysautonomia in cats.
- **Diarrhoea** (the frequent evacuation of watery faeces from the bowel) most commonly has a dietary cause. Other causes include viral diseases such as canine parvovirus and distemper, bacterial infections such as *Campylobacter* and *Salmonella*, colitis, intussusception, EPI, endoparasites and some metabolic diseases.

Both acute and chronic diarrhoea may bring about significant fluid loss and subsequent dehydration of the patient. Therefore, consideration should be given to effective fluid replacement. Metabolic acidosis may also be a consequence, due to loss of bicarbonate ions.

Vomiting

It is essential to assess whether a patient is vomiting or regurgitating.

- **Vomiting (emesis)** is the forceful ejection of stomach contents through the mouth, involving active contraction of the abdominal muscles. It is usually accompanied by hypersalivation and nausea. The most common cause of vomiting is dietary indiscretion. Other causes include infection (viral, bacterial or parasitic), foreign body, neoplasia and abdominal disorders such as peritonitis, pyometra and pyloric stenosis.
- **Regurgitation** is the passive return of food through the mouth. Causes of regurgitation include megaoesophagus.

Excessive vomiting can cause severe extracellular fluid deficits plus the loss of sodium, potassium, chloride and hydrogen ions, potentially leading to metabolic alkalosis.

The volume and frequency of vomitus should be monitored and the specimens examined for blood, mucus or evidence of poisons. It may be valuable to establish whether the sample is digested or undigested food. The incidence of vomiting related to feeding patterns may be of relevance. The veterinary nurse should be able to recognize the various types of vomiting that may be seen in the cat and dog.

Types of vomiting

These include:

- **Projectile vomiting** – forceful vomiting of stomach contents, usually without retching
- **Haematemesis** – vomiting blood
- **Cholemesis** – vomiting bile
- **Cyclic vomiting** – recurring acts of vomiting
- **Stercorous vomiting** – vomiting faecal matter

Retching is an ineffectual attempt to vomit (this may be confused with coughing, especially in cats).

Coughing

This is a reflex response to irritation of the respiratory mucosa and may vary from a dry harsh cough to one that is fluid and productive. There are many possible causes of coughing and its occurrence should be considered in conjunction with the presence of other clinical signs and any circumstantial evidence.

Coughing may be caused by congestive heart failure, pulmonary congestion, canine contagious respiratory disease, canine distemper or bronchitis. Trauma to or malformation of the respiratory tract, laryngeal paralysis or inhalation of noxious or irritant chemicals may also initiate it. Ascarid infestation in young dogs may lead to coughing, as the worm's life cycle involves the larvae wriggling along the trachea from the lungs to be reingested into the oesophagus, thus causing irritation in the pharynx (see Chapter 8).

A slight cough is not uncommon after the removal of an endotracheal tube following general anaesthesia.

Restlessness

This is not uncommon in the hospitalized patient. Fear, loneliness, anxiety and boredom are often the simple causes. However, pain, discomfort, hunger, thirst and the desire to pass urine or faeces may also lead to a restless animal. Restlessness should be investigated to establish the cause and steps should be taken if possible to alleviate distress. Signs include panting, pacing, barking, cowering and an inability to settle.

Pain

The recognition and relief of pain should be considered a priority by the veterinary nurse. This is important not only from the obvious ethical and compassionate perspective but also from the point of view of the patient's recovery. An animal in pain is more likely to develop shock following trauma, a painful chest may interfere with normal respiration and an animal with abdominal pain is less likely to attempt urination or defecation. Mouth pain may diminish an animal's ability and desire to eat and chronic pain may lead to muscle atrophy as the animal carries a painful limb.

Many signs of pain will be obvious, such as carrying a wounded limb or crying out, but others may be less apparent.

Possible signs of pain

- Crying, barking or whining
- Pacing
- Depression
- Anxiety
- Reluctance to be touched
- Lameness
- Reluctance to move
- Aggression
- Reluctance to urinate or defecate
- Inappetence
- Self-mutilation
- Abnormal posture or gait
- Tachycardia or tachypnoea

Many patients, particularly small prey animals, follow their instinct to hide any signs of pain or weakness from potential predators by remaining very still and silent.

In addition to the provision of pain relief as directed by the veterinary surgeon (see Chapters 9 and 22), there are many measures that may be implemented by the veterinary nurse to alleviate the suffering of animals. These include:

- Provision of soft comfortable bedding
- Support for wound and fractures
- Provision of positional support to alleviate laboured breathing and pressure on painful areas
- Placing food and water bowls at a comfortable height and position
- Lubrication or padding to soothe or prevent decubitus ulcers
- Application of cold or heat to affected area
- Clearing of discharges from eyes, ears, nose, rectum and suppurating wounds
- Physiotherapy
- Control of parasites
- Preventing self-mutilation by use of Elizabethan collar or brace.

Temperature, pulse and respiration

These vital signs (Figures 13.2 and 13.3) should be monitored routinely in every hospitalized patient.

Temperature

Thermometers
Various types of thermometer are in common use in veterinary practice.

- The **glass clinical mercury thermometer** is still widely used. This consists of a graduated glass tube with a stubby bulb at one end containing mercury. When the temperature rises, the mercury expands, causing it to travel along the tube. The thermometer has a kink in the bulb end, which prevents the backflow of mercury when it is removed from the animal. This allows an accurate reading of body temperature. Great care should be taken when using and storing the mercury thermometer, as both broken glass and the mercury can be hazardous.
- The **digital thermometer** is also in widespread use. This is safe and hardwearing and provides an accurate digital reading on an integrated screen.
- The **electronic thermometer** is designed for rectal or oesophageal use. It allows continual monitoring of body temperature. The temperature may be read from a digital readout.
- The **subclinical thermometer** may be used to record subnormal temperatures and is valuable for anaesthetized patients and those that are critically ill.

The thermometer may be calibrated in degrees Celsius (°C) or Fahrenheit (°F).

Although the veterinary nurse should be familiar with both readings, Celsius is now the standard unit for measurement of temperature.

Temperature conversions
A Fahrenheit reading may be converted to Celsius by use of the formula:

$°C = (°F - 32) \times 5/9$

For example, a temperature reading of 50°F is converted to Celsius thus:
$(50°F - 32) \times 5/9 = 18 \times 5/9 = 10°C$

Taking an animal's temperature
It is usual and preferable to take the temperature of an animal via the rectal route (see box). If this is not possible because of trauma or pain, the axilla or external ear canal may be used. Generally, the reading from these areas can be expected to be 2°C lower than the rectal reading.

Procedure for taking the temperature via the rectal route using a mercury thermometer

1. Ensure adequate restraint of the patient.
2. Shake down the thermometer to ensure that the mercury returns to the bulb (avoid hard surfaces).
3. Lubricate the bulb with suitable lubricant.
4. Gently insert the thermometer into the rectum with a twisting motion. The anal sphincter of the dog will relax easily but slightly more pressure will be required in the cat to relax the inner sphincter muscle. The thermometer should be directed against the upper wall of the rectum to avoid insertion into the faecal mass.
5. Hold the thermometer in the rectum for the stated time (30 seconds to 1 minute).
6. Gently remove the thermometer and wipe clean with cotton wool.
7. Hold the thermometer horizontally and rotate until the mercury level is visible.
8. Read and record temperature.
9. Clean thermometer carefully using antiseptic solution.

	Temperature (°C)	Pulse (beats/minute)	Respiration (breaths/minute)
Dog	38.3–38.7	60–80	10–30
Cat	38.0–38.5	110–180	20–30

13.2 Normal range of vital signs in the dog and cat.

Species	Body temperature (°C)	Heart rate (beats/minute)	Respiration rate (breaths/minute)
Domestic rabbit	38.5–40.0	130–325 (larger breeds lower rates)	30–60
Mice	37–38	500–600	100–250
Rats	37.6–38.6	260–450	70–150
Gerbils	37.0–38.5	300–400	90–140
Hamsters, Syrian	36.2–37.5	280–412	33–127
Hamsters, Russian	36–38	300–460	60–80
Guinea pigs	37.2–39.5	190–300	90–150
Chinchillas	37–38	120–160	50–60
Chipmunks	37.8–39.6	150–280	60–90
Ferrets	37.8–40.0	200–250	33–36

13.3 Normal range of vital signs in small mammals. (Values taken from *BSAVA Manual of Exotic Pets, 4th edn* (eds A Meredith and S Redrobe) and *Veterinary Nursing of Exotic Pets* (S Girling, Blackwell))

Abnormal temperatures

- **Hyperthermia** – elevated body temperature. Causes include heat stroke, exercise, seizures, infection and pain
- **Pyrexia (fever)** – elevation in body temperature due to infectious causes
- **Hypothermia** – reduced body temperature as seen in hypovolaemic shock, general anaesthesia and impending parturition

Pulse

Monitoring the pulse assists in evaluating the efficacy of the cardiovascular system. The ability to locate and interpret the rate and character of the pulse is a valuable skill that should be mastered by the veterinary nurse. The pulse can be palpated at any point where an artery runs close to the body surface. Each pulsation corresponds with the contraction of the left ventricle of the heart as it pumps blood into the aorta and pulmonary arteries.

Taking the pulse

In the dog and cat, suitable sites for monitoring the pulse include:

- The femoral artery on the medial aspect of the femur (Figure 13.4)
- The digital artery on the palmar aspect of the carpus
- The coccygeal artery on the ventral aspect of the base of the tail.

The lingual artery on the underside of the tongue may be utilized in anaesthetized patients.

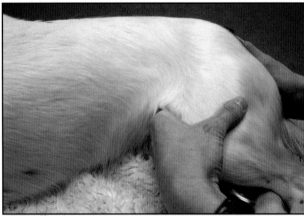

13.4 Locating the femoral pulse by gently sliding the hand into the patient's inguinal region. (Courtesy of A Boag)

Procedure for taking the pulse

1. Ensure adequate patient restraint.
2. Locate the artery with fingertips.
3. Count the pulsations for one minute.
4. Record the rate.

Abnormal pulse rates

In a normal patient, the pulse rate increases on inspiration and decreases on expiration. This variation is known as **sinus arrhythmia**. Possible causes of abnormal pulse rates are as follows.

- **Tachycardia** (raised pulse rate) may occur merely as a result of exercise or excitement but may be indicative of fever, hypotension, pain, stress or the administration of certain drugs such as atropine.
- **Bradycardia** (lowered pulse rate) would be expected in animals that are asleep, unconscious, or anaesthetized. It may also be observed in patients with a debilitating disease or hypokalaemia. Exotic species such as tortoises and hedgehogs that hibernate in the winter will experience a very low pulse rate throughout this period.
- A weak, thready pulse may be indicative of shock or a diminished cardiac output.
- A pulse that is strong and jerky (**hyperkinetic**) is referred to as a 'water hammer' pulse or Corrigan's pulse and may be indicative of certain cardiac anomalies such as patent ductus arteriosus.
- A pulse rate that is lower than a corresponding heart rate is known as a **pulse deficit** and is present in many cardiac arrhythmias.

Respiration

The respiratory rate should be assessed when the patient is at rest but not sleeping or panting. *Either* inspirations *or* expirations should be counted for exactly 1 minute. The depth of respiration, which indicates the volume of air inspired with each breath, should also be assessed.

The rhythm and rate of respiration can be assessed by careful observation of the patient or by gently resting the hands on either side of the chest cavity.

Abnormal respiration

- **Tachypnoea** (increased respiratory rate) may be observed following exercise or excitement. An animal that is in pain, shock or overheated will also exhibit this sign.
- **Bradypnoea** (decreased respiratory rate) is seen normally in sleeping or hibernating animals, but may also be indicative of narcotic or hypnotic poisons, brain trauma or metabolic disorders.
- **Dyspnoea** (difficult or laboured breathing) may be caused by stenosis or obstruction of the respiratory tract, bronchitis or lung disease/damage. Air (pneumothorax) or fluid in the thorax (chylothorax, haemothorax or pyothorax) may also lead to dyspnoea.

Further reading

Aspinall V (2003) *Clinical Procedures in Veterinary Nursing*. Elsevier, Oxford

Moore M (ed.) (2000) *BSAVA Manual of Veterinary Nursing*. BSAVA Publications, Cheltenham

Chapter 14

Essential patient care

Jennifer Seymour and Caroline van der Heiden

Learning objectives

After studying this chapter, students should be able to:

- **Recognize the basic requirements of the hospitalized patient**
- **Apply the knowledge of patient needs to provide care to hospitalized patients**
- **Recognize and describe the use of various items to groom a hospitalized animal**
- **Explain the grooming of an animal, describing the areas requiring particular attention**
- **Describe the equipment and procedure required to bath an animal**
- **Describe the equipment and procedure to clip claws**

General care of the patient

The provision of basic care to hospitalized patients is fundamental and is often the exclusive responsibility of the veterinary nurse. The importance of understanding and attending to the needs of sick, frightened or traumatized animals can never be overstated.

The specific needs of hospitalized patients will obviously be dependent on their condition. However, all patients have five basic requirements: nutrition, warmth, comfort, hygiene and mental stimulation.

Nutrition

Adequate nutrition is vital to the normal metabolic functioning of any animal (see Chapter 16) but the sick, traumatized or convalescing patient has an additional requirement for nutrients to facilitate recovery and tissue repair.

Even the most highly nutritious and balanced diet has no value unless it is consumed by the patient. Consideration should therefore be given to the following factors.

Environment

- Cats are more likely to eat in a secluded peaceful area away from barking dogs.
- Sometimes just the enjoyment of access to sunshine can stimulate a patient's appetite.

Timing of meals

Timing can be significant for some patients and feeding at the animal's normal mealtime is more likely to elicit a positive outcome. Feeding times should be regular and frequent. The amount of food given at each meal should be small and any food not eaten after 15 minutes should be removed.

Food is not normally left with dogs overnight except in the case of difficult or shy feeders. It is often necessary to leave food with cats, as overnight is often the only time that some hospitalized cats will eat.

Diet and presentation

Animals are more likely to eat food that smells, feels and tastes familiar. A cat used to eating dry food will be less likely to attempt to eat a moist meal; a dog routinely fed on a home-made diet is unlikely to be impressed by commercial food from a tin. Food that is the usual size and texture will be more readily accepted. It is useful to discuss the normal feeding regime with the owners, who will often be only too pleased to bring specially prepared tempting morsels from home.

Some animals may be encouraged to eat if they are given strong-smelling extra-tasty food such as pilchards, freshly cooked meat or meat extract. In addition, a wide range of commercial diets is available for the inappetent and convalescing patient.

Cold food and fluids can be unappetizing to patients that are feeling unwell or miserable. Warming food to blood temperature can make a huge difference to palatability.

Food bowls

Some animals are reluctant to eat from dishes made of certain materials, such as metal or plastic, as they can be tainted with an off-putting odour or taste. Animals eating from bowls with high sides may feel vulnerable if they cannot see potential predators (this is particularly pertinent for small mammals).

It is inadvisable to place food and water dishes next to litter trays, as animals do not ordinarily eat in close proximity to urine and faeces.

Patients with restrictive casts or dressings may find it more comfortable to eat from a raised dish.

Encouragement

The ability to smell and taste food has a significant influence on an animal's desire and willingness to eat. Cats, especially, will be more inclined to eat if their nasal passages are clear and free from discharge.

Many animals can be encouraged to eat by stroking, fussing and talking to them while hand-feeding.

Assisted feeding

Ensuring adequate nutritional support is vital to the quick and successful recovery of the hospitalized patient and should be considered a major role of the veterinary nurse. Sufficient time should be allocated within the nursing day to allow this important task to be completed satisfactorily.

Assisted feeding techniques are covered in depth in Chapter 16. Methods used to encourage feeding and to ensure the intake of nutrients include:

- Placing the food on the nose or paws of the patient (this may instigate licking and subsequently stimulate natural feeding)
- Spoon feeding or syringe feeding (this may encourage voluntary eating, but care should be taken to prevent aspiration of food into the respiratory tract)
- Naso-oesophageal tubing
- Percutaneous endoscopically placed gastrostomy tubing (PEG; see Chapter 16).

Warmth

It is important that all patients are kept warm and free from draughts. The temperature of the hospital ward should be kept constant with adequate ventilation. An ambient temperature of 18–20°C is recommended.

Sources of additional warmth

- **Blankets and towels** are often used in the veterinary hospital, but care should be taken that they do not become soaked with urine; this could lead to urine scalds in a recumbent or weak patient.
- **Deep-pile 'veterinary' bedding** (e.g. Vetbed) is ideal for use in the ward. It is comfortable, warm and easily washed. The main advantage is that the base of the bedding absorbs any fluid, thereby ensuring that the patient remains dry.
- **Bubble wrap** is a cheap, readily available material that is particularly suitable for cats, small mammals and birds.
- **Heat lamps** should be used with great care. Animals that are unable to move can easily become overheated, dehydrated and possibly burnt if a lamp is used injudiciously. The heat lamp should be set at a minimum height of 60 cm from the patient and constant observation should be maintained.

▶

- **Hot-water bottles** are a good source of heat for weak patients, but they do have certain disadvantages. They will require refilling at regular intervals and it is possible that the stopper may become loose or that patients may chew the rubber, and scalding may occur as a result. Boiling water should never be used and the bottles should always be covered with a towel or blanket.
- **Heated pads** are useful, but must be used with care. They should be covered with a towel and the patient should be checked and turned at regular intervals. Animals with a tendency to chew should not be allowed heated pads, as chewing the flex could lead to electrocution.

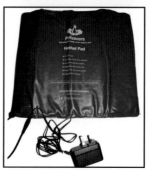

- **Microwave pads/bags** are now commonly used in the veterinary practice. They are quick and easy to use; they have the advantages of staying warm longer than hot-water bottles and having no flex.
- **Incubators** are ideal for smaller critical patients and for neonatal puppies and kittens. The environment can be automatically maintained at the desired temperature. Newborn animals are **poikilothermic** (body temperature varies with ambient temperature) and therefore a constant temperature of 30–33°C should be maintained for these patients.

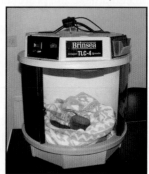

Comfort

Kennels and cages for hospitalized patients should provide adequate space for the animal to stand and lie down comfortably (see Figure 14.1 and Chapter 12). Confinement in a small space may cause animals distress and force them to sleep, eat and excrete in the same vicinity – a situation they would normally avoid. Furthermore, this arrangement will severely restrict a veterinary nurse's attempt to spend quality time in the cage providing the patient with valuable and much appreciated 'TLC'.

Patients should be provided with adequate bedding materials and allowed to assume a position that they find comfortable. Fractured limbs, open wounds and dressings should be kept uppermost and supported with soft padding. Familiar bedding brought in by the owner may provide extra comfort and security.

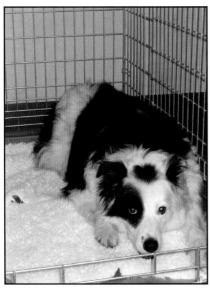

14.1
Hospitalized dog on suitable absorbent bedding.

Recumbent patients

Recumbent animals (see Chapter 15) should be provided with extra padding to prevent the occurrence of decubitus ulcers (pressure sores), especially on bony prominences. The application of a bandage or petroleum jelly to these areas may be beneficial. The recumbent patient should be turned regularly every 2–4 hours to prevent the occurrence of hypostatic pneumonia.

Various physiotherapy techniques may be beneficial for the recumbent patient. These include massage, coupage, application of cold or heat and hydrotherapy. These are covered in depth in Chapter 21.

Hygiene

A high standard of hygiene must be maintained on the hospital ward. Convalescing patients or those suffering trauma or disease have a lowered resistance to the invasion of microorganisms and subsequently are more likely to succumb to nosocomial infections.

All patients should be routinely checked for abnormal secretions, which may cause discomfort or irritation. Nasal, oral, aural and ocular discharges should be gently wiped clean and soothing lotion applied as necessary. Open wounds should be cleaned and covered with a sterile dressing to prevent contamination. Any drains, catheters or feeding tubes should be monitored and kept uncontaminated to prevent invasion of bacteria. Patients soiled with urine and faeces should be bathed and dried immediately to increase morale and prevent scalding of the skin.

Contagious patients, such as cats suffering from feline influenza or dogs with parvovirus, must be isolated and barrier nursing implemented to prevent the spread of infection. Utensils, medical equipment and bedding should be exclusive to these individual patients and not shared with other kennel occupants.

The general cleanliness of the kennel ward should include the routine removal of faeces, urine, vomitus and discharge. A suitable disinfectant, diluted correctly, should be used to disinfect the area following the elimination of organic material (see Chapter 12). Protective clothing should be worn when using these solutions to comply with COSHH regulations (see Chapter 1).

Uneaten food should not be left in the kennel, as it will be unpleasant for the patient and may attract flies in hot weather. Used food bowls and other fomites should be washed thoroughly, or if necessary autoclaved or destroyed. All soiled kennel materials should be disposed of as clinical waste and all reusable bedding thoroughly washed.

Mental stimulation

It is important to maintain the morale of the hospitalized patient. An animal left alone with no company or stimulus will very quickly become dispirited and miserable. Often, very little time and effort is required to cheer a gloomy patient. Simple actions such as talking, fussing, stroking and use of its name will do much to raise an animal's spirits. Patients should, however, be allowed periods when they can sleep and rest without distraction.

Long-stay patients may benefit from visits from the owner, though this may not be advisable in all cases as patient and owner alike may become distressed when parting. Familiar toys and other belongings from home may be allowed at the veterinary surgeon's discretion.

Whenever possible, the patient should be taken outside to enjoy fresh air and a change of environment.

Routine daily care of hospitalized animals

Careful monitoring of patients in the hospital ward will ensure that they are provided with the necessary care they need (Figure 14.2). The daily routine should include the following.

Check	Care routine
General check	All animals are inspected briefly by touring the kennels/cages to establish that there are no urgent problems that require immediate attention
Individual check	Each individual should be looked at for some time, noting the behaviour of the animal compared with its normal (e.g. whether it is lively, aggressive, unresponsive). Its posture should be noted (whether it is standing, lying down or in an abnormal position)
Observations	Respiration should be checked before the animal is disturbed Pulse and temperature may be taken (before exercise)
Soiling	Check for soiling of kennel and record details of quantity and type of eliminations If animal has urinated or defecated: note appearance or amount, assess what has been eaten (if food was left with the animal) and record the observation before removing it
Water bowl	Note how much has been taken and whether any spilling has occurred (if there is spilling, the assessment of intake will be inaccurate)
Physical check on patient	Note and record any abnormalities Inspect wounds Gently remove any discharges

14.2 Care routine for hospitalized animals.

Provision of food and water

Suitable nutrients should be offered when appropriate. Patients should be observed when eating to establish the amount eaten and any evidence of eating abnormalities.

Clean, fresh water should always be available unless otherwise directed by the veterinary surgeon. Recording the amount offered and then calculating the remainder can establish the volume of water intake.

Opportunity for urination and defecation

Cats should be provided with litter trays, which should be replaced when soiled. Many cats prefer to attend to their personal hygiene in privacy, and may benefit from a covered litter tray – easily provided by an upturned box with a cut-out entry hole.

Ideally, dogs should be allowed to urinate and defecate outside, before they are forced to foul their kennel. The belief that they have somehow misbehaved by passing urine and faeces in their kennel can cause them unnecessary anxiety in an already stressful environment.

Urination and defecation should be observed to identify any pain or difficulty. Voided urine and faeces should be monitored for volume, frequency and consistency.

Administration of medication

The veterinary surgeon's instructions regarding the administration of drugs should be followed precisely. The dose and strength of drug, and the time and method of administration must be checked carefully before delivery.

Weighing and recording

All patients should be weighed on admission to the hospital and regularly throughout their stay.

Routine and accurate completion of hospital charts should be carried out. This will ensure precise recording of clinical parameters, bodily functions and administration of medication (Figure 14.3).

Grooming of hospitalized animals

Every effort should be made to keep hospitalized animals in a hygienic and comfortable condition. The grooming of hospitalized dogs should be carried out as part of their general nursing care, unless their condition contraindicates it. There are various reasons why grooming as a normal routine is beneficial (whether the animal is at home or during hospitalization).

Benefits of grooming

- Cleanliness
- Health
- Appearance
- Inspection
- Relationship

The initial letters of these headings form a useful memory aid: CHAIR.

Cleanliness
Keeping the animal clean by the removal of dirt and discharge and assisting in the casting of hair contributes towards the animal's health and well-being. At home, the regular grooming of dogs and cats reduces the amount of hair deposited on furniture and carpets. It is important that animals with dense or long coats are groomed regularly, as their coats rapidly become tangled, matted and soiled.

Health
By keeping the animal's coat clean, grooming assists the condition of the skin and hair and thus contributes to the animal's health.

- Grooming stimulates **anagen** (the hair growth stage) by the removal of dead, shedding hairs.
- The removal of discharge and prevention of matting prevents skin irritation.
- The close inspection of the animal during grooming assists in early recognition of problems.
- During grooming, daily care and attention to any bony prominences, skin folds, feet and claws, eyes and ears, mouth and teeth, anus, vulva and prepuce contribute to the health of the animal.

Animal details		Owner details	Clinical summary
Species Breed		Name	
Age Sex		Address	
Name Weight		Tel no	

Date	Temp	Resp	Pulse	Fed	Ate	Water	Urine	Faeces	Medication	Comments

14.3 Example of hospital chart.

Appearance

Owners usually give this as the first reason for grooming, though it is the least important for the animal itself. Many owners take a pride in the appearance of their animals and this becomes very apparent when a postoperative animal with large areas of denuded skin is returned to an owner who was not forewarned. Owners of pedigree dogs often want their pets to look like the breed as seen at championship dog shows, which means that many dogs are trimmed and clipped by professional groomers, a practice that also assists the owner's daily grooming of the dog. The appearance of the true show dog is of major concern to its owner and show preparation often involves hours of careful grooming and trimming or clipping. Nurses should be careful not to remove hair from show dogs without the owner's consent. This emphasis on appearance needs to be appreciated: many owners, rightly or wrongly, judge the standard of care at the practice or kennels by the appearance of the animal when it is returned to them.

Inspection

The daily inspection of an animal during the grooming routine contributes to its health by presenting an opportunity for early recognition of problems. For example, flea excreta will only be discovered on close examination of the coat. It is recommended that inspection is carried out in a logical daily sequence so that any problems found can be attended to before further damage or discomfort is caused to the animal during the actual grooming (see below).

Relationship and human contact

This is an important reason for grooming. For the dog in the wild state, mutual grooming is part of pack socialization activities. Dogs lower in the pack order submit to grooming by a more dominant member, while dominant dogs make it clear whether or not they consent to being groomed by other members of the pack. When dogs are groomed by their handlers, the activity strengthens the bond between them and confirms to the dog its place in the hierarchy: the handler is the 'pack leader'. The act of grooming, therefore, should assist in the handling and training of the dog.

Grooming can also assist in teaching a dog to sit or stand still whilst the procedure is carried out, which will be of great assistance for veterinary examinations. If a dog resents grooming for no physical reason, it is likely to prove generally difficult to handle.

Introducing an animal to grooming

Ideally the process of grooming should be introduced (to all domesticated species) at a very young age as part of socialization and habituation. Even short-haired puppies and kittens should be handled each day and introduced gently to brushes and combs. The experience should be made pleasant for the animal, with praise given for good behaviour but a firm tone if the animal struggles.

As with all training, grooming should be carried out for a few minutes at a time at first and gradually built up as the animal becomes accustomed to it. Each session should end on a successful note with the animal being praised for compliance.

Owners of long-haired animals should in particular be advised that time spent in the early stages of ownership will ensure that the animal is easier to groom in later years and is less likely to be presented at the veterinary practice for de-matting when an owner is unable to groom the pet because it objects, struggles or even attempts to bite.

Routine grooming

Routine grooming is part of the daily care of a normal healthy animal, but the veterinary nurse can be faced with quite a problem as there are so many different types of coat. In addition, various factors have a direct effect on the coat and it is necessary to have a broad understanding of them so that the coat can be correctly maintained while the animal is in the nurse's care and so that owners' queries regarding grooming at home can be answered.

Hair growth

The major factors affecting hair growth include: environmental temperature and time of year; health and reproductive status; and feeding and nutrition. It should be noted that the average rate of hair growth in the dog is 0.5 mm/day; an average smooth-coat type takes about 6 months to regrow completely. Fine silky long-haired coats take up to 18 months; a similar growth rate can be expected in cats.

Environmental factors

Dogs kept in housing with constantly high environmental temperature (usually with central heating) will often shed hair almost continuously throughout the year but with noticeable increases in spring and autumn. Shedding in dogs kennelled out of doors, or with less environmental heating, tends to be more obviously seasonal: shedding is very noticeable in spring and autumn. This seasonal coat change is a natural process triggered by increasing day length in spring and decreasing day length in autumn.

Seasonal coat changes

Spring = increasing day length →
    Triggering of production of summer coat
    + Increased hair shedding (of winter coat)
    + Coarser coat with reduced density
    + Increased sebaceous gland activity →
    Summer coat (allowing increased air circulation through coat)

Autumn = decreasing day length →
    Triggering of production of winter coat
    + Increased hair shedding (of summer coat)
    + New coat growth
    + Reduced sebaceous gland activity →
    Winter coat (increased coat density = insulation against the cold)

Health and reproductive status

Condition can often be assessed by observing the coat and noting any unseasonable loss or thinning of hair. Thinning during periods of ill-health is due to interruption of the growth cycle: fewer individual hairs are in the growth stage. An animal suffering from ill-health may also have a dull, harsh coat.

The reproductive status of an animal can have an effect on coat growth and this can be quite obvious during pregnancy and lactation, and occasionally after neutering. These and other so-called hormonal alopecias usually involve thinning of hair on certain areas of the body.

Feeding and nutrition

Diet affects hair growth, as it does all other functions. Nutrients required for good health of skin and hair include amino acids, essential fatty acids, zinc and iodine (see Chapter 16).

Type of coat

The type of coat is governed by combinations of individual hair types that make up the coat. These are the rigid primary or **guard** hairs and the soft, thinner secondary or **lanugo** hairs. The various proportions, lengths and weights of these hair types account for the many and varied types of coat seen in dogs and cats. Most coat types can be divided into five broad groups for the purpose of grooming: smooth, wire, double, silky or woolly (Figure 14.4).

Grooming equipment and methods

A fairly wide range of attention and equipment is required to deal with the various types of coat. For the routine maintenance grooming of patients and boarders, it is advisable to stock a range of basic grooming equipment (Figure 14.5).

Although different coats require different attention, a logical general sequence can be adopted for all common breeds to ensure that nothing is missed out during the grooming session:

- Assess the animal's temperament
- Carry out a physical inspection of the animal
- Remove loose hair
- Comb, brush and finish.

Coat group	Coat type	Examples
Smooth coat	Short Intermediate or coarse [a] Dense	Boxer, Dachshund, Chihuahua German Shepherd Dog, Pembroke Corgi
Wire coat		Wire-haired Terrier
Double coat		Rough Collie, Long-Haired German Shepherd Dog
Silky coat	Medium Long fine	Most spaniels, setters and some retrievers Afghan Hounds, Bearded Collies
Woolly coat		Poodle, Bedlington Terrier, Curly-Coated Retriever, Irish Water Spaniel

14.4 Coat types. [a] Wild dogs and wolves have this type and it is therefore sometimes referred to as a 'normal' coat.

Equipment	Types	Features and use
Brushes	Double-sided grooming brush (pins and bristles)	Metal pins with rounded ends. The straight pins are more effective than bristle with silky coats. Used for silky, double coats and feathering to separate hairs and smooth and lay the coat. Not so useful for tangled coats Natural or synthetic bristles. Denser than pin brushes and less able to brush through thick coats for hair separation. The bristles are flexible for removal of dirt deep in the coat this brush is most commonly used for routine grooming of short-coated breeds
	Slicker brush	One-way hooked pins. The hooks assist in pulling out loose hair. Pressure should not be used as the hooks easily damage the dog's skin. Used for removing loose hair from thick coats, grooming silky coats (especially feathering), wire, woolly and double coats
	Hound glove	Flexible, with bristles, small plastic projections or a velvet type surface, often double sided. Used to assist moulting and for the routine grooming of short-coated breeds. Pressure and vigorous use should be avoided with wire bristles
Combs	Metal combs	Handle and non-handle combs. Both are available in various tooth widths. Used for grooming of longer hair behind ears in silky coats etc. Also used for detangling and breaking up small mats
	Rake	Designed for greater pull through dense coats. Used for removal of loose undercoat and breaking up some small mats (with great care as damage can easily be inflicted on the dog's skin)
	De-matting comb with specialized teeth	Only used to cut out mats; it is a much safer way to remove mats than by the use of scissors, allowing the maximum amount of coat to be preserved once the mat is removed
Scissors	Trimming scissors	Long very sharp blades tapering to a point. Different sizes available. Used to trim neatly around the edges of ears, etc.
	Thinning scissors	Specialized blades for thinning without leaving 'steps' in the coat Used to enhance features, e.g. the shoulders, sides of chest

14.5 Grooming and trimming equipment.

Physical inspection routine

Before grooming, a physical inspection should be carried out to assess:

- The state of the animal's coat – and thus the need for the use of non-routine equipment (such as the de-matting comb)
- The state of the animal's health – to ensure close observation of the animal so that lesions normally obscured by the coat are found prior to the use of any equipment that might cause injury to the animal (it is too late to find a wart once the comb's teeth have caused it to bleed).

The inspection should be carried out in a logical sequence. The dog should be checked closely from head to tail, both visually and by running the hands carefully over the animal. Areas requiring special attention, particularly with elderly or hospitalized animals, include:

- Mouth, teeth, gums and lip folds
- Eyes and ears
- Hocks and elbows
- Foot pads and claws
- Body orifices.

Eyes and ears

Discharges should be wiped away with clean damp cotton wool. In some breeds the long hair on the ears (and face) may gather food whilst the animal is eating and this should be removed by washing. The hair may be trimmed carefully to prevent recurrence or, for a pedigree breed where this long hair is a feature, a note should be made to use a feeding 'snood' (snoods hold the long hair and ears back during feeding and are often used for Afghan Hounds) or to provide a narrow deep feeding bowl that allows the long hair and ears to fall on each side of the bowl rather than in the food.

Hocks and elbows

Any pressure sores should be noted and attended to, including making improvements to bedding. If there is hard skin but no sign of breaks in the skin, white petroleum jelly may be applied.

Foot pads and claws

Foot pads may be cracked or, in dogs that pace about continually in hard-surfaced runs, they may be reddened and thin due to the abrasive action of the surface.

Claws should be checked for injury and condition; for example, they may be overgrown when a dog has restricted exercise or is walked only on grass (see 'Claw clipping', below). Some dogs with a long-term abnormal gait may wear their claws away unevenly, so that some of the claws need to be trimmed on a regular basis.

Body orifices

The anus, vulva and prepuce may require regular removal of discharges and soiling. With long-haired animals it may be necessary to trim or clip away some of the surrounding hair to allow easier cleaning of these areas. Any treatment or attention to any abnormalities found should be dealt with at this stage, before grooming is undertaken.

Grooming procedures

Loosening the dead hair

Most coats will benefit from the groomer pulling the fingertips along the skin through the coat, against the lie of the hair. This will help to remove the loose hair and therefore stimulate normal hair growth. Dogs tend to find this procedure pleasant and some will get excited and see it as a game, so firm but friendly handling is required to insist that the dog stays fairly still.

Combing

Using a traditional comb, any tangles can be eased out gently and any loose hair removed from the coat at this stage. The comb is used with the lie of the hair at an angle (usually about 45 degrees). Particular attention should be paid to areas on the longer-haired breeds that have a tendency to tangle and mat, such as behind the ears and feathering between and on the backs of the hindlegs. As the comb is more accurate than a brush and is usually smaller, it can be used with care on areas that are difficult assess, ensuring that no areas are missed or tangles remain underneath a superficially groomed coat.

If mats are found during combing and they are not able to be removed or teased out gently during a traditional comb, a specialized de-matting comb can be used where appropriate to remove the mat (see below), followed by a combing out of the remaining hair gently with the traditional comb. Where a mat has been removed it is important to check the skin underneath it for damage, as the area may be reddened or even suppurating. If the mat has caused irritation to the skin, this should be dealt with depending on the severity.

Brushing

The type of brush used depends on the type of coat, and the action of brushing depends on the brush (Figure 14.6). Great care should be exercised when grooming with pin or slicker brushes, as it is possible to damage the skin with some types if used too vigorously. It is not generally advisable to use this type of brush against the lie of the hair.

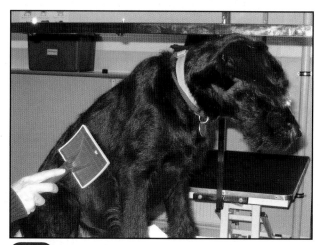

14.6   Grooming a dog with a slicker brush.

Smooth coat brushing technique

1. Once the combing is complete a bristle brush can be used.
2. First it is used on the hair covering the trunk. The brush is used *against* the lie of the hair in short straight strokes. This is begun at the base of the tail and thighs and moves gradually forward as each area is brushed.
3. Brushing against the lie stops at the back of the head and at the base of the skull, leaving the head untouched at this stage.

continues ▶

4. The brush is then used gently on the head *with* the lie of the hair and thereafter working downwards and backwards with short straight strokes, until the entire body and legs have been brushed.
5. Taking hold of the tail, it is carefully brushed, gently but firmly, from base to tip. Care is required when grooming tails, as many dogs are quite sensitive about their tails being groomed and some may react sharply to all but the most gentle brushing.
6. During the brushing phase the brush should be periodically cleaned to remove any build-up of hair. This can be done by drawing a traditional comb through the bristles.

Finishing

After combing and brushing, a smooth or silky medium type of coat can be finished off by using a damp cloth or smooth hound-glove (or a piece of velvet or damp synthetic chamois cloth). The face is gently wiped over, followed by the remainder of the body, working from front to back. This action smoothes down the coat and removes stray hair and dust from the coat surface, giving a sleek shine to a healthy coat. This is not done generally with coats that are of the woolly or wire type, as these are usually required to stand up and are brushed into shape and left.

De-matting

Sometimes the coat of a long-haired animal has been so grossly neglected and become so matted that it would be unkind to try to de-mat it while the animal is conscious. The neglect may have arisen because the animal has been so difficult to groom when conscious anyway.

In such cases the veterinary surgeon might sedate or anaesthetize the animal and request the veterinary nurse to 'de-mat' it. This should be carried out with great care: it is very easy to cut the skin, and scissors should not be used by unskilled nurses. Cats are especially at risk when hair mats are cut away.

Coat clipping and trimming

Under normal circumstances a nurse is unlikely to be involved in the long-term maintenance of a coat that requires clipping or trimming. However, it is essential that all those who care for hospitalized animals should know how to look after a variety of coat types.

The routine clipping or trimming of some areas in long-haired dogs will assist in maintaining cleanliness, but care should be taken. *Do not trim or clip an animal without its owner's consent* – it may be a pedigree show dog which either should not be trimmed or needs specialized clipping and trimming.

The clipping, hand stripping and trimming of specific breeds is generally within the realms of the professional dog groomer and showing kennel. Interested veterinary nurses can attend special courses on this art, but in general practice it is more usual for a nurse to clip or trim a pet dog at its owner's request because the animal is difficult or impossible to groom. This may be due to the animal's temperament, or because the dog is elderly or infirm with perhaps an elderly owner. In the latter case, trimming and clipping may be carried out as part of a geriatric care policy. Where temperament is the problem, it is usually necessary to sedate the dog or, in extreme cases, to anaesthetize it as already discussed for de-matting.

In general practice, the veterinary nurse needs to know how to use common equipment for trimming or clipping a dog neatly and tidily. The regular trimming of some types of coat assists grooming and general hygiene, while clipping can assist in grooming by keeping the coat short enough to be managed easily.

Trimming

Trimming is carried out with special scissors. Areas that are commonly trimmed to assist in grooming are those prone to matting or collection of soiling in breeds, such as some spaniels and setters. This includes the ears, to avoid the collection of food when eating, and the matting of the long silky hair just behind the ears. Feet are trimmed particularly between the toes, where mud can collect and dry on the hair so that it causes discomfort by rubbing and by pushing the toes apart. In bitches, it may be necessary to trim soiled areas after whelping if soiling and staining from whelping fluid cannot be removed easily any other way.

If a dog soils itself or mats easily, grooming will be simplified if hair is judiciously trimmed from the anal area and hindleg feathering – but without being scissor-happy. A balance should be struck between the need to keep the dog hygienic and the owner's need for the dog's appearance to be acceptable.

Clipping

Clipping is by means of special clippers. There are set styles of clip designed to enhance breed features; for example, some of the hair of terrier breeds is removed or thinned out by professional hand stripping. Non-showing owners of breeds with long heavy coats, such as the Old English Sheepdog, may have their animals clipped out for the summer. Dogs such as Poodles do not moult normally and it is essential to clip the coat regularly, otherwise it would become unmanageable for the owner and would cause discomfort and distress to the dog.

Clippers should only be used according to the manufacturer's instructions, as they are easily damaged by misuse. For example, the hair must be completely dry, as wet hair quickly blunts the blades. The blades should not be forced through a thick coat or matting, as they may be clogged by the hair and stop the machine, possibly causing damage to the equipment. If the clippers become hot during use, they should be allowed to cool down before continuing.

Clipping machines should be regularly serviced and maintained. They need to be thoroughly cleaned and oiled after each use and then stored in a dry environment. A variety of blades should be available, with spares of those used most commonly to enable a rotation for regular sharpening.

Bathing

Bathing (Figure 14.7) is carried out for three main reasons:

- To eradicate and control ectoparasites
- To treat skin conditions and apply topical medication
- To cleanse and condition the coat.

Cleansing may be required for various reasons:

- Because the coat is soiled with a substance that cannot be removed by normal grooming
- To remove odours (e.g. when a dog has rolled in excreta)
- To assist in the removal and masking of the scent from a bitch just out of season who is still receiving the attention of male dogs
- To improve the appearance of the coat before a show.

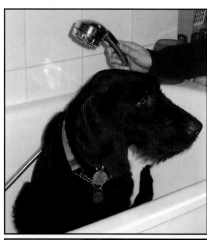

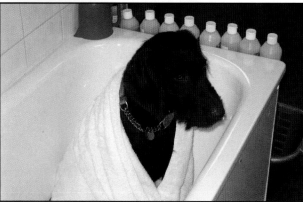

(14.7)

Bathing a dog.

Shampoo

There are many products for shampooing dogs. Some are generally available; others (for specialized medical or antiparasitic use) are only available by prescription. The preparations fall into three categories:

- **Insecticidal** (to eradicate and control parasites, most commonly fleas, lice and ticks)
- **Medicated** (containing some form of antiseptic or other active ingredient and prescribed for dogs with minor skin problems)
- **Cleansing** (general purpose or also for conditioning).

The latter category includes those most widely used – shampoos for general coat cleansing. A conditioning agent is often added to improve the hair texture by lubrication, so that the coat is more manageable for brushing out when dry.

Specialized shampoos are available from the pet trade for different types of coat. The two most notable are the 'mild' shampoo for puppies and dogs with sensitive skins, and 'colour-enhancing' shampoos for particular coats, such as products containing optical whiteners for white coats.

Note that if the shampoo is in a glass bottle the amount required should be decanted into a plastic cup or a similar small unbreakable receptacle before bathing commences. A small amount of water may be added to the shampoo at this stage so that it is easier to distribute when applied to the dog's coat.

Dog baths

The ideal dog bath should:

- Allow the handler to get the dog in and out of the bath easily but also contain the dog safely, deterring escape
- Allow access to all parts of the dog being bathed without the handler having to bend or reach excessively

- Have a non-slip area for the animal to stand on, with the surrounding area also non-slip for the safety of the handler
- Have a flexible shower hose with a spray head
- Have easily adjustable water and heat controls
- Have an easily cleaned surface allowing access for cleaning all parts of the bath.

Many specially designed dog baths are available. In some small establishments, where the bathing of dogs is not carried out regularly, it is possible to modify other installations. For example, non-slip mats can be added to a shower cubicle in which the floor has been raised and the shower-hose and controls lowered, or the mats can be added to a bath designed for a disabled person and fitted with a shower-hose.

The domestic bath

Clients who bath their dogs in a domestic bath should always be advised to use a non-slip mat and that they should not put the plug in the bath. An inexpensive mixer shower-hose can be fitted to the bath taps. Clients should be warned that some modern domestic baths scratch easily and can be damaged by the claws of a scrambling dog.

Drying the dog

Several towels are needed to dry a dog after it has been bathed. It is always advisable to put out at least two extra ones, to save having to search for more towels while a half-dry dog shakes itself and distributes water all around the bathing area.

The number of towels needed can be reduced by first using a synthetic chamois cloth to remove excess water. This can be wrung out several times and re-used before towels finish the drying off.

Dogs that are bathed regularly may be familiar with hairdryers but these can frighten a dog that is new to the experience. Never blow the drier towards the dog's face. Instead, blow towards the hind end from the front, moving towards the rear and directing the hot air along the hair shaft, not directly at the skin. Continuously test the heat by keeping a hand in front of the air jet at the approximate distance of the dog's skin. The same hand can assist the drying process by lifting the dog's hair, running the fingers through to ruffle the coat.

The dog should be sitting comfortably. Panting or shivering would indicate distress or discomfort.

Protective clothing

It should be standard practice for the handler to wear protective clothing when bathing a dog. It not only keeps the handler's clothes dry but may also be required for safety. The usual clothing is:

- Waterproof overall or apron
- Water-resistant boots or shoes with non-slip soles
- Protective gloves where suggested by a shampoo manufacturer (those who have sensitive skin may prefer to wear protective gloves anyway).

Handling and restraint for bathing

All dogs must be adequately restrained during bathing. A large wet dog leaping out of a bath can injure both itself and the handler, and back injuries are not uncommon. A collar and lead, or nylon slip-lead, should be looped over the handler's arm so that it is readily accessible if restraint is required. With a large or boisterous dog, it is advisable to have a second person to steady or restrain it.

Where there are no steps for the dog to be encouraged to walk into the bath, it will require to be lifted. With large dogs, this should be carried out by two people for safety.

⚠ WARNINGS

- **A dog should never be encouraged or allowed to jump into or out of the bath at any time, as it may easily slip on a wet surface and injure itself.**
- **A dog should never be left unattended in a bath, as it may try to jump out, injuring itself if it slips.**
- **A dog should never be tied up in the bath, as it could leap over the side and strangle itself in a few seconds while the handler reaches away.**

Bathing procedure

The procedure for bathing dogs depends to some extent on the reason for the bath.

General procedure for coat cleansing

1. Know why the dog is being bathed.
2. Assess the dog's temperament and arrange assistance if necessary.
3. Assemble all the equipment and prepare the bathing area.
4. Put on protective clothing.
5. Bring the dog into the bathing area and encourage it up steps into the bath, or lift it in (with help if needed).
6. Reassure the dog and start water flow away from the dog, running the water over a hand until a constant acceptable temperature is maintained.
7. Carefully apply the water, soaking the dog well but taking care not to alarm it. Protect the dog's eyes with a hand and do not spray water directly on to its face.
8. Apply shampoo sparingly to the entire coat but avoid sensitive areas such as the face, or into the vulva or sheath. (If the head requires particular attention due to a medical condition, protect the eyes by applying a bland eye ointment or smearing the lids with petroleum jelly.)
9. Massage shampoo into the coat, or use as directed (e.g. leave it on for the recommended time before rinsing).
10. Rinse thoroughly, starting at the upper front and moving in a downwards and backwards sequence so that every part is thoroughly rinsed.
11. Squeeze out excess water; then remove as much water as possible with a synthetic chamois leather cloth, squeezing it out as necessary and reapplying.
12. Remove the dog from the bath, either by encouraging it to step out or by lifting it carefully.
13. Towel dry.
14. Use hairdryer if it is safe to do so (keep electric dryers away from risk of contact with water) and if the dog's temperament permits.
15. Return the dog to a warm kennel to avoid chilling.
16. Record that the bath has been carried out, stating what shampoo has been used.

Dental care (oral hygiene)

Dental disease is one of the most common problems seen in veterinary practice and the veterinary nurse is increasingly involved with client education in this respect. Changes in the consistency of pet food have led to a greater need for routine teeth-cleaning, which is now recognized as necessary for dental health and therefore referred to correctly as 'oral maintenance'. For optimum results, all teeth should be cleaned daily. The procedures are described in detail in Chapter 26.

Toothbrushes

Animal toothbrushes have bristles that are designed to enable the operator to reach and clean under the gum line, and the small spaces that surround each tooth where plaque readily accumulates. Other cleaning methods can be used to accustom the animal to the cleaning routine, such as the use of pads and swabs; these can only remove the plaque above the gum line, therefore brushing is by far superior. The selection of the correct toothbrush is very important. Initially a finger brush can be used for dogs to accustom them to the feel of bristles before progression on to a toothbrush. Toothbrushes specifically designed for dogs are now available, with a long handle and dual ends for easy access to all areas. Cats also require a specially designed toothbrush, as they have very little room between the back teeth and inside of their cheeks.

Introducing the oral hygiene procedure

Advice regarding the introduction of an animal to the tooth-cleaning procedure is offered by the manufacturers of the various products that are now widely available. Some general considerations are as follows.

- Before attempting cleaning, always assess the temperament of the animal and handle accordingly, but always proceed with caution.
- Exercise patience and do not try to proceed too quickly.
- Initially, do not expect the animal to tolerate the brushing for more than a few minutes at a time.
- Incorporate short rest breaks into the routine to avoid the animal becoming uncomfortable and restless.
- Begin by gently handling the animal's mouth daily and praising good behaviour. Increase the handling time to 5 minutes or so after a few days.
- Once the animal tolerates the handling, hold its mouth closed with one hand while opening the mouth on one side with the other hand and gently rub the teeth with a finger.
- When this finger-rubbing stage is tolerated, use a toothbrush on a few teeth and increase the number of teeth brushed as the animal becomes accustomed to the experience.
- When the animal has accepted brushing of the outside of its teeth, gently pull its top jaw upwards to open its mouth. Gently introduce the brush into the mouth to clean the inner surfaces of the teeth, again increasing the number brushed as the animal becomes accustomed to the procedure.

- Fingerstall toothbrushes are useful for cleaning the inside of a dog's teeth. The most effective way of brushing is to point the bristles upwards while brushing the upper teeth and downwards for brushing the lower teeth. This angling allows cleaning of the small space that surrounds each tooth where the gum meets it.

Claw clipping

The average healthy animal does not usually require attention to its claws which, under normal circumstances, wear naturally with everyday use – with the notable exception of the dew claw (though this claw tends to be slow growing). Dogs that have dew claws should be checked regularly for signs of abnormal length or the claw curling into the skin.

Where disease, injury or any type of immobility occurs, the claws may overgrow. This can lead to further immobility if the claws have grown to such an extent that they prevent or restrict the animal's normal gait. In extreme cases the claws may be so long that they curl around and begin to grow in towards the foot pad, causing the animal discomfort or even pain if the skin is penetrated.

Where animals do require some attention, the problem usually arises in one of the categories described in Figure 14.8.

Animals requiring attention	Comments
Animals that are only exercised on soft ground	Dogs exercised on grass only, particularly very lightweight ones, are more likely to require claw clipping than those that do road work or use concrete or similar runs daily
Animals whose normal behaviour or exercise is restricted by their housing and management	This includes most small mammals kept as pets
Elderly animals that are unable to exercise normally	Dogs that are stiff or generally less active due to old age are more likely to require regular attention to their claws
Dogs with immobilized fractured limbs	The nails will not wear on the injured limb and therefore need to be trimmed while the leg is immobile
Animals with injury or disease conditions of the foot or nail	The claws of a foot affected by disease need to be trimmed. A nail that is partly broken off will need to be trimmed
Previous injury to the foot or leg causing abnormal gait	Previous injuries such as fractures or damaged tendons may cause a change in the normal gait, leading to uneven wearing of some of the claws
Puppies in the nest	The claws of nursing puppies are very sharp and grow rapidly, and the bitch's teats can become very sore from their scratches. To prevent or reduce damage to the lactating bitch, clip the puppies' claws weekly
Animals causing damage to property	Cat owners often request claw clipping when a pet damages their furniture (waterbeds are especially at risk). Clipping of cat claws is a controversial issue and only of very short-term usefulness in this situation; instead, owners should be encouraged to provide scratching-posts

14.8 Reasons for claw problems.

Equipment

Essential equipment for claws includes clippers suitable for the size and thickness of the claw. There are various types available. They should be kept sharp and in good working order and should always be used as recommended by the manufacturer.

In case bleeding occurs due to inadvertent cutting of the quick, cotton wool and a silver nitrate pencil should be to hand.

Procedure for claw clipping

1. The animal should be suitably restrained and reassured throughout the procedure.
2. Take the foot firmly. Use thumb or fingers to push up each toe in turn and fully expose the nail.
3. Inspect each nail in turn for damage and length of quick, if it can be seen (if the nail is black the quick will not be seen). A very bright light is helpful.
4. *If the quick is visible*, place the clippers below the quick and cut the nail at an angle. Do this with a rapid action before the animal detects pressure and attempts to withdraw its foot.
5. Take great care not to cut into the quick – it causes pain. An animal that has been caused pain during claw clipping is likely to be very uncooperative and distressed on all future occasions.
6. *If the quick is not visible*, estimate where it should be. Apply slight pressure with the clippers and note the animal's reaction. If necessary, revise the estimated position and cut well below it. Err on the side of caution: it is better to make one or two safe small trial cuts than to make one large cut that causes pain and bleeding.
7. If the animal reacts strongly, watch for bleeding. If bleeding does occur it may be stemmed by pressure from a pad of cotton wool. If bleeding persists, traditional styptics such as friar's balsam can be applied with a cotton bud, but a silver nitrate pencil, *applied with great care*, is more effective. A patient should never be sent out with a bleeding nail, therefore observe closely until all bleeding has subsided.
8. Once each foot is completed, move to the next. Check each time for the presence of a dew claw, which can easily be hidden in long-haired dogs.
9. Once the procedure is over, always praise the animal for compliance. A food reward may be offered at the end.

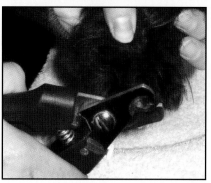

Further reading

Moore M (ed.) (2000) *BSAVA Manual of Veterinary Nursing*. BSAVA Publications, Cheltenham
Taylor R (1992) An introduction to dog grooming (parts 1 and 2). *BVNA Journal*, 7, (5/6), 158–164

Chapter 15

General nursing, the nursing process and nursing models

Sharon Chandler, Jennifer Seymour and Andrea Jeffery

> ### Learning objectives
>
> After studying this chapter, students should be able to:
>
> - **Identify the most appropriate bedding for inpatients**
> - **Select appropriate dressings and materials to bandage any area of the patient's body**
> - **Describe methods for local applications of heat and cold**
> - **Describe the correct methods for drug administration**
> - **Select the equipment for carrying out an enema**
> - **Describe the special nursing requirements for a range of patients, including vomiting, soiled, recumbent, geriatric, critically ill, neonates and the comatose patient**
> - **Describe the procedure for placement of urinary catheters and their management**
> - **Describe the nursing process**

Beds and bedding

Bedding for hospitalized patients may differ from that usually offered by pet owners, especially for the small mammals, where their normal bedding may be inappropriate in relation to their condition.

Dogs

Hospitalized dogs require warm and comfortable bedding. Basic hospital provision should offer bedding that is:

- Easy to clean (e.g. plastic-covered foam beds)
- Easy to wash (e.g. synthetic absorbent 'Vetbed')
- Easy and cheap to dispose of (e.g. newspaper – unshredded).

Combinations of these basic materials are usually used to provide the required level of comfort, but additional materials (e.g. pillows, blankets) may be added, especially for recumbent or recovering animals. Any additional items should only be used if facilities allow repeated frequent washing of these heavier items, as they may otherwise pose an infection risk. All bedding should be *hot* washed between different patients or when soiling has occurred.

It may seem a nice sentiment for the patient to have familiar bedding from home but this should be discouraged, due to the possible introduction of infective agents, dust and dirt. The bedding is also likely to become soiled and possibly damaged by the practice's hot washing.

Cats

The same basic rules apply as for dogs. If the practice kennel size allows, provision of small plastic baskets for cats to curl up in are a good addition, though this may be inappropriate in some cases (e.g. fracture patients with legs bandaged in extension).

Rabbits

For short stays in the hospital a thick layer of newspaper and a small amount of hay are appropriate. Hay should be from a known mite-free source. For recovery or very sick rabbits, 'Vetbed' or light blankets can be used. Organic bedding may be inappropriate when there are open or discharging wounds.

Small mammals

These are best housed in their own cages from home. Owners should be instructed to clean their pet's housing prior to admission. Some bedding may be inappropriate if it interferes with wound healing (e.g. shavings), but this will need to be assessed on an individual basis. Any straw or hay that comes into the practice should be from a known mite-free source. The practice should have in stock approved commercial bedding to replace any that is inappropriate. Most small mammals will be supplied with a separate sleeping area, usually a box or commercial 'house', but simply having a designated area is sufficient.

Bandaging and dressings

The ability to place an effective bandage can make the difference between success and failure for any given surgical or non-surgical wound. Indeed, bandages can *create* wounds, or make existing wounds worse, if applied incorrectly or without due care.

Nurses should be able to:

- Recognize types of wound
- Select correct materials appropriate for the wound
- Apply materials in correct order and manner
- Monitor for and recognize bandage-related problems
- Instruct owners on care and observation of the bandage
- Be familiar and able to assist with application of specialized bandages.

Wound healing

To be able to apply the appropriate dressings and bandages it is essential to have knowledge of the way in which wounds heal, as this will affect how they are managed (see also Chapter 24).

- **First intention healing** occurs when the two edges of a wound are directly apposed; healing is able to occur without complication (e.g. a surgical wound) (Figure 15.1). First intention healing is rapid and gives good cosmetic results.
- **Second intention healing** occurs when wound edges are remote from each other and cannot be apposed, or when infection is a consideration. The wound is left open and allowed to fill by granulation tissue (Figure 15.2). In Figure 15.2(c) the epithelial cells have extended over the granulation tissue. Second intention healing takes far longer to complete and leaves areas of scarring that have less sensation and resistance to injury in the future.

The healing process

When an injury is sustained the healing process begins immediately with haemostasis and activation of inflammatory cells to the area. The order in which cells arrive at the site is:

1. **Granulocytes** – provide non-specific immunity to infection
2. **Macrophages** – critical to repair: release factors within wound to promote healing (these factors cause local cells such as fibroblasts to multiply and endothelial cells to burrow under the basement membrane and form projections of new vessels)
3. **Lymphocytes** – excite reparative reactions.

Reasons to bandage

Bandaging is used to hold dressings in place in any area of the patient. Other reasons for bandaging include:

- Support for:
  - Fractures or dislocations
  - Sprains or strains
  - Healing wounds
- Protection against:
  - Self-mutilation
  - Infection
  - Enviroment
- Pressure to:
  - Arrest haemorrhage
  - Prevent or control swelling
- Immobilization to:
  - Restrict joint movement
  - Restrict movement at fracture site
  - Provide comfort and pain relief.

Basic bandaging formula

- Initial layer – dressing
- Primary layer – padding (comfort/support/absorption)
- Secondary layer – conforming (strength/contouring/security)
- Tertiary layer – protection (conforming/strength)

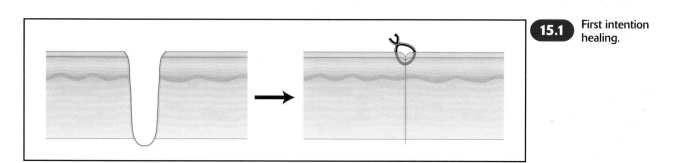

15.1 First intention healing.

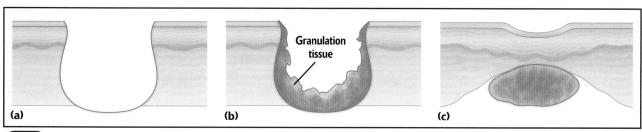

(a) (b) (c)

15.2 Second intention healing.

Granulation tissue

Basic principles of bandaging

- Avoid departing from the basic bandaging formula wherever possible.
- Never leave more than the tips of the toes out on limb bandages.
- Check and change regularly.
- Always attempt to include padding layer to provide comfort.
- Avoid sticking *anything* to the skin (the bandage is likely to slip anyway).
- Never exchange firmness for tightness to achieve aim of bandage.

Dressings

Dressings are applied, before any other materials, directly to the wound. They prevent following layers from sticking to or contaminating the area. They are invariably sterile and need careful handling. There are many different dressings available (Figure 15.3).

Padding, conforming and protective materials

Types of padding material are given in Figure 15.4. Conforming materials (Figure 15.5) are supplied in two basic varieties: those with an elastic component and those without. Every manufacturer has a different design, construction and proportion of elastic. Protective materials may be adhesive or cohesive (Figure 15.6).

Common bandaging techniques

Limb

Limb bandages are commonly encountered in general practice. They can be used for the distal portion (e.g. for cut pads, dew claw removal) or the entire limb (e.g. many surgical procedures or trauma).

Dressing type	Description	Uses
Dry	Plain gauze swabs	Debridement of wounds
Impregnated	Petroleum gel Antibiotic	Superficial open wounds
Semi-occlusive	Usually with a layer of permeable non-stick material on one or both sides and a central absorbent core May have adhesive section round edge to enable accurate, stable placement	Surgical wounds Wounds with mild to moderate discharges
Absorbent	Made of various materials Usually thicker and often with a coloured side that faces the wound May have adhesive section round edge to enable accurate placement	Large wounds where there is a large amount of exudate; helps to remove fluid from wound area whilst preventing drying at the wound surface
Gels	Gel-based; or gels with no base that need to be used in conjunction with other dressings	Where maintenance of moisture is essential (granulating wounds) Where there is a large deficit beneath skin level that is difficult to dress in any other manner
Others	Silver-impregnated Iodine-impregnated	Properties proven to help to prevent infections and encourage speed of healing

15.3 Types of dressing.

Type	Description	Uses/comments
Cotton wool	Natural or man-made absorbent material in rolls	Can be used as sole padding material in most bandages Can be difficult to apply compared with others
Padding bandage	Natural absorbent material supplied in rolls of various sizes	Preferable to cotton wool in most cases due to ease of application Particularly good for limbs
Synthetic padding	Supplied in rolls of various sizes Thinner and lighter	Good where less bulk is needed (e.g. under casts, smaller patients) Can cause sweating and is not so absorbent
Foam	Variety of thicknesses	Useful when external fixators are bandaged or under drains etc.
Cotton wool/gauze	Cotton wool sandwiched between gauze layers Supplied in rolls	Very useful for abdomens and thorax bandages Holes may be cut to accommodate legs and prepuce

15.4 Types of padding.

Type	Description	Uses/comments
Loose open weave	Has no elastic component but loose weave aids conforming property (e.g. Crinx)	Any area of the body to conform padding to body area
Conforming	Has an elastic component	Can be placed too tightly – care needs to be taken during application, especially if not a lot of padding underneath: blood/fluid flow can be compromised, resulting in swelling or death of tissue
Tubular	Bandage supplied in a tube construction	Under casts and on abdomens and thorax Holes can be cut for legs/prepuce etc.
Crepe	Washable cotton fibre material on a role	Not commonly used but may be useful to hold small dressings in place on thorax etc.

15.5 Conforming materials.

Type	Description	Uses/comments
Adhesive	Thick cotton-based material with an adhesive side. Supplied in rolls of various sizes	Good for foot bandages (due to thickness)
Cohesive	Latex-containing material that sticks to itself but not to skin or hair. Supplied in rolls of various sizes and colours	Most commonly used protective material. Conforms well and can be used in any bandaging. *Care needs to be taken as latex component means that the bandage 'tightens' once in place if stretched too much during application*

15.6 Adhesive and cohesive protective materials.

Procedure for limb and foot bandage

1. Ensure the patient is suitably restrained.
2. Place cotton wool padding between the patient's toes, pads and dew claws to absorb sweat and prevent irritation.
3. Apply a layer of cotton wool or soft dressing around the foot.
4. Apply the conforming bandage longitudinally to the cranial and caudal surface of the limb.
5. Wind it around the foot in a figure-of-eight pattern, to ensure even tension throughout the bandage.
6. Continue up the limb.
7. Anchor the bandage over the hock or carpus.
8. Apply an external layer of adhesive tape in the same manner.

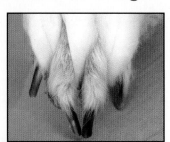
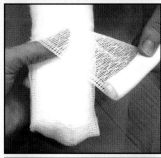
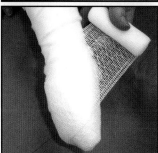

The very tips of the toes can be left out of the bandage to enable peripheral circulation to be monitored. In this case the bandage is simply started by rolling the bandage round the distal limbs and not cranially and caudally over the toes. Either technique is acceptable and effective.

Ear

Ear bandages are used either to help to arrest haemorrhage or to keep dressings in place. They may be used after some surgical procedures (e.g. aural resections), but recent thinking is that surgical ear wounds are best left open to the air. Either one ear or both ears may be bandaged.

Procedure for bandaging a single ear

1. Place a pad of cotton wool on the top of the patient's head.
2. Fold the ear back on to the pad.
3. Apply a dry dressing and place a further pad of cotton wool over the ear.
4. Apply conforming bandage over the ear and then under the chin.
5. Anchor the bandage on either side of the free ear.
6. Cover the bandage with adhesive tape or cohesive bandage.

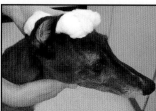
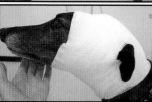
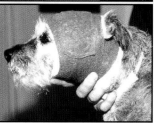

After application the patient should be observed for a few minutes to ensure that the bandage is not too tight and causing breathing difficulties. The aim is to have the bandage as far forward as possible (without interfering with sight), otherwise the bandage will slip backwards and the role of the bandage will be compromised.

Chest and abdomen

The chest bandage is prevented from slipping by passing the bandaging materials between the front legs in a figure-of-eight fashion, resulting in a cross-over of bandages between the forelimbs on the ventral surface (Figure 15.7).

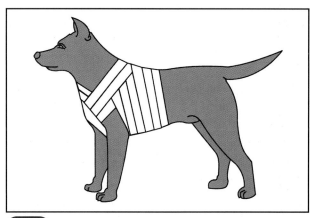

15.7 Chest bandage.

If cohesive bandage is used it must not be placed too tightly, as the patient may have difficulty in breathing easily. Adhesive material should be avoided, as it tends to make the patient very hot and has minimal ability to expand and retract with respiration.

The abdomen is difficult to bandage due to the relative narrowness of the area compared with the thorax. 'Bunching' of material tends to occur and the only way to prevent this is to extend a chest bandage down over the abdomen. Padding layers can simply be laid round the abdomen and secured with conforming and protective layers, or gamgee can be used and secured with tape.

Tail

The tail occasionally needs a *light* bandage to arrest haemorrhage, keep a dressing in place or protect the tail tip from injury (Figure 15.8). Tail bandages are difficult to keep in place. Flicking hair into some turns of the initial layer of bandage can help to hold it in place.

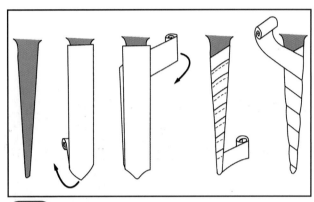

15.8 Tail bandaging.

Specialized bandaging techniques

The three most common special techniques are:

- **Ehmer sling**, to support the hindlimb following reduction of hip luxation
- **Velpeau sling**, to support the shoulder joint following luxation or surgery
- **Robert Jones bandage**, to provide support and immobilization to fractured limbs in a first aid situation or following surgery.

Procedure for Ehmer sling

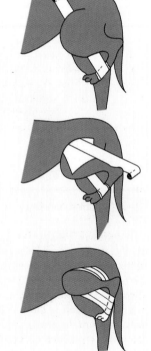

1. Apply padding material to the metatarsus and stifle.
2. Flex the leg and rotate the foot inwards. This will force the hip joint into the acetabulum.
3. Apply conforming bandage to the metatarsus, bringing it medial to the stifle joint.
4. Continue the bandage over the thigh and back to the metatarsus in a figure-of-eight motion.
5. Repeat until full support of the hip is achieved.
6. Hold the bandage in place with adhesive tape.
7. This dressing is usually kept in place for 4–5 days.

Procedure for Velpeau sling

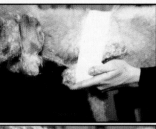
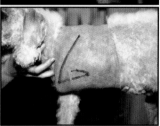

1. Apply a layer of padding material to the foreleg.
2. Apply conforming bandage to the paw.
3. Hold the leg in flexion and apply the bandage over the elbow, then over the shoulder and round the chest.
4. Repeat until full support of the shoulder is achieved.
5. Secure the dressing using adhesive tape.

Procedure for Robert Jones bandage

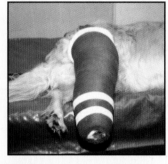

1. Apply zinc oxide traction tapes to the dorsal and ventral surfaces of the foot.
2. Take cotton wool from the roll and wrap it tightly around the leg and foot. A large quantity should be used to support the limb.
3. Apply conforming bandage firmly to the padded leg.
4. Incorporate the traction tapes into the bandage to prevent slipping.
5. Cover the bandage with adhesive tape for protection and extra support.
6. On completion, the foot should be visible so that checks may be made for oedema and temperature. Occasionally the toes are included in the bandage.
7. The bandage may be kept in place for up to 2 weeks.

Spica bandage

This specialized bandage is used to immobilize the elbow joint or associated bones (e.g. scapula, humerus, proximal radius and ulna). It involves taking the bandaging material up and over the cranial thorax, using the opposite leg around which to place a figure-of-eight bandage (Figure 15.9).

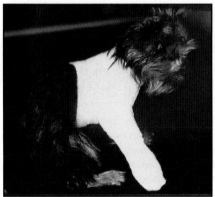

15.9 Spica bandage.

Bandaging assessment

To ensure correct selection and application, three questions should be asked during the bandaging procedure:

- Is the bandage achieving the aim? (e.g. no slipping)
- Is the bandage comfortable? (e.g. no chewing by the patient)
- Is the bandage sensible? (e.g. the patient can move/breathe easily)

Care of bandages and dressings

Once the bandage has been applied, constant checks should be maintained until it is removed.

- The bandage should be checked to ensure that it is not uncomfortable or too tight.
- Any evidence of odour, oedema, discharge, skin irritation, or wetness due to the wound itself (discharges or blood) should be heeded.
- It is important that the dressing does not become soiled or wet from environmental factors (e.g. urine, water, mud). (The dressing should be covered with a plastic bag when the patient is taken outside.)

Constant chewing or licking at the bandage by the patient should be discouraged, but patient interference can indicate that the bandage is uncomfortable, or that there is irritation or pain beneath it, and this should be investigated. If there appears to be nothing wrong and the behaviour persists, one of the following measures may be tried:

- Elizabethan collar (Figure 15.10)
- Discipline
- Provision of toys
- Muzzle
- Application of foul-tasting substance to dressing
- Sedation.

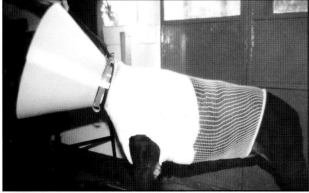

15.10 The Elizabethan collar prevents the dog interfering with the bandage.

Local applications of heat and cold

Heat may be provided by applying cotton wool soaked in hot water or by means of a poultice prepared with medicants such as kaolin. The hot application will cause **vasodilation** and therefore increased blood supply to the affected area. This will provide white blood cells for wound healing and assist in fluid removal from the area.

The application of heat is indicated in cases of:

- Oedema
- Infected wounds
- Abscesses.

Cold may be provided by applying gauze soaked in cold water or an ice pack. Burns and scalds should be flushed with cold water from the tap. The cold application will cause **vasoconstriction**, therefore reducing heat and blood loss. The application of cold is indicated in cases of:

- Pain
- Haemorrhage
- Minor burns and scalds
- Heatstroke.

Administration of medicines

Medicines may be administered via various routes:

- **Orally**
- **Rectally** – in the form of an enema or suppository
- **Parenterally** – by means of hypodermic injection
- **Topically** – to the external surface of the body.

Systemic routes are those by which the drug affects the body as a whole. They include oral, rectal and parenteral routes.

The route should be chosen that is the most appropriate for the patient and for the drug. The classification, dosage and administration of drugs are considered in depth in Chapter 9, but the following factors should be considered before drugs are administered:

- Pharmacological properties
- Rate of absorption
- The patient
- Convenience for the administrator.

Pharmacological properties

It is essential that the drug to be administered is compatible with the chosen route. Some drugs will not be adequately absorbed from the gastrointestinal tract if given orally, whereas others (e.g. pancreatic enzymes extract) must be given via this route as they act on the digestive system. Some drugs may be dangerous if not administered via the recommended route. For example, if thiopental is injected subcutaneously, it causes irritation and sloughing of the skin.

Rate of absorption

The requirements for the onset of action of the administered drug should be considered. In general, an intravenous injection will have the fastest action, followed (in descending order) by intramuscular injection, subcutaneous injection and the oral route.

The patient

The condition and temperament of the patient will influence the route of drug administration. It may not be possible to administer drugs to an aggressive patient via the oral, topical or intravenous routes; therefore an alternative route should be used. Administration of oral drugs to patients with respiratory embarrassment or mouth trauma such as a fractured jaw may cause pain or distress and should be avoided. Continued use of the same injection site may cause soreness and pain and should be minimized if possible.

Convenience for the administrator
Most clients will be able to give drugs orally to their animals and this will allow treatment to be given in the familiar surroundings of home. For the veterinary surgeon or nurse, it may be more convenient to administer drugs parenterally.

Oral administration
Drugs are administered orally in the form of tablets, capsules, liquids, pastes, powders or granules.

Oral administration of tablets and capsules

1. The patient should be restrained as gently as possible.
2. Open the animal's mouth by placing one hand over the muzzle, while the other hand is used to hold the tablet and also to pull down the lower jaw.
3. Place the tablet on the base of the patient's tongue.
4. Close the mouth and stroke the neck to ensure swallowing.

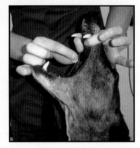

Cytotoxic drugs
It is important to take precautions and wear personal protective clothing (PPC) when administering cytotoxic agents, as the drug may be inhaled or absorbed through the skin, causing toxic effects:

*   Wear gloves, apron and mask
*   Do not dispense on surfaces where food is prepared
*   Protect work surfaces with disposable absorbent sheets
*   Avoid breaking tablets
*   Dispose of packaging in a safe manner to comply with COSHH regulations (see Chapter 1)
*   Wash hands thoroughly after handling.

Oral administration of liquid medication
1. The liquid should be placed in a syringe for ease of administration.
2. The patient's head should be tilted back.
3. Place the syringe into the side of the mouth behind the canine teeth.
4. *Slowly* administer the liquid to the back of the throat. Administering too quickly may cause the liquid to enter the respiratory tract, leading to gagging and other potential complications.
5. Stroke the neck to ensure swallowing.

Rectal administration
The rectal route is not commonly used in small animal practice, but drugs such as liquid paraffin or glycerine may be given in the form of an enema (see below) or suppository.

Parenteral administration
This term describes the administration of medicines via routes not involving the alimentary canal. This may be achieved with hypodermic injections given via the following routes:

*   Subcutaneous
*   Intramuscular
*   Intravenous
*   Intracardiac
*   Intraperitoneal
*   Intrapleural
*   Intra-articular
*   Epidural.

The choice of route should be decided by considering the condition and temperament of the patient, the properties and volume of the drug to be administered, and the desired speed of effect. Hypodermic injections are most commonly administered via the subcutaneous, intramuscular and intravenous routes.

The details given below are for dogs and cats. The subcutaneous, intramuscular and accessible intravenous sites used in small mammals, birds and reptiles are listed in Figure 15.11.

Species	Subcutaneous	Intramuscular	Intravenous
Rabbits	Under the skin over the neck and thorax	Gluteals, quadriceps, triceps, paralumbar	Cephalic, saphenous, marginal ear veins [a]
Small mammals	Under the skin over the neck and thorax	Quadriceps [b]	Lateral tail vein in rats and mice. NB Intraosseous injection is often preferable [c]
Birds	Loose skin of groin and axilla. Small volumes over tibiotarsus [d]	Lower pectorals	Basilic, right jugular, medial tarsometatarsal veins. NB Intraosseous injection is often preferable [e]
Chelonians	Intracoelomic preferred to s.c. [f]	Pectorals, quadriceps femoris	Jugular, dorsal tail veins
Snakes	Along the back. Intracoelomic preferred to s.c.	Paravertebral	Jugular, ventral coccygeal veins

15.11 The subcutaneous, intramuscular and accessible intravenous sites in common exotic pets. [a] Use of local anaesthetic cream recommended. [b] The quadriceps musculature is probably the most accessible muscle mass but it is tightly enveloped in fascia and large injections are therefore likely to prove painful. In rats the maximum volume that can be injected into the quadriceps is approximately 0.2–0.3 ml. This falls to 0.1 ml in hamsters and gerbils, and 0.03 ml in mice. [c] Suitable intraosseous sites in small mammals and reptiles include the proximal femur and proximal tibia. [d] The lower leg is easily extended and accessed for small volume s.c. injections. [e] Intraosseous injections in birds should avoid the aerated bones such as the humerus and femur. Recommended sites include the proximal and distal ulna, together with the proximal tibia. [f] The subcutaneous route is less useful in reptilian patients due to the relative inelasticity of reptile skin, which accounts for the significant leakage of injected material from subcutaneous injection sites. The intracoelomic route is preferred and is comparable to the intraperitoneal route in mammals.

Subcutaneous injection

The loose skin from the back of the neck to the rump is the most common site. This area is suitable because of its poor supply of nerves and large blood vessels. Only non-irritant drugs should be administered via this route, as otherwise there may be irritation or necrosis of tissues. Drug action following subcutaneous injection will take effect after 30–45 minutes.

Subcutaneous injection procedure

1. Select a sterile needle and syringe. Draw up the required volume of drug.
2. Ensure the patient is suitably restrained.
3. Raise a fold of skin from a suitable area.
4. Moisten the skin with a spirit swab to flatten the hair and remove surface dirt. *(Spirit should not be used when injecting a vaccine, as it may inactivate it.)*
5. Insert the needle under the skin and withdraw the syringe plunger slightly. If blood appears in the syringe, a blood vessel has been punctured and a new site must be selected.
6. If no blood appears, the drug may be injected into the patient.
7. Massage the injection site gently to disperse the drug.
8. Make detailed records of the medication given.
9. Dispose of needle and syringe safely (see Chapter 1).

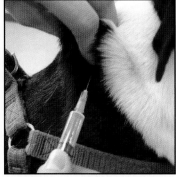

Intramuscular injection

The most common site for intramuscular injection is the quadriceps group of muscles in front of the femur (Figure 15.12). The lumbodorsal and triceps muscles may also be used. The gluteal muscles of the buttocks and the hamstring muscle group should be avoided, as there is a danger of bone or sciatic nerve damage. Because of the density of muscle tissue, large amounts of fluid may be very painful if injected via this route. The maximum administration should be 2 ml in the cat and 5 ml in the dog.

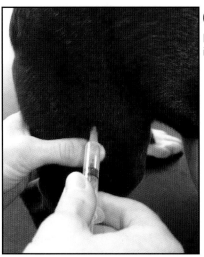

15.12

Intramuscular injection.

The technique is similar to that for the subcutaneous route except that the needle should be inserted at right angles into the muscle mass. Drug action following intramuscular injection will take effect after 20–30 minutes.

Intravenous injection

The common sites for intravenous injection are the cephalic vein in the forelimb, the lateral saphenous vein in the hindlimb, and the jugular vein in the neck. The sublingual vein may be used in an anaesthetized or unconscious patient. Drug action following intravenous injection will take effect in 0–2 minutes.

Cephalic vein injection

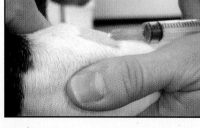

1. The patient, either sitting or in sternal recumbency, should be restrained by an assistant.
2. The assistant should restrain the patient's head with one hand and use the other hand to extend the leg and 'raise' the vein by applying pressure around the elbow joint with the thumb.
3. Clip a 4 x 4 cm area over the cephalic vein, halfway between the carpus and elbow on the cranial aspect of the selected forelimb.
4. Clean the area with a skin antiseptic followed by surgical spirit.
5. The operator should stabilize the vein and insert the needle through the prepared skin into the vein. Blood should flow gently into the syringe.
6. The assistant should then release the pressure on the vein and the operator may gently introduce the drug into the circulation. If large volumes of fluid are to be injected, regular checks should be made to ensure that the needle remains in the vein (by occasionally drawing back a little blood).
7. Once the injection has been administered, the needle may be removed from the vein and pressure applied to the injection site for a minimum of 30 seconds, to prevent haemorrhage.

Topical administration

This refers to the application of medication to the external surfaces of the body – the skin, eyes, ears, nose or mucous membranes.

The skin

Skin treatment may be applied in the form of shampoo, ointment or cream.

The eyes

Eye medication may be applied in the form of drops or ointment. For either medium, the animal's head is tilted back and its eye is held open with the fingers. *When applying any substance to the eye, the surface of the cornea should never be touched by the fingers or by the nozzle of the applicator.*

Drops are applied by dropping liquid on to the centre of the eyeball (Figure 15.13).

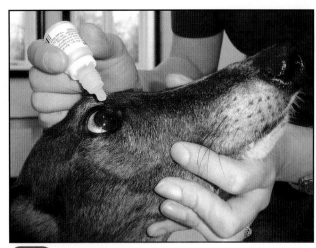

15.13 Application of eyedrops.

Ointment is applied by gently squeezing a line of the drug on to the inner canthus of the eye, taking care not to touch the surface of the eye with the nozzle or finger. It is often best to approach the patient from the side when using eye ointment, rather than a face-to-face confrontational approach.

After the medication has been applied, the patient should be allowed to blink to disperse the drug evenly over the eye.

The ears

Aural medication may be applied in the form of drops or ointment. Ideally the ear should be free from wax and discharge before application, but this is not always possible. The patient should be restrained and its pinna held firmly. The nozzle of the applicator is introduced into the ear canal and the contents gently applied (Figure 15.14). The external auditory meatus should be massaged to ensure maximum coverage.

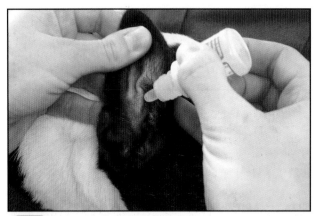

15.14 Application of ear drops.

Assisted feeding

The importance of maintaining nutrition during the recovery of patients from surgery or disease cannot be overemphasized. Convalescent periods can be radically reduced when adequate nutrition is provided. Feeding tubes are readily available and have become more frequently used when oral feeding is impossible or contraindicated. It is essential that the veterinary nurse becomes familiar with the management of these tubes, and this subject is covered in detail in Chapter 16.

Assisted feeding should only be instigated when all attempts to induce the animal to eat voluntarily have failed. Anorexic patients may be tempted to eat by:

- Improving palatability (e.g. warming or wetting the food)
- Feeding by hand
- Offering odorous foods (e.g. pilchards)
- Offering favourite food (liaise with owners)
- Offering freshly cooked food
- Smearing food on lips
- Stroking and providing company
- Feeding in privacy.

Reasons for considering assisted feeding include:

- Failure to entice voluntary eating
- Physical inability (e.g. fractured jaw)
- Following injury or surgery to oral cavity, or where feeding is contraindicated (e.g. oesophageal trauma).

Geriatric nursing

Geriatric nursing involves nursing the ageing animal in both health and disease. Geriatric patients must be treated with extra care; they are less able to adapt to change and they recover more slowly from medical or surgical interference (*for each 5 years of a pet's age, allow 24 hours longer to recover*).

The key to nursing the geriatric patient is good information (history, medication), the provision of security, comfort (soft bedding), the correct type of food and an adequate source of water.

Changes associated with old age

Physical

- Greying (e.g. muzzle)
- Thickening of the skin
- Coarse coat
- Loss of musculature
- Loss of stamina and strength
- Weakening of bone
- Lowered physical tolerance to change
- Loss of sight or hearing
- Poor tolerance to lack of fluid intake
- Impaired temperature regulation
- Arthritis and joint stiffness
- Higher susceptibility to infection

Mental

- Lowered responses to stimuli
- Less adaptable
- Increased fussiness about food
- Development of food preferences
- Less interest in activity
- Less obedient
- Disorientation

Many of the mental alterations are related to physical change; for example, disorientation is made worse when the patient is blind or deaf. Ageing changes and the accumulation of any injuries the patient may have sustained result in a loss of functional reserve: the organs of the body become less capable of dealing with extra demands placed on them for repair of tissue, assimilation of substances, etc.

Changes due to disease must be carefully distinguished from those of old age, though disease can become more obvious or affect a patient more rapidly when they become old. Very few sick, elderly patients suffer from a single disease. Many conditions are subtle and multiple.

Diseases common in geriatric animals

- Cancer
- Chronic renal disease
- Cardiac disease
- Osteoarthritis (degenerative joint disease – DJD)
- Cataracts
- Dental disease
- Constipation
- Incontinence

Apparent **urinary incontinence** is not always due to a total inability to control micturition but rather where patients lose bladder muscle/sphincter tone. This may result in 'leaking' of urine during sleep, relaxation or long periods of confinement. These patients cannot be left alone for long periods without the opportunity to urinate. They urinate in the house or while asleep and may appear to be incontinent to their owners.

Nursing considerations

The patient's history needs to be known. This includes any known medical conditions, current treatment and preferred food. It should be remembered that patients may be suffering from diseases other than those for which they have been admitted. Specific conditions are dealt with in Chapter 21. The following points are general guidelines.

Drugs

All patients should be weighed, but it is particularly important to weigh the geriatric patient so that accurate drug dose calculations can be made. Drug dosage is the veterinary surgeon's responsibility but anaesthetic drugs may well be prepared by nursing staff and accurate calculations are essential. Young patients may have the capacity to survive mild medication overdosage; geriatrics may not.

Feeding

Geriatric patients generally need fewer calories but simply feeding them less can result in a lowered intake of protein, vitamins and minerals.

Dietary considerations in the absence of any disease include a highly digestible, well balanced proprietary food. There are many available and some companies produce diets specifically formulated for the older dog. Cats tend to stay active for longer and special diets are less available. To avoid digestive upsets, any changes in diet should be introduced gradually.

Lack of interest in food is rarely due to true anorexia in the previously appetent hospitalized geriatric patient. It is more likely that the patient is being offered different food, finds the amount offered too great, has dental disease resulting in pain or has difficulty in standing to eat.

Obesity

This is common in the geriatric patient and management is achieved through client education. It needs to be emphasized to the owners that excess weight is potentially dangerous to their pet, extra strain being placed on the heart, kidneys, liver and musculoskeletal system in obese patients. This may help to persuade owners that their pet would be happier and

healthier if it lost weight. Target weights may be suggested, but all diets should be checked with a veterinary surgeon to ensure that increased exercise (if possible) and diet changes are not contraindicated.

Fluid balance (water and urine)

⚠ WARNING
Do not restrict water intake in a geriatric patient unless it is vomiting. This is particularly important in relation to the withdrawal of fluids prior to surgery.

No patient should be deprived of water for more than an hour before induction of anaesthesia. Water does not need to be withdrawn the night before; this can be extremely dangerous. Younger patients will tolerate the insult, but in geriatric patients renal function can be seriously compromised when water intake is restricted.

If the amount of water being consumed by a geriatric is in doubt, it may be necessary to measure fluid intake to ensure that adequate quantities are being provided. Urine output will indicate adequate fluid provision and this too can be measured. Many elderly patients will be suffering from various degrees of renal compromise and may drink and urinate in excess of normal calculated volumes (2 ml urine/kg/day, 40–60 ml maintenance fluids/kg/day). If vomiting is present, intravenous fluids must be administered. Urine should be observed for normal colour and passage (i.e. no straining).

Exercise

Little and often is recommended. Elderly dogs enjoy 'pottering'. Even hospitalized dogs should be given time to wander, maybe in an outside run. Frequent walks will help to exercise stiff joints and ensure plenty of opportunities to urinate (which may save time on cleaning out kennels). Elderly cats often sleep for long periods of time, but encouraging them to move around can be beneficial to circulation and joint health.

Special care should be taken if the patient is blind or deaf.

As many owners will not previously have experienced an elderly pet, considerations should be discussed on discharge or at consultation.

Defecation

Constipation is more common in the elderly dog and cat. Defecation should be observed, where possible, to enable elimination of any suspected tenesmus or difficulty in evacuation of faeces. Faecal examination should be carried out on a regular basis to detect any abnormalities.

Bedding and kennelling

Blankets and soft bedding should be provided, along with foam mattresses for those with osteoarthritis. Geriatrics should be kept out of draughts and if possible somewhere not too noisy. Frequent light exercise should be encouraged, to improve peripheral circulation and maintenance of peripheral temperature. External additional heat sources may be required. Core temperature should be monitored if there is any suspicion that the patient is cold.

Grooming

Elderly patients should be groomed regularly, as they are less likely to keep themselves clean. Grooming helps to give a feeling of well-being and provides an opportunity to check the coat and skin, and to clean discharges from eyes and nose. The human contact is in itself beneficial.

If the patient has lost its sight or hearing, those who care for it should move slowly and talk reassuringly at all times. This will help to prevent the dog biting when suddenly touched or frightened.

Convalescence

This will take more time in geriatric animals than in younger ones. Patience is essential and a longer period for convalescence must be allowed. If patients are discharged before they have fully recovered, the owners should be informed that it will take some time for a pet to complete its recovery.

Maintenance of normal body temperature is especially important pre-, intra- and postoperatively. Thermoregulation in geriatrics is often compromised. Adequate water intake is also very important; patients must be able to reach water bowls, and water may be added to food if necessary. Exercise should be gentle. Physiotherapy, especially massage, may be used to improve circulation to the extremities.

Care of the vomiting patient

Vomiting (**emesis**) is the forcible ejection of contents of the stomach through the mouth. It should not be confused with regurgitation, which is the return of undigested food from the oesophagus (see Chapter 21).

Nursing of the vomiting patient can be very straightforward (e.g. in the case of scavenging) or much more complex (e.g. as a result of metabolic imbalances).

Mechanical and functional disorders

Patients suffering from mechanical or functional disorders are usually admitted for surgical correction of the condition. Dietary management is usually simple.

Foreign bodies

Food is generally withheld until surgery has been carried out. If water induces vomiting, it too should be withheld but replaced by intravenous fluids. Most vomiting patients have some degree of dehydration and in these cases an intravenous drip is set up to provide fluid.

The reintroduction of food and water after surgery will vary in each individual case but the following are basic guidelines.

In some cases nothing will be allowed by mouth for 24–48 hours. Intravenous fluid therapy must continue to supply calculated daily requirements. Feeding during this time should not be neglected and hopefully some form of enteral feeding will be available (see Chapter 16). Tube feeding allows the surgical site a chance to heal whilst still providing a route for nutrition, which is essential to rapid recovery.

If fluids by mouth are allowed, initially small amounts should be offered frequently (50–100 ml every hour). If these are not vomited, then the amounts can be increased over the next 8 hours. Intravenous fluids may be continued during this time, as total fluid requirements will not be achieved initially.

Reintroduction of food begins once fluids are retained, usually over 24–72 hours. Food offered will vary: usually it will be a bland diet of soft small chunks of moist food, offered little and often. Liquidized food may be specified in some cases (e.g. in the management of pyloric stenosis). Bland foods include chicken, fish or a commercially prepared diet.

Feeding of patients after intestinal surgery (enterectomy or enterotomy) should begin immediately after recovery from anaesthesia. This helps to prevent intestinal stasis.

Megaoesophagus

Patients with megaoesophagus regurgitate rather than vomit. Food becomes lodged in the oesophagus cranial to a stricture or narrowing, so that only a limited amount of food reaches the stomach.

Dietary management (even after surgery, if performed) will involve varying degrees of liquidized or semi-solid food fed from a height (Figure 15.15). Feeding from a height helps to prevent regurgitation and the possible development of aspiration pneumonia – gravity helps the passage of food to the stomach. Passage of food can also be aided after feeding by gentle coupage whilst the patient is in an upright position.

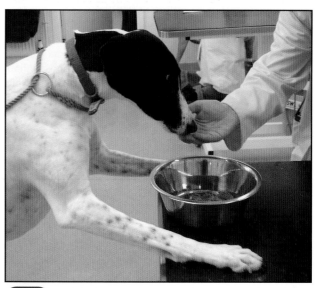

15.15 Feeding from height.

Metabolic disorders

Patients that vomit due to metabolic disorders are generally more challenging to the nurse. If vomiting has been prolonged, they will be dehydrated and require fluid therapy in combination with other treatment. The percentage of dehydration can be estimated clinically (see Chapter 19).

It is pleasant for the patient to have moist cotton wool wiped around the mucous membranes of the mouth, especially if water has been withdrawn. This not only freshens the mouth but also removes excess saliva.

If water is not vomited, oral electrolyte fluids may be useful (see Chapter 19 for details of fluid therapy).

Antiemetic drugs, such as metoclopramide, can be given by intramuscular, subcutaneous or intravenous routes by slow infusion over 24 hours. The oral route is usually contraindicated in these patients. For continuous effect, the veterinary surgeon may request drugs to be placed in the drip fluid.

Water, and then food, can be reintroduced when vomiting ceases.

Reintroduction of food

The following is a general guide for the reintroduction of food to a patient that has been vomiting. It assumes that water does not cause vomiting. If at any stage vomiting reoccurs, return to the previous day's protocol.

- **Day 1**: Offer small amounts of bland food 3–4 times daily. Total amount offered should equal one-quarter to one-half of normal daily kilocalorie requirement.
- **Day 2**: Offer small amounts of bland food frequently, to total one-half to three-quarters of daily requirement.
- **Days 3–6**: As for days 1 and 2 but total amount offered should be equal to normal requirement.
- **Days 7–14**: Reintroduce normal diet by mixing increasing amounts with the bland diet.

Patients that have had a single acute vomiting episode due to scavenging will need to be starved for 24–48 hours before the reintroduction of food. In these cases the above regime can be followed and can also be given as advice to owners over the telephone. Specific types of food may be required, longer periods of starvation necessary or placement of feeding tubes. A veterinary surgeon will give instructions on the course to be followed.

General points

Nausea is unpleasant. It can be identified in dogs and cats by:

- Restlessness
- Salivation
- Repeated swallowing
- Retching.

These signs should be brought to the attention of the veterinary surgeon. Other points that should be remembered in the nursing of the vomiting patient include :

- Clean away any excess vomitus and clean the mouth. If not contraindicated, offer small amounts of cool fresh water (10–15 ml) to allow rinsing of the mouth
- Handle gently. Lift only if absolutely necessary, ensuring that no pressure is placed on the patient's abdomen
- Hand-feeding and encouragement may be required during the recovery period
- If syringe feeding of fluids is instituted at any time, remember the potential for the development of aspiration pneumonia. It is surprisingly easy to cause pneumonia, especially in smaller dogs and cats
- When patients are discharged, give the owners written instructions regarding the type of food, the amounts to be offered, its consistency and the method of feeding.

The soiled patient

Hospitalized patients may become soiled at some time during their stay. It is the nurse's responsibility to ensure that all soiling is cleaned efficiently, effectively and quickly.

Regular walking of inpatients may seem time-consuming but it may conserve time spent in cleaning kennels and soiled patients. Cats must be supplied with litter trays; advice should be sought from the owners regarding types of litter used, as some cats are fussy.

Animals may become soiled by urine, faeces, blood, vomit, other body fluids or food. Reasons for soiling include:

- Confinement to a small area
- Disturbed routine
- Medical or surgical condition
- Puppies not yet house-trained
- Recumbency.

Care of soiled patients

- Clean as quickly as possible.
- Choose shampoos carefully. Take into consideration the patient's coat length, the reason for its hospitalization and the area to be cleaned or bathed. Chlorhexidine gluconate or povidone–iodine are preferable if the patient has any surgical or open wounds. Dry dog shampoos are available, but they are inadequate if soiling has occurred.
- Once the area has been cleaned, dry it thoroughly. Most patients will tolerate a hair dryer after a towel rub-down. All knots in the coat should be removed, since they may harbour faeces. Conditioners will make the process much less tiresome for nursing staff and for the patient (especially in long-haired breeds).
- Whilst grooming, check for any area of soreness, especially if the patient is recumbent. If necessary, clip hair away from these areas.
- It is best to clip heavily contaminated areas, especially if further contamination is expected (e.g. under drainage tubes). Ensure that client permission to clip has been given. White petroleum jelly can be applied around these areas after clipping, to prevent soreness and to make cleaning easier. There are also barrier film sprays (like a plastic skin), e.g. Cavilon (3M), that can be used to protect skin surfaces from urine and faecal scalding.

Cats generally keep themselves very clean. If bathing is necessary, use mild shampoos and avoid products based on coal tar (phenol is poisonous to cats). Regular grooming of hospitalized longhaired cats is essential. Cats with oral lesions or fractured jaws are unable to clean themselves and so regular cleaning of the lips, chin and paws will be required.

Enemas

An enema is a liquid substance placed into the rectum and colon of a patient. The enema is not intended to flush colonic contents but to distend the rectum and distal colon gently, initiating normal expulsive reflexes.

Reasons for administering an enema

Emptying the rectum

- To relieve constipation or impaction
- As preparation for radiographic studies. The colon and rectum overlie abdominal structures and will obscure them if they are not emptied
- As part of a radiographic contrast study
- To enable the administration of drugs
- In preparation for endoscopic examination

As a diagnostic aid

Barium sulphate enemas can be given to outline the rectal and colonic walls. After the radiography the patient will need to evacuate the barium and a quick retreat to the outside is strongly advised.

Administering medication

The colon has a large capacity for absorption. It is therefore a good route for the administration of soluble drugs, but it is rarely used in veterinary medicine due to lack of patient cooperation.

Solutions used

Water

Warm tap water is the preferred solution. It is readily available, non-toxic and non-irritant. In addition, any cleaning of the peri-anal area is reasonably straightforward.

Liquid paraffin

This is readily available and reasonably cheap. Cleaning the patient after the enema can be difficult, since liquid paraffin is oil based and not water soluble. The patient needs to be bathed with shampoo to remove this substance.

Mineral oil

This suffers the same disadvantages as liquid paraffin and is more expensive. However, oil-based substances are an advantage when treating a constipated patient. The oil helps to soften and lubricate the faecal masses and allows easier evacuation of the bowel.

Saline (phosphate enema)

This is usually available as manufactured sachets with phosphate included. They promote defecation by being osmotically active, promoting water retention in the colon. These enemas should be used with care in small (weighing less than 15 kg) and young patients because their excessive use can result in unwanted absorption of certain ions, resulting in system toxicity.

Ready-to-use mini enema

A proprietary brand of miniature enema is introduced into the rectum by an attached nozzle. It is extremely useful in cats, the procedure being no more stressful than using a rectal thermometer.

Gastrointestinal cleaning agents

These are laxatives rather than enemas but can be used for bowel clearance for all the same indications. These agents are given orally and defecation occurs rapidly after administration. Stomach tubing may be required to administer the fluid, as they are flavoured for the human market and dogs are usually unwilling to drink them.

Miscellaneous substances

The following variations are either more expensive or largely outdated and have no advantages over solutions already mentioned: glycerine and water; olive oil and water; obstetric lubricant; and soft soap (may cause mucosal irritation).

Equipment

The basic equipment includes enema solution, gloves, lubricant (e.g. K-Y jelly) and any of the following: can and tubing, Higginson syringe, prepared barium bag, syringe and catheter (Figure 15.16).

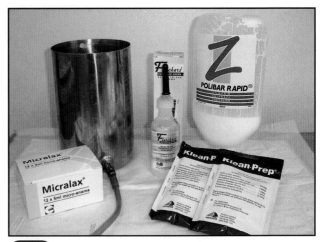

15.16   Equipment for enemas.

Administration of an enema

Figure 15.17 gives guidance on the volumes of solution.

Solution	Volume used (ml/kg)	Frequency
Water	5–10	Every 20–30 minutes if necessary
Liquid paraffin	2–3	Every 1–2 hours
Saline solution	1–2	Do not repeat for 12 hours
Barium sulphate	5–10	Single administration
Klean Prep	20	Single administration
Laxative fluids		Single administration

15.17   Enema solutions and volumes.

Giving an enema to a dog

This method requires two people

1. Prepare all equipment.
2. The assistant restrains the patient in a suitable area, preferably outside where cleaning will be easier.
3. Lubricate the end of the tube or nozzle.
4. Elevate the patient's tail and place the tube into the anus. Rotate gently until access to the rectum is achieved (this is easy in the dog but occasionally more difficult in the cat).
5. Advance the tube into the rectum.
6. Stand to the side of the patient and allow fluid to run into the rectum by gravity, or gently pump in fluid.
7. Allow dogs free exercise to evacuate bowels and supply cats with litter trays and an adequately sized cage.

The recumbent patient

An animal that is lying down and unable to rise is described as **recumbent**. A large number of conditions might result in recumbency, the more common being:

- Fractures (e.g. pelvis, limbs)
- Spinal trauma (e.g. disc protrusion)
- Weakness due to medical disease
- Neurological injury or disease
- Shock.

Kennelling

Size

Previously active animals attempt to drag themselves around (especially fracture and spinal cases in which pain has been relieved). The kennel should be large enough for such a patient to lie in lateral recumbency comfortably, but not so big that it has room to cause damage to itself.

Position

Most recumbent patients benefit from being nursed in a kennel sited in an area of activity. This stimulates them and relieves boredom, since nursing staff inevitably talk to them more frequently. Kennels should not be in direct sunlight, since these patients may be unable to move to a shady area.

Bedding

The patient should be bedded on thick, waterproof (PVC-covered) foam mattresses, with 'Vetbed' or similar on the top. If these are unavailable, thick layers of newspaper with blankets on top may be used. Beanbags, although very comfortable, become soiled very easily and are difficult to clean; they are normally impractical in the hospital situation.

Food and water

Both food and water need to be within easy reach. Patients that are recumbent due to a medical condition may be depressed, and feeding by hand may be necessary. Patients that fail to drink sufficiently can have water added to their food or be encouraged to drink by having water syringed into the side of the mouth.

Most recumbent patients require a concentrated, highly digestible diet to meet the extra nutritional needs of stress due to kennelling or continuing tissue repair. Highly digestible diets have the added advantage of producing less faecal material. The energy requirement supplied by carbohydrates is generally lower during recumbency and the amount of carbohydrates offered may need to be reduced. Sick animals may have an increased nutrient requirement, since these are necessary for tissue repair (i.e. raised protein). If the recumbent patient fails to eat, advice should be sought from the owner regarding the animal's preferences and favourite foods.

Obesity may be an existing problem or weight may be gained during the period of recumbency due to less energy being used. It may be necessary to introduce reducing diets, but only in consultation with the veterinary surgeon.

Urination and defecation

If possible, recumbent patients should be taken outside. The change of environment and fresh air are beneficial to their mental attitude. In addition, natural urination and defecation are always preferable to catheterization and enemata. Patients may need help to stand, since many are unwilling to urinate lying down. Towel support is useful (Figure 15.18); even tetraplegics and quadraplegics can be managed in this way, using crossed towels to support the chest. When an animal is supported, gentle manual pressure may be applied to the bladder to encourage urination (Figure 15.19).

Catheterization

Full details of methods, equipment and complications are given later in this chapter in the section 'Urinary catheterization'.

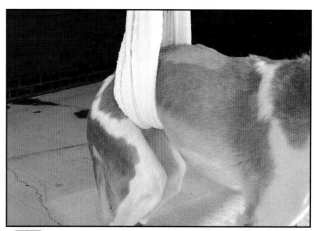

15.18 Assisted walking for the recumbent patient.

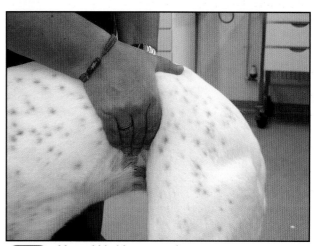

15.19 Manual bladder expression.

Indwelling Foley catheters can be used. They are beneficial in keeping the patient dry by preventing soiling from urine overflow 24 hours a day. Indwelling Foley catheters with a bag attached have the added advantage of enabling urine output to be easily measured.

In dogs, plastic dog catheters can be sutured to the prepuce or catheterization can be carried out 2–3 times daily. There are also Foley catheters made from silicone that can be passed up the male urethra and remain in the bladder in exactly the same manner as the latex Foley. The silicone is so smooth that the catheter advances up the curved male urethra even without the aid of a stylet. Wire-guide stylets are available and may make the procedure even easier.

Cat bladders can generally be expressed manually, or catheterization may be performed.

⚠ WARNING
Placement of urinary catheters is invasive and should not be carried out casually. Antibiotic cover will be required and the potential for temporary bladder function problems after removal of indwelling catheters must be recognized. The raised possibility of urinary tract infections is also a major consideration.

Constipation and diarrhoea

A record of defecation should be kept, as otherwise it is easy for 3–5 days of non-production to go unnoticed. If the patient becomes constipated, a laxative may be required.

Any diarrhoea in the recumbent patient increases the risk of sores, infection in any wounds, fly-strike in the summer and discomfort to the patient. The veterinary surgeon should be informed. Excess hair in the perianal/anal area should be clipped. Cleaning as quickly as possible after contamination occurs is extremely important.

Decubital ulcers and urine scalding

Prevention
It is better to prevent both decubital ulcers (Figure 15.20) and urine scalding, rather than treat them after they have occurred.

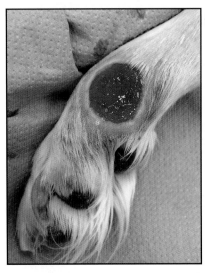

15.20 Decubital ulcer.

- The use of soft **bedding** with absorbable blankets, together with regular **turning** of the patient (every 4 hours), will help to lessen the occurrence of sores.
- Bony prominences are most likely to suffer (e.g. elbows and ischial wings). These areas can be **padded** with foam rings from the top of tablet pots (Figure 15.21) or the patient can be encouraged to lie laterally for short periods. A balance between lateral and sternal recumbency needs to be found (see 'Hypostatic pneumonia', below).

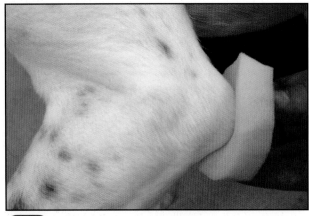

15.21 Padding of bony prominences.

- **Massage** is beneficial and can be performed while the patient is recumbent.
- **Slings** to raise patients for longer periods are used in the US and at larger veterinary establishments in the UK.

- **Catheterization** (indwelling or repeated) enables bladder drainage without soiling. Otherwise assisted walking is essential to provide opportunities for urination.
- **Waterbeds** may be useful but are rarely used in the UK.

Management of urine scalds
Any patient that is dirtied by urine should be checked for the presence of urine scalds. They begin as innocent-looking red patches and are very easily managed if treated at this stage. There is no excuse for their progressing, given proper nursing care.

Urine scalding is relieved by:

- Regular washing with a mild antiseptic shampoo (e.g. dilute chlorhexidine gluconate or povidone–iodine); both must be rinsed off thoroughly
- Clipping hair and the application of soothing healing or barrier creams
- Catheterization.

Catheterization is no longer considered good practice by some clinicians (see warning box above regarding complications of indwelling catheters). Simple urine management is sufficient, unless the patient's condition expressly requires catheterization.

Management of decubital ulcers
Decubital ulcers are far more serious and can be extremely difficult to resolve. Hardening of areas prone to them with spirit is *not* recommended. Treatment is as follows:

1. Clip the area around the sore.
2. Clean with a mild antiseptic solution (e.g. dilute povidone–iodine or chlorhexidine gluconate).
3. Dry thoroughly.
4. Apply an appropriate cream or protective barrier film (e.g. Cavilon (3M)).
5. If it is summer, and the position of the ulcer allows, cover with a dressing to prevent fly-strike and contamination.
6. If on lower limb, consider bandaging.

Hypostatic pneumonia
Hypostatic pneumonia is caused by the pooling of blood and a consequent decrease in viability of the dependent lung. It is more likely to occur in an old, sick and debilitated animal that has been in lateral recumbency for a long period. Signs of hypostatic pneumonia are:

- Rapid shallow breathing
- Increased respiratory effort
- Moist noises when breathing, possibly even gurgling
- Depressed attitude.

If hypostatic pneumonia is suspected, a veterinary surgeon should be informed immediately. Auscultation of the lung fields and radiography may be required to confirm the diagnosis.

Prevention
Turning the patient at least every 4 hours, 24 hours a day, is essential nursing. Sternal recumbency should be encouraged by using sandbags, water/sand-filled containers or radiography cradles (and remember to support the head).

Regular coupage (the external impact massage of the thorax with cupped hands) 4–5 times daily for 5 minutes will improve thoracic circulation. By promoting coughing it also aids removal of secretions that build up in the bronchial tree. A veterinary surgeon should be consulted before coupage is used, to ensure that there are no contraindications such as fractured ribs.

It is important to realize that serious secondary chest infections may result if hypostatic pneumonia is allowed to develop. This alone can cause death.

Treatment

If hypostatic pneumonia with a secondary infection is present, all of the above guidelines for prevention should be continued. In addition, treatment (e.g. antibiotics) will probably be prescribed.

Passive physiotherapy

Physiotherapy helps to maintain and improve peripheral circulation. It is of benefit to all recumbent patients, even if only for the extra human contact and attention. The subject is covered in detail in Chapter 21.

Massage

This is particularly useful for the limbs (see Chapter 21). The patient should be massaged from the toes towards the body to encourage venous return to the heart.

Supported exercise

Towel-walking is the most common (and cheapest) method (see Figure 15.18). Adequate staff need to be available, as both the patient and the staff member can be injured if the patient is heavy. Wheeled total support hoists for walking recumbent patients assist mobility of heavier patients and enable effective active physical therapy with the patient in a normal walking position (Figure 15.22).

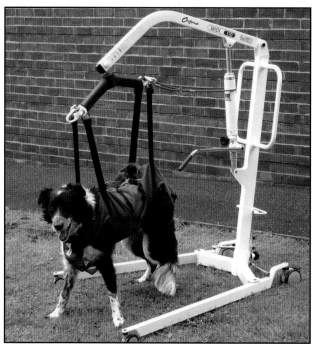

15.22 Wheeled 'total support' hoist for walking recumbent patients.

Hydrotherapy

Swimming is very useful physiotherapy for dogs (cats generally do not appreciate it). Small dogs can be swum in large sinks and baths in the hospital; larger patients need pools. Swimming enables patients to move their limbs freely without weight-bearing forces.

The temperature of the water must be checked before the patient is immersed. Constant support and observation are essential to prevent panic and possible drowning. For full details on hydrotherapy, see Chapter 21.

Passive joint movement

Manually moving joints within their normal range helps to prevent stiffness and improves circulation.

Body temperature

Recumbent patients expend very little energy; therefore heat production is lower than normal. Body temperature may fall to a subnormal level. Blankets to cover the patient may be sufficient. Other heating methods include:

• Veterinary duvet-type covers with reflective filling
• Veterinary instant heat pads, which should be wrapped initially: when activated, they heat to 52°C
• Hot-water bottles, which should be wrapped to prevent burning of the patient
• Heated waterbeds – use only if the patient is very debilitated and will not bite or scratch; they are expensive pieces of equipment to replace if punctured
• Bubble packaging – cheap and effective
• Silver foil – good for extremities but remove if patients become active, especially young ones, as it may be chewed
• Silver reflective survival blankets
• Infrared lamps
• Incubators.

⚠ **WARNING**
Electrically heated beds are not recommended unless the patient is under constant supervision. Some varieties have been implicated in causing serious burns when patients were placed directly on top of them. A blanket should always be between the heated pad and the patient.

Home nursing

Recumbent patients are generally managed in a hospital environment. Some will inevitably be recumbent for a longer period and may be nursed at home. Most owners are quite capable of learning how to nurse their own pet, but tasks that come automatically to a nurse need to be pointed out to an owner. It is helpful to write clear instructions to which owners can refer once they are home. Owners should be assured that they can phone at any time if they are worried. Weekly checks at the surgery should be arranged to monitor for signs of decubital ulcers, urine scalding or hypostatic pneumonia.

The comatose patient

In this context, **comatose** is interpreted as being in a long-term coma rather than unconscious during a routine recovery from anaesthesia. This may occur in conditions such as tetanus, neurological disease or after major convulsions. In reality these patients are rarely nursed in general practice – they really need a critical care unit with 24-hour staffing and expert care (see Chapter 18).

The nursing of a comatose patient is essentially similar to that for a recumbent one and all the nursing points made above for the care of the recumbent patient can be implemented for the comatose patient – with the exception of eating, drinking and exercise. Nutrition is best provided by total parenteral nutrition (TPN) via a jugular catheter or by a jejunostomy tube; fluid is provided intravenously.

In addition, the following points should be considered when nursing the comatose patient:

* Keep a patent airway – pull tongue forward and consider endotracheal intubation
* Clean any secretions from the oral cavity – use suction or swabs and lower the head to encourage drainage by gravity
* Monitor at 15-minute intervals:
  - Temperature, pulse rate and quality, respiratory rate and rhythm
  - Capillary refill time
  - Urine output (30-minute intervals if catheter is in place)
  - Drip rates
  - Drug administration.

Constant 24-hour observation is essential for the comatose patient.

Transport of the unconscious patient

The priority for these patients is maintenance of the airway. All unconscious patients should be transported from one area to another on a firm surface to enable their head and neck to be extended, thus protecting the airway. For cats and small mammals this is usually a basket; for dogs and larger mammals a trolley should be used.

For all patients:

* Extend head and neck
* If possible, pull tongue forward so that it can be seen during transport
* Monitor colour of mucous membranes
* Observe breathing patterns
* Ensure that there are enough people to move the patient safely
* Stop transportation to readjust position of patient if necessary
* Transport patient as rapidly as possible
* Cover patient to maintain heat.

As a general rule patients should *not* be carried in the arms, though in reality this is the method used by many, over small distances. In all cases the head and neck should be supported by a firm surface (e.g. piece of hardboard) to ensure that the airway is not compromised.

The unconscious patient's head should never be allowed to 'flop' towards the floor, nor should the patient be cradled in the arms. Cradling the unconscious patient is bad practice and dangerous: the tongue can fall into the back of the larynx and occlude the airway.

Dogs

Unconscious dogs weighing over 10 kg should be transported on trolleys, for the health and safety of personnel as well as that of the dog. Keeping endotracheal tubes in place during transport of anaesthetized patients can be the best way to protect airways. The dog's head should always be at the end of the trolley where the staff member is facing forward, so that constant observation of breathing can be done with ease.

Cats

Cats are best transported in baskets. It is important that the head and neck are extended during the whole of the transportation period, even if this means 'bunching' the cat's hind end at the opposing end of the basket. If this is not possible, the cat should be transported on a trolley.

Endotracheal tubes can be left in place to protect the airway, but it may be necessary to stop and remove the tube rapidly if the patient regains consciousness.

Rabbits

For the purpose of transport, rabbits can be moved in the same way as the cat. Some of the dwarf varieties may be best treated as for the smaller mammals.

Small mammals

Small mammals often recover rapidly from anaesthesia and are best not transported from the area of anaesthesia until recovered. If transport is essential, small boxes (with the patient's head extended) is the best method. *Small mammals lose heat rapidly and hypothermia may delay recovery. Small pre-warmed containers should be used.*

The critically ill patient

Critically ill patients need to be nursed in a designated area. This should be:

* Quiet
* Well ventilated
* Well lit
* Well served with electrical points for monitors.

There will need to be adequate:

* Monitoring equipment for nursing staff to use effectively
* Staff members (for 24-hour care)
* On-site laboratory facilities.

Management

Nursing care of critically ill patients is time-consuming and demanding. All the care for the recumbent patient and the soiled patient (above) should be applied, with any appropriate adaptations with regard to the individual patient's needs or condition.

Charts should be made up at the beginning of the day, with timed intervals for any given activity. In this way the patient care is documented and it is easy for any member of staff to take over and assess recent progress and protocols. Checks, monitoring, drugs and nutrition are less likely to be missed accidentally if there is clear and accurate timed record keeping. In particular, pain medication needs to be given at accurate time intervals, especially when the patient may be unable to exhibit discomfort. In addition, the areas of intravenous and urinary catheter management, temperature control and tube management need to have the highest consideration.

Intravenous catheter management

This must be exemplary, as many critically ill patients are immunosuppressed and likely to contract infections easily. Washing of hands is mandatory and wearing of gloves advisable. Any spilt blood from around catheter should be cleaned with antiseptic solution and checks should be made to ensure that all tapes securing catheters and dressings are clean.

Catheter patency is maintained by flushing with heparinized saline (4 units heparin per 1 ml of 0.9% saline) every 4–6 hours. Regular changing of peripheral catheters (usually every 3–5 days) should be done in line with instructions from the veterinary surgeon in charge. Jugular lines are rarely changed if they are functioning well. The skin insertion site of jugular catheters demands particular care and should be inspected at least daily, preferably twice daily, with gloved hands, replacing sterile dressing at the site as appropriate.

Urinary catheter management

Placement of urinary catheters holds a high risk of urinary tract infection (UTI). Ensuring that catheters are placed with sterile gloves and equipment will help to reduce the risk, as will keeping the kennel clean. The patient needs to be monitored for signs of infection, as UTIs can initiate a systemic response.

Temperature control

Core temperature should be monitored at least every 30 minutes. The aim is to keep the temperature at a constant level. Warming patients gradually usually prevents inadvertent overheating.

Tube management

These may be chest drainage tubes, active drainage tubes from wounds, feeding tubes or nasal oxygen provision tubes (see also Chapters 16, 19 and 24). The same basic rules apply to all.

- Wash hands and wear gloves on handling.
- Check insertion sites (for some, hourly; others daily).
- Dress sites that involve breaches in the skin with sterile dressings; change the dressings as appropriate but at least daily.
- Bandage so that the tubes are protected but also in a manner that provides patient comfort; ensure that no clamps etc. rub or press into the skin surface.
- Ensure that feeding tubes are flushed thoroughly to prevent blockage.

Patient's mental attitude

The importance of maintaining mental stimulation for patients has been mentioned in the section on care of the recumbent patient (above), but it does need some expansion in the case of the critically ill.

Critically ill patients are often responding to stimuli in a very delayed fashion, or may be unconscious. This does not necessarily mean that they are unaware. Having a radio in the background may help to calm patients, as will sitting with them without carrying out any procedure. These patients tend to have had, and are having, maximum attention but all is related to things being 'done' to them. Stress, whether exhibited by the patient (e.g. by aggression or panic) or not (e.g. in the case of some neurological conditions), will actively delay recovery times. Taking time simply to sit and stroke or talk to the patient is an essential area of good nursing care for these individuals.

Nutrition

The methods for tube feeding are covered in Chapter 16 and apply equally to the critically ill.

Fresh food should be offered to tube-fed patients regularly, as it is preferable for them to eat normally and tube feeding to be stopped as soon as possible. In the seemingly unconscious or mentally 'dull' animal, the smell of food can produce a marked response, which can be a good indicator of improvement.

Critically ill patients should never be starved. They need at least twice their basic energy requirement (see Chapter 16)

due to the stresses to which they are exposed in critical care treatment.

Tube feeding or total parenteral nutrition needs to be started immediately if patients are unable to (or will not) eat for themselves.

Environment

As critically ill patients begin to recover a change in environment can be beneficial, especially if the patient has been distressed during the more critical period. The patient may be moved into a different area, outside if monitoring equipment allows. A change of environment and different sources of stimulation can promote a more rapid recovery.

Neonates

The care of neonates, including those that are critically ill, is considered in detail in Chapter 25.

Neonates can become critically ill very rapidly as a result of almost any insult, whether physiological or mechanical. Whatever the cause of the crisis, there are some basic considerations that must be acted upon:

- Temperature – maintain at 25–30°C
- Fluids – neonates dehydrate quickly; begin intravenous, intraosseous or intraperitoneal administration (see Chapter 19)
- Feed as soon as possible, at least supply some glucose in fluids
- Encourage movement
- If the patient is reluctant to move, massage from periphery towards heart to encourage better perfusion and distribution of fluids and heat.

Once these basics have been performed, the cause of the crisis can be investigated and treated. Even healthy neonates have a very reduced capacity for sudden changes of any kind and can deteriorate very quickly; this is even more so in the critically ill neonate and therefore *constant* monitoring is usually required.

Special considerations

There are a number of special considerations when performing basic procedures in neonates.

- Use antiseptics and spirit carefully – they encourage heat loss. *Careless use can be the difference between survival and demise.*
- Reduce clipping of fur to as small areas as possible, to preserve body heat.
- Accurate dosing of drugs is essential. Use of 1 ml or 100 IU syringes is advisable when drawing up small quantities. Drugs may be diluted *with care*; they must be water-miscible and thorough mixing ensured.
- Move neonates around gently and do not change orientation rapidly – the sudden need for redistribution of circulating blood volume can cause shock that they may not be able to survive.
- Keep the neonate's head slightly below the rest of the body whenever possible, to allow drainage of saliva. This is particularly important if the neonate is semiconscious.

Urinary catheterization

A **catheter** is a tubular instrument (usually flexible) that is passed through body channels for the withdrawal of fluids from (or the introduction of fluids into) a body cavity.

Reasons for urinary catheterization

- To obtain a (sterile) urine sample when:
  - A patient will not urinate when required (this may be because the patient is only at the surgery for short periods, e.g. at consultation, or timed urine samples are required, e.g. water deprivation test)
  - Obtaining a midstream urine sample (MUS) can be very difficult in practice as male dogs usually void little and often during exercise, and culture and sensitivity testing requires urine to be collected in a sterile manner.
- To empty the urinary bladder:
  - Before abdominal, vaginal and urethral surgery
  - Before a pneumocystogram
  - When there is a partial obstruction or inability to urinate but a catheter can be passed into the bladder (e.g. due to prostatic enlargement).
- To introduce contrast agents for radiographic procedures.
- To maintain constant, controlled bladder drainage (indwelling catheters):
  - In the recumbent or incontinent patient to prevent soiling
  - After bladder surgery, to avoid overdistension of the bladder, thereby reducing tension on the suture line and helping to provide optimum healing conditions for the operative site.
- For retrograde flushing (the use of fluid pressure to dislodge particles causing an obstruction: a urinary catheter is placed caudal to the particle and water or sterile saline used to dislodge the calculi from the urethra back into the bladder). Hydropropulsion can be used to relieve a partial blockage in an emergency situation.

- To maintain a patent urethra:
  - In male cats suffering from feline lower urinary tract disease (FLUTD) – a catheter may be placed to maintain bladder drainage whilst treatment or dietary management is initiated; catheter placement also allows flushing of the bladder with solutions that may dissolve struvite crystals (e.g. Walpole's solution, though this is an older technique which is now rarely used)
  - Where dysuria or anuria is present but surgery is delayed due to the patient being in a poor condition for surgery (e.g. raised blood urea levels, electrolyte imbalance etc.).
- To monitor urine output:
  - Essential in patients with renal failure receiving intravenous fluids
  - If the patient is in intensive care
  - After renal surgery to ensure adequate production of urine (*minimum urine output should be 1–2 ml/kg bodyweight/hour*).
- To introduce drugs.

Complications associated with catheterization

Complications that might arise include reactive cystitis, infective cystitis, urethral damage, failure to catheterize the urethra, resistance by the patient, blockage of indwelling catheters or removal of indwelling catheters by the patient. Reasons for these complications are described below. Figure 15.23 outlines methods of preventing them and the action to be taken should they arise.

	Prevention	Action
Infection	Use only new or re-sterilized catheters. Use sterile gloves to handle catheters or employ the 'no touch' technique described for dog catheterization. Use sterile lubricants. Clean penis or vulva thoroughly before catheterization; clip surrounding hair if necessary. Catheterization should be carried out in a clean environment, not in the patient's kennel. Systemic antibiotics may be prescribed by the veterinary surgeon. Patients with indwelling catheters should receive systemic antibiotics whilst catheterized and continue the course for 5–10 days after removal	If infection becomes evident, treatment will consist of systemic antibiotics and, in some cases, soluble antibiotics flushed directly into the bladder
Cystitis after catheterization	Gentle introduction of the catheter – no force should be necessary. Use of lubricants is beneficial – they help to limit the epithelial damage to the urethral mucosa, thereby reducing inflammation. Trauma is less likely if an experienced person catheterizes debilitated patients	With indwelling catheters there is inevitably some degree of cystitis after removal of the catheter. If it is significant: • Encourage the patient to increase its fluid intake, either as water or by adding water to the food • Walk the patient frequently to allow urination; observe colour and amount of urine passed. If catheterization of the cervix does occur, remove the catheter and begin with a new one
Patient resistance		Sedate or, in extreme cases, anaesthetize the patient
Blockage of indwelling catheters	General hygiene and cleaning. Encourage increased water intake (this helps to maintain a continuous flow of urine through the catheter). If bags are attached, check regularly to ensure that urine is able to drain freely	Flush with sterile saline or water
Urethral damage	Never use force. Use adequate lubrication. If an obstruction or difficulty occurs, stop and inform a senior member of staff	If trauma caused by catheterization is suspected, a veterinary surgeon will have to decide what further action is to be taken. Minor trauma may require antibiotic treatment to prevent secondary bacterial infection
Failure to catheterize the urethra in the bitch	The only prevention is to gain experience in bitch catheterization. The easiest way for the student nurse to appreciate the position of the urethral orifice is by the use of a lighted speculum to provide viewed introduction of the catheter	

15.23 Complications associated with catheterization.

Infection

Urinary tract infection (UTI) can easily be caused by catheterization if bacteria present in the urethra are pushed into the bladder by the catheter. In most circumstances the bacteria are rapidly eliminated and cause no further concern. The risk of infection is increased when:

* The bladder is traumatized
* A preputial or vaginal discharge is present
* Indwelling catheters are used or repeated catheterization is carried out
* The patient is immunosuppressed, i.e. its immune system is compromised in some way and the body's natural defences are not operating normally.

The increase in resistance of organisms to antibiotic treatment is well documented. Therefore prophylactic antibiotic cover for catheterization (especially where indwelling catheters are in place) is less acceptable than in the past. As a result many establishments are reluctant to place indwelling catheters, preferring to use frequent visits outside or bladder expression.

Cystitis after catheterization

This is associated with indwelling catheters. It may also be seen where there has been repeated catheterization.

Patient resistance

This is common in bitches, queens and tomcats. Sedation or general anaesthesia may be required.

Removal of indwelling catheters by patients

Adequate suturing (tomcat, dog) and the application of Elizabethan collars should prevent catheter removal by the patient.

Blockage of indwelling catheters

Urine will cease to flow from the catheter. Flushing of catheters at regular intervals (2–3 times per day) is advisable.

Urethral damage

This is most likely to occur in the male dog. Due to the ischial curve of the urethra, some epithelial damage is inevitable as the catheter is passed around the curve. This is why a small amount of blood may be present in the tip of the catheter on removal from the urethra, which should be done gently.

Urethral damage in the bitch is usually due to excess force being used to advance the catheter into the bladder.

Failure to catheterize the urethra

Failure to catheterize the urethra may occur in the bitch if the urethral orifice is passed and the catheter cannot be advanced because it meets the cervix. Catheterization of the cervix is a rare occurrence and is easily identified:

* By viewing the urethral orifice with a lighted speculum
* Because no urine flows through the catheter – but note that catheters can be placed correctly and still not produce urine, due to either an empty bladder or an obstruction to urine flow (e.g. excessive lubricant blocking the drainage holes).

Types of urinary catheter

Most catheters manufactured for the veterinary market (Figures 15.24 and 15.25) are supplied individually, double wrapped, with an inner nylon and outer paper or plastic sleeve. The catheters are ready for use, having been sterilized by either ethylene oxide gas or gamma radiation. Silicone Foley catheters come non-sterile and require sterilization by autoclave or ethylene oxide. Metal bitch catheters (now rarely in use) may be autoclaved.

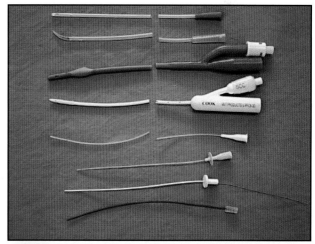

15.25   Urinary catheters. From top to bottom: dog; Tieman's; latex Foley; silicone Foley; cat; Jackson cat; silicone cat; Teflon cat.

Type	Species	Sex	Material	Indwelling	Sizes (FG)	Length (cm)	Luer fitting
Dog catheter	Dog	Male and female	Flexible grade of nylon (polyamide)	No but can be adapted to be indwelling	6–10	50–60	Yes
Silicone Foley	Dog	Male and female	Flexible medical grade silicone	Yes	5–10	30 and 55	No
Tieman's	Dog	Female	PVC (polyvinyl chloride)	No	8–12	43	Yes
Foley	Dog	Female	Teflon-coated latex	Yes	8–16	30–40	No
Cat catheter	Cat	Male and female	Flexible grade of nylon	No	3 and 4	30.5	Yes
Jackson cat catheter	Cat	Male and female	Flexible grade of nylon	Yes	3 and 4	11	Yes
Silicone cat catheter	Cat	Male	Medical grade silicone	Yes	3.5	12	Yes
Slippery Sam catheter	Cat	Male	PTFE (Teflon)	Yes	3–3.5	14 and 11	Yes

15.24   Types of urinary catheter.

With the exception of silicone catheters (which may be re-sterilized in the autoclave), urinary catheters are designed for single use only. The cleaning and reuse of catheters (other than silicone varieties) is not recommended.

Dog catheters

Plastic dog catheters

These have a rounded tip behind which are two oval drainage holes (one at each side). They are designed for single use in the male dog and can be used as indwelling catheters.

The largest gauge appropriate for patient size should be chosen. If the gauge is too small, the tip of the catheter has a tendency to 'catch' in the urethral epithelium and bend. This may cause significant urethral trauma. The only exception is where the urethra is narrowed due to a partial obstruction, such as an enlarged prostate, or a stricture. In these cases, there is no option other than to use a catheter that would otherwise be too small for the patient.

A second disadvantage of using small catheters in large patients is that the patient is stimulated to urinate when the catheter is introduced into the urethra, and urine will flow around the catheter as well as through the lumen.

Many people prefer to use dog catheters to catheterize bitches. They have no curved tip but are much firmer, providing more control for insertion into the urethral orifice, particularly when digital catheterization is used. This extra rigidity far outweighs the advantage of the curved tip of the Tieman's catheter (see also below).

Foley silicone catheter

In design these catheters are exactly the same as a standard latex bitch Foley (see below). For dogs a longer length is obviously selected. The catheter is very flexible but, despite this, will advance up the curved male urethra into the bladder where the retaining balloon can be inflated, thus creating an indwelling male dog catheter. Wire-guide stylets are available that pass up the centre of the catheter, to assist in catheter introduction if required. Silicone catheters have the added advantage of being autoclavable and therefore can be reused (this may make their relatively high cost more acceptable). It is the microscopic 'smoothness' of the medical-grade silicone that enables these catheters to be passed up the male urethra. Silicone is inert and causes no mucosal irritation.

All lubricants are compatible with these catheters.

Bitch catheters

Tieman's catheter

Designed for catheterization of the human male, these catheters became popular for use in the bitch due to their curved tip. The moulded tip was found to be advantageous when placing it into the urethral orifice. However, the rest of the catheter is so soft and flexible that the amount of control over the tip is negligible. This makes placing the catheter into the urethral orifice a very difficult task. The excessive length of the catheter is a further disadvantage.

Latex Foley indwelling bitch catheter

Foley catheters incorporate an inflatable balloon behind the drainage holes at the tip of the catheter. The balloon is inflated after placement of the catheter into the bladder, making it an indwelling catheter.

Foley catheters are produced for the human market, but suitable sizes are available for use in most bitches except very tiny puppies. They cannot be used in cats or the male dog (unless in conjunction with a urethrostomy). The balloon is inflated (usually with sterile water or saline) via a channel built into the wall of the catheter which ends in a side arm and a one-way valve. The catheter is removed by deflating the balloon through the same side arm. These latex catheters must not be reused: the balloon is weakened after use and cannot be relied upon to function correctly if reused.

Latex Foley catheters are very flexible, which provides maximum patient comfort but causes a problem when introducing them. Placement is achieved by the use of a rigid metal stylet or probe laid beside the catheter with the point secured in one of the drainage holes at the catheter's tip (Figure 15.26). The stylet is removed once the balloon is inflated.

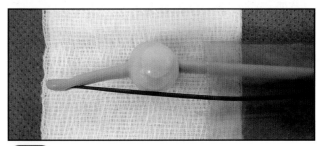

15.26 Tip of Foley catheter.

Latex Foley catheters must not be lubricated with petroleum-based ointments or lubricants, which will damage the latex rubber and so the balloon may burst on inflation.

The absence of a Luer mount in this catheter may cause problems for continuous collection of urine, but urine collection bags with appropriate connectors are available from medical suppliers. If these bags cannot be supplied, the catheter must have an adapter placed so that drip bags can be used for urine collection. Unless 3-litre drip bags are employed, frequent emptying will be required in most dogs. It would be unwise to leave a large dog with only a 1-litre collection bag attached overnight.

An alternative is to bung the catheter and drain the bladder at regular intervals with a spigot or a catheter-tipped 50 ml syringe (Figure 15.27). This method may be acceptable for a recumbent patient but not, for example, after bladder surgery.

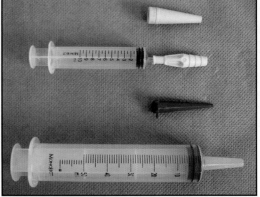

15.27 Spigot and bung.

Silicone indwelling Foley catheter

This can be used in the bitch (at shorter lengths) as for the male. These catheters still require a stylet for correct placement in the bitch. Due to their cost, their use in bitches remains low; the existing latex Foley catheter is adequate in nearly all cases. The silicone Foley is inert, causing little mucosal irritation, and may be preferable for use in patients with wounds near the urethral opening.

Cat catheters

Conventional catheters
These straight catheters with a Luer connection are compatible with all lubricants and are for single use. They are basically a shorter version of the dog catheter.

Jackson catheters
These catheters were designed primarily for use in male cats suffering from feline lower urinary tract disease. They can be used in any male or female cat.

A fine metal stylet, lying in the lumen of the catheter, gives extra rigidity and provides better control for insertion into the urinary bladder. It also helps to displace any loose obstruction (e.g. protein plugs or crystals in the urethra). A normal catheter would be too flexible to achieve this. The stylet is removed once the catheter is in place.

The Jackson is much shorter than the other cat catheters. This is to enable the entire length of the catheter to be placed in the patient, thereby allowing the flange to be sutured to the prepuce. The circular plastic flange is present just behind the Luer fitting of the catheter. In this way the catheter becomes indwelling.

Silicone tomcat catheters
These silicone catheters with distal side holes are very similar in design to a standard Jackson cat catheter. A wire guide is supplied to assist introduction. The proximal fitting enables syringe attachment, and suture holes in the baseplate allow suturing to the prepuce.

Teflon tomcat catheters
In appearance these are very similar to the conventional cat catheter. The very smooth catheter shaft material ensures ease of placement. The material is inert and causes no mucosal irritation. Suture holes in the silicone hub allow securing of the catheter to the prepuce. It is therefore an excellent choice for a 'blocked' cat that requires a longer-term indwelling catheter. Reuse is not recommended; these catheters are designed for single use only. All lubricants are compatible.

Catheter storage and checking

Catheters should be stored in a dry environment and laid flat without any pressure on top of them. Unless a suitably long drawer is available, urinary catheters are best left in their boxes and removed only when required.

All catheters have a shelf-life, after which sterility is no longer guaranteed by the manufacturer. Regular checks should be made, especially if the practice's use of catheters is infrequent.

Cleaning and sterilization of catheters

Practice policy regarding reuse of catheters is rarely the nurse's decision; however, the process of cleaning and sterilization is time-consuming and is not recommended for urinary catheters. Silicone catheters are the only variety marketed as autoclavable.

Cleaning urinary catheters

1. Flush, with force, copious amounts of cold water through the catheter immediately after use. This is usually done with a syringe. Cold water prevents coagulation of any protein that may be present.
2. Remove any blockage with a wire stylet and repeat step (1).
3. Wash the exterior and interior of the catheter with a mild detergent. Rinse thoroughly, as in (1).
4. Check catheter for kinks, holes etc. If any damage is found the catheter must be discarded.
5. Dry in a warm, dust-free atmosphere.

Sterilization
Catheters for sterilization should be packed appropriately (autoclave bags or ethylene oxide). Autoclaving is the best method for nylon catheters. The COSHH Regulations have made the use of ethylene oxide in most practices difficult and expensive. There are no short cuts and therefore it is unlikely that any but the largest of veterinary establishments will continue to sterilize equipment by this method on their own premises.

Other equipment

Specula
A speculum is an instrument that assists in the viewing of cavities. Specula are used to assist catheterization of bitches by holding back the vaginal tissue and allowing good visualization of the urethral orifice. This is of great aid to the student nurse: digital catheterization can be difficult without a visual knowledge of the urethral position.

It is preferable for all specula to be sterile and it is often cheaper in the long run to invest in a metal speculum that can be autoclaved, rather than using the home-made variety that needs gas sterilization. If no specula are available, bitch catheterization is still possible digitally.

There are several varieties of speculum, most of which are not specifically designed for catheterization.

Nasal speculum
There are many slight variations, the adult size being the most appropriate. All have two flat blades that separate when the handles are closed together (Figure 15.28a). Some have a retaining device; others have to be held open. A light source may be attached to one of the blades to illuminate the vagina. If this is not available, a pen torch held by an assistant is an effective alternative.

Rectal speculum
This is used rarely, mainly due to expense. Rectal specula (Figure 15.28b) are conical in shape and, once in place, a section of the conical arm slides out to allow viewing of the urethral orifice. The main problem is to align the removable section with the urethral orifice; this is easy in theory, but difficult in practice.

Auriscope
This is a normal auriscope handle and light, but the attachment used has a section removed from its wall (Figure 15.28c).

Home-made speculum
Monojet syringe packing cases are ideal rigid plastic specula and they are cheap. One section of the cover is removed, the edges are filed smooth and an external light source is used (Figure 15.28d).

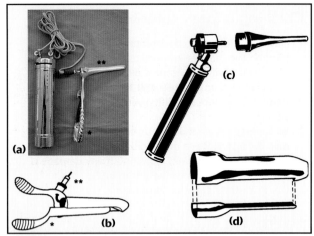

15.28 **(a)** Nasal speculum, suitable for use as a bitch vaginal speculum. Pressing together the handles causes the blades to move apart and open the vestibule. **(b)** Rectal speculum, suitable for use as a bitch speculum. The lower sliding panel is removed after insertion into the vestibule to expose the urethral opening.The lighting attachment, which is connected to a battery, provides a self-contained light source. **(c)** Catheterization speculum for attachment to an auriscope resembles an ear speculum except that a segment of its wall is absent. **(d)** A speculum made from the container of a disposable syringe by cutting away a segment of the plastic. It is important to ensure the edges are smooth.

Batteries and transformers

These should be electrically tested and working correctly. Spare batteries should always be in stock. Transformers do not come into contact with the vulva and do not require sterilization.

Speculum bulbs

These are best stored separately as they break easily. They cannot be sterilized in the autoclave and therefore need gas or, more realistically, chemical sterilization.

Stylets

Stylets can be made or bought. They should be chosen to be long enough for easy use: they need to be at least two-thirds the length of the longest Foley catheter stocked. Stylets can be packed and autoclaved or chemically sterilized.

Metal guide wires are supplied for use with silicone Foleys. These are placed up the centre of the catheter and therefore need to be longer than the length of the Foley. They can be autoclaved.

Urine collection bags

Manufactured varieties are prepacked and sterile; they are designed for single use.

Previously used drip-bags can be used with a giving set attached. The end of the giving set must be thoroughly cleaned and chemically sterilized before being attached to the urinary catheter. A screw attachment bung should be attached to the end of the giving set during storage to keep it clean from dust and dirt.

Bungs and spigots

Plastic bungs are supplied in multi-packs requiring sterilization, or as individually packed sterile units. Chemical sterilization is the only practical method for these bungs. Metal spigots can be autoclaved or placed in chemical sterilizing solution until needed.

Three-way taps

These are invaluable when draining bladders via a catheter. They avoid leakages by controlling urine flow whilst syringes are emptied.

Methods for urinary catheterization

Several general points apply to all methods.

Physical restraint

Most patients will allow urinary catheterization under gentle physical restraint without resistance. If necessary, a muzzle should be used on a dog. The patient should be placed at a comfortable working height.

Dogs and cats may be restrained in a standing position or in lateral recumbency. Bitches may be restrained in dorsal recumbency (Figure 15.29).

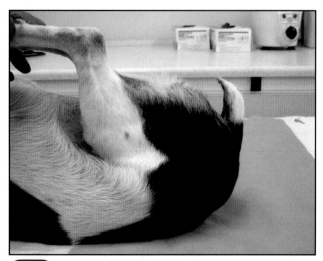

15.29 Bitch in dorsal recumbency for catheterization.

Chemical restraint

Sedation

- Dog: rarely required unless the patient is aggressive or very nervous
- Bitch: most will accept catheterization more readily if lightly sedated, especially if dorsal recumbency is chosen; standing catheterization is best done without sedation, otherwise the patient tends to keep sitting down (which can be tiring for the assistant)
- Cat: catheterization is generally less stressful for all concerned if the cat is sedated.

General anaesthesia

This is rarely indicated or necessary unless the patient has sustained other trauma that makes catheterization under sedation humanely unacceptable (e.g. fractured pelvis, vaginal mass). It is sensible to catheterize during general anaesthesia if this is required for other treatment (e.g. catheterizing a paraplegic patient whilst under general anaesthesia for a myelogram).

Equipment preparation

All equipment should be prepared before restraining the patient. Patient cooperation will be greater if prolonged restraint is avoided.

Lubricants

There is some debate over the necessity for the use of lubricants. Urinary catheterization can be done without, but lubricants aid passage of the catheter and help to avoid abrasive trauma.

- Check contents of lubricants before using them with Foley catheters; most are water based and are compatible with commonly used catheters.
- Make sure that lubricants are sterile.

Cleaning

- Clean the area with an antiseptic solution to remove any discharges and surface dirt.
- Clip around the area if necessary, especially in longhaired breeds (remember to check that permission for this has been obtained from the owner).

Gloves

The use of gloves is recommended for the health and safety of personnel. In general, multiple packs of non-sterile gloves are adequate because the catheter will be fed from its package using a 'no touch' technique. Gloves are therefore used to prevent contamination of staff with urine, rather than protection of the patient from infection.

Sterile gloves will be required when digital catheterization is performed, as the catheter tip is inevitably touched by the finger.

Length of catheter

A dog or cat catheter should be measured against the patient before the catheter is unpacked. This measurement gives a rough estimate of the length of catheter to insert.

Insertion should be stopped once urine starts to flow. Over-insertion can result in the catheter bending and re-entering the urethra or, even worse, knotting in the bladder and requiring surgical removal.

Catheterizing a male dog

Equipment

- Catheter
- Lubricant
- Swabs for cleaning
- Syringe to assist urine drainage
- Three-way tap (if required)
- Sample pot
- Gloves
- Urine bag or a bung
- Kidney dish

If the catheter is to be made indwelling:
- Suture material
- Zinc oxide tape
- For silicone male Foley catheters, water sufficient to fill balloon
- Guide wire
- Syringe

▶

Procedure

1. Wash hands and put on gloves
2. Clean prepuce
3. Extrude penis; if not experienced, get an assistant to do this
4. Clean prepuce

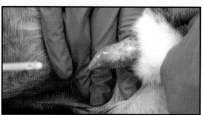

5. Remove catheter from the outer wrapping and cut a feeding sleeve from the inner sterile packaging. This allows easy feeding of the catheter from the packaging into the urethra using a 'no touch' technique. For silicone male Foley catheter placement, feed guide wire up the centre of the catheter

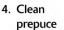
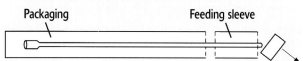

6. Lubricate the catheter and insert the tip into the urethra
7. Advance the catheter up the urethra. Resistance may be met at the os penis, where there is a slight narrowing of the urethra, at the ischial arch and area of the prostate gland if enlarged. Steady but gentle pressure should overcome this resistance. If the catheter cannot be passed, re-evaluate catheter size
8. Inflate balloon once tip of catheter is in bladder if silicone male Foley in use
9. Proceed according to reason for catheterization (e.g. drain bladder, collect sample, hydropropulsion)

To provide an indwelling dog catheter from a polyamide catheter:

1. Place zinc tape around catheter near to prepuce
2. Stitch or stick to prepuce

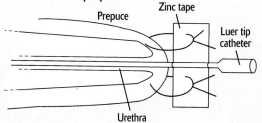

Neither of these options is ideal because dog catheters are not designed to be indwelling. Best to use silicone indwelling male Foley

Catheterizing a bitch: method 1: urethra viewed in dorsal recumbency

Equipment

- Speculum (with or without light source)
- Alternative light source if required
- Catheter
- Lubricant
- Swabs for cleaning
- Gloves

continues ▶

continued

If a Foley catheter is being placed:
- Stylet
- Sterile water/saline to inflate cuff
- Urine bag
- Syringe

Procedure

1. Wash hands and put on gloves
2. Ensure the bitch is in a straight dorsal recumbent position with the hindlimbs flexed and drawn forward. The tail needs to be under control too
3. Clean vulva
4. Remove catheter from outer wrapping and expose tip only from inner sleeve
5. If a Foley catheter is being used, insert the stylet
6. Place lubricated speculum blades between the vulval lips as caudally as possible to avoid the clitoral fossa

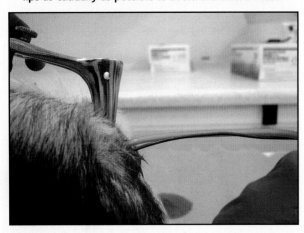

7. Insert *vertically* into the vestibule and turn handles cranially
8. Open the blades of the speculum. The urethral opening will be visible on the cranial side of the vertically oriented vestibule, approximately half way between the vulva and cervix

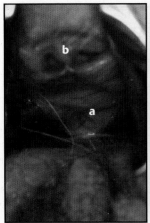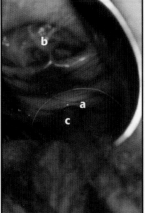

a, the urethral orifice; b, clitoral fossa; c, catheter in position

9. Insert the tip of the catheter into the urethral orifice. **Draw the hindlimbs caudally.** This straightens the urethra, making it easier to push the catheter into the bladder

▶

10. Proceed depending on reason for catheterization. If a Foley catheter is being used, inflate balloon, withdraw stylet, attach bag and place Elizabethan collar

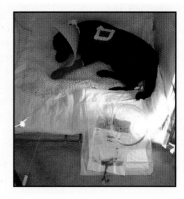

Catheterizing a bitch: method 2: urethra viewed standing

Equipment

As in Method 1
Generally only one assistant is required

Procedure

1. Wash hands and put on gloves
2. Ensure tail is well restrained
3. Clean vulva
4. Place speculum between vulval lips and advance at a slight angle towards the spine, then horizontally
5. Open blades and identify urethral orifice. This will be on the ventral floor of the vestibule
6. Insert catheter at a slightly ventral angle so as to follow the direction of the urethra into the bladder
7. Proceed as for Method 1

Catheterizing a bitch: method 3: digital

Equipment

- Sterile gloves
- Catheter
- Lubricant
- Swabs for cleaning
- Collection pots

If a Foley is being placed:
- Additional equipment is as in Method 1

Procedure

1. Restrain in preferred position, lateral or standing (standing is generally easier)
2. Scrub hands and put on sterile gloves in an aseptic manner
3. Ask an assistant to clean the vulva (gloved person having sterile hands)
4. Assistant removes outer wrapping from catheter and the inner package is removed by the scrubbed person
5. Holding the sterile part of the packaging, place stylet if necessary
6. Lubricate first finger of non-writing hand

▶

7. Place finger into vestibule and feel along ventral surface for a raised pimple
8. Place finger just cranial to this raised area, which is the urethral orifice

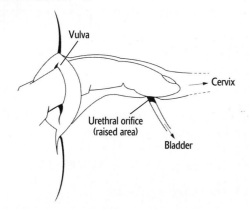

9. Raising hand and finger dorsally, digitally guide catheter, tipped slightly ventrally (as in Method 2) into the urethral orifice

The catheter will run past the fingertip if the orifice is missed

10. Proceed as for Method 1.

The digital method may be difficult or even impossible in smaller breeds

Catheterizing a tomcat

Equipment

As for dog catheterization

Procedure

1. Wash hands and put on gloves
2. Restrain patient and have control of the tail
3. Pull patient's hindlimbs slightly cranially
4. Prepare feeding sleeve as for the dog catheter and lubricate tip
5. With one hand extrude penis by applying gentle pressure each side of the prepuce with two fingers

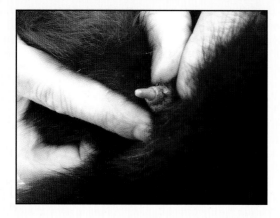

6. Introduce catheter into the urethra gently
7. Collect sample or drain bladder
8. If a Jackson catheter is being placed for continuous drainage, stitch flange to prepuce

Catheterizing a queen

Equipment

As for dog catheterization

Procedure

1. Restrain patient
2. Wash hands and put on gloves
3. Remove outer wrapping and cut a feeding sleeve
4. Lubricate tip of catheter
5. The catheter is placed between the vulval lips and 'blindly' introduced into the urethra. Angle the catheter ventrally, placing gentle pressure until the catheter slips into the urethra
6. The catheter is not designed to be indwelling

Other methods of emptying the urinary bladder

Natural micturition

This is non-invasive and usually easy to achieve with the encouragement of the nurse or owner. In most circumstances it is the preferred method for emptying the bladder but there are several disadvantages:

- The sample is always contaminated and therefore useless for culture and sensitivity evaluation.
- If the patient is unable to urinate normally, another method has to be employed.
- Patients often refuse to produce urine when convenient and required.
- If not required for culture, collection of samples from the environment may be acceptable in some cases. For example, urine can be retrieved from litter trays that have been left empty or filled with non-porous beads (so-called 'washable' litter).

Manual expression of the bladder

This is probably the most common method used for cats. Dogs (especially recumbent patients) can also be encouraged to urinate in this way (see Figure 15.19).

As long as the bladder is of a reasonable size, this task becomes easier with practice. Pressure should be applied steadily and slowly – sudden pressure may cause trauma to the bladder. Generally very little pressure will initiate a free flow of urine. Excessive pressure should never be required, as the bladder can become bruised or even ruptured.

Cystocentesis

This should only be carried out when the bladder is of a palpable size. The technique is fairly straightforward (see Chapter 24) and generally without complications, as long as an aseptic technique is used. It may be the only method available for urine drainage in an obstructive emergency. *As this procedure involves entering a body cavity, it must only be carried out by a veterinary surgeon.*

The nursing process

It is important to emphasize that at the time of writing (2006) veterinary nurses are not autonomous practitioners and are therefore not ultimately responsible for patient care. It is the veterinary surgeon in charge of the case who is responsible.

Qualified Listed veterinary nurses or those enrolled as student nurses with the Royal College of Veterinary Surgeons (RCVS) must act within the remit of Schedule 3 of the Veterinary Surgeons Act and in doing so should only carry out tasks in which they are confident and competent, in accordance with the Act (see Chapter 3).

In order to develop a defined professional role for nurses, one of the first steps is to introduce the Nursing Process and Models of Nursing into the veterinary nursing syllabus to educate veterinary nurses regarding the importance of developing up-to-date evidence-based nursing practice through the implementation of care plans in which veterinary patient nursing care is systematically planned and delivered by nurses. The effectiveness of the care given is then evaluated by the whole team, including the veterinary surgeon.

The Nursing Process is divided into 4 stages and is a cyclical process:

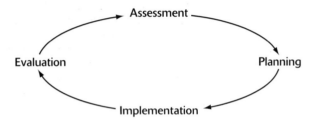

Through carrying out the 'Nursing Process' it will be ensured that nurses have a systematic approach to the delivery of care to every patient that they nurse.

Assessment

Assessment will clearly establish the individual needs of the patient. It is only once a patient assessment has been done that effective care can be given.

1. Collect the information needed via your own observations and via information from the client and other team members.
2. Collect the information systematically and write it down.
3. Review the collected information.
4. Identify actual and potential nursing problems.
5. Identify priorities among the problems.

Assessment: case example

- A Golden Retriever has been brought in by his owner because he is 'not quite himself', he does not want to go on his regular walk and is drinking a lot.
- Additional information is needed from the client and from patient observation to get a fuller history of the dog and his problems.
- Gathering information about a patient is very important. It sets the scene for any action to be taken:

Wrong information → Wrong action
Lack of information → Inadequate action

- We may already know that the Golden Retriever has exercise intolerance and polydipsia but unless we ask we will not find out that he is deaf in his left ear, only eats one meal in the evening, and will only urinate and defecate on concrete and not on grass. All of this information is important for the patient's stay in hospital.
- Upon admission the veterinary surgeon in charge of the case diagnoses diabetes mellitus.

Planning

Once all the information has been gathered during the assessment phase, the next part of the nursing process is the planning stage. This is where the nurse plans what needs to be done about the nursing problems that have been identified.

Planning: aims of nursing

- To solve identified **actual** problems
- To prevent identified **potential** problems becoming actual ones
- To alleviate those problems that cannot be solved
- To help the patient and client to cope positively with those problems that cannot be solved or alleviated
- To prevent recurrence of a treated problem
- To help the patient to be as comfortable as possible even when death is inevitable

Setting goals

A goal has to be set for each actual and potential problem and a distinction should be made between short-term and long-term goals. It is important that any goals set should be stated in terms of outcomes that are able to be observed, measured or tested, so that effective evaluation can then be carried out.

An example of a short-term goal for the Golden Retriever in the case example above would be to ensure that he did not urinate in his kennel; a long-term goal would be for effective management of his diabetes mellitus resulting in normal fluid intake and urinary output. Both of these can be observed and measured.

Nursing plan

A plan is made of all the proposed nursing interventions needed to achieve the goals.

The plan should be written in enough detail that any nurse reading it would know what the plan is.

In order to achieve the short-term goal of ensuring that the dog does not urinate in his kennel, the nursing intervention would be to monitor/measure his fluid intake and to take him outside on concrete every 45–60 minutes.

Implementation

Implementing the nursing plan is the 'doing' stage of the nursing process, otherwise known as the 'nursing intervention'. It is important that nurses make it clear what decision making has taken place in order to justify the nursing intervention. All of this information should be clearly and indelibly recorded on the care plan.

Evaluation

This is a vital part of the nursing process. It is difficult to justify planning and implementing nursing interventions if the outcomes cannot be shown to have benefited either the patient or the client in some way.

Evaluation is a difficult process. A nurse hopes that the evaluation will show that all the nursing goals have been achieved. If this is not the case, the following questions need to be asked:

- Has the goal set for the patient been partially achieved?
- Is more information from the veterinary surgeon or the client required to decide the next step in the nursing care?

- Is a specific problem unchanged and should the nursing intervention be changed or stopped?
- Is there a worsening of the problem and should the goal and nursing intervention be reviewed?
- Was the goal inappropriate when first set?
- Does the goal require interventions from other members of the veterinary team (e.g. veterinary surgeon or physiotherapist)?

By asking these questions, a patient re-evaluation is taking place leading to a revision of the original nursing plan to address the issues that have become apparent during the evaluation. The changes that are required are recorded on the care plan and the whole process begins again.

Models of nursing

The nursing process offers a systematic approach to care but is limited in its function unless it is integrated into a nursing model/framework.

The nursing process (Aggleton and Chalmers, 2000):

- Exhorts nurses to assess but does not tell them what to look for
- Advocates planning but does not say what form the care plan should take
- Talks of intervention but does not specify what might be appropriate interventions
- Calls for evaluation without specifying the standards against which comparisons should be made.

This is where nursing models come in. Nursing models provide the nurse with key pointers regarding patient assessment, care planning, the type of interventions that are appropriate and evaluation. Together with the nursing process they provide detailed guidance for the steps that need to be taken when delivering nursing care.

Models are *systematically constructed*. This means that they have been developed logically and can be adapted to meet specific practice/patient requirements. They also act as guides for *nursing practice* by providing a framework in which to deliver nursing care.

There is a large number of published nursing models developed by nursing theorists (mainly from North America). The model selected here particularly lends itself to veterinary nursing and was developed in the United Kingdom.

The Roper, Logan and Tierney Model of Nursing

The RLT model is made up of five parts:

1. Activities of living
2. The patient's lifespan
3. Dependence–independence continuum
4. Factors influencing the activities of living
5. Individuality in living.

Part One: Activities of living

According to Roper, Logan and Tierney these are the central components of the model. There are 12 activities of living:

- Maintaining a safe environment
- Communicating
- Breathing
- Eating and drinking
- Eliminating
- Personal cleansing and dressing (grooming)
- Controlling body temperature
- Mobilizing
- Working and playing
- Expressing sexuality
- Sleeping
- Dying.

If a client were asked to describe what each day involved for their pet, most people would include some (if not all) of the functions listed above. This is why they are called 'activities of living' (ALs).

Roper reports that when this model was first introduced in 1980 the inclusion of 'expression of sexuality' as an AL was greeted by surprise, but is less likely to cause a problem within the veterinary field. Also the fact that 'Dying' was considered as an AL was unusual at this time, but in veterinary science euthanasia is something that a client can opt for when and if it is needed, which makes this an important activity when this model is applied to veterinary patients.

Part Two: Lifespan

Each animal has a lifespan from birth to death and is likely to have stages along the way of neonate, kitten/puppy, adolescent, adult, senior (geriatric). Some may die before they reach old age.

Within the care plan the 'lifespan' is represented as a diagram showing a unidirectional arrow from birth to death:

Neonate ⟶ Geriatric

It is added at the beginning of the care plan in order that a particular patient's position can be plotted on it and their age can be seen at a glance.

It is important that nurses have a visual reminder of the patient's age when they consider each of the ALs for any particular patient.

Part Three: Dependence–independence continuum

This part of the model is closely related to lifespan and to the ALs:

Total dependence (D) ⟶ Total independence (I)

It acknowledges that there are times in life when a patient cannot perform certain ALs independently.

A patient will have a dependence–independence continuum for each AL and a patient's position could be plotted on each continuum to provide an impression of the degree of dependence or independence in respect of the 12 ALs. Throughout the patient's stay their position on each continuum will be plotted more than once and may change as they move from total dependence to independence as the problem for which they have been admitted resolves.

The completed care plan in Figure 15.30 demonstrates the use of the RLT model of nursing being applied to a veterinary patient.

Patient details:	Kit is a 3-year-old entire male Dalmatian. He has sustained a closed fracture of the left radius and ulna following a road traffic accident.
Patient's position on Lifespan:	Neonate ⟶ Geriatric
Date and Time:	April 24th 2006 2.00pm

Activity of Living	Nursing assessment of patient's ability to carry out Activity of Living	Patient problem (D, dependent; I, independent) D ⟷ I	Potential/ Actual	Nursing goals	Nursing interventions	Evaluation
Maintaining a safe environment	Temperament: Kit likes people but does not like other male dogs Bedding must be provided within the kennel and should be soft and supportive Kit is completely dependent on the veterinary staff to maintain a safe environment	D ⟷ I	Actual	To ensure that Kit has no direct contact with other male dogs Kennel always has soft supportive bedding in place	Kennel away from other males and ensure all staff are aware of his temperament Vetbed and mattress in kennel. Nurses to check bony prominences 4 x daily for signs of pressure	A safe environment was maintained throughout Kit's stay and no problems occurred
Communicating	Kit is able to communicate though vocalization Kit is able to communicate through non-vocal means – facial expression, posture Kit likes people but does not like other male dogs	D ⟷ I	Potential	All nurses dealing with Kit are able to recognize the signs given by Kit in his attempts to communicate	Observe patient before entering kennel Make sure that there are no other male dogs out when Kit is moved from his kennel	Nurses built up a good relationship with Kit during stay No contact with other dogs occurred
Breathing	Currently Kit has a normal respiratory rate and pattern	D ⟷ I	Potential	Patient's respiratory function to remain within normal parameters throughout stay	TPR to be taken 2 x daily in the first instance. Increasing to 4 x daily in the immediate postoperative period Respiration rate to be observed while patient is at rest, before pulse and temperature These should all be taken at same time each day when patient is calm, before exercise and recorded on a chart so that patterns can be seen	Kit's TPR remained within normal parameters throughout stay
Eating and drinking	Diet: Kit eats a low-fat diet as he gets diarrhoea with other types of tinned food He has one meal a day at 6pm Drinking is not a problem as long as Kit can have access to water	D ⟷ I	Potential Potential	Kit's food and fluid intake remain normal throughout stay	Keep on low-fat diet Feed at 6pm	Normal feeding times and diet type were maintained
Eliminating	Kit gets diarrhoea with food other than low-fat diet Normal routine: Kit normally has a walk at 8am, 3.30pm and 8pm	D ⟷ I	Actual Potential	Elimination patterns to remain normal throughout stay Opportunity to urinate and defecate given at same times as home routine	Observe faecal output for any changes Walk at 8am, 3.30pm and 8pm	Kit did not develop diarrhoea Normal routine maintained
Personal cleansing (grooming)	Kit is a short-haired dog and grooming not an issue while hospitalized	D ⟷ I	No problems envisaged	Coat/skin condition not to deteriorate during hospitalization	Check skin over bony prominences daily Check wound 2 x daily during postoperative period	No problems arose

15.30 Nursing Care Plan (Roper, Logan and Tierney model), adapted by A Jeffery and Hilary Orpet).

continues ▶

Activity of Living	Nursing assessment of patient's ability to carry out Activity of Living	Patient problem (D, dependent; I, independent) D ←————→ I	Potential/ Actual	Nursing goals	Nursing interventions	Evaluation
Controlling body temperature	TPR – all within normal range	D ←———┼→ I	Potential	Patient's TPR to remain within normal parameters throughout stay	TPR to be taken 2 x daily in the first instance. Increasing to 4 x daily in the immediate postoperative period Respiration rate to be observed while patient is at rest, before pulse and temperature These should all be taken at the same time each day when patient is calm, before exercise and recorded on a chart so that patterns can be seen	Kit's TPR remained within normal parameters throughout stay
Mobilizing	Kit has a long bone fracture which is very painful He cannot weight bear on his left foreleg	D ←┼———→ I	Actual Actual	Ensure that Kit mobilizes to prevent problems associated with immobility (joint stiffness, muscle wasting, delayed fracture repair)	Provide a kennel large enough for Kit to move around Ensure that the patient is lead walked with support Ensure he has support when urinating and defecating	Kit had difficulty getting up into a standing position but with support managed this The nurses successfully supported him when urinating and defecating
Working and playing	Kit cannot run around outside and play in his usual way	D ←——┼—→ I	Actual	Ensure Kit is able to express normal behaviour within kennel if he wants	Provide nursing contact that does not just involve an intervention 6–8 x daily	Kit built up a good relationship with the nursing team during stay and did not appear to become withdrawn
Expressing sexuality	Kit is an entire 3-year-old male and nurses should consider this when deciding where to hospitalize him (other males, bitches in season)	D ←——┼—→ I	Potential	To be aware of patient's needs	Enable Kit to sniff around in outside run and urinate where he wishes Ensure that Kit is not kennelled next to another young entire male or a bitch in season	Kit was able to express sexuality within the limitations of the hospital environment
Sleeping	Kit may not be able to sleep in an unfamiliar environment or if he is uncomfortable or in pain	D ←┼———→ I	Potential	Kit is secure enough to be able to sleep and rest within his kennel	Ensure pain is managed to enable patient to rest and sleep Keep kennel at an ambient temperature Ensure kennels are quiet and darkened at night to allow sleep Ensure bedding is dry and comfortable	The analgesia given initially in the postoperative period did not keep Kit pain-free, so after reassessment the dose was increased and he became pain-free
Dying	Dying is the final act of living. It is likely that the veterinary staff would need to assist Kit if this were to occur	D ←┼———→ I	Potential	Kit is nursed effectively throughout his stay and is discharged pain-free and weight bearing at the end of the hospitalization period	Ensure that when the owner signs the consent form they are fully aware of the procedure and the surgical/ anaesthetic risks involved Ensure all observations made including pain assessment, TPR , limb and wound checks are clearly recorded Any changes in the patient's condition must be recorded and reported immediately to a veterinary surgeon	Kit was kept pain-free and all nursing interventions carried out as required Kit was discharged 7 days after admission

15.30 *continued* Nursing Care Plan (Roper, Logan and Tierney model), adapted by A Jeffery and Hilary Orpet).

Part Four: Factors influencing the activities of living

Five main factors influence the ALs and should be considered when preparing a care plan for each individual patient:

- Biological
- Psychological
- Sociocultural
- Environmental
- Politicoeconomic.

Biological

It is important that the nurse is aware of the biological state of the body and how that might influence any of the ALs. The veterinary nurse needs to be familiar with the anatomy and physiology of both the healthy and sick animal in order to understand the impact of a disease on an animal within their care.

Psychological

The impact of psychological stresses on the ALs can be significant. For example, a veterinary patient that is suffering separation anxiety from an owner may withdraw from communication, refuse to eat and drink and be unable to sleep – all of which will have a detrimental effect on its health and an impact on the ALs.

Sociocultural

It is important that nurses have knowledge of sociocultural factors and how they may influence ALs. It may appear on first reading that this is not appropriate when nursing veterinary patients, but the relevance becomes apparent when considered in the context of the owner:

- *The client*: In people, response to pain may vary according to ethnic origin. This may influence a client's attitude to their animal's pain.
- *The patient*: Some animals are pack animals. A dog taken from its pack may become lonely.

Environmental

- *The atmosphere – light and sound waves.* For example, bright light can be very tiring for an ill patient, as can the noise of a busy ward with the radio on. Both of these may even prevent the patient from resting or sleeping.
- *The atmosphere – organic and inorganic.* For example, dust may irritate an atopic patient; and pathogenic microorganisms are a risk to all patients, in particular those who are elderly, immunosuppressed or recovering from major surgery.
- *The built environment.* For example, the veterinary practice kennels and all other areas need to be safe in order that the first AL ('maintain a safe environment') can be achieved.

Politicoeconomic

There are two parts to this:

- *Health and economic status.* This relates to the client more than the patient in a veterinary context and it is likely that the economic status of the client may influence the ALs.
- *Health and world economy.* Recession will have an impact on the amount that clients will spend; and veterinary surgeons will invest in staff and equipment that may impact on the care of the veterinary patient.

Part Five: Individuality in living

The ALs are the main concept of this model. Although every patient is likely to carry out these activities, each patient may do them differently, thus expressing themselves as an individual. For example, the way in which a cat will eat may be very different from a dog.

Relationship between the component parts

Figure 15.31 shows how each of the component parts relate to each other and the significance of each in the construction of the Roper, Logan and Tierney Model of Nursing.

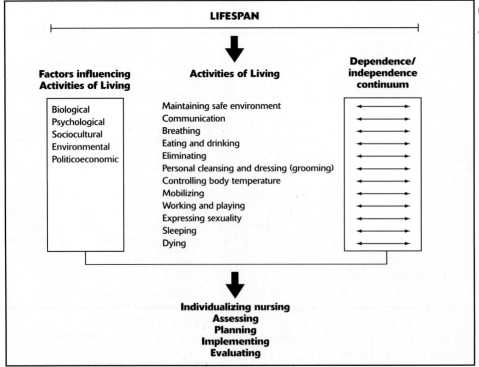

15.31 The Roper, Logan and Tierney Model of Nursing.

Orem's Model of Nursing

Dorothea Orem's views on nursing science are the basis for understanding how empirical nursing evidence is gathered and interpreted. Her quest for greater understanding of the nature of nursing focused on three questions:

1. What *do* nurses do, and what *should* nurses do, as practitioners of nursing?
2. *Why* do nurses do what they do?
3. What are the results of nursing interventions?

Orem's model of nursing focuses on the key idea that an individual is self-caring if they can manage the following effectively:

- Support of life processes and normal functioning
- Maintenance of normal growth and development
- Prevention and control of disease and injury
- Prevention of, or compensation for, disability
- Promotion of well-being.

According to Cavanagh (1991), central to Orem's concept of self-care is that care is being initiated voluntarily and deliberately by an individual. Self-care is the practice of activities that will maintain life and health and will promote well-being.

Universal self-care requisites

Essential to Orem's model are the eight 'universal self-care requisites', which are activities that must be performed in order to achieve self-care:

Orem's universal self-care requisites

- The maintenance of a sufficient intake of air
- The maintenance of a sufficient intake of water
- The maintenance of a sufficient intake of food
- Satisfactory elimination functions
- The maintenance of a balance between activity and rest
- The maintenance of a balance between solitude and social integration
- The prevention of hazards to life, well-being and functioning
- The promotion of functioning and development within social groups and the desire to be normal (normality)

These self-care requisites are essential tasks that an individual must be able to manage in order to care for themselves. As with Roper, Logan and Tierney's ALs, these are all requisites that an animal can achieve, but some of the self-care requisites may be easier for wild animals than domesticated ones. For example, intake of food may be difficult if the domesticated animal is reliant on an owner to feed them and they have no freedom to scavenge (dogs) or hunt (cats).

The idea of balancing demands and abilities (Figure 15.32) is central to Orem's model.

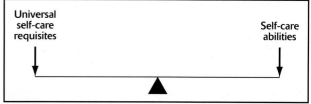

15.32 The Orem model of nursing. A healthy individual: self-care abilities meet self-care requisites.

Developmental self-care requisites

Orem identified a second kind of requisite found in special circumstances associated with development.

Orem's specific developmental self-care requisites

- Interuterine life and birth
- Neonatal life
- Infancy
- The developmental stages of childhood (for which substitute puppy/kittenhood), adolescence and early adulthood
- The developmental stages of adulthood
- Pregnancy

It is at this point that Orem differs from Roper, Logan and Tierney, as the lifespan within the RLT model begins with neonate and does not consider interuterine life as Orem does.

Orem argues that, at each of these stages, universal self-care requisites must also be considered (Figure 15.33). An example of a specific developmental self-care requisite would be a neonate and temperature regulation. An adult may be able to control their own body temperature but a neonate may not.

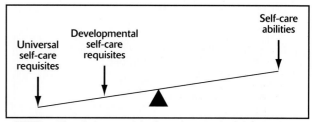

15.33 The Orem model of nursing. An individual with additional developmental self-care requisites is in need of intervention.

Health-deviation self-care requisites

There are times when an individual is ill, becomes injured, has disabilities or is under medical care. In these circumstances, the following additional health-care demands are placed upon them:

- Seeking and securing appropriate medical assistance
- Being aware of and attending to the effects and results of pathological conditions and states
- Effectively carrying out medically prescribed treatment
- Being aware of, and attending to, the discomforting and deleterious effects of medically prescribed treatment

- Modifying self-image in accepting oneself as being in a particular state of health
- Learning to live with the effects of pathological conditions and states.

The owner may act for the animal in order that some of the additional health-care demands are achieved and an individual animal may experience a change in the status of their health but is still able to meet the universal and health deviation self-care requisites (Figure 15.34).

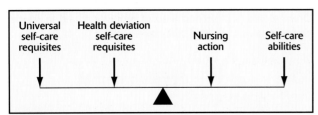

15.34 The Orem model of nursing. An individual able to meet all requisites with nursing assistance.

However, a situation could exist where the total demand placed on an animal exceeds its ability to meet it. In this situation an individual will need nursing intervention in order to enable it to meet its self-care needs. The nurse needs to assess which interventions are needed immediately and which might be needed in the future.

Case example
A cat with a fractured jaw has difficulty with eating, drinking and grooming.

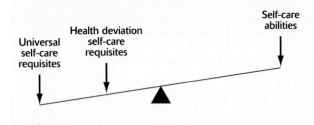

With nursing intervention, the cat can now meet universal and health-deviation self-care requisites.

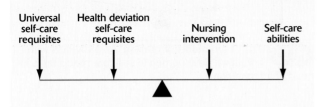

Putting the theory into practice
Cavanagh (1991) suggested that there is no single 'correct' way of setting out a care plan based upon Orem's model. Instead, the nurse must take the ideas that Orem presents and develop a plan to meet the needs of each patient.

This takes confidence as a nurse, but this is a model that can be adapted to meet the needs of veterinary practice while still individualizing care of the patient. If this is the model that is used in practice, it is vital that each stage is recorded to ensure all who read the plan are able to understand and follow it.

The nursing process is a vital part of the model and is the basis of the care plan for any individual patient.

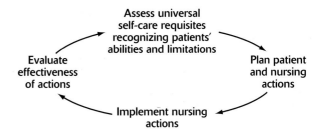

Figure 15.35 is an example of a completed care plan, demonstrating the application of the model within a veterinary context.

Interpretation of language used within Orem's Model

Assessment
Orem does not often refer to 'Assessment' but chooses to use 'nursing history' instead.

Planning
Once the nursing history has been taken, the 'Planning' stage of the nursing process begins. At this stage the nurse will be in discussion with the owner and other professionals within the team regarding the degree to which the nurse will support the patient with their self-care requisites. The following degrees of nursing intervention might be considered.

- *Wholly compensatory* – the patient and client are completely dependent on the nurse (e.g. a tetraplegic dog)
- *Partially compensatory* – the nurse and patient and client working together to meet the self-care requisites (e.g. a dog with a long bone fracture)
- *Supportive/educative* – the nurse is there for support/reassurance (e.g. teaching an owner to inject their pet with insulin).

Implementation
Aggleton and Chalmers (2000) believed that there are six broad ways envisaged by Orem in which care can be implemented:

- Doing or acting for another
- Guiding or directing another
- Providing physical support
- Providing psychological support
- Providing an environment supportive of development
- Teaching another.

Evaluation
Orem refers to this vital part of the Nursing Process as 'case management' (evaluation or audit). In this part of the process she requires the nurse to:

- Plan and control the overall nursing process
- Direct, check and evaluate all aspects of the nursing process
- Ensure that the nursing process is effective and dynamic.

The use of a nursing model in which the nursing process is embedded is vital when delivering nursing care to patients. It ensures that all nurses within the practice are following the same set criteria for any one patient and that there are recorded goals and interventions. Most importantly, because the goals set are able to be measured or observed, it means that an evaluation can be made of the nursing care given, providing a clear evidence base for nursing practice.

Patient details:	12-month-old neutered male, Domestic Short-hair cat			
Reason for admission:	Fractured jaw			
Date and time:				

Universal self-care requisites	Self-care abilities	Self-care limitations	Patient actions	Nursing actions
Maintain intake of air	Breathes without difficulty	Unable to groom/clean therefore food sticks to nose	Breathes well when nostrils clear	Ensure nostrils remain clear during and after feeding Assess respiratory adequacy
Maintain intake of water	Can put mouth down to water bowl and lap water	Difficulty in drinking from a high-sided bowl	Drinking Swallowing	Provide water in a shallow bowl Keep a fluid balance chart Observe for signs of dehydration
Maintain intake of food	Can put mouth down to food bowl	Unable to prehend food	Can swallow when food in mouth	Ensure food is in manageable form Assist with feeding Maintain a record of food eaten
Manage elimination	All	Normally urinates outside in soil	Use litter tray to urinate and defecate	Provide litter tray containing soil Keep a record of urinary/faecal output
Balance activity and rest	Is able to rest and sleep	Unable to have free access	Walk around kennel Rest and sleep on Vetbed	Provide a large kennel Provide an environment for rest/sleep when required
Balance solitude and social intergration	Is able to communicate through body language	Unable to purr or meow due to fracture Unable to communicate with brother		Provide regular nursing attention Organize for family, including children to visit
Prevention of hazards to life, well-being and functioning	Possesses pain sensation Can hear and see	Cannot maintain safety of environment		Monitor vital signs and assess patient for changes in physical and psychological condition
Normalcy	Is able to communicate through body language	Unable to vocalize	Interact with staff, family and other animals	Provide an environment in which he feels at ease

15.35   Nursing Care Plan (Orem model).

References and further reading

Aggleton P and Chalmers H (2000) *Nursing Models and Nursing Practice, 2nd edn.* Palgrave Macmillan, Basingstoke

Cavanagh SJ (1991) *Orem's Model in Action, 3rd edn.* Palgrave Macmillan, Basingstoke

Houlton JEF and Taylor PM (1987) *Trauma Management in the Dog and Cat.* Blackwell Science, Oxford

King L and Boag A (in press) *BSAVA Manual of Canine and Feline Emergency and Critical Care, 2nd edition.* BSAVA Publications, Gloucester

McKenna (2000) *Nursing Theories and Models.* Routledge, London

Moore M (1999) *BSAVA Manual of Veterinary Nursing.* BSAVA Publications, Gloucester

Orem DE (1991) *Nursing: Concepts of Practice, 4th edn.* Mosby, St. Louis (6th edn published 2001)

Roper N, Logan W and Tierney A (2000) *The Roper, Logan and Tierney Model of Nursing.* Churchill Livingstone, Edinburgh

Tomey and Alligood (2002) *Nursing Theorists and their Work, 5th edn.* Mosby, London

Walsh (1997) *Models and Critical Pathways in Clinical Nursing: Conceptual Frameworks for Care Plans.* Baillière Tyndall, London

Chapter 16

Nutrition and feeding

Sandra McCune and Simon J. Girling

Learning objectives

After studying this chapter, students should be able to:

- **Describe the nutritional needs of dogs and cats in a variety of settings and life stages**
- **Describe the organs and their role in digestion, absorption and excretion**
- **Discuss the dietary requirements of a range of small mammals, including rabbits, guinea pigs, rats, mice, hamsters, chinchillas, gerbils, ferrets, reptiles, cage birds, amphibians and ornamental fish**
- **Appreciate the functional benefits of food ingredients**

Introduction

Proper nutrition is essential for the maintenance of optimum health and activity in all living creatures. Wild animals can obtain all the nutrients they need through a combination of hunting, scavenging and foraging but the opportunity for companion animals to access their natural diet has been limited by the process of domestication. It is the responsibility of the owner, therefore, to ensure that the diet they provide meets all the nutritional and behavioural needs of their pet and professional advice in this area is frequently sought.

Failure to provide a nutritionally adequate diet can result in disease or suboptimal performance, but nutritional factors may impact on the health of animals in a number of other ways. Many medical conditions will respond to modification of some aspect of the diet, and nutritional support is particularly important at times of illness or other forms of stress.

Research into the nutritional needs of pets has advanced significantly over the past few decades. Compared to the situation in the 1960s, there is a vastly improved understanding of what should be included in a balanced diet to prevent certain deficiencies, as well as throughout the various life stages and lifestyles of pets as they grow, mature and age. As in human nutrition, attention is now turning towards achieving optimal health through functional foods, i.e. those nutrients that have a health benefit beyond preventing a deficiency, such as antioxidants to boost the function of the immune system, improve cognitive health, decrease cellular damage to DNA and help to slow the progression of ageing. Nutrition plays an essential role in the lifelong health and well-being of both humans and pets and should be an important consideration to discuss with owners at every health check.

Definitions

- **Food** may be defined as any solid or liquid that, when ingested, can supply any or all of the following:
  - Energy-giving materials from which the body can produce movement, heat or other forms of energy
  - Materials for growth, repair or reproduction
  - Substances necessary to initiate or regulate the processes involved in the first two categories.
- **Nutrients** – The components of food that have these functions.
- **Diet** – The foods or food mixtures that are actually eaten.
- **Essential nutrient** – Any nutrient that is required by the animal and cannot be synthesized in the body. If any essential nutrient is lacking or present in insufficient quantity in the diet, then the diet, as a whole, must be considered inadequate.

Energy

In addition to providing specific nutrients, food also supplies energy. Energy is a fundamental requirement of all living species and provides the power for cells to function. The energy content of the diet is derived from carbohydrates, fats and protein, and the amounts of each of these nutrients in a food will determine its energy content. Dietary fat supplies just over twice as much energy as protein or carbohydrate per gram and is therefore a more efficient fuel for metabolism. Water has no energy value and so the energy density of food varies inversely with its moisture content.

Energy intake

Energy intake must be carefully regulated and maintained at a level close to requirements. When maintained over long periods, energy intake in excess of energy expenditure can be detrimental and leads to obesity or, in some young dogs, growth abnormalities. An inadequate energy intake results in poor growth in young animals and weight loss in adults. Although most animals are efficient self-regulators of their energy intake, this ability may be overridden by a number of factors, particularly in dogs.

No animal is able to utilize all the energy from its food. Energy intake is therefore considered at three different levels: gross energy, digestible energy and metabolizable energy.

- **Gross energy (GE)** of ingested food is the maximum amount of energy that can be released by a food and is assessed by bomb calorimetry. Although a substance may have a high GE content, it is of no use unless the animal is able to digest and absorb it.
- **Digestible energy (DE)** is the energy available from a food when it has been absorbed into the body after digestion in the digestive tract and is calculated as GE minus faecal losses.
- **Metabolizable energy (ME)** is the energy that is ultimately utilized by the tissues and is calculated as DE minus urinary losses.

The DE and ME contents of foods depend upon their composition and also upon the species that consumes them. The digestive systems of animals differ markedly between species, and even two fairly similar animals, such as the dog and the cat, show differences in digestibility values when fed the same food. In addition to these species differences, there will be variations between individual animals in their own metabolic efficiency.

Simple formulae have been developed that give reasonable approximations of the ME in a food from its carbohydrate, fat and protein contents, allowing for the losses in absorption and efficiency (Figure 16.1).

Species	Food type and ME equation
Cat	Canned $(P \times 3.9 + F \times 7.7 + C \times 3.0) - 5$
	Dry $(P \times 5.65 + F \times 9.4 + C \times 4.15)\, 0.99 - 126$
	Semi-moist $(P \times 3.7 + F \times 8.8 + C \times 3.3)$
Dog	All $(P \times 3.5 + F \times 8.5 + C \times 3.5)$

16.1 Calculation of metabolizable energy in cat and dog foods in kcal/100 g food. For result in kJ/100 g food, multiply by 4.18. P = protein g/100 g of food; F = fat (acid ether extract) g/100 g of food; C = carbohydrate (calculated by difference) g/100 g of food.

Energy expenditure

Within the body, energy is used to perform muscular work, for basic processes such as breathing and for physical activity to maintain body temperature. There are two components of energy expenditure: basal metabolic rate and thermogenesis.

- **Basal metabolic rate (BMR)** is the amount of energy required to keep the body 'ticking over' and includes processes such as respiration, circulation and kidney function. It may be affected by many factors, including bodyweight and composition, age and hormonal status.
- **Thermogenesis** is simply an increase in metabolic rate over the basal level and includes the costs of digesting, absorbing and utilizing nutrients (the 'thermic effect of food'), muscular work or exercise, stress, and maintenance of body temperature in a cold environment. Unlike BMR, the degree of thermogenesis can vary widely and may cause large variations in daily output.

Energy requirements

Energy requirements of individual animals are based on the weight of actively metabolizing tissue and may be influenced by bodyweight, body surface area, body composition and hair type. Dogs are a unique species in that there is such a wide variation in normal adult bodyweights, and estimations of energy needs are calculated from an allometric equation that relates energy requirements to the animal's metabolic bodyweight, BW $(kg)^{0.75}$ (see 'Feeding healthy dogs and cats'). For other species with a relatively narrow range of bodyweights, including cats, a linear equation that links energy requirements directly to bodyweight is appropriate in most situations (see later). These basic energy requirements may then be modified according to the animal's physiological status (including life stage and state of health or disease), level of activity and environmental conditions (Figures 16.2 and 16.3).

The **energy density** of the diet must be high enough to enable the dog or cat to obtain sufficient calories to maintain **energy balance**. An animal is said to be in energy balance when its expenditure of energy is equal to its intake, with the result that the level of energy stored in the body does not

Physiological state	Stage	MER (kcal/kg BW$^{0.75}$)
Work	Low activity (< 1 hour/day)	100
	Moderate activity (1–3 hours/day)	125
	High activity (3–6 hours/day)	150–175
	Heavy work (e.g. sledge dog, full day)	200–400
Gestation	< 42 days	120–140
	> 42 days	140–225
Lactation	Peak (21–42 days)	*Ad libitum*
Growth, puppies	To 50% of adult weight	210
	From 50% to 80% of adult weight	175
	From 80% to 100% of adult weight	140
Cold	Wind chill factor 8.5°C	125
	Wind chill factor < 0°C	175
Heat	Tropical climates	250

16.2 Estimated energy requirements of healthy dogs in various physiological states (after FEDIAF, 2001). MER, maintenance energy requirement. To calculate MER, multiply bodyweight (kg, raised to power of 0.75) by factor in column. For kJ values, multiply result by 4.18.

Physiological state	Stage	MER (kcal/kg BW)
Adult	Inactive	50–70
	Active	70–90
Gestation		70–90
Lactation		Up to 280
Growth, kittens	To 10 weeks	180–245
	10–20 weeks	80–210
	20–30 weeks	80–100

16.3 Estimated energy requirements of healthy cats in various physiological states (after FEDIAF, 2001). MER, maintenance energy requirement. To calculate MER, multiply bodyweight (kg) by factor in column. For kJ values, multiply result by 4.18.

Amino acid	Dog	Cat
Arginine	✓	✓
Histidine	✓	✓
Isoleucine	✓	✓
Lysine	✓	✓
Methionine	✓	✓
Cystine	✓	✓
Phenylalanine	✓	✓
Tyrosine	✓	✓
Threonine	✓	✓
Tryptophan	✓	✓
Valine	✓	✓
Taurine	✗	✓

16.4 Essential amino acids for dogs and cats. ✓ = essential; ✗ = non-essential.

change. Energy density is the principal factor determining the quantity of food eaten each day and thus the amount of each nutrient ingested by the animal. Nutrient requirements are usually expressed in terms of the ME concentration so that the values are applicable to any type of food or diet regardless of its water content, nutrient content or overall energy value.

Macronutrients

Protein

Proteins are large complex molecules composed of long chains of amino acids linked together by peptide bonds. There are only about 20 amino acids commonly found as protein components but these may be arranged in any combination to give an almost infinite variety of naturally occurring proteins, each with its own characteristic properties. Proteins are essential components of all living cells, where they have several important functions, including regulation of metabolism (as enzymes and some hormones) and a structural role in cell walls and muscle fibre. They are thus an important requirement for tissue growth and repair. Proteins are also a source of energy in the diet.

Protein requirements

Animals need a dietary source of protein to provide the specific amino acids that their tissues cannot synthesize, at a rate sufficient for optimum performance. Amino acids may be classified as either essential (indispensable) or non-essential (dispensable). **Essential amino acids** cannot be synthesized by the body in sufficient amounts and must, therefore, be provided in the diet (Figure 16.4). **Non-essential amino acids** are equally important as components of body proteins, but they can be synthesized from excesses of certain other dietary amino acids or other sources of dietary nitrogen.

Protein is required during normal maintenance to replace protein lost during the natural turnover of epithelial surfaces, hair and other body tissues, and in secretions. Additional protein is needed during periods of growth, pregnancy, lactation and for repair of damaged tissue. It is during these critical stages that protein quality (the amino acid composition of the protein) and digestibility are most important. Animal proteins generally have a more balanced amino acid profile, with a greater proportion of essential amino acids, and better digestibility than plant proteins. The **biological value** of a food

protein is the proportion that can be utilized for synthesizing body tissues and compounds and is not excreted in urine or faeces. Good-quality animal proteins have a higher biological value than plant based proteins.

Protein deficiency and excess

Protein deficiency can result either from insufficient dietary protein or from a shortage of particular amino acids. Signs of protein deficiency include poor growth or weight loss, rough and dull hair coat, anorexia, increased susceptibility to disease, muscle wasting and emaciation, oedema and finally death. Deficiency of a single essential amino acid results in anorexia and subsequent negative nitrogen balance.

Cats exhibit a number of nutritional peculiarities, many of which are reflected in their protein and amino acid requirements. Not only do they have a higher maintenance protein requirement than many other mammals, but they are also particularly sensitive to an arginine-deficient diet and they have a specific dietary need for the amino-sulphonic acid, taurine. **Taurine** is vital to the functioning of a wide range of mammalian organ systems, but, unlike other animals, cats are unable to synthesize sufficient quantities to meet their exceptionally high requirements. A deficiency of taurine in cats results in feline central retinal degeneration and has also been linked to dilated cardiomyopathy, reproductive failure in queens, developmental abnormalities in kittens and impaired immune function.

Dietary protein in excess of the body's requirements is not laid down as muscle but is, instead, converted to fat and stored as adipose tissue.

Fat

Dietary fats consist mainly of mixtures of triglycerides, each triglyceride being a combination of three fatty acids joined by a unit of glycerol. The character of each fat is determined largely by the different fatty acids in each. Fatty acids may be described as **saturated**, where there are no double bonds between carbon atoms, or **unsaturated**, where one or more double bonds are present. Those containing only one double bond are referred to as **monounsaturated**, while those containing more than one double bond are referred to as **polyunsaturated**. Most fats contain all of these types but in widely varying proportions.

There are several families of fatty acid, named according to the position of the first double bond. Fatty acids with the first double bond between the 3rd and 4th carbon are in the n-3 family (e.g. α-linolenic acid, eicosapentaenoic and docosahexaenoic acids), those between the 6th and 7th carbon are the n-6 family (e.g. linoleic acid, γ-linolenic acid and arachidonic acid), and those between the 9th and 10th are the n-9 family (e.g. oleic acid). The n-3 and n-6 families are **essential fatty acids (EFAs)** because they cannot be synthesized *de novo* in mammals, whereas saturated fatty acids and fatty acids of the n-9 series up to 18 carbons can be synthesized *de novo*.

Essential fatty acids

Dietary fat has several roles. It serves as the most concentrated source of energy in the diet and it lends palatability and an acceptable texture to food. However, its most important functions are as a provider of EFAs and as a carrier for the fat-soluble vitamins A, D, E and K. There are currently three recognized EFAs, all of which are polyunsaturated: linoleic, α-linolenic and arachidonic acids. Linoleic and α-linolenic acids are the parent compounds from which the more complex longer-chain compounds (derived EFAs) can be made. The cat is unusual in that it is unable to convert the parent EFAs into longer-chain derivatives and therefore requires a dietary source of arachidonic acid, which in practical terms means a requirement for EFAs of animal origin.

The EFAs are involved in many aspects of health, including kidney function and reproduction. They are essential components of cell membranes and they are necessary for the synthesis of prostaglandins. Signs associated with EFA deficiency in dogs and cats include dull, scurfy coat, hair loss, fatty liver, anaemia and impaired fertility. It should be noted that diets high in polyunsaturated fatty acids may become rancid through oxidation, which can lead to the destruction of other nutrients, particularly vitamin E.

Carbohydrate

Carbohydrates provide the body with energy and may be converted to body fat. This group includes the simple sugars (such as glucose) and the complex sugars (such as starch), which consist of chains of the simpler sugars. All animals have a metabolic requirement for glucose, but provided that the diet contains sufficient glucose precursors (amino acids and glycerol) most animals can synthesize enough to meet their metabolic needs without a dietary source of carbohydrate.

Sugars and cooked starches are economical and easily digested sources of energy, whereas uncooked starches are less readily digested. Some species (some dogs, for example) may find starch palatable, but others, such as the cat, do not respond to the taste of sugar. The value of disaccharides, such as sucrose or lactose, is limited in most animals by the activity of the intestinal disaccharides, such as sucrase and lactase. In particular, the activity of lactase declines with age and an excessive consumption of lactose-containing (dairy) products can lead to the production of diarrhoea.

Dietary fibre

Dietary fibre, or roughage, is the term applied to the group of indigestible polysaccharides such as cellulose, pectin and lignin. They are usually associated with plant material and typically constitute the cell walls of plants. These materials generally escape digestion and pass through the digestive tract relatively unchanged. The role of dietary fibre in the animal depends to a large extent on the physiology of the animal's digestive tract, but in most species a limited amount of dietary fibre may provide bulk to the faeces, regularizing bowel movements and thus helping to prevent constipation or diarrhoea. Soluble and insoluble sources of dietary fibre are used to improve glycaemic control in dogs with diabetes mellitus and in the dietary management of a number of other 'fibre-responsive' diseases.

Micronutrients

Minerals

Minerals are inorganic nutrients, which are sometimes referred to collectively as 'ash'. They may be divided into **macrominerals** (which are required in relatively large amounts) and trace elements or **microminerals** (which are required in relatively small or trace amounts). **Electrolytes** are minerals in their salt form as found in the body tissues and fluids. Figure 16.5 lists the function of the main minerals and Figure 16.6 the dietary requirements.

Element	Function
Macrominerals	
Calcium	Bone and teeth development. Required for blood clotting, nerve and muscle function
Chloride	Maintains osmotic pressure, acid–base and water balance
Magnesium	Bone and teeth development. Energy metabolism
Phosphorus	Bone and teeth development. Required for energy utilization and various enzyme systems
Potassium & Sodium	Maintain osmotic pressure, acid–base and water balance. Required for nerve and muscle function
Microminerals	
Arsenic	Required for growth and red blood cell formation
Chromium	Required for carbohydrate metabolism
Cobalt	Component of vitamin B12
Copper	Required for haemoglobin synthesis, structure of bones and blood vessels, melanin production and various enzyme systems
Fluoride	Bone and teeth development
Iodine	Thyroid hormone production
Iron	Component of haemoglobin and myoglobin. Needed for the utilization of oxygen
Manganese	Required for chondroitin sulphate and cholesterol synthesis. Various enzyme systems associated with carbohydrate and fat metabolism
Molybdenum	Various enzyme systems
Nickel	Function of membranes and nucleic acid metabolism
Selenium	Component of glutathione peroxidase
Silicon	Bone and connective tissue development
Vanadium	Growth, reproduction and fat metabolism
Zinc	Various enzyme systems including alkaline phosphatase, carbonic anhydrase and digestive enzymes. Maintenance of epidermal integrity and immunological homeostasis

16.5 Established functions of minerals in dogs and cats.

Mineral	Cat		Dog	
Calcium	Growth:	110–173 mg/kg BW/day or approximately 160–250 mg/100 kcal (418 kJ) ME	Growth:	320 mg/kg BW/day or approximately 275 mg/100 kcal (418 kJ) ME
	Maintenance:	87–156 mg/kg BW/day or approximately 125–200 mg/100 kcal (418 kJ) ME	Maintenance:	119 mg/kg BW/day or approximately 130–160 mg/100 kcal (418 kJ) ME
Phosphorus	Growth:	90–150 mg/kg BW/day or approximately 120–200 mg/100 kcal (418 kJ) ME	Growth:	240 mg/kg BW/day or approximately 200–225 mg/100 kcal (418 kJ) ME
	Maintenance:	90 mg/kg BW/day or approximately 120 mg/100 kcal (418 kJ) ME	Maintenance:	89 mg/kg BW/day or approximately 120–160 mg/100 kcal (418 kJ) ME
Copper	Growth:	100–160 µg/kg BW/day or approximately 300–460 µg/100 kcal (418 kJ) ME	Growth:	160–500 µg/kg BW/day or approximately 150–440 µg/100 kcal (418 kJ) ME
	Maintenance:	75 µg/kg BW/day or approximately 100 µg/100 kcal (418 kJ) ME	Maintenance:	80 µ/kg BW/day or approximately 150 µg/100 kcal (418 kJ) ME
Iodine	Growth:	20–309 µg/kg BW/day or approximately 27–33 µg/100 kcal (418 kJ) ME	Growth:	30–50 µg/kg BW/day or approximately 16–25 µg/100 kcal (418 kJ) ME
	Maintenance:	7–15 µ/kg BW/day or approximately 10–20 µ/g /100 kcal (418 kJ) ME	Maintenance:	12 µg/kg BW/day or approximately 16–24 µg/100 kcal (418 kJ) ME
Iron	Growth:	4–4.5 mg/kg BW/day or approximately 12–18 mg/100 kcal (418 kJ) ME	Growth:	1.74–2.3 mg/kg BW/day or approximately 1–2 mg/100 kcal (418 kJ) ME
	Maintenance:	1.2 mg/kg BW/day or approximately 1.6 mg/100 kcal (418 kJ) ME	Maintenance:	0.65 mg/kg BW/day or approximately 100–130 mg/100 kcal (418 kJ) ME
Magnesium	Growth:	7.5–9.4 mg/kg BW/day or approximately 10–12.5 mg/100 kcal (418 kJ) ME	Growth:	22 mg/kg BW/day or approximately 25 mg/100 kcal (418 kJ) ME
	Maintenance:	6 mg/kg BW/day or approximately 8 mg/100 kcal (418 kJ) ME	Maintenance:	5.5–8.2 mg/kg BW/day or approximately 11 mg/100 kcal (418 kJ) ME
Manganese	Growth and Maintenance:	80–250 µg/kg BW/day or approximately 100–250 µg/100 kcal (418 kJ) ME	Growth:	280–1000 µg/kg BW/day or approximately 200–600 µg/100 kcal (418 kJ) ME
			Maintenance:	100 µg/kg BW/day or approximately 140–200 µg/100 kcal (418 kJ) ME
Selenium	Growth:	5–13 µg/kg BW/day or approximately 2–5 µg/100 kcal (418 kJ) ME	Growth:	6–13 µg/kg BW/day or approximately 3–8 µg/100 kcal (418 kJ) ME
	Maintenance:	5 µg/kg BW/day or approximately 6 µg/100 kcal (418 kJ) ME	Maintenance:	6 µg/kg BW/day or approximately 7 µg/100 kcal (418 kJ) ME
Sodium	Growth:	15–30 mg/kg BW/day or approximately 20–40 mg/100 kcal (418 kJ) ME	Growth:	30 mg/kg BW/day or approximately 20–25 mg/100 kcal (418 kJ) ME
	Maintenance:	14 mg/kg BW/day or approximately 18 mg/100 kcal (418 kJ) ME	Maintenance:	14 mg/kg BW/day or approximately 18 mg/100 kcal (418 kJ) ME
Chloride	Growth and Maintenance:	29 mg/kg BW/day or approximately 38 mg/100 kcal (418 kJ) ME	Growth:	46 mg/kg BW/day or approximately 40 mg/100 kcal (418 kJ) ME
			Maintenance:	17 mg/kg BW/day or approximately 21–30 mg/100 kcal (418 kJ) ME
Potassium	Growth and Maintenance:	100–125 mg/100 kcal (418 kJ) ME	Growth and Maintenance	100–125 mg/100 kcal (418 kJ) ME
Zinc	Growth and Maintenance:	2.5–3.9 mg/kg BW/day or approximately 1–2 mg/100 kcal (418 kJ) ME	Growth:	1.9–3.3 mg/kg BW/day or approximately 0.97–2 mg/100 kcal (418 kJ) ME
			Maintenance:	0.72 mg/kg BW/day or approximately 0.92–1.200 mg/100 kcal (418 kJ) ME

16.6 Dietary requirements for minerals in dogs and cats.

Macrominerals

Calcium (Ca) and phosphorus (P)

Calcium and phosphorus are closely interrelated nutritionally and will therefore be discussed together. They are the major minerals involved in maintaining the structural rigidity of bones and teeth, and approximately 99% of body calcium and 80% of body phosphorus are stored in the skeletal tissues. Calcium and phosphorus requirements are increased during growth, late pregnancy and lactation. The metabolism of calcium and phosphorus is closely linked with vitamin D.

Calcium is also essential for normal blood clotting and for nerve and muscle function. The level of calcium in the blood plasma is crucial to these functions and is very carefully regulated.

Phosphorus also has many other functions (more than any other mineral) and a complete discussion would require coverage of nearly all the metabolic processes of the body. Phosphorus is involved in many enzyme systems and is also a component of the so-called 'high-energy' organic phosphate compounds. These are mainly responsible for the storage and transfer of energy in the body.

Although the absolute concentrations of these minerals in the diet are of paramount importance, the ratio of calcium to phosphorus is also of great significance. The minimum calcium:phosphorus ratio for growth is generally considered to be about 1:1. For adult animals it is somewhat less critical. Imbalance in this ratio, where calcium is much less than phosphorus, leads to a marked deficiency of calcium in relation to bone formation.

Calcium deficiency (absolute or relative) results in nutritional secondary hyperparathyroidism in which there is increased bone resorption to restore circulating calcium levels. This results in skeletal deformities and lameness in the growing animal. Calcium–phosphorus imbalance may also occur in association with deficiency of vitamin D. This gives rise to rickets in the growing animal or osteomalacia in the adult. Hypocalcaemia in lactating bitches (particularly of the toy breeds) causes eclampsia, with nervous disturbances. This occurs where there is an inability of the calcium regulatory mechanism to compensate for the loss of calcium in milk.

There is evidence that very high levels of calcium and phosphorus or a very high ratio are also harmful. Conditions such as hip dysplasia, osteochondrosis syndrome, enostosis and wobbler syndrome have been related to excessive calcium intake in the growing dog.

Magnesium (Mg)

In association with calcium and phosphorus, magnesium is required for healthy bones and teeth. About 60% of body magnesium is found in skeletal tissue, but it is also to be found in the soft tissues of the body. Heart and skeletal muscle and nervous tissue depend on a proper balance between calcium and magnesium for normal function.

Magnesium is also important in sodium and potassium metabolism and plays a key role in many essential enzyme reactions, particularly those concerned with energy metabolism.

A deficiency of magnesium is characterized by muscular weakness and, in severe cases, convulsions. Nevertheless, a dietary deficiency of magnesium is very unlikely. In contrast, very high intakes of magnesium have been associated with an increased incidence of feline lower urinary tract disease.

Potassium (K)

Potassium is found in high concentrations within cells and is required for acid–base balance and osmoregulation of the body fluids. It is also important for nerve and muscle function and energy metabolism. Potassium is widely distributed in foods and naturally occurring deficiencies are rare; however, its requirement is linked to protein intake, so care may be needed in ensuring that high-protein diets contain adequate potassium.

A potassium deficiency causes muscular weakness, poor growth and lesions of the heart and kidney. In cats, the use of diets containing urinary acidifiers with a marginal potassium content has been associated with hypokalaemia. Potassium excess is rare but results in paresis and bradycardia.

Sodium (Na) and chloride (Cl⁻)

Together, sodium and chloride represent the major electrolytes of the body water and are required for acid–base balance and osmoregulation of the body fluids. Chloride is also an essential component of bile and hydrochloric acid (which is present in gastric juice).

Common salt (NaCl) is the most usual form in which these two minerals are added to food, so the dietary recommendation is often expressed in terms of sodium chloride. As with potassium, salt is widely distributed in normal diets and so deficiencies are rare.

Signs of deficiency may include fatigue, exhaustion, inability to maintain water balance, decreased water intake, retarded growth, dry skin and hair loss. Excess will cause greater than normal fluid intake and it has been suggested that some dogs with hypertension may benefit from a lower sodium diet.

Microminerals

Iron (Fe)

Iron is an essential component of the oxygen-carrying pigments: haemoglobin (in blood) and myoglobin (in muscle). It is also an essential part of many enzymes (haem enzymes) that are involved in respiration at the cellular level.

A deficiency causes anaemia, with the typical clinical picture of weakness and fatigue. Conversely, iron – like most trace elements – is toxic if ingested in excessive amounts and is associated with anorexia and weight loss.

Copper (Cu)

Copper is required for the formation and activity of red blood cells, as a cofactor in many enzyme systems, and for the normal pigmentation of skin and hair. Copper deficiency impairs the absorption and transport of iron and decreases haemoglobin synthesis. Thus a lack of copper in the diet can cause anaemia even when the intake of iron is normal. Bone disorders can also occur as a result of copper deficiency, and in this case the cause is thought to be a reduction in the activity of a copper-containing enzyme, leading to diminished stability and strength of bone collagen. Other signs of deficiency include hair depigmentation, decreased growth, neuromuscular disorders and reproductive failure.

Ironically, excess dietary copper may also cause anaemia, which is thought to result from competition between copper and iron for absorption sites in the intestine. Bedlington Terriers are known to display an unusual defect that results in hepatitis and cirrhosis and appears to be inherited. It has also been identified in other breeds, including West Highland White Terriers and Dobermanns. For these particular breeds, foods with a high copper content and copper-containing mineral supplements should be avoided.

Zinc (Zn)

Zinc is an essential component of many enzyme systems, including those related to protein and carbohydrate metabolism, and is essential for maintaining healthy coat and skin. Zinc is required by all animals, but the zinc requirement is particularly affected by the other components of the diet. For example, a high dietary calcium content or a vegetable protein-based diet can dramatically increase the zinc requirement and this latter effect may be related to that reported for iron absorption.

Zinc deficiency is characterized by poor growth, anorexia, testicular atrophy, emaciation and skin lesions. Although all nutrients are important, the link between zinc and skin and coat condition makes this trace element particularly crucial for the companion animal. This is because a marginal deficiency may occur where an animal is not obviously unwell but its skin or coat condition is suboptimal and significantly detracts from its appearance.

Zinc is relatively non-toxic, but high levels may interfere with the absorption and utilization of iron and copper.

Iodine (I)

Iodine is an essential component of thyroid hormones, which regulate basal metabolism in the body, and this is its only recognized function. Goitre (enlargement of the thyroid gland) is the principal sign of iodine deficiency but other factors may also produce goitre.

Hypothyroidism has been reported in dogs, and iodine deficiency has also been observed in zoo felids, domestic cats, birds and horses. Clinical signs include skin and hair abnormalities, dullness, apathy and drowsiness. There can also be abnormal calcium metabolism and reproductive failure with fetal resorption.

Excessive iodine intakes can be toxic, producing acute effects similar to those of a deficiency. The high doses in some way impair thyroid hormone synthesis and can produce so-called iodine myxoedema or toxic goitre. Anorexia, fever and weight loss may occur in cats.

Selenium (Se)

Selenium is closely interrelated with vitamin E, such that the presence of one nutrient can 'spare' a deficiency of the other and, together, they protect against damage to cell membranes. Nevertheless, it has been shown that selenium cannot be completely replaced by vitamin E and it has a discrete, unique function. Selenium is an obligatory component of glutathione peroxidase, the enzyme that protects cell membranes against damage by oxidizing substances. Selenium may also have other roles, including protection against lead, cadmium and mercury poisoning, and has been implicated as an anticancer agent.

Selenium deficiency has many effects, but one described in dogs is degeneration of skeletal and cardiac muscles. Effects of deficiency in other species include reproductive disorders and oedema.

Selenium is highly toxic in large doses and the difference between the recommended allowance and the toxic dose may be quite small. Effects of excess include vomiting, spasms, staggered gait, salivation and decreased appetite. Injudicious supplementation of foods is therefore particularly dangerous in this respect.

Manganese (Mn)

Manganese is involved in many enzyme-catalysed reactions and is required for carbohydrate and lipid metabolism, cartilage formation, reproduction and cell membrane integrity. A deficiency is characterized by defective growth, reproduction and disturbances in lipid metabolism. Manganese is relatively non-toxic.

Cobalt (Co)

Cobalt is an integral part of the vitamin B12 molecule and a deficiency is unlikely to occur if adequate vitamin B12 is present in the diet.

Other trace elements

A number of trace elements have been demonstrated as necessary for normal health in mammals, though specific requirements have not been established for companion animals. These elements are listed in Figure 16.7 with a brief summary of their functions. It appears that the amounts required in the diet are very low and the likelihood of a deficiency of any of these nutrients in a normal diet is consequently almost non-existent.

Element	Function
Chromium	Carbohydrate metabolism, closely linked with insulin function
Fluoride	Teeth and bone development, possibly some involvement in reproduction
Nickel	Membrane function, possibly involved in metabolism of the nucleic acid RNA
Molybdenum	Constituent of several enzymes, one of which is involved in uric acid metabolism
Silicon	Skeletal development, growth and maintenance of connective tissue
Vanadium	Growth, reproduction and fat metabolism
Arsenic	Growth, also some effect on blood formation, possibly haemoglobin production

16.7 Functions of additional trace elements.

Conversely, as with the majority of the trace elements, these substances are all toxic if fed in large quantities, but the amounts that can be tolerated vary from one element to another. Arsenic, vanadium, fluorine and molybdenum are the most toxic, whereas relatively large amounts of nickel and chromium can be ingested without adverse effects.

Mineral interactions

A large number of mineral–mineral interactions exist. These tend to be of two types:

- **Antagonistic** – the presence of one mineral reduces the transport or biological efficiency of the other.
- **Synergistic** – the two minerals act in a complementary way, either by sparing or substituting for the other mineral, or the two together enhance a biological function.

Most mineral interactions are antagonistic and can occur via a number of different mechanisms. Interactions may happen:

- In the diet during processing and therefore before consumption
- In the digestive tract where there is competition for uptake sites or other cellular mechanisms
- At the tissue level either at storage sites or by inhibition of enzyme activity
- At the time of transport
- In the excretory pathway.

Vitamins

Vitamins are organic compounds that help to regulate the body processes. Most vitamins cannot be synthesized in the body and must therefore be present in the diet. They may be classified as **fat-soluble** (vitamins A, D, E and K) or **water-soluble** (B-complex vitamins and vitamin C). A frequent intake of water-soluble vitamins is necessary since they are poorly stored in the body, with excesses being lost via the urine. The fat-soluble vitamins are stored to a much greater extent and consequently a daily intake is less critical. However, because they are stored, the risk of toxicity arising through excessive intake is far greater with the fat-soluble vitamins. Figures 16.8 and 16.9 list the essential features of vitamins and the dietary requirements of cats and dogs.

Fat-soluble vitamins

Vitamin A

In nature, vitamin A (retinol) is found to a large extent in the form of its precursors, the carotenoids, which are the yellow and orange pigments of most fruits and vegetables. Of these, β-carotene is the most important. Vitamin A is a component of the visual pigments (which transmit light) in the eye and is important for proper vision. It is also concerned with cell differentiation and maintenance of normal cell structure, so it is important for sustaining healthy skin, coat, all mucous membranes and for normal bone and teeth development.

A deficiency of vitamin A may be associated with anorexia, weakness, ataxia, weight loss and abnormalities of the squamous epithelium that are usually manifest as seborrhoeic coat conditions; xerophthalmia (which will ultimately lead to corneal opacity and ulceration); increased susceptibility to microbial infections; crusting lesions of the external nares and accompanying nasal discharge; and epithelial degeneration of the seminiferous tubules and endometrium, leading to infertility.

Vitamin	Feature
A	Fat-soluble. Essential in diet. Found in liver, fats, oils, egg yolks and cereal grain germ. Exists as a pro-vitamin in vegetable sources. Stored in the body. Deficiencies affect vision, hearing, respiratory tract lining, skin and bones. Excesses are toxic
B group	Comprises thiamine (B1), riboflavin (B2), niacin, pyridoxine (B6), pantothenic acid, folic acid, biotin and cobalamin (B12). Water soluble. Many are produced by intestinal bacteria. Found in liver, egg yolks, yeast and whole cereal grains. Exists as the active form in vegetables. Not stored in the body, except vitamin B12 . Deficiencies affect appetite and metabolism. Excesses are not usually toxic
C	Water-soluble. No dietary requirement in healthy dogs and cats. Found in fresh fruit and vegetables. Found as the active form in vegetables. Not stored in the body. Deficiencies affect wound healing and capillary integrity. Excesses are not toxic
D	Fat-soluble. Essential in diet. Found in liver, fats, oils, egg yolks and cereal grain germ. Exists as a pro-vitamin in vegetable sources. Stored in the body. Deficiencies affect bone, teeth and calcium–phosphorus absorption/ utilization. Excesses are toxic
E	Fat-soluble. Essential in diet. Found in liver, fats, oils, egg yolks and cereal grain germ. Found as active form in vegetables. Stored in the body. Deficiencies affect muscle, fat and reproductive ability
K	Fat-soluble. Minimal requirement in diet as it is manufactured by intestinal bacteria. Found in liver, fats, oils, egg yolks and cereal grain germ. Exists as a pro-vitamin in vegetable sources. Not stored in the body. Deficiencies cause a coagulopathy

16.8 Essential features of the major vitamins.

Deficiencies of vitamin A are not common and dogs are able to synthesize vitamin A from plant-derived β-carotene. Cats, however, are unable to perform this conversion and their diet must include a source of preformed vitamin A, which may only be found in animal fat. Excesses of vitamin A are stored in the liver and a toxicity can lead to liver damage. Clinically, the most recognizable signs of hypervitaminosis A are those of a crippling bone disease that results in the formation of bony exostoses and ankylosis of joints, particularly in the cervical vertebrae and the long bones of the forelimb. Cats are particularly susceptible to hypervitaminosis A and the problem usually arises following prolonged oversupplementation of the diet with vitamin A (in cod liver oil, for example) or by feeding large quantities of liver.

Vitamin D

Metabolites of vitamin D stimulate calcium absorption in the intestine and, in conjunction with parathyroid hormone, stimulate resorption of calcium from bone. The requirements for vitamin D are closely linked to the dietary concentrations of calcium and phosphorus. Most mammals are able to synthesize vitamin D3 from lipid compounds in the skin, provided that they have exposure to sunlight and are otherwise well nourished.

There are several compounds that have vitamin D activity but the most important are ergocalciferol (vitamin D2) and cholecalciferol (vitamin D3). Both of these forms are effective as sources of vitamin D activity.

A deficiency of vitamin D is extremely rare but is frequently confounded by a simultaneous calcium and phosphorus imbalance, which causes rickets in the young animal and

Vitamins		Cat			Dog		
			per kg BW/day	per 100 kcal (418 kJ)		per kg BW/day	per 100 kcal (418 kJ)
Vitamin B Choline		Growth: Maintenance:	120–130 mg 120–130 mg	48 mg 48 mg	Growth: Maintenance:	50 mg 25 mg	34 mg 34 mg
Biotin		Growth: Maintenance:	1.5–3 µg 1.5 µg	1.4–3.2 µg 1.4 µg	Growth: Maintenance:	20 µg 20 µg	12.5 µg 12.5 µg
Cobalamin		Growth: Maintenance:	1 µg 0.32 µg	0.4–1.25 µg 0.4–0.5 µg	Growth: Maintenance:	1 µg 0.5 µg	0.7 µg 0.7 µg
Folate		Growth: Maintenance:	25–40 µg 16–20 µg	16–25 µg 27 µg	Growth: Maintenance:	8 µg 4 µg	5.4 µg 5.4 µg
Niacin		Growth: Maintenance:	1.8 mg 0.9 mg	1.8–2.4 mg 1.8 mg	Growth: Maintenance:	0.45 mg 0.225 mg	0.3 mg 0.3–0.45 mg
Pantothenic acid		Growth: Maintenance:	75–180 µg 75–180 µg	100–250 µg 100–250 µg	Growth: Maintenance:	400 µg 200 µg	270–330 µg 270–400 µg
Pyridoxine		Growth: Maintenance:	0.128–0.2 mg 0.07 mg	0.08–0.16 mg 0.08–0.1 mg	Growth: Maintenance:	0.06 mg 0.022 mg	0.03 mg 0.03 mg
Riboflavin		Growth: Maintenance:	150–320 µg 90 µg	130–280 µg 120 µg	Growth: Maintenance:	100 µg 50 µg	68–80 µg 68 µg
Thiamine		Growth: Maintenance:	100–250 µg 80 µg	0.125–0.16 µg 0.1 µg	Growth: Maintenance:	54 µg 20 µg	27–40 µg 27 µg
Vitamin A		Growth: Maintenance: Reproduction:	64–75 IU 64–75 IU 90–100 IU	80–100 IU/kg 80–100 IU/kg 120–140 IU/kg	Growth: Maintenance:	202 IU 75 IU	100–170 IU 100–150 IU
Vitamin D		Growth: Maintenance:	18–22 IU 8 IU	15–25 IU 10 IU	Growth: Maintenance:	22 IU 8 IU	11–18 IU 11–15 IU
Vitamin E		Growth: Maintenance:	1–1.5 IU 0.45 IU	0.9–1 IU 0.6 IU	Growth: Maintenance:	1.4 IU 0.5 IU	1.25 IU 0.6–1 IU
Vitamin K		Growth: Maintenance:	16–60 µg 16–60 µg	2–20 µg 2–20 µg	Growth: Maintenance:	16–60 µg 16–60 µg	2–20 µg 2–20 µg

16.9 Dietary requirements for vitamins in dogs and cats. One international unit (1 IU) of Vitamin D is equivalent to 0.025 mg. One international unit (1 IU) of α-tocopherol is equivalent to 1 mg

osteomalacia in the adult, characterized by a failure of mineralization of newly formed osteoid. In the young animal, endochondral ossification of the growth plates is disturbed, giving rise to the typically enlarged metaphyses, particularly of the radius–ulna and ribs.

Adverse effects of excess vitamin D are generally related to hypercalcaemia which, if prolonged, results in extensive calcification of the soft tissues, lungs, kidneys and stomach. Deformations of the teeth and jaws can also occur and death can result if the intake is particularly high.

Vitamin E

Acting with selenium, vitamin E protects cell membranes against oxidative damage. The requirement for vitamin E is increased when dietary levels of polyunsaturated fatty acids (**PUFAs**), which are easily oxidized, are high. Recent studies of healthy animals have demonstrated an increased immune response to vaccination when the animals were fed diets high in vitamin E and other antioxidants. Given the low potential for toxicity, this work indicates that there are likely added benefits to feeding higher quantities of vitamin E than that required to prevent a deficiency.

In cats, vitamin E deficiency can be induced by feeding diets of oily fish (especially red tuna) which are rich in PUFAs, or feeding rancid oxidized fat. This causes a painful inflammatory condition of body fat (especially subcutaneous fat) known as pansteatitis (yellow fat disease). Vitamin E deficiency in dogs has been associated with skeletal muscle dystrophy, reproductive failure and impairment of the immune response.

In practice, vitamin E toxicity is unlikely to occur. Vitamin E is one of the least toxic vitamins and relatively high doses may be tolerated.

Vitamin K

Vitamin K regulates the formation of several blood-clotting factors (factors VII, IX, X and XII). In normal healthy animals the requirement for vitamin K is met by bacterial synthesis in the intestine and a simple deficiency is unlikely to occur. Hypoprothrombinaemia and haemorrhage may occur in some animals when bacterial synthesis is suppressed, or there are vitamin K antagonists (such as warfarin or other coumarin compounds) in the diet.

Excess vitamin K has low toxicity but very large intakes may produce anaemia and other blood abnormalities in young animals.

Water-soluble vitamins

Water-soluble vitamins are now usually referred to by their chemical names rather than by a letter/number combination.

B-complex

The B-complex vitamins are used to form coenzymes (cofactors) which are involved with normal metabolic function, especially energy metabolism and synthetic pathways.

Thiamine (aneurin, vitamin B1)

Thiamine is involved in carbohydrate metabolism and the requirement for this vitamin is dependent on the carbohydrate content of the diet. Thiamine deficiency can occur in cats as a result of feeding large amounts of certain types of raw fish which contain the enzyme thiaminase. In addition, the vitamin is progressively destroyed by high temperatures and under certain conditions of processing. Most pet food manufacturers supplement their products to compensate for possible losses, but some home-prepared diets may require additional thiamine.

Thiamine deficiency is expressed clinically as anorexia and neurological disorders (especially of the postural mechanisms) followed ultimately by weakness, heart failure and death. Like other water-soluble vitamins, thiamine is of low toxicity when ingested at high levels.

Riboflavin (vitamin B2)

Riboflavin is a constituent of two coenzymes that are essential in a number of oxidative enzyme systems. Cellular growth cannot take place in the absence of riboflavin. Riboflavin deficiency is associated with eye lesions, skin disorders and testicular hypoplasia. Toxicity of this vitamin has not been reported in dogs and cats.

Pantothenic acid

Pantothenic acid is a constituent of coenzyme A, which is essential for carbohydrate, fat and amino acid metabolism. This vitamin is widespread in animal and plant tissues and a deficiency is unlikely to occur in normal circumstances.

Signs of experimentally induced deficiency include depressed growth, fatty liver, gastrointestinal disturbances (including ulcers), convulsions, coma and death. Toxicity has not been reported in any species following ingestion of large doses.

Niacin (nicotinamide and nicotinic acid)

Niacin is a component of two important coenzymes, the nicotinamide adenine dinucleotides, which are required for oxidation–reduction reactions necessary for the utilization of all the major nutrients. In mammalian species, the requirement for niacin is influenced by the dietary level of the amino acid tryptophan, which can be converted to the vitamin. In cats, however, this conversion does not occur because an alternative pathway in the metabolism of tryptophan is favoured, so the dietary requirement for niacin is greater.

A deficiency of niacin causes a condition known as pellagra in humans and blacktongue in dogs and cats, which is characterized by inflammation and ulceration of the oral cavity with thick, blood-stained saliva and foul breath. Both forms of niacin are considered to be of low toxicity.

Pyridoxine (vitamin B6)

This vitamin is involved in a wide range of enzyme systems associated with nitrogen and amino acid metabolism; consequently, increased levels are required as the protein content of the diet increases.

A deficiency of pyridoxine results in anorexia, weight loss and anaemia. In cats, irreversible kidney damage can occur.

Pyridoxine and its derivatives are not considered toxic. Prevalence of pyridoxine toxicity appears to be low. Earliest detectable signs include ataxia and loss of small motor control. Many of the signs of toxicity resemble those of B6 deficiency.

Vitamin B12 (cyanocobalamin)

The function of vitamin B12 is closely linked to that of folic acid. It is also involved in fat and carbohydrate metabolism and in the synthesis of myelin. A deficiency results in pernicious anaemia and neurological signs.

Biotin

Biotin is required for a variety of reactions involving the metabolism of fats and amino acids. The vitamin is important in maintaining the integrity of keratinized structures, such as the skin and hair.

Deficiencies of biotin are unlikely to occur since the daily requirement is normally met by intestinal bacterial synthesis. However, a deficiency may develop following the prolonged use of oral antibiotics that suppress microbial synthesis or the feeding of large amounts of raw egg white, which contains avidin (a protein that binds biotin). Eggs should therefore be cooked if they are to form a significant proportion of the diet.

Signs of biotin deficiency include dry, scaly skin with dull brittle hair, hyperkeratosis, pruritus and skin ulcers. No toxicity has been reported in dogs and cats.

Folic acid (pteroylglutamic acid, folacin)
The folates are important for a number of reactions, including the synthesis of thymidine (an essential component of DNA). Folic acid is essential for normal maturation of red blood cells in bone marrow and the typical signs of folic acid deficiency are anaemia and leucopenia. Deficiencies are unlikely to occur since it is probable that most, if not all, of the daily requirement can be met by intestinal bacterial synthesis. Folic acid is considered to be non-toxic.

Choline
Choline is a constituent of phospholipids, which are essential components of cell membranes, and it is also the precursor of acetylcholine, a neurotransmitter chemical. A dietary deficiency of choline is unlikely to occur, but experimentally it causes fatty infiltration of the liver. No toxicity has been described for dogs and cats.

Ascorbic acid (vitamin C)
Vitamin C is required for many intracellular reactions and protein synthesis, but most mammals are able to synthesize it from glucose. The main exceptions are humans, other primates and the guinea pig. Although there is no dietary requirement for vitamin C in normal healthy companion animals, some researchers believe that a dietary source may be beneficial under certain circumstances (such as stress or high activity levels) or in certain individuals. No signs of either deficiency or excess have been reported in normal cats or dogs.

Vitamin-like compounds
There are substances that exhibit properties similar to those of vitamins, but do not fit the strict definition of a vitamin. These compounds have physiological functionality but can be 'conditionally essential', depending upon the metabolic capacity of the animal. Examples include carnitine, carotenoids, bioflavonoids, ubiquinones and para-aminobenzoic acid (PABA). Research into these nutrients and their functions continues.

Water

An animal's requirement for water is at least as important as that for any other nutrient; life may continue for weeks in the absence of food but only for a few days, or even hours, when water is not available. Water performs many vital functions within the body and the body water content is regulated within quite narrow limits. A daily intake is necessary to replace obligatory water losses from the body, which occur mainly via the urine, faeces, skin and lungs and in productive secretions such as milk.

Water is taken into the body in several forms: as fluid drunk, as a component of food or as metabolic water (that released during the breakdown of protein, fat and carbohydrate). The daily water intake of any individual will depend on a number of factors, including the moisture content of the food, environmental temperature, level of activity and physiological state. A plentiful supply of fresh drinking water should, therefore, always be available.

A balanced diet

In the last several decades much has been learned about the nutritional needs of pets, in particular dogs and cats. With the advent of feeding balanced prepared diets, nutritional deficiencies are a rare occurrence. A diet that is balanced will supply all the key nutrients and energy needed to meet the daily needs of the animal at its particular life stage. Nutrient and energy content are therefore important considerations but other related factors include digestibility and palatability of the food. Animals eat to satisfy their requirement for energy, so if all key nutrients are balanced to the energy content of the diet, then providing the correct quantity of energy also ensures an appropriate intake of essential nutrients. Animals requiring a higher plane of nutrition (as in gestation or lactation) will inevitably receive a higher intake of all key nutrients when they increase the amount of food consumed to meet their energy demands.

Nutrient balance
Nutrient requirements are bounded by a minimum and, in some cases, a maximum value. In other words, the amount of nutrient needed in the diet must lie on a 'plateau' between deficiency on the one hand and toxicity on the other (Figure 16.10).

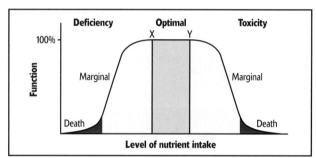

16.10 Relationship of nutrient intake to health.

Nutrient interactions
Deficiencies of a specific nutrient may occur as a result of interactions with other components of the diet, which reduce their bioavailability. For example, excessive amounts of phytate (as is found in cereal-based diets) will interfere with the intestinal absorption of zinc, and high levels of calcium will reduce the absorption of both copper and zinc. The absorption of iron is known to be influenced by a number of factors. Ferrous iron is better absorbed than ferric iron and iron contained in foods of animal origin tends to be better absorbed than that from vegetable sources.

The main criteria for what constitutes a complete diet can be summarized as follows.

- The content of each nutrient must be on the plateau.
- Each nutrient must be present in the correct ratio to the energy content of the diet.
- Each nutrient must be at the correct ratio to other nutrients (where appropriate).
- Each nutrient must be in a form that is usable by the animal for which the diet is made.

Digestibility

The digestibility of a food is a measure of the biological availability of its constituent nutrients to the animal. Although analysis of a particular food may give an indication of its total nutrient content, it is only the portion of nutrients that is actually absorbed from the gut that has any true nutritional value. Factors that affect the digestibility of a substance include the chemical composition of the food, its state of subdivision and its method of preparation or processing.

Palatability

The palatability of food is a complex subject requiring a knowledge of the factors affecting appetite and behaviour, as well as an understanding of taste, smell and texture of food and their interrelationships. The importance of palatability cannot be overemphasized, since a food that is left uneaten, whatever its nutrient content, is of no nutritive value to the animal.

First impressions of a food are always important and food must always be presented in a manner that is appropriate to the size of the animal. Cats and small dogs prefer food in small pieces that are not too sticky, whereas larger dogs are able to eat foods with a much broader spectrum of shape and size.

Smell and taste are necessary sensory components of any meal and animals with poor appetites can often be tempted to eat by providing strong-smelling foods, particularly if the food is warmed to about 35°C. Cats can distinguish between sweet and bitter tastes but do not respond to the addition of glucose in their food. In general, meat is very palatable to dogs and cats and its acceptance can often be further enhanced by the addition of fat, especially animal fat.

Most animals enjoy variety in their diet, though they may be initially suspicious of a food that differs markedly from their previous diet. Above all, it is important to recognize that, like humans, all animals are individuals and each has its own dietary likes and dislikes.

Foods and food types

Prepared pet foods

In the developed countries, the vast majority of dogs and cats are fed commercially prepared pet foods. The enormous range of manufactured pet foods available offers the pet owner a convenient method of feeding their pet; the preparation time involved is minimized and the animal can be provided with a variety of flavours and textures in its diet. All these diets are nutritionally balanced when fed according to the instructions on the label, and are all prepared to the same exacting standards.

Prepared diets for pets may be categorized on the basis of their nutrient content as either complete or complementary and this information should be stated on the product label. A **complete diet** will provide a balanced diet when fed alone, though the specific life stage (such as growth, reproduction or adult maintenance) for which it is designed must be specified. Complete diets require no supplementation except that clean fresh water should always be available. A **complementary diet** is designed to be fed in combination with an additional, specified food source, such as canned meat and biscuit mixer.

There are three main forms in which prepared pet foods are usually presented: dry, moist or semi-moist.

- **Dry foods** have a moisture content of 10–14% and include both complete diets and biscuits. The complete diets are usually a mixture of dry, flaked or crushed cereals and vegetables, and many include a meat-based dry protein concentrate. They may be fed dry or the owner may add gravy or water before feeding. Biscuits are generally made from wheaten flour and may be fed whole or broken and used as a mixer with moist foods.
- **Moist foods** have a moisture content of 60–85%. They are packed in cans, plastic or semirigid aluminium containers, as well as plastic or foil pouches. They tend to have a higher meat content and are filled with gravy or set in jelly, both of which provide important vitamins and minerals and improve the palatability of the product. Moist meat products tend to be the most palatable.
- **Semi-moist foods** have a moisture content of 25–40% and are composed of a meat and cereal mixture which is cooked to a paste and extruded into small, shaped pieces. The main advantage of this type of diet is its convenience.

The product packaging provides useful data (some of which are legally required) that should help the pet owner to make important decisions about how to feed the product. In addition to information that identifies the product and the species for which the food is intended, the pet food label should state:

- The ingredients in descending order of predominance by weight (Figure 16.11)
- The typical (or guaranteed) analysis giving the concentrations of protein, oil, fibre, ash and moisture (if over 14%) in the product
- Whether the food is complete or complementary in respect of the particular life stage for which it is designed
- The manufacturer's directions for use, including feeding recommendations or guidelines.

Dry foods	Canned foods	Semi-moist
Ground cereals (corn, oats, wheat, sorghum)	Ground cereals (corn, oats, wheat, sorghum)	Ground cereals (corn, oats, wheat, sorghum)
Meat and bone meal	Meat and bone meal	Sucrose
Whey	Meat	Meat and bone meal
Soyabean meal	Meat by-products	Wheat bran
Animal fat	Liver	Meat
Iodized salt	Lung	Meat by-products
Vitamin/mineral mix	Corn flour Heart Lard Blood Vitamin/mineral mix	Tallow Milk Soy flour Propylene glycol Iodized salt Vitamin/mineral mix

16.11 Some ingredients used in commercial pet foods.

EC regulations do not currently permit the declaration of energy content on pet food labels, but this may be roughly estimated from its carbohydrate, fat and protein contents (see Figure 16.1). This reinforces the importance of reliable feeding recommendations, but these should always be regarded as guidelines only. Observation of the health, condition and bodyweight of the animal will help to determine whether adjustments are necessary in the amounts fed.

Home-prepared diets

For a variety of reasons, some dog and cat owners prefer to feed their pets on fresh foods prepared at home. However, formulation of a balanced diet for any animal requires a detailed knowledge of:

- The animal's specific nutritional needs
- The nutritive value of different foodstuffs from which the diet is to be prepared (Figures 16.12 and 16.13)
- Dietary interactions
- Methods of preparation and storage which may affect the availability of individual nutrients.

Considerable time, effort and expertise are therefore required to be able to offer the animal a consistent and nutritionally adequate diet. The following foods are common ingredients of home-prepared diets for dogs and cats:

- **Meat**. Lean muscle meat is a poor source of calcium and the feeding of an 'all-meat' diet is the most common cause of nutritional secondary hyperparathyroidism.
- **Offal**. This does not constitute a balanced diet and should not be fed exclusively. In particular, cats may become 'addicted' to liver and risk the development of hypervitaminosis A.

- **Fish**. Care should be taken when feeding raw fish as some types contain thiaminase, leading to thiamine deficiency with prolonged feeding. Large amounts of oily fish, especially red tuna, can precipitate pansteatitis (yellow fat disease) due to vitamin E deficiency.
- **Eggs**. These are a valuable source of good quality protein but should be fed cooked to destroy avidin (which binds biotin).
- **Milk, cheese and other dairy products**. These are a good source of protein, fat, calcium and phosphorus but some individuals may be intolerant of lactose.
- **Cereals and vegetables**. These should be cooked to improve digestibility. High levels of phytate in cereals may reduce the availability of some minerals, especially zinc. Palatability may be low for some dogs and cats and, being obligate carnivores, cats cannot be maintained on an exclusively plant-based diet.

Cooking is advisable for most foods, especially meat, since this will kill most bacteria and parasites and will improve the digestibility of some materials. Overcooking should be avoided, since this will destroy vitamins and reduce the food value of proteins. A minimal amount of cooking water should be used and, if possible, it should fed with the meal in order to conserve vitamins and minerals. Home-prepared diets will almost certainly require careful vitamin and mineral supplementation.

Type of food	Approximate amount (g) required to supply 10 g protein [a]	Ca	P	Na	Cu	Fibre	Fat	BV
Chicken meat	50	L	M	L	L	L	L	H
Chicken skin	62	L	M	L	M	L	H	M
Giblets	47	L	M	L	M	L	L	H
Cod	57	L	M	L	M	L	L	H
Haddock	53	L	M	L	L	L	L	H
Halibut	48	L	M	L	M	L	L	H
Shrimp	55	L	M	H	M	L	L	H
Tuna canned in oil	41	L	M	H	M	L	H	H
Tuna canned in water	36	L	M	L	M	L	L	H
Beef (lean meat)	48	L	M	L	H	L	M	M
Beef (normal meat)	56	L	M	L	H	L	H	M
Beef heart	59	L	M	M	–	L	L	M
Beef kidney	65	L	M	H	–	L	M	M
Beef liver	50	L	M	H	–	L	L	M
Lamb meat	65	L	M	M	–	L	H	M
Cottage cheese (creamed)	74	L	M	H	L	L	L	M
Cottage cheese (non-creamed)	59	L	M	H	L	L	L	M
Cheddar cheese	40	M	M	H	L	L	H	M
Egg (whole)	78	L	L	M	L	L	L	H
Egg white	92	L	L	M	L	L	L	H
Egg yolk	63	L	L	L	L	L	L	H

16.12 Selected common protein sources and quantities required to supply 10 g of protein in home-made diets. [a] The amounts required will vary between products. The amount required to supply 10 g protein can be calculated in the following way: amount required in g = (100 ÷ protein content per 100 g of the food) x 10. Ca, calcium; P, phosphorus; Na, sodium; Cu, copper; BV, protein biological value. L = low levels (provides < 50% of daily requirements on an ME basis). M = medium levels (provides < 50–150% of daily requirements on an ME basis). H = high levels (provides >150% of daily requirements on an ME basis). – = unknown or variable levels. The sodium levels are assuming food is cooked in unsalted water.

Food	Approximate amount (g) required to supply 100 kcal (418 kJ) energy [a]	Ca	P	Na	Cu	Fibre	Fat	BV
Bread white	37	L	L	H	M	H	L	L
Bread whole wheat	41	L	L	H	M	H	L	L
Corn flour	27	L	L	L	–	M	L	L
Corn meal	27	L	L	L	–	M	L	L
Corn flakes (breakfast cereal)	26	L	L	H	M	M	L	L
Macaroni, cooked	75	L	L	L	L	M	L	L
Oatmeal, cooked	181	L	L	L	–	M	L	L
Potato, cooked	133	L	L	L	–	M	L	L
Rice long grain, cooked	80	L	L	L	L	M	L	L
Soybean flour high fat	26	L	M	L	–	–	L	L
Soybean flour low fat	28	L	M	L	–	–	L	L
Spaghetti (quick cook), cooked	77	L	L	L	L	M	L	L
Spaghetti (ordinary), cooked	91	L	L	L	L	M	L	L
Wheat dry	27	L	L	L	–	M	L	L
Wheat cooked	240	L	L	L	–	M	L	L
Wheat flour	30	L	L	L	–	M	L	L
Fat, trimmed from beef	14	L	L	L	L	L	H	0
Lard	11	L	L	L	L	L	H	0
Margarine	14	L	L	H	L	L	H	L
Oils – salad/cooking	12	L	L	L	L	L	H	0

16.13 Selected common carbohydrate and fat sources and quantities required to supply 100 kcal (418 kJ) in home-made diets. [a] The amounts required will vary between products. The amount required to supply 100 kcal can be calculated in the following way: amount required in g to supply 100 kcal = 100 ÷ energy density kcal/g; amount required to supply 418 kJ = 418 ÷ energy density kJ/g. BV, protein biological value. L = low levels (provides < 50% of daily requirements on an ME basis). M = medium levels (provides > 50–150% of daily requirements on an ME basis). H = high levels (provides >150% of daily requirements on an ME basis). – = unknown or variable levels. 0 = does not apply to these ingredients. The sodium levels are assuming food is cooked in unsalted water.

Dietary supplements

Contrary to many advertisements and popular beliefs, young animals and lactating females do not require large quantities of minerals and vitamins. Provided that they are fed a balanced diet appropriate to their life stage, their needs will be met as their food intake increases to meet their energy requirements. However, as knowledge of nutraceuticals and functional foods increases, there is an understanding of the potential benefits of increasing certain types of nutrients that are safe and relatively non-toxic at high levels (see 'Nutraceuticals and functional foods', below).

Non-specific supplementation should be undertaken with care, as this may unbalance an otherwise balanced diet and many nutrient interactions can result in a reduced availability of specific nutrients. This can lead to the possibility of toxicities occurring, as may readily occur with vitamins A and D, for example. Dietary supplementation can be expensive and is unlikely to be of benefit in non-deficient animals. Figure 16.14 lists the deficiencies of foods commonly used in home-prepared diets.

Food	Deficiencies	Excesses
Meat	Calcium, phosphorus, sodium, iron, copper, iodine, vitamins A, D, E	Protein
Fish (bones removed)	Calcium, phosphorus, iodine, vitamins A, D, E	
Fish (including bones) [a]	Iron, vitamins A, D, E	Calcium, phosphorus
Fats and oils		Energy, vitamin D (fish oils)
Eggs	Calcium, phosphorus	Fat, avidin
Milk		Lactose
Cheese, cottage cheese	Calcium, phosphorus	
Liver	Calcium	Vitamin A
Vegetables	Calcium, phosphorus, protein, fat	
Cereals	Calcium, phosphorus	

16.14 Nutrient imbalances of selected foods. [a] Cooked and finely ground fish.

The value of vitamin and mineral supplements used in moderate amounts should not be dismissed. They can act as an insurance for individual animals that may experience difficulties in either absorption or utilization of specific nutrients. Although they are unnecessary when a commercially prepared pet food is fed, supplements are likely to be required in order to produce nutritional balance in home-prepared diets. In addition, they have a psychological benefit for people who need to give what they see as extra care. Nevertheless, in cases of diet-related nutrient deficiencies, it is considered preferable to correct the deficient diet itself rather than to rely on blanket supplementation.

Feeding healthy dogs and cats

Owners tend to treat their dogs and cats as individuals and will develop their own feeding practices, which must take account of the particular circumstances, likes and dislikes of the animal and the owner's view of convenience, cost, variety and suitability of foods. Owners must identify the particular needs of their animal and find a combination of foods to meet them.

The feeding recommendations in the following sections are intended only as guides for the average dog or cat in the usual range of environments found in European households. These guides can be used as a starting point to obtain an approximate estimate of a pet's needs. Then, by observation of the animal to decide whether to feed more or less, and by substitution of one food for another, the owner will be able to arrive at a suitable regimen.

Maintenance

Nutritionally speaking, the stage of adult maintenance is considered to be the period of basal requirements. An adult animal is said to be in maintenance when it is not subjected to the additional physiological stresses of growth, pregnancy or lactation, regular work or high levels of activity, or extremes of environmental temperature. During this period, the diet must provide the correct amount, balance and availability of energy and nutrients required to maintain optimal health and activity and promote peak condition in the animal. Since animals eat to satisfy their requirement for energy, all essential nutrients must be present in the correct amounts relative to the energy content of the diet.

Dogs

Dogs are represented by a wide diversity of breeds of different body types, with adult bodyweights that range over 100-fold from 1 kg to 115 kg. Energy expenditure is directly related to the weight of actively metabolizing tissue. For animals with such widely differing bodyweights, energy requirements are more closely related to the animal's metabolic bodyweight ($BW^{0.75}$) than to bodyweight itself. For typical pet dogs, taking low to moderate amounts of exercise, maintenance energy (ME) requirements may be calculated using the equation:

$$ME \text{ (kcal/day)} = 110 \ BW^{0.75} \text{ (kg)}$$

For more active dogs, the allowance can be increased to $125 \ BW^{0.75}$. Variations in body composition, shape and coat type are complicating factors in determining energy requirements, particularly for the larger breeds. For example, Newfoundlands tend to need less than the predicted amounts whereas Great Danes need more, despite these two breeds being of comparable bodyweight.

The amount of food needed to meet these requirements may then be calculated from a knowledge of the energy values of foods. Feeding recommendations are only ever given as guidelines and are subject to individual variability between dogs and to differences in activity level and environmental conditions. If extra snacks, treats or table scraps are added to the diet, their energy content must be taken into account when calculating the daily food allowance. In addition, spaying may reduce the resting energy requirement of bitches by up to 10%. Regular weighing of the animal allows the owner to monitor the adequacy of the feeding regimen on a quantitative basis.

Although the dog is a member of the order Carnivora, in a nutritional sense it is more accurately defined as omnivorous. Unlike the cat (see below), the dog is able to survive on a diet composed entirely of vegetable material, though a diet based on animal tissue is likely to be preferred.

Most adult dogs in maintenance are able to eat all they require in a single meal and it is perfectly acceptable to adopt a once-a-day feeding regimen. It is usually best to avoid late evening meals since dogs may need to excrete faeces or urine within a few hours of feeding and this can be inconvenient in the middle of the night. There is no disadvantage in feeding more frequently, provided that the total daily intake is limited to the dog's daily needs, and feeding two to three times a day to coincide with family meals is a common practice. Whatever the frequency of feeding, a routine should be established and adhered to as far as possible (Figure 16.15).

Status	Minimum ME density (kcal (kJ)/g)		Digestibility (%)	Protein (%ME)[a]	Fat (%ME)[a]	Fibre (%DM)[b]	Calcium (mg/100 kcal (418kJ))	Phosphate (mg/100 kcal (418kJ))	Sodium (mg/100 kcal (418kJ))
Maintenance	3.5	(14.6)	>75	16–20	30–50	5	130–160	110–160	15
Growth Gestation Lactation	3.9	(16.3)	>80	22–28	30–50	5	280	200–250	23
Geriatric	3.75	(15.7)	>80	14–18	30–50	4	130–150	110–140	15
Stress:									
Environmental Psychological Physical	4.2	(17.6)	>82	20–25	30–50	4 max	150–250	130–230	23

16.15 Recommended nutrient requirements for the dog, according to physiological status. [a] The proportion of metabolizable energy supplied by that nutrient. [b] g/100 g dry matter.

Cats

Domestic cats show a relatively narrow range of adult bodyweights (from 2.5 to 6.5 kg) and their energy requirements may be calculated from a linear relationship. In normal circumstances, an adult cat requires 70–90 kcal/kg bodyweight per day, depending on its level of activity. Large overweight individuals and very inactive or caged cats (such as those in a hospital environment) have lower maintenance energy requirements and allowances should be based on 50–70 kcal/kg bodyweight per day.

Cats have the ability to regulate their energy intake from day to day and they will normally adjust the amount of food they eat to achieve the correct balance, unless they are fed an exceptionally palatable diet or lead a particularly sedentary life.

The cat exhibits a number of nutritional peculiarities that distinguish it from the dog and reflect its naturally predatory lifestyle. Several aspects of feline metabolism have evolved in adaptation to a strictly carnivorous diet that is typically high in protein and low in carbohydrate. In addition, the cat has a dietary requirement for a number of nutrients that are only found naturally in significant quantities in animal tissues. Special nutritional differences of the cat may be summarized as follows.

Nutritional peculiarities of the cat

- A limited ability to regulate amino acid catabolism, resulting in a higher dietary requirement than dogs for **protein** and an inability to adapt to extremely low-protein diets (they also tend to find low-protein diets unpalatable)
- A high dietary requirement for **taurine**, partly because of an inability to conjugate bile acids with glycine instead of taurine and also because of a low rate of taurine synthesis *in vivo*
- A particular sensitivity to **arginine** deficiency
- A limited ability to synthesize **niacin**
- An inability to convert β-carotene to retinol (**vitamin A**), resulting in a dietary requirement for preformed vitamin A
- A limited ability to convert linoleic acid to **arachidonic acid**
- A limited ability to metabolize **carbohydrate**, resulting in an intolerance of high-carbohydrate diets.

Cats may be considered as obligate carnivores, since taurine, preformed vitamin A and arachidonic acid are only found in significant quantities in animal tissues. It is thus essential that the cat is supplied with at least some animal-derived materials in its diet. In view of these nutritional specialties, it should be noted that long-term feeding of dog foods to cats is unacceptable, since these diets may not meet the specific nutritional requirements of the cat.

When allowed continuous access to food, cats tend to adopt a pattern of small, frequent (usually 8–16) meals throughout the whole 24-hour period. However, cats readily adapt to different feeding schedules imposed by their owners and are commonly fed two meals per day. Nevertheless, if feeding time is restricted, sufficient food must be provided to satisfy their daily nutrient and energy requirements.

Environmental factors are known to affect the volume of food a particular animal will eat. Most cats do not relish cold food straight from the refrigerator and prefer to eat food that is close to their own body temperature and that of freshly killed prey. This response may reflect a behavioural strategy in the wild ensuring that only the freshest prey is eaten.

Cats do seek variety in their diet, as long as the new food is not too different from the familiar one, or the palatability too low. However, during times of stress, such as when hospitalized, a familiar diet is preferred. Repeated exposure to fresh supplies of a new food that is not initially acceptable to it may encourage the cat to overcome its reticence. Furthermore, cats can often detect and may reject diets that are deficient in certain nutrients and so it is important that any diet offered is nutritionally complete (Figure 16.16).

Reproduction and lactation

The reproductive life stage is a nutritionally demanding time for the bitch or queen. During this period, her intake of energy and nutrients must be adequate not only to meet her own maintenance requirements but also to support normal growth and development of her offspring during pregnancy and, through milk production, during lactation. At peak lactation her energy and nutrient requirements may rise to up to three or four times the level required for maintenance. This may involve eating large volumes of food but achieving a sufficient intake at times of high demand can be a problem. This may be offset to some extent by feeding a diet that is:

- Concentrated with respect to energy and nutrient density
- Palatable, to encourage feeding
- Highly digestible, to reduce bulk.

The additional requirements imposed by pregnancy are relatively small and can usually be met by simply increasing the amount of the animal's normal food, provided that this is well balanced. In late pregnancy, and particularly if the litter is large, the space occupied by the gravid uterus may be so great that the physical capacity for food intake is limited. In this case, feeding a concentrated diet can help to ensure an adequate intake and offering smaller, more frequent meals can also be beneficial. To meet the high demands of lactation a palatable, highly digestible, concentrated diet should be fed. Milk production is affected by protein quantity and quality in the diet and it is important that the extra food supplied is of good

Status	Minimum ME density (kcal (kJ)/g)		Digestibility (%)	Protein (%ME)[a]	Fat (%ME)[a]	Fibre (%DM)[b]	Calcium (mg/100 kcal (418kJ))	Phosphate (mg/100 kcal (418kJ))	Magnesium (mg/100 kcal (418kJ))	Sodium (mg/100 kcal
Maintenance	3.7	(15.7)	> 75	24–26	> 25	5	130–200	120	80	15
Growth Gestation Lactation	3.9	(16.3)	> 80	30–35	> 40	5	160–250	120–200	150	30
Geriatric	3.75	(15.7)	> 80	24–26	> 34	5	130–150	120	80	15

16.16 Recommended nutrient requirements for the cat, according to physiological status. [a] The proportion of metabolizable energy supplied by that nutrient. [b] g/100 g dry matter.

quality. It is not appropriate simply to increase the dietary energy content by adding fat or carbohydrate sources. Diets formulated for growth or specifically for gestation and lactation are suitable for feeding at this time.

During pregnancy and lactation, the content and balance of nutrients in the diet are critical and must be carefully regulated. Provided that a balanced diet is fed, the increased requirement for nutrients is met when food intake is increased to meet the energy needs of the bitch or queen.

Supplementation with vitamins or minerals is not required and could actually be harmful by causing an imbalance in the diet.

Dogs

The average duration of pregnancy in the bitch is 63 days, but her energy requirements do not increase appreciably until the last third of gestation, when most fetal weight gain occurs. It is important, therefore, to avoid overfeeding in early pregnancy, since this will lead to the deposition of unwanted fat and may predispose the bitch to problems at whelping. A gradual increase in food allowance over the second half of gestation is all that is required and a satisfactory regimen would be to increase the amount of food by 15% of the bitch's maintenance ration each week from the fifth week onwards. During the week before whelping the bitch should, therefore, be eating 60% more than when she was mated. Appetite may be reduced in the later stages of pregnancy, particularly with large litters, and it is sensible to divide the daily allowance into several small meals.

Lactation represents the most nutritionally demanding life stage for the bitch. During the first 4 weeks post whelping, she must eat enough to support both herself and her rapidly growing puppies, which may double their weight within a matter of days. The extra energy and nutrients needed over and above her normal intake depend on the size and age of the litter, but at peak lactation (3–4 weeks after whelping) she may need to eat anything up to four times her normal maintenance allowance. Failure of the diet to meet these demands means that the bitch will nurse her young at the expense of her own body reserves, with a resultant loss of weight and condition.

The food allowance should be increased steadily throughout the first 4 weeks of lactation (in accordance with the bitch's needs):

- A highly palatable, digestible and concentrated food should be offered in several small meals or ad libitum.
- Food should be made available throughout the night.
- An unlimited supply of drinking water should also be provided, to cater for the large volumes involved in milk production.

Weaning of the litter should be accomplished gradually in order to prevent mastitis in the bitch and growth check in the puppies. Most puppies begin to take an interest in solid foods from about 3 to 4 weeks of age and once they are eating well the bitch may be separated from the puppies for progressively longer periods to allow her milk supply to diminish. Weaning may be completed between 6 and 8 weeks of age and it may be advisable to cut the bitch's ration down to half her maintenance level immediately following total separation. Her food allowance may be gradually increased over a period of days. If she has lost condition during lactation, extra food may be introduced as soon as her milk supply has dried up.

If the litter is large, and particularly if the bitch's milk supply seems inadequate, supplementary feeding of the puppies should be encouraged from about 3 weeks.

Eclampsia

Eclampsia (postpuerperal hypocalcaemia) is a condition that can affect lactating bitches (especially of small breeds) with larger litters. Lowered blood calcium concentrations lead to signs that range from restlessness and ataxia to muscle tremors and collapse with tetanic convulsions. Treatment involves oral or intravenous administration of calcium, depending on the severity of signs, and puppies should be removed immediately from affected bitches and hand-reared.

Although some owners give calcium and vitamin D supplements to bitches in late pregnancy and lactation as an 'insurance policy', these do not prevent eclampsia and may, in fact, increase the risk of eclampsia or calcinosis in the bitch and produce developmental abnormalities in the puppies.

Cats

Gestation length in queens is similar to that in bitches and is in the region of 64 days. Unlike dogs and most other mammals, pregnant queens start to eat more and gain weight within a week of conception. By the end of the third week of gestation, the pregnant queen will have gained almost 20% of the extra weight she will carry at term. Following parturition, only about 40% of this extra weight is lost (compared with almost 100% in the bitch) and the remaining 60% is lost during the course of lactation.

This unusual pattern of bodyweight gain in early pregnancy is thought to be due to the extra-uterine deposition of fat and protein reserves that may be mobilized in late pregnancy and lactation, when dietary intake of the queen may be insufficient to meet her greatly increased nutritional demands.

Throughout pregnancy, food intake of the queen rises continuously to fuel her extra weight gain and peaks at around 7–8 weeks of gestation. The food allowance may be gradually increased from 1 week after a successful mating and, since cats rarely overeat, an ad libitum feeding regimen is perfectly acceptable. Voluntary intake may drop slightly just before and immediately after parturition, after which food consumption rises progressively to meet the increased demands of lactation.

As with the bitch, energy requirements of the lactating queen vary with litter size and age and at peak lactation may be anything up to four times her maintenance level. A highly palatable, digestible and concentrated diet should be fed as frequent small meals and ad libitum feeding is preferred, to allow the queen to control her energy intake successfully. Food should be available throughout the night and an unlimited supply of fresh drinking water must be accessible at all times.

It is normal for the queen to lose weight during lactation as her body reserves are used up, but she should achieve her pre-mating weight by the time the kittens are weaned at 6–8 weeks. Although kittens begin to take solid food from about 3–4 weeks of age and demand less of the queen, her energy requirements remain elevated to allow for restoration of her depleted body reserves. After weaning, the additional food allowance can be gradually cut back until the queen is eating her normal amount, or adjusted to compensate for any observed weight loss or gain.

Growth

In relation to bodyweight, growing animals require a much higher plane of nutrition than their adult counterparts. For young animals, the diet must not only supply all the nutrients required for maintenance but also those required to fuel rapid growth and development and to support their active lifestyle. In particular, they have higher demands for energy, protein (which must be digestible and have an amino acid profile appropriate for growth), vitamin E and certain bone-forming minerals, such as calcium and phosphorus. Both the amount and balance of nutrients provided are critical for the growing puppy or kitten and dietary errors at this stage can have damaging effects, particularly on skeletal development, which may be long-lasting and potentially irreversible.

To meet these high demands, young animals must eat large amounts of food relative to their size, but their physical capacity to do so is limited by their small stomach volume. The daily food allowance should therefore be divided into several small meals to compensate for this and the diet itself should meet certain criteria. A suitable diet for growth is formulated to ensure an adequate intake of energy and nutrients in a relatively small volume of food. Diets for growth should be:

- Concentrated
- Nutritionally balanced
- Highly palatable
- Highly digestible.

For the first few weeks of life, all the nutritional needs of the puppy or kitten are met by their mother's milk and no supplementary feeding is necessary, unless the milk supply is inadequate. As their interest in solid food gradually increases, finely chopped soft foods or dry kibble moistened with milk or gravy may be provided in shallow bowls. The food may be the same as that offered to the mother or may be one designed specifically for growth.

Contrary to popular belief, milk is not essential in the diet of weaned puppies or kittens. After weaning, their ability to digest lactose becomes progressively less efficient and feeding large quantities of milk can result in diarrhoea. Nevertheless, milk remains a useful source of nutrients for individuals that can tolerate it, if fed in restricted amounts.

Puppies

Most owners are aware that correct nutrition is fundamental to achieving normal growth and development in the growing dog, but there is a common tendency to overfeed (to produce rapid growth rates) or to oversupplement the diet (to prevent classic deficiency syndromes). Excessive energy intake, however, is likely to cause obesity in the small breeds and rapid growth rates in the large and giant breeds, which may be detrimental to the animal.

The aim should be to allow the puppy to grow sufficiently quickly to enable it to fulfil its genetic potential while the bones are still capable of growth. A more rapid increase in bodyweight can place undue stresses on the juvenile skeleton, particularly in the fast-growing large and giant breeds, and may predispose to a variety of disorders that are characterized by abnormalities of bone growth and development. Examples of these include osteochondrosis syndrome, hip dysplasia, wobbler syndrome and enostosis (panosteitis). In some cases, excessive dietary calcium may also play a major contributory role.

It is therefore unwise to overfeed growing dogs in an attempt to obtain the maximum possible rate of growth and a more advantageous approach is to restrict their intake moderately and allow them to take slightly longer to reach their adult weight.

Supplements

Oversupplementation with fat-soluble vitamins A and D may also result in skeletal and other abnormalities and care should always be exercised with supplements such as cod liver oil, which is a rich source of both these vitamins. A properly balanced diet that is formulated for growth does not need any form of supplementation and careless use of additives can result in serious dietary imbalances with deleterious consequences. This is true even of the large breeds, since their extra needs are catered for by their increased food intake to meet their energy requirements.

Growth rates

All puppies grow very rapidly in the early stages and most breeds will have reached about half their adult weight by 5–6 months of age. Because of the wide variation in adult bodyweight, different breeds continue to mature at different relative rates and, in general, the larger breeds take longer to mature than the smaller breeds. Small and toy breeds may reach their adult weight at 6–9 months of age. Larger breeds will still be growing at this age and take longer to mature. Labrador Retriever or Newfoundland puppies, for example, may not reach their adult weight until 16 months or 2 years, respectively.

Energy and protein requirements

At weaning (between 6 and 8 weeks of age), the puppy's energy requirements are about double those of an adult of the same breed, per unit of bodyweight. As the puppy grows, this requirement declines progressively. By the time it has reached 40% of its mature weight, the energy requirement is only 1.6 times that for adult maintenance. At 80% of its mature weight, the puppy needs only 1.2 times as much energy as an adult per unit of bodyweight.

High levels of high-quality protein are also required for growth. Although it is often thought that large amounts of additional protein in the puppy diet will aid the development of good condition and muscle, this is not the case. Instead, protein eaten in excess of requirements is metabolized to produce energy or stored as fat.

Growth diets

Most puppies can be weaned on to a varied diet or a single complete food when they are between 6 and 8 weeks of age. At this stage, it is better to feed them four small meals a day than to allow continuous access to food. Commercial diets designed specifically for growth are ideal and it is recommended that a growth formulation is fed until the puppy attains at least 75% of its adult weight. Although such diets require no further supplementation, some owners may like to offer alternative foods from time to time. Meat, offal, cheese, eggs and bread are often fed to dogs, but at any one time only a few different food sources should be introduced, gradually, to allow the digestive system to adapt. If alternative foods are to form the major part of a home-prepared diet, food composition tables should be consulted and careful supplementation with vitamins and minerals will almost certainly be required.

Puppies should have their food allowance divided into four or five meals a day until about 10 weeks of age and then three meals a day until they have reached approximately 50% of their expected adult bodyweight. At this stage (5–6 months), the frequency of feeding can be reduced to twice daily. As the puppy approaches its adult weight, the daily food allowance can be gradually incorporated into a single meal, as in the adult. Ad libitum feeding is not recommended for growing dogs, since they tend to overeat and this can lead to obesity or skeletal developmental abnormalities. As a guide, feeding at a level of 85% of ad libitum feeding has been shown to result in optimal growth and body composition in dogs. Precise recommendations on the amounts to feed are difficult to give, because of huge variations in individual requirements and in the caloric densities of the foods themselves. It is important, therefore, that the health and condition of growing dogs is regularly assessed 'by hand and eye' to monitor their progress and allow any necessary dietary adjustments to be made.

Kittens

Kittens weigh between 85 g and 120 g at birth and may gain up to 100 g per week in the early stages of growth. They should weigh between 600 g and 1000 g at weaning. Males grow at a faster rate than females and by 6 weeks of age they are already significantly heavier. At 1 year, male cats can be up to 45% heavier than females from the same litter.

At weaning, the energy requirements of kittens per unit of bodyweight are between three and four times that of an adult and reach a peak at about 10 weeks of age. Unlike puppies, kittens do not tend to overeat and are not prone to the same problems of obesity and skeletal developmental abnormalities as growing dogs. It is usual, therefore, to allow kittens un-restricted access to food during the rapid growth phase, though multiple small feeds throughout the day (at least four or five per day at weaning) may also be offered. Moist food that is left uneaten should be discarded at least twice daily.

Concentrated diets designed for kitten growth are ideal at this stage to ensure an optimal intake of energy, protein, tau-rine and calcium, in particular. Growing kittens tend to have acidic urine, due to the liberation of hydrogen ions during bone growth, and it is important that urine-acidifying diets designed for the management of struvite-associated lower urinary tract diseases are avoided in young cats (up to a year of age).

Although male kittens take slightly longer to mature than females, most kittens will have attained 75% of their ultimate adult bodyweight by 6 months of age. Further weight gains after this are attributable to developmental changes rather than skeletal growth and at this stage the growth diet may be changed to an adult formulation. If desired, the frequency of feeding may be reduced to twice daily, but many people con-tinue to offer multiple feeds throughout the day, even to adult cats. This pattern of feeding fits in well with the cat's natural preference to snack feed during both day and night rather than eat a small number of large meals. Total food intakes continue to rise between 6 and 12 months of age to coincide with continued slow growth, but tend to stabilize at an adult level towards the end of the first year.

Feeding orphaned puppies and kittens

Hand-rearing of puppies and kittens may be necessary if the mother has an inadequate supply of milk, or is sick or if the litter is orphaned. The ideal alternative is to cross-foster the young on to a lactating bitch or queen whose young are old enough to be weaned, but this is not always a practical option. Mother-less puppies and kittens have vital requirements in two main areas: provision of a suitable environment; and nutrition. The care of orphaned puppies and kittens may be summarized as follows:

- Ideally, the environment should be controlled by an incubator. Alternatively, a heating pad with adequate insulation of the pen can be used.
- After they have been fed, the mother would normally provoke reflex defecation and urination in the puppies and kittens by licking the anogenital area. This action can be stimulated by applying a piece of damp cotton wool at the anogenital area or simply by running a dampened forefinger along the abdominal wall.
- At 16–21 days of age, puppies and kittens no longer require stimulation to urinate and defecate. From 28 days of age, when they completely control their body temperature, they begin to explore their surroundings and become more independent.

The food supplied must be a concentrated source of nutri-ents based on the composition of normal bitch or queen's milk. Figure 16.17 shows the average composition of milk from bitches, cows, goats and queens. It is clear that cow's milk and goat's milk are inadequate as a substitute for rearing puppies and kittens, since the protein and fat levels are too low. Cal-cium levels are also considerably lower than that of bitch's milk. Many commercially available milk substitutes are now avail-able for dogs and cats. They are usually based on cow's milk that has been modified to resemble bitch or queen's milk more closely. They can be administered by means of a small syringe or a puppy or kitten feeding bottle.

Dried milk feeds should be reconstituted daily and fed warm (38°C). Food must be given slowly and must not be forced into the animal. Frequent small feeds (at least four) should be of-fered throughout the day. When feeding from a miniature bottle, the hole in the teat may need to be enlarged so that the

Nutrient	% Nutrient as fed (g/100 kcal (418 kJ)) (ME)									
	Bitch's milk		Cow's milk		Queen's milk		Goat's milk		Evaporated milk + water [a]	
Water	77	(0)	88	(0)	81.5	(0)	87	(0)	80	(0)
Protein	8.2	(6.6)	3.2	(5.4)	7.4	(8.4)	3.5	(5.5)	5.3	(5.5)
Fat	9.8	(7.8)	3.7	(6.3)	5.2	(5.9)	4.2	(6.6)	6.1	(6.3)
Lactose	3.6	(2.9)	4.6	(7.8)	5.0	(5.7)	4.5	(7)	7.6	(7.8)
Calcium	0.28	(0.22)	0.12	(0.2)	0.035	(0.04)	0.13	(0.2)	0.19	(0.2)
Phosphorus	0.22	(0.18)	0.1	(0.17)	0.07	(0.08)	0.11	(0.17)	0.15	(0.16)
ME kcal/100 g [b] kJ/100 g [b]	125 522		59 246		88 360		64 267		97 406	

16.17 Nutrient content of milk from different sources. [a] 3 parts whole evaporated milk diluted with 1 part water. [b] ME content as-fed was estimated using nutrient energy densities of 3.5 kcal (14.6 kJ)/g for protein and lactose, and 8.5 kcal (35.6 kJ)/g for fat.

flow is improved and the puppy or kitten does not suck in air. When they begin to explore their surroundings (at 3–4 weeks), a high-quality puppy or kitten food can be introduced. This can be mixed with a milk substitute to begin with and then offered separately.

Senior animals

As a general guideline, dogs and cats may be considered to be geriatric once they have reached the final third of their anticipated lifespan. The aim of feeding elderly but otherwise healthy animals is to slow or prevent the progression of metabolic changes associated with ageing and thus to increase longevity and preserve the quality of life.

Old age is often accompanied by clinical disease for which dietary management may constitute an important component of therapy. Chronic renal failure is a particular problem of middle-aged and old cats, whereas old dogs tend to be more susceptible to heart disease. There is a tendency towards obesity in older animals, especially dogs, and oral hygiene measures have particular significance in old age. Free access to a clean supply of water is essential to prevent dehydration. Figure 16.18 summarizes the age-related changes in dogs and cats and their effect on nutritional status.

Ageing change	Effect on nutritional status
Metabolism	
Reduced sensitivity to thirst	Dehydration
Reduced thermoregulation	Increased energy expenditure with extremes of heat
Reduced immunological competence	Increased susceptibility to infection
Decreased activity and metabolic rate (possibly due to decreased thyroid function)	Decreased energy needs predispose towards obesity
Increased body fat	Predisposes towards obesity
Special senses	
Decreased olfaction	Reduced food intake which may lead to a loss of weight and condition
Decreased ability to taste	
Decreased visual acuity	
Oral cavity	
Dental calculus	
Periodontal disease	Reduced food intake which may lead to a loss of weight and condition
Loss of teeth	
Decreased saliva production	
Gingival hyperplasia	
Urinary system	
Decreased renal function	
Decreased renal blood flow	Decreased protein requirement
Decreased glomerular filtration rate	
Skeletal system	
Osteoarthritis	Decreased mobility reduces energy requirements
Reduced muscle mass	Decreased protein reserves
Cardiovascular system	
Congestive cardiac failure	Decreased salt intake

16.18 Ageing changes in dogs and cats and their effect on nutritional status.

Dogs

Most senior dogs have a maintenance energy requirement that is approximately 20% less than that of a younger adult of equivalent bodyweight. This decline in energy requirement appears to be linked to both a reduction in physical activity and a decrease in basal metabolic rate, which is largely driven by changes in body composition (reduction in lean body tissue and concomitant increase in fat mass). To reduce the risk of obesity, therefore, older dogs should be fed to a lower energy requirement than younger dogs without restricting the intake of other essential nutrients. This means that reducing the amount of food offered is *not* an advisable way to achieve weight loss; reducing total energy intake is the safest practice. The majority of dogs maintain digestive efficiency as they age, making the determination of energy provision to senior dogs relatively straightforward to calculate. Nevertheless, it is probable that some individuals might exhibit a reduction in apparent digestibility of nutrients or have a reduced appetite, and may be underweight if intake does not meet their energy requirements.

High levels of dietary protein may increase the renal workload when kidney function may already be impaired to some extent. Conversely, very low protein diets may be associated with a risk of protein malnutrition and tend to be unpalatable. Historically there has been a belief that reducing protein intake in older animals will relieve 'stress' on their renal function and may help to prevent or slow progression of renal disease. More recent data have shown that this theory cannot be substantiated. Indeed, there is no scientific evidence to support restricting dietary protein in healthy, clinically normal dogs (and cats) as they age.

In general, healthy older dogs should have diets based on their individual needs which will be related to bodyweight, condition and physical activity. Early clinical and biochemical signs of chronic renal failure would support the introduction of a diet with a low phosphorus and moderately reduced protein content. Protein sources for older dogs should be highly digestible and of high biological value.

Although restriction of dietary sodium or phosphorus may be indicated in old dogs with cardiac or renal diseases, respectively, there is no evidence that healthy individuals have altered requirements for these or other minerals. Similarly, vitamin requirements of healthy senior dogs are not thought to differ markedly from those of younger adults.

Cats

In contrast to dogs (and humans), the energy requirements of cats do not change with increasing age. Evidence suggests that there is no apparent change in body composition (lean:fat ratios) with advancing age. This is supported by the fact that obesity is not considered a significant problem in old cats and there is a greater tendency for geriatric cats to be underweight. The maintained lean:fat ratio probably reflects constant activity levels throughout life and suggests that basal metabolic rate probably does not decrease as cats age. Cats show a significant decline in digestive function with age, resulting in a significant decrease in the digestibilities of protein, fat and, hence, energy. Most healthy cats are able to compensate for this effect by increasing their food intake to maintain bodyweight, but in some cases provision of a more energy-dense food may be appropriate. In contrast to dogs, calorie provision to senior cats should not be reduced.

In view of the high protein requirements of the cat and reduced digestive efficiency in old age, and because of the associated risk of protein malnutrition, restriction of dietary protein is not recommended in healthy individuals. Highly digestible protein sources of high biological value should be employed for all healthy, clinically normal older cats. However, in cats with evidence of chronic renal failure, moderate restriction of dietary protein to alleviate clinical signs of uraemia may be implemented, together with dietary phosphorus restriction.

Careful monitoring of food intake is important in the senior cat and may help to identify conditions associated with altered food intake. For example: hyperthyroidism is characterized by weight loss despite an increased appetite; and prolonged inappetence may predispose an obese cat to hepatic lipidosis.

Working dogs

Working dogs perform at a wide range of activity levels and in a variety of environmental conditions, from acting as guide dogs for the blind to pulling sledges in polar regions. The diet and feeding regimen employed in each case varies widely according to the role the dog is asked to perform and its individual work and training schedule. Any increase in physical activity requires extra energy to sustain the increase in muscular work but a further allowance must be made for the element of stress that is associated with strenuous activity. Both physiological and psychological stresses further increase the demand for energy and certain nutrients in hard-working dogs.

Fats and carbohydrates

The main fuels for muscular exercise in the working dog are fats and carbohydrates. Sprinting dogs, such as the racing Greyhound, require short but very intense bursts of energy. In these circumstances, the muscle fibres contract very rapidly and rely mainly on readily available glucose as an energy source. Muscle glycogen stores supply approximately 70–80% of the energy required for this type of exercise, with fats providing the rest. For these working dogs, a diet that provides a relatively large quantity of carbohydrate may be appropriate, since this helps to maximize muscle glycogen reserves. Useful sources of carbohydrate include corn, oat flakes, rice and potatoes.

However, high-carbohydrate diets are not suitable for most other working dogs and may actually reduce performance. They may exacerbate the accumulation of lactic acid in muscles during prolonged exercise, leading to muscle damage and exhaustion. For working dogs that are active for long periods (endurance performers), energy for sustained muscle activity is produced through aerobic fatty acid oxidation with fat providing 70–90% of the energy and carbohydrates providing the rest. Dogs that perform this type of work may benefit from training on a high-fat diet. This also applies to dogs that operate in a hostile environment (such as sledge dogs or avalanche rescue dogs) where extra energy is required to maintain body temperature as well as for increased muscular activity. For most other working dogs, the optimal dietary fat:carbohydrate ratio falls somewhere between these two extremes.

Protein

The protein requirements of hard-working dogs may be slightly increased over maintenance levels, but there is no evidence to suggest that a high-protein diet will promote superior muscle development. Exercise stress may increase the demand for specific amino acids and has been associated with anaemia, so a good-quality protein source is essential for dogs in work. Suitable protein sources include meats, fishmeal, powdered whole egg and casein.

Vitamins and minerals

Little is known about the requirements of hard-working dogs for vitamins and minerals. There may be a higher requirement for iron, because of its involvement in haemoglobin production and oxygen transport. Similarly, vitamin E and selenium requirements may be increased, since they act as antioxidants and protect cell membranes, including red blood cells, from damage. If the diet is nutritionally balanced, however, these increased demands will be met when the dog consumes more to satisfy its energy requirements.

Energy requirements

The amount of extra energy required by working dogs depends on environmental conditions, the amount of exercise and the nature of the work. A dog that travels long distances in the course of its work may need as much as two to three times the normal adult maintenance ration. Despite this, food intake may be reduced in some dogs due to fatigue. To offset this, the diet should be concentrated, palatable and highly digestible. This type of diet is also lower in bulk, which is a significant advantage to the working dog. As well as being an ideal energy source for most working dogs, fat is an excellent means of increasing the energy density of the diet and both fat and protein may be used to enhance palatability.

Where the type of work performed is not overly strenuous, the additional needs may be met by simply feeding more of the dog's nutritionally balanced maintenance diet. At higher levels of performance, a more concentrated source of energy and nutrients is recommended and complete diets formulated for active dogs are ideal. Alternatively, supplementary foods, such as fish or meat, may be added to the maintenance ration, but this strategy will require suitable vitamin and mineral supplementation. On rest or training days, the dietary requirements will differ and the amounts fed must be adjusted accordingly. A smaller allowance of the same meal is most appropriate.

Frequency of feeding

Working dogs should receive only a small concentrated meal before working, as a full stomach limits performance and increases the risk of bloat. If the working period is prolonged, a further small meal may be given during the rest period. The main meal should provide two-thirds of the daily ration and should be reserved until after work. A rest period of about an hour should be allowed before feeding if the work is strenuous. To prevent dehydration, working dogs should be given free access to water.

Feeding exotic pets

Small mammals

Basic energy and macronutrient requirements for rabbits and rodents are given in Figures 16.19 and 16.20.

Rabbits

Rabbits are herbivores with a high dietary requirement for fibre. Many commercial rabbit pelleted diets are available (Figure 16.21), but it is still vitally important that rabbits are encouraged to consume significant quantities of freshly grazed grass or dried grass products and hay. This is to ensure that the correct fibre levels (crude fibre levels of > 18% with indigestible fibre levels of > 12.5% have been quoted) are achieved to encourage normal gastrointestinal motility and dental wear. The silicates present in grasses are particularly abrasive and help to ensure sufficient dental wear. Supervised browsing on other plants may also be encouraged but grass cuttings should not be fed as these may ferment.

	Rabbits	Guinea pigs	Hamsters	Gerbils	Rats and mice
Bodyweight (BW)	0.5–7.0 kg	0.75–1.0 kg	85–140 g	50–60 g	20–800 g
Maintenance	110.00	110.00	110.00	110.00	110.00
Growth	190–210	145.00	145.00	145.00	145.00
Gestation	135–200	145.00	145.00	145.00	145.00
Lactation	300.00	165.00	310.00	440.00	440.00

16.19 Basic energy requirements for rabbits and rodents (ME (kcal/day) = 110–440 $BW^{0.75}$).

	Rabbits	Guinea pigs	Hamsters	Gerbils	Rats and mice
ME (kcal/g)	2–2.4	1.7–2.9	2.5–3.9	2.5–3.7	2.2–3
Protein (%)	12–18	18–20	18–22	17–18	13–20
Fat (%)	2–4	2–4	4–5	6–9	1–5
Fibre (%)	13–24	10–18	4–8	4	4

16.20 Basic macronutrient requirements for rabbits and rodents.

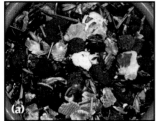
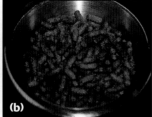

16.21 Commercially available rabbit diets. **(a)** Coarse mix. **(b)** Pelleted diet – this prevents selective feeding. (Reproduced from *BSAVA Manual of Rabbit Medicine and Surgery, 2nd edition*)

Rabbits have an unusual metabolism of calcium whereby they cannot down-regulate the absorption of calcium from their gut. Instead excess calcium is excreted via the kidneys. Excessive dietary calcium can give rise to urolithiasis (usually calcium carbonate), whereas dietary deficiency (often exacerbated by a vitamin D deficiency) is a common cause of osteodystrophy, with associated skeletal and tooth defects. Problems can arise in some rabbits fed 'rabbit mixes' because they are selective feeders and may reject the higher-fibre items (often the pellets and hay) in the ration. Most vitamin and mineral supplements are incorporated in the pelleted portion of the diet and rejection of these can produce a diet that is seriously deficient in calcium, vitamin D and other nutrients. Owners should encourage rabbits to eat all ingredients in the ration by offering smaller quantities and refilling the container only when all food has been consumed.

Rabbits tend to adjust their food intake according to their energy requirements and the energy content of the diet, but adults are likely to eat approximately 30–60 g of dry food/kg bodyweight (BW) per day. Free access to clean water in bowls or suspended bottles should be provided and adults may drink 50–100 ml/kg BW per day.

Guinea pigs
Guinea pigs are herbivorous animals and require a dietary source of vitamin C. A deficiency can result in clinical signs of scurvy that include loss of fur, dental disease, swollen painful joints and lethargy. The main types of feed available are pelleted foods or coarse mixes, but these should be formulated specifically for guinea pigs, i.e. have additional vitamin C in them. Rabbit feeds are unsuitable, since they are lower in protein

and are not supplemented with vitamin C; also some products contain coccidiostats, which can cause liver or kidney damage in guinea pigs. Some pelleted feeds for guinea pigs contain vitamin C at levels that only just meet the minimum requirements, and prolonged storage (over 3 months) can deplete vitamin C levels in the food. Supplementary vitamin C may be administered in the drinking water (1 g/l), or fresh fruit and leafy vegetables, which contain high levels of the vitamin, may be added to the diet. Any dietary changes should take place gradually to avoid gastrointestinal upset. The minimum dietary requirement for vitamin C in the guinea pig is 10 mg/kg/day. This will dramatically increase in situations such as pregnancy, growth and disease.

Relatively high levels of fibre are required and a shortage can lead to dental disease and fur chewing, which may result in the formation of hairballs. Gastrointestinal hypomotility may also occur on diets insufficient in crude fibre and lead to bloat. An adequate supply of good quality hay or dried grass products can usually prevent these conditions. Malocclusion can prevent feeding, drinking and swallowing of saliva (slobbers) and can prove fatal, as guinea pigs often develop metabolic ketoacidosis when they cease feeding, as well as developing hypovitaminosis C (scurvy).

Guinea pigs may eat 5–8 g/100 g BW per day. Food may be provided in open bowls on the cage floor but may become contaminated with excreta.

Average daily water intake is 10 ml/100 g BW but this may increase if no succulent foods are fed. Free access to water should be provided. Open water bowls may become contaminated and so inverted water bottles with a small sipper tube are often suspended from the side of the cage slightly above floor level. Fresh water should be provided daily and the water bottle cleaned.

Rats and mice
Rats and mice are omnivorous and will eat almost anything. Their nutritional requirements are well documented and commercial pelleted foods or coarse mixes are widely available. The basic ration may be supplemented with small quantities of a variety of foods, particularly vegetable-based materials, and offering these may encourage handling by the owner. Most rats and mice will adjust their energy intake to match their requirements but overfeeding of highly palatable foods can lead to obesity. As a guide, adult rats require 10–20 g/day of dry food, whereas adult mice require 5–10 g/day.

It should be noted that rats in particular are prone to obesity and therefore the feeding of sweet biscuits, cake etc. should be avoided. In addition, as with other animals, human chocolate should not be fed to rats, as they are prone to chronic progressive nephrosis in later life which may be exacerbated or induced by the theobromine present in chocolate.

Free access to water should be available from small bowls or suspended water bottles. Adult rats may drink 25–45 ml/day and adult mice may drink 5–7 ml/day.

Hamsters

Hamsters are omnivorous. Specific diets are available but most good-quality rat or mouse diets will meet the requirements of the hamster. Commercial pelleted diets or coarse mixes can be supplemented with treat foods such as washed vegetables, seeds, fruits and nuts. Diets rich in simple sugars (glucose, lactose, sucrose, fructose) are best avoided.

Most adults will eat 5–15 g of pelleted feed and drink 15– 20 ml of water per day, but free access to water should be offered. Food and water should be provided in heavy dishes that are not easily overturned or contaminated; alternatively, hoppers may be used. Stale food should be removed from the cage to prevent hoarding by the hamster.

Gerbils

Gerbils are primarily herbivorous and their natural diet is based on grains and seeds, supplemented with fresh vegetables and roots when these are available. Commercial pelleted foods or seed and grain diets are available for gerbils, or adult gerbils can be fed good-quality rat or mice diets. Some mixes may contain large amounts of sunflower seeds, which are very palatable to gerbils and have a high fat and low calcium content. Gerbils often selectively eat sunflower seeds at the expense of other dietary ingredients but an excessive intake can result in obesity, hypercholesterolaemia (with resultant arterial disease) and calcium deficiency, with associated skeletal problems. The diet should be supplemented with chopped green vegetables, roots and fruit, and if pelleted food is given an appropriate seed mix should also be provided. Average food consumption in the adult is 10–15 g daily.

Like other rodents, gerbils need some hard foods or pieces of wood in their environment to gnaw and so prevent problems with tooth malocclusion. Food dishes should be ceramic, since plastic dishes may be eaten.

Gerbils conserve water efficiently through their ability to concentrate their urine. Most of their water requirement is met from succulent foods and from metabolism of the diet, but free access to clean water should always be provided. Water containers with drinking tubes are best placed outside the cage and should be checked regularly to ensure that they are working. Care should be taken to avoid using water feeders that leak as this leads to increased humidity in the environment, which can encourage skin disease such as red nose in gerbils.

Chinchillas

In the wild, chinchillas eat a wide range of vegetables, but their diet is composed mainly of grasses and seeds. Commercial diets are available but good-quality rabbit or guinea pig diets are also suitable. Good-quality hay should be available ad libitum and the diet may be supplemented with small quantities of dried fruit, nuts, carrot, washed green vegetables and fresh grass. Supplements should be provided in moderation to prevent obesity, bloat, diarrhoea or other gastrointestinal upsets.

Adults may eat approximately 20–40 g/day. Free access to water should be provided from hanging water bottles and it may be advisable to offer an additional water dish until the animal is used to drinking from a bottle.

Ferrets

Ferrets are strict carnivores with high protein and fat requirements. High-fibre diets should be avoided. Ferrets require 35% protein and 20% fat on a dry matter basis, which is higher than for adult cats. Pelleted diets for ferrets are commercially available, or high-quality tinned or dry cat foods may be fed. Dog foods are not appropriate for long-term feeding. Whole carcasses (mice, rabbits, day-old chicks) or chicken heads may occasionally be offered to provide variety or to supplement the diet. If vegetable proteins are fed, urolithiasis and hyperammonaemia with resultant fitting may ensue.

Deficiencies are uncommon if a commercial ferret diet is fed, but some home-mixed diets may result in problems. Examples include a diet based purely on meat, which can lead to calcium deficiencies with resultant skeletal and kidney problems. Ferrets, like cats, require preformed arachidonic acid, vitamin A and taurine in their diets, all of which are found in whole-meat based foods and commercial cat and ferret diets.

Food preferences are established early in life and some individuals may resent dietary change. Ferrets should be fed ad libitum, as they have high metabolic rates and are prone to conditions such as insulinomas in later life. For this reason, and also because dental disease is common in ferrets, feeding a predominantly dry diet is advisable. Water intake is approximately 75–100 ml/kg per day.

Birds

Cagebirds

Passerine bird species, such as the canary and zebra finch, eat a wide variety of fruit and small seeds to obtain a balanced diet in the wild. Captive birds should be fed a mixture of seeds and fruit that mimic the bird's natural feeding ecology. Similarly, psittacine birds (such as parrots, budgerigars, cockatoos, cockatiels, macaws and parakeets) seek out a natural diet containing a wide range of fruit, shoots and seeds, but in captivity they are commonly fed only seed mixes that are composed predominantly of sunflower seeds, which are high in fat but low in calcium and vitamin A. This type of diet may predispose the bird to obesity or nutritional disorders and the problem is compounded in some individuals that become addicted to sunflower seeds.

Commercial diets formulated to meet the needs of different types of bird are available (Figure 16.22) but should still be supplemented with fresh fruit and vegetables. All-seed diets are unlikely to be nutritionally complete for birds and careful vitamin/mineral supplementation will be required. Suitable vegetables include romaine lettuce, chickweed, parsley, watercress, sprouted seeds and root vegetables. Suitable fruits include apples, plums, oranges, grapes (in small amounts), tomatoes, melon, mango, papaya and pears. Many parrots also relish sprouted seeds such as mung beans or barley/rye grass seeds (owners should ensure that these have not been treated with arsenic, as many commercial lawn seeds are treated with this as an antifungal agent). Millet sprays are often fed to adult budgerigars and should be limited, as they are extremely high in fat and encourage obesity.

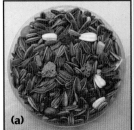 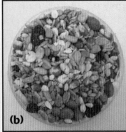 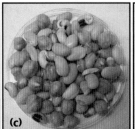 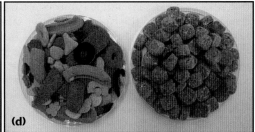

16.22 Commercial cagebird diets. **(a)** Traditional seed diet, with a high proportion of sunflower seed. **(b)** Dehusked seed diet – nutritionally poor. **(c)** Pulse diet, best used as a supplement. **(d)** Two modern pellet feeds for parrots. (Reproduced from *BSAVA Manual of Psittacine Birds, 2nd edition*)

Small birds have high metabolic rates and energy requirements, so it is important that a continuous supply of food is available. Empty husks should be blown from the top of the food on a frequent basis to avoid mistakes in judging how much the bird has actually eaten. Food may be provided in seed hoppers but young birds may be fed from the floor of the cage until they are familiar with alternative feeding systems.

Two types of mineral grit, insoluble and soluble, are frequently offered to companion birds as a dietary supplement. Insoluble grit, such as quartz or other forms of silica, remains in the gizzard where it may assist in the mechanical digestion of food and thus improve digestibility of the diet. Some evidence suggests that captive birds such as parrots that dehusk seeds prior to eating them do not actually require insoluble grit in their diets. Indeed, if the diet is deficient in calcium (as so many all-seed diets are) the parrot may over-consume the insoluble grit in an attempt to correct the deficiency and so develop an impaction of the gizzard. Soluble grit, such as oyster shell or cuttlefish, is usually completely digested by birds and provides a valuable supplementary source of minerals, including calcium and phosphorus.

Fresh water should be available at all times.

Birds of prey

Birds of prey are carnivores and in captivity they are usually fed whole chicks, a diet that provides a complete source of nutrition (as it includes the bones and gut contents), though problems may still arise.

Birds of prey are usually 'worked' by their owners in the summer months and should therefore be weighed regularly (at least once weekly) to ensure that the amount fed to them allows them to maintain a steady bodyweight. In general, the larger the bird of prey, the less prey should be fed as a percentage of the bird's bodyweight.

Some falconers feed wild-caught prey to their raptors. Care should be taken, as two main problems can occur. The first is lead poisoning, from any lead shot remaining in the carcass. The second is associated with feeding wild-bird prey such as pigeons, as these may be infected with protozoal parasites such as *Trichomonas* spp. or nematodes such as *Capillaria* spp. The freezing of any wild-caught pigeons and then their thorough thawing before feeding to a bird of prey helps to reduce the risk of transmission of these parasites, but there is still some risk and of course freezing does not remove the dangers of lead poisoning.

Reptiles

Chelonians

Land tortoises are herbivores, whereas terrapins and many of the soft-shelled turtles are carnivores and scavengers.

Newly hatched tortoises start to feed properly once the yolk sac has been absorbed and may be offered a variety of finely chopped fruits, vegetables and pre-soaked specific tortoise pellets. This diet can be supplemented with vitamins and minerals, and food should be offered ad libitum. Juvenile and adult tortoises may be fed the same range of foods, but the items do not need to be chopped up and the animals can be housed outdoors in summer, with access to grass and other plants. Food intake is reduced or will stop for up to several weeks prior to hibernation, which occurs when ambient temperature and daylight hours begin to decrease.

Although most water requirements are met from their food, tortoises should be provided with regular access to water. The bowl should be deep enough for them to submerge their nose as well as mouth, as they have no hard palate and so must do this to create suction.

Young terrapins feed in water and it is therefore advisable to have a separate feeding tank from their main housing tank, due to the levels of detritus that build up. Their diet includes small insects, small crustaceans and amphibian eggs and larvae. There are several companies that produce commercial aquatic chelonian pelleted diets. Adult terrapins eat amphibians and fish in the wild and so in captivity whole fish or chopped portions of whole fish should be fed to prevent nutritional imbalance. Herring, sprat, whitebait, sardines, minnows, sand eels, tadpoles or froglets, fresh prawns, shrimps and snails are all suitable foods. It is also possible to feed tinned cat or dog foods, hard-boiled eggs, cheese, earthworms or fresh liver or kidney rubbed in a vitamin/mineral supplement occasionally.

The main deficiencies seen in land-based chelonians are in calcium and vitamin D3. These deficiencies are often exacerbated by diets high in protein and by low environmental humidity, all of which have been implicated in the development of shell deformities such as pyramiding. Tortoises should be provided with a vitamin D3 and calcium supplement, and access to a source of ultraviolet light.

In carnivorous chelonians the main deficiencies are associated with vitamin A and calcium, chiefly in individuals fed an all-meat diet with no supplementation. This can result in shell deformities, kidney damage, and xerophthalmia.

Lizards

Lizards eat a wide variety of foods: different species may be insectivorous, carnivorous, herbivorous, frugivorous or omnivorous, and some species may change their feeding requirements as they mature. Insectivores (geckos, chameleons, skinks, anoles, lacertids) feed mainly on mealworms, silk-moth larvae, crickets, locusts and wingless fruit flies. However, these insects are relatively deficient in calcium and the insects themselves must be fed an appropriate nutritional supplement to ensure an adequate intake of supplement in the lizard. Monitors and tegus eat raw eggs, meat, dog food or rodents such as pink mice, mice or rats. Biotin deficiency can occur due to the avidin content of raw eggs, which can act as an anti-vitamin to biotin; therefore care must be taken when feeding hen's eggs.

Vitamin and mineral supplementation is usually required in diets for captive lizards, particularly calcium and vitamin D3 supplementation in lizards such as iguanas, basilisks, chameleons and water dragons. Access to ultraviolet lighting is also essential, UV-B being necessary to facilitate vitamin D3 synthesis in the lizard's skin.

All lizards should have access to fresh water. Some, such as chameleons and a lot of green iguanas, will only drink from water droplets on plants and it is important to mist the tank several times a day. Most lizards should be regularly sprayed with water to prevent skin problems associated with low humidity.

Snakes

Snakes are carnivorous and in captivity will eat rabbits, rats, mice, gerbils, chicks, earthworms, fish, amphibians, lizards or other snakes. The whole carcass is fed, to provide a balanced diet. For humane reasons and to prevent injury to the snake, food is generally offered as dead prey, which may be freshly killed or thawed from frozen. Certain types of fish, including whitebait, have high thiaminase activity and prolonged feeding without thiamine supplementation can result in thiamine deficiencies. This is particularly common in the fish-eating garter snakes (*Thamnophis* spp.). Supplementation may be given at 35mg thiamine/kg food. Cooking the fish to 80°C for 5 minutes will destroy the thiaminases. A garter snake can be converted on to rodent prey by smearing the rodent with the previous fish prey to fool the snake until it regularly accepts the new food.

The quantity of food and frequency of feeding depend on the bodyweight of the snake and surface area of the prey. For example, small garter snakes may require feeding on a daily basis, whereas a large python may require feeding on rabbits once every 2–3 weeks. As a guideline, adult snakes should be fed as often as is required to maintain normal bodyweight. Snakes may not eat for long periods of time and although this is normal at certain times of the year or before a slough, it can result in inanition. Regular weighing is advisable and excessive weight loss may indicate that nutritional support is required. Fluids and easily assimilated foods can be administered by stomach tube.

Water requirements of snakes are low but water should always be provided.

Amphibians

All adult amphibians are carnivores. Amphibian species include frogs, toads, salamanders and newts. Most adults are terrestrial but return to the water to breed and the larval stages are aquatic. Adult amphibians are carnivorous and, since feeding is initiated by the movement of prey, live prey is usually required. Some species may adapt to feeding on dead prey, meat, tinned dog food or even commercial pelleted diets. Raw meat must be supplemented with calcium (10 mg/g of meat). Captive amphibians should be fed two to three times weekly.

Adult frogs and toads feed on insects such as fruit flies, crickets and mealworms; large toads will also eat mice. Aquatic species may eat fish and prepared fish diets.

Salamanders eat earthworms, bloodworms, slugs, insects and prepared fish diets. Larval stages are herbivorous and feed on algae initially, or food sprinkled on the water. As they mature, aquatic prey (small crustaceans such as the water flea or *Daphnia* spp.) and then larger insects or animals are eaten.

Ornamental fish

One of the difficulties in feeding ornamental fish is that, with a few exceptions such as the goldfish, they are rarely kept in a single-species environment. Anatomical differences and variations in feeding strategies complicate the formulation of a single diet that will meet all the requirements of a mixed community, which may include representatives of herbivorous, omnivorous and carnivorous fish species.

An adequate delivery of nutrients is essential for the optimum health of the fish, but in a closed aquatic environment overfeeding and poor diet formulation can have a detrimental effect on conditions in the aquarium. Waste, in the form of uneaten food, undigested food and the excreted metabolic breakdown products of protein, will directly pollute the living environment and can pose a serious threat to the health of aquarium fish. To minimize the risk of pollution-induced stress, the diet must be palatable, easily digested, nutritionally balanced and of high biological value. A number of commercial diets are available for ornamental fish. Nutritionally complete diets are marketed as pellets, flakes and granules; other, complementary, foods include certain pond foods and frozen insect larvae, bloodworms and cockles.

Incomplete foods should be fed with care. Although they are useful 'treats' for aquarium fish, an excessive intake may result in dietary imbalance. Live aquatic food, such as *Daphnia* or *Tubifex* spp., is sometimes offered but may represent a disease risk and pre-frozen packs are considered safer. Fish kept in an established pond may feed on the pond's natural flora and fauna, and so complete diets are seldom required. Species that are kept in relatively bare display ponds, such as koi carp, will require a complete diet.

Of the complete diets available, flake formats offer versatility in that they can be floated on the water for surface feeders or submerged to sink slowly for middle and bottom feeders. Since the flakes are easily broken up into smaller pieces, they provide an excellent single food for a range of species and sizes of fish. Granules offer lower leaching of nutrients, because their surface area to volume ratio is larger, and different granule sizes and densities may be used to target different groups of fish in the aquarium.

As a general guideline, fish kept in a community tank should be fed to satiation two or three times per day. This allows close inspection of the fish and the tank on a regular basis. Feeding to satiation involves the continuous addition of small amounts of food to the aquarium until the fish stop feeding eagerly and is normally achieved in a few minutes or less, depending on the tank size and stocking density.

It should be emphasized that pollution from nitrogenous waste is a considerable threat to the health of fish held in a closed volume of water. Correct diet formulation and feeding regimen can improve protein utilization and help to minimize pollution, but water quality should be maintained through regular water changes or, in the larger aquaria, through the use of filter systems, which must be properly maintained.

Nutraceuticals and functional foods

Nutraceuticals (often referred to as functional foods) are naturally occurring foods or dietary components that provide a health benefit or desirable physiological effect beyond meeting basic nutritional requirements. In parallel with developments in human nutrition, there has been considerable interest in the potential for functional ingredients to improve the health of pets and reduce the likelihood of disease.

Research in dogs and cats has shown that functional ingredients can positively influence a number of body systems and processes, including inflammation and immunity, ageing, the brain, skin and hair coat, musculoskeletal system, oral cavity and gastrointestinal tract. Several functional ingredients are now finding their way into prepared pet foods for healthy dogs and cats, as well as for patients with clinical conditions.

Immune function is improved by supplementation with antioxidants such as vitamins E and C, taurine, lycopene, β-carotene and lutein. Lycopene is a powerful antioxidant abundant in red tomatoes and processed tomato products, whereas lutein (also known as xanthophyll) is a carotenoid pigment found in red peppers, kale, mustard, spinach and egg yolk. These ingredients may promote protective immune function, especially in the young and the old, and dampen inflammation in hypersensitivity reactions.

Omega-3 polyunsaturated fatty acids, which are found in marine fish oils, are commonly used to suppress inflammation, particularly where associated with allergic skin disease and oesteoarthritis. Improvements in the skin and coat condition of dogs, such as increased gloss and softness, decreased scale and better barrier function, are recognized when increased amounts of linoleic acid, zinc, biotin and B vitamins are consumed. Skin inflammation can also be reduced by curcumin (an extract of tumeric) and aloe vera gel, and skin healing can be improved by zinc, vitamins A and C.

Powdered extract from green-lipped mussels (*Perna canaliculus*) contains several constituents – anti-inflammatory fatty acids, chondroitin sulphate (a glycosaminoglycan constituent of cartilage), glutamine, antioxidant and minerals – that can improve joint function. Clinical studies in dogs with osteoarthritis have shown that this powder reduces joint pain and swelling, and improves overall clinical scores.

The omega-3 fatty acid docosahexaenoic acid is important in early development of the brain and retina, as well as for visual function and mental health during life. There is evidence that enriching the diet of pregnant bitches with this fatty acid improves the visual performance and mental development of their puppies. Also, in young and old animals alike, supplementation with antioxidants has been shown to help to maintain cognitive function and learning agility.

Considerable advances in the oral hygiene of dogs and cats have been achieved through the development of products with textures that are abrasive and mimic the teeth-cleaning properties of the wild diet of dogs and cats. The addition of plant extracts, such as eucalyptus and parsley seed oils, can also contribute by reducing oral bacterial loads and promoting fresh breath.

Dietary fibre is added to pet foods to encourage good stool quality and regularize bowel movements. Specific dietary fibres, namely the fructo-oligosaccharides and inulin, promote the growth of so-called friendly bacteria (*Bifidobacterium* and *Lactobacillus* spp.) in the large intestine and are associated with several potential health benefits. These include a reduction in populations of harmful bacteria, increased production of beneficial short-chain fatty acids such as butyrate, increased absorption of some vitamins and minerals, and improved elimination of toxic compounds. Fructo-oligosaccharides and inulin are found naturally in Jerusalem artichoke, burdock, chicory, leeks, onions and asparagus, and can be synthesized from sucrose and lactose.

Clinical nutrition

Nutritional factors may affect the health of any animal in a number of ways. The provision of a nutritionally adequate diet is clearly important in the prevention of disease associated with deficiencies or imbalances of specific nutrients. Nutritional diseases are now rare in companion animals, thanks to the widespread feeding of nutritionally balanced commercial diets, but problems do occasionally arise:

- Where the animal's intake is reduced
- When the diet is poorly formulated or stored
- When an otherwise balanced diet is carelessly oversupplemented
- Where the animal is unable to digest, absorb or utilize the nutrient as a result of disease or genetic factors.

Nutritional support at times of stress, disease or injury is a second area in which nutrition may impact on disease. Failure to consider this aspect of disease management may have a detrimental effect on the animal's recovery. Practices that may adversely affect the nutritional status of sick animals include:

- Failure to record daily weight
- Failure to observe, measure and record the amount of food consumed
- Delay of nutritional support until the patient is in an irreversible state of depletion
- Withholding food for diagnosis procedures
- Failure to recognize and treat increased nutritional needs brought about by injury or illness
- Failure to appreciate the role of nutrition in the prevention of and recovery from infection; unwarranted reliance on drugs
- Prolonged administration of glucose and electrolyte solutions
- Rotation of staff at frequent intervals and confusion of responsibility for patient care
- Inadequate postoperative nutritional support
- Limited availability of laboratory tests to assess nutritional status.

Finally, dietary modification may form an integral part of the management of a variety of clinical conditions.

Nutritional support

The nutritional requirements of the stressed or traumatized patient differ markedly from those of the healthy animal and, coupled with this, there is often a reduced desire or physical ability to eat. Failure to address these altered needs can result in malnutrition of the critical care patient and will have an adverse effect on the animal's recovery.

Conversely, the therapeutic benefits of appropriate nutritional support for these animals may include:

- Increased survival rates
- Improved tolerance to invasive procedures
- Shorter hospitalization periods
- Decreased risk of infection
- Earlier return to mobility
- More rapid wound healing.

Altered nutritional needs of the stressed patient

In the healthy animal, short-term fasting results in a series of adaptive mechanisms that are designed to maintain blood glucose concentrations, preserve lean body tissue and promote survival. Because there is little or no intake of food, the body mobilizes its own tissue reserves to provide essential nutrients and lowers its metabolic rate to reduce energy expenditure.

Most cells adapt to using fatty acids, instead of glucose, as an energy source, and within a few days fat becomes the major source of fuel in the fasting animal. However, the cells of some tissues, such as the brain, kidney and red blood cells, still require a constant supply of glucose for energy. To meet this demand, tissue proteins are broken down to provide amino acids that can then be converted to glucose. In starvation, therefore, fat reserves are used to supply energy, but even in the healthy animal there is inevitably some loss of tissue protein. When feeding is resumed, amino acid mobilization decreases and metabolism returns to normal within 24 hours.

In conditions of stress or trauma, these adaptive mechanisms to food deprivation are overridden. An initial 'ebb' or 'shock' phase lasts for a few hours up to 2 days, during which intravascular fluids are redistributed (**hypovolaemia**) to maintain tissue perfusion. Treatment during this phase is aimed at life-saving procedures. Metabolism may be lowered (**hypometabolism**) during this phase.

This phase is quickly followed by a 'flow' period of accelerated metabolism that is designed to support the healing of wounds and resistance to infection. This stage can last from days to several weeks, depending on the severity of the injury. During this period of **hypermetabolism**, energy requirements increase in accordance with the severity of the injury and are particularly high in cases of head trauma (because the brain has a particularly high energy requirement), septicaemia, extensive burns or following radical surgery. Even healthy animals undergoing minor elective surgery may experience a transient increase in energy requirements of up to 10% above normal.

In stressed animals, glycogen reserves are rapidly depleted and fat becomes the major and preferred energy source. In addition, healing tissues and some tumours require glucose as an energy source and the breakdown of tissue proteins increases markedly in order to maintain blood glucose levels to meet this demand. Nevertheless, high levels of dietary carbohydrate are contraindicated in hypermetabolic patients, since they commonly exhibit a peripheral insulin resistance and are unable to utilize glucose efficiently. An excessive intake of carbohydrate during this period can result in respiratory acidosis and other complications. Unlike the healthy animal, these metabolic changes are not immediately reversed when feeding is resumed.

Protein–energy malnutrition

The cumulative drain on tissues may continue for weeks and, if not corrected, can result in protein-energy malnutrition. During this time, nutritional support becomes a crucial part of the treatment. Protein–energy malnutrition can have a number of adverse effects which, in combination, can delay recovery and increase the patient's susceptibility to infection and shock. The most obvious effects are muscle wasting and weakness, but other side effects include reduced immune function, increased risk of infection and delayed wound healing. Impaired digestive function exacerbates the problem. In extreme cases, death can occur due to sepsis and failure of the heart, lungs and other organs.

Patient assessment

Some form of nutritional support is required for any animal that is unable or unwilling to eat voluntarily, but a thorough veterinary examination is necessary to assess the individual requirements of the patient and the most appropriate method of administering support. Specific nutritional support is indicated if:

- Oral intake is reduced for 3–5 days, or if it is anticipated to be interrupted for this length of time as a result of surgical or other in-hospital procedures
- There is an acute weight loss of > 5–10% of bodyweight (excluding fluid losses)
- Actual weight is 15% or more below ideal bodyweight
- Body condition, as scored on a scale of 1 (cachectic) to 5 (obese), is below the optimal score of 3
- Physical changes are accompanied by hypoalbuminaemia
- Recent trauma, surgery or sepsis is accompanied by anorexia.

Patients who have recently undergone major surgery or trauma, especially when this is associated with head injuries, blood loss, sepsis, severe burns or open wounds, are prime candidates for nutritional support. Another group of patients is those that are physically unable to eat (with jaw fractures, for example, or with oesophageal trauma or surgery to the oral cavity) and those with chronic wasting diseases, such as cancer.

Once an initial assessment has been made, the degree and duration of nutritional support can be estimated and a nutritional plan formulated on an individual basis for each patient. For surgical patients, preoperative assessment is particularly important so that invasive tube placement can be performed at the time of the initial surgery.

Techniques for nutritional support

Nutritional support for small animals may be provided by either the enteral or the parenteral route. **Total parenteral nutrition** is the provision of nutrients by the intravenous route, but this technique is expensive with inherent technical problems and is usually reserved for a small number of patients with gastrointestinal failure.

Where there is a functional gastrointestinal tract, **enteral nutrition** is a more economical and physiologically sound option. Prolonged lack of enteral nutrition can result in intestinal mucosal atrophy, with an associated reduction in functional capacity and risk of intestinal bacterial translocation into the portal blood. A number of techniques are available for enteral feeding, the choice of which depends on various factors, including type of injury, medical condition or surgical procedure, and should be based on individual patient assessment.

If voluntary intake is adequate, nutritional support may simply take the form of providing a more concentrated source of energy and nutrients. Other patients may be encouraged to eat by hand feeding, providing aromatic foods or heating the food offered to stimulate the appetite. Inappetent cats may respond to a pharmacological intervention such as intravenous administration of diazepam, or oral ciproheptadine, but this method of appetite stimulation should not be continued for longer than 3 days and should be used with care (diazepam has been associated with sporadic hepatotoxicity). It is important to check that adequate amounts are actually being consumed.

Where the patient's needs cannot be met through voluntary intake, some form of involuntary tube feeding must be considered. Short-term options include:

- Force feeding by syringe
- Feeding by daily orogastric intubation
- Rolling the food into small balls and 'pilling' the animal.

These methods can be stressful for the patient and may not satisfy the animal's nutritional needs. There is a real risk of aspiration pneumonia with syringe feeding and it is important to ensure that the patient's head is in a natural position (not raised) and that the animal swallows between the administration of each bolus.

With rodents, either oral syringe feeding or the use of straight avian crop tubes (see below) for administration of liquid food is advised but the latter may be stressful, as the rodent must be scruffed prior to administration. Stomach tubing may be performed with care for fish by using a soft rubber tube (premeasured to the level of the stomach, which is usually located just caudal to the pectoral fins) attached to the syringe. With fish species that have pharyngeal teeth (e.g. koi carp), special care must be taken that the teeth are not damaged and, conversely, that the teeth do not damage the feeding tube. The fish's stomach should not be overfilled, as this could lead to passive regurgitation of food with blockage of the gills.

Tube feeding

Crop tubing is one of the easiest and safest ways to give assisted feeding of semi-liquid diets to debilitated birds (Figure 16.23). The avian crop tube for psittacines (which have powerful crushing beaks) is a stainless-steel blunt-ended straight or slightly curved tube with a luer fitting that allows a syringe to be attached. The bird's beak is held open with a gag and the tube is passed from the bird's left side, over the top of the glottis and the airway towards the back of the oropharynx and then down the oesophagus into the crop, which is generally situated at the base of the neck (predominantly on the right side of the midline). For species that do not have crushing beaks, such as raptors and many passerines, crop tubes may be made from drip tubing.

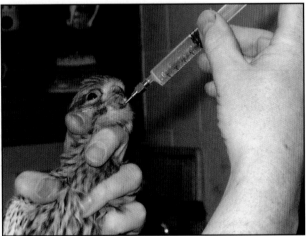

16.23 Passing a crop tube in a female kestrel to provide supplemental nutrition.

For non-avian species, there are several methods of tube feeding (Figure 16.24), including:

- Pharyngostomy tube
- Oesophageal tube
- Naso-oesophageal tube
- Nasogastric tube
- Gastrostomy tube
- Enterostomy tube.

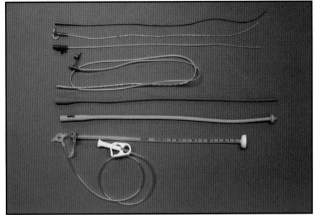

16.24 Multiple sizes and types of feeding tubes available for use in dogs and cats. (Reproduced from the *BSAVA Manual of Canine & Feline Gastroenterology, 2nd edition*)

Surgical placement of a **pharyngostomy** tube has been used successfully for feeding patients with prolonged anorexia and an inability to pick up or chew food. However, because of a high incidence of epiglottic entrapment and interference with the larynx or numerous nerves in this area, the popularity of pharyngostomy tube feeding has recently declined in favour of nasal feeding and oesophagostomy or gastrostomy tubes. It remains a useful method for feeding debilitated reptiles, and care of the tube in these cases is as for nasogastric tubes. **Oesophageal** intubation reportedly has fewer side effects than pharyngostomy tubing but is not commonly used in the UK.

Naso-oesophageal and **nasogastric** intubation require no sedation and either method is well tolerated by most cats and dogs, rabbits and ferrets. (It can be attempted for larger individual guinea pigs and chinchillas but the tubes can be difficult to place, as the epiglottis in these two species is permanently locked above the soft palate.) With nasogastric tubes there appears to be a high incidence of gastric reflux, with resultant oesophagitis and stricture formation, and preference is given to naso-oesophageal tubes (Figure 16.25). These may be left in place for several weeks. Since the tube size is limited this method can only be used for feeding larger animals, but it can be used for long-term administration of fluids to any size of animal. Nasal feeding is recommended as an adjunct to voluntary feeding or where sedation or anaesthesia of the patient poses too great a risk for surgical placement of a gastrostomy tube.

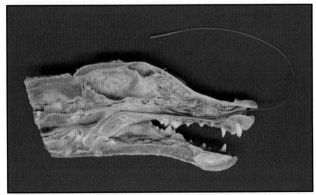

16.25 Anatomical model of canine head, showing correct placement of a naso-oesophageal tube in the ventral meatus. (Reproduced from the *BSAVA Manual of Canine & Feline Gastroenterology, 2nd edition*)

Gastrostomy tube feeding is indicated where long-term involuntary nutritional support is anticipated and the presence of pharyngeal or oesophageal lesions precludes the use of pharyngostomy tubes. The use of gastrostomy tubes is increasing in small-animal medicine thanks to the development of a technique for percutaneous tube placement without the need for laparotomy. Percutaneous endoscopic gastrostomy (PEG; Figure 16.26) is a simple and well tolerated procedure, but requires the use of a flexible endoscope. Alternatively, a large-bore Foley catheter can be placed into the stomach at laparotomy and secured to the abdominal musculature. Complications associated with this method include peritonitis and tube displacement or blockage. Gastrostomy tubes are of wide bore and so will accommodate most types of diet. The tube may be left in place for weeks to months, and tube feeding by this method can be continued by most owners at home.

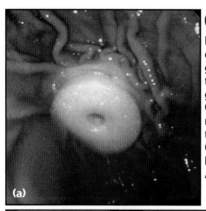

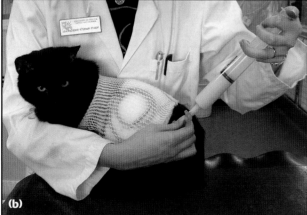

16.26

Percutaneous endoscopic gastrostomy. **(a)** PEG tube in place in the gastric mucosa. **(b)** Supplemental nutrition being given to a cat via a PEG. (a, Courtesy of E Hall; b, courtesy of A Harvey)

Feeding directly into the small intestine by **enterostomy** catheter (either duodenostomy or jejunostomy) may be required when serious conditions of the upper gastrointestinal tract, such as pancreatitis or major gastric or small bowel surgery, are present. Animals fed in this way require liquid elemental diets (simple sugars, amino acid complexes and emulsified fats) that require little digestion and are readily absorbed from the jejunum and ileum. If normal food is supplied by this route, severe digestive tract complications will arise. Parenteral nutrition would be an alternative if small-bowel function was not satisfactory.

Method for tube feeding

The procedure should be started gradually, with food being introduced over 2–3 days. For tubes placed surgically, there are rarely complications feeding 6 hours following placement (though some texts advise delaying use for 24 hours).

Tube feeding

1. Ensure that appropriate connectors and syringes are available.
2. Prepare the total amount of food to be fed at a single feed. Ensure that food is at room temperature, or slightly higher. Cold food may induce vomiting or rapid stomach emptying.
3. Divide one-third of the calculated food requirement into 5–6 feeds and administer one of these portions.
4. Give food slowly.
5. Observe the patient's reaction. It may be experiencing a strange sensation, as the stomach has had no preparation for the arrival of food. It is common for patients to lick their lips – not because the food is tasty but because they feel nauseous.
6. If stomach contents are expelled from the tube prior to a feed, do not feed. The stomach has not emptied sufficiently from the previous feed.
7. If the patient begins to vomit, reduce the volumes of feed.

- If no problems arise after initial feeds, the volumes can be increased to meet calorific requirements.
- The total calculated volume should be administered in at least four separate feeds. Avoid feeding during the night unless absolutely necessary; most patients do not eat continually.

After completion of the procedure, the tube should be flushed with 5–30 ml of water in order to clear debris and maintain patency. Some authorities (though not this author) recommend using carbonated drinks to flush tubes: the bubbles help to loosen any solid food particles that have collected on the inside of the tube. This method should be used with caution, as large amounts of fizzy fluid can make patients feel unwell and possibly induce vomiting.

The area should be cleaned and redressed as required.

Considerations for tube feeding

In smaller patients, or in those that continue to vomit with bolus feeds, some food can be administered through infusion pumps via giving sets. It is important to keep the tube free from blockage. In practice, the complete milks cause the fewest problems and have the added advantage of less preparation time, less mess and higher digestibility. All liquidized foods should be of the consistency of whole-fat milk to ensure easy passage down the tubes. Most tinned foods require the addition of a large amount of water. Special foods are available for tube feeding, which are concentrated and easily digested. This is important, because normal pet food when liquidized becomes bulk limiting, i.e. the amount of fluid food that needs to be given to reach the patient's daily kilocalorie requirement is so substantial that it cannot physically be administered over a 24-hour period without the risk of vomiting.

Energy and nutrient requirements

Daily energy requirements of the hospitalized patient are based on basal energy requirements (BER) or cage-rest maintenance energy requirements (MER) multiplied by an arbitrary factor, the size of which varies according to the severity and nature of the illness (1.2 to 3 times). In some cases, energy requirements may be below normal because the animal is hypometabolic or because it is physically inactive as a result of the injury. MER is calculated using the formulae:

Dog: MER (kcal/day) = 110 x BW$^{0.75}$ (kg)
Cat: MER (kcal/day) = 70 x BW (kg)

For rabbits, rodents and ferrets, in general the requirements for debilitated species vary from 1.5 to 3 times maintenance levels (see Figure 16.19), the lower levels being for mildly injured or infected animals and the upper levels for burns victims, those with serious organ damage or septicaemic cases. The gut contents in herbivorous rodents are voluminous and need to be kept fluid; thus the use of fluid therapy as additional support is essential.

For avian patients, the basal metabolic rate (BMR) = BW$^{0.75}$ (kg) x k, where k is a factor that has been calculated as 129 for passerine species and 78 for psittacine species. The MER for birds is roughly 1.5 x BMR. In addition, for various disease processes the MER is adjusted as the severity of the condition increases (Figure 16.27).

For reptiles, the MER is roughly 1.5 times BMR, where BMR is calculated as for birds but with k = 10; the same disease severity adjustments are made as for birds.

Condition	Energy requirement
Starvation	0.5 x MER
Trauma	1.5 x MER
Sepsis	2.5 x MER
Burns	3–4 x MER

16.27 Energy requirements of birds in various physiological states.

Volume

The volume of food required is calculated by dividing the total daily energy requirement (kcal) by the energy density of the diet (kcal/ml) as recorded on the product label. The total volume required is divided into 4–6 feeds per day, depending on previous oral intake and individual animal tolerance. The normal stomach capacity is no more than 90 ml/kg in dogs and 50 ml/kg in cats.

All dietary transitions should be made slowly and in the initial stages of nutritional support; the calculated amount of nutrients should be approached over a period of 48 hours to avoid vomiting, abdominal discomfort and diarrhoea. For animals that have been inappetent for prolonged periods, slow rates of administration (>10 minutes) are recommended.

For rabbits being fed by nasogastric tube, the volume to be administered at one time varies from 3 ml to 15 ml (depending on the size of the rabbit), given four to six times daily.

For rodents, volumes at any one time vary from 0.5 ml for a mouse up to 2.5 ml for rat, with repeated doses six to eight times daily to ensure correct calorie administration.

For ferrets, suggested volumes at any one time vary from 2 ml to 10 ml, given three to six times daily. It is vitally important than no debilitated ferret goes for longer than 4 hours without nutritional support, as they rapidly become hypoglycaemic.

For birds, the maximum volumes that should be administered at any one time are given in Figure 16.28.

In reptiles, if anorexia has persisted for some time it is essential to rehydrate the patient before attempting to give assisted feeding. Thereafter, initial feeding should be commenced at very low levels (50% of the requirement for the current weight of the reptile). Otherwise excess calories and proteins will cause a rapid uptake of glucose from the bloodstream, taking potassium and phosphorus with it. This can lead to life-threatening hypokalaemia and hypophosphataemia. Blood

Species	Maximum volume (ml)
Budgerigar	1
Cockatiel	3
Conure	5
Cockatoo	7–10
African Grey parrot	8–10
Macaw	10–15

16.28 Maximum volumes of fluid to be administered to birds by crop tube at any one time (Girling, 2003).

phosphorus and potassium should always be monitored when treating chronically anorectic reptiles, whether the species is carnivorous or herbivorous.

Monitoring

Weight and body condition score should be recorded on a daily basis to enable accurate calculation of the patient's energy requirements and to monitor its progress. Adjustments in food allowance can then be made on an individual basis according to observed changes in the animal's bodyweight, body condition and level of activity.

Fat, carbohydrate and protein

Stressed, hypermetabolic patients use fat rather than carbohydrate as their main source of energy and most cells become progressively less able to use glucose efficiently. High levels of carbohydrate in the diet during this period can give rise to serious metabolic disturbances that may lead to respiratory or cardiac failure. High-fat diets are therefore recommended and tend to be more palatable, digestible and calorie-dense, which are advantages for feeding potentially anorexic patients. Protein requirements of the stressed animal are higher than normal, to maintain wound healing and immunity and to compensate for the higher rate of protein breakdown. However, some restriction of dietary protein may be indicated in certain specific conditions, such as chronic kidney or liver disease.

Supplements

Supplementation of the diet with certain amino acids, including glutamine and arginine, may be beneficial in the nutritional management of critical-care patients. There may also be an increased requirement for water-soluble B-complex vitamins, and zinc may have an important role in wound healing. There is further evidence from the human field indicating that antioxidants may be beneficial in preventing the ongoing cellular damage that occurs following a trauma involving ischaemia, hypovolaemia and shock.

It should be noted that guinea pigs have a minimum dietary requirement for vitamin C of 10 mg/kg/day and that this increases during debilitation to levels of around 30 mg/kg/day.

Suitable diets

In selecting a diet for enteral administration, it is important to consider the most appropriate dietary formulation, the caloric density of the diet and, where appropriate, the diameter of the feeding tube. Commercial liquid enteral diets or liquidized canned diets may be used for most purposes. Elemental diets containing amino acids or glucose may be useful if gastrointestinal function is compromised, or to supplement other diets.

Ideally, diets for the critical patient should be highly palatable, highly digestible and nutrient dense in order to ensure an adequate intake of nutrients in a reduced volume of food.

Although healthy dogs (but not cats) can be maintained on a plant-based diet, such diets are unsuitable for the metabolically stressed animal and should be replaced by a meat-based diet for the duration of the dog's illness and convalescence. Following injury, the metabolism of the dog tends to revert to its more carnivorous origins and is more closely aligned with that of the cat. Thus, protein and fat utilization is increased and carbohydrate is used with decreasing efficiency. In addition, plant-based diets are less digestible than meat-based diets and can cause digestive upsets in the stressed patient.

Debilitated rabbits may be supported with oral syringing of vegetable-based baby foods (lactose-free varieties) or, better, with a gruel composed of ground dry rabbit-pellets and water or a commercial small-mammal support formula, as the latter has a better fibre level for gut stimulation. Similar diets are suitable for rodents (using rodent rather than rabbit pellets as gruels where appropriate). Guinea pigs and chinchillas benefit from oral cisapride or parenteral metoclopramide to stimulate gut motility. Ferrets may be supported with nasogastric or oral syringing of meat-based baby foods, or commercially prepared liquid meat-based formulas designed for cats and dogs.

Many semi-liquid diets have been used in avian practice. For granivorous and herbivorous species, diets such as human baby or juvenile foods (preferably the vegetable or fruit versions, and lactose-free as birds cannot digest milk-sugar lactose, which may lead to diarrhoea) have been used for a number of years, but many avian food manufacturers produce semi-liquid nutritional support diets and mashes. Carnivorous species, such as raptors, may be given tinned high-calorie foods such as canine or feline 'a/d diet' (Hills) mixed with previously boiled and cooled water to a consistency suitable for a syringe, or a canine liquid formula such as Reanimyl (Virbac), both of which are also suitable for ferrets. In all avian cases the addition of probiotics to encourage stabilization of gut flora and aid digestion is advisable.

Many foods have been used for debilitated reptiles, including Vetark Professional's Critical Care Formula, which has the benefits of being aqueous, able to pass through small feeding tubes, easily digested and absorbed. Nutritional status can then gradually be built up by using vegetable-based baby foods for herbivorous species, progressing to commercial support formulas with an increased fibre content such as Critical Care for Herbivores (Oxbow) or Science Recovery for Herbivores (Supreme Petfoods). For carnivorous species, the initial aqueous formula can gradually be replaced with baby-food porridges (which are easy to digest and to deliver by stomach tube or gavage) or Hills 'a/d diet' or Reanimyl as for carnivorous birds.

Fish may be tempted to feed by altering food types to live prey such as mealworms or bloodworms for carnivorous species.

Assisted feeding for invertebrates can be difficult. Many arachnids may drink water from soaked cotton-wool balls or from water misted on cage furniture with a plant sprayer. To add essential proteins, sugars and vitamins to the water, it is possible to spray liquid formulations such as those used for reptiles and birds.

Complications of nutritional support

Following a period of food deprivation, all dietary transitions should be made slowly to avoid complications, including the development of potentially serious metabolic derangements (Figure 16.29). In the initial stages of refeeding, vomiting may occur due to gastrointestinal hypomotility, and diarrhoea may result from reduced intestinal surface area and decreased enzyme activity. Normal digestive function is usually restored within a few days of appropriate enteral feeding.

Day	Percent of normal daily food quantity
1	33
2	66
3	100

16.29 Food reintroduction schedule for animals recovering from vomiting, diarrhoea or pancreatitis. Feed small, frequent meals (4–5 day) of a highly digestible, low fat (< 15%; DM; < 30% ME), low fibre (< 2% DDM 0.5 g/100 kcal (418 kJ) ME) diet.

Calorie intake has an important effect on convalescence. An insufficient intake can result in protein–energy malnutrition, but overfeeding can be equally detrimental, particularly when the carbohydrate intake is excessive. In starved hypometabolic patients, excessive carbohydrate can lead to insulin-induced transport of phosphorus and potassium into cells and subsequently hypophosphataemia and hypokalaemia. The resultant respiratory and cardiovascular failure could prove fatal in some cases.

Other complications of nutritional support include mechanical problems or infections related to the feeding tube. Tube obstructions can be minimized by using liquid diets with fine-bore tubes, by sieving liquidized canned diets prior to administration via oesophagostomy or gastrostomy tubes, and by flushing with water after each feed. Occasionally, naso-oesophageal tubes may be regurgitated and pharyngostomy tubes can cause gagging, airway obstruction and related problems. Fewer complications are seen with oesophagostomy tubes.

Dietary sensitivity

The term dietary sensitivity describes any clinically abnormal response to a particular food item and may be further classified as either food intolerance or true food allergy (hypersensitivity). True **dietary hypersensitivity** is an immune-mediated phenomenon whereas **food intolerance** denotes any other clinically abnormal response to a dietary component. Food intolerance can result from an impaired ability to digest the food (often because a specific enzyme is lacking) or from pharmacological, metabolic or toxic reactions. With the exception of certain specific conditions, the clinical signs associated with hypersensitivity reactions are often indistinguishable from those produced by food intolerance, and management protocols are identical for both.

In the dog and cat, dietary sensitivity usually manifests as skin or gastrointestinal disease, and a number of cases will present with signs involving both systems. Pruritus is the most frequently observed presenting sign, which is accompanied by a gradation of clinical signs associated with self-inflicted trauma. Dietary sensitivity has also been implicated in some cases of otitis externa in dogs and of miliary dermatitis and eosinophilic plaque in cats. Certain forms of food intolerance, notably lactose intolerance and gluten-sensitive enteropathy of Irish Setters, usually manifest as diarrhoea. In addition, a number of chronic conditions of the gastrointestinal tract have been reported in which dietary hypersensitivity may play a role, including inflammatory bowel disease in cats and canine idiopathic chronic colitis.

Elimination diets

Food sensitivity may be associated with any dietary ingredient, including additives (although extremely rare), but most reactions are caused by dietary proteins. In cats, reactions to cow's milk and beef account for more than half the reported cases, whereas reactions to cow's milk, beef and cereal (alone or in combination) are most commonly reported in dogs. The successful management of dietary sensitivity involves identification of the offending ingredient and its elimination from the diet. By examining the animal's detailed dietary history, it may be possible to identify foods that the animal has never eaten (or at least within the previous month) and these can be used to form the basis of an elimination diet that is 'hypoallergenic' for that individual. Such restricted diets should contain a minimum number of protein sources which, preferably, are not commonly associated with sensitivity reactions. Elimination diets that have been used successfully in dogs and cats include chicken, lamb, rabbit, duck, venison and a variety of fish species, typically fed with rice, tapioca or potatoes.

The elimination diet should be fed for a minimum of 3 weeks, though a trial period of up to 60 days may be necessary in some animals to achieve a complete remission of signs. Failure to respond within this time suggests that either dietary sensitivity is not involved, other factors may be contributing to the clinical disease or the animal is sensitive to the protein in the elimination diet.

During the diagnostic period there should be no access to any other source of nutrients, including treats, chews or nutritional supplements.

A small number of animals will react to commercially prepared elimination diets but not to home-prepared diets using the same ingredients and it may be preferable to use a home-prepared diet in the initial diagnostic stages.

If clinical improvement occurs, a diagnosis of dietary sensitivity may be confirmed by challenging with the original diet and demonstrating an exacerbation of clinical signs within 1–14 days. Reintroduction of the elimination diet should result in an improvement in signs and, at this stage, it may be possible to introduce a commercially prepared diet with the same ingredients. Individual protein sources can then be introduced at weekly intervals to identify specific dietary allergens that should be avoided.

Management of dietary sensitivity

Once a diagnosis has been established, it is usually possible to manage cases of dietary sensitivity using commercial diets with selected protein sources of high digestibility. Food allergens are usually large glycoproteins and the potential for reaction to these can be further reduced by enzymatic hydrolysis to produce low-molecular-weight proteins. For this reason, several diets designed for the management of dietary sensitivity contain hydrolysed soy isolate protein, which comprises highly digestible (>96%) low-molecular-weight proteins. Alternatively, it may be possible to identify a range of standard products that the animal is able to tolerate.

Obesity management

Obesity is the most common form of malnutrition seen in companion animal practice, with an estimated incidence of 25–33% in dogs and 6–25% in cats. Although cats tend to be more efficient regulators of their energy intake, this ability may be overridden, and recent trends towards the free-choice feeding of palatable dry cat foods together with a more sedentary, indoor lifestyle may have increased the frequency with which feline obesity is observed in some parts of the world.

As well as obesity reducing the animal's enjoyment of life, a number of serious clinical problems have been linked to the condition. These include:

- Osteoarthritis
- Respiratory distress and reduced exercise tolerance
- Diabetes mellitus
- Circulatory problems
- Lowered resistance to infections
- Liver disease (including idiopathic hepatic lipidosis in cats)
- Dermatological problems (which, in cats, may be linked to difficulties in self-grooming)
- Increased risk of feline lower urinary tract disease
- Increased surgical and anaesthetic risk.

Obesity is a consequence of energy intake exceeding requirement at some stage in the animal's life. During this phase, excessive energy intake results in the deposition of fat in adipose tissue and is associated with an increase in fat-cell size (**hypertrophy**) in the adult, or fat cell numbers (**hyperplasia**) in the growing animal. Once fat-cell hyperplasia has occurred, the animal retains a lifelong predisposition for excessive weight gain and it is important that food intake of growing dogs, in particular, is controlled to avoid obesity in the adult. The initial dynamic phase of fat deposition is followed by a static phase in which the animal remains fat but its bodyweight is fairly stable. Appetite may be normal or even reduced and this apparent anomaly may be confusing for the owners.

An animal is considered obese if its bodyweight is 15% or more above the ideal. Breed standards may provide useful guidelines for determining the ideal weight of purebred dogs, but are of little value in crossbred dogs and cats. Practical assessment of the degree of obesity involves subjective evaluation of the animal's appearance and palpation of the subcutaneous fat deposits. In normal animals, the ribs should be palpable but covered with a moderately thin layer of fat and there should be a definite indentation, or waistline, behind the rib cage when viewed from above. Dogs also tend to accumulate fat around the tail head and obese cats may develop an 'apron' of fat in the groin. Accumulation of fat in the abdominal cavity must be differentiated from abdominal enlargement due to other causes, such as ascites, gas, pregnancy or abdominal organ enlargement.

Dietary therapy

Dietary therapy of obesity is aimed at moderate, controlled energy restriction. Rapid weight loss should not be attempted in obese cats, since this can lead to the development of hepatic lipidosis, which is potentially fatal. In general, it is recommended that an initial target weight is set which represents a 15% reduction in bodyweight. Further reductions can then be planned once this target weight has been reached. For dogs, this degree of weight loss can be achieved within 12 weeks by feeding 40–50% of the animal's energy requirement for maintenance at its target weight. In cats, a 15% reduction in weight can be safely achieved over 18 weeks by feeding 60% of the animal's target energy requirements.

Simply feeding less of the normal diet is not recommended, since prepared pet foods are balanced to a normal energy intake. By restricting energy intake, essential nutrients may also be restricted, which can produce deficiency states that may be dangerous. This technique rarely forms part of a structured weight loss programme, and success rates tend to be low.

A more effective strategy is to feed a prepared low-calorie diet that has been specifically formulated to achieve weight loss and ensures an adequate intake of essential nutrients. This is particularly important when the diet is to be fed in the long term. There is emerging evidence that the functional ingredients L-carnitine and conjugated linoleic acids may promote weight loss and assist in obesity management. Dietary therapy should be combined with an increase in physical activity (where possible) and behavioural modifications that aim to produce lifelong habit changes and, therefore, permanent weight loss.

Protocol for weight reduction in dogs and cats

- Counsel the owner on the need to reduce the animal's bodyweight, stressing the medical implications of obesity
- Weigh the dog or cat and set a target weight. The planned reduction should represent no more than 15% of the animal's current weight
- Indicate to the owner how long it is likely to take to reach the target weight safely. The weight loss can usually be achieved in 10–15 weeks in dogs and 16–20 weeks in cats
- Calculate the amount to feed based on 40–50% (dogs) or 60% (cats) of the maintenance energy requirements at target bodyweight
- Stress the concept of feeding the weight reduction diet to the exclusion of all other foods. The discipline and cooperation required of all who come into contact with the animal may be reinforced if they are encouraged to record the total daily food intake on a chart. It may be preferable to confine cats to the home to prevent supplementation from other sources
- Advise weighing the animal carefully on the same scales at the same time every week or fortnight and encourage the owner to record the weight on the chart supplied. Small and steady weight losses are more evident from the weight chart than from simple observation of the animal
- Careful monitoring of cats during weight reduction is recommended. Owners should be questioned to check that food intake matches expectations, and clinical examination should be performed at regular intervals. Periodic haematological and blood biochemical evaluation may also be appropriate
- If satisfactory weight loss is not occurring, then the daily food allowance may be reduced by 10%, whilst keeping a careful watch on the general health of the animal. If such a reduction is necessary, it should be maintained for the rest of the dieting period
- When a satisfactory weight loss has been achieved, the dog or cat should be changed to a normal high-quality diet. It is important to calculate and regularly reassess the daily amount of food required to maintain the target weight
- Follow up after 1 and 3 months, and then at 6-monthly intervals
- At all times, give the owner adequate encouragement

Gastrointestinal disease

Gastrointestinal disorders are common in dogs and cats. In most cases, dietary modification can form an important, sometimes essential, part of managing the condition. Although some acute gastrointestinal disorders can be life-threatening, most cases tend to be self-limiting and respond well to symptomatic treatment. The principle of 'bowel rest' in which food is withheld for 24–72 hours is commonly adopted while fluid and electrolyte status is maintained through the oral or parenteral administration of rehydration fluids. Subsequently, small amounts of a highly digestible bland diet (such as boiled rice, fish or chicken) may be gradually reintroduced. In contrast, chronic conditions that persist for longer than 3–4 weeks are unlikely to be resolved without first identifying a specific cause and implementing the appropriate therapy.

Oesophageal disease

Oesophageal lesions may necessitate feeding via gastrostomy tube to allow the oesophagus to heal; otherwise soft, moist or liquidized foods may be offered. Patients with megaoesophagus should be fed from an elevated position to allow food to enter the stomach with the help of gravity. Traditionally slurries have been used, but many cases are now thought to cope better when fed a more textured diet.

Gastric dilatation–volvulus

Although cereal-based dry foods have previously been linked to this condition in dogs, it is now thought that they may have been falsely incriminated. Gaseous distension of the stomach may result from swallowed air and may be associated with rapid food consumption and excitement or physical activity close to the time of feeding. General dietary recommendations are to feed small frequent meals of a highly digestible, meat-based diet that will encourage gastric emptying and reduce stomach distension. Dogs, particularly those at high risk, should not be fed or allowed to drink large volumes of water within 1 hour of exercise or excitement and should preferably be fed away from other dogs.

Chronic diarrhoea

Diarrhoea may be defined as an increase in frequency, volume or fluidity of faeces, but these characteristics should be considered in the context of the diet being fed. High-fibre diets, for example, will lead to a marked increase in faecal volume and frequency of defecation compared with 'normal' highly digestible foods. Diarrhoea may be classified as 'chronic' if it persists for longer than 3–4 weeks.

Large quantities of water are either consumed or secreted into the gastrointestinal tract every day. In normal circumstances, approximately 95% of this water is reabsorbed from the large intestine. A relatively small decrease in absorption (or increase in secretion) can readily result in increased faecal water content and diarrhoea.

Diarrhoea occurs as the result of one or more mechanisms:

- *Interference with the digestion or absorption of nutrients.* Nutrients retained within the intestinal lumen exert an osmotic effect, leading to the retention of water and diarrhoea (**osmotic diarrhoea**). Osmotic diarrhoea is most commonly seen with nutritional overload, but it is also associated with any condition in which there is a deficiency of enzymes or enterocytes, including exocrine pancreatic insufficiency (EPI), and brush-border enzyme (e.g. lactase) deficiency.
- *Increased secretion of fluid into the intestine by enterocytes* (**secretory diarrhoea**), which may be stimulated by bacterial toxins and by the products of bacterial degradation of bile acids and dietary fat.
- *Increased intestinal permeability due to mucosal damage*, which can result from severe inflammation or as a consequence of other disease processes (e.g. cardiac disease, lymphatic obstruction). If the pore size is large, fluid and plasma proteins escape into the intestinal lumen, creating a protein-losing enteropathy and diarrhoea.
- *Altered intestinal motility.* Contrary to popular belief, most cases are due to a reduction in segmentation contractions rather than increased peristalsis, resulting in stagnation of intestinal contents, bacterial proliferation and degradation of nutrients. The increased faecal volume stimulates secondary peristaltic contractions, which may give the impression of hypermotility.

Small intestinal disease

Diarrhoea of small intestinal origin tends to lead to an increase in faecal volume since this is the main site for digestion and absorption of nutrients. This, in turn, can lead to an increased frequency of defecation. Pale, fatty faeces (**steatorrhoea**) are seen when there is maldigestion or malabsorption of fat, as in EPI and some other small-intestinal disorders. Because nutrients are poorly absorbed into the body, weight loss is common – often despite a marked increase in appetite.

Diet plays an important role in the management of many small-intestinal diseases, generally in conjunction with appropriate pharmacological therapy. Although no single diet is appropriate for every condition, it is generally accepted that diets for the management of conditions involving the small intestine should be highly digestible, since many diseases are likely to interfere with digestive and absorptive function. In most circumstances, therefore, high-fibre diets are contraindicated for the management of small-intestinal disease.

Dietary fat

Restriction of dietary fat is recommended in a range of small-intestinal diseases that disturb fat digestion or absorption, including EPI, small-intestinal bacterial overgrowth (SIBO) and lymphangiectasia. Pancreatic enzymes are reduced or absent with EPI, whereas SIBO adversely affects bile salts. In addition, bacterial metabolism of undigested fat may promote intestinal secretion and further aggravate the diarrhoea.

In some cases, medium-chain triglycerides (MCTs) may form a useful supplemental source of energy, since some MCTs can be absorbed intact from the gastrointestinal tract and can reach the circulation via portal rather than lymphatic channels.

Restriction of dietary fat is less important in the cat than the dog and some diarrhoeic cats appear to fare better on moderate- to high-fat diets.

Protein

Moderate to high quantities of good-quality protein are recommended for small-intestinal diseases, since protein malabsorption or protein-losing enteropathy may be a feature of some cases of chronic small-intestinal diarrhoea. Protein deficiency can further compromise a diseased intestinal tract.

Protein is also important in relation to dietary sensitivity, since most 'allergens' are proteins. Gluten, a protein in wheat and other cereals such as barley (not maize), is responsible for a particular enteropathy of Irish Setters in which poor weight gain or weight loss is usually accompanied by chronic diarrhoea. Where dietary sensitivity is the cause of diarrhoea, sources of dietary protein should be minimized to one or two ingredients that are not normally associated with sensitivity reactions.

Carbohydrate

Carbohydrate digestion and absorption can be impaired in all conditions that damage the lining of the small intestinal wall. Nevertheless, starch presents a relatively low digestive challenge in comparison with fat and may be used to provide a greater contribution to the energy content of diets that are restricted in fat. Highly digestible sources of carbohydrate, such as rice, are recommended. Simple sugars such as lactose (which is found in milk) should be avoided, because the enzymes required for their digestion may be lacking.

Dietary fibre

Although dietary fibre is commonly used in the non-specific treatment of acute diarrhoeas, it is generally not suitable for use in chronic small intestinal diseases. In the short term, fibre may improve faecal consistency, but in chronic cases it may interfere with digestion and absorption, thereby further compromising an impaired gastrointestinal tract. In particular, soluble fibre is contraindicated in EPI since this may interfere with pancreatic enzyme activity.

Vitamins

Several small intestinal diseases can result in deficiencies of water-soluble B-complex vitamins, especially cobalamin (vitamin B12) and folate.

Large intestinal disease

Animals with large intestinal diarrhoea tend to show very frequent defecation and pass small quantities of faeces on each occasion. This may be associated with urgency, straining or pain on defecation. The presence of fresh blood and copious amounts of mucus are also characteristic of large intestinal problems. Although weight loss is not usually a feature of large intestinal disease, it can occur as a secondary problem if appetite is depressed over a long period of time.

Dietary fibre

Dietary fibre may be beneficial in the management of some large intestinal diarrhoeas. Bacterial fermentation of fibres within the large intestine yield short-chain fatty acids, which are important for maintaining the health of cells of the large intestine wall and promote acidification of the contents of the colon. The effects of non-fermentable fibre are primarily related to an increase in faecal bulk. This may help to exercise the smooth muscle of the colon and improve contractility and, in addition, may bind faecal water to produce more formed stools.

Diets containing a mixture of both fermentable and non-fermentable fibres can, therefore, be valuable as non-specific therapy in a number of large-intestinal diseases, including certain infections and 'irritable bowel syndrome', which may be associated with stress.

Protein

Since many cases of colitis and inflammatory bowel disease in dogs and cats are thought to have an immune component, single protein source 'hypoallergenic diets' may be of benefit in their management, at least in the initial stages of therapy.

Constipation

Constipation may be defined as an inability to pass faeces, or difficulty in passing faeces (**tenesmus**). Retained faeces in the rectum and colon become progressively harder as water is reabsorbed and the faecal mass becomes increasingly impacted. High-fibre diets are of benefit in the prevention, but not the treatment, of constipation. Insoluble fibre increases faecal bulk, which is thought to increase colonic motility by stretching colonic muscles, resulting in more forceful, albeit less frequent, contractions. Soluble fibres may add further to faecal bulk, through their ability to retain water in the intestinal lumen. Fibres combining soluble and insoluble properties may be optimal for the prevention of constipation.

Pancreatic disease

Exocrine pancreatic insufficiency

Exocrine pancreatic secretions are reduced or absent in patients with exocrine pancreatic insufficiency (EPI), resulting in an inability to adequately digest fat and, to a lesser extent, protein and carbohydrate in the diet. Because there is poor digestion and malabsorption of nutrients, especially fat, weight loss is common despite a marked increase in appetite, and affected animals produce large volumes of pale, fatty faeces (steatorrhoea).

Although enzyme replacement therapy improves digestibility in patients with EPI, their requirements for energy and nutrients are still higher than in the normal animal. Low-fat diets of high digestibility help to reduce the digestive challenge within the gastrointestinal tract and may reduce the daily requirement for enzyme replacer. Diets high in fibre (particularly soluble fibre) are to be avoided, since they interfere with pancreatic enzyme activity. Requirements for cobalamin (vitamin B12) are often raised with EPI, and those for zinc and copper may be marginally increased. Cobalamin deficiency may also occur with EPI but can be corrected by parenteral supplementation.

Pancreatitis

The initial therapy of acute pancreatitis is aimed at preventing the secretion of proteolytic enzymes from the exocrine pancreas, which promote further tissue damage within the organ. This involves a strict policy of nil by mouth (food and water) for 2–5 days, with the parenteral administration of fluid and electrolytes. If vomiting does not occur for 48 hours, oral electrolyte drinks may be given for 1–2 days before the gradual reintroduction of solid food.

High-carbohydrate foods (such as rice, pasta or potatoes), which have the least stimulating effect on pancreatic secretions, may be offered initially in several small feeds per day. If this is tolerated, a highly digestible, low-fat diet may be offered, in which the protein content is moderately reduced and of high biological value. This type of diet is useful in the recovery period of acute pancreatitis and may also help to prevent recurrent bouts of chronic pancreatitis.

Liver disease

Hepatobiliary disease can lead to derangements in both the metabolism and storage of proteins, fats, carbohydrates and certain micronutrients, as well as in the detoxification of potentially hazardous by-products. Hepatic encephalopathy (HE) can occur where there is either critical loss of functional hepatic tissue (60–70%) or portosystemic shunting. In HE, a number of neurotoxic substances (mainly ammonia) may enter the peripheral and cerebral circulation, giving rise to a complex of neurological signs. These toxins are derived mainly from the alimentary tract, being synthesized by gastrointestinal flora or consumed in the diet, but ammonia is also produced as a by-product of protein catabolism and when amino acids are converted to glucose and energy via gluconeogenesis.

The liver has a large functional reserve and a phenomenal capacity for regeneration following insult. Nutritional support during the period of hepatocellular repair can help to delay or prevent irreversible progression of the disease. For dogs, this can be achieved by modification of the diet in the following ways:

- **Adequate energy provision, using non-protein sources.** This limits ammonia production by avoiding the use of amino acids to provide energy and by preventing muscle wasting.
- **Moderate restriction of dietary protein** to help to limit the amount of ammonia generated both in the intestines and from the use of amino acids for gluconeogenesis.

However, dietary protein intake must be carefully balanced to meet the individual animal's needs, since an inadequate intake will promote the breakdown of structural proteins.

- **High-quality proteins** are recommended since they tend to be highly digestible and are likely to meet the animal's needs with minimal production of ammonia.
- **Careful use of fat as an energy source**, to increase the energy density of the diet and improve palatability. Both these effects are beneficial in the management of dogs with liver disease, since inappetence is a common problem. However, moderate fat restriction is indicated in dogs with an impaired ability to digest fat due to a lack of bile.
- **Provision of complex carbohydrates**, such as starch and fibre, in the diet. This will improve glucose utilization by slowing down the delivery of glucose from the gut to the liver.
- **Inclusion of dietary fibre.** This may assist in the elimination of ammonia and other toxins in the faeces, inhibits ammonia production by bacteria in the colon and prevents constipation, which is also important in the management of HE.
- **Supplementation with water-soluble vitamins (B-complex)** to compensate for impaired synthesis and increased losses of these nutrients. Supplementation with vitamin E may be beneficial in limiting ongoing liver disease.
- **Supplementation with zinc**, which is involved in the detoxification of ammonia. This can help to improve nervous signs associated with HE. Zinc reduces fibrosis and, by reducing the availability of copper, provides protection against liver injury associated with copper accumulation in the liver. This is particularly beneficial in patients with copper storage liver disease.
- **Restriction of dietary copper intake.** Copper accumulates within the liver during chronic liver diseases and contributes to hepatocellular damage, inflammation and fibrosis.
- **Moderate restriction of sodium intake**, especially where liver disease is associated with hypoalbuminaemia or portal hypertension. An excessive intake can precipitate or exacerbate ascites.

Cats

Diets for cats with liver disease must meet the normally high feline requirements for protein and essential amino acids. Protein-restricted diets are *not* recommended unless the disease is accompanied by HE, which is rare in cats. The protein content of these diets should be of high biological value and ensure an adequate intake of arginine, taurine and carnitine. Diets formulated for the management of feline chronic renal failure may be appropriate in this minority of cases.

Most cats with liver disease, particularly those with hepatic lipidosis, may have increased protein requirements and the requirements for B-complex vitamins and fat-soluble vitamins K and E may similarly be raised. High-fat diets may be detrimental in feline hepatic lipidosis and in cats with other forms of hepatic disease. Highly digestible diets with a relatively high protein content, moderately reduced fat content and enhanced levels of zinc and vitamins B, K and E are likely to be of benefit in most cats with hepatic disease. For cats with hepatic lipidosis, enteral tube feeding will almost certainly be required.

Diabetes mellitus

Animals with diabetes mellitus have impaired production or release of insulin, which may be combined with a tissue insensitivity to insulin (insulin resistance). This results in an imbalance in the metabolism of carbohydrate, fat and protein and is characterized by hyperglycaemia and an inability to regulate blood sugar levels. Successful long-term management of diabetes mellitus involves a combination of appropriate insulin replacement therapy and a suitable dietary regimen. The aim is to provide a consistent supply of nutrients to match the activity of exogenous insulin and thereby achieve relatively stable blood glucose levels. Consistency in the feeding regimen is essential and involves standardization of the quantity of food given, the dietary content (energy density and dietary constituents) and the timing of meals. The exercise routine, which may alter the animal's energy requirements, should also be carefully regulated. A schedule should be established that is compatible with the normal household routine. Feeding a patient with diabetes mellitus should incorporate the following.

- **Timing of feeding** should be arranged such that maximal absorption and metabolism of nutrients coincides with maximal activity of administered insulin and may vary with the type of insulin preparation used. Insulins with an intermediate duration of action (such as lente or isophane preparations in dogs and lente or protamine zinc preparations in cats) are commonly used as single or, where insulin metabolism is faster, as twice-daily injections.
- **Increasing the number of meals** daily reduces the degree of postprandial hyperglycaemia and improves glycaemic control, provided that the meals are fed whilst the injected insulin is still active. In most cases, however, the daily food allowance may be divided into two meals. When insulin is injected once daily, one meal may be fed at the time of injection with the second meal given 6–8 hours later. When insulin is given twice daily, meals should be given either at injection times (2 meals/day) or additionally at times of peak insulin activity (3–4 meals/day).

For canine diabetics, modification of the diet can help to improve glycaemic control and may reduce the requirement for replacement insulin therapy:

- **Simple sugars**, such as glucose, sucrose and lactose, are to be avoided (other than in the emergency treatment of hypoglycaemia resulting from insulin overdosage) since they are rapidly absorbed and promote wide fluctuations in blood sugar levels
- **Complex carbohydrates** such as starch are digested relatively slowly and result in a more gradual release of glucose into the circulation over a period of hours
- **Dietary fibre** further slows down the rate of digestion within the gut lumen and therefore slows the rate of postprandial nutrient uptake. When combined with the slow digestion of starch, this effect helps to reduce postprandial glycaemic peaks
- **High-fat diets** should be avoided since diabetics tend to develop hyperlipidaemia and other lipid-related complications

The benefits of high-fibre, high-starch diets have not been clearly demonstrated in diabetic cats, which are poorly adapted to high-carbohydrate diets. Current recommendations are to feed diabetic cats a 'normal' diet, i.e. one that is high in protein and low in carbohydrate. Semi-moist diets, which are rich in simple sugars, are contraindicated.

If the diabetic animal is also obese (which can exacerbate diabetes), weight reduction measures should be incorporated into the diabetic regimen. Dietary therapy for other coexisting disease, such as chronic renal failure, hepatic disease, congestive heart failure or chronic gastrointestinal disease, may take priority over diets designed for improving glycaemic control, but, again, consistency in the feeding regimen is the rule.

Chronic renal failure

Chronic renal failure (CRF) is a relatively common syndrome in older dogs and cats and represents the end stage of a number of renal diseases. It is a progressive condition in which existing renal damage is irreversible, but dietary measures can improve the clinical signs of uraemia associated with CRF and may help to slow progression of the condition.

Clinical signs of CRF are not apparent until at least 65–75% of renal tissue is destroyed. Since many of the clinical signs related to CRF are associated with the accumulation of toxic protein catabolites and failure to excrete phosphorus, the emphasis in dietary therapy is on modification of the phosphorus and protein contents of the diet. Other dietary components to be considered include calcium, sodium, potassium and water-soluble vitamins, together with the dietary energy content and fat. Maintenance of normal hydration is also important, through the provision of unlimited access to drinking water or via fluid replacement in cases of persistent vomiting.

Phosphorus restriction

Dietary phosphorus restriction is an important part of management of CRF and should be initiated early in the course of the disease. This helps to limit renal mineralization and secondary hyperparathyroidism. In cats, feeding a diet low in phosphorus and protein content has been shown to double their lifespan as compared with cats with CRF fed normal diets. In dogs, this type of diet has been shown to slow progression of renal damage.

Protein restriction

Restriction of dietary protein is of clinical benefit in uraemic patients, since this minimizes the accumulation of nitrogenous waste associated with protein breakdown, helps to limit the intake of dietary phosphorus and reduces the protein-related solute load on the failing kidneys, thereby lessening the severity of polydipsia/polyuria. Excessive protein restriction is to be avoided, since it can result in protein malnutrition in both dogs and cats. The protein in diets for patients with CRF should be of high biological value.

Dogs

For dogs with CRF, a staged approach to management is recommended and early cases may benefit from phosphorus restriction whilst maintaining a 'normal' protein intake. More advanced cases that are showing clinical signs of uraemia should be fed diets that are restricted in both phosphorus and protein. Where possible, the degree of protein restriction should be individualized according to the dog's clinical and biochemical status.

Cats

The potential risks of dietary protein reduction are greater in the cat than in the dog. It is currently recommended that well hydrated cats with azotaemia (increased concentrations of urea, creatinine or other non-protein nitrogenous compounds in blood) and hyperphosphataemia (or hypoparathyroidism) should be fed diets that are restricted in phosphorus and moderately restricted in protein.

Energy density

Feeding an energy-dense diet, in which the energy content is derived from non-protein sources, avoids tissue catabolism and helps to reduce nitrogenous waste production. Appetite is often poor in affected animals and so the energy density of the diet should be high, to enable the animal to obtain its nutritional requirements from a relatively small volume of food. Fat is particularly useful in this respect, since it increases energy density and aids palatability of the diet. For this reason, canned diets designed to support dogs and cats with CRF tend to be high in fat.

Potassium, calcium and sodium

Many cats with CRF are hypokalaemic and require some degree of dietary potassium supplementation. However, some cats (often those most severely affected) are hyperkalaemic and so serum potassium levels should be closely monitored in cats with CRF.

Serum calcium levels may be low, normal or high in patients with CRF. Calcium supplementation may be required in hypocalcaemic individuals.

Sodium balance may be disrupted in advanced CRF and systemic hypertension can occur in both dogs and cats. It is currently recommended that dietary sodium levels are either normal or moderately restricted, since excessive sodium restriction may also be detrimental.

Vitamins

Requirements for water-soluble (B-complex) vitamins may be increased in dogs and cats with CRF because of reduced intake (inappetence), increased urinary losses in polyuric cases and higher demands during the recuperative processes.

Urolithiasis

Urolithiasis is the disease that results from the formation of calculi (uroliths) within the urinary tract. Crystals form in urine when the concentrations of its constituents exceed a critical level of supersaturation. Dietary factors can profoundly influence urolith formation, because dietary ingredients and feeding patterns influence the pH, volume and solute concentration of the urine.

Urolithiasis is an important cause of feline lower urinary tract diseases (FLUTD), particularly in obstructed cases. Traditionally, struvite urolithiasis has been of greatest importance but, although the incidence has declined in recent years, calcium oxalate urolithiasis is now seen with increasing frequency. Uroliths that are commonly found in dogs include struvite, calcium oxalate, cystine and ammonium urate. Mixed calculi may also occur in some cases. Various types of urolith may be found in both cats and dogs. In both species magnesium ammonium phosphate (struvite) and calcium oxalate form most frequently.

Struvite

Factors that decrease the risk of struvite (magnesium ammonium phosphate) crystal formation in urine include:

- Acidification of the urine (to between pH 6.0 and 6.5 in cats and between pH 5.5 and 6.0 in dogs)
- Increased urine volume to dilute solute concentrations and increase the frequency of urination
- Moderate restriction of dietary magnesium and phosphorus.

Diets that achieve these goals may be used to dissolve struvite uroliths in situ or to prevent recurrence of the condition. Initial relief of obstructed cases may require surgical intervention.

Commercial diets are available that have been designed to achieve urinary undersaturation with struvite, but urinary acidifiers may be added to an animal's normal diet to achieve the appropriate effect. Diets of high moisture content and high digestibility are preferred, but water may also be added to dry foods if necessary. Moderate supplementation with sodium chloride (salt) may stimulate thirst and promote increased water turnover. Acidified diets are not appropriate for feeding to young animals or to pregnant or lactating females. Furthermore, levels of taurine and potassium should be enhanced when acidified diets are fed to cats.

The main difference between canine and feline struvite urolithiasis is that, in dogs, struvite uroliths are usually associated with urinary tract infection, whereas most feline struvite uroliths are sterile. Urease-producing bacteria such as staphylococci and *Proteus* spp. create an increasingly alkaline environment and conditions that are ideal for the formation of struvite and, occasionally, other types of urolith. Where infection is present, prolonged antibiotic therapy is essential in addition to dietary and other measures. Dietary protein restriction may also be beneficial in these cases, since this reduces the available substrate in urine for urease-producing bacteria.

Calcium oxalate

It is not possible to dissolve calcium oxalate uroliths in situ by dietary or any other means, and surgery is currently the only method of removing them in dogs and cats. Nevertheless, dietary manipulation can help to prevent recurrence of the condition. The goal is to reduce urinary saturation with calcium oxalate. Diets designed for the management of calcium oxalate urolithiasis should promote increased urine volume, preferably through the addition of water to the food. Although restriction of dietary calcium and oxalate may be beneficial, restriction of only one of these components may increase intestinal absorption of the other. Increased magnesium intake is sometimes recommended in the prevention of calcium oxalate urolithiasis, but care should be taken to ensure that this does not predispose the animal to struvite urolith formation.

Cystine

Cystine urolithiasis occurs in dogs with an inherited defect in cystine metabolism, resulting in impaired reabsorption of the amino acid from the proximal tubule of the kidney and, hence, cystinuria. This leads to cystine urolith formation since cystine is relatively insoluble, particularly in acidic urine. Dissolution and prevention of recurrence of cystine uroliths can be achieved through:

- Increasing water intake to increase urine volume
- Reduction of dietary protein to reduce cystine excretion
- Alkalinization of urine (with bicarbonate or citrate) to increase cystine solubility
- Administration of compounds such as D-penicillamine or 2-mercaptopropionylglycine (2-MPG), which convert cystine to a more soluble compound.

Ammonium urate

Urate uroliths occur mostly in Dalmatians and in patients with portosystemic shunts, when hepatic conversion of uric acid (a product of purine metabolism) to allantoin is impaired. Allantoin is highly soluble but increased urinary excretion of uric acid may predispose the dog to urolith formation.

Surgical relief of obstruction may be required in some cases. In others, dissolution and prevention of recurrence of urate uroliths may be achieved by:

- Restriction of dietary protein to limit purine intake
- Supplementation with potassium citrate to promote neutral or slightly alkaline urine
- Increased water intake
- Administration of allopurinol, which inhibits uric acid production.

Idiopathic cystitis in cats

For a significant proportion of cats with non-obstructive lower urinary tract disease, a specific cause cannot be identified for this clinical sign and the condition is classified as 'idiopathic'. Although clinical signs resolve spontaneously within 5–7 days, many cases recur after a variable period. Studies have shown that the rate of recurrence can be reduced by feeding a canned diet formulated for the production of acidic urine, although the equivalent dry formulation has no impact on the biological behaviour of the disease.

Skin disease

Deficiencies in essential fatty acids, protein, zinc, vitamins A and E and certain B-complex vitamins may give rise to skin disease. In addition, supplementation with supraphysiological doses of certain nutrients, including vitamin A and essential fatty acids, have been used in the treatment of specific skin conditions where no apparent dietary deficiency exists. Essential fatty acids, particularly those of the omega 3 series found in marine fish oils, are currently thought to be of greatest value in the management of pruritic skin diseases associated with hypersensitivity reactions. Another area in which diet is related to skin disease is that of dietary sensitivity which, in dogs and cats, is commonly manifest as a pruritic skin disorder.

Cardiac disease

Early-stage heart disease

Dogs with early or low-grade heart disease, i.e. those with little or no limitation of physical activity, can benefit from dietary modifications to slow the progression of disease and delay the occurrence of congestive heart failure and end-stage disease. Supplementation with arginine, carnitine and taurine may improve heart muscle function, blood flow and exercise tolerance. Sodium should be mildly restricted and levels of potassium and magnesium controlled to correct for losses associated with heart failure and any drug therapies (see 'Congestive heart failure' below).

Congestive heart failure

Congestive heart failure is associated with retention of sodium and water. Restriction of dietary sodium is a useful dietary strategy that helps to decrease fluid retention. Renal function is often compromised in cardiac failure and so the transition to a low-sodium diet should take place gradually (over at least 5 days) to allow the kidneys to adapt.

Weight loss is common in cardiac patients (cardiac cachexia) as a consequence of a number of factors. Patients are often anorectic and malabsorption may occur as a result of reduced intestinal perfusion. Furthermore, energy requirements may be increased, which can accelerate the wasting process. It is essential to ensure an adequate energy intake and some form of nutritional support is necessary if voluntary intake is reduced.

Fat may improve palatability and increase the energy density of the diet, but high-fat diets may not be appropriate in all cases. Some cardiac patients may be obese; for these, controlled weight reduction can help to improve clinical status.

Some degree of renal and hepatic dysfunction is often associated with congestive heart failure. Diets in which the protein content is moderately restricted and of high biological value should be introduced for these patients, but in other patients with protein energy malnutrition an increase in protein intake may be necessary.

Diuretic agents can have a marked effect on nutritional requirements, particularly for sodium and potassium, and may increase urinary losses of water-soluble vitamins (B-complex). Long-term use of furosemide or thiazide diuretics may cause potassium depletion and may also promote urinary magnesium loss. Conversely, spironolactone tends to conserve potassium but sodium excretion is enhanced, and in this case low-sodium diets should be avoided. Low-salt diets should also be used with care when vasodilators such as captopril and enalapril are administered, since these drugs are also associated with sodium loss and potassium retention.

Dilated cardiomyopathy

Low myocardial concentrations of carnitine have been associated with dilated cardiomyopathy in some dogs, notably Boxers, and dietary supplementation with L-carnitine (not D-carnitine or a mixture of D- and L-carnitine) is recommended as an adjunct to conventional medical therapy. In cats, many cases of dilated cardiomyopathy have been linked to taurine deficiency and so plasma taurine status should be determined in all cases, prior to supplementation. Where appropriate, the deficient diet should be replaced with a feline diet of adequate taurine content and additional taurine supplementation should be provided as necessary, usually for a period of 12–16 weeks.

Further reading

Agar S (2001) *Small Animal Nutrition*. Butterworth Heinemann, Oxford

Burger I (1993) *The Waltham Book of Companion Animal Nutrition*. Pergamon Press, Oxford

Calvert I (2004) Nutrition. In: *BSAVA Manual of Reptiles, 2nd edn* (eds SJ Girling and P Raiti), pp. 18–39. BSAVA Publications, Gloucester

FEDIAF (2001) *Guideline for complete and complementary pet food for cats and dogs*. FEDIAF, Bruxelles, Belgium

Girling S (2003) *Veterinary Nursing of Exotic Pets*. Blackwell Publishing, Oxford

Hand MS, Thatcher CD, Remillard RL and Roudebush P (2000) *Small Animal Clinical Nutrition, 4th edn*, Mark Morris Institute, Kansas

Harcourt-Brown F (2002) Diet and husbandry. In: *Textbook of Rabbit Medicine*, pp. 19–51. Butterworth Heinemann, Oxford

Harper EJ and Skinner ND (1998) Clinical nutrition of small psittacines and passerines. *Seminars in Avian and Exotic Pet Medicine*, **7**(3), 116–127

Kelly N and Wills J (1996) *BSAVA Manual of Companion Animal Nutrition and Feeding*. BSAVA Publications, Gloucester

Markwell PJ (1994) *Applied Clinical Nutrition of the Dog and Cat*. Waltham Centre for Pet Nutrition, Melton Mowbray

Meredith A and Redrobe S (2002) *BSAVA Manual of Exotic Pets, 4th edn*. BSAVA Publications, Cheltenham

Thorne C (1992) *The Waltham Book of Dog and Cat Behaviour*. Pergamon Press, Oxford

Wildgoose W (2001) *BSAVA Manual of Ornamental Fish, 2nd edn*. BSAVA Publications, Gloucester

Wills J and Simpson KW (eds) (1994) *The Waltham Book of Clinical Nutrition of the Dog and Cat*. Pergamon Press, Oxford

Chapter 17

Laboratory diagnostic aids

Anne Ward and Donald Mactaggart

Learning objectives

After studying this chapter, students should be able to:

- Identify the requirements of a veterinary practice laboratory
- List the essential equipment used in the practice laboratory
- Collect and prepare specimens for submission to an external laboratory
- Identify the procedures for performing haematology, biochemistry, urinalysis and faecal and skin examinations
- State the key legislation pertaining to the laboratory

The veterinary practice laboratory

The requirement to have improved and accessible laboratory diagnosis within the veterinary practice is increasing every day. Veterinarians depend on this vital service, whether it is for the preoperative general screening of an animal's health or for the critically ill animal rushed to the practice in the middle of the night. In both circumstances, the requirement is there for immediate and reliable results that will enhance the treatment and care being provided for that animal.

Health and safety

It is necessary that all general health and safety principles are maintained, especially when dealing with hazardous or biological specimens (see Chapter 1). Strict rules must be followed when working within the laboratory, and the recommended health and safety guidelines must be adhered to at all times.

Staff are reminded that they are responsible not only for their own health and safety but also for that of others who may be affected by their actions.

Recommended health and safety guidelines for laboratory work

- Read the practice Local Rules relating to risks in the laboratory.
- Read the practice COSHH assessments for the laboratory.
- Switch off all mobile phones before entering the laboratory.
- Personal Protective Equipment (PPE) is to be worn at all times in the laboratory. Do not wear your laboratory coat outside the laboratory.
- Wear gloves when carrying out any laboratory procedure.
- Keep long hair tied back.
- Be aware of potential zoonotic risks. Women should be particularly aware of the possibility of *Toxoplasma* infection when working with cat faeces and the implications to themselves.
- Containers must be clearly labelled with their contents and dilution rates. Never put substances into or use substances from unmarked containers.
- Return equipment to its storage point at the end of every session.
- Dispose of all normal, clinical, special and glass waste in the correct manner.
- All contaminated 'sharps' and syringes must be placed into the appropriate clinical waste containers provided in the laboratory.
- Wash your hands at the start and end of each laboratory session.
- Dress appropriately; do not wear any materials or jewellery that may dangle down.
- No smoking, eating (including chewing gum) or drinking is allowed in the laboratory at any time.
- Keep work areas tidy and disinfected prior to and at the conclusion of each laboratory task.
- Know where the first aid kit is and what actions to take in the event of an accident. Be familiar with the accident book routine.

continues ▶

continued
- All chemical spillages/accidents must be reported to the appropriate member of staff at once. Immediately wipe up any liquid spilt on the floor and ensure safe footwear.
- Any accident, however trivial, should be reported to the appropriate member of staff.

Legal Acts and Regulations of particular importance to the laboratory include:

- Health and Safety at Work etc., Act 1974
- Control of Substances Hazardous to Health (COSHH) 2002
- Control of Pollution (Special Waste) (Amendment) Regulations 1988
- Collection and Disposal of Waste Regulations 1988
- Hazardous Waste (England and Wales) Regulations 2005
- Scientific Procedures Act 1986 (amended 1993)
- Environmental Protection Act 1990
- Reporting of Diseases and Dangerous Occurrences Regulations (RIDDOR) 1995
- First Aid at Work Regulations 1981.

Legislation may vary within the United Kingdom. For more information refer to Chapter 1 and the Health and Safety Executive website http://www.hse.gov.uk .

Risks and hazards

Infection
Some pathogens (e.g. *Salmonella*) present a higher risk than others. Pregnant women should avoid handling any specimens that may contain *Chlamydophila* (e.g. feline eye or avian tissues) or *Toxoplasma* (cat faeces) because of the dangers that could pass to a developing fetus.

Chemicals
Many chemicals in the laboratory are toxic, corrosive or flammable and should be handled with care (Figure 17.1).

Equipment
Maintenance of laboratory equipment should be carried out routinely. Instructions for its use should be clearly displayed and the manufacturer's instructions followed.

Classification and abbreviation	Sign	Description of hazard	Precautions
Explosive (E)		Chemicals that explode	Use only as directed Keep tightly closed, cool and in a ventilated place Keep away from sources of heat or ignition Dispose of safely and as directed
Oxidizing (O)		Chemicals that react exothermically (releases heat) with other chemicals	Use only as directed Keep tightly closed and in a ventilated place Keep away from sources of heat or ignition This material and its container must be disposed of in a safe way
Extremely flammable (F+) / Highly flammable (F)		Chemicals that may catch fire in contact with air, only need brief contact with an ignition source, have a very low flash point or evolve highly flammable gases in contact with water	Keep container tightly closed Keep away from sources of heat or ignition Do not breathe vapour or spray Take precautionary measures against static discharges
Very toxic (T+) / Toxic (T)		May cause death or acute or chronic damage to health when inhaled, swallowed or absorbed through the skin	Wear suitable protective clothing, gloves and eye/face protection After contact with skin, wash immediately with plenty of water In case of contact with eyes, rinse immediately with plenty of water and seek medical advice In case of accident or if you feel unwell, seek medical advice immediately
Corrosive (C)		Chemicals that may destroy living tissue on contact	Wear suitable gloves and eye/face protection Take off all contaminated clothing immediately In case of contact with skin, wash immediately with plenty of water In case of contact with eyes, rinse immediately (for 15 minutes) with plenty of water and seek medical advice
Harmful (Xn) (Xi)		Chemicals that may cause damage to health (Xn) or may cause inflammation to the skin or other mucous membranes (Xi)	Do not breathe vapour, spray or dust Avoid contact with skin Wash hands thoroughly before you eat, drink or smoke In case of contact, rinse immediately with plenty of water and seek advice
Dangerous for the environment (N)		Presents or may present an immediate or delayed danger for one or more parts of the environment	Do not empty into drains Keep away from food, drink and animal feeding stuffs This material and its container must be disposed of in a safe way

17.1   'Dangerous substances': common health hazards in the laboratory.   *continues* ▶

Classification and abbreviation	Sign	Description of hazard	Precautions
Carcinogenic (Carc), Mutagenic (Muta)		Chemicals that may induce cancer (Carc) or heritable genetic defects (Muta) or increase their incidence if inhaled, ingested or allowed to penetrate the skin	Wear suitable protective clothing, gloves and eye/face protection In case of contact with skin, wash immediately with plenty of water In case of contact with eyes, rinse immediately (for 15 minutes) with plenty of water and seek medical advice In case of accident or if you feel unwell, seek medical advice immediately
Reproduction (Repr)		Chemicals that produce or increase the incidence of non-heritable adverse affects in the progeny and/or impairment of male or female reproductive functions of capacity	Wear suitable protective clothing, gloves and eye/face protection In case of contact with skin, wash immediately with plenty of water In case of contact with eyes, rinse immediately (for 15 minutes) with plenty of water and seek medical advice In case of accident or if you feel unwell, seek medical advice immediately

17.1 *continued* 'Dangerous substances': common health hazards in the laboratory.

Laboratory equipment

The correct management of equipment and materials found in the laboratory is critical in ensuring accuracy, reliability and safe usage. It is important to identify any faults that may occur, such as damage or contamination, and how these should then be handled, along with the necessary procedures that may be required for control of infection.

Glassware

Laboratory glassware includes flasks, beakers, watch-glasses, test tubes and centrifuge test tubes.

Care and cleaning of laboratory glassware

1. Wear gloves.
2. Place used glassware into disinfectant as soon as possible.
3. Remove gross dirt with a soft-bristled brush.
4. Clean glassware in a fresh solution of detergent.
5. Leave to soak, or clean ultrasonically (if available).
6. Rinse in distilled or deionized water.
7. Repeat rinsing 2–3 times or until all of the detergent has been rinsed away.
8. Allow to drain.
9. Air dry or place inside a drying cabinet or oven.
10. Store in a clean, dry and dust-free environment.

The microscope

A comfortable workstation with a good microscope is a necessity. The microscope is an optical instrument made up of several elements (Figure 17.2).

The total magnification of the microscope is the product of the objective magnification multiplied by the ocular magnification. Thus, a x40 objective lens with a x10 ocular lens provides a total magnification of 400 times the original specimen.

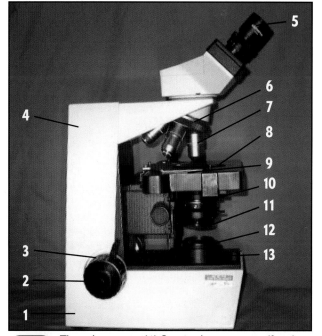

17.2 The microscope. (**1**) Supporting structure (foot/base, limb and body). (**2**) Fine focus knob (used for racking stage up and down slowly). (**3**) Coarse focus knob (used for racking stage up and down more quickly). (**4**) Limb (main body of microscope). (**5**) Eyepiece (usually x6 or x10 lens). (**6**) Nosepiece (holds objectives). (**7**) Objectives (containing several lenses, engraved with each magnification; x100 for use with oil immersion only, letters OI may be used, oil increases resolution; magnification produced by objective and by eyepieces). (**8**) Stage (holds microscope slide in place). (**9**) Vernier scale (recording apparatus allowing particular position of microscope slide to be relocated exactly). (**10**) Substage condenser (allows focus of light source on object, giving good resolution and consistent illumination). (**11**) Substage iris diaphragm (adjusts amount of light to condenser and increases resolution). (**12**) Lamp iris diaphragm (reduces glare, thus improving contrast). (**13**) Rheostat (modifies intensity of light source).

Care and cleaning of a light microscope

- Do not place near a window (because of increased heat or moisture).
- Do not place near vibrations (i.e. doors, centrifuge), liquids or draughts.
- Keep microscope free from dust and oil; always replace dust cover when not in use.
- When carrying a microscope, always hold at the 'limb' and support under the 'base/foot'.
- Keep stage clean; always wipe the underneath surface of a slide before placing on the stage.
- Oil any moving parts as necessary.
- Use special lens cleaning tissue or a soft brush to clean the eyepiece lens or objectives. (Never use alcohol to clean the lens, as it may soften the mounting material.)
- Remove oil from the objective using lens paper (oil can seep into the objective and damage the lens).
- Keep objectives and eyepieces in their containers when not in use.
- Always remove samples when not in use.
- When replacing a bulb, the microscope must be switched off and unplugged. Once the bulb has cooled, it can be removed and replaced.
- If the microscope is used frequently during the day, leave the light on continuously as this will extend the life of the bulb compared with switching it off and on each time it is used.

Using a light microscope

1. Remove dust cover and plug the lead into the electrical socket.
2. Lower the stage to its lowest point.
3. Check that the rheostat is turned down low.
4. Switch on the light; turn the rheostat up to increase the light further.
5. Inspect the eyepieces, objectives and condenser lens and clean with lens-cleaning tissue if necessary.
6. Place the slide or counting chamber on the stage with the appropriate side up and frosted edge or identification detail to the left.
7. Move the lowest objective (x4) into position by turning the turret or nose piece (not the objective lens) and ensure that the lens clicks firmly into place.
8. Without looking down the eyepieces, rack the stage up as high as it can go so that it is almost (but not actually) touching the slide. *Never rack the stage up when viewing through the eyepiece (the slide might be broken and the microscope could be damaged).*
9. Looking through the eyepieces, adjust the distance between them so that each field appears almost identical and the two fields can be viewed as one.
10. Slowly rack down whilst looking down the eyepieces, using the coarse focus knob (CFK).
11. Once an image is in view, use the fine focus knob (FFK) to refine the detail further.
12. Adjust the condenser and diaphragms according to the manufacturer's instructions to provide optimal light.

▶

13. When using the x10 objective:
    - Look for a suitable examination area using the x4 (low-power) objective
    - Swing the x10 objective into place.
    - The FFK is now used to bring the image into view.
14. When using the x40 (high-dry) objective:
    - Complete the steps using the x4 and the x10 objective before rotating the x40 objective into place
    - Use the FFK to refine the image.
15. Do not use oil on the slide when using a x4, x10 or x40 objective.
16. When using the x100 (oil) objective (to view blood smears and bacteria), follow these steps:
    i. Fully open the iris diaphragm
    ii. Set the condenser at its highest point
    iii. Rack the stage down so that you can place a drop of oil on the area that is to be viewed
    iv. Rotate the oil immersion objective into place
    v. Without looking down the eyepieces, rack the stage up until the objective passes through the oil and almost comes into contact with the slide
    vi. Very slowly rack down the CFK until an image appears and use the FFK to refine this image further
    vii. If the objective comes out of the oil it has been racked too far; therefore repeat the process in raising the stage then viewing by racking slowly down again, first using the CFK then the FFK
    viii. Once in focus the objective will slide across the surface of the slide as you look for cells
    ix. The oil acts as an extension to the lens
    x. Immediately clean the oil off the x100 objective with appropriate lens tissue.
17. Once an image is in view, use the **battlement technique** to scan the slide thoroughly.

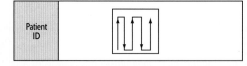

18. To work out the magnification, multiply the eyepiece magnification by the objective magnification.
19. When finished:
    i. Turn the light down
    ii. Lower the stage completely, using the CFK
    iii. Remove the slide or counting chamber
    iv. Rotate the nosepiece to the lowest objective again
    v. Check and clean the oil immersion lens again, if necessary
    vi. Rack the stage as high as it can go
    vii. Switch off at the plug before removing
    viii. Replace dust cover
    ix. Place microscope back into its allocated storage point.

The Vernier scale

On a microscope there are two main scales. The vertical main scale reads from 0 to 40 and the horizontal main scales reads from 40 to 100, which means that the two readings will not become confused. Each main scale has a vernier scale attached, reading from 0 to 10, to provide two readings for the exact location on a microscope slide if required later for relocation. A measurement is made by combining the readings from the two scales (Figure 17.3).

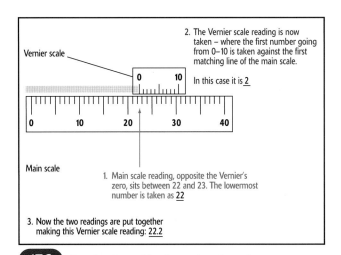

Vernier scale

2. The Vernier scale reading is now taken – where the first number going from 0–10 is taken against the first matching line of the main scale.

0   10

In this case it is <u>2</u>

0   10   20   30   40

Main scale

1. Main scale reading, opposite the Vernier's zero, sits between 22 and 23. The lowermost number is taken as <u>22</u>

3. Now the two readings are put together making this Vernier scale reading: <u>22.2</u>

17.3 Reading from Vernier and main scales.

Centrifuges

A centrifuge is an essential piece of equipment that spins a substance in order to separate the fluid portion from the solid content using centrifugal force (Figure 17.4). The soluble liquid portion of a sample following centrifugation is known as the **supernatant**; the material settling at the bottom of the liquid is the **sediment**. Usually an electric motor drives the rotary motion of the sample. The principles behind the use, care and maintenance of the different centrifuges are relatively generic.

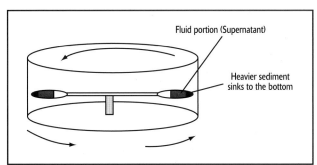

Fluid portion (Supernatant)

Heavier sediment sinks to the bottom

17.4 Swing-out style of centrifuge, demonstrating the separation of a substance under centrifugal force.

The inner bowl of the centrifuge is a solid piece of metal designed as a guard to retain the rotor buckets and samples should they become detached. Modern centrifuges have a number of built-in safety devices, including a lid-lock that cannot be opened until spinning has finished and that will not operate unless correctly loaded. A safety plate is present either as a separate screw-on lid or as a built-in part of the main lid. Samples are placed into buckets that have rubber cushions at the bottom to prevent breakages.

The **microhaematocrit centrifuge** has a special type of rotor consisting of an almost flat horizontal surface with slots for capillary tubes (Figure 17.5). There is a rubber cushion on the outside of the lip of the rotor and a safety plate is screwed down to hold the tubes firmly in place. With this type of centrifuge it is possible to remove the microhaematocrit plate and replace with a plate that can accommodate centrifuge containers for blood samples undergoing plasma or serum estimations.

It is important that appropriate quality checks are put in place to ensure standardization and control of results.

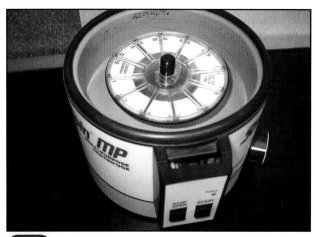

17.5 Microhaematocrit centrifuge.

Speeds and times

The style of buckets within the centrifuge or the actual size of the centrifuge will determine the type of container for the sample. Once the sample has been secured in place, a determined time and speed appropriate to the sample being centrifuged are selected. This selection differs according to the variance in viscosity and cell content of the substance. As a guideline, speeds and times for different substances are as follows:

- Blood: 10,000 rpm for 5 minutes
- Urine: 2000 rpm for 5 minutes
- Faeces: 1000–1500 rpm for 3 minutes.

Rules for using a centrifuge

- Always balance out the samples – try to spin four samples in total, so that results can be compared and a mean result taken.
- Build up speed slowly and avoid using the brake for slowing the speed down.
- Always place on a flat sturdy surface.
- Never lift up the lid when in use.
- Make sure that the safety lid is secured in place if spinning micro/haematocrit tubes.
- Clean up any spillages immediately.
- Service regularly.
- Clean routinely: the entire head, bowl, rubber cushion and safety plate should be wiped out, cleaned and disinfected.

The Bunsen burner

A diagram of a gas Bunsen burner is shown in Figure 17.6.

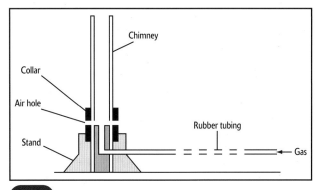

Chimney

Collar

Air hole

Stand

Rubber tubing

Gas

17.6 The Bunsen burner.

Using a Bunsen burner

- Keep long hair tied back.
- The air hole *must* be closed prior to lighting the chimney.
- When flame is not being used, always return to a gold flame by closing the air hole.
- Blue flames should only be used when heating directly.
- Be aware of the location of the emergency switch to turn off the gas supply if needed.

Incubator

The incubator is a heated cabinet used during the culture of bacteria or fungi. It has a temperature range of 25–100°C but is usually kept at 37°C to mimic normal body temperature. An inner glass door allows contents to be checked without lowering the temperature. Plates are placed lid-side down in the incubator, to reduce condensation on agar surfaces.

Analysers

Many different types of analyser are available and each comes with guidelines and instructions that should be read thoroughly before using the equipment. Most manufacturers also provide training during installation.

With analysers in the correct hands, an up-to-date laboratory can provide immediate information on blood chemistry, electrolytes, hormones, haematology and blood gases. A thorough and accurate picture of a patient's health status can be obtained quickly.

Advantages of an in-house analyser

- Provision of general health profiles and pre-anaesthetic screening
- Fast diagnosis for emergency cases
- Revenue for the practice
- Single-test or panel-testing flexibility
- Rapid response to patients' needs
- Simple to use and to maintain
- Simple reports
- Quality assurance tests available to check accuracy
- Reliable and comprehensive technical and educational support available from the equipment provider

Collection and storage of specimens

Laboratory tests play a key role in determining the health status of an animal. Whether the sample is tested in-house or by an external laboratory, the reliability of the results depends on how the sample was collected, how it was transported and how it was processed within the laboratory.

With the increasing risk of litigation, it is essential that tests are recorded accurately and clearly in case they are needed as evidence. There is also a legal obligation to maintain patient records for a minimum of 7 years.

The reason that a sample is being tested (e.g. haematology, parasitology, differential count, biochemistry, toxicology or DNA studies) will determine the appropriate method of collection. External laboratories will have a protocol describing how a particular sample should be obtained.

Species variation also needs to be considered. For example, a blood sample from a bird requires a lithium heparin anticoagulant, whilst ethylene diamine tetra-acetic acid (EDTA) is usually used for mammalian samples.

Samples that may need to be collected include:

- Blood and bone marrow
- Urine
- Faeces
- Skin or hair
- Sperm
- Other body fluids
- Tissue
- Specimens for bacterial or viral diagnosis
- Necropsy or post-mortem samples.

PRACTICAL TIP
The sample container must be labelled *immediately* with patient identification, date and time of sample taking, and any preservatives that may have been used.

Blood sampling

Blood for analysis can be obtained in dogs and cats by venepuncture from the jugular, cephalic, lingual (anaesthetized only), femoral or lateral saphenous vein. The most common sites are the jugular and cephalic veins. Collection sites in other species are shown in Figure 17.7.

Species	Comments
Rat	No more than 10% of blood volume (2–4 ml for 300–500 g bodyweight) Lateral tail vein or saphenous vein
Mouse	Bodyweight 25–40 g: 0.2–0.3 ml Lateral tail vein or saphenous vein
Hamster	Cephalic vein with a 27 gauge needle, use tourniquet and a capillary tube (0.2–0.3 ml); or lateral saphenous vein using a 25 gauge needle; capillary tube or blood tube for larger volumes
Gerbil	Lateral tail vein and saphenous vein
Chipmunk	Jugular vein under anaesthetic
Guinea pig Degu	Jugular vein under anaesthetic
Chinchilla	Jugular vein under anaesthetic
Rabbit	Marginal ear vein, jugular vein, cephalic vein, saphenous vein Use EMLA™ cream Take up to 1% of bodyweight
Ferret	Vena cava under anaesthesia (toenail clipping, cardiac and periorbital no longer done) Lateral saphenous or cephalic vein up to 1ml; or jugular/vena cava; larger amounts using 26 gauge needle, up to 2 ml
Hedgehog	Saphenous or cephalic vein up to 0.5 ml, jugular if skinny. Cranial vena cava can be used for larger amounts
Birds	*Macaw:* brachial vein or jugular vein, 25–27 gauge needle. Larger birds: use metatarsal vein. Clipping toenails no longer done *Pigeon:* jugular, cutaneous ulnar or medial metatarsal vein. EDTA only, as heparin clumps cells *Birds of prey:* right jugular vein (may need to be obtained under anaesthesia) or brachial vein

17.7 Blood collection sites in exotic species.   *continues* ▶

Species	Comments
Tortoise Turtle	Jugular or subcarapacial (upper), cardiac or dorsal tail vein – may need chemical restraint if aggressive or awkward
Snake	Pre-heparinized syringe, 0.2–0.4 ml. Cardiocentesis preferred (using a Doppler to locate heart; best sedated) or coccygeal vein in larger snakes
Lizard	Ventral coccygeal vein preferred, or ventral abdominal/ cardiac puncture
Amphibian	Cardiac puncture preferred, central ventral abdominal vein
Fish	Medial caudal vein

17.7 *continued* Blood collection sites in exotic species.

Patient preparation

Fasting for 8–12 hours will help to reduce the risk of the sample becoming lipaemic, which could affect the results. Some tests, however, may require the animal being fed (**post-prandial**; if assessing bile acids for liver dysfunction) or rested and stress-free (glucose estimation).

Equipment

- Electronic clippers with a no. 40 clipping blade
- Skin cleanser (i.e. chlorhexidine)
- Surgical spirit
- Needle of suitable size
- Syringe of suitable size
- Appropriate blood container for the test
- 'Plaster' following venepuncture

Blood sample tubes

Blood samples may be collected in plastic or glass tubes. **Vacutainers** are blood containers that are sealed under pressure; although they are more expensive and require larger volumes of blood, they have the advantage of maintaining sterility.

Once blood is outside the body, clotting will normally occur within a couple of minutes unless an **anticoagulant** is added to prevent this. Various types of containers with anticoagulants already added are available for different uses (Figure 17.8). An incorrect blood:anticoagulant ratio may result in inaccurate results and the side of the blood tube should be checked to ensure that the correct amount is collected. Laboratories may differ in their tube preference, depending on their own diagnostic equipment.

Storage

If a blood sample needs to be preserved prior to dispatch or examination, it must be clearly labelled on the outside of the collection pot with the name of the patient and of the client, the date and time of sampling and the type of sample contained. The sample should then be refrigerated at 2–4°C.

Blood samples for culture

Bacteraemia or septicaemia can be confirmed by culture from aseptically obtained blood samples. The skin is prepared aseptically for a jugular vein sample. Sterile gloves should be worn during collection. Two or three samples of 5–10 ml each are taken over 24 hours, as bacteraemia may be intermittent. The top of the culture bottle should be swabbed and allowed to dry before the sample is injected into it. Incubation is for 7 days.

Bone marrow sampling

Bone marrow aspiration is performed to identify haematological disorders such as non-regenerative anaemias, hypoplastic anaemias, neoplastic disease and immune-mediated destruction of the red cell precursors.

Equipment

- 18 gauge Jamshidi disposable bone marrow needle
- Petri dish
- Microscope slides
- Pipette
- 2–3% EDTA/isotonic saline solution:
  - A 2 ml EDTA vacutainer tube is filled with isotonic (0.9%) saline and mixed well
  - 2 ml of the resulting EDTA solution is added to 5–8 ml of sterile isotonic saline in a serum vacutainer

Patient preparation

Samples are most commonly collected from the iliac crest in large dogs or the trochanteric fossa of the femur in small dogs and cats. Other sites include the proximal humerus. The animal is anaesthetized or heavily sedated and is restrained in either sternal or lateral recumbency. The skin area over the bone marrow site is clipped and surgically scrubbed. The tendency for haemorrhage after collection is very small, even in thrombocytopenic animals.

Procedure

Half of the microscope slides need to be placed at an angle (e.g. on a sandbag). The other slides are placed nearby to be used for smearing.

Colour code		Additive	Use
Plastic blood tubes	**Vacutainers**		
Pink	Lilac	EDTA (ethylenediamine tetra-acetic acid)	General haematology
Dark purple	Light blue 1:9 Black 1:4	Sodium citrate	Clotting disorders
White	Red	Plain	All serum tests
Orange	Green	Lithium heparin	Biochemistry Plasma tests Haematology (birds only)
Yellow	Grey	Sodium fluoride, potassium oxalate	Blood glucose estimations

17.8 Types of blood container.

A small incision is made in the skin and the bone marrow sample is taken. From this point the sample needs to be processed quickly so that it does not clot (see 'Bone marrow squash preparation' in the 'Processing samples' section, later).

Urine collection

If possible a morning sample should be obtained, as this tends to be when urine is at its most concentrated, thus increasing the chances of finding abnormalities. The sample should be examined within 1 hour of collection; alternatively it may be refrigerated at 4–8°C (up to 6 hours maximum; ensure that the sample returns to room temperature before urinalysis) or a preservative may be added. If the sample is to be cultured it should be stored at room temperature. Chilling may reduce the chances of recovering any bacteria that may be present.

Equipment

Containers

Bacterial contamination will alter pH levels and accelerate the disintegration of some components, such as urinary casts. Urine for microbial examination should be transferred into a container with boric acid, which will reduce the growth of any contaminating bacteria during transit to the laboratory. Containers must therefore be thoroughly clean, dry and preferably sterile (Figure 17.9). Washed-out jam jars, ice-cream tubs etc. should not be used, because of the possible presence of glucose or other reducing substances. Owners should always be given a sterile pot (and a pair of disposable gloves) for collecting samples at home.

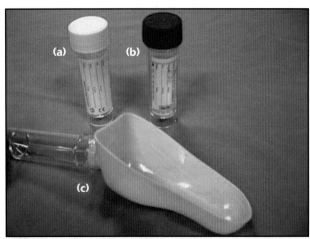

17.9 Urine sample containers. **(a)** Sterile universal container. **(b)** Universal container with boric acid added. **(c)** Commercial collection funnel with sample container attached.

Types of containers include:

- Sterile kidney dish
- Plain sterile 20 ml universal container or 60 ml container
- Sterile universal container with boric acid preservative added (the required amount of urine must be collected as indicated on the container so that the ratio of preservative:sample is correct).

The container should be labelled immediately after sample collection with patient identification, date and time of collection, 'urine' (to identify the type of sample collected) and identification of any preservatives used (including the actual amount added to the sample).

Preservatives

It is always best to examine urine immediately, or if necessary refrigerate, but if this is not possible preservatives can be used to prevent bacterial growth or chemical decomposition for up to 2 days. Types of urine preservative that can be used include:

- Toluene – add enough to have a thin film on top
- Formalin 10% – 1 drop to 2.5 ml urine
- Thymol – 1 mg/ml urine
- Boric acid – 0.5 g/28 ml urine (most commonly used preservative; if for culture, analyse within 8 hours).

Methods of collection

Methods of collection include:

- Mid-stream free collection (non-sterile – unsuitable for culture)
- Manual expression of the bladder (non-sterile – unsuitable for culture)
- Catheterization
- Cystocentesis.

Advantages and disadvantages of each method are set out in Figure 17.10. Equipment and procedures for catheterization and cystocentesis are described in detail in Chapter 15.

Collection method	Advantages	Disadvantages
Mid-stream	Easy to perform Non-traumatic Quite sterile in cats, though considered non-sterile in dogs Good sample for haematuria investigation as no iatrogenesis	Contamination from collection chamber or urethra Requires patient cooperation Heavier sediment (such as blood cells, crystals and malignant cells) may not be dispelled until bladder almost empty
Manual	Easy to perform Non-traumatic Quite sterile in cats, though considered non-sterile in dogs	Contamination from urethra Bladder rupture, tissue damage or haematuria due to trauma associated with expression Cannot be used for bacteriological analysis Patient must be relaxed Cannot be used on patients with poor skin structure (e.g. hyperadrenocorticism)
Catheterization	Relatively sterile Used as part of a contrast imaging procedure Used to monitor urine output Can maintain urethral patency if required	Sedation or general anaesthetic may be required Iatrogenic infection (cystitis) or damage to urethra Increased cost to client Iatrogenic haematuria
Cystocentesis	Quick Relatively non-painful Sterile No urethral contamination Decreased iatrogenic haematuria Iatrogenic infection uncommon Easy to perform in cats Preferred method for bacterial culture	Sedation or general anaesthetic may be required Experience required Contraindicated with a distended bladder

17.10 Advantages and disadvantages of different urine collection methods.

Faecal samples

Strict hygiene must be adhered to at all times. Preparation of the appropriate equipment and materials beforehand is essential in ensuring the safety of the person collecting the sample and also to minimize potential contamination or degradation of the sample being collected.

A number of the endoparasites are **zoonotic**. *Samples in suspected cases should be treated with the utmost respect and care.*

Equipment

- Suitable container (some have a spoon to reduce contamination)
- Rubber/plastic gloves
- Wooden spatula
- Preservative if required (10% formalin)
- Means of sample identification

A sterile or clean pot should be used, with a screw cap. Universal containers with a spoon attached to the lid may be used for transferring the faeces in a safe and controlled manner (Figure 17.11). The size of the pot may depend on the dexterity of the collector.

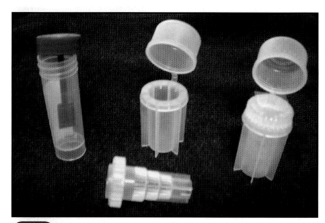

17.11 Faecal sample containers.

Patient preparation

When testing for the presence of blood the patient should be on a meat-free diet for 3 days, though this is not always practical. Some antidiarrhoeal preparations – such as mineral oil, oral contrast material (barium), bismuth or kaolin – may float and could interfere with the examination of worm eggs. This will also occur with some antibiotics. It is recommended that medication is withdrawn for 5–10 days prior to testing.

Collection methods

Samples can be obtained directly from the ground or rectally from the animal. Whichever method is used, it is essential that contamination is avoided and that the pot is filled completely, as this will help to minimize any changes. Desiccation (drying out) of the sample will be avoided by ensuring that the pot is airtight and secured appropriately. Analysis of faeces should be carried out as soon as practicably possible.

Ground collection

Ideally the area for defecation should have been disinfected in advance. Alternatively, only the top portion of an evacuated sample should be taken.

- Use a glove, spoon or spatula to transfer the sample into the container.
- Label the pot as usual and send or store immediately.

Rectal collection

- Use the glove as the container, by turning it inside out once a sample has been obtained and then tying the end of the glove securely.
- Label the glove as usual, using a permanent pen, and send or store immediately.

Storage

Worm eggs embryonate quickly and can continue to do so outside the host's body. The sample should be refrigerated (for up to 7 days only), but if examining for live larvae the examination must be carried out immediately. Samples should never be frozen. If examination will be delayed for more than 24 hours after collection, the faeces should be diluted with 10% formalin, but this will render any microbiological testing impossible.

Complications

Complications or false negatives/positives may occur due to any of the following:

- Incorrect patient preparation
- Incorrect sample collection technique
- Incorrect handling, containment or storage of the sample prior to testing
- Contamination
- Time scale between evacuation and examination
- Incorrect materials or test methods
- Operator error.

Skin and hair sampling

The skin should be examined carefully for ectoparasites and lesions that are suitable for sampling. Some ectoparasites can be seen macroscopically (i.e. with the naked eye) whilst others (e.g. mites) are only visible using a microscope. Care must be taken when collecting specimens, as some skin conditions can be zoonotic, including all of the dermatophytes (fungi) and several of the ectoparasites (e.g. fleas and several mite species).

The samples collected depend on clinical signs. Techniques appropriate for identification of different organisms are suggested in Figure 17.12.

Organism suspected	Techniques for collection and examination
Bacteria	Swab for cytology; stain, then oil immersion microscopy Sterile swab for bacterial culture and antibiotic sensitivity testing
Dermatophytes	Wood's lamp examination of animal Low-power microscopy of hair pluck or skin scrape (unstained) Fungal culture
Malassezia yeast	Tape strip from skin or ear swab for cytology; stain, then oil immersion microscopy Fungal culture
Fleas and flea faeces	Direct removal – catch flea with fingers or tape strip Coat brushing

17.12 Collection and examination methods for suspected skin pathogens. *continues* ▶

Organism suspected	Techniques for collection and examination
Tick	Direct removal
Lice	Direct removal; low-power microscopy Coat brushing; low-power microscopy
Cheyletiella mite	Coat brushing; low-power microscopy Tape strip; low-power microscopy Skin scrape (superficial) ; low-power microscopy
Demodex mite	Skin scrape (deep); low-power microscopy Hair pluck; low-power microscopy Impression smear of pustule (unstained); low-power microscopy
Sarcoptes/Notoedres mites	Skin scraping (deep); low-power microscopy
Otodectes (ear) mite	Cotton swab to collect ear cerumen (wax); low-power microscopy
Trombicula (harvest) mite	Tape strip; low-power microscopy

17.12 *continued* Collection and examination methods for suspected skin pathogens.

Skin scraping

This technique is used to collect skin for microscopic examination for ectoparasites such as *Sarcoptes* and *Demodex* mites. It is always best to take several skin scrapings, from different sites, as some mites can be difficult to find.

Skin scrape procedure

1. Choose a suitable area. The various mites tend to affect different areas of the body and so the area chosen will depend on which parasite is being sought. For example, *Sarcoptes* often affects the pinnae, *Cheyletiella* the dorsum and *Demodex* the feet. Try to avoid areas that have been severely traumatized, as mites may be difficult to find in these areas.
2. Gently clip hair from the area to be scraped.
3. Apply a drop of liquid paraffin to the microscope slide, the skin surface and a no. 10 scalpel blade. Some people prefer to use 10% potassium hydroxide (KOH) as this helps to clear the background keratin of the skin and hair, making identification of the parasites easier. However, liquid paraffin keeps the parasite alive and mobile, making locating them far easier.
4. Use a blunted blade, to avoid cutting the skin surface if the animal struggles. Sedation may be required for scraping sensitive areas such as the face and feet.
5. Squeeze the skin between the fingers, which helps to bring deeper parasites such as *Demodex* to the surface.
6. Gently scrape the top layer of the skin surface until capillary oozing of blood occurs. Transfer to the microscope slide.
7. Place a cover slip over the top and examine under low-power (x4) objective microscopy. Then use higher power (x10) to examine in more detail.
8. Scan slide using the 'battlement' technique (see earlier) to ensure that all the sample has been examined.

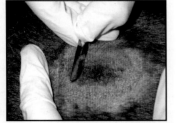

Coat brushings

Brushings may reveal fleas and/or their faeces, lice and eggs, and *Cheyletiella* mites and eggs.

Coat brushing procedure

1. Stand the patient on top of a large sheet of white paper.
2. Briskly brush the coat with the fingers or brush for several minutes.
3. Collect the dislodged material from the paper using clear adhesive tape and stick directly on to a microscope slide.
4. Examine under the microscope in the same way as a skin scrape.

Wet paper test

1. Wet a small wad of cotton wool and squeeze out all the excess moisture.
2. Dab the wad over the sample left on the white paper after coat brushing.
3. Flea faeces may be confirmed by blood-tinged marks on the cotton wool or paper, giving an orange halo around the flea faeces.

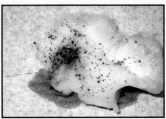

Hair plucks

Hair plucks may be examined for the presence of fungal spores (dermatophytosis), *Demodex* mites (which live in the hair follicle), or louse and *Cheyletiella* eggs (which are attached to the hair shaft).

Small amounts of hair are plucked from the affected area and placed on a microscope slide, with some liquid paraffin if examining for eggs. A coverslip is placed and the sample examined with low-power microscopy. Negative findings do not rule out demodicosis or dermatophytosis.

Hair pluck samples may also be used for culture (see later).

Tape strips

Clear adhesive tape can be used to detect fleas, lice, *Cheyletiella* and harvest mites. The area to be tested is chosen and, if necessary, hairs separated to allow access to the skin below. A length of clear adhesive tape is pressed firmly on to the area. This is repeated several times and the tape laid sticky side down on to a microscope slide. Low-power microscopy is used to examine for ectoparasites. Strips can also be stained for cytology (see below).

McKenzie brushing technique

If a person in a household has suspected ringworm, the McKenzie technique can be used to take samples from animals that are not showing any obvious signs of fungal infection but are suspected 'carriers' of infection. Because the method covers the whole area of the coat, it increases the chances of sampling infected hairs.

A sterile toothbrush is used to comb through the entire coat for several minutes. It is good to brush *against* the natural flow of hairs. The toothbrush head is touched on to a culture plate several times. The plate is observed for growth of dermatophytes.

Impression smears
These are made by applying a microscope slide directly on to the area of interest. The slide is then stained and examined under high-power microscopy for cells and microbes.

Fine-needle aspiration
This is mainly used to examine cutaneous masses to determine whether they are inflammatory, cystic or neoplastic (see 'Tissue sampling') but it can also be used to examine most areas of the body, including the abdomen, thorax and joints.

'Stab' technique
This is an alternative to fine-needle aspiration. A needle is held in the fingers and inserted into the mass several times by the veterinary surgeon. It is then removed and attached to an air-filled syringe before being expressed on to a microscope slide.

Bacteriological sampling of the skin
The commonest bacterial pathogen of the skin is *Staphylococcus intermedius*. Bacterial culture is useful to check the antibiotic sensitivity of the bacteria. Topical and systemic antibiotics should be stopped at least 3 days before sample collection.

Hair over a pustule is removed with scissors. Pustules are thin and so should not be swabbed with alcohol, as this may be absorbed into the pustule and result in no bacterial growth. The pustule is lanced with a sterile 23 gauge needle and the contents squeezed on to a bacterial swab. Samples are usually sent to an external laboratory for culture and antibiotic sensitivity testing, using transport medium to protect the sample. Instructions for packing and posting pathological specimens must be followed (see Chapter 1).

Ear wax
Wax (cerumen) can be collected using a damp cotton swab. For examination for *Otodectes* mites the wax sample is added to a microscope slide, mixed with liquid paraffin, covered with a cover slip and examined under low-power microscopy. For cytological examination, the wax is gently rolled on to a microscope slide, allowed to air dry, stained with a commercial Wright's stain (e.g. *RAPIDIFF®*) and examined with high-power microscopy for the presence of cells, yeast or bacteria.

Sperm collection
Sperm may be collected for fertility testing from dogs, cats and rabbits by digital manipulation (see Chapter 25).

Storage
After a semen sample has been collected, it is placed on a warming block maintained at 37°C. Semen samples are highly viscous directly after collection and are therefore kept at this temperature until they become liquefied. The sample is then either examined immediately or it can be frozen. Before freezing, the sample is mixed with a freezing medium in a 1:1 ratio so that the semen is protected during the process of freezing and storage.

Other body fluids
With all of the following procedures for collecting samples of other body fluids, which will be performed by veterinary surgeons, it is important to ensure that full preparation is made so that equipment and materials are ready at the appropriate times. The patient must be correctly prepared and suitably positioned. If the patient is conscious, it is important to provide a quiet, calm and controlled environment, because even a small movement at the wrong moment with any of these procedures can have serious implications.

If the sample needs to be preserved prior to dispatch or examination, the collection pot should be clearly labelled with the name of the animal and of the client, the date and time of collection and the type of sample contained. The sample should then be refrigerated at 2–4°C.

Cerebrospinal fluid
Cerebrospinal fluid (CSF) is collected by the veterinary surgeon with the patient under general anaesthesia. Collection is from the cisterna magna or L5–L6 lumbar space in the dog or L6–L7 in the cat. A CSF sample may be collected from a neurological patient or just prior to myelography, when a contrast agent is injected into the same space as where the CSF fluid is located for imaging the spinal cord for possible trauma or neoplasia.

Sample collection
Strict asepsis must be maintained. A meningal infection could have disastrous consequences. The CSF is produced within the ventricles of the brain and found in the subarachnoid layer of the meninges, which is between the arachnoid and pia mater layers. This fluid is essential in providing nutrients to the tissues that it surrounds. It also acts as a protective 'shock-absorber' to the delicate tissues of the brain and spinal cord.

The skin is prepared as it would be for a surgical procedure and the patient is anaesthetized and intubated so that the patient and the rate of their ventilation may be controlled. There are two methods by which CSF can be obtained, depending on the size of the patient and on the veterinary surgeon's preference: cisternal puncture or lumbar puncture.

The endotracheal (ET) tube may be compromised due to the positioning of the patient's neck. To avoid this it is recommended that either a specially reinforced ET tube or a deflated cuffed tube be used, so that the patient may at least breathe around the tube if kinking should occur. It is also important to ensure that a large ET tube is used. The anaesthetist must ensure that the patient is in a moderate to deep plane of anaesthesia, due to the stimulation that may occur on penetration of the dura mater. The patient must be kept extremely still whilst the needle is in place.

Equipment
- Sterile 5 ml plain container and an EDTA container
- 22–19 gauge x 1–3.5-inch spinal needle
- Skin preparation solutions
- Sterile gloves
- Surgical drape
- Special reinforced ET tube of a large size for the patient, with a syringe to deflate and inflate the cuff of the ET tube as necessary. Suitable depth of anaesthesia before the procedure is performed

Collection by cisternal puncture
The patient is positioned on its left side for right-handed veterinary surgeons, and on its right side for left-handed veterinary surgeons. It is essential that the patient's collar is removed and that its nose remains parallel to the table. The animal's head is flexed to make an angle of 90 degrees with the vertebral column, so that the sample can be collected from the cisterna magna at the atlanto-occipital articulation. Once scrubbed, gowned and gloved, the surgeon prepares the area and slowly inserts the spinal needle within the centre of the triangle (Figure 17.13).

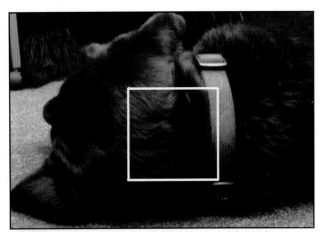

17.13 Cisternal puncture. Area that would require clipping. Collars should always be removed prior to this procedure.

Care must be taken, as insertion of the needle beyond the subarachnoid space may result in temporary or permanent paralysis of the patient.

The needle is advanced slowly through the skin and the stylet is removed. The needle is further advanced slowly until CSF appears. A 'pop' sensation may be detected as the needle penetrates the dura mater (no twitch should be observed as seen with the lumbar puncture technique). CSF should be allowed to drip slowly into plain and EDTA collection pots without alteration of the needle position. The needle should be kept still and parallel to the table at all times. Negative pressure should not be used to withdraw the CSF. The needle should be carefully removed in the exact position that it was introduced.

Collection by lumbar puncture

CSF is collected by the veterinary surgeon from the anaesthetized animal by percutaneous insertion of a spinal needle into the lumbar area and into the subarachnoid space of the spinal column. A free-flow sample is collected with the animal in either lateral or sternal recumbency. It is important that the patient is restrained securely until the end of the procedure.

The area is clipped and surgically prepared. If the patient is in a lateral position, its hindlimbs are pulled cranially under the abdomen. If the patient is in sternal position, its legs should be lifted up towards the ceiling position to open the spaces between the lumbar vertebrae. In dogs, the site is between L5–L6 and the needle is inserted alongside the spinous process of L6. In the cat L6–L7 is used.

The needle must penetrate through the ligamentum flavum, which can be quite tough. A 'pop' sensation may be detected. The stylet is removed intermittently to check progress as the needle is slowly inserted. The needle is inserted until the ventral surface of the needle touches the ventral surface of the vertebral canal, then withdrawn about 1 mm to be located within the subarachnoid space. When the needle penetrates through the cauda equina, the patient will 'twitch'. This is an excellent indicator that the needle is in the correct place. Collection of CSF from the lumbar region is slower than that from a cisternal puncture. Blood contamination must be avoided as it will impair the results. Respiratory and cardiac rates may increase.

Synovial fluid collection – arthrocentesis

Synovial fluid analysis consists of a white blood cell count and differential (cytology) smear, total protein assay and bacteriology. A separate sample is required for each test to

be performed. Arthrocentesis is performed by the veterinary surgeon, usually using general anaesthesia. An area approximately 2–3 cm² in size is surgically prepared for either a lateral, medial or ventral approach, depending on the joint in question and operator preference. Slow and careful insertion of the needle is required to reduce trauma to the surrounding tissues or haemorrhage into the sample. Once the needle is inside the joint capsule, slow but careful aspiration should be performed. Only a few drops will be collected, unless inflammation is present.

Equipment

- Sterile EDTA tube (one per test)
- Surgical gloves
- Surgical drape
- Skin preparation solutions
- Usually a 1 ml or 2 ml syringe (5 ml syringe if inflammation present)
- 18–23 gauge x 1-inch needle

Thoracic fluid collection – thoracocentesis

Thoracocentesis can be performed by the veterinary surgeon on a conscious or anaesthetized patient to remove air or fluid from the pleural space (see Chapter 21 for technique). Strict asepsis must be maintained throughout the procedure. An oblique approach is usually taken with small-chested animals, whereas a lateral approach is adopted for the deeper-chested patient. A butterfly needle is often preferred, due to the sensation felt by the operator when the needle tip comes into contact with tissues. A specific thoracocentesis catheter is available, which has the combination of a butterfly needle with a Teflon-styleted catheter, which helps to deflect the lung tissue with which it may come into contact. The stylet is removed once inside the pleural space and then the syringe and three-way tap are attached. This type of catheter reduces the likelihood of damaging any surrounding tissues.

Abdominal paracentesis

This technique is performed by the veterinary surgeon to remove fluid from the abdominal cavity. The animal is usually sedated or anaesthetized and placed into right lateral recumbency. An area 5–8 cm² to one side of the linea alba (midline between the umbilical and bladder) is surgically prepared; strict asepsis must be maintained at all times. If the patient is sedated a local analgesic may be required beforehand to reduce the likelihood of patient movement.

A needle (18–19 gauge x 1–2 inch) or a butterfly catheter (14–16 gauge) with a three-way tap is inserted and the fluid gently drawn out using a 10–20 ml syringe. Repositioning of the needle may be required due to the surrounding omentum. The sample is collected into either a plain or an EDTA pot. The amount aspirated is measured.

Pericardiocentesis

Excess fluid within the pericardium may be extracted by the veterinary surgeon using pericardiocentesis (see Chapter 21 for technique). Strict asepsis is employed. The patient is either sedated and given a local analgesic or is given a general anaesthetic. Risks associated with the procedure include infection, perforation of a major artery, and trauma to the lung or liver. It is therefore essential that both the equipment and the patient are prepared properly.

Tissue sampling

Types of lumps or masses that may require analysis include:

- Tumours
- Cysts
- Abscesses
- Haematomas
- Foreign bodies
- Allergic reactions.

Fine-needle aspiration

If the sample is being collected from a cavity, surgical preparation of the patient should be performed. If the skin is being sampled, swabbing with alcohol should be sufficient.

Equipment

This should include a 21–25 gauge needle with a 3–20 ml syringe. The consistency of the tissue being aspirated will influence the choice of syringe. For example, a softer tissue such as a lymph node should be successfully aspirated using a 3 ml syringe, whereas a firmer tissue would require a larger syringe to provide adequate suction in the collection of cells suitable for cytological examination.

Fine-needle aspiration technique

1. Hold the mass firmly.
2. Attach a syringe to the needle.
3. Introduce the needle into the centre of the mass with strong negative pressure being applied by drawing back on the plunger to about three-quarters of the syringe.
4. Sample several areas of the mass. Avoid contamination with other tissues close to the mass.
5. Release the negative pressure before withdrawing from the mass, so that the cells stay within the needle rather than being sucked into the syringe and lost.
6. Remove the needle from the syringe and draw air into the syringe.
7. Replace the needle on to the syringe and expel the contents on to the middle of a microscope slide by rapidly depressing the plunger.
8. Spread the sample for examination, applying the technique used for blood smears (see later). The sample is then air dried, stained and examined using high-power microscopy.

Tissue biopsy

Techniques for obtaining a solid biopsy sample include:

- Intracapsular – lump removed without the capsule of surrounding tissue
- Marginal – removal of the mass and capsule only
- Wide – mass removed with a zone of normal tissue
- Radical – mass removal with entire surrounding tissue compartment (i.e. muscle, fascia).

The inclusion of normal tissue around the edge of a mass will allow the histologist to compare normal and abnormal tissue and to assess whether all the tumorous tissue has been removed. Diagrams of the size and site of the mass removed will be helpful for the laboratory.

Samples should be placed in an appropriate pot with 10% neutral buffered formalin (10:1 fixative to sample). A wide-mouthed jar should be used in case the tissue swells during transit (Figure 17.14). It is important to follow the directions of the external laboratory.

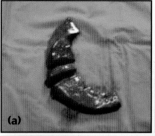
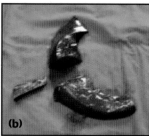
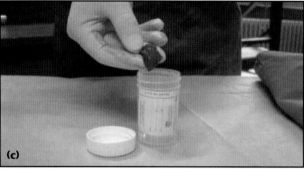

17.14 Preparing a sample from an excised mass. **(a)** A slice is taken from the central point of the excised tissue. **(b)** The slice is removed from the remaining mass and sent for analysis. **(c)** A wide-mouthed container is used, to facilitate removal of the sample slice from the pot at the laboratory should the sample have become swollen or rigid.

Tissue may also be applied to a clean slide and pressed gently along its length to give a series of impression smears that can be stained for cytology.

Sample collection for bacteriology

Samples should be:

- Taken from a living or recently dead animal (within 4 hours)
- Taken from the affected site as early as possible following the onset of clinical signs
- Taken from the edges of lesions, where infection is most active
- Collected as aseptically as possible
- Collected prior to any form of treatment
- Submitted in generous amounts
- Submitted in appropriate transport media and containers
- Submitted individually in separate watertight containers. Screw-capped jars should be clearly marked indicating sample enclosed, animal identification and date of collection
- Delivered speedily to the laboratory (avoiding specimens sitting in the local post office over a weekend)
- Refrigerated at 4°C as soon as possible after collection if transportation is delayed.

Sample collection for viral diagnosis

The laboratory will advise on the appropriate transport medium. It is essential that samples are collected at a time of virus excretion. Faeces, skin scrapings, body fluids, tissue or blood with anticoagulant should be placed into bijoux bottles, containing the viral transport medium, and transported to the laboratory as soon as possible.

Necropsy or post-mortem samples

Necropsy or post-mortem samples are taken from dead animals. If a cadaver is being sent for a post-mortem investigation, the following points need to be borne in mind (see also Chapter 1).

- All animals autolyse very quickly (especially birds and fish). Reptiles, dogs and cats need to be examined within 72 hours of death.
- Bird feathers tend to insulate the bird, therefore the cadaver should be soaked in a detergent such as chlorhexidine solution. This will dampen the bird and allow immediate chilling (water alone will just run off).
- Avoid placing the cadaver next to any heat or chemical sources and store in a designated fridge.
- Seal in a plastic bag, protect with wadding and pack into a box that is surrounded by ice for preservation.
- *Do not freeze* or allow ice to contact any of the tissue directly, as ice crystals will disrupt the structure of the cells.
- Send by registered courier (if not being transported by the owner), using the fastest route available.

Toxicological examinations might include:

- Contents of stomach, intestines
- Samples of the liver and kidneys
- Samples of blood, urine, faeces and vomit (if available).

Each specimen should be sealed and carefully identified.

Packing and dispatching samples to external laboratories

The essential requirement in sending samples to an external laboratory is that the samples should arrive at the laboratory in good condition. The following should be taken into account during preparation, storage, packaging and dispatching of samples:

- The rate of cell/tissue breakdown (**autolysis**) is increased by humidity and increased temperature, therefore these should be minimized
- Freezing or fixing can reduce autolysis
- The sample should be preserved, in the correct sample pot
- Blood should be separated into serum or plasma (if required) before posting
- Whole blood, serum and plasma should be packed to prevent variations in temperature and physical damage
- Forms must be completed giving all necessary details
- Each sample should be clearly labelled
- Samples should be packaged and sealed correctly
- Records should be kept of all samples taken, where sent and the results received.

Packing the laboratory sample

1. Before handling samples, put on gloves and an apron.
2. Check that the sample is correct.
3. Check that the sample is hermetically sealed (i.e. the container is air-tight and moisture-proof). Do not place tape around the top of the container, as this may make it difficult to open at the receiving laboratory.
4. Check that the outside of the container is clean.
5. Label correctly with:
   i. Animal's name
   ii. Species
   iii. Breed
   iv. Age
   v. Sex
   vi. Owner's name and address and reference number
   vii. Date and time of collection
   viii. How the sample was obtained and storage methods used
   ix. Any preservatives used
   x. Name of attending clinician
   xi. Practice address and telephone number
   xii. Tests required
   xiii. Full history of the patient, including any recent medications administered and the diet currently being fed
   xiv. Clinician's differential diagnosis.
6. Wrap the sample in sufficient amount of absorbent material to prevent leakage.
7. Place sample into a padded 'jiffy' bag.
8. Fill out a laboratory form and place into a separate polythene or 'jiffy' bag.
9. Place the sample and laboratory form in a cardboard box or similar.
10. Place the box into a padded envelope (preferably a pre-paid one supplied by the laboratory).
11. Clearly label the outside of the package with the *full* name of the laboratory to which it is being sent, including the postal code.
12. Label the package appropriately, e.g.: 'PATHOLOGICAL SPECIMEN'; 'FRAGILE, HANDLE WITH CARE'; 'VETERINARY PATHOLOGICAL SAMPLE' (see Chapter 1).
13. Label the back of the packaging with the *full* name and address of the sender.
14. Send samples via courier or by first-class post, preferably using a Royal Mail Safebox.
15. Make sure that the sample will arrive on a working day.

NOTE: Incorrect packaging could lead to the specimen being destroyed or prosecution by the carrier.

Safebox
The Royal Mail's tough and resilient Safebox is a convenient method for sending and receiving diagnostic specimens through the post. The Safebox provides prepaid postage, separate compartments for the specimen and documentation, and a tamper-evident seal to eliminate any risk to users. It is designed to make leakage almost impossible and is fully compliant with Packaging Instruction 650 and the requirements of UN3373, as well as meeting all the performance tests of Packaging Instruction 602.

Transport of bacterial samples

Streptococcus spp. are especially susceptible to desiccation (drying out) when collected with a dry swab. To avoid this, a commercial swab with transport medium should be used. Ideally all swabs are submerged in the transport medium unless they are to be processed immediately. Anaerobic transport media are available. Different pathogens suit different media, and laboratories may have specific requirements.

Processing samples

All preparations made from original samples must be clearly labelled.

Blood smears

Microscopic examination of the structure and shape of the blood cells (morphological assessment) will provide information on conditions such as anaemia, infection, inflammation and other abnormalities. Even if a sample is to be sent away to an external laboratory for automated cell counts, it is still an essential part of any haematological examination to view the cells with a microscope first.

Equipment

- Microscope slides
- Spreader (slide with one corner taken off)
- Blood (EDTA)

Blood smear preparation

1. Ensure that the microscope slide is dry, and free from dust and grease.
2. Place slide on a pale background.
3. Place a small drop of blood near one end of the slide.
4. Place the spreader just in front of the blood at an angle of 45 degrees.

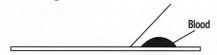

5. Move the spreader *back into* the blood until the blood runs along the edge of the spreader.

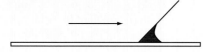

6. Move the spreader *forward* in a single smooth rapid motion.

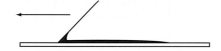

7. Air dry the smear.
8. Either stain when dry, or fix in absolute methanol for 5 minutes and stain within 3 days.

Faults

- Smear too long – too much blood or blood is anaemic or spreader angle too small
- Smear too short – too little blood or spreader angle too great
- Alternate thick/thin bands – uneven spreader edge or jerky motion when spreading
- Areas of no blood – grease on the slide
- Smear thick and narrow – blood has not had time to spread along the spreader

Staining blood smears

The most commonly used stains for haematological examination are from the **Romanowsky** group. The stain allows visualization of the otherwise normally colourless leucocytes (white blood cells). Romanowsky stains include:

- Leishman's (common in UK)
- Giemsa (used for identifying particular cells and parasites, e.g. *Haemobartonella felis*)
- *RAPI*DIFF® stains (quick and easy, though not as sensitive as Leishman's).

Staining procedures

Equipment
- Dish
- Rack
- Stain
- Distilled water
- Blotting paper

Leishman's

1. Place slide on rack, smear uppermost.
2. Cover with Leishman's stain and leave 1–2 minutes to fix smear.
3. Cover the slide with twice the volume of buffered distilled water (pH 6.8).
4. Gently rock the slide from side to side to mix solution evenly; leave for 10–15 minutes.
5. Wash off the slide with the buffered distilled water. Flood the slide for 1 minute until pinkish tinge just appears.
6. Pour off water and stand slide upright on blotting paper to dry.
7. Once the smear is dry, examine under low-power objective to check focus and then use oil immersion objective.

Giemsa
Make up fresh solutions of Giemsa daily and allow 2 ml per slide.

1. Dip slide in methanol for a few seconds to fix the cells.
2. Flood the slide with Giemsa and leave for 30 minutes.
3. Rinse the slide with distilled water and leave upright to dry.

*RAPI*DIFF®

1. Dip slide into solution A – fixative (methanol) light blue – 5 times.
2. Remove and dip into solution B – stain (eosin) red – 5 times.
3. Remove and dip into solution C – stain (methylene blue dye) purple – 7 times (this helps to stain the platelets if left slightly longer).
4. Rinse the slide with distilled water and leave upright to air dry.

Coverslips

Once the slide is dry, a coverslip can be applied to protect the sample. Place the edge of the cover slip against the microscope slide at an angle of 45 degrees and let it drop down; this will help to push any bubbles to the side.

Bone marrow squash preparation

Squash preparations can be made from aspirated samples (Figure 17.15). A drop of the sample is placed on an angled slide so that the blood can drain down. A second slide is used to smear the sample gently. To ensure an adequate sample before sending to the laboratory, a slide can be stained with *RAPIDIFF®* and examined under the practice microscope. Small flecks (spicules) should be visible.

Cytological smear preparation

Two spreading techniques that allow particularly fragile tissues to remain intact for the evaluation of cells are illustrated in Figures 17.16 and 17.17. Once dried, the smears can be stained with *RAPIDIFF®* and examined using oil immersion microscopy.

Bacterial culture

Bacteria will only grow when in a suitable environment (see Chapter 7):

- The correct nutrient and water requirements for its survival must be available
- Optimum growth temperature is usually 37°C (normal body temperature)
- The pH is best kept at 7–7.4
- The correct gaseous environment should be provided, e.g. with or without oxygen, or increased or decreased amounts of oxygen.

The rate of growth varies between bacterial species. For example, *Escherichia coli* grows and reproduces in 15 minutes, whereas *Mycobacterium tuberculosis* takes 48 hours before it can reproduce; this time scale is known as the **generation time**.

Media for growing microorganisms

To allow bacteria to grow, a culture medium is used to provide the organisms with the essential nutrients they require. There

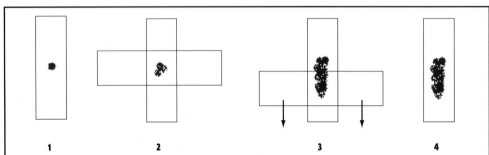

17.15 Four-step method of squash preparation of aspirated material on a slide.

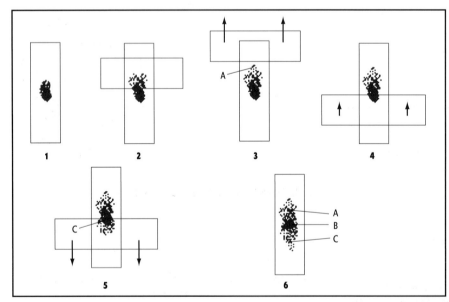

17.16 Cytological smear preparation. **(1)** A portion of the aspirate is expelled on to a glass slide. **(2,3)** A second glass slide is placed over about one-third of the preparation area (A) and gentle pressure is applied to aid spreading. The spreader slide is slid forwards smoothly and removed. **(4,5)** The edge of a tilted glass microscope slide (second spreader slide) is slid forwards from the end opposite the squash preparation until it contacts about one-third of the expelled aspirate (area C). The spreader slide is then slid rapidly and smoothly backwards. These steps produce an area that is spread with mechanical forces (as for a blood smear preparation). **(6)** The middle area (B) is left untouched and contains a high concentration of cells.

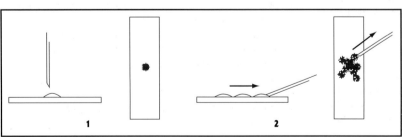

17.17 Needle spread or 'starfish' preparation. **(1)** A portion of the aspirate is expelled on to a glass microscope slide. **(2)** The tip of a needle is placed in the aspirate and moved peripherally, pulling a trail of sample with it. This procedure is repeated in several directions, resulting in a preparation with multiple projections.

are two types: liquid medium, or broth; and a solid medium that is hardened to a jelly-like consistency by adding agar. The medium may be simple, enriched, or selective/differential.

Simple media

These are also known as simple agar or nutrient agar. They provide basic nutrients, in the form of a nutrient broth or nutrient agar, for the growth of less fastidious bacteria.

Enriched media

These are for more fastidious bacteria that require additives such as blood, serum or egg. **Blood agar** contains 5–10% of actual blood; it supports the growth of most mammalian pathogens and may be used to detect haemolysis. **Chocolate agar** is blood agar that has been heated to 80°C; this causes the blood cells to rupture, releasing haemoglobin, which makes the medium more nutritious.

Enrichment broths are liquid media that are selective for a particular bacterium; for example, **selenite broth** is selective for the growth of salmonellae. Unlike the selective media described below, an enrichment broth has no inhibitory agent to prevent the growth of other organisms; instead, it favours the growth of the target species, allowing it to outgrow other organisms. This is especially helpful where small numbers of the target organism are present.

Selective/differential media

These are made for a particular bacterium or a group of bacteria and they contain inhibitory substances that prevent the growth of unwanted bacterial species. Some of the media can also change colour, which indicates the presence of a type of organism; these are referred to as **indicator media**.

Biochemical agar distinguishes between different bacteria because of their different reactions with the agar: sugar fermented by the bacterium, or by enzymes produced by the bacterium, may cause the indicator agar to change colour.

Examples of selective media include:

- **MacConkey's agar** – contains bile salts, which stops most non-enteric bacterial growth but allows enteric bacterial growth. Lactose-fermenting bacteria such as *Escherichia coli* produce red colonies, as they are able to ferment lactose, producing acids that lower the pH of the medium, causing the pH indicator medium to turn red. *Salmonella* colonies remain colourless
- **Sabouraud's agar** – has high glucose content and low pH (5.6), ideal for fungal growth. It turns from yellow to red as an indication of fungal growth (though this should be confirmed by examining spore growth under a microscope)
- **Deoxycholate-citrate agar** (DCA) – inhibits non-enteric bacteria whilst *Salmonella* spp. thrive on it.

Transport agar

This is used for temporary storage and transport (swabs) of a specimen by acting as a maintenance agar. It ensures the *survival* of any organism, rather than promoting its growth, until further examination can be carried out.

Inoculating the agar plate

The aim is to obtain single bacterial colonies for observing colonial morphology, for antibiotic susceptibility testing and for biochemical identification. The **quadrant streak** method, using the whole plate, is usually employed for most diagnostic specimens.

Equipment

- Petri dish with suitable agar (sterile). Agar plates should be stored at 4°C in the dark and upside down (to reduce the risk of condensation)
- Acetate pen or chinagraph pencil
- Inoculating loop (**nichrome**)
- Bunsen burner

Plate inoculation procedure

1. Mark the agar plate on the underside. This will act as the point for the initial inoculation ('well').
2. Sterilize the inoculation loop by passing it through the hot flame of a Bunsen burner; 'flame' it until it is red hot. Allow it to cool before use.
3. Use the inoculating loop to obtain the sample from agar (keeping the loop parallel to the plate) or from broth (scoop with the loop). The neck of the broth bottle should be sterilized before and after removing the inoculum by passing it quickly through the flame of a Bunsen burner.
4. Place the sample on the agar above the labelled point and, using the inoculating loop, spread it over a portion of the agar (A).
5. 'Flame' the loop again and allow it to cool. Touch it to the uninoculated agar to allow it to cool.
6. Dip the loop into the edge of area A and streak this on to area B in a zigzag fashion.
7. Repeat step 5.
8. Dip the loop into the edge of area B and streak this on to area C in a zigzag fashion.
9. Repeat step 5.
10. Dip the loop into the edge of area C and streak this on to area D in a zigzag fashion.
11. Put the lid on and place the plate, lid-side down, into an incubator at 37°C for 24 hours.

NOTE: Incinerate the plate after use as clinical waste.

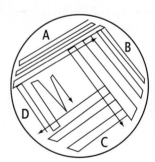

From bacterial culture to smear

Smear preparation

1. Prepare slide: clean with alcohol and allow to dry; label the slide.
2. Pass the slide through the Bunsen flame to remove any grease residue, or clean using alcohol.
3. Place one drop of water on to the centre of the slide, using a sterile inoculating loop.
4. Using the sterile inoculating loop, transfer the microbes from one of the colonies to the slide.
5. Mix with water on the slide to emulsify and then spread *thinly*.
6. Sterilize the loop.
7. Allow smears to dry thoroughly before proceeding further.

continues ▶

continued

Fixing

Samples are 'fixed' to kill any bacteria (whilst preserving cell morphology) and ensure that the material is firmly fixed to the slide. To do this, the slide is passed through a Bunsen flame (smear side up) two or three times. *Be careful not to overheat – just enough to warm.*

Bacterial stains

Most microbial cells are colourless or contain very little pigment, which makes them difficult to identify under a microscope. Identification is made easier if cells are killed, by fixing them with heat as explained above, and then died with a stain. Once the stain has been rinsed off, the dye remains in and around the cells and colours them against the clear background.

- **Simple stains** (e.g. methylene blue) colour the cell or the background in a way that enables the size, shape and arrangement of the cells to be observed.
- **Differential stains** (e.g. Gram stain, acid-fast stains) reveal more detail and can be used to differentiate between cell types. This requires a combination of two dyes, referred to as the **primary stain** and the **counter-stain**.
- **Structural stains** are used to dye only certain parts of the cell.

Methylene blue staining

This stain shows up the shapes of the bacteria, e.g. rod, coccus, vibrio, spirochaete (see Chapter 7).

1. Flood the slide with 1% methylene blue.
2. Leave for 2 minutes.
3. Wash off with distilled water.
4. Dry and examine under high-power (oil immersion) microscope.

Gram stain

The Gram stain is the most commonly used differential stain for determining cell morphology. The technique divides most clinically significant bacteria into two main groups (Gram-positive and Gram-negative) as the first step in bacterial identification (see Chapter 7). There are four steps in the Gram staining technique:

- Crystal violet (primary stain) – stains both types of bacteria violet
- Iodine (mordant) – fixes violet stain (Lugol's iodine is weaker than Gram's iodine, which makes the latter the stain of choice for this procedure)
- Acetone (decolorizer) – Gram-negative organism loses colour
- Carbol fuschin (counter-stain) – Gram-negative organism stains red.

Gram staining procedure

1. Flood slides with methyl violet or crystal violet for 30 seconds.
2. Wash in tap water.
3. Flood slide with Gram's iodine for 60 seconds.
4. Wash in tap water.
5. Rinse with acetone for 3 seconds.
6. Wash quickly in tap water.
7. Counter-stain with dilute carbol fuchsin for 30 seconds.
8. Wash well with water
9. Blot dry and examine.   ▶

NOTES:
- **Once staining has begun, smears should never be allowed to dry**
- **Used slides should be placed in a container of disinfectant**

Results
- Gram-positive organisms stain dark violet
- Gram-negative organisms stain pink
- Tissue cells stain pink
- Fibrin strands stain violet

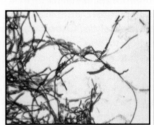   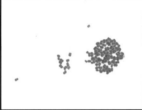

Gram-positive bacilli   Gram-negative bacilli

Ziehl–Neelsen (ZN) or acid-fast stain

This stain differentiates acid-fast from non-acid-fast bacteria. The technique uses a primary stain of lipid (fat)-soluble carbol fuchsin, with steam heat acting as mordant to drive the stain into the cell.

Ziehl–Neelsen staining procedure

1. Flood the slide with ZN carbol fuchsin solution and apply gentle heat until steam rises. *Do not boil* and *do not allow the stain to dry on the slide.* Leave for 5 minutes.
2. Wash well in tap water.
3. Decolorize with acid alcohol for at least 1 minute.
4. Wash in tap water and repeat decolorization until the film is very pale pink.
5. Counter-stain with Loeffler's alkaline methylene blue (LAMB). Leave for 2–3 minutes.
6. Wash with water.
7. Blot dry and examine.

Results
Acid-fast bacteria stain bright red on a blue background; all other organisms stain blue.

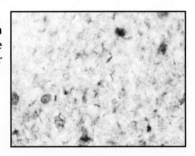

Haematology

Blood analysis may indicate disease, dysfunction, infection or a variety of systemic disorders, or may be performed as a general screening protocol in preparation for a procedure such as anaesthesia or surgery. Some abnormal results may indicate a patient's unsuitability for a procedure. Routine screening can allow early detection of a problem.

Components of blood

- **Plasma** is the fluid portion of the blood, which is clear and straw-coloured.
- **Serum** is plasma from which fibrinogen (a plasma protein) and prothrombin (a precursor of thrombin) have been removed. It is obtained from a clotted sample, which releases the serum portion from the cell when it clots.
- Within the plasma are:
  - **Erythrocytes**, or **red blood cells** (RBCs)
  - **Leucocytes**, or **white blood cells** (WBCs)
  - **Thrombocytes**, or **platelets**.

Blood cell morphology

The normal morphology of blood cells in dogs and cats is described and illustrated below. The cells are measured in micrometres (also called microns), written as μm (μ stands for micro and is pronounced 'mu'); 1000 μm = 1 millimetre (mm).

Cells with pointed cell margins (**crenation**) may be the result of a delay in drying the blood smear or an old sample.

Erythrocytes

- Round/biconcave corpuscle (Figure 17.18)
- Anuclear when mature
- Stain reddish/orange and exhibit prominent central pallor
- Size: in dog 7 μm, in cat 6 μm.

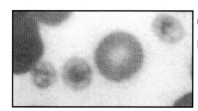

17.18 Erythrocyte and three platelets (paler).

Erythrocytes contain a protein called **haemoglobin**, which carries oxygen around the body and carbon dioxide to the lungs. An oxygenated erythrocyte will be bright red and a deoxygenated one will appear a darker red. **Heinz bodies** are round structures representing denatured haemoglobin, caused by certain oxidant drugs or chemicals. They are seen normally in the cat, though increased numbers are associated with diseases such as lymphosarcoma, hyperthyroidism and diabetes mellitus. Figure 17.19 defines some of the terms associated with the examination of erythrocytes and explains their significance.

Leucocytes

Leucocytes are subdivided into two categories: **granulocytes** (polymorphonuclear) – neutrophils, eosinophils and basophils; and **agranulocytes** (mononuclear) – lymphocytes and monocytes.

- **Neutrophils** have a diameter of 10–12 μm. They are principally involved with phagocytosis and have a lifespan of 5–10 hours.
- **Eosinophils** are similar in size to neutrophils, or slightly larger.
- **Basophils** are the least common granulocytes, and are similar in size to neutrophils, or slightly larger.
- **Lymphocytes** are round cells, slightly smaller than a neutrophil. They can be small, medium or large, with small and medium sizes predominant. They are produced by the lymph nodes and lymphatic tissue of the spleen

Term	Definition and significance
Anisocytosis	Marked variation in red cell size
Autoagglutination	'Grape-like' clusters of red cells more easily seen in the thicker part of the film
Basophilic stippling	Presence of small dark-blue bodies within the erythrocyte. Common in immature RBCs in cats during a response to anaemia; usually a characteristic of lead poisoning when seen in dogs
Howell–Jolly bodies	Spherical or ovoid eccentrically located granules, approximately 1 mm in diameter, occasionally observed in stroma of circulating erythrocytes, especially in stained preparations (as compared with wet unstained films); probably represent nuclear remnants, inasmuch as can be stained with dyes rather specific for chromatin. Significance of the bodies not exactly known; occur most frequently after splenectomy or in megaloblastic or severe haemolytic anaemia or steatorrhoea
Hypochromasia	Reduced cellular haemoglobin giving paler appearance and increased area of central pallor
Microcytosis	Overall smaller red cell size
Oligocythaemia	Decrease in RBCs – could indicate anaemia
Poikilocytosis	Abnormality of shape, often seen in association with hypochromia
Polychromasia	Many larger bluer red cells. These are slightly immature red cells and represent a regenerative response
Polycythaemia	Increased RBC count, could indicate dehydration
Reticulocyte	An immature RBC, enucleated; cytoplasm contains fine threads. May occur in cases of regenerative anaemia following acute haemorrhage
Rouleaux formation	Formation in which red cells settle in long chains or stacks when blood spread on glass slide. This field shows a few doublets and triplets of proper thickness for evaluation; background shows faint blue colour due to precipitated plasma proteins that have been stained; one small mature lymphocyte and one monocyte are in the field
Schistocyte	Red blood cell fragment
Spherocytes	Ball-like cells that appear smaller and darker stained, with no area of central pallor
Supra vital staining	The staining of live cells by incubating them with the stain *in vitro*; used to stain reticulocytes

17.19 Descriptive terms used in the examination of erythrocytes.

and liver. There are two types, B cells and T cells, which are indistinguishable by microscopic examination.

- **Monocytes** are generally the largest of the mature leucocyte blood cells (diameter 15–20 μm).

Figures 17.20 and 17.21 describe and illustrate the morphological features likely to be seen under the microscope. Figure 17.22 defines some of the terms associated with the examination of leucocytes and explains their significance.

Cell	Nucleus	Nuclear chromatin	Cytoplasm	Granules	Vacuoles
Neutrophil	Single, long and narrow with 3–5 lobes or segments resembling beads on string Nuclear membrane irregular Purple when stained	Large very dark-stained areas separated by smaller lighter-stained areas (Figure 17.21a)	Pale blue or grey	Invisible Purple when stained	
Eosinophil	Monolobed or segmented; lobes often fewer and not as well defined as in neutrophil Purple when stained but partially obscured by red granules (Figure 17.21b)	Less dense than in neutrophil Increase in number during allergic reactions, injury sites (against bacteria) or in response to nematode infection	Pale to light blue or grey	Round, variable in size and number Do not usually fill cytoplasm Colour similar to or slightly darker than RBC Best observed when less compact in cytoplasm or freely dispersed by cell rupture	Small clear observed occasionally
Basophil	Irregular, bilobed or segmented but often not to degree seen in mature neutrophil Purple when stained		Light grey	Round to oval, variable in number and staining intensity Reddish purple to dark purple	
Lymphocyte	Large and round to oval Agranular within cytoplasm Slight indentation (kidney-shaped) Almost fills the cell (Figure 17.21c)	Smooth areas mixed with clumped deeply stained areas	Light blue Limited in amount, in crescent at one side of nucleus		
Monocyte	Extremely variable in shape: oval, sometimes resembling kidney bean (Figure 17.21d), with single or multiple indentations and lobulations (e.g. shaped like bean, butterfly wing or horseshoe)	Fine granular, lacy, with few clumped areas	Blue-grey, denser stained than neutrophil cytoplasm Moderate amount		Multiple, variable sizes, clustered at one side of cell or spread along cell periphery giving foamy appearance

17.20 Morphology of leucocytes.

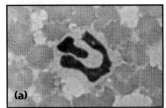 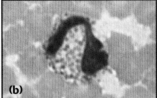 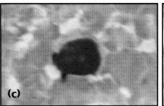 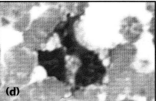

17.21 Leucocytes: **(a)** neutrophil; **(b)** canine eosinophil; **(c)** canine lymphocyte; **(d)** canine monocyte.

Term	Definition	Causes/indications
Basopenia	↓ Basophils	Rarely recorded
Basophilia	↑ Basophils	Rare but sometimes seen with types of leukaemia
Eosinopenia	↓ Eosinophils	Due to increased adrenal activity, corticosteroids, pneumonia or distemper
Eosinophilia	↑ Eosinophils	Due to an allergic reaction, tissue injury, neoplasm, oestrus or severe parasitism
Left-shift neutrophilia	Increased number of immature neutrophils (band forms)	Suggests acute inflammation
Leucocytosis	↑ WBCs	
Leucopenia	Reduction in one type of blood cell	
Lymphocytosis	↑ Lymphocytes	Could indicate chronic disease, recovery from a viral infection and possibly hypoadrenocorticism
Lymphopenia	↓ Lymphocytes	Due to increase in adrenal activity, or side effect of corticosteroids
Monopenia	↓ Monocytes	Rarely recorded
Monocytosis	↑ Monocytes	Could indicate chronic disease or acute inflammation
Myelocyte	Immature leucocyte	
Neutropenia	↓ Neutrophils	Due to bacterial infection (severe) or early viral infections
Neutrophilia	↑ Neutrophils	Due to bacterial infection, rapidly growing neoplasms or anaemia
Panleucopenia	Reduction in all types of white blood cells	Possibly due to early stage of viral infection

17.22 Descriptive terms used in the examination of leucocytes.

Thrombocytes

Platelets are small, round to oval, and anuclear, with pink to purple cytoplasmic granules. They appear on a blood film as non-nucleated fragments of variable shape (see Figure 17.18). The round platelets measure about 2–4 μm in diameter and the oval about 3.5 μm in length. Clumping of platelets occurs more in the cat, compared with the dog, and is usually seen on the thinner end of the slide.

Blood cell counts

Normal values for erythrocytes, leucocytes and other haematological counts are given in Figure 17.23. The most common of the leucocytes are the neutrophils, which should be counted in at least 10 fields (x40 lens) and the average calculated. An average of 4–6 neutrophils in the fields is the equivalent of approximately 7,000–10,000/m³.

Lymphocytes are the second most common leucocytes, but their numbers decrease with age – immature dogs have higher counts than adult dogs.

Platelets (thrombocytes) can be examined in a Romanowsky-stained blood smear, which should show approximately 3–25 platelets in a x400 objective field. A thrombocytopenic sample (i.e. with a decreased platelet count) may be indicative of leukaemia.

Figure 17.24 describes some typical haematological tests and illustrates their significance.

Packed cell volume

Packed cell volume (PCV), also known as **haematocrit**, is the percentage of blood that is occupied by the RBCs.

Equipment

Blood can be collected directly into a microhaematocrit tube or Wintrobe haematocrit tube or placed into an EDTA blood tube/vacutainer. There are different sizes of haematocrit and microhaematocrit tubes, depending on the centrifuge machine being used. There are two types of tube, depending on the type of blood sample collected:

- Red mark – coated with heparin (if from a non-anticoagulated sample)
- Blue mark – plain (if from an anticoagulated sample).

Method

1. Fill the (micro-)haematocrit tube to three-quarters full with blood (anticoagulated).
2. Seal the end of the tube and wipe the outside.
3. Centrifuge for 5 minutes at 10,000 rpm, ensuring that the open end points inwards.

Centrifugation will separate blood into three different layers (Figure 17.25):

	Dog	Cat
RBC (10^{12}/l)	5.5–8.5	5–10
PCV (l/l)	37–55% (hounds 45–65%)	24–45%
WBC (10^9/l)	6–17	5.5–19.5
Neutrophils (10^9/l)	6–18	5.5–19.5
Neutrophils (% WBC)	70%	60%
Eosinophils (% WBC)	4%	5%
Basophils (% WBC)	1%	1%
Lymphocytes (% WBC)	20%	32%
Monocytes (% WBC)	5%	3%
Thrombocytes (10^9/l)	200 (1 platelet/35 RBCs)	200 (1 platelet/35 RBCs)
Erythrocyte sedimentation rate (ESR) (mm/h)	0–5	4–13
Haemoglobin (Hb) (g/100 ml)	12–18	9–17
MCV (mean cell volume) (fl)	60–70	39–55
MCHC (mean cell haemoglobin concentration) (g/dl)	32–36	30–36

17.23 Normal values for haematological tests.

Test	Definition	Significance of results	
		Increased	Decreased
Complete blood count (CBC)	A number of tests used to determine RBC, WBC and platelet levels	WBC: leukaemia, stress, inflammation, inability to fight infection	Platelets: haemostasis problem
Haemoglobin (Hb)	A complex protein (pigment) molecule contained within an RBC, responsible for its colour and the transportation of oxygen to the tissues and cells	Dehydration	Anaemia
Mean corpuscular volume (MCV)	Mean volume for a group of erythrocytes	Regenerative anaemia	Liver disease
Mean haemoglobin concentration (MCHC)	Concentration of haemoglobin in the average erythrocyte (or ratio of weight in haemoglobin to volume in which it is contained)	Not indicative	Iron deficiency

17.24 Significance of haematological test results.

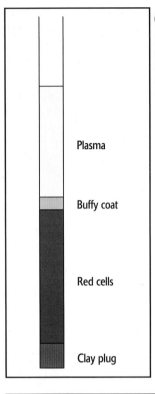

17.25 Layers of a centrifuged sample in a haematocrit tube for PCV evaluation. (Reproduced from *BSAVA Manual of Canine and Feline Clinical Pathology, 2nd edition*)

1. **Plasma** – should be colourless in the normal animal
2. **Buffy coat** – contains white blood cells and platelets
3. **Red blood cells** – located at the bottom of the column.

Reading a PCV

Methods of reading a PCV include:

- Hand-held scale (Figure 17.26)
- Hawksley reader (Figure 17.27)
- Scale on lid of centrifuge (if available)
- Measuring with a ruler. Use the following calculation if measuring PCV with a ruler:

PCV (mm) = [(height of RBCs)/(total column height)] x 100

Three samples should be assessed and the average calculated.

Results

Normal PCV values are:

- Dog – 37–55% (mean 45%) (sight hounds 45–65%)
- Cat – 24–45% (mean 35%).

An increased PCV may indicate dehydration (reduced plasma levels). A decreased PCV may indicate anaemia, but a haemoglobin test should be carried out to confirm this.

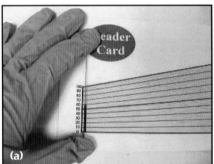
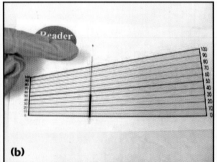
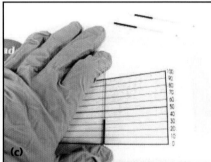

17.26 Reading a PCV with a hand-held scale. **(a)** The top of the bung is set in line with zero on the scale. **(b)** The sample is moved along the scale until the top of the *plasma* is in line with the top line, which is 100 on the scale (not the top of the haematocrit tube). **(c)** The PCV reading is taken from the top of the RBCs and a percentage reading is taken for the buffy coat, as an increase or decrease from normal values could be indicative of a disease, condition or infection.

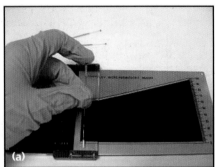
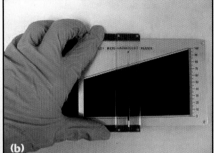
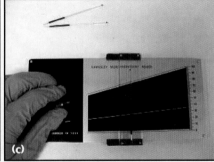

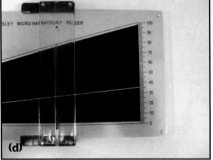

17.27 Reading a PCV with the Hawksley haematocrit reader. **(a)** The Microhaematocrit is loaded into a groove within a plastic holder at the front of the Hawksley reader. The top of the bung is set in line with the baseline of the scale. **(b)** The plastic holder is moved across the scale until the top of the plasma is in line with 100 on the Hawksley reader scale. **(c)** The lever to the left is lifted until the line is at the top of the RBC column (not including the buffy coat or plasma); the line will then indicate the percentage for this sample. **(d)** The lever is used again to assess the percentage of the buffy coat layer (without counting either the RBC column or the plasma portion).

Plasma layer

- Straw-coloured – normal
- Pink – haemolysis of the sample
- White – lipaemic (increased fat content of plasma)
- Yellow – icteric (presence of bilirubin, possibly indicating a liver problem)

Buffy coat layer

The colour should be whitish, though if pink it could indicate the presence of immature RBCs. Abnormal levels include:

- 1.2% – leucocytosis
- < 0.5% – leucopenia.

Blood clotting

Thrombocytes are important for blood coagulation (clotting) and for haemostasis, by repairing breaches in the walls of blood vessels. Under the influence of the protein **thromboplastin** released by platelets, **prothrombin** is converted to **thrombin**, which acts on **fibrinogen** to produce **fibrin**, a binding agent that forms a meshwork in the presence of calcium, resulting in clotting.

Normal clotting times are usually 1–2 minutes. An increase in clotting time may be caused by: a haemorrhagic disorder such as haemophilia; prothrombin deficiency; liver disease; infectious canine hepatitis; warfarin poisoning; or anaemia. The activated coagulation (clotting) time (ACT), bleeding time or a platelet count test can be used to check the clotting levels of the blood.

Whole-blood ACT

1. Put 1 ml of whole blood into a small glass tube.
2. Put the tube into a water bath at 37°C.
3. Record the time from aspiration to the time when the first tube clots.

The normal value for dogs is <10 minutes.

Bleeding time

1. Make two small nicks in the skin, gum or ear pinna, using a commercial bleeding test kit and start a stopwatch.
2. Gently wipe away any trickles of blood from the wound but avoid touching the wound itself.
3. Note when the wound stops bleeding and stop the watch.

Blood groups

Dogs have 11 different blood groups, identified as **dog erythrocyte antigens** (DEA), but only six are of clinical relevance: DEA 1.1, 1.2, 3, 4, 5 and 7.

Blood transfusions are becoming more commonplace in general practice for the treatment of severe blood loss, anaemia, bleeding disorders, acute pancreatitis and hypoalbuminaemia. The ideal canine blood donor would be DEA 4, as this group is classed as a universal donor to all other blood groups, but blood typing to assess a patient's actual group is recommended wherever possible.

Cats have A, B and AB groups but no universal donor. Transfusion with the wrong blood group could result in a life-threatening haemolytic reaction.

Canine blood group determination assay

Agglutination test cards (Figure 17.28a) are each labelled with an expiry date. The cards are stable for a period of 18 months from date of manufacture if refrigerated. It is not necessary to bring the card to room temperature prior to use. Directions for use are found within the manufacturer's guidelines and should be followed closely, noting that there are different assay methods and kits for the cat and the dog.

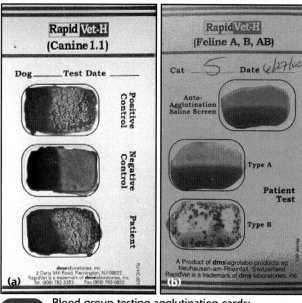

17.28 Blood group testing agglutination cards: **(a)** canine; **(b)** feline (DMS Laboratories).

Feline blood group determination assay

Agglutination of the patient's sample in either the well that is marked 'Type A' or the well marked 'Type B' indicates that the cat's blood group is A or B, respectively (Figure 17.28b). If the sample shows agglutination in both wells, the cat's blood group is AB.

Biochemistry

Biochemical estimations are usually carried out on serum or plasma. 'Normal' (reference) values depend on the test or equipment being used and it is important to refer to equipment manuals or the manufacturer's values. Figure 17.29 gives some

Substance and units	Dog	Cat
Albumin (g/l)	25–40	25–40
Alanine aminotransferase (IU/l)	10–75	35–134
Alkaline phosphatase (IU/l)	0–80	15–96
Blood urea nitrogen (mmol/l)	2.5–7	5–11
Calcium (mmol/l)	2–3	1.8–3
Cholesterol (mmol/l)	2.5–8	2–6.5
Creatinine (mmol/l)	40–130	40–130
Glucose (mmol/l)	3.3–6	3.3–6
Pancreatic amylase (IU/l)	350–1200	515–2210
Phosphate (mmol/l)	0.8–1.6	1.3–2.6
Total bilirubin (mmol/l)	1.7–10	2–5
Total protein (g/l)	54–71	54–78

17.29 Normal reference ranges for biochemical tests. It should be remembered that reference levels will vary between laboratories.

reference ranges for normal values, but these must be interpreted with care as 'normal' reference values vary between analysers and between laboratories.

A variety of tests can be performed on blood, involving:

- Direct biochemical levels
- Commercial test strips
- Electrolytes
- Commercial in-house test kits for viral, protozoal, nematode and hormonal levels.

Biochemical levels and commercial test strips

ACTH (adrenocorticotrophic hormone) stimulation test

The ACTH stimulation test measures blood cortisol values before and after stimulation of the adrenal glands with synthetic ACTH (tetracosactide). A high result after stimulation is suggestive of hyperadrenocorticism (Cushing's disease). A low level before and after stimulation is suggestive of hypoadrenocorticism (Addison's disease).

Cats: Assay cortisol levels at 0, 60 and 120–180 minutes. Inject tetracosactide (Synacthen) at 0.125 mg i.v. after basal level measured at 0 minutes.

Dogs: Assay cortisol levels at 0 and 2 hours. Inject tetracosactide (Synacthen) at 0.125 mg i.v. (<5 kg bodyweight) or 0.25 mg i.v. (>5 kg bodyweight) after basal level measured at 0 hours.

Albumin

This protein is produced by the liver. Reduced levels may indicate problems or disease in the liver, kidneys or intestinal tract.

Alanine aminotransferase (ALT)

This enzyme may be an indicator of liver disease or injury.

Alkaline phosphatase (ALP)

This enzyme is present in a number of tissues, including liver and bone. Elevated levels may indicate liver disease, Cushing's syndrome (hyperadrenocorticism) or steroid therapy.

Ammonia (NH₃)

Ammonia is a product of metabolism that should be excreted. If present in high levels, it can be associated with a portal shunt and can cause neurological problems known as hepatoencephalopathy.

Bile acid stimulation test

This test is a useful indicator for hepatic function or disease; it is a diagnostic test for portosystemic shunts in the dog and cat.

After a fatty meal the gallbladder contracts, releasing bile acids into the duodenum to allow emulsification and absorption of the fats. In normal animals, hepatic clearance of bile acids is very efficient, with only low levels being present in peripheral blood postprandially. Significant hepatocellular dysfunction reduces hepatic functional mass or shunting of blood away from the liver. This can give rise to high levels of bile acid.

1. Fast the animal for 12 hours.
2. Take about 1–2 ml blood into a plain/gel tube.
3. Administer fatty meal or vegetable oil.
4. Take a second sample of blood 2 hours after eating.
5. Label tubes with name and time of sample.
6. Submit tubes and request form to the laboratory.

The exact form of fatty meal administered for this test is not critical, provided that it induces gallbladder contraction. Proprietary paediatric diets are recommended. In anorexic animals, administration of vegetable oil orally can be used.

Blood urea nitrogen (BUN)

BUN is produced by the liver and then excreted by the kidneys as a waste product. An elevated BUN could indicate renal insufficiency or dehydration. A decreased BUN could be associated with liver disease.

Azostix (Ames) test strips can be used on whole blood to assess for BUN levels:

1. Apply a drop of blood to the test strip.
2. Wait 60 seconds and wash off with water.
3. Read immediately against the colour guide found on the actual test strip container.

Calcium (Ca²⁺)

Increased levels of calcium may indicate parathyroid gland disease, renal disease or some types of tumours.

Cholesterol

An increase may indicate a variety of disorders, including hypothyroidism, diabetes mellitus, liver disease, renal disease or hyperadrenocorticism.

Creatinine

This byproduct of muscle metabolism is excreted by the kidneys. Elevated results could indicate renal insufficiency, urinary tract obstruction or dehydration.

Dexamethasone suppression tests

Dexamethasone suppression tests (DSTs) are used for the investigation of hyperadrenocorticism (Cushing's disease). They measure blood cortisol values before and after suppression of the adrenal glands with the synthetic corticosteroid dexamethasone. The low-dose DST (LDDST) can be used instead of, or in addition to, the ACTH stimulation test (see above) for the diagnosis of hyperadrenocorticism. Once the diagnosis of hyperadrenocorticism is made, the high-dose DST (HDDST) is used to try and differentiate between the two causes of hyperadrenocorticism – pituitary-dependent or adrenal tumour – but it is unreliable.

LDDST: Assess blood cortisol at 0, 3 and 8 hours. Give 0.01–0.015 mg/kg dexamethasone i.v. after the 0 hour sample. Failure to suppress at 3 and 8 hours indicates hyperadrenocorticism (some cases show partial suppression at 3 hours).

HDDST: Assess blood cortisol at 0, 3 and 8 hours. Give 1.0 mg/kg dexamethasone i.v. after the 0 hour sample.

Pituitary-dependent: most cases suppress after 3 and 8 hours.

Adrenal tumours: Most fail to suppress or show partial suppression at 3 hours.

Glucose

Elevated levels of glucose may indicate diabetes mellitus, or Cushing's disease (hyperadrenocorticism) if the sample was taken just after a meal following exercise, or may be due to stress (especially in cats). Low levels may indicate liver disease, infection, insulin overdose, septicaemia or certain tumours.

Test strips are available that can test for glucose specifically.

Serial blood glucose typing (canine and feline)

Serial blood glucose testing is used to assess insulin responsiveness, peak activity, duration and the extent of glycaemic control over a 24-hour period. This test can be used early in therapy to allow optimum feeding and insulin administration for the individual case. It is also helpful where glycaemic control is deteriorating or is very unstable.

Results of this test can be profoundly affected by stress at sampling, inappetence and exercise. To minimize artefacts, the taking of samples through an indwelling catheter is preferred over repeated venepuncture.

Shortened tests run over the normal working day can miss significant hyperglycaemia overnight. At a minimum, a 2–3-hour postprandial sample should be taken after the evening meal, with 2-hourly sampling being the ideal. During the test, dogs should be managed as usual in relation to the timing of insulin and feeding.

1. Take baseline blood (1 ml) sample into fluoride oxalate anticoagulant. Mix the sample and check for the presence of any clotting. Label with time and owner's name.
2. Store this and subsequent samples in the fridge prior to despatch.
3. Insert indwelling intravenous catheter. Flush the cap with heparinized saline in the normal manner.
4. Diabetic management and feeding regime should as far as possible be normal for the patient.
5. Take further samples into fluoride oxalate as above at 2–3-hourly intervals.

Pancreatic amylase

This enzyme is produced by the pancreas, which secretes amylase to aid in digestion. Elevated blood levels can indicate pancreatic disease or pancreatitis.

Phosphate

Increased levels of phosphate may indicate renal insufficiency.

Thyroxine

Thyroxine (T4) is produced in the thyroid gland. A raised T4 level can indicate hyperthyroidism (cats) and a low T4 level is seen in hypothyroidism (dogs). Unfortunately, many other factors can also lower T4 levels (illness, several medications) so a low T4 level on its own is unreliable for the diagnosis of hypothyroidism. Dynamic tests are more reliable for the diagnosis of hypothyroidism. In these tests, T4 levels are compared before and after stimulation of the thyroid gland with either thyroid stimulating hormone (TSH stimulation test; TSH only available in UK if imported with a Special Treatment Authorization) or, more commonly, thyrotropin releasing hormone (TRH stimulation test).

Total bilirubin (TBIL)

Bilirubin is a breakdown product of haemoglobin as well as a component of bile. High levels may indicate liver disease, anaemia or a biliary obstruction (possibly due to neoplasia).

Total protein (TP)

Levels of total protein may indicate various conditions, including dehydration, liver disease, renal disease or intestinal disease. TP levels can also be obtained using a refractometer, sometimes combined with urine specific gravity estimations – it is important to read from the correct graph.

Electrolytes

Electrolytes are the main salts of the body (see Chapter 19). They are maintained at optimum levels in the healthy animal and any alteration in their balance can be life-threatening. They should be analysed in cases of gastrointestinal tract, urinary, cardiac or certain endocrine diseases (e.g. hypoadrenocorticism).

- **Sodium (Na⁺)** – normal values 140–155 mmol/l (dog), 145–157 mmol/l (cat); increased levels may indicate intestinal or kidney disease; decreased levels may indicate intestinal disease or hypoadrenocorticism
- **Potassium (K⁺)** – normal values 3.6–5.8 mmol/l (dog), 3.6–555 mmol/l (cat); increased levels may indicate hypoadrenocorticism or renal disease; decreased levels may indicate intestinal disease
- **Chloride (Cl⁻)** – blood chloride levels play an important role in maintenance of water distribution, osmotic pressure and normal anion:cation ratio. Normal levels in the dog: 54–55 IU. Levels may be elevated in renal disease.

In-house test kits

A number of in-house test kits are now available for quick and reliable diagnosis. They are simple to use; instructions provided by the manufacturer should be followed. High specificity and sensitivity are associated with these tests, reducing the risk of false positives occurring.

Kits are available for detection of the following:

- Feline leukaemia virus (FeLV) infection (antibodies)
- Feline immunodeficiency virus (FIV) infection (antibodies)
- Giardiasis
- Heartworm
- Leishmaniasis
- Canine parvovirus
- Thyroxine (radioimmunoassay)

Urinalysis

Urinalysis is the chemical and microscopic analysis of urine. It is non-invasive and simple and can assist the veterinary clinician in the diagnosis of many conditions affecting the urinary and other systems of the body (Figure 17.30).

Term	Definition
Bilirubinuria	Presence of bilirubin in the urine
Calculi (*sing.* calculus)	Abnormal concretions occurring within the animal body and usually composed of mineral salts
Glucosuria	Glucose in the urine; a characteristic of diabetes
Haematuria	Presence of blood in the urine
Ketonuria	Presence of ketone bodies in the urine; a characteristic of diabetes
Proteinuria	Excessive protein in the urine
Urobilinuria	Presence in the urine of urobilins in excessive amount, formed mainly from haemoglobin
Urochrome	A yellowy urinary pigment normally present in urine
Urolith	Urinary calculus (stone)

17.30 Descriptive terms used in urinalysis.

Most urinalysis techniques involve the use of just a few inexpensive items of laboratory equipment that are easy to use. The most important factor is to ensure the correct usage of such equipment by appropriate care, maintenance and training of all personnel involved with it. This will help to ensure the longevity of the equipment and the reliability of the test results.

Care must be taken when handling urine, due to the potential hazard with certain zoonotic organisms such as *Leptospira*. Gloves must be worn at all times when collecting and handling urine samples.

Physical tests

Physical urinalysis tests examine the appearance, volume and specific gravity of the urine.

Appearance

Points to consider include colour, turbidity, odour and any deposits. Normal appearances for these factors are described in Figure 17.31; abnormalities are described in Figure 17.32.

Feature	Normal appearance
Colour	Pale yellow (due to presence of pigment, urochrome) Rabbits have porphyrin pigments that produce a red coloration (not to be confused with blood)
Turbidity	Transparent in cats and dogs Cloudy in birds and rabbits Old urine samples may also appear cloudy
Odour	Slight sour smell in dogs Can be quite putrid in tomcats (due to presence of pheromones) Certain diets (e.g. volatile fatty acids, fish) can add strength to odour
Sediment	Little or none

17.31 Normal physical appearance of urine.

Urine volume

Normal urine production is a good indicator of kidney function, hydration status and body fluid balance. Normal urine production is approximately 1–2 ml/kg/hour for both dogs (24–40 ml/kg/day) and cats (22–30 ml/kg/day). Volume can be measured via the collection of voided urine, use of a metabolism cage or an indwelling catheter and urine collection system.

Good fluid balance ensures optimal bodily performance and plays a major role in the recovery of sick animals. A decrease in urine volume and an increase in specific gravity (see below) may be indicative of dehydration or systemic illness. An increased amount may indicate renal disease, endocrine disorders, hepatic disease or drug therapy (e.g. diuretics, glucocorticoids).

Specific gravity

Specific gravity (SG) is the density or weight of a known volume of fluid compared with an equal amount of distilled water:

$$SG = \frac{\text{Weight of a certain volume of a liquid}}{\text{Weight of the same volume of water}}$$

The SG of distilled water is 1.000. Normal SG values for urine are 1.015–1.045 for the dog and 1.020–1.050 for the cat. A decrease in SG may be indicative of chronic renal failure, diabetes insipidus, some liver disorders, increased thirst (polydipsia) or the use of corticosteroids or fluid therapy. An increase in SG may indicate acute renal failure, shock, dehydration or fluid loss.

Measurement of urine SG can be performed using a refractometer (Figure 17.33).

Feature	Abnormality	Possible causes of abnormal appearance
Colour	Pale/clear	Polyuric/polydipsic conditions
	Darker yellow/orange	Dehydration due to fever, fluid losses through vomiting or diarrhoea, or water deprivation
	Orange/brown	Bilirubin content (? liver problem) Concentration due to dehydration
	Red, brown or black	Blood (haematuria) Blood pigments Certain drugs (e.g. phenothiazines can change urine colour to red)
	Green/yellow	Biliverdin content (on standing, bilirubin oxidizes to green, i.e. biliverdin)
	Fluorescent green	Artificial colourings that can be found in canned dog food
	Blue or green tinged	Certain drugs (e.g. methylene blue)
Turbidity	Cloudy	Contamination by semen or pus (leucocytes) Number of bacteria Amount of mucus Deterioration due to incorrect storage Suspended crystals
Odour	Sweet/fruity	Ketones (e.g. diabetes mellitus)
	Ammonia	Indicative of an older sample In fresh urine: number of bacteria (e.g. cystitis)
	Foul	Excess protein (e.g. cystitis)
Sediment	Cellular deposit	Damage to part of the urinary tract

17.32 Abnormalities in physical characteristics of urine.

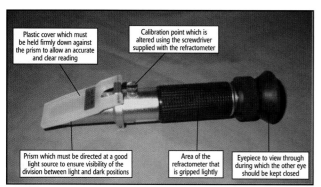

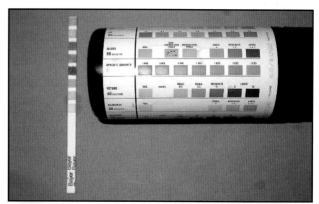

Labels on figure 17.33:
- Plastic cover which must be held firmly down against the prism to allow an accurate and clear reading
- Calibration point which is altered using the screwdriver supplied with the refractometer
- Prism which must be directed at a good light source to ensure visibility of the division between light and dark positions
- Area of the refractometer that is gripped lightly
- Eyepiece to view through during which the other eye should be kept closed

17.33 Refractometer for measuring specific gravity of urine.

Using a refractometer

1. Open the prism cover.
2. Check calibration of the refractometer using distilled water, which should read 1.000. If not reading 1.000, recalibrate as follows.
   i. Unscrew the fixation nut of the calibration screw
   ii. Turn the calibration screw downwards to bring the scale up or unscrew this screw to bring the scale down until it reads 1.000
   iii. Reaffix the calibration nut
   iv. Wipe clean with soft tissue or a lens cleaning wipe.
3. To view, hold the refractometer horizontally in the direction of a good light source, preferably a natural light source.
4. Wearing gloves, place 1–2 drops of urine on the face of the lower prism and view through the eyepiece. Note where colour boundary line is and read against specific gravity scale.
5. After use, clean the prism and cover very carefully with a wet soft cloth or damp lens wipe.

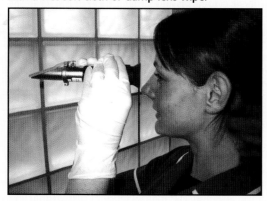

Chemical tests

Chemical tests are useful tools in the evaluation of urine. Using commercial dipsticks, they are quick, easy to perform and inexpensive. The test strips are kept in an air-tight container. The expiry date should be checked before the test is carried out. Dipstick tests are not a reliable method for measuring specific gravity.

When the strips are dipped in urine, a chemical reaction takes place and the colour of the pads may change over time. The colour change is compared with the colour-coded chart on the strip container (Figure 17.34). Fresh urine should be used and it is essential to compare the reading on each pad at the exact time stated on the strip container. It is useful to list

the chemicals on a separate piece of paper before starting the test, so that the results can be recorded at the specified time.

Dipsticks are available to measure pH, proteins, glucose, ketones, bilirubin, urobilinogen, nitrite and blood in urine. Normal values and possible causes of abnormal levels are given in Figure 17.35.

17.34 Commercial dipstick used for chemical testing of urine samples. The colour change is compared with the colour-coded chart on the strip container.

	Normal values	Possible causes of abnormal levels	
		Increased levels	Decreased levels
pH	Dog 5–7 Cat 7–9	Bacterial infection Cystitis Alkalosis Old urine sample	Fever Starvation Diabetes mellitus Chronic renal failure Acidosis
Proteins	Small amount	Renal failure Haemorrhage Inflammatory disease Pyrexia	
Glucose	None	Stress Excitement Diabetes mellitus Inappropriate collection (false-positive)	
Ketones	None	Diabetes mellitus Carbohydrate metabolism Hypoglycaemia Prolonged starvation Pyrexia	
Bilirubin (bile pigment)	Trace to ++	Liver disease or damage Haemolytic or obstructive jaundice	
Urobilinogen (bile salts)	Small amounts	Liver dysfunction	Liver dysfunction
Nitrite	None	Bacterial infection (especially Gram-negative rods, e.g. E. coli)	

17.35 Normal and abnormal values in chemical urinalysis.

Blood in urine (haematuria)

Blood is not normally present in urine. Contamination of a urine sample may occur, for example, when damage is caused by a urinary catheter, or from the genital tract of a bitch in pro-oestrus. If the blood is non-haemolysed this suggests haem-orrhage within the lower urogenital tract, whereas a haemo-lysed sample suggests damage in the upper urinary tract.

An increased level of red blood cells may indicate haemor-rhage, inflammatory reaction, urolithiasis, trauma, poor sam-ple collection, toxins, infection, metabolic disorder, traumatic or neoplastic conditions.

An increased level of white blood cells may arise in response to damage of the urinary tract. Large numbers may indicate an inflammatory condition of the urinary system.

Microscopic examination of urine sediment

Normal urine contains little sediment, but low levels of epithe-lial cells, mucus, blood cells and contaminating bacteria may be present. Centrifugation allows concentration of crystals, bacteria and cells, which can be a useful diagnostic tool.

Equipment

- Urine sample
- Centrifuge tube
- Centrifuge
- Dropping pipette
- Microscope slide and cover slip
- Sedistain, also Leishman's or Gram stain if examining for bacteria

Preparation of urine sediment

Centrifugation

1. Fill the tube with the urine sample, using a sterile pipette.
2. Centrifuge the sample (5 minutes at 1000–2000 rpm); balance the centrifuge.
3. Remove the supernatant fluid, leaving a few drops in which to re-suspend the sample.
4. 'Flick' the tube to re-suspend the sediment with the last couple of drops of urine and dye.

Wet preparation

To make a wet preparation of the centrifuged sediment for examination of crystals and casts, place a few drops on a microscope slide and apply a cover slip at an angle of 45 degrees to avoid any air bubbles.

Examine under low power and low illumination (by clos-ing iris and racking down the substage condenser). This pro-duces a greater contrast between transparent deposits.

Smear

To prepare a smear for examination of cells and bacteria:

1. Place a small drop of the centrifuged sediment on a miscroscope slide and make a smear, using the same method as for blood (see above). Alternatively, use a bacteriological loop to spread the drop evenly over the slide.
2. Allow the smear to air dry.
3. Sedistain or Leishman's stain may be used to show cells present. Stain with Gram's stain to identify bacteria.

Examine under low power and low illumination: low power first, followed by a higher power. For bacteria, use of the oil x100 objective will be required.

Examination of cells

The following might be found in the sediment (Figure 17.36).

- **Blood cells**
  - Erythrocytes – haematuria (blood in urine, oestrus, trauma from catheterization
  - Leucocytes – inflammatory reaction in urogenital tract (cystitis)
- **Epithelial cells**
  - Squamous cells (lower urethra, vaginal, prepuce) – large granular cells with nucleus
  - Transitional cells (bladder) – smaller than squamous cells
  - Renal epithelial cells (kidney) – smallest cell type, round or comma-shaped, seen in acute renal failure
- **Spermatozoa** – seen in male dogs, less common in tomcats
- **Worm eggs** – rare; bladder worm (*Capillaria plica*)
- **Yeast cells** – non-nucleated round or oval bodies; due to contamination
- **Bacteria** – always present to some degree; culture and sensitivity tests
- **Faecal material** – contamination
- **Mucus** – may indicate kidney damage, recent surgery, retrograde ejaculate (if male).

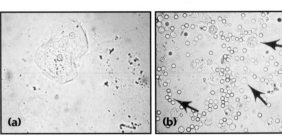

17.36 Cells that might be visible in microscopic urinalysis: **(a)** Squamous epithelial cells in canine urine sediment. Note their angular borders, abundant translucent cytoplasm and single condensed nucleus. (Unstained; original magnification X400). **(b)** Size comparison of cells in an active canine urine sediment. Erythrocytes are the smallest cells (left arrow), leucocytes are larger than erythrocytes (middle arrow) and transitional epithelial cells are larger than leucocytes (right arrow). Squamous epithelial cells are the largest cells (not pictured). (Unstained; original magnification X400). (Reproduced from *BSAVA Manual of Canine and Feline Nephrology and Neurology, 2nd edition*)

Examination of crystals

Urine crystals can be seen in urolithiasis, cystitis, haematuria and also in normal animals. Identification of the crystal is essen-tial for the diagnosis and management of each patient. The main types of crystal that may be found are composed of struvite, cystine, calcium oxalate and ammonium urate (see Chapter 16).

Crystals may aggregate together to form large **uroliths** or **calculi** ('stones') (Figure 17.37). If these crystals damage the urinary tract the disease is known as **urolithiasis**.

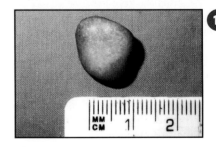

17.37 Urolith.

Struvite (triple phosphate)

These crystals are shaped like a coffin lid (Figure 17.38a) and may be found in alkaline urine, commonly in conjunction with urinary tract infections. They may also be found in animals that are clinically normal.

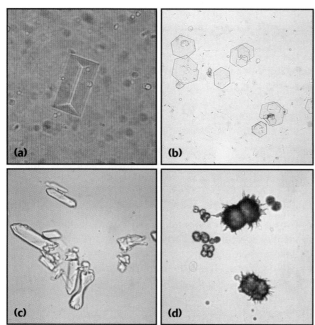

17.38 Crystals found in urine sediment: **(a)** struvite; **(b)** cystine; **(c)** calcium oxalate monohydrate; **(d)** ammonium biurate. Magnifications vary. (Reproduced from *BSAVA Manual of Canine and Feline Nephrology and Neurology, 2nd edition*)

Quantitative calculi analysis and incidence may be more indicative of urolithiasis. This can be confirmed with radiography, as most struvite uroliths are radiopaque. Of uroliths analysed in cats, 82–90% are struvite, with 80–97% occurrence in bitches and immature male dogs, and a rate of 50–75% in mature male dogs.

Cystine

These thin hexagonal-shaped structures (Figure 17.38b) may be found in acidic urine in adult male dogs. Cystine uroliths are moderately radiopaque.

Calcium oxalate

These envelope-shaped crystals (Figure 17.38c) may be found in acidic or neutral pH urine. Certain breeds are prone to oxalate due to a genetic defect; they include Miniature Schnauzer, Yorkshire Terrier, Lhaso Apso, Miniature Poodle and, in cats, Burmese, Himalayan and Persian. They are not usually a problem unless calculi formation occurs.

Calcium oxalate crystals are also found in animals that ingest antifreeze (ethylene glycol). They are radiopaque and are responsible for 10–20% of the urolith cases occurring in adult male dogs.

Ammonium urate

These crystals, found in acidic and neutral urine, may be shaped like thorn-apples, spindles or rosettes (Figure 17.38d) – almost like sand. Their presence in the urine of Dalmatians is normal, due to the way that this breed metabolizes and excretes protein. Ammonium urate crystals may also be found in dogs that have portosystemic shunts or liver disease.

Examination of casts

Casts are formed in the distal tubules and collecting tubules of the kidneys. They are composed of albumin/protein material. Their presence in large numbers suggests proteinuria and may indicate renal disease. The presence of bilirubin will stain the casts yellow.

Casts might be confused with hairs, fibres or strands of mucus under the microscope. Casts generally have straight parallel sides and tend to get pushed to the edge of the cover slip.

There are five types of cast:

* **Hyaline** – protein precipitates, casts dissolve rapidly in alkaline urine; due to fever or exercise
* **Cellular** – WBCs or pus, epithelial cells, RBCs; due to acute renal failure or pyelonephritis
* **Granular** – degeneration of other cells or casts; commonly associated with acute renal failure in the dog (where small quantities of highly concentrated urine is passed containing many casts); chronic renal failure results in more dilute urine, decreased specific gravity, larger volumes of urine with fewer casts
* **Waxy** – final stage of degeneration of granular casts; indicates extensive renal damage
* **Fatty** – rarely seen; stain with Sudan III.

Faecal analysis

Faecal testing may aid in the diagnosis relating to impaired digestion, bacterial or yeast infections. Evidence of internal protozoal and helminth parasites may also be detected, but there may be negative results due to the migratory behaviour of parasites through tissues or organs, intermittent shedding of the parasite from the animal, different developmental stages of the parasite or just a low infestation number. Negative results do not necessarily mean there is no parasitosis.

It is vitally important to ensure strict hygiene is maintained at all times in the handling of faecal samples. Some of the organisms have a serious zoonotic potential, e.g. *Salmonella, Campylobacter, Cryptosporidium, Toxoplasma gondii*.

The following may be found in a normal faecal sample:

* Water (60–80%)
* Undigested food in small amounts
* Enzymes (trypsin)
* Bile products (biliverdin) – pigments produce the colour brown
* Small amounts of mucus from the colon
* Bacteria
* A few epithelial cells
* Some blood (particularly if the animal is fed meat)
* Hair.

Macroscopic examination

Macroscopic examination should include appraisal of the appearance, colour, consistency and odour of the faeces.

Appearance and colour

Some conditions may be seen with the naked eye. For example, whole ascarid worms are spaghetti-like (see Chapter 8), whereas smaller segments resembling rice or cucumber seeds might indicate a tapeworm. Other material that may be visible includes grass, string, odd fragments of prey and undigested foodstuff.

The animal's diet may affect the colour of faeces, but the normal colour is a light to dark brown. Colours that would be considered abnormal are described in Figure 17.39.

Abnormality	Possible causes
Dark brown/ black (melaena)	Increased red meat in diet Upper intestinal haemorrhage, i.e. from the stomach or small intestines as haemorrhage slightly digested
Pink	Hepatic dysfunction, i.e. biliary obstruction
Red/bloody	Fresh blood on the faeces indicative of lower intestinal haemorrhage Fresh blood seen within faeces is more suggestive of bleeding higher up the gastrointestinal tract, possibly due to enteritis or parasitosis
White (steatorrhoea)	Increased fat in diet Feeding of bones within diet Metabolic problem, e.g. undigested fat (EPI)
Blue	Suspected warfarin poisoning
Yellow	Increased bile pigment content, may be suggestive of liver problem or disorder
Mucous	Mucus on faeces may indicate lower alimentary tract problem such as bowel disease Mucus within faeces may be suggestive of ileac problem

17.39 Abnormal faecal colour or consistency.

Consistency and odour

Consistency may vary from normal to constipation (hard, dry) or diarrhoea (soft, wet).

Odour depends on diet, but the following points should be considered:

- Increased fat levels in the diet produce a rancid smell
- A very rich diet may produce a strong smell
- Some conditions carry a characteristic smell (e.g. parvovirus infection).

Microscopic examination

Microscopic analysis could detect any of the following:

- Fat/starch or muscle fibres (impaired digestion)
- Bacterial or yeast infection
- Parasitosis – adult worms, segments or eggs, and protozoan cells

- Artefacts, e.g. plant cells, pollen grains, grass, air bubbles, bone, wood, fibres from clothing.

Baermann technique

Faeces are suspended in muslin at the top of a column of water (often constructed from a funnel with a piece of tubing attached; the end of the tubing is sealed with a clip). The sample is left overnight, during which time any larvae that leave the faecal deposit will fall to the bottom of the water column. In the morning the clip is released and about 15 ml of water collected into a test tube. The test tube is then left to stand or is centrifuged so that any larvae drop to the bottom of the tube. The supernatant is removed and the sediment is placed on a microscope slide and viewed.

Analysis of skin and hair samples

The main reason for laboratory examination of skin samples is to identify ectoparasites, bacteria, fungi and yeasts. Care must be taken when handling specimens, as some skin conditions may be zoonotic. The tests to be carried out will depend on the clinical signs of the patient.

Ectoparasites

Ectoparasites fall into two groups: insects (fleas, lice, flies) and arachnids (mites, ticks) (see Chapter 8). The main methods of collecting ectoparasites are skin scrapings, coat brushings, hair plucks and adhesive tape strips (see above).

Microscopic examination

Using low-power (x4 objective) microscopy should be sufficient to examine the ectoparasites that are visible to the naked eye. Higher power (x10, x40) should be used for the microscopic mites (*Sarcoptes* spp., *Demodex* spp.) and for examining in closer detail for identification purposes (Figure 17.40).

- **Insects** (fleas, lice) – adult has three pairs of legs, three parts to the body (head, thorax, abdomen) and one pair of antennae
- **Arachnids** (mites, ticks) – adult has four pairs of legs, two parts to the body (cephalothorax, abdomen) and no antennae.

Species	Size V = visible to naked eye M = microscopic	Colour	Body shape	Legs L = long S = short (posterior two pairs do not project beyond body)	Other identifying features
Ctenocephalides spp. (fleas)	2–3 mm V	Black	Wingless Laterally flattened	L (hind)	Species can be identified by the shape of the head and variations in the number and shape of combs on the head
Trichodectes canis (dog biting louse)	2 mm V	Yellow-brown	Dorsoventrally flattened	L	Head similar width to body
Linognathus setosus (dog sucking louse)	2 mm V	Blue-black	Dorsoventrally flattened	L	Head narrow compared with body
Felicola subrostratus (cat biting louse)	1 mm V	Yellow	Dorsoventrally flattened	L	Triangular head similar width to body

17.40 Identification of ectoparasites in small mammals.

continues ▶

Species	Size V = visible to naked eye M = microscopic	Colour	Body shape	Legs L = long S = short (posterior two pairs do not project beyond body)	Other identifying features
Dipteran fly larva (blue, green and blackbottle maggots)	5–10 mm V	White	Tubular	S	Wormlike
Ixodes spp. (commonest tick)	2–10 mm V	Grey/blue	Pear	L	Tightly attached to host
Sarcoptes scabiei	0.2–0.4 mm M	–	Round/oval	S	Y-shaped joined apodeme at base head Anterior legs have suckers Posterior short legs do not extend beyond body Terminal anus (allows to distinguish from Notoedres)
Notoedres cati (Very rare UK)	0.1 mm M	–	Round/oval	S	As Sarcoptes but smaller and anus is dorsal
Cheyletiella spp. (walking dandruff)	0.4 mm V (only just)	White	Saddle shaped with 'waist'	L	Hooked mouthparts (pedipalps) on head
Otodectes cynotis (ear mite)	0.3 mm M (although visible with otoscope)	White	Oval	L	Unjoined apodeme at base head Posterior long legs
Demodex canis (Demodex cati – rare)	0.2 mm M	–	Cigar shaped	S (very)	Long cigar shape is unique
Neotrombicula autumnalis (harvest mite)	0.4 mm V (only just)	Orange	Oval	L (3 pairs as larval stage)	Orange colour and 3 pairs hairy legs is unique

17.40 *continued* Identification of ectoparasites in small mammals.

Fungi

Dermatophyte infections affect the superficial skin, hair and occasionally the nails. Typical lesions that are useful for sampling are broken hairs, scale and crusts. *All dermatophytes are zoonotic and therefore protective clothing and gloves should be worn.* The three main dermatophyte (ringworm) species found on dogs and cats are *Microsporum canis* (which, despite its name, mainly affects cats), *Microsporum gypseum* and *Trichophyton mentagrophytes* (see Chapter 7).

Diagnostic methods for examining dermatophytes include:

- Wood's lamp examination
- Microscopy of hair plucks
- Fungal culture (this is the most reliable method).

Wood's lamp

The Wood's lamp (Figure 17.41), which delivers an ultraviolet wavelength of 365–366 nm, should be warmed up for 5 minutes before use. *Care must be taken to avoid prolonged exposure to UV light and gloves should also be worn because of the zoonotic risk.*

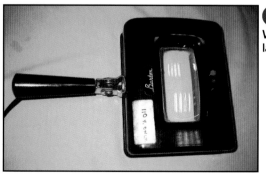

17.41 Wood's lamp.

When growing on hair and skin, *M. canis* produces a certain tryptophane metabolite that fluoresces a vivid apple-green under the UV light of a Wood's lamp. However, it is estimated that only 50% of *M. canis* infections fluoresce and therefore a negative result *cannot* be used alone to rule out dermatophytosis. *M. gypseum* occasionally fluoresces yellow-green, but *T. mentagrophytes* never fluoresces. Non-specific bluish-white fluorescence is not due to ringworm but is commonly found due to scales of flaky skin, mud, dirt, detergent solution, maize starch (from gloves) or paraffin oil.

Microscope examination of hair plucks

Plucked hairs can be examined microscopically for the presence of fungal spores (Figure 17.42). The ideal hairs to examine are those that fluoresce under the Wood's lamp. The hairs are

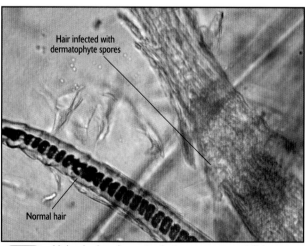

Hair infected with dermatophyte spores

Normal hair

17.42 Hair plucks: dermatophyte spores are visible on the hair on the right.

placed on a microscope slide with potassium hydroxide (KOH) and examined under low or medium power. This method is *not very reliable* for detecting dermatophytosis.

Fungal culture

This is the most reliable method for detecting ringworm fungi. A small sample of hair or skin crust is placed on a fungal culture plate. Sabouraud's agar is the medium most commonly used to grow dermatophytes. It normally takes 7–10 days for colonies to grow.

Identification of the species of dermatophyte is made by examining the colony characteristics (colour/texture) and by microscope examination of the colony for **macroconidia** (the predominant spore form that will be seen – large, single and multicellular), which are unique to each species. If no growth occurs after 3 weeks, the sample is considered negative.

- *Microsporum canis* grows as a whitish, coarsely fluffy spreading colony, which develops a deep yellow pigment on the underside. This pigment appears during the first week of growth, but becomes dark and dull with ageing. The macroconidia have thick walls and >6 cells.
- *Microsporum gypseum* characteristically has rapidly spreading colonies whose surface is a rich cinnamon–buff with the texture of chamois. The underside is a light buff.
 The macroconidia have thin symmetrical walls and <6 cells.
- *Trichophyton mentagrophytes* has two colony types. The zoophilic form produces a flat colony with a yellowish buff or cream-coloured powdery surface. The powder appears to be sprinkled in concentric rings or rays. The underside may be tan or dark brown. The anthropophilic form consists of a dense, downy white colony. The macroconidia are cigar-shaped, with thin walls and defined cells.

Fungal identification techniques

- If fluoresces under Wood's lamp – probably *Microsporum canis*.
- Culture a sample of hair/crust on Sabouraud's agar or an in-house culture plate e.g. dermatophyte test medium (DTM) which contains a colour indicator that turns the plate from yellow to red if dermatophytes 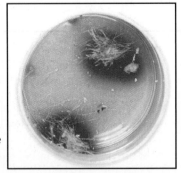 are present. Plates are kept at room temperature for 3 weeks and checked daily for growth and colour change.
- Macroconidia identification. The colony can be lifted with an acetate strip and stained with lactophenol or methylene blue and examined under high-power microscopy. Each species of dermatophyte has differently shaped macroconidia (see above).

Fungal identification can be difficult and so samples may be sent to an external laboratory for examination. The sample should be placed in a loose container or paper envelope, avoiding airtight jars as dermatophytes require air to survive.

Cytology

Cytology is the examination of cells with the microscope. It is probably underused in veterinary practice and can provide rapid results with minimum costs. Cytology can be used to examine every system in the body. With experience, the clinician can become familiar with basic cytology, e.g. differentiating inflammation from neoplasia or bacteria from yeast infection. However, detailed cytological interpretation such as the examination of neoplasia requires the experience of a trained cytopathologist.

Skin and ears

Cytology is most frequently carried out for microbial examination of ears and skin and for examination of cutaneous 'lumps'. Samples are usually collected by tape strips, fine-needle aspiration or impression smears (see above).

To examine tape strips for microbes, a few drops of methylene blue (Solution C in commercial *RAP*/DIFF® stain) are placed on the microscope slide before the tape strip is applied. Examination is with high-power oil immersion. Bacterial cocci appear as small purple dots and some may be seen phagocytosed within neutrophils in bacterial infection (pyoderma). *Malassezia* are budding yeasts and appear as purple 'Russian doll' or 'footprint' shapes (Figure 17.43).

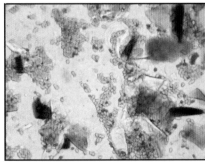

17.43
Classic 'footprints in the snow' appearance of *Malassezia* yeast.

Cerebrospinal fluid

A CSF sample should be slightly viscous, clear and colourless. Anything else should be considered abnormal:

- Cloudy – an increased cellular count
- Pink – haemorrhage (traumatic, pathogenic)
- Yellow (xanthochromic) – indicative of CNS inflammation or vascular disorder.

Cytological analysis of CSF must be performed within 30 minutes of collection (granulocytes in particular will begin to degenerate, invalidating the results). The following tests may be performed during CSF analysis (Figure 17.44):

Findings	Possible causes
Blood cells (RBCs, WBCs, differential count)	Abscess Haemorrhage (possibly due to poor technique in sample collection) Fungal infection Inflammation Viral infection Post vaccination
Protein	Inflammation (intrathecal membrane) Toxic/metabolic imbalances Vascular disease (immune disorders) Neoplastic disease

17.44   Results of cerebrospinal fluid analysis.   *continues* ▶

Findings	Possible causes
Titres for infectious disease in the dog	Viral: canine distemper Bacterial: Lyme disease Protozoal: *Toxoplasma, Neospora* Rickettsial: *Ehrlichia canis*, Rocky Mountain spotted fever Fungal: *Aspergillus, Cryptococcus*
Titres for infectious disease in the cat	Viral: FeLV, FIV, FIP Protozoal: *Toxoplasma* Fungal: *Cryptococcus*

17.44   *continued*   Results of cerebrospinal fluid analysis.

- Red blood cell, white blood cell and differential counts
- Protein content
- Antibody titres for infectious disease
- Bacteriology.

Other body fluids

Thoracic fluid

The following abnormal substances may be withdrawn from this site, indicating different conditions:

- Blood – haemothorax
- Chyle – chylothorax
- Air – pneumothorax
- Pus – pyothorax (empyema).

Abdominal fluid

The appearance of the fluid may suggest various conditions (Figure 17.45). A comparison of exudates and transudates is given in Figure 17.46. (See also Chapter 24.)

Colour	Description	Possible causes
Clear	True transudate	Hyperproteinaemia results from malnutrition, hepatic, cardiac or renal failure and protein-losing enteropathy. Thoracic fluid or oedema
Pink	Modified transudate	Can vary from clear to yellow; due to hypertension; portal hypertension; tumours obstructing venous flow; cardiac disease (right-sided heart failure)
Red	Exudate or blood	*Exudate*: may be turbid; occasionally yellow High cell and protein; peritoneal cavity infection; nocardiosis (bacterial lung infection); FIP *Blood*: haem; trauma, ruptured spleen; neoplasia (haemangiosarcoma); clotting disorder (warfarin poisoning)
Turbid White	Chyle	Contains chylomicrons (lipoprotein) from intestines via lymphatic system to systemic circulation via the thoracic duct High cell and protein content; lymphatic vessel rupture; possible trauma, neoplasia or inflammation; or cardiac disease
Brown	Gut contents	Perforation of the alimentary tract; trauma; pressure necrosis from a foreign body, ulceration or neoplasia
Yellow	Urine	Paracentesis into the bladder; bladder rupture; trauma; hyperadrenocorticism or other associated skin disorders; urine flow obstruction; ruptured renal pelvis or ureter
Green	Bile	Gall bladder rupture; RTA; cholelith (biliary stone) or tumour obstructing/perforating bile duct; liver puncture from biopsy

17.45   Types of abdominal fluid.

Exudate	Transudate
Protein-rich SG >1.020 Inflammatory fluid containing leucocytes and lysosomes Turbid (possible blood) May clot due to an increased fibrinogen content	Protein-poor SG <1.012 Non-inflammatory fluid Clear and pale Does not clot

17.46   Characteristics of exudates and transudates.

Bacteriology

Bacterial types

Culture of bacteria requires a knowledge of the oxygen requirements for growth (see Chapter 7):

- **Aerobic** bacteria need oxygen to grow
  - **Obligatory** aerobes need oxygen all the time (e.g. *Pseudomonas, Salmonella*)
- **Anaerobic** bacteria only grow if oxygen is absent (e.g. most species of *Clostridium*)
  - **Facultative** anaerobes grow whether oxygen is absent or present (e.g. *Staphylococcus*)
- **Microaerophilic** bacteria need only minute quantities of oxygen (e.g. *Campylobacter*).

Colony formation

Identifying and categorizing isolated bacterial colonies based upon their varied appearance and morphology (form and structure) will permit the selection and transfer of different species from a mixed culture, and allow transfer of a single colony to a sterile medium for cultivation of a pure culture.

When a single bacterial cell is deposited on the surface of a nutritive medium, it begins to divide exponentially. After thousands (up to billions) of cells have been formed, a visible mass appears. This mass of cells is called a **colony.** Each species of bacterial (or fungal) organism will exhibit colony characteristics, including:

- **Size** – e.g. punctiform (tiny)
- **Shape** – e.g. round, irregular or regular
- **Colour** (pigment) – opaque, translucent, shiny or dull
- **Elevation** – convex, umbonate (uneven), flat or raised
- **Margin** (edges) – entire (smooth), undulate (wavy) or lobate (lobed)
- **Surface texture** – moist, mucoid, dry or rough
- **Consistency** – viscous or watery.

Antibiotic sensitivity testing (Kirby–Bauer method)

This is a useful indicator for identifying the most appropriate antibiotic to treat an infection. The test can be used for a variety of antibacterial agents, such as sulphonamides, and for synthetic chemotherapeutic agents when dealing with microorganisms other than bacteria.

A layer of pure culture of the infective organism is spread evenly over the surface of an agar plate. Disks impregnated with various antimicrobial agents are then placed on the surface of the agar and the plate is incubated.

Resistance or susceptibility to an antimicrobial agent is shown by the growth pattern around the discs. Where the organism grows freely, it is not susceptible to the agent in the disc. Discs with no growth near them indicate that the organisms is **sensitive** to that agent (Figure 17.47). The *diameter* of the **zone of inhibition** (no growth) around the disc gives a measure of the degree of susceptibility/resistance. The zone size varies between antimicrobials and can be compared with a known standard for a susceptible bacterium.

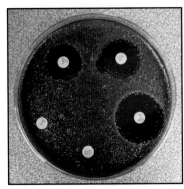

17.47 Antibacterial sensitivity plate: the organism was sensitive to three of the antibiotics (no growth zone around the disc) but resistant to the other two (no zone of inhibition).

Further reading

Ford RB and Mazzaferro E (2006) *Kirk and Bistner's Handbook of Veterinary Procedures and Emergency Treatment, 8th edn.* Saunders, Philadelphia

Hendrix C (2002) *Laboratory Procedures for Veterinary Technicians, 4th edn.* Mosby

Hotston Moore A (2000) *BSAVA Manual of Advanced Veterinary Nursing.* BSAVA Publications, Cheltenham

Mactaggart D (2004) Practice microscope – toy or tool? *In Practice* **26**, 397–399

Orpet H and Welsh P (2002) *Handbook of Veterinary Nursing.* Blackwell Science, Oxford

Quinn PJ, Donnelly WJ, Markey BK, Carter, ME and Leonard FC (2002) *Veterinary Microbiology and Microbial Diseases.* Blackwell Publishing, Oxford

Shaw S and Day M (2005) *Arthropod-borne Infectious Diseases of the Dog and Cat.* Manson, London

Villiers E and Blackwood L (2005) *BSAVA Manual of Canine and Feline Clinical Pathology, 2nd edn.* BSAVA Publications, Gloucester

Willard M, Tvedten H and Turnwald GH (1999) *Small Animal Clinical Diagnosis by Laboratory Method, 3rd edn.* WB Saunders, Philadelphia

Chapter 18

First aid and emergencies

Amanda Boag and Kate Nichols

Learning objectives

After studying this chapter, students should be able to:

- **Define a veterinary emergency and provide advice on emergency care over the telephone**
- **Recognize the severity of an emergency and perform appropriate triage**
- **Describe the approach to the assessment of the emergency patient**
- **List the major body systems and understand their importance in the evaluation of the emergency patient**
- **Describe the procedure to follow if a patient undergoes cardiopulmonary arrest**
- **Explain the veterinary nurse's role when evaluating emergency patients and understand professional limitations**
- **List common veterinary emergencies, their presenting signs and their initial stabilization and treatment**

Introduction

Veterinary emergency medicine is a rapidly developing area of the profession. In general, an **emergency** can be classified as any illness or injury where the animal's owner or guardian perceives that urgent veterinary attention is needed. The Royal College of Veterinary Surgeons (RCVS) requires that all veterinary surgeons take steps to provide 24-hour emergency cover for their patients. **Emergency cover** is defined in the *RCVS Guide to Professional Conduct* as 'the provision of immediate first aid and pain relief to deal promptly with emergencies'.

Historically most practices have provided their own cover, but the RCVS now states that 'veterinary surgeons are encouraged to co-operate with each other in the provision of 24-hour emergency cover. Such co-operation may be between groups of local practices. Alternatively, 24-hour emergency cover may be provided by a dedicated 24-hour emergency service clinic.'

Increasingly practices are working together to provide out-of-hours care or are using one of the dedicated emergency service clinics that have opened in the last few years.

While veterinary surgeons and nurses are now able to develop a special interest in this field, it is vital that *all* members of nursing staff are confident and competent in dealing with emergencies. These can present at any time, including during routine daily clinics, and some practices (especially in rural areas) will continue to provide their own out-of-hours cover.

This chapter will outline the general approach to the veterinary emergency patient and the role of the nurse and will summarize some of the common clinical conditions seen in an emergency practice. Emergency work is *always* a team effort and the emergency nurse is a vital part of the veterinary team. A successful outcome for the patient depends on:

- Early recognition of the severity and nature of the problem
- Good communication with the owner and with other members of the team
- Implementation of appropriate treatment
- Careful and diligent monitoring.

Although a veterinary surgeon will examine each patient, the experienced emergency nurse should be able to assess the severity of illness of each animal. This allows cases to be prioritized on the basis of clinical need and determines the optimal order in which they should be treated. The goal is to ensure a successful outcome for as many patients as possible, but the decision to euthanase some patients will sometimes need to be made.

Rules for emergency practice

- Remain calm
- Be prepared
- Do not put yourself, the owner or other staff members at risk
- Ensure that the animal is at no further risk
- Assess severity of injury/illness
- Contact the veterinary surgeon as soon as possible

Types of emergency

Veterinary emergencies comprise a wide range of clinical problems ranging from those that are imminently life-threatening to minor injuries and ailments. **Triage** is the process of rapidly classifying patients on the basis of their clinical priority, allowing identification of those patients that need urgent life-saving help and ensuring that this occurs immediately and before patients with less severe problems are dealt with.

In emergency practice, one of the nurse's major roles is to perform triage so that the veterinary surgeon can focus their attention on the patients that need them the most. The process of triage involves assessing information from the patient's history and initial clinical examination, in particular an assessment of their major body systems.

- **Severe life-threatening emergencies** are those that involve significant disturbances in the major body systems where there is the potential for rapid deterioration and death.
- The list of **minor emergencies** is long but includes problems such as minor wounds, mild vomiting or diarrhoea, polydipsia, skin lesions/scratching and weight-bearing lameness. Although these animals may be dealt with on an emergency basis, their full evaluation and treatment can be delayed until after the needs of those patients with life-threatening emergencies have been addressed.

Telephone calls

This form of communication is often the first contact the practice will have with a client and their pet during an emergency. Understandably, clients may be very distressed and concerned at this time. Owners may not understand why certain questions need to be asked and may become upset. It is vital that the veterinary nurse or receptionist remains sympathetic, calm and patient and shows that they understand that the client is distressed. The client needs to be reassured that the questions being asked are in order that the best advice and help can be provided for them and their pet.

The immediate aim of the telephone conversation is to establish whether the pet has a life-threatening problem. If this is the case, the owner should be advised that the pet should be brought to the practice as soon as possible. Further questioning at this point will only delay the pet's arrival at the practice and may have a negative impact on its chances of survival.

Emergencies where examination at a veterinary practice should be advised without delay

- Respiratory distress
- Severe bleeding, either from wounds or from body orifices
- Collapse or unconsciousness
- Rapid and progressive abdominal distension
- Inability to urinate
- Sudden onset of severe neurological abnormalities
- Protracted vomiting, especially if animal is also depressed
- Severe diarrhoea, especially if haemorrhagic
- Witnessed ingestion of toxin
- Severe weakness or inability to stand   ▶

- Extreme pain
- Fracture with bone ends visible or wounds in close proximity to fracture site
- Dystocia

In other situations, further questioning may be needed to determine whether the animal needs to be seen immediately or whether an appointment can be made. Examples of this include:

- Mild to moderate vomiting
- Non-haemorrhagic diarrhoea
- Small wounds with minimal blood loss
- Discomfort on urinating but urine is being passed
- Polyuria/polydipsia
- Weight-bearing lameness.

Questions to be asked if the emergency is not life-threatening

- What is the breed, age and sex of the pet?
- Is it on any medication? If so, what, and when was it last given?
- What is the exact nature of the problem?
- When did the problem start and has it been progressive?
- Has the animal ever had this problem before? If so, when? Was it treated?
- Does the animal seem depressed or lethargic?
- Does the animal have any other signs or symptoms?

In general, questions should be asked about the nature of the problem before asking for owner details such as name and address. It can be frustrating for a distressed owner to be asked administrative questions before being asked about their pet's problem. To gain maximum information, questions should be specific and concise. To avoid misunderstanding, it is preferable to speak directly to the owner rather than a third party.

Occasionally telephone advice is sought when the pet seems relatively normal but a serious incident has recently occurred. It is recommended that the following advice is given.

- **Recent trauma** (e.g. glancing blow from a car, fall from a height) has occurred and the animal appears to have recovered.
  - In this situation a full clinical examination by a veterinary surgeon should be recommended. It is possible that the animal has internal injuries. A veterinary surgeon may be able to identify these injuries, allowing early treatment. If the owners are unwilling to bring the pet to the practice, they should be asked to observe the pet closely and call back immediately if any unusual signs (especially respiratory distress, weakness and pale mucous membranes) are observed.
- An animal has suffered a **seizure** but it has stopped by the time the owner contacts the veterinary practice.
  - It is recommended that the animal be seen as soon as possible. Although many seizures are single incidents, an underlying medical problem may be identified.

Owners will often ask if there is any treatment or first aid they can give at home. Any advice should be given with caution. Very few owners have medical training and their interpretation of clinical signs may be misleading. If in doubt, it is always advisable to recommend that a pet is seen at the practice in order that it may be examined by a trained professional.

In some situations, first aid provided by the owner before reaching the practice may be helpful:

- With **haemorrhage**, owners should be advised to apply pressure directly over an area of profuse bleeding, using a clean towel or cloth, whilst the animal is transported to the clinic.
- In rare cases where a **foreign object** is present in the wound, the owner should be instructed *not* to remove it but to transport the animal to the practice with the object in place. It may be possible to apply pressure around the foreign object. Removing the object can potentially make the bleeding much worse.
- On rare occasions, either as a result of trauma or if a surgical wound has broken down, owners may report being able to see **internal organs** (often fat or intestines) protruding through the wound. The owners should be advised to cover the pet's abdomen lightly (not tightly) with a clean bath towel for transportation and prevent the animal from licking the area.

The owner's personal safety is paramount and it may not be possible for first aid measures to be carried out on animals with painful wounds.

Rules for telephone conversations

- Always answer the phone by introducing yourself and your practice. A panicking owner needs to know that they have contacted their vet.
- Always be polite.
- Ascertain as quickly as possible whether the problem is life-threatening.
- Be able to provide clear directions to the practice.
- Be able to offer alternative means of transport (local pet ambulances, taxi firms) in case the owner has transport difficulties.
- Obtain an estimated time of arrival.
- Obtain the owner's contact details, including a mobile telephone number if possible. Repeat this information back to the caller to ensure that it is correct.
- Give the owner a financial quote for an emergency consultation.
- Check whether the pet regularly attends a veterinary surgery and, if so, which one.

Practices should consider having a telephone log book where details of emergency telephone calls can be recorded. This book can also contain useful information such as pet ambulance numbers.

When an emergency call is taken the veterinary nurse or receptionist should inform the rest of the team about the nature of the emergency and its expected arrival time. The surgery should be prepared to receive the patient. This may include preparing equipment for oxygen administration, intravenous fluid administration or wound dressings.

Handling and transport of emergency patients

Emergency patients generally have the same considerations regarding handling and transportation as other patients (see Chapter 10). Importantly, emergency patients may be shocked and in pain. Dogs and cats that are normally considered to be friendly and placid may become aggressive when injured and in pain. Veterinary staff should be cautious when approaching these animals and should use a muzzle or other restraint if concerned. Analgesia should be given at the earliest possible opportunity; this will facilitate further handling. Owners should also be reminded that they should be cautious even when handling their own pet.

The dyspnoeic patient, especially the dyspnoeic cat, warrants special consideration These patients may already be stressed due to their underlying disease and the journey to the practice. Further handling of these patients on arrival, especially if they struggle, may precipitate cardiopulmonary arrest. Dyspnoeic animals should be placed in an oxygen-enriched environment and given time to settle after arrival before a full examination or further procedures (e.g. catheter placement, radiography) are carried out.

Arrival at the surgery

The key to successfully treating emergencies is to be prepared. As much paperwork as possible, including a consent form, should be prepared in advance. All practices, including both general practices and practices that predominantly carry out emergency or out-of-hours work, should have a designated area for dealing with emergency patients. This emergency area or room should be easily accessible from as many other areas of the building as possible, including the client entry area/consulting rooms and areas with diagnostic equipment such as the laboratory and radiography room. Oxygen and anaesthetic equipment should be readily available. In most practices, the preparation area or induction room is best suited as it is usually fitted with most of the emergency equipment required. Figure 18.1 gives a suggested list of equipment and drugs that should be readily available.

Emergency equipment

Endotracheal tubes (varying sizes)
Laryngoscope
Oxygen supply
Anaesthetic circuits
Intravenous catheters (varying sizes)
Tape for tying in ET tube
Tape for securing IV catheters
ECG machine
Assortment of syringes and needles
Suction machine/bulb syringe
Dog urinary catheter (for difficult intubations)
Good light source
Drug dosage chart
Fluid administration equipment
Scalpel blades/suture material

Emergency drugs

Adrenaline (epinephrine)
Atropine
Lidocaine (lignocaine)
Diazepam
Calcium gluconate (10%)
Dextrose solution (50%)
Furosemide
Dexamethasone
Propofol
Nitroglycerine paste
Opioid analgesics
Intravenous fluids – replacement crystalloid
Intravenous fluids – colloid
Mannitol

18.1 Emergency equipment and drugs that should be readily available in the designated emergency area.

All staff (veterinary surgeons, veterinary nurses, other patient care staff and reception staff) should know that this area is where emergencies should be taken. The area should be well lit and spacious with items and equipment stored tidily.

There should be a mobile crash box or trolley that is fully stocked and ready for use at all times (Figure 18.2). It should be the responsibility of one person in the practice (usually a veterinary nurse) to ensure that it is checked after every use and at least once weekly. Any patient with a potentially life-threatening condition should be taken immediately to the designated emergency area on arrival at the practice, for a primary survey.

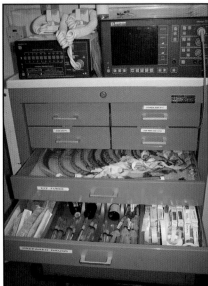

18.2

Example of crash trolley from large veterinary hospital and crash box from smaller veterinary practice. Note presence of large variety of endotracheal tubes, intravenous catheters, drugs and monitoring equipment.

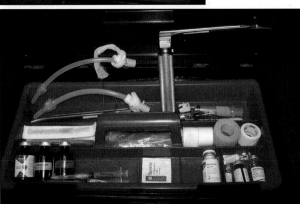

Primary survey

This starts with an assessment of whether the animal has just undergone or is likely to undergo imminent cardiopulmonary arrest. The mnemonic ABC should be followed:

- **Airway** – does the patient have a patent airway?
- **Breathing** – is the patient making useful breathing efforts?
- **Circulation** – does the patient have evidence of spontaneous circulation (heartbeat, pulses)?

It should also be determined whether the patient is conscious or unconscious.

The primary survey should take approximately 30 seconds to perform. Once this assessment has been carried out and it is established that the patient is unlikely to undergo cardio-respiratory arrest, the triage nurse should carry out a major

body systems assessment. If the nurse has any concerns at all that the patient has arrested, the veterinary surgeon should be called and cardiopulmonary resuscitation should be started.

Major body system assessment

The three major body systems are considered to be:

- Cardiovascular
- Respiratory
- Neurological.

When triaging a patient, these systems should always be examined first, regardless of any other injuries. Dysfunction in any of these systems is potentially life-threatening. If a patient dies, it is always the result of failure of one of these systems.

Although other injuries may be more obvious, they are unlikely to kill the patient unless they have a secondary effect on one of the major body systems. For example, consider a dog that has been hit by a car, resulting in a fracture of the femur with a large open wound. Although this injury may appear dramatic, on its own it will not lead to the dog's death. However, the haemorrhage from the fracture site may lead to hypovolaemic shock, cardiovascular system compromise and death. The shock will be detected by examination of the cardiovascular system.

The major body system assessment provides a means of assessing whether the patient's injuries are life-threatening. All parameters should be recorded at the time they are measured.

Parameters that should be recorded during a primary survey

- Heart rate
- Pulse quality
- Mucous membrane colour
- Capillary refill time
- Respiratory rate
- Respiratory effort
- Gait
- Mentation
- Temperature

Cardiovascular system

Information from the cardiovascular system examination is the best way the veterinary surgeon has of quickly assessing the degree and type of shock. Repeat cardiovascular system examination, as the animal receives treatment for shock, is the best way of easily and cheaply monitoring the animal's response to treatment. The information provided by the nurse has a vitally important role in the outcome of the case.

The cardiovascular system examination involves assessment of a patient's heart rate, pulse quality, mucous membrane colour and capillary refill time.

Heart rate

Heart rate should be measured while auscultating the patient's heart with a stethoscope and should be compared with the patient's pulse rate. The heart and pulse rates should be the same. If they are not, the veterinary surgeon should be alerted.

Pulse

A **pulse deficit** occurs when a heart beat is heard but there is no corresponding pulse. Thus, the pulse rate measured will be lower than the heart rate. Pulse deficits are a sign of arrhythmia.

The easiest pulse to feel is the femoral pulse. It is felt by sliding the fingers gently into the inguinal region (see Chapter 13). In some patients (e.g. those with femoral or pelvic fractures, heavily muscled or obese animals) this pulse can be difficult to feel and palpation of a metatarsal pulse on the dorsomedial aspect of the metatarsus may be easier (Figure 18.3).

With practice, **pulse quality** can be assessed. Pulse quality can be classified as: normal; tall and narrow (bounding or hyperkinetic); or weak (thready). Information on the quality of the pulse should be recorded each time it is felt.

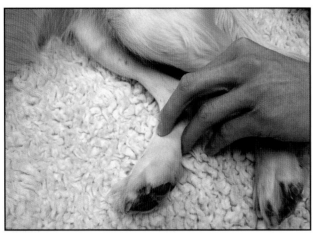

18.3 Locating the metatarsal pulse. Palpation of this pulse is especially useful in patients with pelvic or femoral fractures.

Mucous membrane colour

The normal colour is pale pink (paler in cats than dogs). It should be remembered that some breeds (e.g. Chow-Chow) have pigmented dark mucous membranes. Some disease states will cause abnormalities of mucous membrane colour; for example, they may be pale or white in hypovolaemic shock with anaemia, bright red in distributive shock, or blue with hypoxia.

The **capillary refill time** (CRT) is checked by applying firm pressure with the thumb on the gingival mucosa to blanch the mucous membranes (see Chapter 13) and timing how quickly the colour returns. A normal refill time is 1–2 seconds. The CRT may be rapid (<1 second) in early shock or slow (>2.5 seconds) in late shock.

Respiratory system

Respiratory system assessment involves evaluation of the animal's respiratory rate and effort. It is useful to record whether there are any audible noises associated with the respiratory effort and, if possible, whether inspiration (breathing in) or expiration (breathing out) involves the most effort. This information can assist the veterinary surgeon in diagnosing the cause of the breathing difficulty.

Findings that suggest severe respiratory distress

- Cyanotic (blue) mucous membranes
- Open-mouth breathing (especially in cats)
- Abducted elbows
- Extended neck
- Paradoxical abdominal movement (abdomen moves in while chest moves out)
- Dilated pupils
- Anxious facial expression

Oxygen should always be supplied while a dyspnoeic animal is being examined (Figures 18.4, 18.5 and 18.6). Care should be taken that the method of oxygen supplementation does not distress the patient further.

Method of oxygen supplementation	Advantages	Disadvantages
Flow-by (hold oxygen source close to patient's nose or mouth)	Cheap Easy Well tolerated	Does not allow high inspired concentration of oxygen
Mask	Cheap Easy	Not tolerated by some patients Does not allow high inspired concentration of oxygen
Nasal prongs	Cheap	Not tolerated by some patients Tend to fall out frequently (designed for human noses) May cause sneezing
Nasal catheter (Figure 18.5)	Cheap Catheter easy to place with practice	May require sedation for placement of catheter Catheter irritates some patients May cause sneezing
Transtracheal catheter	May be useful in patients with upper airway problems	Difficult to maintain and use in conscious patient Not tolerated by some patients
Improvised oxygen cage (e.g. Elizabethan collar with cling-film)	Cheap Widely available	Patients rapidly become hot Can get CO_2 build-up
Oxygen cage/ incubator (Figure 18.6)	Allows delivery of up to 90% oxygen Minimal stress May allow temperature and humidity control	Not widely available Expensive
Intubation and ventilation	Allows 100% oxygen delivery Allows control of breathing	Requires anaesthesia Not possible long term except in specialist institutions

18.4 Methods of oxygen supplementation.

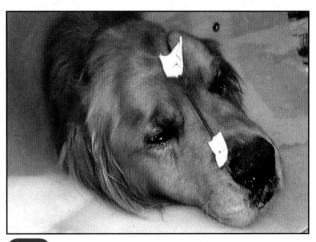

18.5 Nasal oxygen catheter in place.

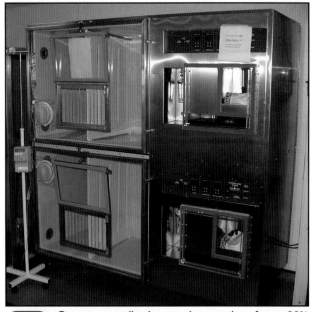

18.6 Oxygen cage allowing supplementation of up to 90% oxygen, with temperature and humidity control.

Nervous system

Initial evaluation of the nervous system involves an assessment of the patient's gait and mentation.

Gait

During assessment of gait, the following terms are used:

- **Paresis** – weakness
- **Plegia** – paralysis (unable to move)
- **Quadriplegia** – paralysis of all four limbs
- **Paraplegia** – paralysis of any two limbs
- **Hemiplegia** – paralysis of one side of the body
- **Hypermetria** – exaggerated limb movements.

In a paralysed animal it is important to note whether the animal can feel its limbs (e.g. turns its head towards the handler when its toes are squeezed) even though it is unable to move them.

Mentation

The animal's mentation may be classified as:

- **Alert**
- **Obtunded** (mentally dull)
- **Stuporous** (semi-conscious, able to be roused only by a painful stimulus)
- **Coma** (unconscious and unable to be roused).

Other neurological features to note include:

- Pupil size and symmetry
- Presence or absence of pupillary light reflexes
- Presence or absence of palpebral reflex
- Facial asymmetry and any head tilt
- Nystagmus (abnormal flicking eye movements)
- Presence of gag reflex (in stuporous or comatose patients only)
- Anal tone (may be assessed when taking temperature).

Body temperature

Once the major body system assessment has been completed, the animal's temperature can be taken and recorded. These points should be noted:

- Any faecal staining of the perineum
- Any blood or melaena on the thermometer
- Whether normal anal tone was present.

After the primary survey has been completed, any major body system conditions can be prioritized and stabilization started as soon as possible.

Secondary survey

A secondary survey to establish other abnormalities can be performed once the primary survey is complete and treatment for any major body system abnormalities has been started. A head-to-tail approach is recommended to ensure that a systematic examination is performed.

Nose

Note any discharge (serous, purulent, haemorrhagic) and whether it is unilateral or bilateral. Note any swellings or asymmetry that may suggest nasal fractures or tumours.

Mouth

Note the colour of the mucous membranes. Initial examination of mucous membrane colour and capillary refill time (CRT) should have been performed as part of the major body systems assessment (see above). Normal mucous membranes are pale pink in colour.

Abnormal mucous membrane colours

- Pale – suggestive of anaemia or hypovolaemic shock
- Red – suggestive of distributive shock or localized inflammation (gingivitis)
- Cyanotic (blue) – suggestive of severe hypoxia
- Jaundiced (yellow) – suggestive of liver disease or haemolytic anaemia
- Cherry red – suggestive of carbon monoxide poisoning. (This is rare. Red mucous membranes are much more likely to be seen with distributive shock)

The oral cavity should be examined for any signs of haemorrhage, including both gross haemorrhage and petechial (pinprick) haemorrhages in the mucosa.

The moistness of the mucous membranes can be assessed. Dry mucous membranes are suggestive of dehydration.

Any ulcers on either the mucosa or the tongue should be noted.

The hard palate should be assessed to see if it is split (a common injury in cats with head trauma).

The mouth should be closed and an assessment made of whether the jaw closes properly or whether there is any asymmetry that may suggest a fracture.

Excessive salivation should be noted.

Eyes

The eyes should be assessed for any discharge (serous or purulent) and whether it is unilateral or bilateral.

The symmetry of the eyes should be assessed and any blepharospasm (indicative of ocular pain) noted.

If there is no obvious ocular injury, the conjunctival mucous membranes should be assessed for their colour and the presence of haemorrhage.

The position of the eyeball should be noted. An abnormal position is known as **strabismus** and the direction of the strabismus should be noted. Abnormal ocular movements **(nystagmus)** should be noted and the direction of the fast component of the movement should be recorded.

The pupil size and symmetry should be noted. The presence of asymmetrical pupils is known as **anisocoria** and it should be noted which pupil is larger.

The palpebral reflex and pupillary light response should be checked.

Ears

Both ears should be checked for any discharge and the nature of the discharge noted. The pinnae should be observed for any petechial haemorrhages.

Limbs

Any obvious wounds should be noted.

The limbs should be gently palpated and any swellings, pain or crepitus should be recorded. If a limb is clearly being held at an abnormal angle and a fracture is suspected, this limb should not be palpated but the veterinary surgeon should be alerted. Try to prevent the animal using this limb until the veterinary surgeon has examined it.

If the animal is ambulatory, it should be noted if it is lame and if so on which limb(s) it is lame and how severe the lameness is.

It is important to note if the neurological function of each limb is intact. If the animal is moving the limb voluntarily, there must be some functioning nerve supply. If there are concerns that an animal cannot move or feel a limb, the toes on that foot should be pinched. Withdrawal of the limb implies that local nerve reflexes are intact but does not necessarily mean that the spinal cord is functioning normally. The animal should be closely observed to see whether there is pain sensation accompanying the reflex. This may involve vocalizing, turning its head towards the limb or attempting to bite. Loss of conscious pain perception in a limb indicates a poor prognosis.

Thorax

Any external wounds or swellings should be noted. If there is any evidence of a penetrating chest wound (e.g. a piece of skin sucked in and out as the animal breathes, often accompanied by a gentle hissing sound) it should be covered with a sterile adherent dressing until it can be examined by the veterinary surgeon.

Thoracic auscultation is a useful skill for the emergency nurse to develop. When auscultating the chest, the nurse should listen to whether the lung sounds are abnormally quiet or loud. The distribution (e.g. left vs. right, dorsal vs. ventral) of any abnormal sounds should be recorded.

Abdomen

The hands should be run gently over the abdomen. Any wounds, swellings or bruising should be noted.

Deep abdominal palpation is a skill that can take years to develop. The ability to palpate the bladder in the caudal abdomen is a useful skill for the emergency nurse to master. An obstructed bladder or urethra is a common emergency. Distended bladders feel firm, hard and enlarged. If this condition is suspected, the nurse should *not* attempt to express the bladder as there is a chance it may rupture.

External genitalia

In both sexes, the external genitalia should be checked for any discharge or discoloration of the mucous membranes. Any evidence of urine scalding should be noted, as this could be evidence of a more chronic urinary problem.

Tail

Any wounds should be noted.

It should also be noted whether the animal can move its tail. Neurological injuries to the tail are common in cats following trauma.

Capsule history

A 'capsule history' should be obtained from the owners of all emergency patients. This history focuses on the essential information that could alter the early management of the patient. A more detailed history may be taken once the patient is more stable.

Important questions to ask for a capsule history

- What is the age, sex and neutering status of the animal?
- If an entire female, when was her last season or litter?
- Is the animal on any medications?
- Has the animal been diagnosed with any long-term medical problems?
- Does the animal have any known allergies?
- Has the animal had access to any known toxins?
- When was the last time the animal ate and drank?
- When was the last time the animal passed faeces and urinated and was it normal?
- How long has the animal been showing signs of its current problem?
- Has this problem got better, worse or stayed the same since it was first noticed?

General nursing care

The stabilization of life-threatening medical conditions must take priority but, having addressed these, the patient's general physical comfort and level of psychological stress should be considered.

Mental welfare

Many emergency patients are distressed, in pain or confused. Being in the unfamiliar environment of the veterinary practice surrounded by strangers can serve to make this worse.

- Be kind and gentle with the patient. Talk softly and use the patient's name as much as possible.
- Be aware if the patient has any physical disabilities, such as being blind, deaf or recumbent, that may make the situation more unsettling.

- Always approach the patient slowly and perform any procedures with the minimum handling necessary. Some patients may benefit from a period in a kennel or basket without being handled whilst they become accustomed to the environment.
- Emergency patients should *never* be covered from view.
- Be aware that some patients may find the presence of other animals stressful and organize kennelling to reduce this if possible.

Physical comfort

The patient should be given a warm and comfortable bed. If the patient is recumbent, it should be turned regularly and at least every 4 hours.

If the patient is able to stand and walk, then it should be allowed to do this. Critically ill patients should not walk long distances but the benefit of standing and walking around the room should not be underestimated, especially in older patients who may have concurrent chronic orthopaedic disease (e.g. arthritis). Patients that are able to walk outside will benefit from the fresh air and sunshine.

Toileting needs

The necessity for the patient to urinate and defecate should be considered. Although it may not be possible or advisable for critically sick dogs to be walked outside, they should be allowed to leave their kennel regularly for toileting purposes. If they are recumbent, a urinary catheter should be considered. If a patient soils itself or its bedding, it should be cleaned immediately. In patients with diarrhoea, clipping the perineal and caudal thigh region should be considered and a barrier cream applied. A tail bandage may be beneficial, and should be replaced regularly. Cats should be provided with a litter tray, containing a familiar type of litter if possible.

Dressings, catheter sites and tube sites

All dressings and catheter or tube insertion sites should be checked regularly. Any dressings that become soiled or displaced should be changed as soon as possible. All catheter sites should be unwrapped and checked at least once daily, and more frequently if the site appears to cause discomfort. Other tubes (e.g. oesophagostomy tubes, gastrostomy tubes) should be checked and rewrapped on the advice of the veterinary surgeon.

A record should be made each time dressings are replaced; the necessity for frequent dressing changes may indicate a worsening situation.

Oral food and water

The decision to offer food and water should be made by the veterinary surgeon and is dependent on the underlying disease process. The nurse should be proactive in ascertaining when food and water can be offered.

If food can be offered, small amounts of fresh food should be placed in the patient's kennel. If the patient does not want to eat, the food should be removed after 1 hour and more fresh food offered at a later time. The presence of stale food in the patient's kennel may act as an adverse stimulus and decrease the patient's appetite. Some patients may have trouble moving to their water or food bowl and may benefit from hand-feeding.

Monitoring

The nurse is responsible for monitoring the patient. Although many advanced monitoring techniques are now available in veterinary practice, the most important monitoring tool is the serial clinical examination.

The following parameters should be recorded at regular intervals (up to every 15 minutes in unstable patients; every 6–8 hours in stable patients).

Regular monitoring

- Pulse rate
- Pulse quality
- Mucous membrane colour
- Capillary refill time
- Respiratory rate
- Respiratory effort
- Temperature
- Demeanour
- Bodyweight (every 12 hours)

Other monitoring techniques that can be considered include:

- Urine output
- Urine specific gravity
- Blood pressure
- Pulse oximetry
- ECG
- Central venous pressure
- Serial electrolyte and blood gas parameters.

It is vital that any parameter monitored is recorded accurately. Successful management of emergency patients often involves several members of staff and it is essential that the patient's status is accurately communicated between staff members. Emergency patients often require a great deal of effort but can be some of the most rewarding patients to nurse.

Cardiopulmonary arrest, resuscitation and death

Early recognition of cardiopulmonary arrest or impending cardiopulmonary arrest is vital.

Signs of impending or actual cardiac arrest

- Agonal (gasping) breathing pattern *or* absence of useful respiratory movements
- Absence of a heartbeat and pulse *or* weak and rapid pulses that will usually slow rapidly and dramatically shortly prior to arrest
- Loss of consciousness
- Fixed dilated pupils and lack of a palpebral and corneal reflex

Patients that have suffered cardiopulmonary arrest shortly before arrival at the practice will be identified during the primary survey and resuscitation attempts should be started immediately. The longer the time from arrest to return of spontaneous circulation, the worse the prognosis is likely to be. If in doubt, resuscitation procedures should always be started. It may be necessary to do this before the veterinary surgeon arrives and before speaking to the owner.

Mucous membrane colour and capillary refill time may remain normal for a brief period after cessation of effective circulation. If the patient is being monitored by an ECG, this may also remain relatively normal for several minutes after cessation of cardiac contractions.

Cardiopulmonary–cerebral resuscitation

Cardiopulmonary–cerebral resuscitation (**CPCR**) is the provision of artificial support of ventilation and circulation (**basic life support**) until spontaneous circulation and breathing are restored and sustained. Basic life support (see below) is based around the familiar ABC mnemonic:

- Airway
- Breathing
- Circulation.

Advanced life support (see below) refers to the administration of drugs or other treatments to restart and maintain spontaneous circulation.

Cardiopulmonary–cerebral resuscitation procedure

All members of staff should be trained in basic CPCR, including student veterinary nurses, animal nursing assistants and receptionists. They can all be trained to carry out one or more tasks. Successful CPCR requires a team approach. Planning and practice is the key. The minimum number of people for CPCR is three, but more (four to six) is ideal.

Following recognition that a patient has undergone cardiopulmonary arrest, the following tasks should be carried out as quickly and smoothly as possible:

- Placement and securing (tying in) of an endotracheal tube
- Provision of oxygen and ventilation
- Provision of external cardiac compressions
- Placement and securing of an intravenous catheter
- Placement of an ECG to assist the veterinary surgeon in making decisions on appropriate medication.

These tasks are usually carried out in the order listed above, but this may change depending both on the patient and the number and experience of staff present. The patient is typically placed in right lateral recumbency.

It is vital that a person is nominated to 'run the crash' as soon as possible. This person would usually be a veterinary surgeon but an experienced nurse may need to fulfil this role until a veterinary surgeon arrives. It is this person's responsibility to direct the other members of the team and ensure all tasks are being carried out.

Depending on the number and training of staff present the following roles are usually assigned:

- One person to provide adequate ventilation
- One person to undertake chest compressions
- One person to monitor the patient, including palpating for the presence of pulses
- One person to draw up drugs as requested and record all medications given as well as any other interventions.

All practices should have regular CPCR training sessions where all can practise their responsibilities. Various veterinary CPCR models are available but even stuffed toys of various sizes can be used to imitate patients. Different scenarios should

be considered. After the practice session, or after a real CPCR, there should be a review and evaluation to encourage and facilitate ongoing improvements.

Basic life support

Airway

An airway is best provided by an endotracheal tube that is tied securely in place. On rare occasions an animal will have undergone cardiopulmonary arrest because of an obstructed airway. If airway obstruction is suspected, a variety of endotracheal tubes should be available including some much smaller than would normally be chosen for the size of patient. A stiff male dog urinary catheter is also useful as it can be placed through the larynx and passed beyond the obstruction. It can then be used to deliver oxygen while the obstruction is addressed.

Very rarely an endotracheal tube cannot be placed and an emergency tracheotomy must be carried out. The patient should be rolled into dorsal recumbency with hyperextension of the neck. An area over the trachea in the mid cervical region is rapidly clipped and a brief surgical preparation is performed. The veterinary surgeon will rapidly make an incision through the subcutaneous tissues of the neck and then between the tracheal rings. Ideally a specially designed tracheostomy tube is placed through the tracheal incision into the airway, but if this is not available a standard endotracheal tube can be used.

Breathing

Ventilation is usually provided by connecting the endotracheal tube to an anaesthetic circuit (preferably a Bain) or an Ambu bag (Figure 18.7). The respiration rate should be 6–12 breaths per minute. The volume of air per breath should be judged so that the chest wall can be seen to rise only a small amount. In an arrest situation it is very easy either to ventilate too quickly or to overinflate on each breath. This has the potential to damage the lungs by causing barotrauma and so caution must be exercised.

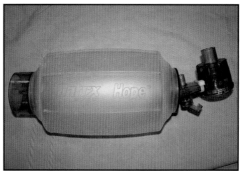

18.7 Ambu bag, designed to be attached to an endotracheal tube and used to ventilate patients.

Circulation

Circulation is maintained by chest compressions. In dogs and cats, effective chest compression is best accomplished with the animal in right lateral recumbency. In cats and small dogs, pressure should be applied using the heel of the hand directly over the heart (rib spaces 4 to 6). In cats it may be most effective to hold the thorax within the hand so pressure can be applied directly across the heart. In larger dogs, pressure should be applied, again using the heel of the hand, at the highest point on the thoracic wall (Figure 18.8). Chest compressions should be given at a rate of approximately 100 per minute with an equal time for compression and relaxation. If chest compressions are successful, a palpable femoral pulse is generated.

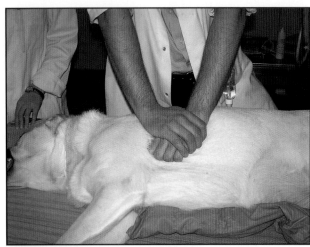

18.8 Position for administering external cardiac compression to a large dog.

Abdominal counter-pressure

If there is a large number of people (more than four) present for CPCR, it may be helpful for someone to perform abdominal counter-pressure. This involves pressing down firmly on the abdomen between chest compressions. It acts to increase venous return to the chest and improves blood pressure and cerebral and myocardial perfusion.

Advanced life support

Once ECG monitoring has started, the veterinary surgeon may wish to administer drugs to return the heart to a normal rhythm. Although a veterinary nurse does not need to understand fully the mechanism of action of each drug, having an understanding of which drug is appropriate and why can make both the veterinary nurse's and the veterinary surgeon's job quicker and easier. An experienced nurse can start to prepare drugs that are likely to be necessary, so that they can be administered as soon as they are requested.

The three common cardiac arrest rhythms in dogs and cats (Figure 18.9) are:

* Pulseless electrical activity (PEA)
* Asystole
* Ventricular fibrillation.

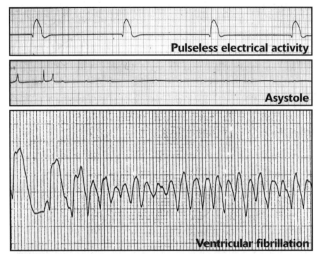

18.9 Common ECG rhythms seen with cardiac arrest in dogs and cats. (Courtesy of V Luis Fuentes)

The three drugs used most commonly during resuscitation are:

* **Adrenaline (epinephrine)**, a peripheral vasoconstrictor that acts to increase blood flow to the heart and brain. It is used in asystole and PEA.
* **Atropine**, an anticholinergic drug used to reduce vagal tone. It is used to control severe bradycardia which may lead to asystole or PEA.
* **Lidocaine (lignocaine)**, an antiarrhythmic drug. It is used for the treatment of ventricular arrhythmias such as fast ventricular tachycardia. It may be used as a chemical defibrillator but is rarely successful in this situation.

Electrical defibrillation

Electrical defibrillation is occasionally used to shock the heart from chaotic non-pulse-producing electrical activity (commonly ventricular fibrillation) to normal sinus rhythm. A large electrical charge is passed through the heart, with the aim of causing the cardiac cells to depolarize and then repolarize synchronously.

Defibrillation is only useful in cases where arrest has been caused by ventricular fibrillation or rapid ventricular tachycardia. The most common arrhythmia in human cardiopulmonary arrest is ventricular fibrillation and this is why defibrillators are so readily available and commonly used in human medicine. It is, however, a rare cause of arrest in dogs and cats. The earlier a heart is defibrillated, the better chance the patient will have of survival. The energy necessary for external defibrillation is approximately 5 joules/kg. Excessive energy levels and repeated defibrillation can cause myocardial damage; therefore it is advisable to start at the lower energy levels and increase as needed.

Extreme caution must be exercised whenever a defibrillator is being used. One person who is trained to operate the machine should be in charge and should instruct all other personnel to 'Clear' before discharging the defibrillator. To prevent risk of serious injury, all personnel must be clear of the patient *and* the table on which the patient is lying before the defibrillator is discharged. Defibrillators should never be used by untrained personnel. Alcohol-based solvents should never be used in the proximity of the defibrillator.

Collapse and unconsciousness

Many emergency patients will present because of collapse. The term collapse is used when an animal is unable or unwilling to stand and walk but remains aware of its surroundings. During the initial major body systems assessment, it should be ascertained whether an animal is:

* An **alert** collapsed animal with normal mentation
* A **depressed** collapsed animal that is quiet but will respond to stimuli such as calling its name or clapping hands behind its head
* An **obtunded** collapsed animal with a decreased level of consciousness that will only respond to painful stimuli such as squeezing hard on its toes or touching a painful area
* An **unconscious** (comatose) collapsed animal that does not respond to stimuli but has a palpable pulse and heart rate.

Animals are considered to be dead when they do not respond to stimuli and have no heartbeat on thoracic auscultation. If they are still making breathing movements, death may only just have occurred and resuscitation efforts should be started.

In an unconscious collapsed patient the airway may become blocked or narrowed due to the position of the neck and the tongue. The patient's muscles will tend to relax and can occlude the pharyngeal region especially in breeds with a large amount of soft tissue in this area, such as Bulldogs. It is vital that the airway is clear and open to allow adequate ventilation and oxygen delivery to the lungs.

Unconscious patients should be placed in lateral recumbency with their heads tilted dorsally (up), their mouths held gently open and the tongue gently pulled out. The airway should be examined to ensure that it is clear, but caution should be exercised and the safety of veterinary personnel must not be compromised.

There are many potential causes of collapse. The most common groups are summarized in Figure 18.10.

Presentation	Possible causes of collapse
Alert collapsed animal	Orthopaedic disease Peripheral neurological disease
Depressed collapsed animal	Mild to moderate shock Pain
Obtunded collapsed animal	Moderate to severe shock
Unconscious collapsed animal with very fast or slow heart rate	Severe shock – cardiopulmonary arrest imminent
Unconscious collapsed animal with normal heart rate	Neurological disease Metabolic disease (e.g. hypoglycaemia)

18.10 Groups of differential diagnoses to be considered in a collapsed animal.

Shock

Shock is defined as a state of acute circulatory collapse where the circulation is unable to transport sufficient oxygen to meet the tissues' needs. The consequences of untreated shock are severe, as a lack of oxygen supply to the tissues will have significant effects on all organs, especially the brain, heart and kidneys. If the state of shock is prolonged, it may lead to organ failure and death.

The lack of tissue oxygen supply may be secondary to a number of circulatory system problems. Four major types of shock are recognized and are described in Figure 18.11. The distinction between the types of shock is important, as the treatment strategy varies. In most situations, the different types of shock can be distinguished by a careful and thorough physical examination focusing on the cardiovascular system and, most importantly, the perfusion parameters (heart rate, pulse quality, mucous membrane colour and capillary refill time).

Hypovolaemic shock

Hypovolaemic shock is the most common form of shock seen in veterinary patients.

Characteristics of severe hypovolaemic shock

- Tachycardia (up to 220 beats per minute (bpm) in dogs and 250 bpm in cats)
- Prolonged capillary refill time
- Pale mucous membranes
- Poor pulse quality
- Low blood pressure

Fluid replacement

As hypovolaemic shock occurs due to reduced circulating blood volume, treatment revolves around replacing the fluid deficit. The fluid used to restore the deficit is dependent on the type of fluid loss (e.g. haemorrhage, vomiting, diarrhoea). The commonest fluids used are isotonic replacement crystalloid fluids, such as Hartmann's solution, but occasionally it is necessary to use colloids or whole blood.

When treating shock, the fluid is given intravenously (or rarely via the intraosseous route). Initially the fluid is given at a fast rate over a relatively short period. The dose (or bolus) of fluid used varies, with a full shock dose of crystalloid being 60–90 ml/kg bodyweight in the dog and 40–60 ml/kg in the cat. Depending on the severity of the shock, this dose may be given over a period as short as 30 minutes (see Chapter 19).

Arrest of haemorrhage

If there is an obvious cause of the shock such as haemorrhage, efforts should be made to arrest it.

Methods of arresting haemorrhage

- **Direct digital pressure** – ensure that gloves are worn and apply pressure for at least 5 minutes.
- **Artery forceps** (haemostats) – if the bleeding vessel can be visualized it may be possible to clamp it directly with artery forceps.
- **Pressure dressing** – apply direct pressure over the bleeding area using an absorbent pad and cohesive bandage. If blood seeps through, reapply another layer. Do not remove the initial layer as a clot may be dislodged. Monitor mucous membrane colour of toes if a pressure dressing is used.

Type of shock	Description	Common causes
Hypovolaemic	Decreased circulating blood volume	Haemorrhage Severe vomiting and diarrhoea Third spacing (loss of fluid into body cavities, e.g. abdomen)
Distributive (includes anaphylactic, toxic and septic shock)	Abnormal distribution of body fluids secondary to body-wide dilation of all blood vessels	Sepsis Systemic inflammatory response syndrome (e.g. severe pancreatitis) Severe allergic reaction
Cardiogenic	Failure of the heart to act as an effective pump	Dilated cardiomyopathy Severe arrhythmias
Obstructive	Physical obstruction to blood flow within the vascular system	Pulmonary thromboembolism Pericardial effusion

18.11 Different forms of shock.

Distributive shock

This type of shock occurs when the body suffers an insult (often severe infection or inflammation) that causes the generalized release of inflammatory mediators (cytokines) that promote peripheral vasodilation. The body can no longer properly control where the blood volume is distributed. The peripheral tissues may have an increased blood supply to the detriment of the more important internal organs. Anaphylactic, toxic and septic shock are all forms of distributive shock.

Hallmarks of distributive shock

- Tachycardia
- Poor pulse quality
- *Red* mucous membranes
- Capillary refill time initially rapid, progressing to slow.

As the body is unable to constrict its blood vessels normally, the mucous membranes appear abnormally red. It is the presence of these inappropriately red mucous membranes that should alert the nurse to the presence of distributive shock.

The successful treatment of distributive shock involves rapidly identifying and treating the underlying cause. In some cases this is relatively straightforward (e.g. anaphylactic shock), in others (e.g. ruptured pyometra) it may require more invasive procedures. Fluid therapy is important but can be difficult, as these patients frequently have inflamed and leaky blood vessels. They are predisposed to the development of peripheral oedema if a large volume of crystalloid fluid is used.

In anaphylactic shock (e.g. insect stings) the patient can be treated with adrenaline, corticosteroids, antihistamines and fluid therapy if seen soon after exposure to the allergen.

Cardiogenic shock

This is seen in conditions where the heart can no longer pump effectively. It is most commonly seen in degenerative conditions of the heart muscle such as dilated cardiomyopathy or in severe arrhythmias. The findings on physical examination depend on the nature of the heart disease but may include heart murmurs, irregular pulses (especially if pulse deficits are present) and either very fast (>240 bpm) or very slow heart rates. Treatment depends on the underlying heart disease and is covered in the cardiovascular emergencies section. Fluid therapy is generally contraindicated in this form of shock.

Obstructive shock

This is the rarest form of shock in veterinary medicine. It may be seen in pericardial effusion and pulmonary thromboembolism. These conditions are covered under the cardiovascular and respiratory emergencies sections, respectively.

General treatments for shock

Patients with shock are likely to benefit from oxygen supplementation and being hospitalized in a comfortable stress-free environment. They may have a reduced body temperature and should be rewarmed slowly, but only after fluid therapy has started. Patients with shock require careful and close monitoring, especially in the first few hours after presentation.

Other markers of shock

Blood pressure

A drop in blood pressure is a late change in shock, as the body has a number of mechanisms to maintain blood pressure. A mean arterial blood pressure below 60 mmHg (mercury) is serious, as there may be damage to vital organs such as the brain, heart and kidneys.

Urine output

When monitoring a patient in shock, measurement of urine output (in ml/kg bodyweight/h) is useful as it is a non-invasive method of evaluating blood supply (perfusion) to the kidneys. If the animal is producing plenty of urine (>2 ml/kg/h) the kidneys are likely to be well perfused. Normal urine production is 1–2 ml/kg/h. Serial measurements of urine output are a useful and cheap monitoring tool that can be used in most practice situations.

Lactate

Lactate is generated secondary to anaerobic respiration in the tissues and is the best objective marker of shock. Until recently it could not easily be measured in veterinary patients. Normal lactate values are <2.5 mmol/l and values >6 mmol/l imply severe shock. Lactate values should return rapidly to normal if the shock is treated successfully.

Cardiovascular emergencies

Many emergency patients present with cardiovascular system abnormalities on examination (e.g. tachycardia, poor pulse quality). In many cases these abnormalities represent the cardiovascular response to shock and are not indicative of primary cardiovascular system disease. This section focuses on those emergencies that are primarily cardiovascular in nature.

Acute congestive heart failure (CHF)

CHF may occur secondary to a number of heart conditions. The most common are:

- Chronic mitral valve disease in small-breed dogs
- Dilated cardiomyopathy (weakness of the heart muscle) in large-breed dogs
- Hypertrophic cardiomyopathy (thickening and stiffening of the heart muscle) in cats.

CHF is usually seen in older patients but can occur in younger animals. Whatever the underlying cause, the clinical signs and emergency stabilization procedures are the same.

Clinical signs

- Cough, especially at night
- Dyspnoea/tachypnoea
- Reluctance to exercise
- Tachycardia
- Poor pulse quality
- Pale mucous membranes
- Cyanosis
- Heart murmur or gallop rhythm on cardiac auscultation

Diagnostic aids

If the patient is stable:

- Thoracic radiograph
- ECG
- Echocardiogram (ultrasonogram of the heart)

Treatment

- Do not stress
- Oxygen therapy
- Medical intervention, including:
  - Thoracocentesis if pleural effusion (commoner in cats)
  - Loop diuretic, e.g. furosemide intravenously or intramuscularly
  - Glyceryl trinitrate paste on skin, most commonly ear or groin as it is well absorbed from these areas. Use non-latex gloves to apply
- Once stabilized, medical therapy including ACE (angiotensin-converting enzyme) inhibitors, diuretics, pimobendan, digoxin, calcium-channel blockers may be used depending on the nature of the underlying disease

Pericardial effusion

This condition is principally seen in older large-breed dogs where the pericardial sac becomes full of fluid. This puts pressure on the heart so that it cannot fill properly and leads to signs of right-sided congestive heart failure.

Clinical signs

- Exercise intolerance
- Dyspnoea/tachypnoea
- Ascites (fluid in the abdomen)
- Muffled heart sounds on cardiac auscultation
- Tachycardia
- Poor pulse quality

Diagnostic aids

- Echocardiography (ultrasonography of the heart)
- Thoracic radiography
- ECG – electrical alternans (height of QRS complex alters from beat to beat) due to fluid in the pericardial sac

Treatment

- Pericardiocentesis (a needle is used to drain the fluid from the pericardial sac)
- Placement of intravenous catheter in case emergency treatment with lidocaine is necessary due to arrhythmias during pericardiocentesis
- In recurrent cases, surgery to remove the pericardial sac may be necessary
- Medical therapy is not effective

Aortic thromboembolism

This is a relatively common condition in cats but a rare condition in dogs. A thrombus (clot) blocks the aorta, disrupting blood flow to the hindlimbs. In cats it usually occurs secondary to underlying heart disease, whereas in dogs it usually occurs secondary to abnormal blood clotting. Rarely, thrombi can occur at other sites.

Clinical signs

- Extreme pain (vocalizing)
- Unilateral or bilateral paresis or paralysis of the hindlimb
- Cold hindlimb(s) with non palpable pulse(s)
- In the cat, dyspnoea or tachypnoea (signs of underlying cardiomyopathy)
- History of heart disease

Diagnostic aids

Diagnosis is usually based on a physical examination; supportive tests may be useful, especially in dogs, where an underlying medical disease is often the precipitating factor.

- Haematology and biochemistry
- Urinalysis
- Abdominal ultrasonography
- Echocardiography
- Thoracic radiography
- Blood pressure
- Endocrine testing

Treatment

- Prognosis poor
- Oxygen therapy
- Analgesia
- Environmental comfort
- Treatment of underlying disease
- Thrombolytic drugs – these include streptokinase and tissue plasminogen activator. There is limited experience of their use in veterinary medicine. They are very expensive and associated with a number of side effects, including bleeding. If used, they are more effective within hours of the clot first forming
- Anti-thrombotic drugs (e.g. aspirin, heparin) – these may help to reduce the risk of further clots forming but will not break down clots that are already present

Arrhythmia – tachycardia

Animals present with an abnormal heart rhythm that is so fast that the heart does not have time to fill properly with blood between beats. This is a rare emergency but needs to be identified quickly or heart failure can follow.

Clinical signs

- Collapse or syncope
- Exercise intolerance
- Severe tachycardia (>240 bpm)
- Poor or intermittent pulses

Diagnostic aids

- ECG

Treatment

- Medical therapy with anti-arrhythmic drugs
- Therapy is challenging as the drugs used have side effects, including the potential to worsen the arrhythmia

Arrhythmia – bradycardia

Animals present with an abnormally slow heart rate, leading to collapse. This is rare. Medical causes such as hyperkalaemia should be ruled out at an early stage.

Clinical signs

- Collapse or syncope
- Exercise intolerance
- Marked bradycardia (usually <60 bpm)

Diagnostic aids

- ECG
- Serum potassium level
- Other medical tests dependent on potassium level

Treatment

- If serum potassium level high, this should be treated urgently (see 'Metabolic emergencies')
- Cage rest
- Medical therapy unlikely to be effective unless patient is hyperkalaemic
- Pacemaker implantation may be necessary

Respiratory emergencies

Respiratory emergencies are very common and can be challenging to treat successfully. Several treatment strategies can be used irrespective of the cause of the dyspnoea, notably:

- Oxygen therapy
- Stress-free cool (but not cold) environment
- Maintain in sternal recumbency.

Upper airway disease

Upper airway problems generally present as dyspnoea associated with an audible noise (stridor or stertor). The emergency treatment of upper airway disease involves oxygen therapy and calming and cooling the patient. If the patient is in severe distress, it may be necessary to bypass the upper airway temporarily by anaesthetizing and intubating the patient. Emergency tracheotomies rarely need to be performed.

Common causes of upper airway dyspnoea are discussed in more detail below. Rarer causes include laryngeal masses, severe trauma to the upper airway and airway foreign bodies.

Laryngeal paralysis

This is a common cause of dyspnoea in older large-breed dogs. The muscles that hold the larynx open during inspiration become paralysed and the larynx collapses as the dog tries to breathe in.

Clinical signs

- Marked dyspnoea, often with paradoxical abdominal movement
- Stridor (audible whistling noise) on inspiration
- Exercise intolerance
- History of change in bark
- Cyanosis
- Hyperthermia

Diagnostic aids

The diagnosis is often suspected on the basis of the history and physical examination.

- Laryngoscopy under a light plane of anaesthesia is confirmatory

Treatment

- Oxygen therapy
- Sedation (commonly low doses of acepromazine) to reduce stress and inspiratory effort
- Cooling
- If severe, the patient may need to be anaesthetized and intubated. The patient can then be cooled and allowed to recover slowly from the anaesthetic. Rarely, a tracheostomy needs to be performed
- Long-term treatment requires surgery (usually a 'tie-back' procedure) but this is not commonly done on an emergency basis

Brachycephalic obstructive airway syndrome (BOAS)

This is a common disease in brachycephalic breeds such as Bulldogs and Pugs. It can be seen in brachycephalic cats such as Persians, but is less severe in this species. The dyspnoea is caused by airway obstruction secondary to the abnormal anatomy of these breeds. It is considered to include several components:

- Stenotic nares
- Long soft palate
- Everted laryngeal saccules
- Hypoplastic (narrow) trachea.

Clinical signs

- Dyspnoea
- Exercise intolerance
- Stertorous (snoring) breathing sounds
- Collapse/syncope
- Cyanosis

Diagnostic aids

Diagnosis is usually made on the basis of compatible clinical signs, breed and physical examination. Anaesthesia and examination of the upper airway confirms the diagnosis.

Treatment

- Oxygen therapy
- Sedation (commonly acepromazine)
- Cooling
- If severe, the patient may need to be anaesthetized and intubated. The patient can then be cooled and allowed to recover slowly from the anaesthesic. Rarely, a tracheostomy needs to be performed
- If severe, surgery may be needed to correct the anatomical abnormality, but this surgery is not commonly done on an emergency basis

Tracheal collapse

This condition typically occurs in small-breed dogs where the cartilaginous tracheal rings are abnormal or degenerate and the trachea collapses as the animal breathes in and out.

Clinical signs

- Cough (goose-honk) and dyspnoea commonly occur with stress or excitement
- Cyanosis
- Collapse/syncope

Diagnostic aids

Diagnosis is usually made on history, clinical signs and examination.

- Thoracic radiography
- Tracheal endoscopy

Treatment

- Oxygen therapy
- Stress-free environment and strict rest
- Sedation if necessary
- If severe, the patient may need to be anaesthetized and intubated. This should be avoided if possible as the endotracheal tube will cause further irritation to the trachea and the patient may be worse following an anaesthetic
- Long-term medical management includes weight loss and drug therapy but is rarely curative
- Surgical options are available but have a variable success rate

Pleural space disease

Animals with dyspnoea secondary to pleural space disease commonly present with short shallow respiration and dull lung sounds on thoracic auscultation.

Pleural effusion

This occurs when fluid accumulates in the pleural space. There are a number of types of fluid but the emergency treatment is the same.

Types of fluid

- **Transudate** – secondary to severe hypoalbuminaemia (low blood protein)
- **Modified transudate** – secondary to heart failure
- **Neoplastic exudate** – secondary to neoplasia within the chest, commonly lymphoma in cats
- **Pyothorax** – infected purulent fluid in the chest
- **Haemothorax** – blood in the chest secondary to trauma or a clotting disorder
- **Chylothorax** – a milky fluid that builds up due to problems with lymphatic drainage in the chest or rupture of the thoracic duct.

Clinical signs

- Dyspnoea and tachypnoea
- Dull lung sounds on auscultation
- Inappetence
- Weight loss

Diagnostic aids

- Thoracocentesis – this is therapeutic as well. Any fluid obtained should be kept for analysis
- Thoracic radiography – only if stable. Thoracocentesis should generally be performed before thoracic radiography
- Thoracic ultrasonography

Treatment

- Oxygen therapy
- Thoracocentesis

- Treatment of the underlying cause – this may be medical or surgical
- Occasionally it is necessary to place thoracostomy (chest) tubes to allow frequent drainage

Pneumothorax

This occurs when air accumulates in the pleural space. Causes include:

- Trauma
- Inhaled foreign body
- Idiopathic (especially in large-breed dogs)
- External penetrating wound (open pneumothorax).

Clinical signs

- Dyspnoea with short shallow respirations
- Dull lung sounds on auscultation
- External wound (open pneumothorax)
- Cyanosis

Diagnostic aids

- Oxygen therapy
- Thoracocentesis – this is therapeutic as well as diagnostic
- Thoracic radiography

Treatment

- Thoracocentesis
- In non-traumatic cases, surgical exploration of the chest
- Thoracostomy tubes placed if large volumes of air produced
- With open pneumothorax, a sterile adherent dressing should be placed over the wound until the patient is stable for surgery

Feline asthma

This is the only lower airway disease of importance in veterinary emergency patients.

Clinical signs

- Dyspnoea principally on expiration
- Wheezes on auscultation
- Abdominal effort on expiration

Diagnostic aids

- Physical examination
- Thoracic radiography
- Cytology on wash samples taken from the airways

Treatment

- Oxygen therapy
- Medical treatment:
  - Corticosteroids
  - Bronchodilators
  - Inhaled medications (Figure 18.12)

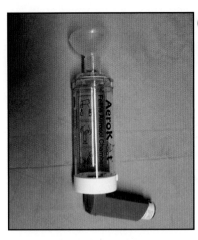

18.12 Aerokat inhaler used for administration of inhaled medications.

Parenchymal disease

Parenchymal disease develops when the alveoli become infiltrated with either fluid or tissue.

Common causes are:

- Heart failure (pulmonary oedema)
- Pneumonia (bacterial or parasitic)
- Neoplasia
- Non-cardiogenic oedema (e.g. secondary to head trauma, airway obstructions, severe systemic illness)
- Pulmonary contusions (bleeding into lung following trauma)
- Pulmonary thromboembolism.

Clinical signs

- Dyspnoea
- Cyanosis
- Crackles on auscultation of the lungs
- Inappetence

Diagnostic aids

- Thoracic radiography
- Haematology and biochemistry
- Urinalysis
- Bronchoscopy with airway washes in some patients
- Echocardiography (heart ultrasonography)

Treatment

- Oxygen therapy
- Medical treatment of the underlying disease may include:
  - Diuretics (e.g. furosemide)
  - Antibiotics
  - Anthelmintics

Neurological emergencies

Head trauma

Head trauma is a common emergency in both dogs and cats. It can occur secondary to road traffic accidents, falling from a height or being attacked by other animals (bitten by dog or cat, kicked by large animal). Clinical signs can be variable, depending on whether the brain has been damaged and, if so, which part.

Clinical signs

- Depression
- Anisocoria (variation in pupil size)
- Nystagmus
- Strabismus
- Cranial nerve deficits
- Epistaxis
- Bruising or swelling of face
- Asymmetry of face or jaw
- Inability to close mouth properly (mandibular or maxillary fractures)
- Ocular haemorrhage (scleral or within eye)
- Bradycardia
- Abnormal breathing pattern
- Seizures
- Coma
- Signs of trauma in other body areas (especially thorax or limb fractures)

Diagnostic aids

- Frequent neurological examination
- Haematology and biochemistry
- Blood pressure
- Skull radiographs
- Advanced imaging techniques (CT scan, MRI scan)

Treatment

- Ensuring patent airway
- Supplementing oxygen (take care that this does not cause stress)
- Intravenous fluid therapy to maintain blood pressure
- Head elevated at 30 degrees to reduce intracranial pressure
- Avoidance of any techniques that may increase intracranial pressure, such as jugular venepuncture
- Monitoring and maintaining body temperature
- If recumbent, turning every 4 hours
- Monitoring bladder size and catheterization or expression if necessary
- Medical therapies to reduce intracranial pressure (e.g. mannitol)
- Analgesia
- Treat concurrent injuries

Seizures

Seizures occur relatively commonly in dogs and rarely in cats. They represent an acute and usually brief disturbance of normal electrical activity in the brain and can be very distressing for both the patient and the owner. Most seizures are short (less than 2 minutes) and owners often only manage to telephone for veterinary advice once the seizure is over. As seizures can sometimes occur close together, it is always best to advise that the animal is examined by a veterinary surgeon as soon as practical even if the seizure has stopped.

Seizures are often described as having a pre-ictal, ictal and post-ictal phase. During the pre-ictal phase the animal may show mild behaviour changes, though these are not always recognised by owners. The ictal phase represents the seizure itself and the post-ictal phase a period after the seizure where the animal displays abnormal neurological signs.

Status epilepticus is a condition where seizures are prolonged (>5 minutes) or where there are multiple seizures in a short space of time (e.g. 30 minutes) and the animal does not recover completely between them. Animals with status epilepticus should be seen immediately, as prolonged or very frequent seizures may cause permanent brain damage.

Clinical signs

Ictal phase

- Loss of motor coordination with paddling of the limbs
- Rigid collapse
- Loss of consciousness
- Hypersalivation and abnormal chewing movements
- Defecation
- Urination
- Signs are usually generalized but, rarely, partial seizures are seen where the animal does not lose consciousness totally but becomes less aware, with focal twitching of the face or a single limb

Post-ictal phase

- Confusion
- Depression/listlessness
- Ataxia
- Visual disturbances, including blindness.

The post-ictal phase may last for several hours after a seizure episode.

Causes

- Idiopathic epilepsy
- Brain tumour (neoplasia)
- Trauma
- Infection
- Inflammation
- Toxin
- Metabolic problems (hypoglycaemia, hepatic encephalopathy)

Diagnostic tests

- Blood glucose level
- Haematology and biochemistry
- Full neurological examination
- Cerebrospinal fluid (CSF) tap
- Brain imaging (CT, MRI) if available

Treatment

If the animal is having a seizure when it arrives at the practice, or starts to do so whilst hospitalized, medications should be given to control the seizure. Although most seizures are short, longer seizures (especially if lasting more than 5 minutes) can lead to further brain damage. Drugs used to treat seizures include:

- Diazepam (valium) – intravenous or per rectum
- Phenobarbital – intravenous or oral
- Potassium bromide – oral or per rectum.

The drug of choice for acute control of seizures is diazepam given by the intravenous route, but the rectal route can be used if intravenous access cannot be obtained. Phenobarbital and potassium bromide are more commonly used as oral medications for the longer-term control of seizures.

If a seizuring animal develops respiratory distress or cyanosis, it is important to secure an airway. However, drugs (sedation or anaesthetic) must be given to allow this to happen safely. ***Never* put your hand in the mouth of a seizuring dog.**

Nursing care

- Monitor body temperature and cool if hyperthermic.
- Monitor heart rate and respiratory rate.
- Ensure patent intravenous access in case further seizures occur.
- Turn patient every 4 hours.
- Monitor bladder size and catheterize or express if necessary.
- Lubricate eyes.
- Maintain a calm environment. However, it is *not* necessary to maintain a dark room and this can in fact be detrimental, as it can compromise the ability to monitor the patient

Spinal cord disease

Causes

- Intervertebral disc disease
- Direct trauma (e.g. road traffic accident)
- Anatomical abnormalities (e.g. 'wobbler' dogs)
- Vascular disease (e.g. fibrocartilaginous emboli)
- Spinal cord haemorrhage
- Spinal cord neoplasia
- Infection
- Degenerative spinal cord disease (e.g. degenerative myelopathy)

Clinical signs

These will be variable depending on the site and severity of the spinal cord injury. In general, cervical spinal cord disease has signs involving all four limbs, whereas thoracolumbar spinal cord disease has signs involving the hindlimbs only. It is very important to assess whether the animal can feel pain in each of its legs, which is usually done by squeezing firmly on one of the animal's toes. It should be remembered that the animal simply withdrawing its leg when the toe is squeezed is a local reflex arc and does not necessarily mean that the animal is aware and feeling the sensation. Signs that the animal can feel the sensation include vocalization, turning the head to look at the leg or pupillary dilation at the time the toe is squeezed. If deep pain sensation is lost, the animal's prognosis, in terms of the likelihood of it walking again, is much worse.

Clinical signs may include:

- Limb weakness (paresis) and proprioceptive deficits (mild disease)
- Ataxia (mild disease)
- Paralysis (severe disease)
- Recumbency/inability to walk (severe disease)
- Pain on palpation of spine
- Urinary incontinence
- Lack of anal tone
- Loss of deep pain sensation (severe disease)
- Change (either decrease or increase dependent on location of lesion) of the strength of the local reflexes (e.g. patellar reflex)
- Normal mentation and cranial nerve examination.

Rarely, severe thoracolumbar spinal cord disease will cause the Schiff–Sherrington phenomenon, where the forelimbs are rigid and the hindlimbs flaccid. This is most often seen following trauma and has a poor prognosis.

Treatment

- Analgesia
- Cage rest
- Monitoring bladder size and expression or catheterization if necessary
- Maintaining warm and comfortable environment
- Turning regularly (every 4 hours) if recumbent
- Surgical treatment required for most causes of acute spinal cord disease
- Use of corticosteroids (e.g. methylprednisolone, dexamethasone) is no longer recommended.

If a spinal fracture is suspected, great care must be taken when moving the patient. If possible, the animal should be strapped to something rigid during transport to the practice. A specially designed animal stretcher is ideal but other rigid objects may be used in an emergency.

Vestibular disease

The vestibular system controls balance and the animal's awareness of its body position in space. Vestibular disease may occur at the level of the inner ear, where the sense organs of balance are located (known as peripheral vestibular disease), or within the brain (known as central vestibular disease).

Causes

- Infection (e.g. otitis media)
- Inflammation
- Neoplasia
- Benign polyps (especially young cats)
- Idiopathic ('old dog' vestibular disease)
- Trauma
- Toxic (including drugs, e.g. high doses of metronidazole)
- Postsurgical (e.g. following ear surgery)

Clinical signs

- Nystagmus (abnormal eye movements)
- Strabismus
- Ataxia
- Mental depression
- Other neurological signs
- Horner's syndrome (constricted pupil, flaccid eyelids, enophthalmos, third eyelid protrusion)
- Nausea
- Signs of external ear disease

Figure 18.13 summarizes the clinical signs that can help to distinguish peripheral from central vestibular disease.

Clinical sign	Peripheral	Central
Nystagmus	Usually horizontal	Can be vertical or rotatory
Horner's syndrome	May be present	Absent
Mentation	Normal	May be depressed
Hemiparesis	Absent	Possible

18.13 Clinical findings that can help to differentiate between peripheral and central vestibular disease.

Treatment

- Treatment of underlying cause (medical or surgical)
- Maintaining in a comfortable padded environment
- May need intravenous fluids and/or nutritional support as may be unable to eat or drink
- Time

Reproductive emergencies

Dystocia

Dystocia refers to problems during the parturition (birthing) process (see Chapter 25). There are a large number of causes of dystocia but some of the more common ones are:

- Primary uterine inertia (i.e. failure of uterus to contract)
- Secondary uterine inertia after prolonged straining
- Fetal malpresentation
- Maternal–fetal disproportion (common in breeds such as Bulldogs)
- Maternal pelvic abnormalities (e.g. previous fractured pelvis)
- Fetal death.

Clinical signs

If the bitch is showing any of the following signs, veterinary advice should be urgently sought:

- She has been straining unproductively for more than 1 hour from the onset of stage II labour without producing a puppy.
- She has been straining unproductively for more than 30 minutes without producing subsequent puppies.
- She has a green-brown vaginal discharge or fetal fluids are seen and 2 hours have elapsed without producing a puppy.
- She rests for more than 4 hours between puppies without straining.
- She appears unwell or depressed.
- A puppy can be seen stuck in the birth canal.

For queens, the interval between kittens may be much longer and the entire parturition process may take up to 24 hours. If concerned, it is better to err on the side of caution and recommend that the pet is examined for signs of fetal or maternal distress.

Diagnostic aids

- Digital vaginal examination
- Abdominal radiography
- Abdominal ultrasonography

Treatment

- Keep the bitch in a warm and comfortable environment
- If a puppy is visible in the birth canal, manually assisted delivery may be attempted
- Medical therapy (e.g. oxytocin)
- Surgical delivery (caesarean operation)

Nursing care for caesarean operation

For a successful outcome, the time taken for the anaesthesia and surgical procedure should be minimized. The bitch may be clipped and an initial surgical preparation carried out prior to anaesthesia. All instruments for the surgery and for neonatal resuscitation and care should be prepared before the procedure.

Neonatal resuscitation

Equipment that should be prepared prior to delivery includes:

- A warm environment (incubator) or box with heat lamp
- Plenty of soft, dry, warm towels
- Haemostats for clamping the umbilical cord
- Suture material
- Suction bulb syringe for clearing oral secretions
- Emergency drugs (adrenaline, naloxone).

The following procedures should start once the neonate has been handed over to the nurse:

- Clean the fetal membranes from the puppy's mouth and gently suction the oral cavity (check for cleft palate when doing this).
- Clamp the umbilical cord 1–2 cm from the umbilicus.
- Stimulate and dry the neonate by rubbing with a warm towel.
- Check that the puppy is breathing and has a heartbeat (using digital palpation).

If the puppy is not breathing or does not have a heartbeat:

- Supply oxygen via a tight-fitting face mask or endotracheal tube.
- Continue vigorously rubbing the puppy to stimulate respiration.
- Doxapram drops may be used.
- 'Swinging' puppies is no longer recommended, due to the potential for causing brain damage.
- If there is no heartbeat, start gentle external compressions and administer adrenaline.

Pyometra

This is an infection of the uterus that is common in older entire female dogs. It occurs secondary to hormonally induced changes and is commonest about 5–6 weeks after a season.

Clinical signs

- Vomiting
- Polyuria/polydipsia
- Weakness and lethargy
- Purulent vaginal discharge (not always present)
- Abdominal pain
- Shock.

Diagnostic aids

- Haematology and biochemistry
- Urinalysis
- Vaginal swab
- Abdominal radiography
- Abdominal ultrasonography.

Treatment

- Intravenous fluid therapy
- Antibiotic therapy
- Surgery to remove the infected tissue.

Eclampsia

This is hypocalcaemia secondary to pregnancy or more commonly lactation. It is most often seen in small-breed dogs within two weeks of parturition.

Clinical signs

- Restlessness and anxiety
- Panting
- Hypersalivation
- Twitching/muscle spasms
- Hyperthermia
- Tachycardia
- Collapse.

Diagnostic aids

- Blood calcium level.

Treatment

- Slow intravenous infusion of 10% calcium gluconate (monitor heart rate while doing this)
- Oral calcium supplementation
- Wean the puppies.

Paraphimosis

This is an inability to retract the penis into the prepuce. It commonly occurs in entire male small-breed dogs following an episode of sexual excitement.

Clinical signs

- Engorged protruding penis often dry and may be necrotic
- Dysuria
- Pain and excessive licking associated with penile region.

Treatment

- Analgesia
- Gentle cleaning of penis with warm water or saline solution
- Topical hyperosmolar solution to reduce swelling
- Manual replacement of penis within prepuce (commonly requires heavy sedation or anaesthesia)
- Surgical correction, especially if situation recurs.

For further information, see Chapter 25.

Paediatric emergencies

Young puppies and kittens may present in a collapsed state. Diagnosis is often challenging but the two most common problems are:

- Hypoglycaemia
- Hypothermia

Clinical signs

- Weakness or collapse
- Persistent crying
- Decreased feeding
- Decreased movement

Due to patient size, diagnostic tests and treatment are challenging but the following guidelines should be used:

- Monitor body temperature and warm if hypothermic.
- Measure blood glucose.
- Supplement glucose:
  - Intravenous – a standard intravenous catheter may be used in the jugular vein in paediatric patients
  - Intraosseous – easy to place in paediatric patients and can be life saving
  - Oral – much less effective.
- Supplement fluids.
- Once normothermic, initiate oral feeding regime.

Nursing the paediatric patient

- Ensure warm and comfortable environment.
- Feed regularly by bottle or stomach tube:
  - Every 2 hours in puppies and kittens less than 5 days old
  - Every 4 hours in puppies and kittens more than 5 days old.
- Use a commercial hand-rearing formula to supply patient's needs.
- After feeding, stimulate patient to defecate by gently rubbing the perineum with a damp cotton bud (this function is usually undertaken by the mother).

For further information, see Chapter 25.

Urological emergencies

Urethral obstruction

This occurs when there is a blockage in the urethra and therefore the animal cannot pass urine. As urine cannot be voided from the body, waste products (especially potassium, urea and creatinine) build up rapidly in the bloodstream and can cause life-threatening signs within 24 hours of the obstruction occurring. It occurs most commonly in overweight male neutered cats, but some dog breeds (e.g. Dalmatian) are also predisposed. It is very rare in female animals, as they have a much shorter wider urethra.

Causes

- Urethral calculi (stones)
- Urethral plug (consists of crystals and a mucoid material)
- Urethral neoplasia (cancer) (rare)
- Urethral stricture (may occur secondary to previous obstruction with stones or a plug)

Clinical signs

- Stranguria (straining to urinate without passing any urine)
- Frequent visits to litter tray with no urine produced
- Vocalization (pain) when attempting to urinate
- Licking at urethra

- Depression (dependent on duration of blockage, but most animals are markedly depressed by 24–36 hours after the blockage occurs)
- Anorexia
- Bradycardia (secondary to potassium build-up in bloodstream)
- Distended painful bladder on palpation of the abdomen
- Vomiting
- Collapse

Urethral blockage must be distinguished from cystitis, where the bladder is inflamed but not blocked. Animals with cystitis may also strain to urinate, urinate frequently and show pain when urinating, but they will pass small amounts of urine. Cystitis is more common in female animals. Cystitis is an uncomfortable condition but, as the animal can still void urine, it is not life-threatening in the way that urinary obstruction is.

Diagnostic aids

- Palpation and gentle expression of the bladder
- Blood tests, especially blood potassium level
- ECG – can help to identify signs of hyperkalaemia (high blood potassium).

Once the patient has had the obstruction relieved (been 'unblocked'), the following tests can be carried out:

- Urinalysis and culture
- Ultrasonography of the bladder
- Radiography, including retrograde urethrography

Treatment

- Fluid therapy
- Treatment for hyperkalaemia if present (see 'Metabolic emergencies')
- Urinary catheterization – commonly requires sedation and should be done once the animal has been stabilized with fluid therapy
- Urinary catheter may be left in place for 24–72 hours after decompression and urine production should be monitored during this time
- Analgesia/anti-inflammatories
- If bladder stones are present, surgery may be required to remove them

Uroabdomen

This condition occurs when urine leaks into the abdominal cavity, often secondary to a tear in the bladder wall (ruptured bladder). As in urethral obstruction, urine is not voided from the patient and high levels of potassium, urea and creatinine can build up in the blood, leading to severe clinical signs.

Causes

- Trauma
- Following cystocentesis (this is most often a concern when a cystocentesis is performed while the urethra is blocked)
- Bladder neoplasia (cancer)

Clinical signs

- Distended and/or painful abdomen
- Depression
- Anorexia

- Vomiting
- Bradycardia
- Lack of urination (as urine is leaking into abdomen). If the tear in the bladder wall is small, it is possible that the animal may still be able to void small amounts of urine via the urethra

Diagnostic aids

- Blood tests (especially potassium, urea and creatinine levels)
- Abdominal ultrasonography
- Analysis of fluid collected from the abdominal cavity by abdominocentesis
- Radiography, including contrast studies

Treatment

- Intravenous fluid therapy
- Treatment for hyperkalaemia if present (see 'Metabolic emergencies')
- Surgical repair of the rupture.

Acute renal failure

This can happen if the kidneys suddenly fail. It is much less common than chronic renal failure in veterinary patients.

Causes

- Shock with significant reduction of blood supply to kidneys (most commonly prolonged hypovolaemic shock)
- Infection (e.g. leptospirosis, bacterial pyelonephritis)
- Toxic damage (e.g. ethylene glycol)
- Metabolic (e.g. prolonged hypercalcaemia)
- Drug therapy (e.g. non-steroidal anti-inflammatory drugs, especially if given while the patient is in shock)
- Blood clots in arteries supplying kidneys (rare)
- Progression of chronic renal failure

Clinical signs

- Depression
- Anorexia
- Vomiting
- Uraemia (may be smelled on animal's breath)
- Abnormality in urine production, most commonly reduced (anuria/oliguria) but occasionally massively increased (polyuria)

Diagnostic aids

- Haematology and biochemistry
- Urinalysis, including urine culture
- Abdominal ultrasonography
- Abdominal radiography
- Serology (blood tests for infectious agents such as leptospirosis)

Treatment

- Intravenous fluid therapy
- Treatment for underlying cause, if known (e.g. antibiotics for infection, specific treatment for hypercalcaemia)
- Drugs to encourage urine production (furosemide, mannitol)
- Peritoneal dialysis
- Monitor urine production and blood tests

Metabolic emergencies

Hypoglycaemia

This is a low level of blood glucose (sugar). It is the commonest reversible cause of collapse in neonatal/paediatric patients but can occur in older animals.

Causes

- Young patient, especially toy breeds of dog
- Insulin overdose in diabetic patients
- Insulinoma (functional cancer of pancreas)
- Hypoadrenocorticism (Addison's disease)
- Liver failure
- Sepsis or severe infection

Clinical signs

- Weakness
- Exercise intolerance
- Collapse
- Seizures
- Coma

Diagnostic aids

- Blood glucose level (glucometer)
- Haematology and biochemistry

Treatment

- Intravenous (or intraosseous) glucose supplementation
- Food offered as soon as able to eat
- Rub glucose syrup on oral mucous membranes – unlikely to be effective if animal is severely hypoglycaemic, but may be attempted whilst intravenous access is obtained

Hyperkalaemia

This is an increased blood potassium level. The level of normal potassium in blood is approximately 3.5–5.5 mmol/l. Levels >8.0 mmol/l may be fatal.

Causes

- Urethral obstruction
- Acute renal failure
- Uroabdomen
- Hypoadrenocorticism (Addison's disease)
- Reperfusion injury

Clinical signs

- Bradycardia (slow heart rate)
- Poor pulse quality
- ECG changes
- Other signs dependent on cause of hyperkalaemia

Diagnostic aids

- Serum potassium level
- ECG
- Other tests dependent on underlying cause

Treatment

Ultimately, successful treatment depends on identifying and treating the underlying cause of the hyperkalaemia. However, as it may be immediately life-threatening, the following therapies may be used to stabilize the animal whatever the cause of the hyperkalaemia:

- Intravenous calcium gluconate
- Intravenous insulin and dextrose supplementation
- Intravenous fluid therapy.

Hypercalcaemia

This is an increased level of blood calcium.

Causes

- Neoplasia (cancer), especially lymphoma and anal sac carcinoma
- Toxicity (e.g. human psoriasis cream, some rat poisons)
- Primary hyperparathyroidism (hormonal disease)
- Hypoadrenocorticism (Addison's disease)
- Granulomatous infections (e.g. lungworm, fungal disease)

Clinical signs

- Inappetence/anorexia
- Polyuria/polydipsia
- Depression
- Vomiting
- Tremors
- Renal failure if prolonged

Diagnostic aids

- Haematology and biochemistry
- Urinalysis
- Imaging studies (radiography, ultrasonography)

Treatment

As with hyperkalaemia, successful treatment requires identification and treatment of the underlying disease. However, while diagnostic tests are being carried out to allow this, the following medical treatments can be used to lower the calcium level and reduce the risk of renal damage:

- Intravenous fluid therapy with 0.9% NaCl
- Furosemide
- Bisphosphonates
- Calcitonin.

Hypoadrenocorticism (Addison's disease)

This is a disease where there is impaired secretion of hormones from the adrenal cortex. The animal becomes deficient in a number of hormones, most importantly aldosterone (a mineralocorticoid) and cortisol (a glucocorticoid). Aldosterone is a hormone that helps the body to maintain electrolyte balance (especially potassium) and cortisol is a hormone that helps the animal to maintain normal blood pressure and gastrointestinal tract function and to cope with stress. It is most commonly diagnosed in young to middle-aged female dogs and is very rare in cats.

Clinical signs

- Collapse
- Weakness
- Depression/lethargy
- Polyuria/polydipsia
- Intermittent gastrointestinal signs (vomiting, diarrhoea, inappetence)
- Bradycardia
- Poor pulse quality
- Pale mucous membranes with a prolonged capillary refill time

Diagnostic aids

- Haematology and biochemistry
- Urinalysis
- ACTH stimulation test (this is the only way to make a certain diagnosis)
- ECG

Treatment

- Intravenous fluid therapy
- Treatment of hyperkalaemia if severe (see section above on hyperkalaemia)
- Hormone replacement therapy (both mineralocorticoid and glucocorticoid)

Diabetic ketoacidosis

This is a complication of diabetes mellitus where the body starts to produce ketones as an energy source. As these ketones are organic acids, if produced in large quantities they can cause the blood to become acidic, with severe systemic effects. Diabetic ketoacidosis may occur both in previously undiagnosed diabetics and in diabetic animals that have been on insulin treatment for some time.

Clinical signs

- Collapse
- Inappetence/anorexia
- Vomiting
- Polyuria/polydipsia
- Dehydration
- Signs of shock (tachycardia, poor pulses)
- Tachypnoea (increased breathing rate)
- Ketones may be smelled on the breath (pear drop smell)

Diagnostic aids

- Haematology and biochemistry
- Blood gas analysis (allows quantification of how acidic the blood is)
- Urinalysis and culture
- Abdominal ultrasonography

Treatment

- Intravenous fluid therapy
- Insulin therapy – generally using a short-acting insulin by intravenous or intramuscular route for initial stabilization. A longer-term protocol of subcutaneous insulin for use at home can be introduced once the patient is stable

- Antiemetics
- Antibiotics
- Careful monitoring of electrolytes with supplementation if necessary. Potassium, phosphorus and magnesium may all need supplementing

Disseminated intravascular coagulation (DIC)

During DIC, the clotting system of the body becomes overactivated. This leads to consumption of the patient's clotting factors and the development of a generalized bleeding tendency. DIC always occurs secondary to a severe underlying problem such as septic shock, pancreatitis or heat stroke. It is a serious complication but can be reversible.

Clinical signs

- Petechiation/ecchymoses
- Excesssive bleeding from catheter or venepuncture sites
- Haemorrhage at mucosal surfaces
- Presence of a severe underlying disease

Diagnosis

- Platelet count (will be low with DIC)
- Clotting times (will be prolonged with DIC)
- Other clotting parameters such as D-dimers or fibrinogen degradation products

Treatment

- Treatment of underlying disease
- Fluid therapy to maintain tissue blood flow
- Fresh frozen plasma transfusions
- Medical treatment such as with heparin may be used dependent on the stage and severity of DIC

Gastrointestinal and abdominal emergencies

Pharyngeal or oesophageal fishhook

Dogs, or less commonly cats, may ingest fishhooks either directly or by eating fish or bait attached to them. The fishhook commonly lodges in the pharynx or proximal oesophagus but occasionally lodges more distally. If there is still line attached to the hook, the owners should be instructed neither to pull it, as this may cause further damage, nor to cut the line, as it may help the veterinary surgeon locate the hook.

Clinical signs

- Drooling, possibly with blood-tinged saliva
- Dysphagia (difficulty eating)
- Facial/pharyngeal discomfort (pawing at face)
- It is possible that the animal may display no clinical signs but simply be observed to have eaten the hook

Diagnostic aids

- Radiography

Treatment

- Removal of hook, usually under general anaesthesia

The ease with which the hook can be removed depends both on its location (e.g. hooks lodged in the pharynx are easier to remove than oesophageal ones) and the number of barbs the hook has. Hooks with multiple barbs embedded in the wall of the oesophagus may require careful manipulation to remove. Occasionally surgical removal is necessary.

Oesophageal foreign body

This occurs most commonly in terrier breeds, especially West Highland White Terriers. The foreign body is most commonly a bone.

Clinical signs

- Witnessed ingestion of a foreign object (often fed to dog by owners)
- Regurgitation
- Retching/coughing
- Hypersalivation
- Inappetence
- Depression
- Pain or discomfort on eating

Diagnostic aids

- Radiography
- Endoscopy

Treatment

- Removal of foreign object via mouth, aided by endoscopy
- Removal of foreign object via mouth, aided by fluoroscopy
- Pushing foreign object into stomach and either removal by laparotomy and gastrotomy or left to be destroyed by gastric acid
- Rarely, surgical removal of the object via thoracotomy and oesophagotomy

Complications

- Aspiration pneumonia
- Oesophageal rupture
- Oesophageal stricture (may occur up to several weeks later)

Megaoesophagus

This is a condition where the oesophageal muscle cannot contract normally and loses its tone, meaning that food is no longer pushed normally from the mouth to the stomach following swallowing. It can be congenital but is more commonly an acquired condition in older dogs and less commonly cats. Its main clinical sign is regurgitation, which is the *passive* process whereby food that remains in the oesophagus is brought back. Although a chronic condition, these patients commonly present as an emergency either as the disease worsens or if the patient develops pneumonia.

Clinical signs

- Regurgitation (may occur for up to several hours after eating)
- Weight loss
- Commonly a good appetite maintained
- Coughing/dyspnoea due to secondary aspiration pneumonia

Diagnostic aids

- Radiography
- Haematology, biochemistry and other blood tests to try to identify an underlying cause

Treatment

- Treatment of underlying cause
- Nutrition – often necessary to feed directly into the stomach via gastrotomy tube
- Treatment of concurrent aspiration pneumonia with antibiotics

Vomiting

This is the active expulsion of gastric contents (compared with passive regurgitation). There are many causes of vomiting but they can be subdivided according to whether the origin of the problem is within the gastrointestinal (GI) tract or outside it.

Causes of vomiting

Primary gastrointestinal causes

- GI infection (viral, bacterial, parasitic)
- Dietary indiscretion
- Gastrointestinal foreign body
- Intussusception
- Gastrointestinal neoplasia
- Pancreatitis

Secondary causes

- Renal disease
- Liver disease
- Infection (e.g. pyometra)
- Endocrine disease (e.g. hypoadrenocorticism)
- Neurological disaease
- Drug therapy

Vomiting is commonly (but not always) accompanied by diarrhoea. Vomiting and diarrhoea vary a lot in their severity: some patients with vomiting require emergency evaluation and treatment, whereas others patients have much milder signs where emergency treatment is not necessary. When dealing with an owner whose pet is vomiting, the following questions should be asked and can be used to make an assessment of the severity of the problem and whether the animal should be seen on an emergency basis:

- How many times has the pet vomited in the last 12 hours?
- Is there any blood in the vomit? How much?
- Is the pet still keen to eat and drink? And are they able to keep anything they eat down?
- Is the pet significantly depressed?
- Does the pet have any other signs of abdominal pain (e.g. vocalization, abnormal position)?
- Has the pet been witnessed to eat any toxins or drugs or any objects of a size that might have become stuck in the GI tract?

Diagnostic aids

- Thorough history, including vaccination status and worming history
- Physical examination

- Haematology and biochemistry, including in-house blood smear evaluation to assess for neutropenia (low white blood cell count seen with severe GI infections, especially parvovirus)
- Urinalysis
- Faecal analysis (both for parasites and culture)
- Abdominal radiography
- Abdominal ultrasonography
- Serological testing of both blood and faeces for infectious disease

Treatment

- Intravenous fluid therapy
- Treatment of underlying cause (may be medical or surgical)
- Nil per mouth until diagnosis made
- Antiemetic therapy unless GI obstruction suspected
- Good nursing care – warm comfortable environment

Diarrhoea

Diarrhoea refers to the voiding of abnormal liquid faeces. Patients with diarrhoea may present as an emergency if the diarrhoea is severe (with significant fluid loss), if there is a large amount of blood in the faeces or if it is accompanied by marked vomiting and depression. Diarrhoea is commonly split into:

- **Small-bowel** – large volumes of watery faeces passed with a relatively low frequency
- **Large-bowel** – small volumes of semi-solid faeces passed frequently with straining. A small amount of fresh blood may be present.

Small-bowel diarrhoea is more commonly an emergency than large-bowel diarrhoea, especially if melaena (digested blood presenting as black, sticky or tarry faeces) is present.

Diagnostic aids

- Thorough history, including vaccination status and worming history
- Physical examination
- Haematology and biochemistry, including in-house blood smear evaluation to assess for neutropenia (low white blood cell count seen with severe GI infections, especially parvovirus)
- Urinalysis
- Faecal analysis (both for parasites and culture)
- Abdominal radiography
- Abdominal ultrasonography
- Serological testing of both blood and faeces for infectious disease

Treatment

- Intravenous fluid therapy
- Treatment of underlying cause (may be medical or surgical treatment)
- Nil per mouth until diagnosis made
- Good nursing care – ensure perineal area does not become sore or inflamed. This may require frequent bathing, clipping of hair in this region or a tail bandage

Gastrointestinal obstruction

Patients with GI obstruction most often present with vomiting and sometimes diarrhoea. They also commonly show signs of both hypovolaemic shock and dehydration. The obstruction may be complete or partial. Animals with complete obstructions have more severe and rapidly progressive signs than those with partial obstructions.

Obstructions may occur secondary to:

- Foreign body ingestion
- Intussusceptions (telescoping of the bowel)
- GI neoplasia
- Incarceration

Clinical signs

- Vomiting, sometimes with blood
- Anorexia
- Depression
- Abdominal pain
- Palpable abdominal mass (classically intussusceptions are sausage shaped)
- Hypovolaemic shock
- Dehydration
- Weight loss – especially with partial obstructions
- Diarrhoea/melaena (digested blood in stool), especially with partial obstructions.

Diagnostic aids

- Abdominal radiography
- Abdominal ultrasonography
- Haematology and biochemistry
- Electrolyte and blood gas analysis
- Urinalysis
- Faecal analysis

Treatment

- Intravenous fluid therapy for stabilization
- Surgical removal of the obstruction – this may require resection of a portion of the bowel
- Endoscopic removal may be attempted for gastric foreign bodies

Postoperative monitoring and nursing care

This is crucial for a successful outcome. Patients should initially be maintained on intravenous fluids, with gradual reintroduction of water and then food over the 12–48 hours after surgery. Breakdown (dehiscence) of the incision in the bowel can occur for several days after surgery. Postoperative monitoring should include:

- Perfusion parameters (heart rate, pulse quality, mucous membrane colour and capillary refill time)
- Urine output
- Any vomiting or regurgitation
- Any faeces passed
- Body weight
- Hydration status.

Gastric dilatation–volvulus

GDV is a condition of principally large-breed deep-chested dogs. The stomach becomes dilated with gas and then twists along its long axis. It causes a sudden onset of severe clinical signs.

Clinical signs

- Collapse
- Severe hypovolaemic shock
- Unproductive retching
- Distended tympanic abdomen (though this can be hard to see in some of the most deep-chested dogs where the distended stomach is hidden under the rib cage)
- Tachycardia, possibly with arrhythmia
- Pale mucous membranes with prolonged capillary refill time
- Restlessness in early stages
- Hypersalivation
- Tachypnoea

Diagnostic aids

- Abdominal radiography – right lateral view is most important
- Haematology and biochemistry
- Electrolyte and blood gas including lactate level.
- ECG

Treatment

- Intravenous fluid therapy for stabilization – shock doses of fluid via large-bore catheter are often required
- Gastric decompression via stomach tube – this is not always possible and a stomach tube should never be forced in as this may result in tearing of the oesophagus at the oesophageal gastric junction (cardia)
- Gastric decompression via percutaneous trocharization – a needle or catheter is inserted through the abdominal body wall in the area where tympany is detected, with the aim of entering the stomach and allowing gas to escape
- Surgery – this is the definitive treatment and would usually occur as soon as the patient has been stabilized for anaesthesia with fluid therapy. The stomach is derotated and then emptied (usually by passing a stomach tube following derotation). A gastropexy should then be performed. This involves anchoring the stomach in the correct position by suturing the stomach to the body wall
- Good postoperative care is essential – the monitoring is similar as for the patient with GI obstruction

Pancreatitis

This is a generalized inflammation of the pancreas. In most cases, it is unknown why it happens but it may be associated with obesity, a high-fat diet and certain diseases such as hyper-adrenocorticism. One of the functions of the pancreas is to make the digestive enzymes. When the pancreas becomes inflamed, these enzymes are released into the circulation and can cause severe systemic signs, including shock and death.

Clinical signs

- Vomiting – may be severe
- Anorexia
- Collapse
- Tachycardia
- Severe abdominal pain – dogs may show the 'praying position'
- Dehydration
- Diarrhoea

Diagnostic aids

- Haematology and biochemistry
- Specific pancreatic blood tests such as trypsinogen-like (TLI) and canine pancreatic lipase (cPLI) immunoreactivity
- Abdominal ultrasonography
- Abdominal fluid analysis (if present)
- Abdominal radiographs

Treatment

- Intravenous fluid therapy
- Antiemetics
- Analgesia
- Nil per mouth until vomiting has ceased
- Antibiotics

Haemoabdomen

This occurs when an abdominal organ ruptures and the animal bleeds into its abdominal cavity. The spleen is the most common organ to rupture, often because there is a splenic tumour.

Clinical signs

- Collapse
- Tachycardia
- Poor pulse quality
- Pale mucous membranes
- Abdominal distension with a fluid thrill

Diagnostic aids

- Haematology and biochemistry
- Clotting profile
- Abdominal ultrasonography
- Abdominal fluid analysis
- Thoracic radiographs to look for signs of metastasis (spread of cancer) to the chest
- Abdominal radiographs

Treatment

- Intravenous fluid therapy
- Blood transfusion
- Abdominal pressure wrap (Figure 18.14)
- Surgery to identify and remove the bleeding organ

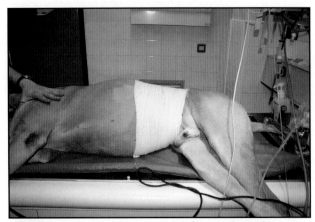

18.14 Abdominal pressure wrap for a patient with haemoabdomen. (Courtesy of D Hughes)

Septic peritonitis

This is a condition where a septic (infected) fluid builds up in the abdominal cavity. The infection most commonly gains entry to the abdominal cavity from a ruptured GI tract, but other sources (e.g. ruptured urogenital or biliary tract) are possible.

Clinical signs

- Collapse
- Tachycardia
- Poor pulse quality
- Red mucous membranes
- Abdominal pain
- Abdominal distension
- Vomiting
- Diarrhoea
- Anorexia

Diagnostic aids

- Haematology and biochemistry
- Clotting profile
- Abdominal radiography
- Abdominal ultrasonography
- Abdominal fluid analysis (cytology, biochemistry and culture)
- Urinalysis

Treatment

- Intravenous fluid therapy
- Intravenous antibiotic therapy
- Analgesia
- Exploratory surgery to lavage (flush) the abdomen and identify and treat the source of infection

Nursing care

Postoperative nursing care is vital to a successful outcome. Parameters to be monitored should include:

- Heart rate
- Pulse quality
- Mucous membrane colour
- Blood pressure
- Urine output
- Degree of pain.

These parameters can be used to guide postoperative fluid and analgesia requirements.

Hepatic failure

Causes

- Infection (e.g. leptospirosis)
- Toxin
- Inflammation
- Neoplasia

Clinical signs

- Weakness
- Inappetence
- Weight loss
- Vomiting, including haematemesis

- Neurological signs (seizures, unusual behaviour, blindness)
- Jaundiced mucous membranes
- Increased tendency to bleed

Diagnostic aids

- Haematology and biochemistry
- Clotting profile
- Liver function tests (bile acid stimulation tests, ammonia level)
- Abdominal ultrasonography
- Aspirate or biopsy of the liver
- Urinalysis

Treatment

- Intravenous fluid therapy
- Antibiotics
- Glucose supplementation
- Lactulose to treat neurological signs (hepatic encephalopathy)
- Blood or plasma transfusion
- Treatment of primary cause

Ocular emergencies

Ocular emergencies are relatively common. Although they are rarely life-threatening, prompt action may need to be taken to prevent loss of sight in the eye. They are also often particularly distressing to owners, as they can look very dramatic, and it is recommended that the animal is admitted to the practice as soon as possible. As even minor ocular problems have the potential to deteriorate rapidly with the possibility of loss of vision, all animals showing a sudden onset of signs related to the eye should be seen urgently.

With all ocular emergencies the following rules can be applied:

- Assess condition of patient – abnormalities in the major body systems should always be addressed first, no matter how severe the injury to the eye
- Assess extent of ocular injury
- Prevent self-trauma (place Elizabethan collar)
- Give analgesia
- Keep eye moist with a false-tear solution
- Keep patient in a quiet dimly lit environment.

Traumatic proptosis

This represents the forward displacement of the entire globe, with entrapment of the eyelids behind the equator of the globe. It is most commonly seen following trauma and in breeds with shallow orbits, such as the Pekingese.

Clinical signs

- Anteriorly displaced globe
- Swelling around orbit
- Signs of other head injuries (e.g. bleeding, bruising)

Treatment

The globe should be replaced into its correct position as quickly as possible if the animal is to regain vision in that eye; however, any concurrent injuries must be considered when deciding if immediate replacement of the globe is the correct course of action.

- Sterile saline-soaked swab over the proptosed globe to keep eye moist – the saline may be slightly cooled to help to reduce periorbital swelling.
- Prevention of self-trauma.
- Analgesia.
- Sedation/anaesthesia with replacement of globe. Following replacement, the eyelids are commonly sutured closed for a period of time.

Ocular foreign body

Clinical signs

- Foreign body visible or may be trapped under eyelids or third eyelid (Figure 18.15)
- Blepharospasm
- Rubbing eye or face
- Epiphora (excess tear production)
- Chemosis (conjunctival swelling)
- Photophobia

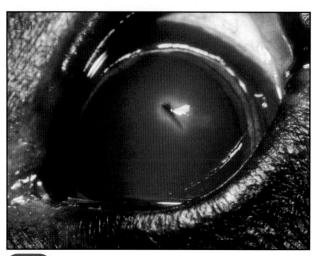

18.15 Corneal foreign body. (Courtesy of D Moore)

Treatment

- Prevention of self-trauma (Elizabethan collar)
- Topical local anaesthesia
- Flushing eye with large volume of sterile saline
- Sedation or anaesthesia if foreign object lodged (especially under third eyelid)
- If foreign object does not appear to have penetrated the cornea, it should be gently grasped and removed
- If foreign object has clearly penetrated the cornea, it should be left in place until it can be removed by a specialist veterinary ophthalmologist.
- Topical antibiotics

Corneal scratch/laceration

This is where the surface of the cornea is damaged. It occurs most commonly secondary to scratches from other animals or damage from vegetation.

Clinical signs

- Ocular pain
- Blepharospasm
- Photophobia
- Epiphora

- Squinting
- Rubbing eye or face
- Visible disruption of the corneal surface
- Corneal oedema (blue discoloration of cornea) (Figure 18.16)
- If cornea is penetrated, there may be anterior uveitis (see below) or prolapse of the iris into or through the corneal wound

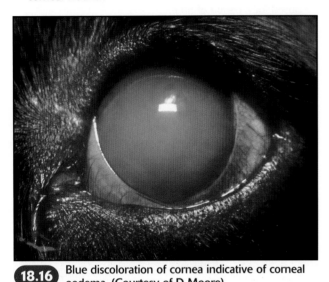

18.16   Blue discoloration of cornea indicative of corneal oedema. (Courtesy of D Moore)

Diagnostic aids

- Fluorescein stain of the eye – areas where the corneal epithelium is damaged will take up the stain

Treatment

- Prevention of self-trauma
- Topical local anaesthesia for analgesia and to allow a full examination
- Topical medical treatment (antibiotics, treatment for uveitis if present)
- Deep scratches, especially if the cornea is penetrated, may require surgery

Corneal ulcer

Causes

- Corneal trauma
- Anatomical (e.g. exophthalmos, abnormal eyelashes)
- Breed-related (e.g. Boxers)
- Infectious
- Lack of tear production
- Chemical injury

Clinical signs

- Ocular pain
- Blepharospasm
- Photophobia
- Epiphora
- Squinting
- Rubbing eye or face
- Purulent ocular discharge
- Corneal oedema (blue discoloration of cornea) (see Figure 18.16)
- Secondary uveitis

Diagnostic aids

- Fluorescein stain eye – ulcerated areas will take up the fluorescein stain, unless the ulcer is very deep with exposure of Descemet's membrane

Treatment

- Prevention of self-trauma
- Topical medical treatment (*not* corticosteroid)
- Treatment of underlying cause
- Severe rapidly progressive ulcers (known as melting ulcers) may require surgical therapy

Uveitis

This refers to inflammation of the uveal tract, which includes the iris, ciliary body and choroid layer. It may occur as a localized ocular problem or may be seen with a wide range of systemic infectious or inflammatory diseases.

Causes

- Ocular trauma
- Infection
- Inflammation
- Neoplasia
- Secondary to problems with the lens

Clinical signs

- Ocular pain
- Blepharospasm
- Photophobia
- Rubbing eye or face
- Squinting
- Miotic (constricted) pupil
- Aqueous flare (cloudiness to anterior chamber)
- Secondary corneal oedema (blue discoloration of cornea) (see Figure 18.16)

Diagnostic aids

- Full ophthalmological examination
- Careful full physical examination for signs of systemic disease
- Haematology and biochemistry
- Urinalysis

Treatment

- Treatment of underlying cause
- Analgesia (topical and/or systemic)
- Prevention of self-trauma
- Topical anti-inflammatory
- Topical mydriatic

Glaucoma

This represents an increased intraocular pressure (i.e. pressure within the eyeball). It can be very painful and if not treated quickly can lead to permanent blindness in that eye. It is an inherited condition in some breeds (e.g. Cocker Spaniel, Springer Spaniel) due to anatomical abnormalities that predispose to poor outflow of the aqueous humour. This is known as primary glaucoma. Secondary glaucoma may occur in any breed and happens secondary to a number of other ocular problems (e.g. lens luxation).

Clinical signs

- Often unilateral, sudden onset, severe ocular pain
- Reduced or absent vision
- Episcleral vascular congestion
- Corneal oedema (blue discoloration to cornea) (Figure 18.19)
- Dilated unresponsive pupil
- Elevated intraocular pressure.

Diagnostic aids

- Measurement of intraocular pressure using:
  - Indentation tonometry (Schiotz tonomoter)
  - Applanation tonometry (Tonopen)

Treatment

- Prevention of self-trauma
- Analgesia (topical or systemic)
- Topical treatment to:
  - Reduce production of aqueous humour
  - Improve outflow of aqueous humour
- Systemic treatment to reduce pressure within globe (e.g. mannitol)
- Surgical intervention by a specialist ophthalmologist may be necessary
- If the eye remains non-visual but painful, enucleation can be considered

Hyphaema

This refers to bleeding within the anterior chamber.

Causes

- Trauma
- Coagulation disorder
- Hypertension
- Neoplasia
- Inflammation

Clinical signs

- Blood visible in anterior chamber (Figure 18.17)
- Disturbed vision
- Secondary uveitis

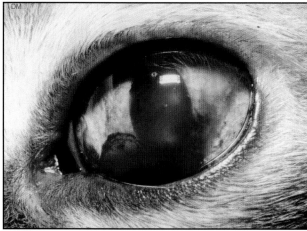

18.17 Hyphaema, with blood visible in the anterior chamber. (Courtesy of D Moore)

Diagnostic aids

- Full clinical examination
- Full ophthalmological examination
- Haematology and biochemistry
- Clotting profile

Treatment

- Treatment of underlying cause
- Treatment of uveitis symptomatically if present

Sudden-onset blindness

Animals that suddenly become blind may appear disoriented or confused or may become depressed and withdrawn. If the eyes appear outwardly normal, owners may not immediately realize their pet has become blind.

Causes

- Chorioretinitis (inflammation of the choroid and retina)
- Retinal detachment secondary to:
  - Hypertension (especially in cats)
  - Trauma
- Retinal degeneration (e.g. SARDS in dogs)
- Optic neuritis (inflammation of the optic nerve)
- Intracranial disease (e.g. pituitary tumour)
- Glaucoma (although eye is usually painful)

Clinical signs

- Blindness
- Bumping into things, especially in a new environment
- Depression and unwillingness to move (especially cats)
- Inappetence/anorexia
- Dilated non-responsive pupils

Diagnostic aids

- Full ophthalmological examination
- Full neurological examination
- Blood pressure measurement (especially cats)
- Haematology and biochemistry
- Urinalysis

Treatment

- Treatment of underlying cause

The animal may be very anxious, especially in a strange environment. To reduce its anxiety:

- Always use animal's name whenever handling it
- Maintain familiar smell if possible
- Reassure animal verbally with a calm tone of voice as much as possible
- Move slowly and gently when handling the animal.

Nasal emergencies

Epistaxis

This refers to bleeding from the nostrils. It may be bilateral or unilateral. Although the volume of blood produced may seem to be large, it is rare for dogs or cats to become significantly anaemic or hypovolaemic following nasal bleeding.

Causes

- Trauma
- Nasal tumour
- Infection, especially aspergillosis
- Nasal foreign body
- Coagulation disorder
- Hypertension

Clinical signs

- Nasal bleeding – always note if it is unilateral or bilateral
- Stertorous breathing
- Open-mouth breathing
- Sneezing
- Melaena (if blood is being swallowed)

Diagnostic aids

- Haematology and biochemistry
- Clotting profile
- Blood pressure
- Nasal radiography
- Nasal endoscopy plus biopsy

Treatment

- Maintain a calm environment
- Sedation
- Cold compress externally
- Topical application of adrenaline (either squirted into nostril or soaked on to a swab and placed in nostril)
- Absorbent dressing within nostril (e.g. tampon). It is vital to keep a record of the number of swabs/tampons used so it can be ensured that all are retrieved
- Monitor for signs of hypovolaemia, which may occur if epistaxis is severe and/or prolonged. Treat with fluid therapy if it occurs

Nasal foreign body

The commonest nasal foreign bodies are grass seeds, blades of grass or small pieces of wood.

Clinical signs

- Sneezing, may be paroxysmal
- Nasal discharge, usually unilateral, occasionally blood tinged
- Rubbing or pawing at nose

Treatment

Removal of foreign body by:

- Endoscopy
- Flushing.

Nasal foreign bodies can be particularly hard to identify. They are rarely seen on radiographs. Endoscopy may be useful but, especially in small patients, the size of the endoscope often precludes a thorough and complete search of the entire nasal chamber. If a foreign body cannot be seen and retrieved under direct visualization, nasal flushing should be performed.

Nasal flush procedure

1. Ensure that a cuffed endotracheal tube is in place, with cuff inflated.
2. Pack pharynx with swabs – count swabs and record. It is vital to double check that all swabs are removed before animal is recovered from anaesthesia.
3. Place animal in sternal recumbency with rostral end of nose tipped downward.
4. Fill 60 ml syringe with saline (20 ml for a cat).
5. Place nozzle of syringe up nostril that is most likely to be affected and squeeze both nostrils shut around.
6. Empty syringe with moderate force into nostril.
7. Hold empty bowl beneath nostril to catch any fluid.
8. Repeat multiple times and with both nostrils (recommend using at least 1 litre saline for a 20 kg dog).
9. Ensure that all swabs are retrieved from pharynx before patient is recovered from anaesthesia – the foreign material may sometimes be found on these swabs when they are removed.

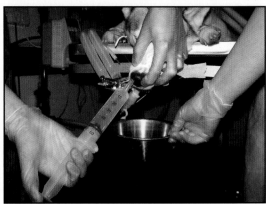

If foreign material is not found, it is possible that it had already been sneezed out before the animal reached the practice. However, it is also possible that it may remain *in situ*. This is unlikely to be dangerous for the animal, but a chronic nasal discharge may develop if any foreign material has been left behind. Owners should be warned of this possibility.

Aural emergencies

Although emergencies involving the ear are very rarely life-threatening, they can cause some distress to both the patient and the owner.

Aural foreign body

Clinical signs

- Head shaking
- Rubbing or scratching ear
- Pain on touching of head or aural region
- Visualization of foreign body on auroscopic examination

Treatment

- Removal of foreign body – invariably requires sedation

Otitis externa and media

This is an infection of the external ear canal (otitis externa) or middle ear (otitis media).

Clinical signs

- Head shaking
- Rubbing of head or scratching of ear
- Self-trauma of aural region
- Vestibular signs (with otitis media – see Neurological emergencies)
- Aural discharge – may be waxy or foul smelling
- Auroscopic examination confirms aural inflammation

Treatment

- Emergency treatment rarely necessary unless neurological signs develop
- Antibiotics (topical and systemic)
- Analgesia
- Aural flush under anaesthesia

Aural haematoma

This is a haematoma of the pinna. Although these swellings are never life-threatening, patients may present as an emergency as they can develop quite rapidly and be quite large.

Causes

- Head shaking
- Self-trauma

Clinical signs

- Soft non-painful swelling of the pinna
- Scratching of the ear
- History of head shaking or aural trauma

Treatment

- Drainage of the haematoma
- Bandaging of the ear following drainage (has been recommended but is very difficult to achieve)
- Injection of corticosteroids following drainage (sometimes used but is discouraged as it delays healing)
- Surgical techniques to maintain pressure across pinna whilst healing occurs
- Reassurance to owners that it is not a life-threatening problem

Environmental emergencies

Hyperthermia (heat stroke)

The normal body temperature of both the dog and cat is approximately 38.5°C. If an animal is placed in a hot environment it will activate cooling mechanisms (e.g. panting, drinking cold water, moving to a cooler place) that act to keep the body temperature close to this normal value. If these cooling mechanisms fail, then the animal's body temperature increases and can reach dangerously high levels (>41°C) and cause heat stroke. Heatstroke *must* be distinguished from the other major cause of an elevated body temperature, which is pyrexia. In pyrexia, the animal's elevated body temperature is an appropriate response to an infection or inflammatory process and is actually a protective mechanism.

- In **hyperthermia**, cooling the animal is a vitally important part of treatment.
- In **pyrexia**, cooling the animal can place the patient under additional physiological stress.

Whenever an increased body temperature is found on examination, it must be decided whether it is elevated due to hyperthermia (in which case external cooling measures are appropriate) or pyrexia (in which case external cooling measures are inappropriate). Heatstroke is very rare in cats.

Causes

- Overexposure to a hot environment that the animal cannot remove itself from (e.g. locked in a car on a hot day, tied up outside in direct sunlight)
- Excessive exercise
- Seizures (uncontrollable excessive muscle activity)
- Upper airway obstruction (inability to hyperventilate and thus loss of one of the dog's major cooling mechanisms)

Clinical signs

- Restlessness
- Panting (or attempts to pant)
- Tachypnoea
- Tachycardia
- Poor pulse quality
- Red mucous membranes
- Markedly elevated body temperature (>41°C)
- Vomiting and diarrhoea
- Ataxia
- Collapse, coma, death

Treatment

- Rapid-rate intravenous fluid therapy with fluids either at room temperature or slightly chilled
- Active external cooling:
  - Wet animal's haircoat (running water will cool more efficiently than still water)
  - Clip animal's haircoat
  - Fan
- Cold-water enema
- Peritoneal lavage with cooled (not cold) fluids

Aggressive cooling measures should be discontinued when the patient's body temperature reaches 40.5°C to avoid overcooling and the development of hypothermia. Frequent and regular (every 10 minutes) monitoring of body temperature should then be performed in conjunction with less aggressive cooling measures until body temperature reaches 39.5°C.

A number of very serious complications can result from heatstroke, especially if the rise in body temperature has been prolonged. Once cooled, animals should be closely monitored for the development of:

- Disseminated intravascular coagulation
- Hypoglycaemia
- 'Shock gut' – with sloughing of the GI tract mucosa and development of haemorrhagic vomiting and diarrhoea
- Acute renal failure
- Cardiac dysrhythmias
- Pulmonary dysfunction.

If these develop, they should be treated symptomatically.

Hypothermia

This refers to a subnormal body temperature. Severe hypothermia is considered to be a body temperature below 28°C and is rare. Mild to moderate hypothermia is common. Smaller animals are more prone to becoming hypothermic, due to their high ratio of surface area to weight. Younger animals are also prone to hypothermia, as they are not yet able to generate body heat in the same way as adults.

Causes

- Severe disease/shock – especially common in cats
- Sedation/anaesthesia
- Prolonged exposure to low environmental temperatures

Clinical signs

- Shivering
- Depression
- Slow breathing rate
- Cardiac arrhythmias
- Coma
- Death

Treatment

- Warmed intravenous fluids
- Rewarming should only start once cardiovascular support (intravenous fluids) has been initiated
- Passive rewarming – maintain warm ambient environment
- Surface rewarming with circulating warm water or air blankets (Figure 18.18)
- If temperature less than 30°C, consider active core rewarming with warm peritoneal dialysis
- Electric heating pads and heating lamps not recommended, due to potential for causing burns
- Care should be taken not to warm the patient too rapidly, especially if they are also in shock. Rapid rewarming can worsen the signs of shock

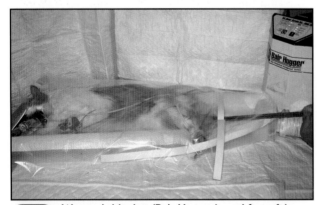

18.18 Warm-air blanket (Bair Hugger) used for safely rewarming patients.

Burns

Burns result when intense heat (or rarely cold) damages the skin and subcutaneous tissues. Serum leaking from the damaged areas may lead to blister formation. Most burns seen in veterinary patients are iatrogenic (i.e. caused by veterinary intervention – notably heat pads).

Burns can be classified by:

- Cause (Figure 18.19)
- Depth
  - Superficial – affecting only outermost layer of skin
  - Partial thickness – affecting slightly deeper layers of skin; blistering common
  - Full thickness – affecting all layers of skin
- Percentage of body surface affected.

Type of burn	Potential causes
Dry	Hot objects, flames, friction, heat pads
Scald	Hot liquid, steam
Cold	Very cold objects, especially metals
Electrical	Chewing on electric cables
Radiation	Sun
Chemical	Caustic soda, paint stripper

18.19 Burns and potential causes.

Clinical signs

- Red, moist skin
- Charred, leathery skin (seen with full-thickness burns)
- Pain (full-thickness burns are less painful, as nerve endings are destroyed)
- Heat
- Signs of shock

Treatment

- Removal of source of the problem, or moving patient away from source (take care no risk to humans)
- Dousing area in cold water for minimum of 10 minutes (care should be taken not to overcool the patient and cause hypothermia)
- Very gently clipping the fur over a large area around the burn (burns can often be much larger than first thought)
- Covering the area, once cooled, with sterile non-adherent dressing or cling film
- Analgesia
- Elizabethan collar to prevent further self-trauma
- Intravenous fluid therapy to treat concurrent shock

> ⚠ **WARNING**
> With electrical burns or electrocution, ensure that the electrical source is **turned off** before approaching patient. **Do not** put yourself at risk of being electrocuted – remember that both metal and water are good conductors of electricity.

Smoke inhalation

Animals are occasionally seen for evaluation and treatment of smoke inhalation after being trapped in fires.

Clinical signs

- Cough
- Dyspnoea
- Nasal discharge
- Singed whiskers/evidence of burns
- Brick-red mucous membranes if carbon monoxide has been inhaled
- Neurological signs – may occur up to several days after smoke inhalation

Diagnostic aids

- Arterial blood gas analysis
- Co-oximetry
- Thoracic radiographs
- Pulse oximetry less useful

Treatment

- Oxygen therapy
- Supportive care

Toxicological emergencies

A large number of substances may poison animals. Owners of animals with an acute onset of clinical signs often query whether their animal could have been poisoned. Although this may occur, poisoning (especially malicious poisoning) is rare.

Due to the large number of potential toxins and the wide variety of clinical signs exhibited, poisoning is a differential diagnosis for many emergency patients.

All substances have the potential to be toxic if given in the wrong amount or at the wrong time. Figure 18.20 summarizes the types of toxins that may be encountered.

Toxins are most commonly ingested but may also be inhaled (e.g. carbon monoxide) or absorbed through the skin.

Type of toxin	Examples
Veterinary prescription drugs	Insulin, NSAIDs, phenobarbital
Human prescription drugs	NSAIDs, human chemotherapy drugs, contraceptive medication, human heart or asthma medication
Human recreational drugs	Cannabis, Ecstasy, cocaine
Human foodstuffs	Chocolate, onions, raisins
Household chemicals	Bleach, oven cleaner, antifreeze, paint
Garden chemicals	Herbicides, pesticides, molluscicides, rodenticides
Plants	Easter lily, foxglove

18.20 Categories of common toxicities, with examples.

History taking for the suspected poisoned patient

Poisoning is more likely to be seen in certain groups of patients:

- Young dogs (due to their tendency to eat indiscriminately)
- Cats (many chemicals and drugs are not adequately detoxified by the liver)
- Animals that are free ranging on farmland or wasteland where chemicals are stored or used.

Sensitive questioning is required as some owners may not wish to reveal what substances their pet has had access to or may not even know that a substance was toxic to their pet. If poisoning is suspected, the following questions should be asked.

Questions for suspected poisonings

- Is the pet on any medication? If so, when did it receive its last dose? How much did it receive?
- Has the pet been given any human medications? If so, what and how much?
- Has the pet had access to any human medications? If so, what?
- What chemical products are kept in the home? Garage? Garden? Is there any way the pet could have had access to them?
- Does the pet have access to any farmland, parkland or industrial land? Can it be checked whether any chemicals are stored or used regularly there?
- Has the pet had any access to illegal substances? (Reassure the owner that this information is given in confidence.)
- Has there been any building work or decorating at home with any unusual substances left around?
- Has the pet eaten anything unusual recently?
- Has there been anything on the pet's coat recently that it may have ingested whilst grooming?

If an owner has witnessed a pet eating a potential toxin, they should be asked to bring as much information as possible about the toxin to the practice. This could include any packaging and an idea of how much of the substance might have been ingested.

Veterinary Poisons Information Service

The VPIS is a 24-hour helpline that supplies clinical information on possible animal toxicities. Practices must be registered to use the service and on calling will be asked for an identification number before information is supplied. The more detail it is possible to give the helpline, the more likely they are to be able to provide an accurate answer concerning possible complications and treatment for the toxicity.

Clinical signs

Toxicities can lead to a huge variety of different clinical presentations, but common clinical signs of poisoning include:

- Gastrointestinal signs
  - Profuse salivation
  - Vomiting
  - Diarrhoea

- Neurological signs
  - Behavioural change
  - Ataxia
  - Seizures
  - Collapse and coma
- Bleeding
- Unconsciousness and death.

The clinical signs and suggested treatments for some of the more common toxicities seen in the UK are summarized in Figure 18.21.

Diagnostic aids

- Haematology and biochemistry
- Urinalysis (especially sediment examination)
- Clotting profile (for suspected rodenticide)
- Any vomit, faeces and urine produced should be kept and frozen in case it is required for future toxicological investigation

Stabilization and treatment

The key aims in initial stabilization of any poisoned patient are to:

- Identify the poison and the amount ingested as accurately as possible
- Prevent further absorption of the poison
- Treat any signs that develop symptomatically
- Administer any antidote or specific treatment (under the direction of a veterinary surgeon).

Preventing further absorption

Emetics

If an owner suspects that their animal has been poisoned, they should be asked to bring it to the practice immediately so that vomiting can be induced in a safe environment. Some owners may wish to try and induce vomiting at home but this is not recommended. Vomiting can be induced using a number of different emetics (Figure 18.22) under the direction of a veterinary surgeon.

Toxin	Toxic dose (if known)	Principal clinical signs	Suggested treatment
Paracetamol	Cat 50–100 mg/kg Dog > 200 mg/kg	Cyanosis (muddy mucous membranes) Respiratory distress Facial swelling (cat) Liver failure (especially dog)	Induction of emesis N-acetylcysteine orally or i.v. Ascorbic acid orally Cimetidine i.v.
Ibuprofen	GI signs: Cat >50 mg/kg Dog >100 mg/kg Renal signs: > 300 mg/kg	Gastric ulceration Vomiting Renal failure	Induction of emesis Activated charcoal Intravenous fluid therapy Gastroprotectant drugs (e.g. H_2-blockers, omeprazole)
Anticoagulant rodenticides	Variable, depending on product	Haemorrhage – commonly starts 5–7 days following ingestion of toxin	Induction of emesis Activated charcoal Vitamin K (s.c. or orally) Whole blood or plasma transfusion
Metaldehyde (slug bait)	Median lethal dose (LD$_{50}$): Dog 210–600 mg/kg Cat 207 mg/kg	Severe seizures Depression Vomiting and diarrhoea Hyperthermia Metabolic acidosis	Gastric lavage Activated charcoal Control seizures Cool
Organophosphates/ carbamate insecticides	Variable, depending on product	Salivation Lacrimation Urination Vomiting and diarrhoea Muscle tetany (twitching) Depression	Activated charcoal Prevent further grooming Bathe (if topical exposure) Atropine 2-PAM
Ethylene glycol (antifreeze)	Cat: 1.5 ml/kg Dog: 6.6 ml/kg	Vomiting Depression Ataxia Dehydration Oliguric renal failure	Induction of emesis Intravenous fluid therapy Administration of ethanol (alcohol) 4-methylpyrazole (specific antidote for use in dogs)
Theobromine (chocolate)	Dog: 250–500 mg/kg NB: 2.25 oz (64 g) cooking chocolate or 20 oz (560 g) of milk chocolate may be toxic in a 10 kg dog	Restlessness Panting Vomiting Tachycardia Cardiac arrhythmias	Induction of emesis Activated charcoal Arrhythmia treatment
Paraquat (weedkiller)	LD$_{50}$ 25–50 mg/kg	Vomiting Renal and hepatic signs Dyspnoea (pulmonary fibrosis)	No specific treatment Supportive care
Easter lily	Unknown – toxic to cat	Acute renal failure	Supportive care

18.21 Toxic dose, clinical signs and suggested treatments for some of the commoner toxicities seen in small animals in the UK.

Agent	Species	Dose	Route
Apomorphine	Dog	0.04–0.08 mg/kg	In conjunctival sac, s.c., i.m. or i.v.
Xylazine	Cat	1.1 mg/kg	i.m.
Washing soda crystals	Dog	1 crystal in small dog; 2 crystals in medium to large dog	Oral

18.22 Recommended compounds for induction of emesis.

Contraindications to emetics

Situations where vomiting should *not* be induced include:

- Where the toxin is a caustic or acidic substance or a volatile petroleum product that could cause further damage to tissues when it is vomited
- Where the patient is depressed or seizuring when there is a high risk of aspiration.
- In species unable to vomit (e.g. rat).

When the administration of an emetic is contraindicated, gastric lavage may be employed. The animal is anaesthetized and the airway protected with a cuffed endotracheal tube.

Activated charcoal

Activated charcoal is administered in many patients following induction of emesis, as it adsorbs many toxins within the gastro-intestinal tract and prevents further absorption of any remaining toxin. Some dogs will willingly eat activated charcoal mixed with food; in other patients the activated charcoal may have to be delivered by stomach tube. With some toxins, it is recommended that a dose of activated charcoal is repeated every 6 hours for 2–3 days.

Topical toxins

In patients where the toxin is on the skin (e.g. flea products, paint, creosote), the following steps should be followed:

- Inform the veterinary surgeon (drug treatments may be available for the toxicity seen with some flea products)
- Fit the patient with an Elizabethan collar to prevent any grooming and possible ingestion of the toxin
- Treat any systemic signs symptomatically
- Wear gloves
- Remove the contamination with a combination of grooming, clipping and bathing. Do not cool the patient too much while bathing it. Rinse the patient with copious amounts of warmed water. Swarfega is useful for the removal of oily compounds such as creosote.

Symptomatic treatment

Most patients are treated symptomatically. The patient's cardiovascular, respiratory and neurological status and body temperature should be carefully monitored. Key treatments include:

- Intravenous fluid therapy to maintain intravascular volume and prevent dehydration
- Maintenance of normal body temperature
- Sedative or anti-seizure medication if neurological signs present.

Specific treatment

Specific treatments (antidotes) are available for only a small number of toxins. Some examples are given in Figure 18.21. It is only recommended that they are used if it is *known* that the toxin has been ingested. Antidotes may be expensive and may not be easily available in veterinary general practice.

Adder bites

The adder (*Viperis berus*) is the only native venomous snake present within the UK. Depending on geographical location, adder bites are not uncommon in dogs, especially in the warmer summer weather. Most bites occur on the limbs or muzzle. The incident is rarely witnessed by the owners as adders are very shy. The bites are rarely fatal.

Clinical signs

- Rapid swelling of bitten area
- Fang marks may be present but often difficult to identify
- Depression
- Rarely, distributive (anaphylactic) shock may occur

Treatment

- Wound management – the adder bite should be treated as any other puncture wound
- Fluid therapy if signs of shock are present
- Medical treatment such as antihistamines
- Cage rest
- Antivenom if available
- Techniques such as tourniquets, cutting the wound or attempting to suck the venom out are not recommended

Insect stings (including bee and wasp)

Insect stings are a relatively common emergency. Although not life-threatening, they can be intensely irritating to the pet and distressing to the owner. They occur most commonly on the limbs or in the oral region. Rarely, if an animal is stung deep within the oropharynx, the associated swelling causes a degree of respiratory tract obstruction that may require emergency intervention.

Clinical signs

- Swelling and redness of bitten area
- Pain
- Pawing at mouth or chewing at limb
- Development of distributive (anaphylactic) shock:
  - Tachycardia
  - Collapse
  - Dyspnoea
  - Vomiting
  - Seizures

Treatment

- Local application of ice to reduce swelling
- Antihistamines
- Corticosteroids
- Intravenous fluid therapy if signs of shock are present

Toad poisoning

Toad poisoning that may be fatal occurs in the southern United States. In the UK, dogs will occasionally pick up and chew toads but, whilst this may result in local oral irritation and hypersalivation, it is not a life-threatening toxicity and is self-limiting. If the patient will allow, the mouth may be flushed with saline to speed resolution of signs.

Traumatic emergencies

Haemorrhage

Haemorrhage is defined as a copious loss of blood from the vessels. If haemorrhage is severe it leads to hypovolaemic shock and death. It is difficult to judge the severity of the haemorrhage simply from observing the amount of blood lost. The severity of the situation is best assessed by examining the animal's cardiovascular system parameters and assessing the patient for signs of shock.

Haemorrhage may be classified both by its location and by the type of vessel damaged:

- **External** haemorrhage occurs from wounds and is easily visible
- **Internal** haemorrhage may not be immediately obvious. Internal haemorrhage can occur in the thoracic or abdominal cavities, the gastrointestinal or urinary tract or in the muscle around a fracture site. Internal haemorrhage may be seen with:
  - Trauma
  - Clotting problems
  - Abnormalities of the internal organs, especially tumours.

Haemorrhage may occur from arteries, veins or capillaries:

- **Arterial bleeding** consists of bright red blood that spurts from the wound. It requires prompt recognition and urgent action to prevent significant blood loss
- **Venous and capillary bleeding** both consist of darker red blood that oozes rather than spurts from the wound.

Although the differentiation between venous and capillary bleeding may be made, it is not a clinically useful distinction. Rather, the more important evaluation considers the volume and rate of blood loss and the effect that this is having on the cardiovascular system (hypovolaemic shock). In practice, most haemorrhage is a mixture of bleeding from different types of vessels. Haemorrhage from a major artery is seen uncommonly but can result in rapid blood loss and death.

Haemorrhage may also be classified by when it occurs relative to the time of injury:

- In emergency practice most haemorrhage is **primary** and results from damage to the blood vessel wall. This may be accidental (e.g. with trauma) or surgical.
- Delayed or **secondary** haemorrhage may be seen in postoperative patients hours to days after surgery if the ligature or clot is disrupted or destroyed by infection.

Clinical signs

- Visible external blood loss
- Bruising
- Swelling of abdomen (if haemorrhage into peritoneal cavity)
- Dyspnoea (if haemorrhage into or around lungs)
- Melaena/haematemesis (if haemorrhage into GI tract)
- Signs of shock dependent on severity of haemorrhage

Treatment

- Control of haemorrhage
- Intravenous fluids
- Blood transfusion

Control of haemorrhage

- **Direct digital pressure** – ensure gloves are worn and apply pressure for at least 5 minutes.
- **Artery forceps (haemostats)** – if the bleeding vessel can be visualized it may be possible to clamp it directly with artery forceps.
- **Pressure dressing** – apply direct pressure over the bleeding area using an absorbent pad and cohesive bandage.
- **Abdominal pressure wrap** – if the patient is bleeding into the peritoneal cavity, an abdominal pressure wrap ('belly wrap') can be placed (see Figure 18.17). The increase in intra-abdominal pressure can aid haemostasis.
- **Pressure points** – firm pressure can be applied directly over an artery. With enough pressure, flow through the artery will temporarily stop and bleeding distal to this point will be reduced. Three potential pressure points are described although they are used rarely:
  - Brachial artery on medial aspect of proximal humerus
  - Femoral artery on medial aspect of femur
  - Coccygeal artery on ventral aspect of tail.
- **Tourniquets** – with severe arterial haemorrhage in a limb it may be necessary to apply a tourniquet *temporarily* while the bleeding artery is located and ligated by the veterinary surgeon. Tourniquets can be applied anywhere on the limb proximal to the site of bleeding. Patients with tourniquets must be continually monitored and the tourniquet removed as soon as possible. If left in place there is a risk the limb may suffer significant compromise. A Penrose drain may be used as a tourniquet if a custom-made one is not available.

Wounds

Wounds are common emergencies. Most wounds are minor and do not put the animal at significant risk. However, some wounds can be life-threatening, especially if they are associated with significant blood loss or if they occur to the chest or abdomen and cause significant damage to underlying structures. The seriousness of a wound can be difficult to judge from its external appearance. An assessment of the animal's cardiovascular and respiratory systems gives a better indication of how life-threatening a wound is. Wounds can be described as shown in Figure 18.23 (see also Chapter 24).

Clinical signs

- Visible disruption of skin
- Pain
- Swelling
- Haemorrhage
- Shock

Treatment

- *Always* treat shock or any other major body system condition first
- Cover wound with sterile dressing to prevent further contamination whilst patient is being stabilized
- Control haemorrhage
- Analgesia

Classification	Description	Notes
Incised	Clean cut caused by sharp object (e.g. glass, scalpel blade)	Bleeding may be profuse, especially if wound is large or deep
Lacerated	Wound causing tearing of tissue and uneven edges (e.g. barbed wire)	Bleeding likely to be less severe than with incised wound but more likely to be contaminated
Abrasion (graze)	Superficial wound where full skin thickness is not penetrated	Embedded dirt or foreign bodies may be present
Contusion (bruise)	Blunt blow that has ruptured capillaries below surface	May be associated with deeper injuries (e.g. fracture)
Puncture	Small external wound but often associated with significant deeper damage	Often caused by dog or cat bites
Gunshot	Nature of wound depends on type of gun	Entry wound may be small but associated with possible significant internal damage

18.23 Wound classifications.

- Once patient is stable:
  - Clip *wide* area around wound (especially bite wounds)
  - Remove any contaminating material
  - Flush wound copiously with sterile saline
  - Dress or suture wound (depending on nature of wound)
- Antibiosis

If any large foreign bodies are present in the wound or if there is a chance the wound penetrates the thoracic or abdominal cavity, the patient will require anaesthesia to explore the wound safely and all possible complications can be dealt with if they arise. Similarly some bite wounds may require surgical exploration. A tooth wound may have caused minimal skin damage but there can be extensive damage to underlying tissues. The animal should be stabilized before surgical exploration.

Fractures

A fracture occurs when there is a break in the continuity of the bone. It most often occurs after trauma, but pathological fractures may be seen. Pathological fractures are fractures that occur with minimal trauma, due to an underlying weakness in the bone. They are most often seen with bone tumours and metabolic bone disease.

For classification of fractures, fracture healing and fracture management see Chapter 24.

Clinical signs

- Lameness (usually non-weight-bearing)
- Swelling
- Pain
- Bruising over fracture site
- Wound (if open fracture)
- Abnormal orientation to limb
- Crepitus

Diagnostic aids

Radiographs are necessary to classify the fracture and decide on a definitive treatment plan, but the diagnosis can generally be made after the physical examination.

Treatment

Fractures most commonly occur following trauma but are rarely life-threatening. Concurrent injuries to the patient affecting the major body systems should *always* be addressed before specific treatment for the fracture is considered.

As the pain caused by the fracture is related to movement of the broken ends of the bone, the emergency management is based on:

- Analgesia
- Immobilization of fracture site
  - Cage rest
  - Dressing – this should be applied as soon as possible to limit pain and further damage. The dressing *must* include the joint *both above and below* the fracture site. If it is not possible to place this dressing with the animal conscious or lightly sedated, strict cage rest should be employed until the patient can be anaesthetized to allow safe placement of the dressing or fracture repair. Further information on dressings can be found in Chapter 15.
- Preventing further patient interference with fracture site
- Ensuring patient comfort
  - If limited mobility, consider placement of urinary catheter.

Luxations

A luxation or dislocation occurs when the normal anatomy of a joint is disrupted so that the articular surfaces are no longer aligned normally. They generally occur secondary to trauma. Any joint can be affected, but luxations of the hip, elbow, carpus and tarsus are most commonly seen.

For classification of luxations, treatment and complications, see Chapter 24.

Clinical signs

- Pain
- Swelling of joint
- Lameness
- Abnormal angulation of the limb

Treatment

- Provide analgesia
- Limit patient movement
- Do not attempt to reduce with patient conscious
- Inform veterinary surgeon as soon as possible. Patients usually require general anaesthesia for reduction of the luxation, but reduction may be easier if the procedure is attempted soon after the injury

Further reading

Battaglia AM (2001) *Small Animal Emergency and Critical Care*. WB Saunders, Philadelphia

Hackett T and Mazzaferro E (2006) *Veterinary Emergency and Critical Care Procedures*. Iowa State University Press, Ames, Iowa

King L and Boag A (eds) (in press) *BSAVA Manual of Canine and Feline Emergency and Critical Care, 2nd edition*. BSAVA Publications, Cheltenham

Macintire DK, Drobatz KJ, Haskins SC and Saxon WD (2005) *Manual of Small Animal Emergency and Critical Care Medicine*. Lipincott, Williams & Wilkins, Philadelphia

Peterson ME and Talcott PA (2001) *Small Animal Toxicology*. WB Saunders, Philadelphia

Wingfield WE (2001) *Veterinary Emergency Medicine Secrets*. Hanlet & Belfus, Philadelphia

Chapter 19

Fluid therapy and shock

Elizabeth Welsh and Simon J. Girling

Learning objectives

After studying this chapter, students should be able to:

- **Define terms used to describe the concentration and movement of fluids**
- **Explain the routes by which dogs and cats gain and lose water from the body and how the body regulates body water**
- **Describe the distribution of water within the body and the differences in composition between intracellular and extracellular fluid**
- **Discuss the different methods used to assess dehydration**
- **Calculate maintenance and replacement fluid requirements for dogs and cats**
- **Discuss the advantages and disadvantages of different routes for fluid replacement therapy and describe one method used to place an over-the-needle intravenous catheter and to prime an administration set**
- **Describe the different methods used to monitor patients receiving intravenous fluids**
- **Define shock, describing common clinical signs associated with the syndrome, and explain why fluid therapy plays an important role in treatment**

Introduction

Many medical and surgical conditions and interventions cause disturbances of fluid, electrolyte and acid–base balance within the body, and knowledge of the homeostatic mechanisms that normally govern these physiological processes is essential if disturbances within this system are to be identified, and rectified, in a logical and effective manner. This chapter will review the physiology of body fluid, electrolyte and acid–base balance and examine how to determine whether fluid therapy is required, what the most appropriate fluids and routes of administration are, and how to assess patients' responses to treatment.

It is important to be familiar with the various methods of measurement of fluids and electrolytes within the body, and to understand the units that describe them.

Definitions

Solution – a solute dissolved in a solvent. For example, saline solution comprises a solute (sodium chloride) dissolved in a solvent (water). In the body, water is the main solvent

Electrolyte – a substance that yields ions when dissolved. For example, sodium chloride yields sodium and chloride ions in solution (dissociated) in water

Ion – a small water-soluble particle of atomic or molecular size which carries one or more positive or negative charge(s). An atom losing or gaining one electron becomes a univalent ion (e.g. Na^+, Cl^-). Losing or gaining 2 electrons results in divalent ions (e.g. Ca^{2+})

Cations – ions carrying one or more positive charge(s). Examples: sodium (Na^+), calcium (Ca^{2+})

Anions – ions carrying one or more negative charge(s). Examples: chloride (Cl^-), bicarbonate (HCO_3^-), phosphate (PO_4^{3-}). *Mnemonic:* anion = **a** negative **ion**

Chemical symbols

C = carbon	Mg = magnesium
Ca = calcium	Mg^{2+} = magnesium ion
Ca^{2+} = calcium ion	N = nitrogen
Cl = chlorine	Na = sodium
Cl^- = chloride ion	Na^+ = sodium ion
CO_2 = carbon dioxide	NaCl = sodium chloride
H = hydrogen	O = oxygen
H^+ = hydrogen ion	P = phosphorus
HCO_3^- = bicarbonate ion	PO_4^{3-} = phosphate ion
K = potassium	SO_4^{2-} = sulphate ion
K^+ = potassium ion	

Fluid strength

Frequently, the strength of biological solutions is measured in terms of their molecular, electrostatic or osmotic composition.

Molar concentration

Molecular composition is described by the molar concentration, measured in the number of moles per litre. However, since biological fluids are very dilute, it is more convenient to measure concentrations in millimoles per litre, that is one thousandth of a mole (1 millimole = 1/1000 mole). Molar concentration is determined as follows:

Molar concentration (mmol/l) =
Concentration (g%) x 100/Molecular weight.

For example, a 0.9% solution of sodium chloride (molecular weight 58.5) contains approximately 154 mmol/l.

Equivalence

The equivalence system is an older system of measurement that is still often used in physiology and in clinical practice, as it gives an indication of the ionic composition of a fluid. It is related to the molecular weight and the valency:

Equivalent weight = Molecular weight/valency

When the valency is 1 (univalent), the equivalent concentration in milliequivalents per litre (mEq/l) is the same as the molar concentration in millimoles per litre. Where the valency is 2 (divalent), the equivalent concentration is twice the molar concentration. In a solution, the sum of the equivalent weights of the cations must be balanced by the anions to ensure electroneutrality.

Concentration

The **concentration of a solution** is measured by the mass of solute that is dissolved in a volume of solvent. The gram per cent (gram % or g/dl) unit describes the number of grams of solute in 100 ml of solvent. Therefore, a 1% solution has 1 g of solute in 100 ml of solvent (or 10 g per litre).

Osmotic pressure

Osmosis is the process by which pure solvent (water) moves from a region of low solute concentration to a region of high solute concentration when separated by a **semi-permeable membrane**, to equalize or at least minimize the difference in concentrations (see Chapter 4a). Semi-permeable membranes are very common in the body and are effectively permeable to solvents but not to solutes. Osmosis is a specialized form of diffusion.

The **osmotic pressure** of a solution is the pressure needed to prevent osmosis from happening and it is proportional to the **number of particles** (not the size of the particles), both ions and undissociated molecules (e.g. protein), in the solution.

Definitions

Isotonic – an isotonic solution exerts equal osmotic pressure to body fluid. Example: 0.9% NaCl (normal saline)
Hypertonic – a hypertonic solution exerts greater osmotic pressure than body fluid. Examples: 7.2% NaCl; 10% dextrose
Hypotonic – a hypotonic solution exerts lower osmotic pressure than body fluid. Examples: sterile water; 0.45% NaCl

In general, **isotonic** solutions are used for parenteral administration, though hypertonic solutions are occasionally given intravenously. When fluids are administered to an animal, by whatever route, they initially enter the extracellular fluid (ECF), (see below). If **hypertonic** solutions are added to the ECF, water will be drawn out of the cells into the ECF, causing cells to shrink in size and resulting in cellular dehydration. Conversely, if **hypotonic** solutions are added to the ECF, water may move into the cells, resulting in cellular swelling and possible lysis of the cells.

Protein molecules contribute to the osmotic pressure of certain body fluids, because they cannot diffuse freely across semi-permeable or cell membranes due to their large size. In contrast, both water and salts can move freely across biological membranes by osmosis and diffusion. Consequently, there is a steady osmotic pressure exerted by the protein that is referred to as the **effective osmotic pressure** (also called the colloid osmotic pressure or oncotic pressure). The osmotic pressure exerted by the blood proteins, primarily albumin, maintains the difference between the osmotic pressure of the plasma and the interstitial fluid. This difference is important in maintaining an adequate volume of fluid within the blood vessels. Similarly, non-diffusible proteins within the cells contribute to the effective intracellular osmotic pressure.

Body water

On average, the water content of the adult body is 60% by weight, ranging from 50% to 70% in normal healthy animals (see also Chapter 4a). The water content of the body varies with age and with nutritional status.

Age

The water content of the body of young animals may be as much as 70–80%, while in older animals it may be as little as 50–55% of bodyweight. Such details highlight the importance of prompt and adequate fluid therapy in neonatal and young animals suffering from excessive fluid losses, especially as their kidneys are less efficient at producing concentrated urine.

Nutritional status

The body water content is affected by the proportion of fat to lean tissue in the body, since fatty tissue contains a much smaller amount of water than do other organs and soft tissues. To avoid the danger of overhydration, fluid therapy in obese animals should be based on the requirement of their ideal bodyweight, as they will have a slightly lower requirement than that calculated from their actual bodyweight.

Body water distribution

Almost two-thirds of the total body water is located inside the cells of the tissues (**intracellular fluid** (ICF), while the remaining one-third is located outside the cells (**extracellular fluid**) (ECF). The ECF may be further divided into: **intravascular fluid** (IVF), which is the water contained within the blood vessels; **interstitial fluid** (ISF), which is present in the spaces between the cells (also within dense connective tissue, bone, cartilage); and **transcellular fluids** (TCF), which are specialized fluids formed by active secretory mechanisms but comprising only a very small proportion of the ECF (e.g. cerebrospinal fluid, gastrointestinal secretions). The distribution of body water into its principal compartments is shown in Figure 19.1.

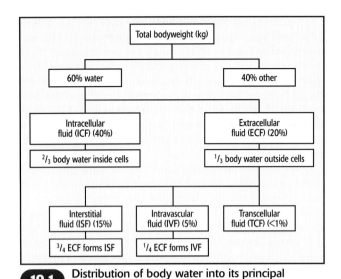

19.1 Distribution of body water into its principal compartments.

The composition of body fluids

The intracellular fluid (ICF) and the extracellular fluid (ECF) differ both in composition and in function, but the interstitial fluid (ISF) and the intravascular (IVF) fluid are similar in composition (Figures 19.2 and 19.3). Transcellular fluid (TCF) composition reflects its specialized function and may bear no resemblance to any other body fluid.

Fluid compartment	Main cations	Main anions
Extracellular fluid (ECF)	Sodium, calcium	Chloride, bicarbonate
Interstitial fluid (ISF)	Sodium, calcium	Chloride, bicarbonate
Intravascular fluid (IVF or plasma water)	Sodium, calcium	Chloride, bicarbonate
Intracellular fluid (ICF)	Potassium, magnesium	Phosphate

19.2 Main cations and anions of body fluids.

Ions	Intravascular fluid	Interstitial fluid	Intracellular fluid
Cations			
Sodium	138	130	10
Potassium	4	4	110
Calcium	2.5	1.5	–
Magnesium	1	1	15
Anions			
Chloride	102	110	10
Bicarbonate	27	27	10
Phosphate	1	1	26
Protein	17	–	50

19.3 Approximate composition of intravascular fluid, interstitial fluid and intracellular fluid (mmol/l).

Plasma contains sodium (Na^+) as the main cation, with smaller amounts of potassium (K^+), calcium (Ca^{2+}) and magnesium (Mg^{2+}) ions. Chloride (Cl^-) and bicarbonate (HCO_3^-) are the main anions, with small amounts of phosphate (PO_4^{3-}) ions. In all body fluids the number of positive charges must equal the number of negative charges so that an electrical gradient does not exist.

Normal blood capillaries have only a limited permeability and the large protein molecules cannot pass easily through this barrier. Therefore, ISF is an **ultrafiltrate** of plasma and contains everything found in plasma except proteins.

The ICF has potassium (K^+) and magnesium (Mg^{2+}) as its main cations and relatively small amounts of sodium ions. The major anion is phosphate (PO_4^{3-}). There is also some bicarbonate (HCO_3^-) and chloride (Cl^-) in the ICF.

Sodium is sometimes referred to as the 'osmotic skeleton' of the ECF, maintaining the volume of the ECF against the osmotic pull of the ICF. Protein (primarily albumin) acts in a similar manner within the blood vessels. Blood pressure (also known as hydrostatic pressure) tends to force fluid out of the arteriole end of capillaries and into the ISF, while the protein within the plasma acts to pull this fluid back into the capillaries at the venule end. Excess fluid in the interstitium is transported back into the intravascular space via the lymphatic system.

Body water and electrolyte balance

Dogs and cats require the following nutrients (in varying quantities) in order to live: water, protein, carbohydrate, fat, vitamins and minerals.

Water is often neglected as an essential nutritional requirement because of its ready availability in the UK. However, the majority of the bodyweight in dogs and cats is attributable to water (Figure 19.1). Functions of water in the body include:

- Solvent
- Transport (of solutes, cells and gases)
- Temperature regulation
- Digestion (many substances are digested by hydrolysis, which requires water).

The water content within the body is a balance of the amount of water that is acquired by the body against the amount of water lost by the body. The normal healthy animal is able to match efficiently the intake and output of water and principal electrolytes. Water is acquired and lost in a number of different ways.

To maintain a normal water balance in a healthy dog or cat, a daily total of approximately 50 ml of fluid/kg bodyweight is required (range 40–60 ml/kg/day) (Figure 19.4).

Source of fluid loss	Volume of fluid loss (average) (ml/kg/24 hours)
Respiratory/cutaneous losses	20
Urinary loss (normal range)	20
Faecal loss (normal faeces)	10
Total	**50**

19.4 Fluid loss.

Water intake

The main methods by which animals gain fluids normally are through drinking, eating and metabolism of food. The majority of fluid is acquired through drinking and eating. Metabolic water contributes only a small amount.

Drinking water or other fluids

Dogs and cats drink when they are thirsty. Thirst is the physiological urge to drink water and is controlled by the hypothalamus within the brain. It is also under voluntary control. The four major stimuli to thirst are:

- **Hypertonicity** detected through osmoreceptors in the hypothalamus (the osmoreceptors responsible for thirst are the same as those responsible for the release of antidiuretic hormone)
- **Hypovolaemia** detected by low-pressure baroreceptors in the great veins and right atrium
- **Hypotension** detected by high-pressure baroreceptors in the carotid sinus and aorta
- **Angiotensin II** released in response to renal hypotension.

Eating

Most moist or wet diets have significant water content. Dry diets may contain as little as 6–10% water.

Metabolism

Metabolism of food within the body releases water as a by-product (providing 10–20% of total fluid intake). Hydrogen within foods (protein, fat and carbohydrate) combines with oxygen to produce water. The amount of water produced depends on the type of food and how completely metabolized the food is; for example, oxidation of fat produces more water than carbohydrate, which in turn produces more water than protein.

Fluid therapy

Animals are occasionally administered fluid parenterally.

Water loss

The main methods by which dogs and cats lose water from the body normally are urination, defecation, respiration and sweating. The fluid lost from the body by urination is sometimes referred to as sensible fluid loss. Because the water lost by other means (respiration and sweating) is not seen, this is referred to as insensible or inevitable fluid loss.

Urination

The normal kidney is able to regulate water loss. Fluid and electrolytes are lost.

Defecation

The amount of fluid lost in faeces is surprisingly small. This is because the normal gastrointestinal tract has very efficient mechanisms for reabsorption of water. Fluid and electrolytes are lost.

Respiration

Water is lost from the respiratory tract by evaporation. This happens normally during breathing and panting because air is humidified as it passes along the tracheobronchial tree and nasal passages. Fluid is lost.

Sweating

Although sweating can cause significant water loss in some species, this is not the case in dogs and cats, which sweat from the footpads only. The amount of fluid lost via this route is influenced by ambient temperature, humidity, activity and fever. Fluid and electrolytes are lost.

Abnormal fluid intake and loss

In many situations an animal's ability to control body fluid balance will be compromised.

Causes of abnormal water intake

- Change in diet
- Metabolic disorders
- Anaesthesia (preoperative fasting/general anaesthesia/recovery)
- Systemic illness
- Mechanical difficulty (fractured jaw)
- Water deprivation

Cause of abnormal fluid loss

- Altered urine production (e.g. renal disease)
- Altered faecal losses (e.g. diarrhoea – an additional 4 ml/kg per stool or up to 200 ml/kg per day in severe cases)
- Vomiting (e.g. an additional 4 ml/kg per incident)
- Increased respiratory losses (e.g. excessive panting due to respiratory disease)
- Transudates, modified transudates and exudates (pyometra, burns, open wounds, peritonitis)
- Surgery (increased evaporative fluid losses from surgical sites)
- Blood loss
- Lactation

Regulation by the kidney

Although the inevitable water losses from the respiratory tract and skin cannot be regulated, within the body the kidneys play an important role in the regulation of not only water and electrolytes but also acid–base balance. At times of reduced intake or increased loss of water, the osmotic concentration of the body fluids increases and the volume of the ECF – more specifically the IVF – is depleted. This has two effects on the animal. Firstly, the animal will become thirsty because of stimulation of thirst centres within the hypothalamus. Secondly, the increase in plasma osmotic concentration will be detected by **osmoreceptors** (cells that are sensitive to osmotic changes in the IVF). These stimulate the release of **antidiuretic hormone** (ADH), which is stored in the posterior pituitary. Release of ADH promotes the reabsorption of water from the renal tubules and this will increase the concentration of the urine that is voided. Conversely, if the osmotic concentration of the plasma is reduced, less ADH will be released and less water will be reabsorbed within the kidney, the urine becoming more dilute.

In addition, a reduction in IVF will be detected directly by the kidneys as a reduction in renal perfusion. This stimulates the release of a kidney hormone, **renin**, generating **angiotensin** in the blood. In turn, angiotensin stimulates the release of **aldosterone** from the adrenal cortex. Aldosterone acts on the kidney to increase the reabsorption of sodium within the distal convoluted tubule, and thence water, resulting in more concentrated urine (Figure 19.5).

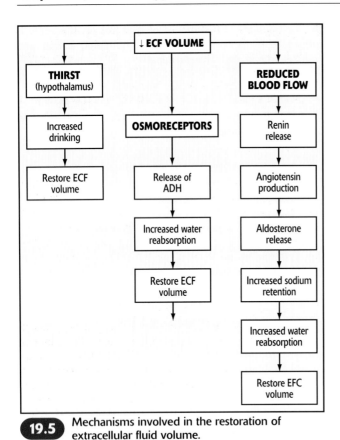

19.5 Mechanisms involved in the restoration of extracellular fluid volume.

Urine specific gravity

Urine specific gravity (USG) is a measure of the solute concentration in urine and is related to the ability of the renal tubules to concentrate or dilute the glomerular filtrate. USG gives the density of urine compared with pure water. It is influenced by the number of molecules in urine, as well as their molecular weight and size; therefore it only approximates solute concentration. It may be measured by a refractometer, urinometer or dipstick.

The specific gravity of distilled water is 1.000. In dogs a USG of >1.030 or in cats >1.035 indicates adequate renal tubular concentrating ability.

Urine specific gravity is affected by:

- Antidiuretic hormone and aldosterone concentrations
- Temperature (USG decreases with increasing temperatures)
- Urinary concentrations of:
  - Glucose
  - Protein
  - Sodium chloride and other crystalloids
  - Blood urea nitrogen (BUN)
- Drug administration (corticosteroids)
- Systemic illness (e.g. diabetes insipidus, hypoadrenocorticism (Addison's disease), hepatopathy).

Definitions

- **Isosthenuria** – urine specific gravity and osmolality are equal to that of the glomerular filtrate/plasma (1.008–1.015). If the animal is azotaemic or dehydrated, isosthenuria is abnormal and indicates altered renal function
- **Hyposthenuria** – decreased urine specific gravity and osmolality, USG <1.015
- **Hypersthenuria** – USG >1.015

Loss of electrolytes

The management of water balance is probably more important than the regulation of electrolyte status. However, electrolytes too are delicately balanced within the body, and the balance of sodium, potassium, chloride and bicarbonate ions is most important. Conditions that cause an increased loss of water may also cause loss of electrolytes. In the normal animal the daily requirement for sodium is approximately 1 mmol/kg per day and for potassium 2 mmol/kg/day.

Recording fluid intake and loss

Recording the daily intake and loss of fluid in veterinary patients is an important part of patient care, especially in those animals suffering from water and electrolyte imbalances. Recording methods range from simply monitoring the drinking and urinary habits of elective surgical patients, to accurate observations of volumes of fluid consumed orally and administered parenterally, measurement of urine and faecal output, and recording of abnormal losses. Ideally, water balance should be recorded on a chart detailing route of administration, type and volume of fluid given and also details of fluid losses. Each page would represent a 24-hour period and a glance at the chart would then be a useful guide to each animal's fluid status (Figure 19.6).

FLUID THERAPY MONITORING CHART

OWNER'S NAME		ANIMAL'S NAME		
ADDRESS		BREED		
CONTACT TEL.		SEX	AGE	WEIGHT

DATE   VET NAME

REASON FOR ADMISSION   FLUID FOR INITIAL INFUSION

MAINTENANCE REQUIREMENT   _____

DEFICIT (dehydration/losses)   _____

TOTAL REQUIREMENT   _____

TO BE INFUSED OVER   _____ HOURS

DRIP FACTOR: 20 drops/ml or 60 drops/ml or Blood at 15 drops/ml. (Circle as appropriate)

CALCULATION: total requirement (mls) x DRIP FACTOR (drops/ml) divided by time of infusion in minutes

Time	Bag size	Fluid type	Due to finish	Drip rate	Fluid total

MONITORING & COMMENTS					OUTPUT			
Patient weight	T	P	R	COMMENTS	V+	D+	Urine	Discharges

19.6 Example of fluid therapy monitoring chart. (Courtesy of Wendy Busby)

Disturbances of water and/or electrolyte balance

Many medical conditions and surgical interventions can disrupt the body's water and/or electrolyte status. Such conditions arise through altered intake or output of water and/or electrolytes.

Dehydration is the term used to describe a reduction in the total body water and the signs and symptoms associated with such a loss. Dehydration can be caused by a loss of water only, which is known as **primary water depletion**. This is common where water intake is reduced or absent because of continued inevitable water losses, e.g. during excessive panting or when an animal is deprived of drinking water. In addition, certain disease states (e.g. diabetes insipidus) can cause a primary water depletion.

More commonly, water losses are accompanied by loss of electrolytes, especially sodium, which is the main cation of the ECF, and this is referred to as **mixed water/electrolyte depletion**. The losses that are incurred during vomiting and diarrhoea include water, sodium, chloride and bicarbonate depletion. If diarrhoea is prolonged, potassium is also lost. In haemorrhage, protein, haemoglobin, platelets and clotting factors are lost in addition to water and electrolytes.

In conditions where urinary output has failed (e.g. blocked urethra, ruptured urinary bladder and acute renal failure), metabolites and electrolytes that are normally excreted in the urine accumulate within the body. In addition, insensible losses lead to water depletion. Therefore, the fluid imbalance that is present is very complicated and relates mainly to water loss, elevated serum potassium levels and acidosis.

A list of the common diseases and the principal fluid disorders they cause are given in Figure 19.7.

Assessing fluid requirements

It is important to assess the degree of dehydration and the state of the circulation prior to initiating fluid therapy. There are a number of clinical and laboratory methods that may be used to establish the amount of fluid required by an individual animal.

History

A good history enables an accurate assessment of fluid deficits to be made. Questions about food and water consumption (anorexia, polydipsia), any gastrointestinal losses (vomiting, diarrhoea), urinary losses (polyuria, oliguria), abnormal discharges (open pyometra) and traumatic losses (blood loss, burns) should be sought from the owner.

Physical examination

Clinical signs are a useful, though not always accurate, means of assessing dehydration. Signs such as loss of skin elasticity and sunken eye do not start to appear until the animal is approximately 5% dehydrated. Animals that are 15% dehydrated are moribund. When assessing the elasticity of the skin, it is important to remember that in cachectic animals it is generally reduced, even when they are not dehydrated, whereas overweight animals will lose their skin elasticity when more severely dehydrated than an animal of normal weight. Intermediate changes are described in Figure 19.8.

Percentage dehydration can be related to the fluid deficit (Figure 19.9).

Primary water depletion
Prolonged inappetence (fractured jaw, head or neck injury, etc.)
Water unavailable (forgetful/neglectful owners)
Unconsciousness (coma)
Fever or excessive panting
Diabetes insipidus

Water and electrolyte depletion
Vomiting
Diarrhoea
'Third space' losses (intestinal obstruction, peritonitis)
Pyometra
Wound drainage

Whole blood loss
Internal haemorrhage
External haemorrhage
Surgical losses

Potassium depletion
Prolonged inappetence (starvation)
Vomiting
Prolonged diarrhoea
Prolonged diuretic therapy

Potassium accumulation
Ruptured urinary bladder
Urethral obstruction
Acute renal failure
Hypoadrenocorticism (Addison's disease)

19.7 Causes of principal fluid abnormalities.

Percentage dehydration	Clinical signs
<5	No detectable clinical signs Increasing urine concentration
5–6	Subtle loss of skin elasticity (skin tent)
6–8	Marked loss of skin elasticity Slightly prolonged capillary refill time Slightly sunken eyes Dry mucous membranes
10–12	Tented skin stands in place Prolonged capillary refill time (2 seconds) Sunken eyes/protrusion of third eyelid Dry mucous membranes Early signs of shock (see later)
12–15	Signs of shock Moribund Death imminent

19.8 Clinical signs associated with dehydration.

Dehydration (%)	Fluid deficit (ml per kg bodyweight)
5 (≤ = mild)	50
8 (≤ 8 = moderate)	80
10 (≤ 10 = marked)	100
12 (≥ 10 = shock)	120

19.9 Dehydration and fluid deficit.

Example: *to calculate the fluid deficit in a 20 kg dog with 10% dehydration*

The entry for 10% dehydration in Figure 19.9 shows that 10% dehydration is equivalent to a fluid deficit of 100 ml/kg bodyweight. Thus in this case:

Fluid deficit = 100 ml x 20 = 2000 ml

It is important to realize that the percentage loss is relative to bodyweight, not to body water.

Laboratory analyses

The following simple laboratory tests can be helpful in estimating fluid losses.

Packed cell volume (PCV)

PCV is an inexpensive but revealing parameter. For each 1% increase in PCV, a fluid loss of approximately 10 ml/kg bodyweight has occurred. Rarely will the normal PCV of the patient be known, and therefore an estimate of 45% is made in dogs and 35% in cats. For example, if a 20 kg dog was found to have a PCV of 55%, the deficit should be calculated thus:

20 kg x 10 ml/kg/% x (55–45%) = 2000 ml

The equation is unreliable where pre-existing anaemia is present, unless the PCV prior to fluid loss is known. Similarly, acute blood loss cannot be evaluated by the PCV unless compensation has taken place or fluid has already been administered to replace the loss.

Haemoglobin

Dehydration will also result in an increase in the haemoglobin concentration of the blood but care must be taken when interpreting results from an anaemic animal.

Total plasma protein (TPP)

Dehydration will cause a rise in TPP. Care must be taken, because a dehydrated hypoproteinaemic animal may present with an apparently normal TPP. It is useful to assess both TPP and PCV in an animal that has been diagnosed clinically as dehydrated, because only rarely will pre-existing disease result in an elevation of both these parameters.

Blood urea and creatinine

Blood urea and creatinine levels rise in the dehydrated animal (pre-renal azotaemia), but it is important to consider the possibility of renal disease, which can also result in an elevation in these two parameters. Consequently, these parameters should be interpreted in the light of the urine specific gravity.

Plasma electrolytes

Estimation of the plasma electrolyte level (e.g. Na^+, K^+, Cl^-) is possible but is frequently of limited value, as recorded values are not always an accurate reflection of the total body content of the individual ion. However, determination of serum potassium concentration is of value, because a marked deficit of this ion can result in severe muscle weakness and cardiac disturbances; equally, an excess of this ion can also result in fatal cardiac dysrhythmias.

Acid–base estimations

For details of assessment of acid–base balance, see later.

Clinical assessment

These measurements can be used to estimate fluid deficits, but are more frequently used to monitor progress of fluid therapy and response to treatment in intensive care patients.

Bodyweight

Bodyweight is easily measured and acute losses may be due to fluid loss or catabolism (expected daily weight loss in an anorexic animal is 0.5–0.1% bodyweight). Acute increases in bodyweight are nearly always caused by increased fluid content.

Central venous pressure (CVP)

CVP is a useful means of estimating the need for fluids in any situation, but especially in congestive cardiac failure or where circulatory overload may be a problem (acute renal failure). Following severe, acute haemorrhage and in shock, CVP is invaluable in determining the adequacy of replacement fluid therapy.

CVP is a measurement of the pressure in the right atrium, i.e. the chamber of the heart to which all the venous blood is returned. A long catheter is placed aseptically in a jugular vein and advanced until the tip of the catheter lies within the chest. Ideally, the catheter tip should lie in the right atrium, but it is often located within the cranial vena cava, where pressure changes in the right atrium are reflected. The catheter is connected to a water manometer and the CVP is measured in centimetres of water (cm H_2O).

Urinary output

Measuring urinary output is a useful means of assessing the adequacy of fluid replacement. As already discussed, urine output is low during dehydration (oliguria), and the return of normal urine output signifies that replacement is adequate. Urine output can be monitored casually by observation, but placing an indwelling urinary catheter allows accurate measurement of output (Figure 19.10). Normal urine output is 1–2 ml/kg/hour. A urine output of less than 0.5 ml/kg/hour is defined as oliguria. If fluid therapy fails to improve the urine output in an oliguric animal, the possibility of acute renal failure should be considered.

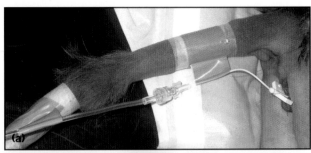

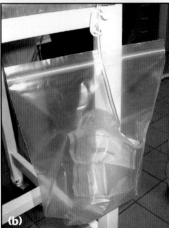

19.10 (a) Indwelling urinary catheter secured to the prepuce and tail of a cat. (b) Closed urinary collection system. Note that the collection bag is below the level of the patient and is protected from environmental contamination by double bagging.

Acid–base balance

In a similar way to water and electrolyte balance, acid–base balance is a closely guarded parameter that can be upset at times of disease. Within the body, hydrogen ions are produced as a result of normal metabolic activity, and the body's acid–base status is a measure of the hydrogen ion concentration within its tissues. Hydrogen ions are measured according to the pH scale. The **pH** value is defined as the negative logarithm (to the base 10) of the hydrogen ion concentration. The pH scale has a range of 1–14 and a pH value of 7 is regarded as neutral, while values above 7 are alkaline and those below 7 are acidic.

In the normal animal, blood is slightly alkaline – it has a normal range of pH 7.35–7.45. When the pH of the blood falls below 7.35 a state of **acidaemia** is said to exist, whereas when the pH of the blood is above 7.45 a state of **alkalaemia** is said to exist. **Acidosis** and **alkalosis** describe abnormal processes and conditions that cause acidaemia or alkalaemia, respectively, if there are no secondary (or compensatory) changes in response to these processes and conditions.

Acidosis and alkalosis can exist without producing acidaemia and alkalaemia, because of the body's secondary compensatory mechanisms. Acidosis and alkalosis may be either **metabolic** or **respiratory**, depending on their origin (see 'Acid–base abnormalities', below).

It is essential for proper cellular function that the blood pH is kept within the normal range. Large changes in pH may result in the animal becoming depressed and may ultimately lead to its death. Therefore the body has efficient mechanisms for dealing with the hydrogen ions that are produced within the body to prevent dramatic fluctuations of pH. There are three principal means of dealing with hydrogen ions, and these systems work in sequence to try to limit the effects of changes in hydrogen ion concentration. **Buffers** are the first to respond to alterations in the pH, followed by a **respiratory response** and finally a **renal response**.

Buffering

Buffers are able to react with acids and bases and reduce the extent of the pH change that they would normally produce. In the body, buffers act by trapping H^+ ions rather than eliminating them from the body. Buffers are required to keep pH within narrow limits until the H^+ ions can be delivered to either the lungs or the kidneys, where they can be removed from the body. In general, buffers are weak acids or proteins. Because weak acids do not dissociate completely in water (unlike strong acids such as hydrochloric acid, HCl) they restrict the number of H^+ ions in solution, whereas proteins (such as haemoglobin) act as anions and have many sites to which cations such as H^+ ions may bind. Most buffering that occurs within the body occurs within cells, and proteins are among the most important intracellular buffers. Extracellular buffers include bicarbonate (HCO_3^-) and hydrogen phosphate (HPO_4^{2-}).

The reaction that converts bicarbonate to carbonic acid (H_2CO_3) (see below) does not become saturated in the same way as the hydrogen phosphate reaction, because the action of the enzyme carbonic anhydrase upon the carbonic acid results in the formation of carbon dioxide and water, both of which can be expelled from the body (or, in the case of water, incorporated in the body water).

Conversions of bicarbonate and hydrogen phosphate:

$$H^+ + HCO_3^- \leftrightarrow \underset{\substack{\text{Carbonic} \\ \text{acid}}}{H_2CO_3} \underset{\substack{\textit{Carbonic} \\ \textit{anhydrase}}}{\leftrightarrow} CO_2 + H_2O$$

$$H^+ + HPO_4^{2-} \leftrightarrow H_2PO_4^-$$

Generation of bicarbonate:

$$CO_2 + H_2O \leftrightarrow H_2CO_3 \leftrightarrow H^+ + HCO_3^-$$

Respiratory system

The respiratory system controls the level of carbon dioxide within the body. Carbon dioxide is in equilibrium with carbonic acid in solution in the body fluids. Increasing respiration will remove carbon dioxide from the body and therefore reduce acidity. Decreasing respiration will retain carbon dioxide and therefore increase acidity.

It has already been noted that the reaction that converts bicarbonate (HCO_3^-) to carbonic acid (H_2CO_3) does not become saturated because of a build-up of water and carbon dioxide (see above); however, the reaction may be limited by the amount of available bicarbonate.

Renal system

Bicarbonate can be generated within the cells of the kidney by a reversal of the reaction that results in the formation of water and carbon dioxide (see above). The bicarbonate that is generated enters the ECF pool, while the H^+ ions that are generated are excreted.

The pH of the body fluids is dependent upon the concentration of carbon dioxide and bicarbonate ions within the body:

$$pH = [HCO_3^-] / pCO_2$$

Therefore, the pH will fall if there is an increase in the concentration of carbon dioxide within the body or a fall of bicarbonate ions within the body, or if H^+ ions are added to the system. Conversely, increasing the concentration of bicarbonate ions within the body or removing H^+ ions will cause an increase in the pH.

Acid–base abnormalities

To estimate acid–base balance an arterial blood sample is required, though venous blood samples can provide useful information if an arterial sample cannot be taken. In dogs and cats, arterial blood is generally taken from either the femoral artery or a superficial branch of the femoral artery. The anticoagulant that is used is heparin, and the sample should be drawn anaerobically. If the arterial blood is not analysed immediately, it should be stored on ice, or at 4°C, until analysis. Analysis of the blood will give the pH of the sample, the bicarbonate ion concentration and the carbon dioxide tension (a measure of the amount of carbon dioxide within the sample), and from this information the clinician will be able to establish what deficits are present.

Acid–base abnormalities are not uncommon during disease and Figure 19.11 shows the four major disturbances that can occur and the situations in which they are likely to arise.

Cause	Examples
Metabolic acidosis	
Accumulation of H⁺	Shock Ruptured bladder/blocked urethra Diabetic keto-acidosis Aspirin/ethylene glycol poisoning
Loss of base (bicarbonate)	Chronic renal failure Chronic diarrhoea
Metabolic alkalosis	
Loss of H⁺	Prepyloric vomiting
Accumulation of base (bicarbonate)	Overadministration of sodium bicarbonate
Respiratory acidosis	
Impaired ventilation	General anaesthesia CNS injuries (cerebral oedema) Severe lung damage Certain nerve/muscle diseases
Inspired carbon dioxide	Anaesthetic equipment
Increased carbon dioxide production	Malignant hyperthermia
Respiratory alkalosis	
Overventilation	Mechanical/manual ventilation Apprehensive/pain/fear

19.11 Causes of acid–base abnormalities.

- **Respiratory acidosis** arises through inadequate ventilation, or a failure of the respiratory system to respond to increased levels of carbon dioxide that are characteristic of rebreathing or increased production. Buffers will lessen the pH disturbance but renal compensation will only occur when the condition becomes long standing.
- **Respiratory alkalosis** occurs much less frequently than respiratory acidosis in veterinary practice.
- **Metabolic acidosis** arises when acid metabolites are retained within the body or when the loss of buffer is marked. Respiratory compensation is rapid but incomplete, and ultimately the kidneys must restore balance, by either excreting hydrogen ions, retaining bicarbonate, or both.
- **Metabolic alkalosis** again occurs much less frequently.

The treatment of the various acid–base abnormalities should be directed at the source of the problem initially. Respiratory acidosis and alkalosis require therapy aimed at correcting the ventilatory disturbance. Metabolic acidosis can be ameliorated by providing extra buffer in the form of sodium bicarbonate. Often, reduced renal perfusion is the cause of a metabolic acidosis and using fluid therapy to restore renal perfusion will be sufficient to correct the abnormality.

Objectives of fluid therapy

The purpose of fluid therapy is to replace deficits from previous losses, improve and maintain renal function, supply maintenance fluid requirements, and provide for ongoing losses.

The most important initial treatment is to restore an adequate circulating volume, as severely dehydrated animals may be showing signs of shock (see later). After this, the remaining deficit can be replaced more slowly. In general, existing deficits should be replaced within the first 24 hours after admission. Thereafter it is important to remember that, while the animal is undergoing treatment, provision must be made to replace the continued inevitable and urinary losses as well as any continuing abnormal losses (e.g. diarrhoea).

Routes of administration of fluids

Oral administration

If an animal is willing to drink, is not vomiting and does not have an intestinal obstruction, the oral route of fluid administration is a simple, cheap and painless method to treat an animal with mild dehydration. In addition, it is an ideal route by which to supply daily maintenance fluid requirements after initial deficits have been replaced. Moreover, the animal does not need to be hospitalized, allowing the owner to take the animal home.

The intestine acts as a barrier for selective absorption of water and electrolytes, providing a wide margin of safety. However, there are a number of disadvantages and the oral route is not the route of choice if an animal is severely dehydrated. Although administering fluid orally does not require absolute sterility, only a limited range of fluids can be given (it is inappropriate for whole blood or plasma expanders such as dextrans), and it can be time-consuming.

Where prehension is limited or impossible, oral therapy is not ruled out and fluid may be administered by either naso-oesophageal tube, pharyngostomy tube, oesophagostomy tube or gastrostomy tube. In general, enteral feeding tubes are well tolerated by animals.

Enteral feeding tubes

- A **naso-oesophageal tube** may be passed via the nostril to the distal oesophagus, and fluids given directly.
- A **pharyngostomy tube** must be placed under anaesthesia via an incision in the skin of the neck. The tube is introduced via the pharynx into the oesophagus, allowing fluid and food to be administered.
- A **gastrostomy tube** again must be positioned under general anaesthesia, and is placed directly into the stomach via an incision in the left flank. Again, fluid and food may be administered through this tube.
- **Oesophagostomy tubes** are becoming more popular and are simpler to place than gastrostomy tubes.

Isotonic or hypotonic fluids are recommended for oral administration to prevent the movement of water out of the ECF and into the bowel. A solution containing sodium chloride at 120 mmol/l in 2% glucose will produce enhanced absorption of sodium and increased uptake of water. This can be prepared by mixing a teaspoonful of salt and a dessertspoon of glucose in 2 pints of water. There are many commercially available oral rehydration solutions. In general they use a similar principle to that described, though some include glycine to further promote electrolyte and water absorption.

Gastric capacity

Dog: the gastric capacity is 90 ml/kg

Cat: the gastric capacity varies with bodyweight, as follows:
* 0.5–1.0 kg: 100 ml/kg
* 1.0–1.5 kg: 70 ml/kg
* 1.5–4.0 kg: 60 ml/kg
* 4.0–6.0 kg: 45 ml/kg

Subcutaneous administration (hypodermoclysis)

Subcutaneous administration of fluids is practical in small animals, where the animal is only mildly dehydrated and fluids cannot be administered orally. Because absorption from this route tends to be slow, especially where peripheral vaso-constriction is present, it is unsuitable for severely dehydrated animals. Only sterile isotonic electrolyte solutions (e.g. Hartmann's) should be administered subcutaneously, and only small volumes should be given at one time (10–20 ml/kg per site). Complete absorption of the fluid may take 6–8 hours. If fluid is not completely absorbed within this time an alternative route of fluid administration should be selected (e.g. intra-venous). Repeated administration can be painful, and in addition there is a risk of skin infection or skin slough.

Intraperitoneal administration

The intraperitoneal route of fluid administration shares many of the advantages and disadvantages of the subcutaneous route, and should only be used where the animal is mildly dehy-drated and fluids cannot be administered orally. It is best suited to neonatal dogs and cats and small mammals, where intra-venous access may be difficult. Hypotonic or isotonic electro-lyte solutions may be administered intraperitoneally. The large adsorptive capacity of the peritoneum makes it an efficient route of administration, but absorption is reduced during shock. Because of the risk of infection it is important that all manipu-lations are carried out aseptically, and great care must be taken not to puncture any of the abdominal organs.

To administer fluids intraperitoneally the animal is held al-most vertically, with its hindlimbs on the table. A second per-son aseptically introduces a short needle or catheter into the abdomen, just behind the umbilicus and in a cranial direction.

Intravenous fluid therapy

The advantages and disadvantages of intravenous fluid therapy are shown in Figure 19.12.

Advantages
Rapid administration of fluids intravascularly
Large volumes of fluid may be administered
Hypertonic solutions may be administered
Plasma expanders may be administered
Blood products may be administered

Disadvantages
Risk of side effects (phlebitis, thrombophlebitis, bacteraemia, thrombosis)
Specialized equipment necessary
Training in technique required
Risk of overhydration
Patient interference

19.12 Intravenous fluid therapy: advantages and disadvantages.

The choice of veins that may be used to administer fluids intravenously includes:

* Cephalic and accessory cephalic
* Lateral saphenous
* Medial saphenous (particularly useful in cats)
* External jugular
* Auricular (particularly useful in rabbits).

Administering fluids intravenously

* **Needles** are inexpensive but are unsuitable for intravenous fluid administration. They are dislodged easily, and the sharp point will not only irritate the wall of the vein but also can penetrate the other side of the vein, thus delivering the fluid perivenously (extravasation).
* **Butterfly needles** (scalp vein sets) are safer, because they can be secured to the limb more easily and are less likely to become dislodged. However, the sharp point of the needle may still irritate the wall of the vein. They are not suitable for long-term fluid administration.
* **Over-the-needle catheters** or cannulae are extremely useful in peripheral veins and they can also be used in the jugular vein of small dogs and cats. They can be secured to the limb and are less likely to become dislodged than needles. Moreover, the smooth tip of the catheter is less likely to cause phlebitis than needles or butterfly needles.
* **Through-the-needle catheters** or cannulae are longer and therefore more appropriate for use in the external jugular vein.

Placing an over-the-needle intravenous catheter

An assistant is required for this procedure, to restrain the ani-mal and raise the vein, as appropriate. Equipment required includes the following.

Hand-washing facilities and gloves
Hands should be washed before commencing skin preparation and again before placement of the catheter. Disposable gloves should be worn during skin preparation, then discarded and replaced following hand washing prior to catheter placement.

Electric clippers
Hair should be clipped liberally from the site of catheter place-ment, ensuring that the barrel of the catheter will not contact contaminated hair or skin during insertion. In addition, fenes-trated drapes may be used to limit contamination during place-ment of jugular catheters.

Preparation
* **Chlorhexidine**, or povidone–iodine-based surgical scrub
* **Sterile water** or spirit (70%)
* **Cotton wool** or surgical swabs: the skin should be cleansed and prepared in a similar manner to a surgical site.

Sterile no. 11 scalpel blade
To minimize the chances of catheter tip flaring during inser-tion, a small full-thickness skin incision may be created directly over the point of catheter insertion.

Suitable intravenous catheter

Fluid flows most rapidly through short, large-gauge catheters. Before catheter placement, the catheter may be primed with either sterile saline or heparinized saline. In any case the catheter plug or stopper should remain in place during catheterization.

Practical tips

- Ensure that the bevel tip of the stylet extends beyond the end of the catheter.
- Just as when performing an intravenous injection, the bevel of the stylet should be facing upwards as it is passed through the skin and into the lumen of the vein.
- Avoid touching the barrel of the catheter or the site of insertion directly.
- When the stylet enters the lumen of the vein, blood will appear in the clear flashback chamber (hub) at the distal end of the catheter. At this time the stylet is held steady as the catheter is advanced off the stylet and into the vein. There should be no resistance to this movement.
- Do not be tempted to pull the catheter back on to the stylet, as this may cause the tip of the catheter to be sheared off and create a catheter embolus.
- Discard any catheters that develop flared or otherwise damaged tips.

Because the tip of the stylet remains within the lumen of the catheter distally, blood spillage should be minimal. Over-the-needle catheters should be replaced every 48–72 hours, as required.

Following insertion of the catheter, one of the following is placed to prevent blood flowing out of the catheter:

- Injection cap
- Three-way tap
- T-piece connector
- Primed administration set.

These devices should be swabbed with alcochol (which is allowed to dry) before needle introduction or syringe attachment.

Syringe containing saline

A syringe containing either sterile saline or heparinized saline (Figure 19.13) for intravenous injection may be used both to confirm correct placement of the catheter and to flush the catheter following placement. Indwelling catheters used for intermittent drug administration or blood sampling should be flushed through with heparinized saline (2–10 IU/ml) two to four times daily to maintain patency.

Tape and bandaging materials

Once secured with tape, the catheter and attachments are protected from patient interference by applying a soft dressing. It is important that the dressing is not constrictive. Bandages should be changed at least daily, or more frequently if soiled by saliva, faeces, urine, vomit and discharges or if they otherwise become wet. At each bandage change, the site of insertion of the catheter should be inspected for signs of inflammation or infection. If unattended, many patients may in addition need Elizabethan collars or similar devices to limit interference with the catheter site.

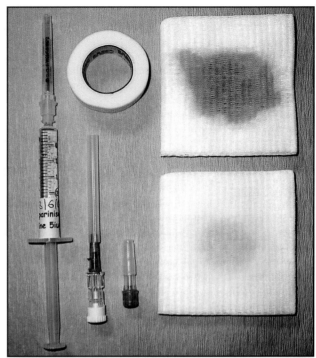

19.13 Preparing for intravenous catheterization using an over-the-needle catheter. Clockwise from top right: surgical scrub (chlorhexidine); alcohol swab; injection stopper; intravenous catheter; syringe of heparinized saline (labelled); adhesive tape.

Monitoring

Animals receiving fluid therapy should have their physiological responses (temperature, pulse and respiration) monitored on a regular basis. Patients with indwelling intravenous catheters require twice daily evaluation. In the event of unexpected pyrexia, the possibility of catheter-related sepsis should be considered.

Indwelling intravenous catheters may be used for a number of other purposes in addition to fluid administration. These include:

- Drug administration
- Blood sampling
- Central venous pressure measurement
- Administration of total peripheral or parenteral nutrition.

Equipment for priming a fluid administration set

Hands should be washed before commencing procedure, and gloves should be worn.

Fluid for infusion

An appropriate fluid (e.g. Hartmann's, 500 ml or 1000 ml) should be chosen. It is important to check that the fluid bag selected contains the appropriate fluid and is still within the manufacturer's 'use by' date, that it is contained within sealed outer packaging and that the fluid within the bag is clear with no obvious contamination. The fluid bag (or collapsible bottle) should then be removed from the outer packaging and hung from the drip stand. Fluid may be warmed prior to administration.

Fluid administration set

There are three main types of drip set (giving set or administration set) available. A normal administration set gives approximately 20 drops/ml. For smaller patients, a mini-drip fluid administration set (paediatric set) giving 60 drops/ml is useful, because it allows more accurate administration of small volumes. A burette is often incorporated into this type of set. This is useful when only small volumes of fluid are required, helping to prevent accidental overhydration. When blood is to be administered, a special blood administration set is required, which incorporates a nylon net filter to remove any aggregated red blood cells or other coagulation debris. A blood administration set gives approximately 15 drops/ml. Giving sets are supplied in sterile packaging and the number of drops per millilitre that they deliver will be written on the packaging and should be checked prior to calculating the drip rate.

A variety of automated infusion pumps (Figure 19.14) and syringe drivers are available, which can be used to deliver a set amount of fluid over a defined period of time. These devices are usually fitted with an alarm system that will alert the nurse or clinician when the fluid line is obstructed, or when the fluid bag or syringe is empty. If infusion devices are used, it is important to remember that they are not a substitute for careful patient monitoring. In addition to infusion pumps and syringe drivers, drip rate counters may be purchased.

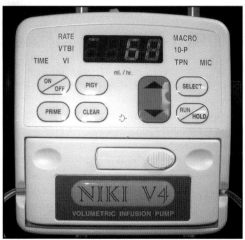

19.14 Volumetric infusion pump.

Drip stand

Extension tubing is available to lengthen the administration line and several extension sets may be used in sequence if required. A number of devices are also available to minimize kinking of the administration line tubing.

Priming a fluid administration set

1. Select an appropriate fluid administration set (e.g. 60 drops/ml for smaller patients or filter administration set for blood products) and remove from the outer packaging.
2. Position the roller clamp as required and place to the closed position.
3. Prepare the fluid bag or bottle by removing the rip tab covering the port through which the stylet of the administration set is placed.
4. Remove the cover from the administration set stylet and, without touching the stylet either with hands or to the outside of the fluid bag, insert the stylet into the appropriate port on the fluid bag or bottle.
5. Squeeze the drip chamber to allow fluid to flow into it and half fill it. The top drip chamber in filter administration sets should be filled completely, the second lower chamber being filled halfway.

▶

6. Without removing the protective cover from the patient end of the administration set, adjust the roller clamp and allow fluid to flow gently down the tubing until it reaches the patient end, ensuring that no bubbles are present.
7. Close the roller clamp. The administration set is now primed and ready to use.

Calculation of fluid flow rate: an example

A 3 kg cat requires a total of 60 ml of fluid. The fluid is to be administered at 5 ml/kg/hour intravenously. A paediatric giving set that delivers 60 drops/ml is available. What flow rate (drops per minute) will be required?

(60 drops/ml x 5 ml x 3 kg)/60 minutes

= 15 drops per minute

= 1 drop per 4 seconds

Other methods of fluid administration

Rectal administration

This route should not be used if an animal is suffering from diarrhoea, nor is it suitable in severely dehydrated patients. Both isotonic and hypotonic fluids may be administered via this route, and sterility of fluid and equipment is not essential. It is important that the fluid is instilled into the colon and not into the rectum, or an enema will result.

Intraosseous administration

Intraosseous needles may be used if it is difficult to place indwelling intravenous catheters (e.g. for puppies, kittens, birds, adults with collapsed veins). Fluid is generally administered by gravity flow into the medullary cavity of the chosen bone. The risk of severe infection must be considered.

A number of bone sites are suitable for placement of intraosseous needles, including:

- Intertrochanteric fossa of the femur
- Tibial crest
- Greater tubercle of the humerus
- Ilium.

Solutions commonly used in fluid therapy

Whole blood

Blood collected from donor animals is generally used within a short period of time after collection. Blood for transfusion should be collected only from fit, healthy adult animals that have not previously been transfused (donor cats should be negative for FeLV, FIV and *Haemobartonella* negative). Approximately 10 ml blood/kg may be collected from a donor dog, and a total of 30–40 ml from a cat. Animals should not be bled more than once in every 2–3 months.

It is important that strict asepsis is observed when collecting the blood. Blood from a donor animal may be collected in commercially available collection sets containing an anticoagulant – either acid citrate dextrose (ACD) or citrate phosphate dextrose (CPD) – to prevent the blood from clotting. If the blood is to be used immediately, heparin or EDTA may be used as an anticoagulant. In cats, blood is generally collected into a syringe containing anticoagulant (0.14 ml CPD/ml blood or heparin 2 IU/ml blood).

Blood is collected from the jugular vein in both dogs and cats, either by gravity flow or by slow aspiration. As blood collects in the collection bag it must be agitated gently to prevent clotting. The volume of blood collected may be estimated by weighing the blood collection bag (1 g = 1 ml).

Commercially available blood collection units contain sufficient anticoagulant for 450 ml of blood, and the blood may be stored in these bags in the refrigerator until required. When ACD is used as the anticoagulant the blood may be stored at 4°C for a period of 3 weeks, whereas when CPD is used the blood may be stored for 4 weeks. Blood in which EDTA or heparin has been used as the anticoagulant should not be stored. When blood has been stored in the refrigerator, it should be warmed gently to a temperature of 37°C (and not more than 40°C) prior to transfusion. Blood that has been stored in this manner is useful for replacement of red blood cells; however, where platelets are required (e.g. clotting abnormalities) blood must be given to the recipient immediately after collection.

Before infusion into the recipient animal, cross-matching (Figure 19.15) and/or blood typing will have been carried out to ensure that the blood is compatible for transfusion. Although initial transfusion reactions are unusual, the A antigen is the most important factor in canine blood typing and, ideally, donor dogs should be DEA1.1-negative.

Most cats are type A, and there is an approximately 40% chance of an incompatible reaction occurring if the blood is not typed prior to transfusion. Blood samples can be taken from both the donor and recipient animals for cross-matching to ensure compatibility before obtaining a large volume of blood from the donor. In-house blood-typing kits are now available for dogs and cats (see Chapter 17).

Indications for transfusion

- Haemorrhage – acute/chronic/internal/external
- Anaemia – acute and chronic
- Specific deficiencies – platelets, clotting factors

Dangers associated with transfusion

- **Transfusion reactions** (Figure 19.16) – transfusion reactions occur when incompatible blood is administered to an animal
- **Pyrogenic** reactions – fever due to pyrogens or bacteria in the blood or transfusion equipment. It is also possible to transfer viral and other agents, especially in cats
- **Acidosis** (metabolic) – after administration of stored blood
- **Overadministration** – causes circulatory overload (overhydration)
- **Air emboli** – occur infrequently when plastic blood-collection bags are used, but are possible when blood is withdrawn using a syringe
- **Citrate toxicity** – hypocalcaemia
- **Hypothermia** – blood for transfusion should be administered at 37°C. Failure to do so may cause hypothermia in the recipient

Blood products

Plasma

If fresh blood can be obtained from donors, plasma may be extracted for immediate use. Blood should be centrifuged immediately after collection, and the plasma separated from the red blood cells. Plasma is a useful replacement fluid in hypovolaemic animals and is suitable for animals that are hypoproteinaemic. Because plasma does not contain any red blood cells, there is less risk of incompatibility reactions occurring.

Cross-match type	Donor	Recipient	Significance of agglutination or haemolysis
Major cross-match	Red blood cells	Serum	Immediate transfusion reaction likely. Delayed transfusion reaction possible
Minor cross-match	Serum	Red blood cells	Immediate transfusion reaction possible

19.15   Blood cross-matching.

Reaction type	Timing	Clinical signs	Cause	Treatment	Prevention
Immediate immune-mediated haemolytic	Immediate (minutes – hours)	Pyrexia, salivation, vomiting, tachycardia, tachypnoea, muscle tremors, hypotension, prostration and haemoglobinuria	Recipient serum contains antibodies to donor red blood cells	Stop transfusion immediately. Fluid therapy to support vascular system	Cross-matching or blood typing
Immediate immune-mediated non-haemolytic	Immediate (minutes – hours)	Urticaria, pruritus, erythema, hypotension, bronchoconstriction, i.e. anaphylactic shock	Hypersensitivity reaction	Stop transfusion immediately. Antihistamines. Corticosteroids. Fluid therapy to support vascular system	Pre-treatment of recipient with antihistamines and corticosteroids has been used
Delayed immune-mediated	3 days to 3 weeks post-transfusion	Pyrexia, anorexia, jaundice	Recipient mounts immune response to donor red blood cells producing antibodies	No specific treatment	Blood typing

19.16   Transfusion reactions.

Packed red blood cells

Separated red cells (e.g. following the collection of plasma) can be given to animals that require red cell replacement. The red cells should be resuspended in an isotonic replacement fluid that does not contain calcium (e.g. 0.9% NaCl), because calcium reacts with the citrate used to prevent clotting.

Plasma replacement fluids – colloids

When whole blood or plasma is unavailable, commercial plasma replacement fluids (colloids, plasma substitutes, plasma volume expanders) may be used. These fluids contain large molecules that will remain within the circulation, thus increasing the plasma's effective osmotic pressure and expanding plasma volume. These fluids may be used where there has been haemorrhage (although they will not replace red blood cells), or where the plasma volume is reduced for other reasons, e.g. fluid and electrolyte depletion. Figure 19.17 summarizes the principal constituents and some of the major indications for these fluids.

Gelatins

The gelatin solutions (e.g. Haemaccel, Gelofusin) are derived from collagen and are isotonic with plasma. They are non-antigenic and do not interfere with cross-matching tests for blood. The solutions will remain in the circulation for about 6 hours and the kidneys rapidly excrete them.

Dextrans

These are hypertonic solutions containing high-molecular-weight glucose polymers in either 0.9% NaCl or 5% dextrose. The solutions are classified by the molecular weight (MW) of the glucose polymer; for example, the MW of dextran 70 (6% solution) is 70,000. They remain in the circulation for times ranging from 2 to 24 hours, depending on their MW. Unfortunately, these solutions tend to interfere with the red cells, some solutions promoting clumping of cells and others producing haemolysis.

In addition, they interfere with the interpretation of cross-matching reactions. The raised plasma osmotic pressure caused by the dextrans will tend to draw water from the cells and ISF space into the blood vessels. Therefore, crystalloids (see below) should be administered at the same time as dextrans to avoid cellular dehydration.

Etherified starch

Etherified starch is derived from amylopectin. Hespan 6% contains hetastarch; it has a high molecular weight (450,000) and a duration of action of 24 hours.

Haemoglobin glutamer-200 (bovine) (Oxyglobin)

Oxyglobin is a haemoglobin-based oxygen carrier. It is compatible with all blood types and has a similar effect on intravascular blood volume, as other colloids.

Crystalloids

In contrast to plasma-volume expanders, crystalloids are non-colloidal substances that pass readily through cell membranes. This means that they will not remain within the ECF compartment but will equilibrate with the ICF compartment and, if renal function is normal, will be excreted in the urine. The most commonly used solutions in general practice are as follows.

Commonly used crystalloids

- **0.9% sodium chloride (NaCl)**, also called **normal saline**. Useful for replacing water and electrolyte losses, especially in vomiting, urinary obstruction, hepatopathy and hypoadrenocorticism. This is an acidifying solution.
- **5% dextrose (glucose) in water.** The dextrose in the solution is rapidly metabolized; therefore these solutions effectively provide free water that can be used to replace primary water deficits.
- **0.18% sodium chloride in 4% dextrose**, also called **glucose or dextrose saline**. Used to replace primary water deficits, and to replace the inevitable losses of sodium and water occurring on a daily basis (maintenance requirements). Potassium will also be required during long-term administration.
- **Ringer's solution**, also called **compound sodium chloride solution.** Used to replace water and electrolyte losses, especially where the losses are pre-pyloric (e.g. gastric vomiting). Contains potassium chloride and calcium chloride in addition to sodium chloride.
- **Lactated Ringer's solution**, also called **Hartmann's solution.** Useful for replacing water and electrolyte losses, especially where the losses are postgastric (e.g. diarrhoea or intestinal foreign body). Contains lactate that is metabolized by the liver to form bicarbonate, i.e. it is alkalinizing.

continues ▶

Solution		Na⁺	K⁺	Ca²⁺	Cl⁻	Others	Indications
Haemaccel	Isotonic	143	5	3	154	Gelatins	Restore circulating volume
Dextrans	Hypertonic Hypertonic	154 –	– –	– –	154 –	– 5% dextrose	Restore circulating volume
0.9% NaCl	Isotonic	154	–	–	154	–	Replace ECF. Gastric losses from vomiting
Hartmann's solution (Ringer's lactate)	Isotonic	131	5	2	111	Lactate	Replace ECF. Especially from diarrhoea and post-gastric losses
Ringer's solution	Isotonic	147	4	2.5	156	–	Replace ECF. Gastric losses from vomiting
5% dextrose	Isotonic	–	–	–	–	5% dextrose	Primary water deficit replacement
0.18% NaCl + 4% dextrose	Isotonic	30	–	–	30	4% dextrose	Maintenance requirements. Primary water deficit replacement. Neonatal ECF replacement

19.17 Principal constituents (in mmol/l) and some of the major indications for commonly used intravenous fluids.

continued

- **Potassium chloride (KCl)**. Can be used when potassium supplementation is needed. If supplementary potassium is added to a crystalloid solution, it is important that the bag is clearly labelled to avoid possible over-administration (relative or absolute).
- **7.2% sodium chloride (NaCl)**: also called **hypertonic saline**. This is a hypertonic solution that can be used for rapid intravascular volume resuscitation. However, it has a very short duration of action. Only very small volumes are required (e.g. 4–7 ml/kg in dogs). It is important that this crystalloid solution is not mistaken for 0.9% NaCl. It is contraindicated in cases of simple dehydration, uncontrolled haemorrhage and cardiac disease.
- **Sodium bicarbonate 8.4%**. Used to treat severe acidosis. It may be injected intravenously but frequently is added to intravenous infusions. However, bicarbonate should not be added to any fluids that contain calcium, as a precipitate will be formed. Again, if sodium bicarbonate is added to a crystalloid solution, it is important that the bag is clearly labelled to avoid possible over-administration (relative or absolute).

Volume and rate of fluid infusion

Replacement volume can be calculated from the history, clinical signs and simple laboratory tests, as described earlier. Usually, this volume can be replaced within the first 24 hours of treatment, with half of the replacement being made in the first 6–8 hours. In addition to replacing existing deficits, the animal has maintenance requirements for fluids that must be met and 0.18% NaCl with 4% dextrose (supplemented with additional potassium chloride) should be given at approximately 50 ml/kg/day to replace normal losses. It is important that potassium should not be administered at a rate greater than 0.5 mmol/kg/hour.

Fluid requirement = losses + maintenance + ongoing losses

The rate of fluid replacement often poses problems. Factors that govern how fast the fluids can be given include:

- Rate of loss
- Health of patient (cardiac and renal disease are of particular note)
- Type of fluid administered
- Response by the patient to therapy.

During active severe haemorrhage and shock, fluids have to be administered rapidly (see 'Treatment of shock').

Overhydration

Overzealous fluid administration may result in the circulatory system becoming overloaded, or the body overhydrated. This is particularly a problem in smaller cats and dogs. Typically, excess of a colloid leads to circulatory overload with right-sided heart failure and, ultimately, congestive cardiac failure. Too much crystalloid, on the other hand, will initially stimulate diuresis (via inhibition of ADH release), but as the electrolyte solution moves from the circulation into the remainder of the extra-cellular space, signs of oedema may develop, i.e. fluid will accumulate in the ISF space. Most seriously, pulmonary oedema may develop, which will initially impair oxygenation and can ultimately result in the death of the patient.

Overinfusion is most likely to occur with:

- Reduced cardiac output (e.g. congestive heart failure)
- Renal/urinary conditions (e.g. acute renal failure, ruptured bladder)
- Inadequate monitoring (this is especially true of smaller patients)
- Fluid administration to normovolaemic animals (e.g. blood given in chronic anaemia).

Clinical signs associated with overhydration

- Serous nasal discharge
- Restlessness
- Chemosis
- Respiratory distress caused by pulmonary congestion and oedema.

Monitoring during fluid therapy

Monitoring during fluid administration should include:

- **Cardiovascular system**: pulse (rate, rhythm, strength), mucous membrane colour, capillary refill time, jugular distension. In addition: central venous pressure, direct or indirect arterial blood pressure, chest auscultation (cardiac arrhythmias, pulmonary oedema)
- **Respiratory system**: respiratory rate and depth, chest auscultation (pulmonary oedema). In addition: arterial blood-gas analysis
- **Temperature**: core body and peripheral
- **Urine output** (1–2 ml/kg/hour).

The following checks should also be made:

- **Catheter site**: signs of inflammation, extravasation, sepsis
- **Administration set**: kinking (devices are available to minimize kinking of administration set tubing)
- **Bandages**: soiling and comfort. Check for distal limb oedema and patient interference or self-mutilation
- **General**: peripheral oedema, bodyweight, skin turgor; and check that fluid is flowing.

Shock

Classification and aetiology

Cells within the body require oxygen and nutrients to function normally (aerobic metabolism). Shock is an imbalance between the delivery of oxygen and nutrients to cells and utilization of oxygen and nutrients by cells. When insufficient oxygen is supplied, cells change from aerobic to anaerobic metabolism. Anaerobic metabolism is an inefficient method of producing energy for cellular function and in addition results in the production of lactic acid. Lactic acid alters the acid–base balance within the body.

Shock may occur as a consequence of any syndrome, disease state or injury that causes a critical decrease in effective blood flow with altered cell metabolism with or without cell death. It may be divided into the following classifications:

- Hypovolaemic shock
- Distributive shock
- Cardiogenic shock
- Obstructive shock.

The following descriptions of these different forms of shock tend to suggest that each form occurs independently of the other. This is not the case. Many shocked animals will have components of more than one, or all, forms of shock.

Hypovolaemic shock

Hypovolaemic shock represents absolute fluid loss and may occur following:

- Haemorrhage
  - External
  - Internal (chest, abdomen, osseofascial)
- Plasma loss
- Third space losses (pyometra, peritonitis, ileus)
- Fluid depletion
  - Mixed water and electrolyte losses (vomiting and diarrhoea)
  - Water losses (deprivation, diuresis).

Distributive shock

Distributive shock represents relative fluid loss. Distributive shock was previously referred to as **vasogenic** or **vasculogenic** shock. This form of shock occurs mainly following the release of naturally occurring vasoactive chemicals within the body. The primary changes are increased capillary permeability and increased vascular capacitance (i.e. there is an increased amount of blood within the venous system). There are a number of causes of distributive shock, including:

- Endotoxaemia (**endotoxic shock**). Endotoxins are formed from the cell walls of principally Gram-negative bacteria, and act to release endogenous vasoactive substances. An initial rise in cardiac output may occur, but it does not compensate for the disturbance of the distribution of blood to the tissues and the increased vascular permeability
- Anaphylaxis (**anaphylactic shock**)
- Neurogenic causes (**neurogenic shock**), e.g. vasomotor paralysis following spinal cord injury or overdose of general anaesthetic agents
- Trauma.

Administration of drugs that have an effect on the capacity of the blood vessels (e.g. acetylpromazine) can induce distributive shock after absolute or relative overdose.

Cardiogenic and obstructive shock

Cardiogenic shock is generally regarded as failure of the heart as an effective pump. Shock may also occur following obstructive problems:

- Cardiomyopathy
- Valvular abnormalities
- Arrhythmias
- Obstructive shock
  - Pericardial tamponade
  - Intracardiac neoplasia
  - Aortic/pulmonary thromboembolism.

Pathophysiology

The pathophysiology of hypovolaemic shock can be used as an example of the pathophysiological changes that occur in shock in general.

Initial responses

Initially, in response to falling blood volume a number of compensatory responses are triggered. These include the following.

Stimulation of the sympathetic nervous system

Loss of blood, or effective circulating volume, reduces the venous return to the right side of the heart, and the output from the left side of the heart falls (cardiac output falls). Pressure-sensitive baroreceptors in the aorta and carotid artery detect the drop in blood pressure (hypotension) secondary to the fall in cardiac output. Centres within the medulla of the brain initiate compensatory mechanisms to restore blood pressure to normal. These compensatory mechanisms involve the sympathetic nervous system and stimulation of the adrenal medulla. Adrenaline and noradrenaline are released and cause the blood vessels of the skin, intestine, kidneys and muscles to constrict, i.e. there is an increase in peripheral vasoconstriction (increase in total peripheral resistance). This causes a direct increase in blood pressure and promotes increased venous return to the heart. At this stage, blood flow to the vital organs (heart, lungs and brain) is maintained. In association with these changes the heart rate increases and there is an increase in the force of contraction of the myocardium (heart muscle).

Endocrine influences

Release of the hormones aldosterone and ADH promote salt and water retention by the kidneys.

Extracellular fluid shift

Capillary hydrostatic pressure is reduced and water moves from the interstitial fluid space into the vascular space as the effective osmotic pressure of the plasma proteins predominates.

Consequences

These early responses occur to compensate for the fall in vascular volume and aim to restore vascular volume and blood pressure and to improve oxygen delivery to the tissues. If volume depletion is severe, the mechanisms that are normally life saving can lead to the animal's death. Prolonged vasoconstriction and low perfusion cause continued tissue hypoxia, anaerobic metabolism and acidosis. Consequently, the peripheral vessels dilate and become engorged with blood. Moreover, cells in the capillary wall become non-functional and fluid is lost from the capillaries into the ISF space. Both of these mechanisms act to reduce the blood returning to the heart even further. The blood soon becomes viscous and slow moving, platelets may start to aggregate, and ultimately the blood will clot within the vessels. This effectively blocks the capillaries. If it is widespread, all the clotting factors will be used up resulting in a bleeding state known as disseminated intravascular coagulation (DIC).

The tissues most susceptible to hypoxia include:

- **Brain** – brain cells are extremely sensitive to hypoxia.
- **Myocardium** – the heart is depressed by hypoxia, acidosis and the presence of the toxins.
- **Kidneys** – when blood flow to the kidneys is reduced, urine output falls. Hypoxia causes the renal tubules to become damaged.
- **Gastrointestinal tract** – mucosal damage allows the invasion of bacteria, and bacterial toxins are absorbed.
- **Liver**.

In the lungs, although there is an initial increase in ventilation, eventually microthrombi and other factors cause the lung to become very inefficient. Ultimately, a state of multiple organ failure develops and the animal dies.

Clinical signs

Hypovolaemic, cardiogenic and late distributive shock all share common clinical signs.

Clinical signs of shock

- Weak rapid pulse
- Increased heart rate (tachycardia) with quiet heart sounds (due to poor cardiac filling)
- Pale mucous membranes (due to vasoconstriction)
- Prolonged capillary refill time (> 2 seconds) (due to vasoconstriction)
- Increased ventilation (due to metabolic acidosis)
- Slow jugular refill and collapsed peripheral veins
- Hypothermia and cold extremities (due to reduced metabolic rate and vasoconstriction)
- Depressed level of consciousness (due to reduced blood flow to brain)
- Muscle weakness (due to hypoxia, vasoconstriction etc.)
- Reduced renal output (oliguria, anuria) (due to reduced blood flow to kidneys)
- Low CVP and low mean arterial blood pressure
- Elevated PCV, haemoglobin (Hb), total protein, urea and creatinine (a blood sample should be obtained prior to fluid administration)

Treatment of shock

Fluid replacement

Adequate volume replacement is the single most important measure in the treatment of shock. However, fluids should be administered with care in cardiogenic shock, which is primarily a failure of the heart to pump fluid effectively around the body, rather than volume depletion.

After clinical assessment of the animal, at least one intravenous catheter should be inserted. If the peripheral veins are collapsed and difficult to catheterize, a jugular catheter may be used (Figure 19.18) or fluids administered intraosseously.

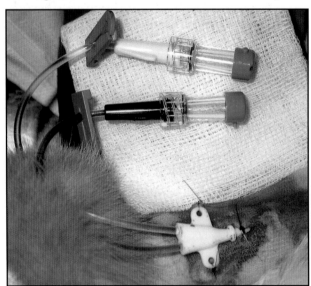

19.18 Double lumen jugular catheter in a cat.

To facilitate administration of large volumes of fluid over a short period of time, large-gauge catheters are required, or more than one intravenous line should be established.

All fluids are given to effect and the volumes required might be very large because of vasodilation or because of contraction of the ISF, which also must be replaced. Frequently, fluid replacement will be the only treatment required to promote recovery. Because fluid administration rates in shock are initially very high (Figure 19.19), it is essential that the animal be monitored closely to avoid overhydration. Fluid rates are adjusted according to the patient's response.

Solution	Rate of fluid infusion (ml/kg)	
	Dog	Cat
Isotonic crystalloid [a]	60–90	40–60
Colloid	10–20	8–12
Hypertonic saline (7.2%)	4–7	2–4

19.19 Rates of fluid infusion for shock. [a] 5% dextrose and 0.18% NaCl/4% dextrose are not suitable for treatment of shock.

Oxygen

It is important to ensure that shocked animals have a patent airway and are breathing efficiently. Because one of the problems in shocked patients is poor delivery of oxygen to tissues, the patient must be adequately oxygenated and administration of supplemental oxygen is a sensible measure. This may be achieved in a number of ways (e.g. flow-by, face-mask, nasal oxygen, incubator, tracheotomy tube, endotracheal tube; see Chapter 18).

Antibiotics

Antibiotics should be administered in all cases of shock either prophylactically or therapeutically. Intravenous broad-spectrum bactericidal agents should be used.

Glucocorticoids

There is much controversy over the use of steroids in shock. The administration of glucocorticoids tends to cause an improvement in the clinical state of the patient but will not necessarily decrease mortality. The greatest advantage will be seen if steroids are administered early in the course of shock and at high doses. Both methylprednisolone sodium succinate and dexamethasone sodium phosphate are suitable agents and are administered intravenously.

Antiprostaglandins

The release of endogenous inflammatory mediators during shock can exacerbate the condition. Administration of drugs that help to block this reaction, such as non-steroidal anti-inflammatory drugs (NSAIDs), would therefore appear logical. Unfortunately, administration of these agents will also block production of prostaglandins essential to maintain renal blood flow and gastric mucosal integrity. Concurrent administration of NSAIDs and glucocorticoids is contra-indicated, and NSAIDs should only ever be given following effective intravascular resuscitation.

Sympathomimetics

Where fluid therapy alone fails to improve cellular blood supply and oxygenation, the use of sympathomimetic drugs (e.g. dopamine, dobutamine, isoprenaline) should be considered. These agents are useful in cardiogenic shock and in advanced shock where myocardial depression is present. They are administered as infusions because of their short half-lives within the circulation. Dopamine also will act to increase renal blood flow.

Sodium bicarbonate

Metabolic acidosis is common in shock, mainly as a result of excess production of lactic acid. In general, administration of intravenous fluids to improve perfusion will allow excess lactate to be metabolized. If facilities are available to measure arterial blood gases and the blood pH falls to 7.2, administration of sodium bicarbonate may be considered.

General measures

If there is an obvious source of blood loss this should be stemmed if possible. Frequently, animals that are in shock will be, or will become, hypothermic. Although it is inadvisable to warm a hypothermic animal rapidly because vasodilation will occur, further loss of body heat can be prevented by ensuring a reasonable ambient temperature, avoiding draughts, lying the animal on an insulated surface, covering the animal and warming fluids to body temperature prior to administration.

Monitoring during shock

The monitoring procedures that are used in fluid therapy also apply to animals that are in shock. Perhaps one of the most useful parameters that can be monitored is the CVP. This gives an indication of the adequacy of fluid replacement and also serves as a useful indicator of the continuing fluid requirements of the animal.

Fluid therapy in small mammals

Maintenance fluids

Maintenance fluid quantities in most small mammals are estimated as nearly double those recommended for cats and dogs (Figure 19.20). This is due to the larger lung and body surface area in relation to mass of small mammals, in addition to their higher metabolic rates. Lactated Ringer's solution is the fluid of choice, but in some instances (e.g. pregnancy toxaemia in guinea pigs) the use of glucose-containing solutions is useful.

Species	Fluid maintenance values (ml/kg/day)
Rabbit	80–100
Guinea pig	100
Chinchilla	100
Rodents	90–100
Ferret	75–100

19.20 Daily fluid maintenance values for selected small mammals.

Assessing fluid requirements

As with cats and dogs, a 1% dehydration equates to a 10 ml/kg bodyweight fluid replacement requirement in addition to the maintenance requirements. An assessment is made of the degree of dehydration of the small mammal. Levels of dehydration can be related to clinical signs, as outlined in Figure 19.21.

Dehydration (%)	Clinical signs
< 5	Not detectable
5–6	Slightly decreased skin turgor
6–8	Slight tenting of skin Slightly pronged capillary refill time Tacky mucous membrane
8–10	Obvious tenting of skin Sunken eyes Prolonged capillary refill time
10–12	Tented skin stands in place Oliguria Signs of shock develop
> 12	Shock Coma Death

19.21 Clinical signs of dehydration levels in small mammals.

The total protein levels and packed red cell volume may also be used to assess levels of dehydration, but it is necessary to know the normal values prior to measurement (Figure 19.22).

Species	PCV range (l/l)	Total protein (g/l)
Ferret	0.44–0.6	51–74
Rabbit	0.36–0.48	54–75
Guinea pig	0.37–0.48	46–62
Chinchilla	0.32–0.46	50–60
Rats	0.36–0.48	56–76
Mice	0.39–0.49	35–72
Gerbil	0.43–0.49	43–85
Hamsters[a]	0.36–0.55	45–75

19.22 Comparison of packed cell volumes and total protein in small mammals. [a] Average for Syrian and Russian species.

Routes of administration

When administering intravenous or intraosseous fluids to small mammals, an infusion device such as a syringe driver that is calibrated accurately for small volumes is advisable. Due to the animals' small size, even small errors in fluid administration may be significant and care should be taken to prevent overinfusion.

Rabbits

Oral

This route is restricted to small volumes, with a maximum of 10 ml/kg administered at any one time.

Subcutaneous

The scruff area or lateral thorax area are ideal sites. This route is useful for the postoperative administration of fluids for longer-recovery patients undergoing minor surgical procedures such as spaying or castration. It is possible to give a maximum of 30–60 ml divided between two or more sites, depending on the size of rabbit.

Intraperitoneal

To perform this it is necessary to tilt the rabbit's head downwards whilst it is in dorsal recumbency so as to allow the gut contents to fall out of the injection zone. The needle is inserted in the lower right quadrant of the ventral abdomen (Figure 19.23). It is inserted just through the abdominal wall and the plunger is drawn back on the syringe to ensure that no puncture of the bladder or gut has occurred. If positioned correctly there should be no resistance to injection. A maximum volume of 20–30 ml may be given at one time, depending on the rabbit's size. Any greater levels of fluids may lead to increased abdominal pressure on the diaphragm, which can lead to increased inspiratory effort.

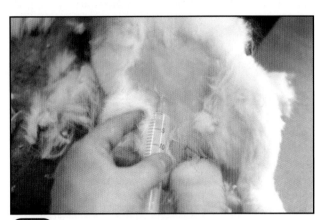

19.23 Intraperitoneal administration of fluid to a rabbit.

Intravenous

There are three vessels commonly used in rabbits. The best tolerated and arguably easiest to use is the lateral ear vein (Figure 19.24). It is preferable to apply a local anaesthetic cream (e.g. EMLA) to the skin surface over the ear vein 10–15 minutes before venepuncture to reduce flinching when catheterization occurs. Smaller rabbits require a 25 gauge over-the-needle or butterfly catheter; for larger rabbits (> 2.5 kg) a 23 gauge catheter is often used. The catheter may be taped to the ear and drip tubing attached to a syringe driver or other infusion device. It is advisable to prime the catheter with heparinized solution prior to insertion to prevent a blockage occurring.

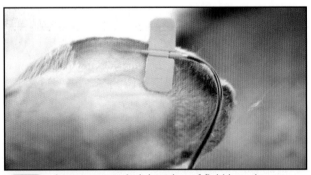

19.24 Intravenous administration of fluid into the marginal ear vein of a rabbit.

The cephalic vein may also be used, as in the cat and dog. This vein may be paired in some rabbits. A 25–27 gauge over-the-needle or butterfly catheter may be used for access and taped in, as in cats and dogs.

For the saphenous vein a 25–27 gauge butterfly catheter is preferred, as the vein is relatively fragile. It runs in the same position as in the cat and dog over the lateral aspect of the hock and is easily visible. Local anaesthetic cream may need to be applied and the limb warmed with a hot-water bottle or a lamp in order to allow venous dilation.

All of these routes can be used for intravenous boluses of up to 10 ml for larger rabbits and 5 ml for smaller Netherland dwarfs, but for continuous therapy a syringe driver is required.

Intraosseous

The proximal femur is the preferred bone to use. The landmark to aim for is the fossa between the hip joint and the greater trochanter. A 20–23 gauge hypodermic needle or spinal needle is used, and sedation is usually required except in depressed patients. The site should be surgically prepared and it may be necessary to cut down through the skin with a sterile scalpel blade. The femur is grasped in one hand and the needle/catheter is screwed through the fossa and then the medullary cavity. Radiographs of the leg may be performed to confirm the correct siting of the catheter. The use of a spinal needle reduces the risk of plugging the needle. This method will require a syringe driver perfusion device.

It is possible to use the proximal tibia but this is less well tolerated, due to interference with the stifle joint.

There is often a need for tubing guards or Elizabethan collars for all intravenous and intraosseous techniques.

Small rodents

Oral

Gavage tubes or avian straight crop tubes can be used to place fluids directly into the oesophagus. The rodent needs to be firmly scruffed in order to restrain the patient adequately and to keep the head and oesophagus in a straight line. This method is often stressful for the rodent. The alternative is to syringe fluids into the mouth, but this frequently does not work as rodents can close off the back of the mouth with the cheek folds. This is a normal anatomical function allowing rodents to gnaw structures without ingesting fragments of the material they are gnawing. Maximum volumes that can be given via the oral route in rodents vary from 5 to 10 ml/kg bodyweight. Naso-oesophageal/gastric tubes are not a viable option in rodents, due to their small size.

Subcutaneous

The scruff area is easily utilized for volumes of 3–4 ml of fluids for smaller rodents and up to 10 ml at any one time for rats. A 25 gauge needle is recommended. This route is not useful for severely shocked or hypovolaemic animals, as with other species.

Intraperitoneal

The positioning is the same as for rabbits (for Figure 19.23). A 25 gauge or smaller needle is used. A maximal volume of 1–4 ml in the smaller rodents and up to 10 ml in large rats may be given.

Intravenous

This route can be difficult, especially in conscious animals. Hamsters and gerbils are extremely difficult, as they have few peripheral veins, and the tail veins in gerbils are dangerous to use due to the risk of causing tail separation. In mice and rats, the lateral tail veins may be attempted and an intravenous bolus of fluids can be given using a 25–27 gauge insulin needle or by insertion of a butterfly catheter. It is possible to perform a cut-down jugular catheterization, but this requires anaesthesia. Warming the tail, applying local anaesthetic cream and sedation will help to dilate the vessels and make venepuncture easier. Volumes of 0.2 ml in mice up to 0.5 ml in rats as a bolus may be given.

Intraosseous

In larger rats the proximal femur may be tolerated, as for rabbits, but smaller species often have too small a medullary cavity for needles to be inserted safely.

Ferrets, guinea pigs and chinchillas

Oral

Naso-oesophageal/gastric tubes may be inserted and doses of 10 ml/kg may be administered at any one time. Ferrets, guinea pigs and chinchillas are more likely to regurgitate than rabbits, especially when debilitated, and so care is needed.

Subcutaneous

This is an easily used route for postoperative fluids and mild dehydration in these species. The scruff area or lateral thorax are preferred sites. However, the subcutaneous route may be painful for guinea pigs – especially over the scruff region, which is a site of brown fat deposition and highly innervated. Doses of 25–30 ml may be given at any one time, preferably at two or more sites. It is worth watching out for fur slip in chinchillas.

Intraperitoneal

Similar principles apply for this route as in rabbits and rodents. Doses of 15–20 ml at any one time are well tolerated for all species. This is a good route for more serious cases as intravenous fluids are not so well tolerated, particularly in chinchillas and guinea pigs.

Intravenous

The cephalic and saphenous veins may be utilized but generally these are very small and difficult to catheterize as well as being poorly tolerated, especially in guinea pigs and chinchillas. Ferrets are also quite uncooperative to this technique when fully conscious. Movement once consciousness has been regained frequently dislodges these catheters, and ferrets will often chew the dressings off; therefore plenty of excess dressing is required to allow time for the fluids to be administered.

Intraosseous

This is the preferred route for severely dehydrated chinchillas and guinea pigs. Site and administration are as described for rabbits. Catheters of 23 gauge are usually sufficient.

Fluid therapy in birds

Maintenance fluids

Maintenance fluid requirements in birds are estimated to be 50 ml/kg/day. The fluid of choice in the majority of cases is lactated Ringer's solution, but glucose-containing solutions may be preferable in smaller debilitated hypoglycaemic avian patients or those with renal failure and high potassium levels.

Assessing fluid requirements

The percentage dehydration of an avian patient is assessed in a similar way to small mammals. A critically ill avian patient is assumed to be at least 5–10% dehydrated. Debilitated avian patients may also be anaemic, and so dehydration factors can be difficult to calculate on the PCV alone; therefore total protein levels should also be measured. In addition, uric acid

levels may be measured as these will often increase in cases of moderate to severe dehydration. Figure 19.25 shows a selection of PCV ranges and total protein values for some commonly seen birds.

Species	PCV range (l/l)	Total protein (g/l)
Budgerigar	0.45–0.57	20–30
Amazon parrot	0.41–0.53	33–53
African Grey parrot	0.42–0.52	26–49
Macaw	0.43–0.54	25–44
Cockatoo	0.42–0.54	28–43
Cockatiel	0.43–0.57	31–44
Mallard	0.42–0.56	32–45
Canada goose	0.35–0.49	37–56
Mute swan	0.32–0.5	36–55
Chicken	0.24–0.43	33–55
Pheasant	0.28–0.42	42–72
Pigeon	0.36–0.48	21–35
Peregrine falcon	0.37–0.53	25–40
Barn owl	0.42–0.51	29–48
Tawny owl	0.36–0.47	27–46

19.25 Average PCV and total protein values for selected healthy birds.

Routes of administration

Oral

This is recommended for seriously debilitated birds but is also useful where crop feeding tubes can be used. It carries the risk of regurgitation and aspiration pneumonia, particularly in waterfowl. It may be useful for mild cases of dehydration where owners wish to treat their pet at home. The crop, where present, is situated at the base of the neck, predominantly on the right-hand side. This route is restricted to small volumes (Figure 19.26).

Species	Volume (ml)
Finch	0.5
Budgerigar	1
Cockatiel	2
Conure	6
Amazon parrot	8
Owl	10
Cockatoo	14
Buzzard	12–14
Macaw	14
Swan	25–30

19.26 Maximum volume of fluids that may be safely administered by crop tube to various birds.

Subcutaneous

The inguinal skin flap area or lateral axillary area are ideal sites. This is a good technique for routine postoperative administration of fluids for longer-recovery patients undergoing minor surgical procedures. It is possible to give a maximum of 10–15 ml at any one site in the larger species, or 1–2 ml in budgerigars.

Intravenous

Where an intravenous catheter is placed, continuous perfusion may be performed using syringe drivers of infusion pumps. However, in some active patients or those where catheter placement is not possible, repeated boluses of fluids may be administered during the course of treatment. Avian vessels are more fragile than mammalian vessels and catheterization is advisable where repeated doses of fluids are necessary.

Three vessels are commonly used in birds: the right jugular vein, the basilic vein or the ulnar vein. The best tolerated and easiest to use is the right jugular vein, which is also the least likely to collapse or develop a haematoma in birds such as the parrot family. It is not easy to locate in some birds of prey and some long-necked waterfowl. Where the vessel is obvious it may be catheterized using a 23 gauge over-the-needle catheter in birds the size of an African Grey parrot (~ 0.5 kg). The vein is mobile but easily seen in the area of non-feathered skin that runs from the ear to the base of the neck. The catheter should be inserted from cranial to caudal and may be stitched in place by applying silk tape to the catheter and suturing this to the skin of the neck with nylon.

The basilic vein runs along the ventral aspect of the wing, caudal to the humerus. It may be catheterized with a 23–27 gauge butterfly catheter in species from macaws to cockatiels. This vessel is mobile and ruptures easily, leaving large haematomas.

The ulnar vein runs along the ventral aspect of the wing, caudal to the ulna bone. It is of narrower diameter than the basilic vein and more mobile, having less soft tissue support. It is therefore more difficult to catheterize and ruptures more easily. Generally a 25–27 gauge needle is required in the larger parrots or a 23 gauge in some of the larger birds of prey. This vein is not useful for birds smaller than conures.

In addition, the medial metatarsal veins are very robust in most geese, ducks and swans and will allow catheterization for a number of days without rupturing. These catheters are also relatively well tolerated. Alternatively, boluses of fluids may be administered via temporary butterfly catheters.

Intraosseous

The proximal tibiotarsus is probably the easiest bone to use. The landmark to aim for is the tibial crest just below the stifle joint. A 20–23 gauge hypodermic needle or spinal needle is used in parrots heavier than 300 g; a 25–27 gauge is used in smaller birds. It is advisable to sedate the bird except in the most depressed patients. The needle is screwed into position in the same direction as the long axis of the tibiotarsus after plucking the area and surgically preparing the site. It may be necessary to cut down through the skin with a sterile scalpel blade in some cases. This method will allow intermittent boluses of fluids, or in severely debilitated cases a syringe driver perfusion device may be used.

It is possible to use the distal or proximal ulna, which is also relatively well tolerated. Again continuous perfusion by way of a syringe driver or intermittent boluses of fluids may be administered via this route, although the latter is restricted in volume still further due to the smaller size of the ulna in relation to the tibiotarsus bone. The distal ulna bone is accessed by flexing the carpal joint maximally. This allows a 21–25 gauge spinal catheter or hypodermic needle to be screwed into the caudally situated ulna bone. Radiography can be used to confirm correct siting of the needle or catheter.

There is often a need for tubing guards or Elizabethan collars for all intravenous or intraosseous techniques where continuous perfusion occurs.

Fluid therapy in reptiles

Maintenance fluids

There is evidence to suggest that reptiles do not have the same extracellular fluid tonicity as mammals. Reported values for reptiles suggest a tonicity of 0.8% (compared with 0.9% in mammals). There is therefore a suggestion that fluids used for mammals should be diluted prior to use in reptiles. For example:

- One-third 5% glucose with 0.9% saline, one-third lactated Ringer's solution, one-third sterile water; or
- Nine-tenths 5% glucose with 0.9% saline, one-tenth sterile water.

Some texts still advise that undiluted lactated Ringer's solution or 4% glucose with 0.18% saline may be used.

Assessing fluid requirements

These may be calculated as for cats and dogs. Fluid replacement rates in reptiles have been the subject of relatively little research. It has been recommended that levels of 20–25 ml/kg bodyweight per day be used for hydration purposes in reptiles, and current literature suggests that rates across several species vary from 10 to 50 ml/kg/day.

There is a restriction on the rate of administration. Most fluids are given intracoelomically in the debilitated reptile, but intravenous and intraosseous routes may also be used. Reptiles and amphibians do not possess true diaphragms, and as such the thorax and abdomen are all interconnected as a **coelom**. When fluids are placed in this cavity it is equivalent to giving intraperitoneal fluids in a mammal, but as there is no diaphragm these fluids can affect the lungs and excessive fluids may severely compromise respiration. Excessive fluids may also overload the circulation, cause pulmonary oedema, result in cardiac and renal overperfusion, or cause solute wash-out, with potassium in particular being excreted and with the increased diuresis causing development of a hypokalaemic crisis. This may manifest initially as an anorectic reptile but will progress to cardiac arrhythmias, coma and death.

The percentage dehydration of a reptilian patient is assessed in a similar way to small mammals (Figure 19.27). Assessments of thirst and urate (the chalky uric acid waste output of the kidneys) output can be made over 24 hours and provide additional information.

Dehydration (%)	Clinical signs
3	Increased thirst Slight lethargy Decreased urates
7	Increased thirst Anorexia Dullness Tenting of the skin and slow return to normal 'Dull corneas' Loss of skin turgor of spectacles in snakes
10	Dull to comatose Skin remains tented after pinching Desiccating mucous membranes Sunken eyeballs No urate/urine output

19.27 Clinical signs of dehydration levels in reptiles.

Packed cell volumes and total protein levels may also be used to assess dehydration, with each 1% increase in PCV suggesting a 10 ml/kg fluid replacement requirement (Figure 19.28).

Species	PCV range (l/l)	Total protein (g/l)
Testudo spp. tortoise	0.19–0.4	32–50
Green iguana	0.25–0.38	28–69
Ratsnake	0.2–0.3	30–60
Boa constrictor	0.2–0.32	46–60

19.28 Average PCV and total protein values for selected reptile species.

In working out the fluid deficits, it is still important not to exceed levels of 25–30 ml/kg/day, for reasons mentioned above, and so rehydration of severely debilitated reptiles may take days to weeks.

Routes of administration

Chelonians

Oral

This route can be used as for lizards and snakes. A pharyngostomy tube may be inserted and fluid levels of 10 ml/kg at any one time can be administered. Alternatively a stomach tube may be inserted each time it is needed. The feeding tube is first measured to correspond with the length from the tip of the extended nose to the line where the pectoral and abdominal ventral scutes connect. It can then be lubricated and passed after extending the animal's head and gently prising the mouth open with a wooden or plastic speculum.

Subcutaneous

This is a frequently used route for postoperative fluids and mild dehydration in these species. It may be given in the area just cranial to the hindlimbs, or in the skin folds just lateral to the neck. Relatively large volumes may be given via this route.

Intracoelomic

A maximum rate of 20–25 ml/kg/day only can be given by this route, otherwise fluid will exert excessive pressure on the lung fields due to the restriction placed by the shell. There are two main access sites. The area cranial to the hindlimbs is the same site as that for subcutaneous administration, but the insertion is deeper. The concern with this route is that the bladder lies in this area, and if full may be punctured. The other access site is cranial and is located lateral to the neck and medial to the forelimb. The needle is kept close and parallel to the plastron and a ³/₄ inch needle may be inserted to the level of the hub.

Intravenous

There are two main routes that may be used: the dorsal tail vein and the jugular vein.

- The **dorsal tail vein** is a plexus of veins. It is not possible to give large volumes of fluids via this route and it is certainly not possible to place a catheter. The access lies in the midline, on the dorsal aspect of the tail. The needle is inserted at an angle of 90 degrees until it touches the coccygeal vertebra. The needle is then pulled back whilst applying negative pressure until blood flows into the hub.

- The **jugular veins** may be accessed for catheter placement in the sedated or anaesthetized tortoise. The neck is extended and the head tilted away from the operator, giving access to the neck. The jugular vein runs from the dorsal aspect of the eardrum along the dorsal aspect of the neck. An over-the-needle catheter may be placed directly, or in thick-skinned animals a cut-down technique employed.

Intraosseous

Two main sites can be used.

- The **plastro-carapacial junction/pillar** is the pillar of shell that connects the plastron to the carapace. It is approached from the caudal aspect, just cranial to one of the hindlimbs (Figure 19.29). The spinal or hypodermic needle (21–23 gauge) is screwed into the shell while attempting to keep the angle of insertion parallel with the outer wall of the shell, thus entering the medullary cavity. In larger older species, the shell may be too tough to allow penetration by this method.
- The **proximal tibia** may be approached in the same way as for lizards. The area is thoroughly scrubbed and the hypodermic or spinal needle is screwed into the tibial crest in the direction of the long axis of the distal tibia.

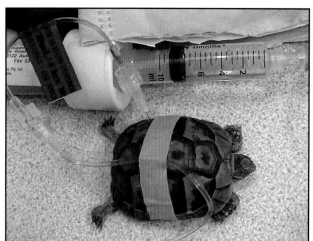

19.29 Intraosseous fluid administration into a septicaemic hatchling tortoise. (Courtesy of M Jessop)

Lizards

Oral

Gavage tubes or avian straight crop tubes or feeding tubes can be used to place fluids directly into the oesophagus/stomach. The reptile needs to be firmly restrained to keep the head and oesophagus in a straight line. The mouth is opened with a plastic or wooden tongue depressor and the tube is inserted to the level of the caudal aspect of the sternum that approximates to one-third to one-half of the body cavity length of the reptile. This method is often stressful for the reptile. The alternative is to syringe fluids into the mouth but there is a risk of inhalation in a debilitated reptile. A pharyngostomy tube may be placed for nutritional support and so may be used for fluid therapy.

Subcutaneous

The lateral thoracic area is easily utilized for smaller volumes of fluids. There is a risk of the lizard developing a darkened pigmented area over the injection site, particularly in the chameleon family.

Intracoelomic

The lizard is placed in dorsal recumbency in a similar manner as that described in peritoneal administration in small mammals. The needle, 25 gauge or smaller, is advanced slowly until it just pops through the abdominal wall in the lower right ventral quadrant. The plunger is pulled back to ensure that no organ penetration had been achieved, and the fluids can be administered without any resistance.

Intravenous

This route can be difficult in small lizards and frequently requires sedation or anaesthesia. Several routes may be used.

- The **cephalic vein** is accessed in the anaesthetized lizard using a cut-down technique. The incision is made through the skin on the cranial aspect in the middle of the antebrachium, in a perpendicular angle to the long axis of the radius and ulna. The vessel may then be catheterized using an over-the-needle catheter and sutured in place. This technique is only really useful for lizards over 0.25 kg in weight.
- The **jugular vein** may be accessed via a cut-down technique in the anaesthetized or sedated lizard. An incision is made in a craniocaudal manner starting 2.5 cm caudal to the angle of the jaw. An over-the-needle catheter may then be sutured in place.
- The **ventral tail vein** is a plexus of veins. It is accessed from the ventral aspect of the tail in the conscious lizard. It is only suitable for single bolus injections, and special care should be taken with species that exhibit autotomy (spontaneous tail shedding) such as day geckos and green iguanas. The needle is inserted at an angle of 90 degrees and advanced until it touches the coccygeal vertebra. The needle is then withdrawn slightly, with negative pressure applied to the syringe. When blood flows into the syringe, the infusion may begin.

Intraosseous

This is a good route in the smaller species of lizards where venous access is restricted or difficult. There are several access points that may be used. Hypodermic or spinal needles of 23–25 gauge may be used.

- The **proximal femur** may be accessed from the fossa created between the greater trochanter and the hip joint. This route may be difficult due to the 90 degree angle that the femur often forms with the pelvis.
- The **distal femur** is relatively easy to access from the stifle joint. It does provide restriction of movement in the stifle joint, but it is easy to bandage the catheter at this site and access to the medullary cavity of the femur is easier via this route. Sedation or anaesthesia is required.
- The **proximal tibia** is possible in the larger species. Anaesthesia and sedation are needed, and the spinal needle or hypodermic needle may be screwed into the tibial crest region in a proximodistal manner.

Snakes

Oral

This is not suitable for seriously debilitated animals or those with pre-existing gut pathology. It is useful in mild cases of dehydration where a pharyngostomy feeding tube is in place, or if the owner is experienced in stomach tubing and wishes to treat their pet at home. A stomach tube is easily passed by restraining the snake's head gently but firmly and then inserting a plastic/wooden tongue depressor to open the mouth. A lubricated feeding tube is then passed through the labial notch (the area at the most rostral aspect of the mouth without teeth) and down to a distance of one-third of the snake's length.

Subcutaneous

The ideal site is the lateral aspect of the dorsum of the snake in the caudal third of its body. This is a good route for use as routine postoperative administration of fluids for longer-recovery patients undergoing minor surgical procedures. There is a lymph sinus that runs just lateral to the epaxial muscles on both sides and moderately large volumes of fluid can be given if administered subcutaneously over these sinuses. However, it may still be necessary to use several sites.

Intracoelomic

This route is good for more seriously dehydrated reptiles, as there is a large vasculature at this site for absorption. The needle or butterfly catheter is inserted at a point two rows of lateral scales dorsal to the ventral scales in the caudal third of the snake, but cranial to the vent. The needle is inserted so that it just penetrates the body wall; the plunger of the syringe is pulled back to ensure that no organ puncture has occurred and the fluids are administered. If correctly inserted there will be no resistance to the injection.

Intravenous

There are no major vessels in snakes that are easily accessible. If intravenous administration is required, one of the following routes may be used.

- The **ventral tail vein** is a plexus of veins, and may be accessed from the ventrum. The needle is inserted midline, one-third of the tail length from the vent, and advanced until it touches the coccygeal vertebrae at a 90 degree angle. The needle is then retracted slightly whilst applying negative pressure to the syringe until blood flows into the hub. Fluids may then be given.
- The **palatine vein** is present on the roof of the mouth, as its name suggests, and is paired. Cannulation may be performed with a 25–27 gauge butterfly catheter and frequently the snake has to be sedated or anaesthetized to gain access.
- The **intracardiac** route can be used in emergencies. The heart is catheterized under sedation or anaesthesia. The heart may be seen to beat against the ventral scale, approximately one-quarter of its length from the snout when the snake is placed in dorsal recumbency. A 25–27 gauge over-the-needle catheter may be inserted between the scales in a caudocranial manner at 30 degrees to the body wall into the single ventricle. A bolus may be administered, or the catheter may be taped, glued or sutured in place for 24–48 hours.
- **Jugular veins** can also only be accessed in an anaesthetized or sedated snake. A full-thickness skin cut-down procedure may be made 50–75 mm caudal to the angle of the jaw two rows of scales dorsal to the ventral scales to gain access. The jugular vein can then be seen medial to the ribs. An over-the-needle catheter with plastic wings is advised and this should be sutured in place.

Intraosseous

This route is not possible for snakes.

Fluid therapy in amphibians

Maintenance fluids

A maximum fluid rate of 20–25 ml/kg/day, similar to reptiles, may safely be given. Potassium-containing fluids should be avoided initially as many dehydrated amphibians develop hyperkalaemia; glucose–saline combinations are preferred.

Routes of administration

Cutaneous

This route can be used in mildly dehydrated amphibians. Only dechlorinated water should be used. It should be warmed to the amphibian's preferred body temperature and be well oxygenated. Absorption will occur across the skin membranes where there is no evidence of skin disease.

Oral

This route can be used for hypotonic fluid therapy via a small feeding tube inserted orally. The procedure is stressful and trauma may easily occur during restraint and opening of the amphibian's mouth.

Intracoelomic

Fluid is easily given by this route via the right lower ventral quadrant of the 'abdomen'. The amphibian should be placed in dorsal recumbency with the head down to allow coelom contents to fall away from the injection site.

Intravenous

In the larger anurans, and some salamanders, the midline ventral abdominal vein may be used for bolus fluids or blood transfusions. The vessel lies midline, just below the skin surface, and runs from the pubis area of the pelvis to the xiphoid of the sternum. A 25–27 gauge insulin needle may be used to gain access, but the vessel is very fragile and care should be taken not to rupture it.

Fluid therapy in fish

Dehydration may be seen in marine species, especially where skin lesions cause a break in the barrier between the hypotonic tissue fluids and hypertonic sea water, creating an osmotic potential. This is unlikely to occur in freshwater species.

Mild fluid deficits may be replaced via gastric intubation using freshwater or hypotonic saline. In larger species it may be possible to access the ventral tail vein caudal to the vent, as would be performed for blood sampling, and administer a bolus of intravenous hypotonic fluids. This author (SG) has administered volumes of 5–10 ml/kg by this technique.

Fluid therapy in invertebrates

Dehydration is seen in invertebrates and may manifest itself as weakness, collapse and dysecdysis (incomplete shedding of skin) in those invertebrates that shed their skin (e.g. many arachnids) and death. Fluids may be administered orally by soaking cotton wool or other absorbent material for the invertebrate to consume water droplets from, as bowls of water are rarely used.

With care, it is possible in large arachnids to inject fluids or perform a haemolymph transfusion into the cardiac sinus chamber (the invertebrate equivalent of the heart). A 24–26 gauge over-the-needle catheter is carefully inserted in a caudocranial manner through the dorsal surface of the abdomen at an angle of 30–45 degrees where it will easily enter the cardiac sinus chamber. The hole in the exoskeleton may be sealed using sterile tissue glue. Care must be taken to minimize the trauma to the exoskeleton and not to overinfuse, as this will lead to increased internal pressure and circulatory compromise.

Further reading

Cannon M (2000) Fluid therapy for cats 1. Providing fluids to the feline patient. *In Practice*, **22**, 242–251

Cannon M (2000) Fluid therapy for cats 2. Restoring fluid and electrolyte balance. *In Practice*, **22**, 317–326

College of Animal Welfare (2000) *300 Questions and Answers in Anatomy and Physiology*. Butterworth Heinemann, Oxford

Frye F (1991) Pathological conditions related to the captive environment. In: *Biomedical and Surgical Aspects of Captive Reptile Husbandry*, pp. 161–182. Krieger Publishing, Malabar, Florida

Francis-Floyd R and Wildgoose W (2001) Behavioural changes. In: *Manual of Ornamental Fish, 2nd edn*, pp. 155–161. BSAVA Publications, Gloucester

Girling SJ (2002) *Veterinary Nursing of Exotic Pets*. Blackwell Publishing, Oxford

Hansen BD (2001) Intravenous catheters. *Waltham Focus*, **11**, 4–10

Haskins SC (1988) A simple fluid therapy planning guide. *Seminars in Veterinary Medicine and Surgery*, **3**, 227–236

Klingenberg R (1996) Therapeutics. In: *Reptile Medicine and Surgery*, (ed. D Mader), pp. 299–321. WB Saunders, Philadelphia

Knottenbelt C and Mackin A (1998) Blood transfusions in the dog and cat. *In Practice*, **20**, 110–113 and 191–199

Rudloff E and Kirby R (2001) Resuscitation from hypovolaemic shock. *Waltham Focus*, **11**, 11–22

Chapter 20

Diagnostic imaging

Ruth Dennis, Anna Williams and Philip Lhermette

Learning objectives

After studying this chapter, students should be able to:

- **Understand the physical principles of diagnostic radiography**
- **Have a sound working knowledge of radiographic equipment, procedures and safety**
- **Know how to perform basic radiographic studies and to prepare for and assist in more complex investigations**
- **Identify faults in radiography and know how to correct them**
- **Understand the principles of diagnostic ultrasonography and know how to assist in ultrasound examinations**
- **Understand the basic principles of MRI, CT, scintigraphy and endoscopy**
- **Understand specific considerations for imaging exotic pets**

Introduction

Radiography is a fundamental part of veterinary practice and is a procedure in which most nurses become actively involved. The production of diagnostic films requires skill in the use of radiographic equipment, in patient positioning and in the processing of the films. At the same time the procedure must be carried out safely without hazard to the handlers or patient.

Basic principles of radiography

X-rays are produced by X-ray machines when electricity from the mains is transformed to a high-voltage current, converting some of the energy in the current to X-ray energy. The intensity and penetrating power of the emergent X-ray beam varies with the size and complexity of the apparatus and the exposure settings used; portable X-ray machines are capable of only a relatively low output, whereas larger machines are far more powerful.

X-rays travel in straight lines and can be focused into an area called the **primary beam**, which is directed at the patient. Within the patient's tissues some of the X-rays are absorbed; the remainder pass through and are detected by photographic X-ray film, producing a hidden image. When the film is processed chemically a permanent picture or radiograph is produced and the image may be viewed.

Production and properties of X-rays

X-rays are members of the **electromagnetic spectrum**, a group of types of radiation that have some similar properties but differ from each other in their **wavelength** and **frequency** (Figure 20.1).

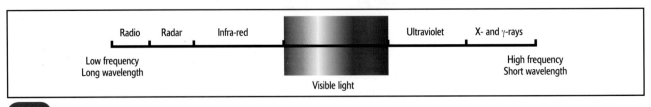

| Radio | Radar | Infra-red | Ultraviolet | X- and γ-rays |

Low frequency
Long wavelength

High frequency
Short wavelength

Visible light

20.1 The electromagnetic spectrum.

The energy in a given type of radiation is directly proportional to the frequency of the radiation and inversely proportional to its wavelength. X-rays and gamma rays are similar types of electromagnetic radiation that have high frequency, short wavelength and therefore high energy. X-rays are produced by X-ray machines and gamma rays by the decay of radioactive materials.

Members of the electromagnetic spectrum have the following common features:

* They do not require a medium for transmission and can pass through a vacuum.
* They travel in straight lines.
* They travel at the same speed: 3×10^8 m/s in a vacuum.
* They interact with matter by being absorbed or scattered.

X-rays have some additional properties which mean that they can be used to produce images of the internal structures of people and animals; they are also used in engineering for detecting flaws in pipes and construction materials.

* **Penetration:** Because of their high energy, X-rays can penetrate substances that are opaque to visible ('white') light. The X-ray photons are absorbed to varying degrees, depending on the nature of the substance penetrated and the power of the photons themselves, and some may pass right through the patient, emerging at the other side. The shorter its wavelength, the higher is the energy of the X-ray photon and the greater its penetrating ability.
* **Effect on photographic film:** X-rays have the ability to produce a hidden or latent image on photographic film, which can be rendered visible by processing (film in cameras is damaged by exposure to X-radiation).
* **Fluorescence:** X-rays cause crystals of certain substances to fluoresce (emit visible light) and this property is utilized in the composition of intensifying screens, which are used in the recording of the image.

X-rays also produce biological changes in living tissues by altering the structure of atoms or molecules or by causing chemical reactions. Some of these effects can be used beneficially in the radiotherapy of tumours, but they are harmful to normal tissues and constitute a safety hazard. Aspects of radiation safety are considered later in the chapter.

Production of X-rays

X-ray photons or quanta are tiny packets of energy that are released whenever rapidly moving electrons are slowed down or stopped. Electrons are present in the atoms of all elements and in order to grasp the fundamentals of simple radiation physics it is necessary to understand the structure of an atom (Figure 20.2). Atoms contains the following particles:

* **Protons** – positively charged particles contained in the centre or nucleus of the atom
* **Neutrons** – particles of similar size to protons that are also found in the nucleus but carry no electrical charge
* **Electrons** – smaller, negatively charged particles that orbit around the nucleus in different planes or 'shells'.

The number of electrons normally equals the number of protons and so the atom as a whole is electrically neutral. The number of protons and electrons is unique to the atoms of each element and is called the **atomic number**. If an atom loses one or more

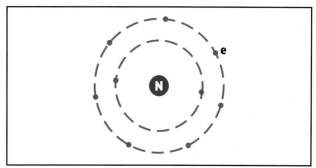

20.2 Structure of an atom. N = nucleus (protons and neutrons); e = electron (dotted lines represent electron 'shells').

electrons it becomes positively charged and may be written as X^+ (where X is the symbol for that element). If an atom gains electrons it becomes negatively charged (X^-). Atoms with charges are called **ions** or are said to be ionized. **Compounds** are combinations of two or more elements and usually consist of positive ions of one element in combination with negative ions of another; for example, silver bromide (in X-ray film emulsion) consists of silver Ag^+ and bromide Br^- ions.

In an X-ray tube head, X-ray photons are produced by collisions between fast-moving electrons and the atoms of a 'target' element. Electrons that are completely halted by the target atoms give up all of their energy to form an X-ray photon, whereas those that are merely decelerated give up smaller and variable amounts of energy, producing lower-energy X-ray photons. The X-ray beam produced therefore contains photons of a range of energies and is said to be **polychromatic**. If the number of incident electrons is increased, more X-ray photons are produced and the intensity of the X-ray beam increases. If the incident electrons are faster-moving, they have more energy to lose and so the X-ray photons produced are more energetic; the X-ray beam's quality is therefore increased and it has greater penetrating power.

The intensity and quality of an X-ray beam can be altered by adjusting the settings on the machine, and the practical effect of this will be discussed in greater detail later.

The X-ray tube head

The X-ray tube head is the part of the machine where the X-rays are generated. A diagram of the simplest type of X-ray tube, a **stationary** or **fixed anode** tube, is shown in Figure 20.3.

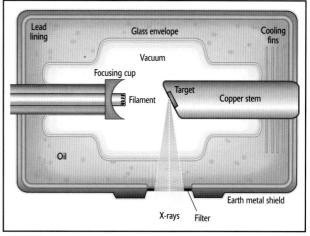

20.3 A stationary or fixed anode X-ray tube.

The X-ray tube head contains two electrodes: the negatively charged **cathode** and the positively charged **anode**. Electrons are produced at the cathode, which is a coiled wire filament. When a small electrical current is passed through the filament it becomes hot and releases a cloud of electrons by a process called **thermionic emission**. Tungsten is used as the filament material because:

- It has a high atomic number, 74, and therefore has many electrons
- It has a very high melting point of 3380°C and so can safely be heated
- It has helpful mechanical properties which mean that fine, coiled filaments can be made.

The current required to heat the filament is small and so the mains current to the filament is reduced by a **step-down** or **filament transformer**, which is wired into the X-ray machine (a transformer is a device for increasing or decreasing an electric current).

Next, the cloud of electrons needs to be made to travel at high speed across the short distance to the target. This is done by applying a high electrical potential difference between the filament and the target so that the filament becomes negative (and therefore repels the electrons) and the target becomes positive (and attracts them). The filament therefore becomes a cathode and the target an anode. The electrons are formed into a narrow beam by the fact that the filament sits in a nickel or molybdenum **focusing cup**, which is also at a negative potential and so repels the electrons. The electron beam constitutes a weak electric current across the tube, which is measured in **milliamperes (mA)**.

The potential difference applied between the filament and the target needs to be very high and many times the voltage of the mains supply, which is 240 volts. In fact it is measured in thousands of volts, or **kilovolts (kV)**, and is created from the mains in a second electrical circuit using a **step-up** or **high-tension transformer**, which is also part of the electrical circuitry of the X-ray machine.

The stream of electrons strikes the target or anode at very high speed. Tungsten or rhenium–tungsten alloy is used as the target material because its high atomic number renders it a relatively efficient producer of X-rays. Unfortunately the process is still very inefficient and more than 99% of the energy lost by the electrons is converted to heat, so the anode must be able to withstand very high temperatures without melting or cracking. Tungsten's high melting point is therefore useful in the target as well as in the filament.

In a simple type of X-ray tube as shown in Figure 20.3, the target is a small rectangle of tungsten about 3 mm thick set in a copper block. Copper is a good conductor of heat and so the heat is removed from the target by conduction along the copper stem to cooling fins radiating into the surrounding oil bath, which can absorb much heat.

The target is set at an angle of about 20 degrees to the vertical (Figure 20.4). This is so that the area of the target which the electrons strike (and therefore the area over which heat is produced) is as large as possible. This area is called the **actual focal spot**. At the same time the angulation of the target means that the X-ray beam appears to originate from a much smaller area and this is called the **effective focal spot**. The importance of having a small effective focal spot – ideally a point source – is discussed later in the chapter with regard to image definition. The design of the target to maximize actual focal spot size whilst minimizing the effective focal spot is known as the 'line focus principle'.

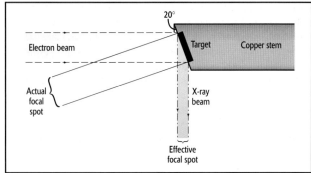

20.4 How angulation of target produces a large actual focal spot and a small effective focal spot.

Some X-ray machines allow a choice of focal spot size using two different-sized filaments at the cathode:

- The smaller filament produces an electron beam with a smaller cross-sectional area and hence smaller effective and actual focal spots. This is known as **fine focus**. The emergent X-ray beam arises from a tiny area and will produce very fine radiographic definition. However, the heat generated is concentrated over a very small area of the target and so the exposure factors that can be used are limited.
- The larger filament produces a wider electron beam with larger effective and actual focal spot sizes – the **coarse** or **broad focus**. Higher exposures can be used but the image definition will be slightly less sharp due to the **penumbra effect**, a blurring of margins related to the geometry of the beam (Figure 20.5).

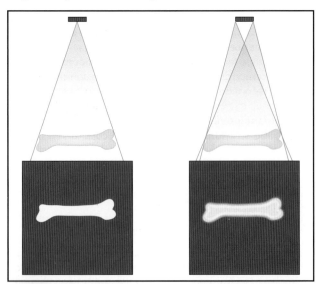

20.5 Effect of focal-spot size. (A) The spot is a pinpoint and the projected image is sharp. (B) The rays from a focal spot of large dimensions cause a penumbra effect, which blurs the projected image.

In practice, fine focus is selected for small parts when fine definition is required (e.g. the limbs), and coarse focus when thicker areas are to be radiographed (e.g. the chest and abdomen); these require higher exposure factors and so the heat generated at the target is higher.

The cathode, anode and part of the copper stem are enclosed in a **glass envelope**. Within the envelope is a vacuum, which prevents the moving electrons from colliding with air molecules and losing speed. The glass envelope is bathed in oil which acts both as a heat sink and as an electrical insulator, and the whole is encased in an earthed, lead-lined **metal** casing. X-rays are produced in all directions by the target but only one narrow beam of X-rays is required, and this emerges through a window in the casing, placed beneath the angled target. This beam is called the **primary** or **useful beam**. X-rays produced in other directions are absorbed by the casing.

Within the X-ray beam are some low-energy or 'soft' X-ray photons, which are not powerful enough to pass through the patient but which may be absorbed or scattered by the patient and therefore represent a safety hazard. They are removed from the beam by an **aluminium filter** placed across the tube window; these filters are legally required as a safety precaution and must not be removed.

In stationary anode X-ray tubes the X-ray output is limited by the amount of heat generated at the target. Overheating the target would produce melting and surface irregularity, which would reduce the efficiency of the tube; in modern machines automatic 'overload' devices prevent such high exposures from being used. Stationary anode X-ray tubes are found in low-powered, portable X-ray machines. These have limited ability to produce short exposure times for thoracic radiography or high output for large patients. More powerful machines require a more efficient way of removing the heat and this is accomplished using a **rotating anode** (Figure 20.6). In such tubes the target area is the bevelled rim of a metal disc of about 10 cm diameter whose rim is set at about 20 degrees, as in a stationary anode X-ray tube. The target area is again tungsten or rhenium–tungsten. During the exposure the disc rotates rapidly so that the target area upon which the electrons impinge is constantly changing. The actual focal spot is therefore the whole circumference of the disc and so is many times greater than in a stationary anode X-ray tube. The heat generated is spread over a much bigger area, allowing larger exposures to be made, whilst the effective focal spot remains the same. The disc is mounted on a molybdenum rod and is rotated at speeds of up to 10,000 rpm by an induction motor at the other end of the rod. Molybdenum is used because it is a poor conductor of heat and therefore prevents the motor from overheating. Heat generated in the anode is lost by radiation through the vacuum and the glass envelope into the oil bath.

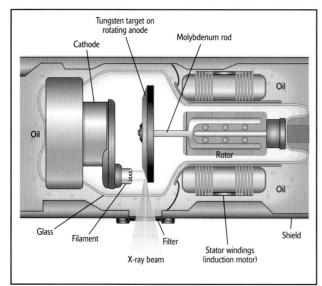

Tungsten target on rotating anode
Molybdenum rod
Cathode
Oil
Oil
Rotor
Oil
Glass
Filament
Filter
Shield
X-ray beam
Stator windings (induction motor)

20.6 A rotating anode X-ray tube.

The size of the emerging X-ray beam must be controlled for safety reasons, otherwise it will spread out over a very large area. This is achieved using a **collimation device**, preferably a light beam diaphragm. Methods of collimation are described later.

The X-ray control panel

X-ray machine control panels vary in their complexity, but some or all of the following controls will be present.

On/off switch

As well as switching the machine on at the mains socket, there will be an on/off switch or key on the control panel. Sometimes the line voltage compensator (see below) is incorporated into the on/off switch, which therefore performs both functions. When the machine is switched on a warning light on the control panel will indicate that it is ready to produce X-rays or, in the case of panels with digital displays, the numbers will be illuminated. In some old machines the filament is heated continually whilst the machine is on and may burn out. Such machines should always be turned off when the exposure is terminated. X-ray machines must always be switched off when not in use, so that accidental exposure cannot occur when unprotected people are in the room.

Line voltage compensator

Fluctuations in the normal mains electricity output may occur, resulting in an inconsistent output of X-rays. The images produced may appear under- or overexposed despite using normal exposure factors. In some machines these fluctuations are automatically corrected by an **auto-transformer** wired into the circuit, but in others it is controlled manually. A voltmeter dial on the control panel will indicate the incoming voltage, which can be adjusted until it is satisfactory. In such machines the line voltage should be checked before each session of radiography.

Kilovoltage (kV) control

The kilovoltage control selects the **kilovoltage** (potential difference) that is applied across the tube during the instant of exposure. It determines the speed and energy with which the electrons bombard the target and hence the quality or penetrating power of the X-ray beam produced. Depending on the power and sophistication of the X-ray machine, the kilovoltage is controlled in various ways. Ideally it is controlled quite independently of the milliamperage, often in increments of 1 kV, and the kilovoltage meter is either a dial or a digital display.

In smaller machines the kilovoltage is linked to the milliamperage so that if a higher milliamperage is selected only lower kilovoltages can be used. Often there is a single control knob for both kilovoltage and milliamperage and as the kilovoltage is increased the milliamperage available drops. This is not ideal since, for larger patients, a high kilovoltage and high milliamperage may be required at the same time, meaning that long exposure times are needed. In very basic machines the kilovoltage and milliamperage are fixed, and only the time can be altered.

Milliamperage (mA) control

The **milliamperage** is a measure of the quantity of electrons crossing the tube during the exposure (the 'tube current') and is directly related to the quantity of X-rays produced. Moving electrons constitute an electrical current, which is measured in amperes, but the tube current is very small and is measured in 1/1000 amperes or milliamperes (mA). Adjusting the milliamperage control alters the degree of heating of the filament and hence the number of electrons released by thermionic emission, the tube current and the intensity of the X-ray beam.

Timer

The quantity of X-rays produced depends not only on the milliamperage but also on the length of the exposure, and so a composite term, the **milliampere-seconds** or **mAs**, is often used. A given rate of mAs may be obtained using a high milliamperage with a short time, or vice versa. The two numbers are multiplied together. For example, 30 mAs = 300 mA for 0.1 s or 30 mA for 1.0 s. The effect on the film is the same except that the longer the exposure the more likely it is that movement blur will occur. One should always therefore use the largest milliamperage allowed by the machine for that kilovoltage setting, in order to minimize the exposure time. It will now be appreciated why the type of machine in which kilovoltage and milliamperage are inversely linked is less than ideal.

The timer is usually electronic and is usually another dial on the control panel, giving a choice of a wide range of exposure times up to several seconds long. Release of the exposure button terminates the exposure even when long times have been selected. In larger machines an automatic display of the resulting mAs is also present. At one time, X-ray machines relied on clockwork timers in hand-sets that also incorporated the exposure button. A dial was 'wound up' to an appropriate time setting and ran back to zero whilst the exposure button was depressed. The time had to be reset between exposures. These timers were not only inaccurate and noisy but also they did not allow the exposure to be aborted if necessary. Some modern machines with a digital display have a single control for mAs which automatically selects the shortest exposure time for the selected mAs.

Exposure button

The exposure button must be at the end of a cable that can stretch to more than 2 m to enable radiographers to distance themselves from the primary beam during the exposure. Alternatively, the button may be on the control panel itself, provided that the panel is at least 2 m from the tube head or is separated from it by a lead screen. Most exposure buttons are two-stage devices: depression of the button to a halfway stage ('prepping') heats the filament and rotates the anode if a rotating anode is present; after a brief pause, further depression of the button causes application of the kilovoltage to the tube and an instantaneous exposure to be made. In some machines only a single-stage exposure button is present; in this case there is slight delay between depression of the button and exposure, during which time the patient may move. In old machines with single-stage exposure buttons the filament may be constantly heated while the machine is switched on and in these there is a risk of burning out the filament.

Types of X-ray machine

X-ray machines can conveniently be divided into three broad types: portable, mobile and fixed.

Portable machines

These are the commonest type of machine found in general practice (Figure 20.7). As their name suggests, they are relatively easy to move from site to site for large animal radiography and many come with a special carrying case. The largest ones weigh about 20 kg. The electrical transformers are located in the tube head, which is usually supported on a wheeled metal stand though some may be wall-mounted. The tube head must never be held for radiography, as this is very hazardous to the person holding. The controls may be either on a separate panel or else on the head itself. Portable

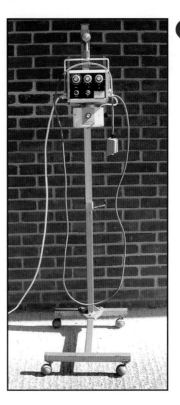

20.7 Portable X-ray machine.

machines are low powered, producing only about 20–60 mA and often less. In most the kilovoltage and milliamperage are inversely linked. Although portable machines are widely used, their relatively low output means that longer exposure times are needed, and chest and abdomen radiographs of larger dogs are often degraded by the effects of movement blur.

Mobile machines

These are larger and more powerful than portable machines but can still be moved from room to room on wheels (Figure 20.8), some having battery-operated motors. The transformers are bulkier and encased in a large box, which is an integral part of the tube stand. Mobile machines usually have outputs of up to 300 mA and are likely to produce good radiographs of most small animal patients. Although they are more expensive to buy new, they can sometimes be obtained second-hand from hospitals, where they will have had relatively little use yet

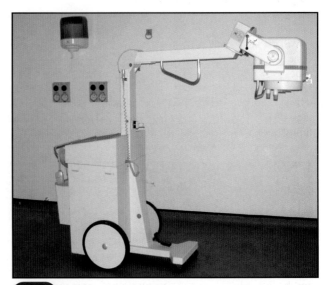

20.8 Mobile X-ray machine.

been well cared for, having been used mainly for bedridden patients. They are not usually suitable for equine radiography since the tube head will not reach to the floor, but special tube arm adaptors can be fitted. If used for equine radiography the horse should be restrained in stocks since the X-ray machine cannot be moved away quickly if the patient moves.

Fixed machines

The most powerful X-ray machines are built into the X-ray room, being screwed to the floor or being mounted on rails or overhead gantries (Figure 20.9). The tube head is usually quite mobile on its mounting and can be moved in several directions, which is especially valuable for equine radiography. The transformers are situated in cabinets some distance from the machine itself, and connected to it by high-tension cables. The largest fixed machines can produce up to 1250 mA and produce excellent radiographs of all patients, but because of the high cost of purchase, installation and maintenance they are rarely found outside veterinary institutions and large equine practices. However, several companies are now producing smaller, fixed X-ray machines especially for the veterinary market which are much more affordable. Fixed X-ray machines are often linked electronically to a floating table top and moving grid.

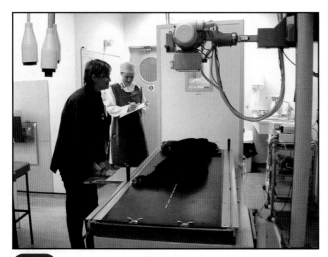

20.9 Fixed X-ray machine.

High-frequency machines

Many older X-ray machines, in particular portable machines, generate X-rays from a pulsating voltage supply. Most modern machines, including portables, use high-frequency generators to produce a stable high voltage supply to the X-ray tube. They do this by increasing the frequency of the waveform of the standard mains supply from 50 cycles per second (Hz) up to thousands of cycles per second (kHz). The advantage of this is that machines are capable of shorter exposure times, higher exposures, and improved efficiency.

Formation of the X-ray image

The X-ray picture is essentially a 'shadowgraph', or a picture in black, white and varying shades of grey, caused by differences in the amount of absorption of the beam by different tissues and hence in differences in the amount of radiation reaching the X-ray film and causing blackening (Figure 20.10).

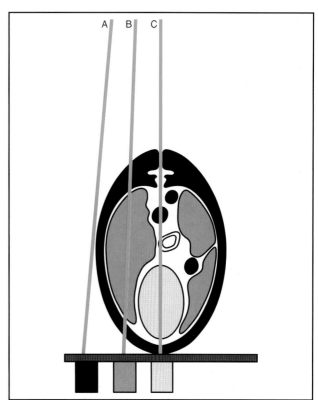

20.10 Cross-section of a thorax to show formation of an X-ray shadowgraph. X-ray photons passing along path C are largely absorbed, resulting in white areas on the radiograph. X-ray photons passing along path B are partly absorbed, producing intermediate shades of grey on the radiograph. X-ray photons passing along path A are outside the patient and so are not absorbed, producing black areas on the radiograph.

The degree of absorption by a given tissue depends on three factors:

- The **atomic number** (*Z*) of the tissue, or the average of the different atomic numbers present (the 'effective' atomic number).
- The **specific gravity** of the tissue
- The **thickness** of the tissue.

Bone has a higher effective atomic number than soft tissue and so absorbs more X-ray photons, producing whiter areas on the radiograph. Similarly, soft tissue has a higher effective atomic number than fat.

Specific gravity is the density or mass per unit volume. Bone has a high specific gravity, soft tissue a medium specific gravity and gas a very low specific gravity; hence gas-filled areas absorb few X-rays and appear nearly black on the radiograph.

The combination of effective atomic number and specific gravity produces five characteristic shades to be seen on a radiograph:

- Gas – very dark
- Fat – dark grey
- Soft tissue or fluid – mid grey
- Bone – nearly white
- Metal – white (as all X-rays absorbed).

It should noted that solid soft tissue and fluid produce the same radiographic appearance; therefore fluid within a soft tissue viscus (e.g. urine in the bladder or blood in the heart) cannot be differentiated from the tissue that surrounds it. Fat is less radio-opaque (darker) than soft tissue and fluid, so fat in the abdomen is helpful in surrounding and outlining the various organs.

Overlap in the ranges of grey shades on the radiograph occurs due to the fact that thicker areas of tissue absorb more X-ray photons than thinner areas; hence a very thick area of soft tissue may actually appear more radio-opaque (whiter) than a thin area of bone.

Selection of exposure factors

Kilovoltage

The kilovoltage (kV) controls the **penetrating power** of the X-ray beam. A higher kV is required for tissues that have a higher atomic number or specific gravity, or are very thick. Both the nature and depth of the tissue being X-rayed must therefore be taken into consideration when selecting the appropriate kV setting. A range of about 40–100 kV is used in veterinary radiography. The kV affects both the scale of **contrast** on the image (the number of grey shades) and the **radiographic density** (the degree of blackening of the film).

Increasing the kV will cause greater penetration of all tissues and hence a blacker film. Too high a kV will over-penetrate tissues, resulting in a dark film with few different shades; this is called a **flat** film or is said to be 'lacking in contrast'. Too low a kV will under-penetrate tissue (especially bone), which will appear white, on a black or dark grey background. This type of appearance is sometimes called **soot and white-wash**; its contrast is too high. Figure 20.11 shows the effect of alterations in the kilovoltage.

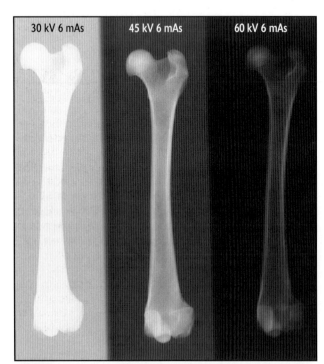

20.11 Effect on subject penetration of altering the kilovoltage but keeping the mAs constant. With low kV there is little penetration of the subject; with high kV there is too much.

Milliamperage and time

The milliamperage (mA) setting determines the tube current and therefore the quantity of X-rays per second in the emergent beam, also known as its **intensity**. Altering the mA will not affect the penetrating power of the beam (i.e. the contrast of the image) but *will* change the degree of blackening of the film under the areas that are penetrated (the radiographic density).

The product of milliamperage and length of the exposure produces the milliampere-seconds (mAs) factor or total quantity of X-rays used for that particular exposure. Normally the maximum mA and shortest time possible are used for the chest, in order to reduce the effects of movement blur (times of less than 0.05 s are preferred).

Increasing the mAs will produce more X-ray photons to blacken the film, though they have no more penetrating ability. The contrast between adjacent tissues (the difference in shades of grey) will not change, but the overall picture will be darker. Figure 20.12 shows the effect of alterations in the mAs.

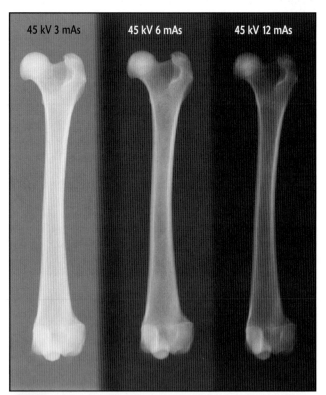

20.12 Effect on film blackening of altering the mAs but keeping the kilovoltage constant. The patient penetration (internal detail) is similar in each case but the image is darker with higher mAs.

Although kV and mAs can be seen to govern different parameters of the X-ray beam, in the diagnostic range of exposures they are linked, in that pictures which appear similar can be produced by raising the kV and at the same time lowering the mAs, or vice versa. A useful and simple rule is that for every 10 kV increase, the mAs can be halved (Figure 20.13). Conversely, if the mAs is doubled, the kV must be reduced by 10. In practice, the time factor is usually paramount and so it is normal to work with as high a kV as possible, allowing the mAs to be kept low.

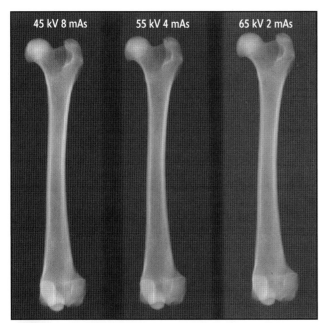

45 kV 8 mAs   55 kV 4 mAs   65 kV 2 mAs

20.13 Interplay between kilovoltage and mAs. If the kilovoltage is increased by 10 and the mAs is halved, the effect on the film is almost identical.

Focal–film distance (FFD)

The FFD is the total distance between the focal spot and the X-ray film. It is important because, although the quality of the X-ray beam remains constant as it travels from the tube head, the intensity falls with increasing distance as the beam spreads out over a larger area. Figure 20.14 shows that if the FFD is doubled, the intensity of the beam over a given area is reduced to one-quarter and the film will appear underexposed unless the mAs is raised. Conversely, if the FFD is reduced the film will appear overexposed. The rule governing this effect is called the **inverse square law**, which states that *the intensity of the primary beam projected on to an X-ray film is reduced to one-quarter by doubling the distance from the X-ray film.* Thus a long FFD requires a higher mAs than a short FFD and the exact figure can be calculated mathematically from the equation:

$$\text{New mAs} = \text{Old mAs} \times (\text{New distance}^2/\text{Old distance}^2)$$

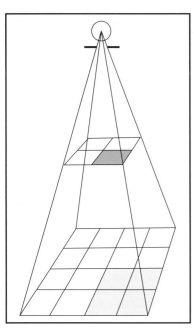

20.14 Inverse square law. The intensity of the beam falling on a given area is reduced to one-quarter by doubling the distance from the point of source.

Longer FFDs require a higher mAs to be used, but image definition will be improved due to a reduction in the penumbra effect. It is normal practice to work always at the same FFD for a given X-ray machine; a suitable distance for a portable X-ray machine is 75 cm, whilst 100 cm is normally used for more powerful X-ray machines that produce a higher milliamperage.

Exposure charts

In order to avoid wastage of film and time in repeating radiographs, it is necessary to build up an exposure chart for each machine. An exposure chart is a list of the kV and mAs required for radiography of various areas of different-sized patients. For the exposure chart to be accurate all other parameters must be kept constant and given on the chart (i.e. line voltage, FFD, film–screen combination, use of a grid and quality of processing). The chart may be compiled for patients of different types (e.g. cats and small, medium, large and giant dogs) or may be made more accurate still by measuring the thickness of the part to be X-rayed using callipers. The exposure chart can be built up over a period of time by recording all exposures made in the X-ray day book, with comments.

Exposure charts are not usually interchangeable between types of machine and may not even be accurate for other machines of the same make and model, because of the varying factors listed above.

X-ray tube rating

The maximum kV and mAs produced by an X-ray tube are determined by the amount of heat production that it can withstand. If this heat production is exceeded, the tube is said to be 'overloaded' and damage may occur. The majority of X-ray machines have built-in fail-safe mechanisms that prevent these limits from being exceeded; and if too high an exposure combination is selected a warning light will come on and the machine will fail to expose. This may not be the case in old machines and so care should be taken to work within the machine's capabilities by consulting the manufacturer's details of maximum safe combinations of kV, mA and time. These details are known as **ratings charts**.

Scattered radiation

Although most of the X-ray photons entering the patient during the exposure are either completely absorbed or pass straight through, a certain proportion undergo a process known as scattering. Scattering occurs when incident photons interact with the tissues, losing some of their energy and 'bouncing' off in random directions as photons of lower energy (Figure 20.15). At lower kilovoltages and when thin areas of tissue are being radiographed, the production of **scattered** or **secondary radiation** is small and most is reabsorbed within the patient. Scatter is therefore not a problem when cats, small dogs and the skull and limbs of larger dogs are being radiographed. However, when higher kilovoltages are required in order to penetrate thicker or denser tissues, the amount and energy of the scattered radiation increases and substantial amounts may exit from the patient's body. The problems associated with this scattered radiation are two-fold:

- Scatter is a potential hazard to the radiographers, as it travels in all directions and may also ricochet back off the tabletop or the floor or walls of the room. This remains a problem in the radiographic examination of equine limbs,

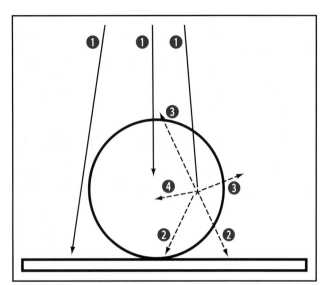

20.15 Formation of scattered radiation. (1) Photons of the primary beam. (2) Scatter in a forwards direction causing film fogging. (3) Scatter in a backwards direction, which is a safety hazard. (4) Some scatter is absorbed by the patient.

but it should be less serious in small animal radiography where patients are usually artificially restrained and the radiographer stands further away.

- Scattered radiation will cause a uniform blackening of the X-ray film unrelated to the radiographic image, and will detract from the film's contrast and definition. The blurring that results is called **fogging.**

Scatter production increases with higher kV, thicker or denser tissues, and larger field sizes of the primary beam. The amount of scattered radiation produced may be reduced in several ways.

Reducing scattered radiation

- **Reduction of the kilovoltage factor** will reduce scattered radiation and the lowest practicable kilovoltage should be selected. This is not always feasible, as in lower-powered X-ray machines the priority is usually to keep exposure time down using a low mAs factor and hence a large kV.
- **Collimation of the primary beam** (i.e. restriction in the size of the primary beam, using a device such as a light beam diaphragm) has a very large effect on the production of scatter. The primary beam should therefore cover only the area of interest, and tight collimation on to very small lesions (such as areas of bone pathology) will greatly improve the quality of the finished radiograph.
- **Reduction of back-scatter** from the tabletop can be achieved by covering it with a 1 mm thick lead sheet.
- **Compression** of a large abdomen using a broad radiolucent compression band will reduce the thickness of tissue being radiographed and will also reduce the amount of scattered radiation produced. Compression band devices may be attached to X-ray tables but should be used with caution in animals with abdominal pathology such as uterine or bladder distension. Compression techniques are no longer widely used in veterinary practice.

The use of grids

Even when the above precautions are taken, scattered radiation is still often a significant problem. The amount of scatter reaching the film can be greatly reduced by using a device known as a grid, which is a flat plate placed between the patient and the cassette. A grid consists of a series of thin strips of lead alternating with strips of a material that allows X-rays through, such as plastic or aluminium. The whole is encased in a protective aluminium cover. X-ray photons that have passed undeflected through a patient will pass through the radiolucent plastic or aluminium strips ('interspaces') but obliquely moving scattered radiation will largely be absorbed by the lead strips (Figure 20.16). Thus there will be a reduction in the degree of film fogging and an improvement in the image quality, though with coarse grids the grid lines will be visible. Significant amounts of scattered radiation are produced from depths of solid tissue greater than 10 cm (or a 15 cm depth of chest, which contains much air) and so the use of a grid is usually recommended for areas thicker than this. Various types of grid are available, and there are two broad groups: stationary grids and moving grids.

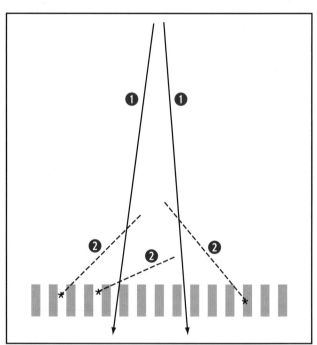

20.16 Effect of a grid. (1) Most primary beam X-ray photons pass through the grid. (2) Obliquely moving scattered radiation is absorbed by the strips of lead.

Stationary grids

Stationary grids are either separate pieces of equipment or are built into the front of special cassettes. Various sizes are available, but it is advisable to buy a grid large enough to cover the biggest cassette used in the practice. Grids are expensive and fragile and should be treated with care, as the strips may be broken if the grid is dropped.

Parallel grids

A parallel grid is the simplest and cheapest type of grid. The strips are vertical, and parallel to each other (Figure 20.17). This means that, since the X-ray beam is diverging from its very small source, the X-ray photons at the edge of the primary beam may also be absorbed by the lead strips, as well as scatter. There may therefore be some reduction in the quality of the film around the edges; this is called **grid cut-off.**

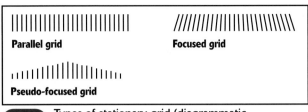

20.17 Types of stationary grid (diagrammatic cross-sections).

Focused grids
A focused grid should prevent grid cut-off, as the central strips are vertical but those on either side slope gradually, to take into account the divergence of the primary beam (Figure 20.17). A focused grid must be used at its correct focal–film distance and should not be used upside down. The X-ray beam must be centred correctly over the grid, at right angles to it.

Pseudo-focused grids
A pseudo-focused grid is intermediate between a parallel and a focused grid in efficiency and price. The strips are vertical but get progressively shorter towards the edges, so reducing the amount of primary beam absorbed (Figure 20.17). Pseudo-focused grids should also be used at the correct focal–film distance and should not be used upside down.

Crossed grids
Most grids contain strips aligned only in one direction and therefore scattered radiation travelling in line with the strips will not be absorbed. Crossed grids contain strips running in both directions and so remove much more scattered radiation. The strips may either be parallel or focused. Crossed grids are expensive and are likely only be used in establishments routinely radiographing equine spines, chests and pelvises.

Moving grids
The use of a stationary grid results in the presence of visible parallel lines on the radiograph. These lines may be eliminated by the use of a grid that oscillates slightly during the exposure. This requires an electronic connection between the X-ray machine and the moving grid or 'Potter–Bucky diaphragm', which is built into the X-ray table. Moving grids are used in larger veterinary institutions and moving grid tables may sometimes be available for purchase second-hand from human hospitals.

Grid parameters

Grid factor
The use of a grid means that, as well as scattered radiation, the grid will absorb some of the useful, primary beam. The mAs factor must therefore be increased when using a grid (to increase the number of X-ray photons in the beam) by an amount known as the grid factor. This is usually 2.5–3 times, but will be specified for each grid. In most cases it will require that a longer exposure time is used, as the X-ray machine will probably be already set at its maximum mA output. The increase in time may increase the risk of movement blur on the film, and the radiographer will have to decide whether or not this is outweighed by the advantages of using a grid.

Lines per centimetre
The greater the number of lines per centimetre, the finer are the grid lines on the film and the less is the disruption to the image (coarse grid lines may be very distracting). The usual number is about 24 lines/cm for grids used in general practice. Grids with finer lines are more expensive.

Grid ratio
The grid ratio is the ratio of the height of the strips to the width of the radiolucent interspace. The higher the grid ratio, the more efficient it is at absorbing scatter, but the more expensive the grid and the larger the grid factor. Practice grids usually have a ratio of 5:1 to 10:1. Grids used with more powerful machines may have a ratio of 16:1.

Recording the X-ray image

Once the X-ray beam has passed through the subject and undergone differential absorption by the tissues, it must be recorded in order to produce a visible and permanent image. The conventional way of doing this is by using X-ray film, which has some properties in common with photographic film – including its sensitivity to white (visible) light. It must therefore be enclosed in a light-proof container (either a metal or plastic cassette or a thick paper envelope) and handled only in conditions of special subdued 'safe-lighting' until after processing. Images can also now be recorded electronically using computed or digital radiography equipment.

Structure of X-ray film
The part of the film that is responsible for producing the image is the **emulsion**, which usually coats the film base on both sides in a thin, uniform layer. The emulsion gives unexposed film an apple green, fawn or mauve colour when examined in daylight (obviously an unexposed film examined in this way will then be ruined for X-ray purposes). The emulsion consists of gelatin in which are suspended tiny grains of silver bromide. The silver bromide molecules are sensitive to X-ray photons and to visible light, both of which change their chemical structure slightly. During a radiographic exposure, X-ray photons passing through the patient will cause this invisible chemical change in the underlying film emulsion, but the picture is not visible to the naked eye and the film will still be spoilt by blackening ('fogging') if exposed to white light. The picture is therefore a hidden or 'latent' image and must be rendered visible to the eye by chemical processing or development. When the film is developed the chemical change in the emulsion continues until those silver bromide grains that were exposed lose their bromine and become grains of pure silver, appearing black when the film is viewed.

The emulsion layers are attached to the transparent polyester film base by a sticky 'subbing' layer and the outer surfaces are protected by a supercoat (Figure 20.18).

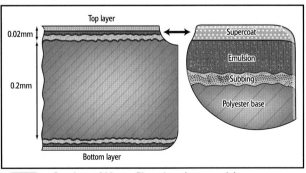

20.18 Section of X-ray film, showing emulsion coats bound to the base by subbing layers and protected by supercoats.

Intensifying screens and cassettes

Unfortunately, X-ray film used alone requires a very large exposure to produce an image and the use of film in this way is unacceptable in most circumstances. However, it was discovered many years ago that the exposure time could be greatly reduced for the same degree of blackening if some of the X-ray photons emerging from the patient were converted into visible light photons by using crystals of phosphorescent material coating flat sheets held against the X-ray film. These devices are known as **intensifying screens** (because they *intensify* the effect of the X-rays on the film) and for many years the commonest phosphor used in the construction of intensifying screens was **calcium tungstate**, which emits blue light when stimulated by X-rays. More recently a new group of phosphors has been used in intensifying screens; these are the **rare-earth** phosphors, which produce blue, green or ultraviolet light. It is important that the X-ray film being used is sensitive primarily to the right colour of light and for this reason some film–screen combinations are incompatible. One advantage of rare-earth screens is that they are more efficient at converting X-radiation into light than are calcium tungstate screens and so exposure factors can be markedly reduced, producing less scattered radiation and images with less movement blur. Additionally, they produce finer image definition. Often the trade name of the screen is embossed along its edge and can be seen on the edge of films exposed in that cassette.

The main benefits of screens are therefore that they:

- Allow much lower mAs settings to be used and so reduce movement blur, scatter production and patient exposure
- Prolong the life of the X-ray tube
- Increase radiographic contrast.

Screens consist of a stiff plastic base covered with a white reflecting surface and then with a layer of the phosphor. Over the top is a protective supercoat layer. The screens are usually used in pairs and are enclosed in a light-proof metal, plastic or carbon fibre box known as a **cassette** (Figure 20.19) with the film sandwiched between. Occasionally a single screen is used together with single-sided emulsion film used for human mammography; such a combination produces images of higher definition but requires slightly larger exposures. These systems are especially popular for equine orthopaedic radiography. For

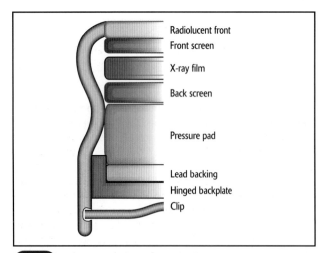

20.19 Cross-section through an X-ray cassette.

Labels in figure:
- Radiolucent front
- Front screen
- X-ray film
- Back screen
- Pressure pad
- Lead backing
- Hinged backplate
- Clip

good detail the film and screens must be in close contact and so the cassette contains a thick felt or foam pad between the back plate and the back screen. Poor screen–film contact causes blurring in that part of the film. The top of the cassette must be radiolucent (i.e. allow X-rays through), and the bottom may be lead-lined to absorb remaining X-rays and prevent back-scatter, though this is uncommon with modern cassettes. The cassette must be fully light-proof with secure fastenings and should be robust. Recently, small flexible plastic cassettes containing one or two screens have become available for small animal intraoral radiography.

Care of intensifying screens and cassettes

Intensifying screens are expensive and fairly delicate and should be treated gently. Scratches or abrasions will damage the phosphor layer permanently, resulting in white (unexposed) marks on all subsequent radiographs produced in that cassette. Screens should not be splashed with chemicals or touched with dirty or greasy fingers. Any dust particles or hairs falling on the screens when the cassette is open in the darkroom will prevent light from reaching the film and will produce fine white specks or lines on the image (even minute particles will prevent the visible light from the intensifying screens from blackening the film in that area, though they will not, of course, interfere with the passage of X-rays). Screens should therefore be cleaned periodically by wiping them gently with lint in a circular motion using a proprietary antistatic screen-cleaning liquid. The cassettes are then propped open in a dust-free environment in a vertical position to allow the screens to dry naturally. If they are reloaded whilst the screens are still damp, the film will stick to the screens and damage them.

Cassettes should be handled carefully and never dropped. They should be kept clean, as stains on the front may produce artefactual shadows on the radiograph and fluids seeping in will mark the screens. The catches must not be strained by closing the cassette when a film is trapped along the edges.

Types of X-ray film

Non-screen film

Non-screen film is film designed for use without intensifying screens, i.e. the image is solely due to X-rays. This requires a very large mAs (long exposure time) but produces extremely fine image definition. The film comes wrapped in thick, light-proof paper rather than being used in a cassette. Non-screen film is now only available as small dental film, which is used for dental radiography and other intraoral views in cats and small dogs. The patient will be anaesthetized for this type of study and so the very high exposure required is not a problem, as the radiographer can retire to a safe distance, and movement blur should not occur. The 13 x 18 cm film that was previously popular for intraoral radiography of dogs and for radiography of small exotic species is no longer manufactured; it has been replaced by flexible plastic cassettes of the same size containing one or two high-detail screens that can be inserted into the mouth of an animal for intraoral radiography. Image quality is inferior to that which is obtained with non-screen film. The flexible nature of these 'cassettes' means that image blurring due to poor screen–film contact will occur if the device is bent in the mouth, but they can be reinforced by taping thick cardboard to them. Care should be taken that the patient's teeth do not damage the device and so an appropriate level of anaesthesia is needed.

Screen film

Screen film is designed for use in cassettes and is used for all other studies. The detail produced is less than with non-screen film, as the visible light produced by the phosphor crystals spreads out in all directions and will result in blackening of a larger number of silver halide grains than the initial X-ray photon would have done – an effect called **screen unsharpness** (Figure 20.20). **Monochromatic** or blue-sensitive film is for use with calcium tungstate or blue light-emitting rare-earth screens; it is sensitive only to visible light in the blue part of the spectrum. For use with green light-emitting rare-earth screens the sensitivity of the film emulsion is extended to include green as well as blue light; this is called **orthochromatic** film. It can therefore be appreciated that whilst green-sensitive film can be used with blue light-emitting screens as well (since it is sensitive to both colours), blue-sensitive film can only be used with blue light-emitting screens. One manufacturer produces ultraviolet light-emitting screens, which should therefore be used only with the same brand of film.

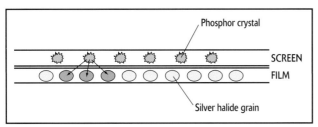

20.20 Screen unsharpness. The arrows show how visible light emitted from each phosphor crystal may affect several silver halide grains, resulting in some loss of definition of the image.

Most types of film are duplitized or double-sided, i.e. there is a layer of emulsion on both sides of the base, which doubles the efficiency of the film and the contrast and density of the image. However, this does result in some loss of definition, due to the superimposition of two slightly different images, and so single-sided emulsion film has become quite popular, especially for equine limb radiography. Human mammography film is used and gives very finely detailed images with good soft tissue and bone detail; it is used in a cassette containing a single green light-emitting screen. The main disadvantages are that the system requires about 5 times more exposure and the film cannot be processed in glutaraldehyde-free developer.

Film and screen speed

The speed of a film, a screen or a screen–film combination describes the exposure required for a given degree of blackening of the film. The speed is due to the size and shape of the phosphor crystals in the screens and the silver bromide grains in the film emulsion, as well as to the thickness of the layers. Fast film–screen combinations require less exposure but produce poorer image definition (the image is more blurred) whereas slow film–screen combinations produce finer detail and are often called **high definition**. In practice, a medium-speed system is usually the best compromise for keeping exposure times down and still getting reasonable quality images. Rare-earth systems give better definition at the same speed. Different manufacturers describe their various films and screens with different terms, which makes it difficult to make comparisons, but most produce several speeds of film and screen, e.g. slow (high detail), medium and fast. If a choice of speeds of film–screen combinations is available in the practice, then a slow high-definition combination may be used where

exposure times are not a problem (e.g. for bone detail in limbs and skulls) but a faster combination should be used where it is important to keep exposure times short in order to reduce movement blur (e.g. for the chest and abdomen), especially if a grid is used.

Films, screens and cassettes come in a range of sizes from 13 x 18 cm to 35 x 43 cm. It is wise to have several different sizes available so as not to waste film by radiographing small areas on large cassettes, though multiple exposures can be made on the same film. Hangers of corresponding size must be available if the films are processed manually.

Storage of X-ray film

As has already been mentioned, unexposed X-ray film is sensitive to light and so must be stored in a light-proof container. This may be either the original film box or a light-proof hopper. Film boxes and loaded cassettes should be kept away from the X-ray area in case they are fogged by scattered radiation; they may be kept in lead-lined cupboards if stored near a source of radiation.

Films are also sensitive to certain chemical fumes and of course to chemical splashes, so good darkroom technique is essential. They may be damaged by pressure or folding and so should be stored upright and handled carefully without being bent or scratched. In hot climates high temperature or humidity may be a problem and so film should be refrigerated. This is not usually necessary in the UK. Film has a finite shelf-life which varies with the type of film. It is therefore wise to date the film boxes on arrival and use them in sequence, within the expiry date shown on the box.

Radiographic processing

The invisible or latent image on the exposed X-ray film is rendered visible and permanent by a series of chemical reactions known as processing. As with photographic film, this must be carried out under conditions of relative darkness as the X-ray film is sensitive to blackening by white light (fogging) until processing is complete.

Although most people now use automatic processors, an understanding of the principles of manual processing is necessary as automatic processors operate on the same principles. This will also permit identification of processing faults, which will appear similar whether caused by problems with manual or automatic processing.

Manual processing

There are five stages in the procedure of manual film processing: development, intermediate rinsing, fixing, washing and drying.

Development

The main active ingredient in the developing solution is either **phenidone-hydroquinone** or **metol-hydroquinone**. These chemicals convert the exposed crystals of silver bromide into minute grains of black metallic silver whilst the bromide ions are released into the solution. This process is known as **reduction** and the developer acts as a **reducing agent**. The length of time for which the film is immersed in the developer (usually 3–5 minutes) is critical, since longer development times will allow some of the unexposed silver bromide crystals to be converted to black metallic silver as well, causing uniform darkening of the film (**chemical** or **development fog**: see section on film faults). The developer must also be used at a constant and uniform temperature (usually 20°C/68°F) and ways of achieving this will be considered later. Precise times and temperatures for developing films are given in the manufacturer's instructions along with some indication of how the development time may be altered to compensate for unavoidable changes in the temperature of the solution.

Other chemicals present in the developing solution include an **accelerator** and a **buffer**, to produce and maintain the alkalinity of the solution necessary for efficient development, and a **restrainer** to reduce the amount of development fog.

X-ray developing solutions are purchased as concentrated liquids. Skin irritation may be observed after handling processing solutions. This may be due to an allergic reaction or due to the alkaline nature of the developer. Gloves should be worn when the chemicals are handled. If the problem is marked, the person's doctor should be consulted and informed of the chemicals involved.

During the development of each film a certain quantity of the developer will be absorbed into the film emulsion and so the level in the developer tank will gradually fall. On no account should the solution be topped up with water, as this will cause dilution and subsequent underdevelopment of films. The original developer solution is also unsuitable for topping up, as the proportions of the different chemical constituents of the developer change with each film that is developed and the solution becomes imbalanced. Instead, special **developer replenisher** solutions should be used, which take into account, and compensate for, this imbalance. Eventually, the developer will become exhausted as the active ingredients are used up and the solution becomes saturated with bromide ions.

Developer will also deteriorate with time by the process of **oxidation**, which will again result in underdevelopment of films. This process can be slowed by keeping the developer tank covered; in larger replenishment tanks there may also be a floating lid on the surface of the solution. Whether or not the developer is used, it is therefore unlikely to be fit for use after 3 months and so the general rule is to change the developer completely either every 3 months or when an equal volume of replenisher has been used, whichever is the sooner.

Rinsing

After the appropriate development time the film and hanger are removed from the solution and quickly transferred to the rinse water tank. Surplus developer should not be allowed to drain back into the developer tank, because it will be saturated with bromide ions and will contribute to developer exhaustion. The film should be rinsed for about 10 seconds to remove excess developer solution and prevent carryover into the fixer tank. Ideally the rinse tank will be situated between the developer and the fixer to prevent splashes of developer falling into the fixer.

Fixing

Following immersion in the developer, development is halted and the image is rendered permanent by a process known as **fixing**. The fixer is acidic and this neutralizes the developer, preventing further development of the emulsion. The fixer also removes the unexposed silver halide crystals, leaving a metallic silver image that can be viewed in normal light, a process known as **clearing**. The fixer contains **sodium** or **ammonium thiosulphate**, which dissolves the unexposed silver halide, causing the emulsion to take on a milky-white appearance until the process is complete. The time taken for the removal of all of the unexposed halide is called the **clearing time** and depends on the thickness of the film emulsion, the temperature and

concentration of the solution and the degree of exhaustion of the fixer. The fixer becomes exhausted as the amount of dissolved silver halide builds up within it, and exhaustion of fixer will occur more quickly than exhaustion of developer.

Fixer temperature is not critical but warm fixer will clear a film faster than cold fixer. However, staining may occur above 21°C/70°F and so the fixer should not be overheated. Fixing can also be speeded up by agitating the film slightly in the fixer. After 30 seconds' immersion in the fixer it is safe to switch on the darkroom light, and the film may be viewed once the milky appearance has cleared. The total fixing time should be at least twice the clearing time, a total of about 10 minutes.

A third function of the fixer bath is to harden the film emulsion (a process known as **tanning**) to prevent the film from being scratched when handled.

As well as the fixing agent (thiosulphate) and the **hardener**, the fixer solution contains a **weak acid** (to neutralize any remaining developer), a **buffer** (to maintain the acidity) and a **preservative**.

Fixing solutions are normally made up from concentrated liquids by the addition of water, according to manufacturer's instructions, as are developing solutions. They should be changed when the clearing time has doubled.

Washing

Following development and fixing, the film must be washed thoroughly to remove residual chemicals which would cause fading and yellow-brown staining of the film. Washing is best achieved by immersion of the film and hanger in a tank with a constant circulation of water, using at least 3 litres per minute so that the film is properly rinsed; static water tanks are much less satisfactory. Washing time should be 15–30 minutes.

Drying

Following adequate washing the films should be removed from their hangers for drying. Films left in hangers of the channel type will not dry adequately around the edges. The usual method is to clip the films to a taut line over a sink, taking care that they do not touch each other. The atmosphere should be dust-free with a good air circulation. Drying frames and warm-air drying cabinets are also available and are useful if film throughput is high.

Manual processing procedure

In order to ensure that no mistakes are made a strict protocol should be adhered to and all those involved in film processing must be familiar with it. The following steps should be carried out.

Preparation

1. Check that the developer and fixer are at the correct level. Check that the developer is at the required temperature and is adequately stirred.
2. Ensure that hands are clean and dry.
3. Select a suitable film hanger and check that new films for reloading the cassette are available.
4. Lock the door, switch on the safe-light and switch off the main light.

Unloading the cassette

1. Open the cassette and take hold of the film gently in one corner between finger and thumb. Shaking the cassette gently first may help to dislodge the film.
2. Remove the film and close the cassette to prevent dirt falling into it.

Identifying the film

If labelling has not been performed during radiography, label the film using a **light marker** if available. These simple devices allow details written or typed on a thin piece of paper to be imprinted on to the corner of the film before processing, using a small flash of light. Often, cassettes contain small lead blockers in one corner to prevent that part of the film being exposed to X-rays and preserving it for the light-marking identification. The paper slips can be overprinted with the practice's name, which adds a professional touch.

Loading the hanger

Load the film into the hanger, handling it as little as possible and touching it only at the edges.

Processing the film

The processing stages are illustrated in Figure 20.21.

1. Remove the developer tank lid, insert the film and hanger and agitate gently to remove air bubbles from the film's surface.
2. Close the lid and commence timing. The lid is kept on for two reasons: firstly it reduces the amount of oxidation of the developer by the atmosphere; and secondly the developing film is still sensitive to fogging by prolonged exposure to the safe-light.
3. The film may be agitated periodically during development to bring fresh developer into contact with the film surface and prevent streaking.
4. At the end of the development period, remove the film and transfer quickly to the rinse tank.
5. Immerse and agitate the film in the rinse water for about 10 seconds.
6. Transfer the film to the fixing tank. After 30 seconds the light may be switched on or the door opened. The film may be examined briefly once the milky appearance has cleared but it should be fixed for at least 10 minutes to allow hardening to take place.
7. Wash in running water for half an hour. (If running water is not available in the darkroom, the film may be washed elsewhere.)
8. Dry the film by hanging it on a taut wire in a dust-free atmosphere. Films in channel hangers must be removed first and hung by clips. Films must not touch each other during drying.

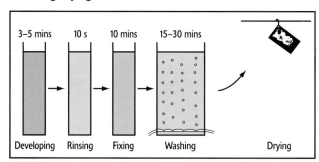

20.21 Processing routine.

Reloading the cassette

This stage may be performed whilst the film is developing.

1. Ensure hands are clean and dry.
2. Open the cassette.
3. Remove a new film from the film box or hopper. Handle carefully without excessive pressure or bending, as unprocessed films are susceptible to damage by pressure.

4. Lay the film in the cassette and, with a fingertip, ensure that it is seated correctly and will not be trapped when the cassette is closed.

Manual processing of non-screen film

As the emulsion of non-screen film is thicker than that of screen film, it takes longer for the developing and fixing chemicals to penetrate the emulsion and act on the silver halide crystals. Development time should normally be increased by about 1 minute and clearing time in the fixer will be several minutes longer.

Automatic processing

Automatic film processing has several advantages over systems of manual film development, as it saves considerable time and effort and produces a dry radiograph that is ready to interpret in a very short space of time (as little as 90 seconds with some machines). In addition, the films are processed to a consistently high standard.

Automatic processors are now widely used in general practice. A darkroom is still required to unload and reload the cassettes, but only a dry bench is necessary. The processor may be entirely within the darkroom, or the feed tray may pass through the darkroom wall to a processor that is located outside.

An alternative is a daylight processor such as may be used in a human hospital; these automatically unload and process the exposed film and then reload the cassette. Daylight processors do not require a darkroom but do require special cassettes and need regular servicing. An alternative found in some practices is a small automatic processor with light-proof sleeves into which the forearms are inserted, manipulating the cassette inside a dark area and feeding the film into the machine by feel.

Construction of an automatic processor

An automatic processor consists of a light-proof container enclosing a series of rollers that pass the film through developer, fixer, wash water and warm air (Figures 20.22 and 20.23). The intermediate rinse is omitted, as excess developer is removed from the films by squeegee rollers. The chemicals are used at a higher temperature (about 28°C/82°F) to speed up the process, and the solutions are pumped in afresh for each film at a predetermined rate; there is therefore no risk of poor processing due to the use of exhausted chemicals. A considerable amount of water needs to flow through the unit for the final rinse and so there must be an adequate water supply and adequate drainage. Finally, the films are dried by a flow of warm air. If the film throughput is high, a silver recovery unit may be attached to the processor to retrieve silver from waste chemicals.

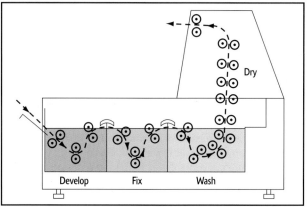

20.22 Essential features of an automatic processor. (Reproduced from Douglas *et al.*, 1987, with permission from Elsevier)

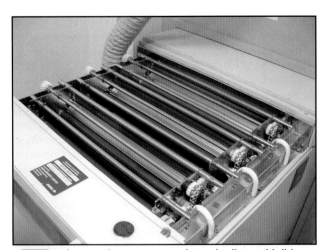

20.23 Automatic processor tanks and rollers, with lid removed.

Maintenance of the automatic processor

Automatic processors usually require a warm-up period of 10–20 minutes prior to use (longer in cold weather). Films processed before the machine has reached its operating temperature will be underdeveloped. After the warm-up period a piece of unexposed film should be passed through to check the correct functioning of the processor and to remove any dried-on chemicals from the rollers by adherence to the unhardened emulsion. At least 10 films per day should be put through the processor to ensure adequate replenishment of the chemicals in the tanks; if necessary these may be old films. At the end of the working day the machine should be switched off and the superficial rollers wiped or rinsed to remove any chemical scum.

Once a week the machine may be given a more thorough clean according to the manufacturer's instructions. This requires a deep sink so that the whole roller assembly for each of the three tanks can be removed and thoroughly cleaned. An old toothbrush is useful for cleaning around the cogs. The tanks also need to be cleaned once the chemicals have been drained out. An algicide solution such as 'Milton' can be added to the wash tank to help to remove algae from the tank walls and roller assembly. Care should be taken when handling chemical solutions as they contain substances that are classified as irritant and can also lead to sensitization from cumulative exposure. Cleaning and mixing tasks should therefore always be undertaken using appropriate eye protection and protective clothing.

The chemicals required are produced specially for automatic processors and are not usually interchangeable with solutions for manual processing as they are formulated for use at higher temperatures. Since fresh chemicals are pumped in for each film and then discarded, there is no need for developer replenisher solution. The chemicals are made up by mixing concentrated solutions thoroughly with water; in the case of the developer there are three concentrates, one acting as a 'starter' solution; for fixer there are two. The constituents must be mixed in the correct order and with the correct amount of water. The developer and fixer solutions are mixed and then stored in tanks ready to be pumped into the processor.

An alternative means of mixing chemicals for automatic processors is by automatic mixer unit. This method provides a safer and more convenient way of mixing and storing chemical solutions. Chemical concentrates for automatic processors are packaged in bottles with plastic seals and screw caps. Mixing is achieved by removing the screw cap and placing the upturned bottle on to the seal opener of the mixing unit; the seal is automatically broken and the contents flow into the tank below, where the correct amount of water is then added. The prepared chemicals can be pumped directly from the mixer unit tanks into the processor.

The automatic processor should be serviced regularly by the manufacturer's engineers as breakdowns can be very inconvenient. Most engineers will also operate an emergency service but nevertheless it may be wise to have the facility to process by hand, should the occasion arise.

Film quality with automatic processing

Although automatic processing will produce films of a consistently good standard, there is always a slight loss of contrast compared with the best that can be achieved by perfect hand processing. The latter is not often achieved and so the automatic processor is usually of great benefit to the practice and likely to increase the enthusiasm of the staff for radiography.

Automatic processing of non-screen film

Non-screen film may be put through the automatic processor but will usually require subsequent manual fixing and further washing and drying to finish the clearing process in the thicker emulsion layers. A small amount of the fixer solution placed in a small plastic box is adequate for this. Depending on the size of the film and the nature of the processor, some non-screen film may be too small to pass through the roller system and will need complete manual development.

Film faults

Radiographic quality is often degraded by faults arising during exposure or processing of the film. It is important to be able to recognize the cause of film faults in order to correct them. Sometimes there may be several possible causes for a given fault. Common film faults, their causes and remedies are discussed in detail in the section 'Assessing radiographic quality' below (see Figure 20.26).

Disposal of waste chemicals

Spent chemical solutions should not be poured into the normal drainage system as they are environmentally damaging. Solutions should be collected and disposed of by a licensed waste disposal company. It is now a legal requirement that the Environment Agency must be notified when hazardous waste, such as spent developer and fixer, is produced or removed from any premises. Records of types and quantities of hazardous waste must then be kept for at least 3 years. Certain types of premises, including veterinary surgeries, are exempt from having to notify the Environment Agency provided that less than 200 kg of hazardous waste are produced per year.

Fixer solution can be collected and reused several times in automatic processors, using dipsticks to test it for activity and to show when it is exhausted. To retrieve the silver content of waste fixer it can then be passed through a silver recovery system, though the cost-effectiveness of this depends upon the world price of silver. Another alternative may be to take fixer to a local hospital to pass through their silver recovery unit.

Darkroom design and maintenance

Requirements

The darkroom is an important part of the radiography set-up within each practice (Figure 20.24). The following factors should be considered in its construction.

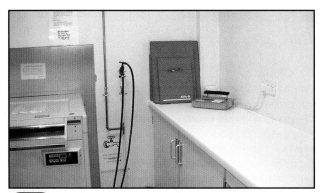

20.24 A darkroom for an automatic processor.

Size
Ideally it should be of a reasonable size to allow for satisfactory working conditions, and should not be used for any other purpose.

Light-proofing
The darkroom must be completely light-proof, and this must be checked by standing inside the darkroom for about 5 minutes until the eyes becomes dark-adapted, as small chinks of light entering may otherwise go unnoticed. The room must be lockable from the inside to prevent the door being opened inadvertently whilst films are being processed. Light-proof maze entrances or revolving cylindrical doors are used in busy hospital departments so that radiographers have free access to the darkroom.

Services
There usually needs to be a supply of electricity and mains water and a drain, though some tabletop processors use water in bottles rather than mains water. Access to a sink for cleaning the processor also needs to be considered when designing the room.

Ventilation
Due to the presence of chemical fumes, some form of light-proofed ventilation is essential.

Walls, floor and ceiling
The walls and ceiling should be painted white or cream (not black) so as to reflect the subdued lighting, making it easier for those working inside to see what they are doing. The walls and floor should be washable and resistant to chemical splashes; it may be wise to tile any wall areas likely to be splashed.

Safe lighting
Since X-ray film is sensitive to white light until the fixing stage, illumination must be achieved using light of low intensity and a specific colour from **safe-lights,** which are boxes containing low-wattage bulbs behind brown or dark red filters. The colour of light produced must be safe for the type of film being processed, as green-sensitive films require different filters to blue-sensitive films. If the wrong filter is used, the films will become uniformly fogged whilst being handled in the darkroom. Safe-light filters must be checked carefully for flaws and damage, as even small pinpricks will allow light leakage; this includes the top filter of an indirect safe-light.

The efficiency of the safe-lights may be checked by laying a pair of scissors or a bunch of keys on an unexposed film on the work bench for periods of up to 2 minutes and then processing it. If significant fogging is occurring, the metal object will be visible on the film. It should be noted that no safe-light is completely safe if the films are exposed for too long or if the safe-light is too close to the handling area. Film manufacturers will advise on the correct filter colour needed for particular types of film.

Two types of safe-light are available: **direct safe-lights** shine directly over the working area and **indirect safe-lights** produce light upwards which is reflected from the ceiling. The number of safe-lights required varies with the size of the room but should be sufficient to allow efficient film handling without fumbling.

Dry and wet areas
If manual processing is used the darkroom should be divided into two working areas: the **dry area** and the **wet area**. If the room is large enough these areas may be separated by being on opposite sides of the room, but where this is not possible they must be separated by a partition to prevent splashes from the wet area reaching the dry bench and damaging the films or contaminating the intensifying screens.

- In the **dry area** the films are stored in boxes (preferably in cupboards) or in film hoppers, loaded into and out of cassettes and placed in the film hangers prior to processing. Sometimes films are also labelled at this stage. Dry film hangers should be stored on a rack above the dry bench and there may also be a storage area for cassettes.
- In the **wet area**, the processing chemicals are kept and used. There should be a viewing box with a drip tray for initial examination of the films, a wall rack for wet hangers and some arrangement for allowing films to dry without dripping over the floor or other working areas.

Usually, the processing solutions are contained in tanks. The **developer tank** should have a well fitting lid to slow down the rate of deterioration of the developer due to oxidation by the atmosphere. Ideally the intermediate **rinse water** is held in a separate tank situated between the developer and the fixer so as to prevent splashes of developer falling into the fixer. The rinse water should be changed frequently. The final **wash tank** should contain running water if possible and should be at least 4 times the size of the developer tank.

In a busy radiography unit the tanks should be housed together in a larger container filled with water and maintained at a constant temperature (usually 20°C/68°F). This **water bath** ensures that the chemicals are always at the correct, uniform temperature for processing and saves time, as well as helping to avoid underdevelopment of films. It is not essential to heat the fixer but inclusion in the water bath will prevent fixing from slowing down in very cold weather. Water bath arrangements may be purchased as special units or may be self-constructed, using an immersion heater and a thermostat.

If a water bath is not available the tanks should sit in a shallow sink to prevent wetting the floor. In this case the developer must be heated prior to use using an immersion heater with a thermostat or a thermometer (the latter requires constant checking). The solution must not be allowed to overheat and must be thoroughly mixed before the film is placed in the tank, as an uneven temperature in the solution will result in patchy development and a mottled appearance to the film.

If few radiographs are processed, the chemicals may be kept in dark, stoppered bottles and poured into shallow dishes for use (as in photography). It may also be necessary to employ this technique should the automatic processor break down or for small dental film that cannot be put through an automatic processor. Unused cat litter trays make ideal processing dishes for radiographs. The correct development temperature is achieved either by heating the solution prior to use or by placing the dish on an electric heating pad. The solutions are usually discarded after use as the developer oxidizes rapidly.

Other darkroom equipment

Film hangers are required for manual processing and are available in two types: **channel hangers** and **clip hangers**. Each type has its advantages and disadvantages. Channel hangers are easier to load but may result in poor development of the edges of the film. Films must be removed for drying and attached to the drying line using clips. The hangers should be washed after the films are removed, as chemicals may otherwise build up in the channels, causing staining of subsequent films. Very large films may not be held securely in channel hangers. Clip hangers avoid these disadvantages but are more fragile and more cumbersome to use and they may tear the films if not used correctly.

A **timer** with a bell should be present in the darkroom so that the period of development can be timed accurately. The timer should ideally be capable of being pre-set to a given time.

A **hand towel** and a **waste-paper bin** are also useful additions to the darkroom.

General care of the darkroom

Most film faults arise during processing and often radiographs that have been carefully taken are spoilt by careless darkroom technique. Competent handling of the films during this stage is therefore vital to the success of radiography within the practice and it is a duty usually delegated to the veterinary nurse. Film faults can also arise during automatic processing.

The darkroom should be kept tidy, clean and uncluttered, with all the equipment in its correct place. Cleanliness is particularly important, as undeveloped films handled with fingers that are dirty or contaminated with developer, fixer or water will show permanent fingerprints. Splashes of liquid falling on to undeveloped films result in black (developer), grey (water) or white (fixer) patches on subsequent films due to interference with light emission. Dust and dirt falling into open cassettes will result in small white screen marks on the radiographs.

With manual processing, attention must also be paid to the maintenance of the processing solutions, as underdevelopment is a common film fault. The tanks should be topped up when the fluid levels fall and the chemicals should be changed regularly, with a record being kept of the date on which they are changed. Developer should be renewed every 90 days or when it has been replenished by the same volume as the original solution, whichever is sooner. Whether using manual or automatic processing, separate mixing rods should be used for making up developer and fixer and should be cleaned after use. Chemicals splashing on to the walls or the floor should be wiped up, as they produce dust when dry and they may stain or corrode the surfaces. The chemical solutions may also damage clothing and so aprons should be worn while they are being mixed. The temperature of the solutions for manual processing should be checked regularly and the heater or thermostat adjusted if necessary.

Other important points are to ensure that the cassettes are always reloaded ready for use when the previous film is removed and to check that a sufficient number of film hangers are always clean and dry.

Other image recording methods

With modern technological advances new methods of acquiring and viewing radiographic images have become available. These methods are based on digital acquisition of the image where the radiographer is still required to position the animal accurately and select the appropriate exposure factors, but the acquired image is viewed on a computer monitor and may be printed to produce a hard copy.

Two main systems currently exist: computed radiography and digital radiography.

Computed radiography (CR)

CR replaces the conventional film and cassette with an imaging plate (IP) containing a photostimulable storage phosphor that can be used in conjunction with conventional X-ray generating apparatus. IPs look very similar to conventional cassettes and are available in the same sizes but are lighter in weight. The radiographic image is recorded on the storage phosphor, which is usually made from barium fluorohalide crystals coated with europium. To process the image the exposed IP is placed in a reader unit, where it is read by laser and digitized by computer (Figure 20.25); the image can then be viewed on a workstation monitor and may be stored on disc or printed by laser printer. IPs are reusable and are erased and reset within the reader unit ready to be used again.

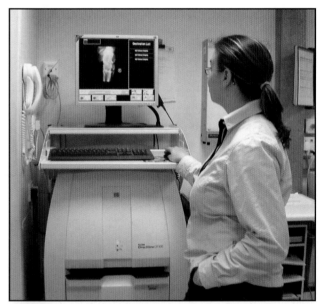

20.25 Reader unit for computed radiography.

Digital radiography (DR)

DR systems record X-ray images using flat panel detectors (FPDs) instead of conventional film and cassettes. FPDs are connected to the image processor by cable linkage and are available in a wide range of sizes from as large as 50 x 50 cm down to small sizes suitable for dental radiography. There are two DR systems available that employ different technologies to create digital radiographs; these are indirect DR (IDR) and direct DR (DDR). Both IDR and DDR systems require dedicated X-ray generating equipment and cannot be used with conventional equipment.

IDR uses FPDs that contain intensifying screens which convert X-rays to light, which is then converted to electrical charge by a device known as a charge coupled device (CCD). Each element of the CCD translates light photons into an electrical charge proportional to the light intensity received. Information from the CCD is processed by computer and the resulting image is displayed on a workstation monitor.

DDR uses FPDs that convert X-rays directly into electrical charge with the use of crystals such as amorphous selenium. Electrical charges are stored in capacitors that are 'read' and processed by computer; the resultant radiograph is displayed on the workstation screen.

Viewing the radiograph

Although the radiograph may be examined whilst it is still wet (for technical quality, a provisional diagnosis or the need for a contrast study), the image will be somewhat blurred due to swelling of the two layers of wet emulsion. Full examination must be delayed until the film has dried, when the emulsion will have shrunk and the image is clearer. Films should be examined on clean viewing boxes (not held up to a window) in a dim area to allow the eyes to pick out detail on the film without distracting glare from elsewhere. If the film is small, the rest of the viewer may be masked off with a black card – a simple procedure that will allow very much more detail to be appreciated. Relatively overexposed areas should be examined with a special bright light, and a magnifying glass may be useful to look for fine detail.

Assessing radiographic quality

Films must be of high technical quality if a radiographic examination is to produce maximum information about the patient. Errors can arise both during radiography and in the darkroom and the radiographer should be able to assess the film for its quality, recognize any faults and know how to correct them (Figure 20.26). Before film faults can be recognized, it is necessary to understand the terms **density**, **contrast** and **definition**.

Density

Radiographic density is the degree of blackening of the film and is determined by two factors: the **exposure** used and the **processing technique**:

Exposure

Film blackening is affected by the quantity of X-rays passing through the patient and reaching the film. It is influenced by the kilovoltage, the mAs and the FFD. If the patient's image is generally too dark, then the film is **overexposed** and the exposure factors should be reduced or the FFD increased; conversely, if it is too light, then it is **underexposed** and the exposure factors should be increased or the FFD reduced. Usually, corrections are made to the exposure factors; the FFD should remain constant unless it has been inadvertently altered.

Processing

Radiographic density can also be affected by processing. **Underdevelopment**, due to the use of diluted, exhausted or cold developer or development for too short a time, will cause all areas of the film to be too light, including the background. Development can be tested by performing the **finger test**, i.e. putting a finger between the film and the light viewer in an area where the film was not covered by the patient and which should therefore be completely black. If the finger is visible, the film is underdeveloped. Underdevelopment is the commonest film fault arising with manual processing, and should be corrected by topping up the developer with replenisher (not water), by changing the solution regularly and by ensuring that it is used at the correct temperature and for the correct length of time. Underdevelopment may also occur with automatic processing, if the machine is not working at the correct temperature. **Overdevelopment** may occur if the developer is too hot or if the film is inadvertently left in the solution for too long. In this case some of the *un*exposed silver halide crystals will be converted to black metallic silver, leading to uniform darkening of the film or **development fog**.

Overexposure and **overdevelopment** may be hard to differentiate, as both will cause an increased radiographic density. However, areas covered by metal markers during the exposure will remain white if the fault is overexposure but will darken if the film is overdeveloped.

Underexposure and **underdevelopment** can usually be easily differentiated. Underdevelopment will produce a grey background using the finger test; with underexposure the background should still be black but the area covered by the patient will be too pale.

In general, films that are too dark are to be preferred to those that are too light, as they may still yield adequate information when examined under a bright light.

Contrast

Contrast is the difference between various radiographic densities (shades of grey) seen on the radiograph. A medium contrast film with a reasonable number of grey shades as well as white and black on the image is desirable, as it will yield most information. A film that shows a white image on a black background with few intermediate grey shades has too high a contrast ('soot and whitewash') and is due to the use of too low a kilovoltage with insufficient penetrating power. A film without extremes of density, showing mainly grey shades, has a very low contrast and is called a 'flat' film. Poor contrast is usually due to underdevelopment, in which case the background will be grey (use the finger test). Overexposure, overdevelopment and various types of fogging will also produce a flat film but in this case the background density will be black and the remainder of the film will also be very dark.

Definition

Definition refers to the sharpness and clarity of the structures visible on a radiograph. Good definition is usually essential if the film is to be diagnostic. Definition may be affected by a number of factors, as follows.

Movement blur

This is the most common cause of poor definition on chest and abdomen radiographs and is usually due to respiration or struggling by the patient. It may also occur if the tube stand is unstable or if the cassette moves (the latter is applicable only to equine radiography). Patient movement is minimized by the use of sedation or general anaesthesia and by adequate artificial restraint using sandbags etc. The exposure time should be kept as low as possible.

Scattered radiation

Scattered radiation produced when thick or dense areas of tissue are X-rayed will produce random darkening of the film, resulting in loss of definition and contrast. Its effects may be reduced by collimating the beam and by the use of a grid.

Fault	Cause	Remedy
Film too dark	Overexposure	Reduce exposure factors; check thickness of patient; check correct film/screen combination used
	Overdevelopment	Check developer temperature; time development accurately; check automatic processor cycle and thermostat
	FFD too short	Increase FFD
	Fogging	See below for causes and remedies
Film too pale	Underexposure (background black but image too light)	Increase exposure factors; check thickness of patient; check correct film/screen combination used
	Underdevelopment (background pale only)	Check developer temperature; time development accurately; check automatic processor cycle and thermostat; change developer
	FFD too long	Decrease FFD
Patchy film density	Developer not stirred; film not agitated in developer	Correct the development technique
Contrast too high ('soot and whitewash film')	kV too low	Increase kV
Contrast too low ('flat film')	Overexposure	Reduce exposure factors
	Underdevelopment	Correct the development technique
	Overdevelopment	Correct the development technique
	Fogging	See below for causes and remedies
Fogging	Scattered radiation from patient	Collimate the beam; use a grid
	Scattered radiation from elsewhere	Change storage area for films and cassettes
	Exposure to white light before fixing stage	Check darkroom and safe-lights, film hoppers, lids on film boxes, keep lid on developer whilst film in the tank
	Storage fog	Use films before expiry date
	Chemical or development fog	Avoid overdevelopment
Image blurring	Patient movement Tube head movement Cassette movement Scattered radiation Fogging Poor film–screen contact Large object–film distance (OFD) Double exposure	Depends on the cause
Extraneous marks:		
small, bright marks	Dirt on the intensifying screens	Clean the screens
black patches	Developer splashes on film	Careful processing
white patches	Fixer splashes on film	Careful processing
grey patches	Water splashes on film	Careful processing
	Chemical splashes on intensifying screens	Careful processing
scratches	Careless handling of unprocessed film	Clean the screens
	Guideshoes of automatic processor malaligned	Handle unprocessed film carefully
crescentic black crimp marks	Bending of unprocessed film	Handle unprocessed film carefully
fingerprints	Handling of unprocessed film with dirty hands	Wash and dry hands before processing
branching black marks	Static electricity	Handle unprocessed film carefully; use antistatic screen cleaner
parallel marks on film	Roller marks	Check seating and cleanliness of rollers
scum on surface	Scale or algae in processor	Clean processor; use water softener or anti-algal agents
Chemical stains:		
yellowing/browning on storage	Insufficient fixing or washing	Correct fixing/washing
areas of film supposed to be clear are grey and opaque	Insufficient fixing	Increase fixing time; change fixer
borders around films	Dirty channel hangers	Clean the hangers
Grid lines too coarse	X-ray beam not perpendicular to grid; focused or pseudo-focused grid used upside down	Correct alignment of beam and grid
Damp films for automatic processor	Thermostat malfunction	Call service engineer
	Dryer temperature too low	Call service engineer
	Insufficient fixing	Change fixer

20.26 Common faults and their remedies.

Fog

Fogging is darkening of the film unrelated to the radiographic image and has a number of causes. These include: scattered radiation; accidental exposure of the film to radiation or white light prior to or during processing; the use of an unsuitable safe-light filter; prolonged storage; and overdevelopment. The result is a loss of definition and contrast.

Poor film–screen contact

Poor contact between the intensifying screen and the film within the cassette due to shrinkage of the felt or foam pad will cause blurring of the image in the affected area. It will be present in the same place on all films taken in that cassette.

Film and screen speed

Fast film–screen combinations require a lower exposure for a given degree of film blackening than do slower combinations, but the definition of the image is poorer due to the larger size of the phosphor crystals in the intensifying screens and to the characteristics of the film emulsion.

Focal spot size

Some machines allow a choice of focal spot size. **Fine focus** produces finer radiographic detail but the exposure factors available are limited. **Coarse focus** allows higher exposure factors but, since the effective focal spot is larger, some detail is lost by the penumbra effect (see Figure 20.5). The penumbra effect is reduced by keeping the object–film distance as small as possible and by using a reasonably long focus–film distance.

Magnification and object–film distance (OFD)

Since the X-ray beam diverges from the focal spot, the geometry of the X-ray beam results in some degree of magnification of the image. Magnified images will usually also be blurred, because the penumbra effect increases with increasing OFD. In order to reduce this effect, the part being radiographed should always be positioned as close as possible to the film, with the focal–film distance as long as is practicable for that machine (Figure 20.27).

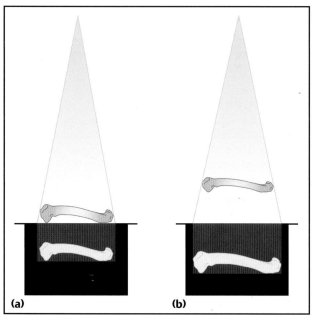

20.27 Magnification and object–film distance (OFD). **(a)** Object close to film, so reproduced accurately on radiograph. **(b)** Object not close to film, so image is magnified.

Labelling, storage and filing of radiographs

Labelling

All radiographs should be permanently labelled with the case identification (name or number), the date, a right or left marker if appropriate and any other relevant details (e.g. time after administration of a contrast medium). Labelling of the paper sleeve or film envelope only is inadequate and liable to cause mix-ups, especially on busy days. Films can be labelled at one of three stages: during exposure, in the darkroom or on dry film after processing.

Labelling during exposure

Films can be identified during radiography by placing lead letters on the cassette or by writing details on special graphite tape, which is then stuck to the cassette. Care should be taken to ensure that the whole of the information appears on the film after processing and is neither lost on the edge of the film nor overexposed. Right or left markers should be used at this stage (and not substituted for by the use of personal codes such as scissors or keys).

Labelling in the darkroom

Films may also be identified by labelling in the darkroom prior to processing. The most efficient method is to use a light marker, which is a small device that prints information, written or typed on paper, on to the corner of the film, using white light. A small rectangular area in the corner of the film must therefore be protected from exposure to X-rays by the incorporation of a piece of lead in the cassette to act as a blocker and leave a space on the film on which these details may be printed. There are also special cassettes available with a movable window which can be inserted into a light-marking camera for imprinting the details; this can be done in daylight outside the darkroom.

Labelling of the dry film

Information may be written on the film after processing using a white 'Chinagraph' pencil, white ink or a black felt-tip pen. Such identification may not be acceptable for films used in legal cases, and so labelling after processing is not good practice.

Identification of radiographs for the BVA/KC scoring schemes

The requirement for submission of films to the BVA/KC Hip and Elbow Dysplasia Scoring Schemes is that they must be identified with the dog's Kennel Club number during radiography, i.e. using lead letters or tape or by a light marker before processing. Labelling after processing is not acceptable. The date and right or left markers as appropriate must also be present.

Storing and filing radiographs

Radiographs may be required for retrospective study or as legal documents and so should be clearly labelled and carefully filed. Many films can accumulate within a short space of time in a busy practice and the filing system must be simple and foolproof.

Films processed manually must be completely dry before filing, otherwise they will be damaged by sticking to paper. Films may be stored in their original paper folders or in special X-ray envelopes, with case details (e.g. owner's name, patient information and date) marked clearly on the outside. These may then be kept in film boxes, filing cabinets or on shelving depending on the number of films involved. Films may be stored either chronologically or in alphabetical order of owner's name, with films from each year usually being kept separately. Films of special interest and good examples of normal anatomy should be noted for future reference.

Viewing and storage of digital radiographs

Viewing

Images acquired on CR and DR systems are viewed on a video monitor and may be post-processed by the user to enhance the image and improve their diagnostic value. Typical post-processing techniques include **subtraction** for improving prominence of the anatomical area of interest by removing superimposed structures, **edge enhancement** for improving visibility of small high-contrast structures (e.g. foreign bodies in soft tissue) and **brightness and contrast enhancement** to enable the user to improve the image subjectively. Other post-processing tools allow the image to be magnified, annotated and mirrored. Post-processed images can be stored, printed by laser printer and transmitted to other monitors within the same facility or to other premises where compatible viewing equipment is available (**teleradiology**).

Storage

Storage of digitally acquired radiographs usually takes two forms: **on-line** and **off-line** storage. On-line is for storage of images in the short-term and data can be stored on hard disc drive or RAID (Redundant Array of Independent Disks) unit, both methods enabling digital data to be stored and retrieved rapidly (in seconds).

For long-term storage and archiving there are three main storage media: magnetic discs, magnetic tape and optical discs.

Magnetic media

Magnetic discs and magnetic tape work in a similar way to videocassette tape and must therefore be protected from strong magnetic fields or environmental extremes.

Optical discs

Optical discs consist of a glass disc coated thinly with metal alloy and contained within a protective cartridge. Digital data are 'burned' on to the disc by laser writer, resulting in a permanent data record. This type of disc is also known as a WORM (Write Once Read Many) disc because once data have been stored they are non-erasable but may be retrieved repeatedly. Optical discs have larger data storage capacity than magnetic media and provide a reliable non-corruptible medium for archiving digital radiographs.

Radiation protection

Dangers associated with radiography

Exposure of the human or animal body to radiation is not without hazard, because of the biological effects that X-rays have on living tissues via cellular chemical reactions. X-rays have four properties that mean that the danger from them may be seriously underestimated:

- They are **invisible**.
- They are **painless**.
- The effects are **latent**, i.e. they are not evident immediately and may not manifest until some time later – even several decades in some cases.
- Their effects are **cumulative** and so repeated very low doses may be as hazardous as a single large exposure.

Large doses are unlikely to occur in human or veterinary radiography but may be seen after nuclear accidents. It is the danger arising from repeated exposure to small amounts of radiation that concerns people working with veterinary radiography. Despite these hazards, it is possible to perform radiography in veterinary practice with no significant risk to any of the people involved, provided that adequate precautions are taken.

The adverse effects of radiation on the body may be divided into three groups: somatic, carcinogenic and genetic.

Somatic effects

These are direct changes in body tissues that usually occur soon after exposure. They include skin reddening and cracking, blood disorders, baldness, cataract formation and digestive upsets. The latter cause severe dehydration, which is the usual cause of death following nuclear accidents or bombs. Different tissues vary in their susceptibility to this type of damage, with the developing fetus being particularly susceptible. The somatic effect is used to advantage in the radiotherapy of tumours, since tumour cells are often more sensitive to radiation damage than are normal cells.

Carcinogenic effects

These are the induction of tumours in tissues that have been exposed to radiation. There may be a considerable time lag before these tumours arise; it may be as long as 20–30 years in the case of leukaemia.

Genetic effects

These occur when gonads (ovaries and testes) are irradiated and mutations are induced in the chromosomes of germ cells. The mutations may give rise to inherited abnormalities in the offspring.

Sources of radiation hazard

During an exposure, there are three potential sources of X-rays that may be hazardous to the radiographers: the tube head, the primary beam and secondary or scattered radiation (Figure 20.28).

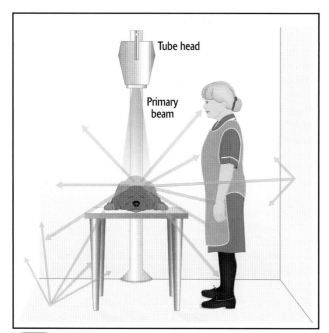

20.28 Spread of scattered radiation.

Tube head

Although the tube head is lead-lined (except at the window where the primary beam emerges), older machines may have suffered cracks in the casing, which allows X-rays to escape in other directions. For this reason the tube head should never be held or touched during an exposure. Checks on the efficiency of the casing can be made by taping envelope-wrapped non-screen film to the tube head, leaving it for a few exposures and then processing it. Any cracks in the casing will cause black lines to appear on the film, where it has been exposed.

Primary beam

The beam of X-rays produced at the anode is directed out of the tube head through the window. This primary beam consti-tutes the greatest safety hazard, since it consists of high-energy X-rays. It may be visualized using a **light beam dia-phragm**, a device attached to the tube head that produces a light over the area covered by the X-ray beam (Figure 20.29). The light beam diaphragm usually contains crossed wires that produce a shadow in the illuminated area, showing the posi-tion of the centre of the beam (the **central ray**). Movable metal

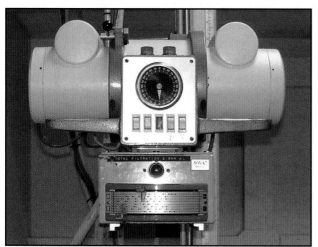

20.29 A light beam diaphragm attached to an X-ray tube head.

plates operated by knobs allow the area covered to be ad-justed to the size required, a procedure known as **collimation**. Collimation should always be as 'tight' as possible (i.e. to as small an area as possible) and the accuracy of the light beam diaphragm should be checked periodically. This can be done by arranging pairs of coins along each margin of the light beam with their edges touching, so that one of each pair lies inside and one outside the light beam, and making an exposure. After processing, the image should show four coins inside the black area and the other four coins outside, if the light beam diaphragm was accurate.

An alternative but now uncommon method of collimation is to use conical or cylindrical devices or **cones** attached to the tube window to produce a circular primary beam of varying diameter. Cones are much less satisfactory than light beam diaphragms, since the area covered by the primary beam is not seen. Whichever method of collimation is used, the area covered by the primary beam should be no larger than the size of the cassette, and so the borders of the beam should be visible on the processed radiograph.

No part of any handler should come within the primary beam, even if protected by lead rubber clothing. In the rare cases where animals have to be held for radiography, a light beam diaphragm *must* be used to ensure that the primary beam is safely colli-mated. To prevent the primary beam from passing through the table and scattering off the floor or irradiating the feet of any handlers, the tabletop should be covered with lead or else a lead sheet should be placed underneath the cassette.

The use of a horizontal X-ray beam is especially hazardous, as the primary beam will pass with little attenuation through doors, windows and thin walls. This procedure should only be performed with great care, with the primary beam directed only towards a thick wall. The procedure for the use of hori-zontal beam radiography should be described in the practice's Local Rules (see below).

Secondary or scattered radiation

Scattered radiation is produced in all directions when the pri-mary beam strikes a solid object, and so it arises from the patient and the cassette. It is produced by the table or floor if the tabletop is not lead-lined; it can also bounce off walls and ceil-ings and travel in unexpected directions. It is, however, of much lower energy than the primary beam and is absorbed by pro-tective clothing. Its intensity falls off rapidly with distance from the source (due to the inverse square law). The best protection against scatter is to stand as far from the X-ray machine and patient as possible – a minimum of 2m, and better still behind a lead-lined screen.

Ways of reducing the amount of scatter produced (as al-ready discussed in the section on scattered radiation, above) include tight collimation of the primary beam, compression of large areas of soft tissue, reduction in the kilovoltage where possible and the use of lead-backed cassettes and a lead-topped table. Protection against scatter is also afforded by protective clothing. The rotation of staff involved in large-animal radio-graphy is advisable, since personnel may of necessity stand closer to the primary beam. With small-animal radiography and non-manual restraint, rotation of staff is less important.

Legislation

In 1985 the law governing the use of radiation and radioactive materials was revised and updated with the publication of The Ionizing Radiations Regulations (IRR) 1985, since updated as the Ionizing Radiations Regulations (revised) 1999. This legal document covers all uses of radiation and radioactive materials, including veterinary radiography. As it is written in legal terms and is somewhat lengthy, a second booklet was published at the same time which attempted to explain the Regulations and is called the Approved Code of Practice for the Protection of Persons against Ionizing Radiation arising from any Work Activity. The Code of Practice does contain some specific references to veterinary radiography but is also rather long-winded and so guidance notes explaining the law as it applies to veterinary radiography were published by the BVA in 2002 (Veterinary Guidance Notes for the Ionizing Radiations Regulations 1999). These cover premises, equipment, personnel and procedures and aim to minimize radiation doses received by veterinary staff. A summary of the legislation is given in the following paragraphs.

Principles of radiation protection

Protection follows three basic principles:

- Radiography should only be undertaken if there is definite clinical justification for the use of the procedure
- Any exposure of personnel should be kept to a minimum. The three words to remember are: Time, Distance, Shielding (i.e. reduce the need for repeat exposures, stand well back and wear protective clothing or stand behind a lead screen)
- No dose limit should be exceeded.

The aim is to avoid exposure at all times, but failing this a high standard of protection will exist if the advice contained in the Guidance Notes is followed.

Local Rules and written arrangements

The **Local Rules** are a set of instructions drawn up by the practice's Radiation Protection Adviser which set down details of equipment, procedures and restriction of access to the controlled area for that practice. The **written arrangements** are part of the Local Rules and include the sequence of actions to be followed for each exposure, including the method of restraint of patients for radiography and the precautions to be taken should manual restraint be necessary. A copy of the Local Rules should be given to anyone involved in radiography (including the nurses) and should also be displayed in the X-ray room.

Radiation Protection Supervisor (RPS)

An RPS must be appointed within the practice and will usually be the principal or a senior partner, although may be the Head Nurse in some practices. The RPS is responsible for ensuring that radiography is carried out safely and in accordance with the Regulations, and that the Local Rules are obeyed, but the person need not be present at every radiographic examination.

Radiation Protection Adviser (RPA)

Most practices will also need to appoint an external RPA. RPAs must hold a certificate of competence issued by an appropriate body stating that they have the knowledge, experience and competence required to act as a veterinary RPA. They are usually medical physicists, though holders of the RCVD Diploma in Veterinary Radiology who have undertaken appropriate further training may also be eligible. The RPA will give advice on all aspects of radiation protection, the demarcation of the controlled area and will advise on drawing up the Local Rules and instructions for safe working.

The controlled area

A specific room should be identified for small-animal radiography and should have sufficiently thick walls that no part of the controlled area extends outside it (single brick is usually adequate; thin walls may be reinforced with lead ply or barium plaster). The room should be large enough to allow people remaining in the room to stand at least 2 m from the primary beam. If this is not possible, a protective lead screen should be provided, unless the radiographer can routinely step outside the room and stand behind a brick wall during the exposure. Unshielded doors and windows may be acceptable if the work load is low and the room is large enough. Special recommendations are made for flooring in cases where there may be an occupied area below the radiography room.

Technically, the **controlled area** is the area around the primary beam within which the average dose rate of exposure exceeds a given limit (laid down in the Regulations). The controlled area for a typical practice is within a 2 m radius from the beam but usually needs to be defined by the RPA. Since the controlled area must be physically demarcated and clearly labelled, it is usually simpler to designate the whole X-ray room as a controlled area and to place warning notices on its doors to exclude people not involved in radiography. When the radiographic examination is completed the X-ray machine must be disconnected from the power supply; the room then ceases to be a controlled area and may be entered freely.

A **warning sign** should be placed at the entrance to the X-ray room, consisting of the radiation warning symbol and a simple legend (see Chapter 1). For permanently installed equipment there should also be an automatic signal at the room entrance indicating when the X-ray machine is in a state of readiness to produce X-rays. This signal usually takes the form of a red light or an illuminated sign. Whilst not a legal requirement for portable and mobile X-ray machines (which comprise the majority of practice X-ray machines), many practitioners have installed red lights outside their radiography rooms to warn when radiography is in progress and prevent accidental entry, and this is to be recommended.

In addition, all X-ray machines should have lights visible from the control panel indicating (a) when they are switched on at the mains and (b) when exposure is taking place. Sometimes (b) is instead a noise such as a beep or buzz.

X-ray equipment

Radiation safety features of the X-ray machine should be regularly checked by a qualified engineer. Leakage radiation from the tube housing must not exceed a certain level and the beam filtration must be equivalent to not less than 2.5 mm aluminium. All machines must be fitted with a collimation device, preferably a light beam diaphragm. The exposure button must allow the radiographer to stand at least 2 m from the primary beam, which means either that it must be at the end of a sufficiently long cable or else that it should be on the control panel which is placed well away from the tube head. The timer should be electronic rather than clockwork, as exposures cannot usually be aborted with the latter, should the patient move.

Suppliers of X-ray machines have a responsibility to ensure that they are safe and functioning correctly, and they should provide a report to this effect when installing the equipment. *Servicing of X-ray machines is a legal requirement and should be carried out at least once a year.*

The X-ray table must be lead-lined, or else a sheet of lead 1 mm thick and larger than the maximum size of the beam should be placed on the table and beneath the cassette to absorb the residual primary beam and reduce scatter. Many practices now use purpose-built X-ray tables that are not only lead-lined but also fitted with hooks to aid in patient positioning.

Practices performing equine radiography also require cassette holders with long handles for supporting cassettes during limb radiography, and various types of wooden blocks for positioning the lower limbs with the minimum of manual restraint.

Film and film processing

The Regulations recommend the use of fast film–screen combinations in order to reduce exposure times. They stress the importance of correct processing techniques in order to minimize the number of non-diagnostic films and avoid the need for repeat exposures.

Recording exposures

It is necessary to record each radiographic exposure made and this is done using a daybook for radiography including the following details for each exposure: date; patient identity and description; exposure factors used; quality of image; and means of restraint. If the animal has had to be held during radiography, the name(s) of the person(s) doing so must be recorded.

Protective clothing

Protective clothing consists of aprons, gloves and sleeves and is usually made of plastic or rubber impregnated with lead. The thickness and efficiency of the garment is described in millimetres of lead equivalent (LE), i.e. the thickness of pure lead that would afford the same protection. It is important to remember that *protective clothing is only effective against scatter and does not protect against the primary beam.*

Lead aprons should be worn by any person who needs to be present in the X-ray room during the exposure. They are designed to cover the trunk (especially the gonads) and should reach at least to mid-thigh level. Their thickness should be at least 0.25 mm LE; many are 0.35 or even 0.5 mm LE, though the latter are rather heavy to wear. Single-sided aprons covering the front of the body but with straps at the back are cheaper but provide less protection than double-sided aprons covering both front and back and are also less comfortable to wear for long periods. Aprons are expensive items and should be handled carefully; when not in use they should be stored on coat hangers or on rails and they must never be folded as this can lead to undetected cracking of the material (Figure 20.30).

Lead gloves, open-palm mitts and hand shields must be available for use in those cases where manual restraint of the patient is unavoidable. They are also required for equine radiography when a limb or a cassette holder may need to be held.

Lead sleeves are tubes of lead rubber into which the hands and forearms may be inserted as an alternative to gloves. Single sheets of lead rubber draped over the hands are not adequate as they do not protect against back-scatter.

Gloves, hand shields and sleeves should be at least 0.35 mm LE and must never appear in the primary beam, since they offer inadequate protection against high-energy X-rays. It is important to remember that, although a lead glove may appear completely opaque on a radiograph, the film is being protected by two layers of lead rubber but the hand by only one (Figure 20.31). Lead rubber **neck guards** for protection of the thyroid gland may also be used.

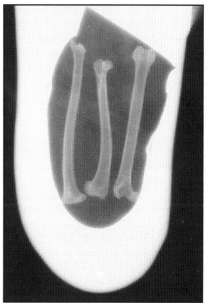

20.31
Radiograph of bones covered by a single thickness of lead rubber: compare with the edge, where there are two layers of lead rubber.

All items of protective clothing should be checked frequently for signs of cracking. A small defect may not allow many X-rays through but will always be over the same area of skin. If in doubt, the garment may be X-rayed to check for cracks (Figure 20.32). Mobile lead screens with lead glass windows are also useful as the radiographer can stand behind them during the exposure and still see the patient. Unfortunately they are very expensive.

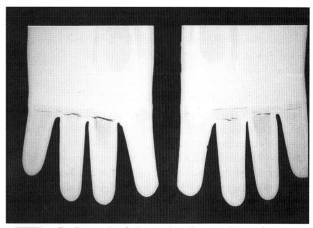

20.30 Correct storage of lead aprons and gloves.

20.32 Radiograph of gloves showing cracking of the lead rubber at the usual site – the base of the fingers.

Dosimetry

All persons who are involved in radiography should wear small monitoring devices or **dosemeters** to record any radiation to which they are exposed. Dosemeters should be worn on the trunk beneath the lead apron, though an extra dosemeter may be worn on the collar or sleeve to monitor the levels of radiation received by unprotected parts of the body. Each dosemeter should be worn only by the person to whom it is issued and it must neither be left in the X-ray room whilst not being worn nor exposed to heat or sunlight. Two types of dosemeter are available:

- **Film badges** contain small pieces of X-ray film and are usually blue. They contain small metal filters that allow assessment of the type of radiation to which the badge has been exposed.
- **Thermoluminescent dosemeters** (TLDs) contain radiation-sensitive lithium fluoride crystals and are usually orange. On exposure to radiation the electrons in the crystals are rearranged, thus storing energy. During the reading process the crystals are heated and give off light in proportion to the amount of energy that they have stored – this gives a quantitative reading.

Dosemeters are obtained from dosimetry services such as the National Radiological Protection Board (RPA) and they should be sent off for reading every 1–3 months, depending on the radiographic caseload. If animals are likely to be held for radiography (e.g. equine work), special finger badges may be worn inside the lead gloves to monitor the dose to the hands.

Dosemeters may also be used to monitor radiation levels in the X-ray room or in adjacent rooms by mounting them on the wall. They can be used to check the adequacy of protection offered by internal walls and doors. The exact arrangement for dosimetry in the practice will be made in consultation with the RPA, and the records must be filed for easy retrieval. Anyone whose badge reveals a reading should be informed, so that the cause can be identified if possible and working practices adjusted accordingly.

Dose limits

Dose limits are amounts of radiation that are thought not to constitute a greater risk to health than those encountered in everyday life. Legal limits have been laid down for various categories of person and for different parts of the body. Maximum permitted doses (MPDs) are laid down for the whole body, for individual organs, for the lens of the eye and for pregnancy. 'Classified' persons are those working with radiation who are likely to receive more than 30% of any relevant MPD. However, in veterinary practice these levels should not be reached and so veterinary workers rarely need to be designated as classified persons, provided that they are working under written arrangements (see above).

Staff involved in radiography

The Local Rules will include a list of names of designated persons authorized to carry out exposures. It should be remembered that nurses and other lay staff aged 16 or 17 have a lower MPD than do adults aged 18 or over and therefore their involvement in radiography should be limited. Young people under 16 years of age should not be present during radiography under any circumstances. Owners should not routinely be present as they are members of the general public and are neither trained in radiography nor wearing dosemeters, although their presence may be necessary in emergency

situations. The Local Rules should ensure that doses to pregnant women are well within the legal limit, but nevertheless it is wise to avoid the involvement of pregnant women in radiography whenever possible.

The general rule is that the minimum number of people should be present during radiography. When, as is usual, the patient is artificially restrained, only the person making the exposure need be present and this should be the case in the majority of radiographic studies. Often the radiographer will be able to stand outside the room during the exposure.

Radiographic procedures and restraint

Whenever possible, the beam should be directed vertically downwards on to an X-ray table. The minimum number of people should remain in the room and they should either stand behind lead screens or wear protective clothing. All those present must obey the instructions given by the person operating the X-ray machine. The beam must be collimated to the smallest size practicable and must be entirely within the borders of the film. Grids should only be used when the part being X-rayed is more than 10 cm thick, as their use necessitates an increase in the exposure.

The method of restraint of the patient is of paramount importance. Many practices previously held all their patients for radiography but this should now be discontinued: it is not only dangerous but also illegal. The Approved Code of Practice states that 'only in exceptional circumstances should a patient or animal undergoing a diagnostic examination be supported or manipulated by hand'. These exceptional circumstances may include severely ill or injured animals for whom a diagnosis requires radiography but for whom sedation, anaesthesia or restraint with sandbags is dangerous (e.g. congestive heart failure; ruptured diaphragm or other severe traumatic injuries). In these cases the animal may be held, provided that those restraining it are fully protected and provided that no part of their hands (even in gloves) enters the primary beam. A light beam diaphragm is essential for manual restraint. The majority of patients may be positioned and restrained artificially under varying degrees of sedation or general anaesthesia, and sometimes with no chemical restraint at all.

Large animals

Special consideration is given to large animal radiography using a horizontal beam. The investigation may need to be undertaken outside the X-ray room, when it should preferably take place in a walled or fenced area with the primary beam directed at a wall of double brick. The extent of the controlled area should be identified using portable warning signs, in order to prevent people not involved from being accidentally irradiated. Everyone taking part in radiography must wear protective clothing and dosemeters. The extra hazards posed by the use of a horizontal beam must be remembered and care must be taken not to irradiate the legs of anyone assisting in the procedure. Collimation must be tight and accurate, especially if a limb or cassette holder is being held by a gloved hand close to the primary beam.

Positioning

In order to produce radiographs of maximum diagnostic value it is necessary to position the patient carefully and to centre and collimate the beam accurately. Poor positioning, with rotation or obliquity of the area being radiographed, will result in a film that is hard to interpret or misleading or that fails to demonstrate the lesion. There are several general rules that should be adhered to when positioning the patient.

Patient positioning

- Use a large enough cassette to cover the whole area of interest, such as the chest or abdomen in a large dog – it is very difficult to interpret images that are made up of a mosaic of smaller radiographs.
- Place the area of interest as close to the film as possible in order to minimize magnification and blurring and to produce an accurate image.
- Centre over the area of interest, especially if it is a joint or a disc space.
- Ensure that the central ray of the primary beam is perpendicular to the film otherwise distortion and non-uniform exposure of the structures will result. If a grid is being used, accurate alignment of the primary beam is essential to prevent grid faults.
- Collimate the beam to as small an area as possible, to reduce the amount of scattered radiation produced.
- Since a radiograph is a two-dimensional image of a three-dimensional structure, it is usually necessary to take two radiographs at right angles to each other in order to visualize the area fully. Oblique views may then be taken to highlight lesions seen on the initial films if appropriate.

Restraint

Small animals should be held for radiography *only in exceptional circumstances*, when a radiograph is essential for a diagnosis but their condition renders other means of restraint unsafe. In practice, patients rarely need to be held and most views may be achieved using a combination of chemical restraint and positioning aids.

Simple lateral views of chest, abdomen and limbs may be possible on placid animals without any form of sedation. Other views require varying degrees of sedation or general anaesthesia and the positioning requirements and the temperament of the patient must be taken into consideration when assessing the depth of sedation required. It is also important to handle patients gently, calmly and firmly during radiography, and to reassure them with touch and voice.

Positioning aids

With the skilful use of positioning aids and the correct degree of chemical restraint, almost any radiographic view may be achieved without the need to hold the animal. The following positioning aids should be present in the practice.

Positioning aids

- **Troughs:** Radiolucent plastic or foam-filled troughs are essential for restraining animals on their backs. They are available in a variety of sizes.
- **Foam wedges:** When lateral views are required, these are placed under the chest, skull or spine to prevent rotation and to ensure that a true lateral view is achieved. They are also useful for accurate limb positioning. They are radiolucent and may therefore be used in the primary beam. It is useful to have several, in different shapes and sizes, and to cover them with plastic for easy cleaning. ▶

- **Sandbags:** Long, thin sandbags of various sizes may be wrapped around limbs or placed over the neck for restraint. They should only be loosely filled with sand, so that they can be bent and twisted. As they are radio-opaque they should not be used in the primary beam. They should be plastic-covered for easy cleaning.
- **Tapes:** Cotton tapes are looped around limbs and may then be tied to hooks on the edge of the table or wrapped around sandbags, for positioning of the limbs. Sticky tape may also be useful at times.
- **Velcro bands:** Fabric bands with Velcro fastenings are especially useful for ventrodorsal hip radiographs, as they can be placed around the stifles to align the femora correctly. Non-stick elasticated bandage can also be used.
- **Wooden blocks:** These are used to raise the cassette to the area of interest for certain views (e.g. dorsoventral skull). They are radio-opaque and so should not be placed between the patient and the film.

Nomenclature

Each radiographic projection is named by a composite term describing first the point of entry and then the point of exit of the beam. For example, a **dorsoventral (DV)** view of the chest involves the X-ray beam entering through the spine (**dorsally**) and emerging through the sternum (**ventrally**). An exception is the lateromedial or mediolateral view, which is commonly just called the **lateral** view. A standardized nomenclature has been devised for veterinary radiology and the naming of the various body regions is illustrated in Chapter 4. The correct terminology will be used throughout this section.

Note that the terms anterior and posterior are no longer used in veterinary radiography as they are not appropriate to four-legged creatures. Instead, anteroposterior (AP) and postero-anterior (PA) views of the limbs are called:

- **Craniocaudal (CrCd)** or **caudocranial (CdCr)** above the radiocarpal and tibiotarsal joints
- **Dorsopalmar (Dpa)/palmarodorsal (PaD)** or **dorsoplantar (DPl)/plantarodorsal (PlD)** below.

Dorsal recumbency describes an animal lying on its back and **sternal recumbency** describes the crouching position.

Positioning for common views

The following notes describe in brief the positioning for the more common views performed in veterinary practice. Further details are found in *Principles of Veterinary Radiography* (Douglas *et al.*, 1987). Anatomy texts and radiological atlases should be consulted for identification of normal anatomical structures.

Thorax

The right lateral recumbent position is usually preferred to the left lateral for a single screening film, as the heart outline is more consistent in shape. When assessing the lungs it is useful to perform the left lateral view too, as the uppermost lung field is better aerated in lateral recumbency and is therefore more likely to show pathology. When investigating known or suspected lung disease (such as a search for metastases) right and left lateral radiographs with or without a DV or VD should always be obtained. For cardiac examination a right lateral and DV are recommended.

If performing radiography under general anaesthesia, the animal should be radiographed as soon as possible after induction, as collapse of the dependent lung area occurs quickly and can mimic pathology. Ideally, the patient should be kept in sternal recumbency until the lateral radiograph is to be taken. Manual inflation of the chest (taking all necessary safety precautions for the person doing this) will be of great benefit in aerating the lungs and improving the image. The kV should be reduced slightly, by about 2–5 kV.

Lateral view

1. Place a foam pad under the sternum to raise it to the same height above the tabletop as the spine (Figure 20.33).
2. Draw the forelimbs forwards with tapes or sandbags to prevent them from obscuring the cranial thorax.
3. Restrain the hindlimbs with a sandbag; place a further sandbag carefully over the neck if the animal is not anaesthetized.
4. Centre on the middle of the fifth rib and level with the caudal border of the scapula.
5. Collimate to include lung fields and expose on inspiration for maximum aeration.

The trachea, heart, aorta, caudal vena cava, diaphragm, bronchovascular lung markings and skeletal structures can be identified on a lateral view. The oesophagus is not normally visible on plain films.

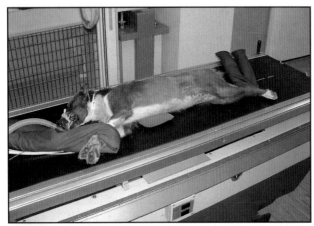

20.33 Positioning for lateral chest/abdomen views.

Dorsoventral view

The dorsoventral (DV) view and not the ventrodorsal must be used for assessment of the heart, because in the latter position the heart may tip to one side.

1. Position the patient in sternal recumbency, crouching symmetrically (Figure 20.34).
2. Push the elbows laterally to 'prop' up the dog or cat.
3. Drape a sandbag over the neck to keep the head down, shaking the sand into either end to produce a sparsely filled area in the middle of the sandbag. It may be useful to rest the patient's chin on a foam pad or wooden block.
4. Centre in the midline between the tips of the scapulae. Collimate to include the lung fields and expose on inspiration.

The trachea, heart, aorta, caudal vena cava, diaphragm, bronchovascular lung markings and skeletal structures can be identified on a DV view. The oesophagus is not normally visible on plain films.

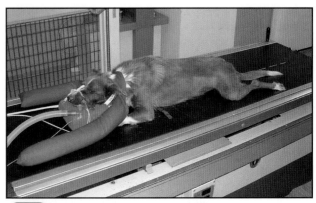

20.34 Positioning for dorsoventral chest view.

Ventrodorsal view

⚠ **WARNING**

Patients must never be placed on their backs if pleural fluid, pneumothorax or a ruptured diaphragm is suspected, as this may cause respiratory embarrassment.

1. Position in dorsal recumbency using a radiolucent trough or sandbags around the hind end (Figure 20.35).
2. Ensure that the patient is lying straight and not tipped to one side.
3. Draw the forelimbs forwards with tapes or by placing a sandbag gently over them. Secure the hindlimbs too if necessary.
4. Centre on the mid-point of the sternum, collimate to the lung field and expose on inspiration.

The trachea, heart, aorta, caudal vena cava, diaphragm, bronchovascular lung markings and skeletal structures can be identified on a VD view. The oesophagus is not normally visible on plain films.

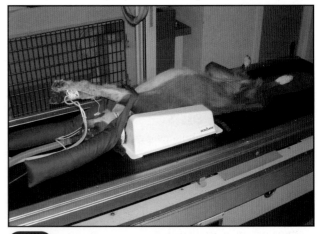

20.35 Positioning for ventrodorsal chest/abdomen view.

Abdomen

Lateral view

1. Position the patient in lateral recumbency and pad up the sternum if necessary (see Figure 20.33).
2. Restrain the fore- and hindlimbs with sandbags, ensuring that the hindlimbs are pulled well back so that they do not obscure the caudal abdomen.

3. Place a further sandbag over the neck (sometimes one end of the sandbag placed around the forelimbs can be used for this).
4. Centre over the area of interest and collimate as necessary.
5. Expose on expiration to give a more 'spread out' view of the abdominal viscera.

The liver, spleen, kidneys, bladder, stomach, small and large intestine, and skeletal structures can be identified on a lateral view.

Ventrodorsal view

1. Position in dorsal recumbency using a trough, or by placing sandbags on either side of the chest (see Figure 20.35).
2. Sandbag or tape the fore- and hindlimbs if necessary.
3. Centre and collimate as required and expose on expiration.

The liver, spleen, kidneys, bladder, stomach, small and large intestine, and skeletal structures can be identified on a VD view.

Dorsoventral views of the abdomen are rarely taken, as the viscera are usually compressed and distorted, but they may be all that is possible if the patient is dyspnoeic and cannot be placed on its back.

Skull
Skull views generally require general anaesthesia, as accurate positioning cannot otherwise be achieved.

Lateral view

1. Position the animal in lateral recumbency, using foam wedges under the nose and mandible to ensure that the line between the eyes is vertical and that the midline is horizontal and parallel to the table. The degree of padding depends on the shape of the patient's skull.
2. It may also be necessary to pad the neck and sternum.
3. Centre and collimate as required.

The cranium, frontal sinuses, nasal chambers, teeth, mandibles and tympanic bullae can be identified on a lateral view.

Dorsoventral view

1. Place the animal in a crouching position, with the chin resting on a wooden or foam block, on which is placed the cassette.
2. Secure the head with a sandbag over the neck if necessary. Ensure that the line between the eyes is horizontal.
3. Centre and collimate as required.
4. If an endotracheal tube is being used, it may require removal before exposure so as not to obscure any structures in the midline.

Ventrodorsal view

1. Place the animal in dorsal recumbency in a trough, with the head and neck extended.
2. Put foam pads under the neck and nose.
3. Hold the nose down using a tape placed behind the upper canine teeth, or using sticky tape.

Lateral oblique view for tympanic bullae

1. Place the animal in lateral recumbency with the side to be radiographed down.
2. Using foam pads, rotate the skull about 20 degrees around its long axis, towards the VD position (this will skyline the tympanic bulla nearest the table).

3. Centre and collimate by palpation of the bulla.
4. It is usually necessary to repeat the procedure for the other bulla, either to give a normal for comparison or to check if it is also affected. Care should be taken to ensure that the positioning is the same for the two sides.

Intra-oral DV (occlusal) view for nasal chambers
This view always requires general anaesthesia.

1. Place the animal in sternal recumbency with the chin resting on a wooden or foam block.
2. Insert a non-screen film or flexible plastic cassette into the mouth above the tongue, placing it corner first so as to get it as far back in the mouth as possible.
3. Ensure that the head is level.
4. Centre and collimate over the nasal chambers.

Other views
Many other views of the skull are possible but their description is beyond the scope of this chapter. They include the intra-oral VD for the mandibles, special obliques for temporo-mandibular joints, obliques for dental arcades and the frontal sinuses, skyline views of the frontal sinuses and cranium and the open-mouth view for tympanic bullae and the odontoid peg of C2. (See *BSAVA Manual of Canine and Feline Musculoskeletal Imaging*.)

Vertebral column
Spinal pathology is often undramatic and therefore requires particularly careful positioning, especially if disc spaces are under scrutiny. General anaesthesia is usually required in order to obtain diagnostic radiographs. Great care should be taken with patients that may have spinal fractures or dislocations in case positioning for radiography causes displacement of the fragments; in such cases the use of a horizontal beam for VD views could be considered as this will remove the need to roll the patient on to its back.

It is not possible to get an accurate picture of the entire spine on one film, since the X-ray beam is diverging and will not equally penetrate all disc spaces, and so it is usually necessary to take serial radiographs of small areas. In medium and large dogs, up to six films may be required for a spinal survey, as follows: cervical C1–C6; cervicothoracic C6–T3; thoracic T3–T11; thoracolumbar T11–L3; lumbar L1–L7; sacral and caudal (coccygeal) L6–Cd4.

Once a lesion is suspected, collimated views taken over the area of interest should be made. For disc disease, only the few disc spaces in the centre of the film are fully assessable (Figure 20.36).

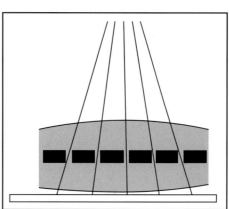

20.36 Radiography of disc spaces.

Lateral view

Ample use of foam pads is required to prevent the spine sagging or rotating (Figure 20.37) and to ensure that it forms a straight line parallel to the tabletop. It is necessary to centre and collimate to the area of interest by the palpation of bony landmarks (in obese animals the spine may be some distance below the skin surface).

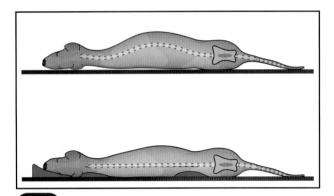

20.37 Use of foam pads for spinal radiography.

Ventrodorsal (VD) views

1. Place the animal in symmetrical dorsal recumbency, using a trough or sandbags.
2. Secure the limbs as appropriate.
3. Centre and collimate over the area of interest.
4. For VD views of the cervical spine and cervicothoracic junction, the X-ray beam must be angled 15–20 degrees towards the patient's head in order to pass through the disc spaces.

Forelimbs

Although many diagnoses may be possible from a single view (usually the mediolateral) it is often necessary to obtain the orthogonal view too (i.e. the view at right-angles to this). For investigation of suspected joint disease, centre over the joint of interest. Some joint diseases, such as osteochondrosis (OCD), are commonly bilateral and so the opposite limb should be radiographed as well. For long bones, the beam should be centred over the middle of the bone but include the joints above and below, with the long bone parallel to the film. If there is any doubt about the significance of a lesion or if the normal length of a bone must be known for fracture repair, then the opposite limb will serve as a useful control.

Mediolateral (ML) scapula

1. With the animal lying on the affected side, pull the lower limb caudally and the upper limb cranially, flexing it towards the head and securing it with a tape. It may also be pushed slightly dorsally so that it lies above the level of the spine.
2. Centre and collimate to the lower scapula by palpation.

Caudocranial (CdCr) scapula

1. Place the animal on its back in a trough, tipping it slightly over to the side that is not under investigation.
2. Draw the limb cranially and secure in maximum extension with a tape.
3. Centre and collimate by palpation.

Mediolateral shoulder

1. With the animal lying on the affected side (Figure 20.38), draw the lower limb cranially and secure it; pull the upper limb well back out of the way.
2. Extend the head and neck.
3. Centre and collimate to the shoulder joint by palpation.

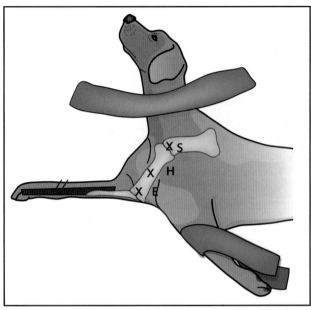

20.38 Positioning for lateral forelimb view. X = centring points, S = shoulder; H = humerus; E = elbow.

Caudocranial shoulder

As for caudocranial scapula but centred on the shoulder joint.

Cranioproximal–craniodistal (CrPr–CrDi) shoulder

This special oblique view is used to skyline the bicipital groove in cases of suspected shoulder tenosynovitis.

1. Place the patient in sternal recumbency (as for a DV chest) and flex the affected forelimb at the shoulder and elbow, the opposite side of the body being raised on a sandbag and the head displaced away from the shoulder under investigation.
2. Support the cassette on the forearm beneath the shoulder joint.
3. Centre and collimate to the shoulder joint.

Mediolateral humerus

As for the lateral shoulder (see Figure 20.38) but centred on the humerus.

Caudocranial humerus

As for the caudocranial scapula but centred on the humerus.

Craniocaudal humerus

An alternative view. The animal is placed on its back and the affected limb pulled caudally, securing with a tape. The humerus should lie parallel to the film. It may not be possible to use a trough for this view.

Mediolateral elbow

Extended view: as for mediolateral shoulder (see Figure 20.38) but centred on the elbow.

Flexed view (more useful for assessing degenerative joint disease): as for mediolateral shoulder but with the lower limb flexed at the elbow so that the paw comes up to the patient's chin. Secured with a tape or sandbag (Figure 20.39a).

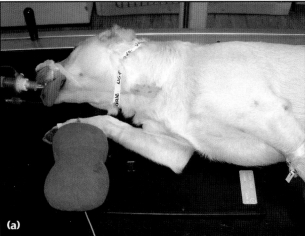

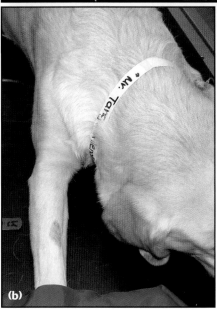

20.39
(a) Positioning for flexed lateral elbow view.
(b) Positioning for craniocaudal elbow view.

Craniocaudal elbow

1. Position the animal in sternal recumbency with both forelimbs extended and pulled cranially.
2. Turn the head and neck to the non-affected side and restrain by draping a sandbag over the neck. Take care that the affected elbow does not slide sideways.
3. Centre on the elbow joint, angling the beam about 10 degrees towards the patient's tail (Figure 20.39b).

Caudocranial elbow

An alternative view: as for caudocranial shoulder but centred on the elbow joint.

Mediolateral forearm (radius and ulna), carpus and paw

1. With the animal lying on the affected side, draw the lower limb cranially and the upper limb caudally out of the way (see Figure 20.38).
2. Ensure that a lateral position is achieved, using foam pads or sticky tape.

3. Centre and collimate to the appropriate area.
4. For individual toes, it may be useful to separate them by drawing the affected one forwards and the others backwards with tapes.

Craniocaudal forearm and dorsopalmar (DPa) carpus and paw

As for craniocaudal elbow, but centred and collimated to the appropriate area and using a vertical beam.

Hindlimbs

Lateral pelvis

The animal is positioned on its side, using foam pads under the spine and sternum to achieve a true lateral position. The beam is centred on the hip joints.

Ventrodorsal (VD) pelvis: extended hip position

This position is described in some detail as it is required for official assessment of hip dysplasia in dogs. It requires general anaesthesia or a reasonable degree of sedation.

1. Place the animal on its back in a trough, ensuring that it is perfectly upright and not tipped to either side.
2. Extend the forelimbs cranially and secure them with tapes; a sandbag may also be draped over the sternum, taking care not to impair respiration.
3. Extend the hindlimbs caudally, using tapes looped just above the hocks and tied to hooks on the edge of the table. The femora should be parallel to each other and to the tabletop, and the stifles should be rotated inwards by means of a further tape or bandage tied firmly around them (Figure 20.40).
4. Centre on the pubic symphysis. Perfect positioning may be achieved in this way without the need for manual restraint.

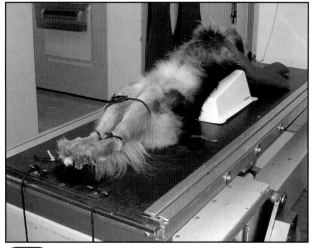

20.40 Positioning for assessment of hip dysplasia.

For submission to the BVA/KC Hip Dysplasia Scoring Scheme (see Chapter 5), the film must be permanently identified with the patient's Kennel Club number (or other identification if the dog is unregistered), the date and a right or left marker before processing. Radiographs labelled after processing will not be accepted by the scheme.

The various anatomical areas of the hip joint assessed under the scoring scheme can be identified.

VD pelvis: flexed or frog-legged view

This view allows some assessment of the hips but is not as satisfactory as the extended view. The hindlimbs are flexed and allowed to fall to either side. Sandbags may be used to steady the hind paws.

VD pelvis: dorsal acetabular rim (DAR) view

This is used to provide measurements prior to triple pelvic osteotomy surgery. The exposure needs to be increased by about 5–10 kV from that used for the extended VD projection.

1. Position the dog in sternal recumbency with a trough under its chest.
2. Pull the hindlimbs forwards so that the pelvis is rotated towards a more vertical position and the hocks are raised on sandbags.
3. Palpate the pelvis to ensure that it is symmetrical and the tail is extended caudally.
4. Centre at the base of the tail.

Mediolateral femur

Two methods are used, both requiring the animal to lie on the affected side. In the first method the uppermost limb is pulled upwards so that it is roughly vertical, and is secured with tapes or sandbags. It may be difficult to prevent superimposition of part of this limb over the femur under investigation and so an alternative is to pull the lower hindlimb cranially and the upper hindlimb back. In this case the lower femur is radiographed through the soft tissues of the abdomen.

Craniocaudal femur

As for the extended view of the hips, but centring and collimating to the femur. It may help to tilt the animal slightly away from the side being radiographed. The beam is centred on the mid-femur and includes the hip and stifle.

Caudocranial femur

This is an alternative to the CrCd projection.

1. With the dog in dorsal recumbency, support the thorax in a trough and drape sandbags over the forelimbs.
2. Using a tie around the hock of the affected leg, pull the leg cranially and secure the tie around cleats at the head of the table.
3. The femur should be parallel to the tabletop and may be held away from the dog's body using a foam wedge. This projection shows the head of the femur very well, with no superimposition of the pelvis or tail.

Mediolateral stifle

1. Position the animal with the affected side down (Figure 20.41a).
2. Move the other hindlimb upwards or caudally so that it is not superimposed over the lower stifle.
3. Ensure that a true lateral projection is obtained by placing a small pad under the hock.
4. In obese animals, the mammary tissue or sheath may obscure the stifle joint; this may be prevented by tying a tape around the caudal abdomen to act like a corset.
5. Centre and collimate on the stifle by palpation.

Craniocaudal stifle

This is similar to the VD pelvic (extended) view.

1. Position the animal in dorsal recumbency and extend the affected limb.
2. The other hindlimb may be left free.
3. It may be useful to tilt the animal slightly away from the affected side to ensure a true craniocaudal view.

Caudocranial stifle

An alternative view (Figure 20.41b), with the animal positioned in sternal recumbency and with the affected limb extended caudally. The opposite side of the animal may need to be raised on sandbags to obtain a true CdCr position.

Mediolateral tibia, hock and paw

1. With the patient lying on the affected side, draw the upper limb cranially or caudally to prevent superimposition.
2. Use foam wedges to achieve a true lateral position if necessary.
3. Centre and collimate to the required area.

Craniocaudal tibia and dorsoplantar hock

As for craniocaudal stifle, but centred and collimated to the appropriate area. For the hock, the tape is looped around the paw. To reduce the object–film distance for the hock view, it may be necessary to raise the cassette from the table with a wooden block.

Dorsoplantar paw

Two methods are available. The patient may be positioned as for craniocaudal stifle, but with the paw held down to the cassette with strong radiolucent tape. Alternatively, the animal may crouch, with the affected paw pulled slightly outwards and resting on the cassette.

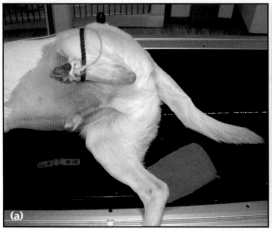
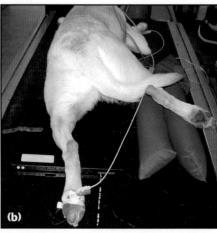

20.41 (a) Positioning for lateral stifle view. (b) Positioning for caudocranial stifle view.

Radiographic contrast studies

Although much information about soft tissues can be gained from good-quality radiographs, certain structures may be unclear either because they are radiolucent or because they are masked by other structures. In addition, the inner lining (the mucosal surface) of hollow fluid-filled organs cannot be assessed, because it is of the same radiographic density as the fluid contained within the organ. A good example is the urinary bladder, which appears simply as a homogeneous pear-shaped structure of soft tissue/fluid density.

Contrast studies aim to render these structures and organs more apparent and to outline the mucosal surface where appropriate, either by changing the radio-opacity of the structure itself or by altering that of the surrounding tissue. Both procedures increase the contrast between the structure of interest and the surrounding tissues, allowing assessment of its position, size, shape and internal architecture. If serial films are taken over a period, it may also be possible to gain some idea of the function of the organ (e.g. rate of stomach emptying).

Many contrast techniques are possible, but only those of most relevance to veterinary radiography will be discussed.

Types of contrast media

Two broad groups of contrast media exist: positive and negative.

Positive contrast agents

Positive contrast agents contain elements of high atomic number that absorb a large proportion of the X-ray beam and are therefore relatively radio-opaque, appearing whiter on radiographs than do normal tissues. They are said to provide **positive contrast** with soft tissues. The agents most commonly used are components of barium (atomic number 56) and iodine (atomic number 53).

Barium sulphate preparations

Barium sulphate is a white, chalky material which may be mixed with water to produce a fine colloidal suspension. It is available as a liquid, a paste or a powder that is made up to the desired thickness by the addition of water. It is used almost exclusively in the gut and is not suitable for injection into blood vessels. Being inert, it is non-toxic and well tolerated by the patient and it produces excellent contrast. Its main disadvantages are that if it is aspirated it may cause pneumonia and if it leaks through a perforated area of gut into the thoracic or abdominal cavities it may provoke the formation of granulomas or adhesions. Barium should not be given to constipated patients as it will exacerbate the condition.

Water-soluble iodine preparations

The iodine compounds are water-soluble and may therefore be injected into the bloodstream. However, anaphylaxis is a possibility (although it is extremely rare) and so an emergency protocol for such an eventuality should be in place. The compounds are excreted by the kidney and outline the upper urinary tract. They are also safe to use in many other parts of the body. Intravascular injection of these media usually causes nausea and retching and so the patient must be heavily sedated or anaesthetized. Despite being radio-opaque, they appear as clear solutions to the eye (unlike barium).

Being water-soluble, the iodine preparations are absorbed by the body and so should be used in the gut in preference to barium if there is a possibility of perforation. However, due to their high osmotic pressure they absorb fluid during their passage through the gut, with the result that they become progressively diluted and so the pictures they produce have much less contrast than those obtained using barium; there is also a risk of collapse in a dehydrated patient. They are therefore not routinely used for gut studies.

Many different water-soluble iodine preparations are available but most contain diatrizoate, metrizoate or iothalamate as the active ingredients. For myelography special iodine media with lower osmotic pressures must be used to avoid irritation of the spinal cord and these are iohexol and iopamidol.

Negative contrast agents

These are gases which, because of their low density, appear relatively radiolucent or black on radiographs, providing **negative contrast** with soft tissues. Room air is usually used in veterinary radiography.

Double-contrast studies

Studies on hollow organs may utilize both a positive and a negative agent in a **double-contrast study**. In these cases a small amount of positive contrast agent is used to coat the inner lining of the organ, which is then distended with gas. This provides excellent mucosal detail and prevents the obliteration of small filling defects, such as calculi, by large volumes of positive contrast. Examples of commonly performed studies are double-contrast cystography (bladder) and double-contrast gastrography (stomach).

Patient preparation

Adequate patient preparation is essential before many of the contrast studies. Prior to a barium study of the stomach or small intestine, the animal must be starved for at least 24 hours to empty the gut of residual ingesta. If food remains in the gut it will mix with the barium, mimicking pathology. Patients should also be starved prior to studies on the kidneys, as a full stomach may obscure the renal shadows. However, most patients are anaesthetized for these studies and so will have been starved anyway.

The presence of faeces in the colon will also obscure much abdominal detail and so an enema is often required prior to the contrast study. This is particularly important before investigations of the urinary tract as faeces may obscure or distort the kidneys, ureters, bladder or urethra. The colon must be completely empty of faeces if a barium enema is to be performed as even a small amount of faecal material will produce filling defects, giving the appearance of severe pathology. The patient should therefore be starved for 24 hours and the colon must be thoroughly washed out with tepid saline or water.

Plain radiographs must *always* be taken and examined before the contrast study commences. They are assessed for the following factors:

- Any pathology previously overlooked
- Correct exposure factors, to avoid the need to repeat films after the contrast study has begun
- Adequacy of patient preparation
- Assessment of the amount of contrast medium required
- Comparison with subsequent radiographs (to show whether any shadows on the images are due to contrast media or were already present).

A brief description of common contrast studies is given below. More detailed information can be found in Chapter 13 of *Principles of Veterinary Radiography* (Douglas *et al.*, 1987) and in Chapter 7 of the *BSAVA Manual of Small Animal Diagnostic Imaging* (see 'Further reading').

Gastrointestinal tract

Oesophagus (barium swallow)

Indications
Regurgitation, retching, dysphagia (difficulty in swallowing).

Preparation
No patient preparation required; plain radiographs.

Equipment

- Barium paste is usually preferred since it is sticky and adheres to the oesophageal mucosa for several minutes.
- Barium liquid may be used if paste is not available (5–50 ml, depending on patient size).
- Oral water-soluble iodine preparations should be used if a perforation is suspected.
- Liquid barium mixed with tinned meat should be used if a megaoesophagus is suspected clinically or on plain radiographs, as paste or liquid alone may fail to demonstrate the full extent of the oesophagus.

Restraint
Moderate sedation. (Heavy sedation or general anaesthesia is contraindicated because of the possibility of regurgitation and aspiration.)

Technique
Barium paste is deposited on the back of the tongue. Barium or iodine liquids should be given slowly by syringe into the buccal pouch, allowing the patient to swallow a small amount at a time to avoid aspiration. Barium/meat mixture is usually eaten voluntarily, as animals with megaoesophagus tend to be hungry.

Radiographs are taken immediately after administration of the contrast medium. Lateral views are usually sufficient but ventrodorsal views may also occasionally be indicated. Two separate radiographs may be needed to cover the cervical and thoracic areas of the oesophagus.

Stomach (gastrogram)
Two techniques are used: barium only, or barium and air (double-contrast gastrogram). The latter gives better mucosal detail.

Indications
Persistent vomiting, haematemesis, displacement of stomach, assessment of liver size.

Preparation
24 hours of starvation; enema if necessary; plain radiographs.

Equipment

- Barium liquid (20–100 ml, depending on patient size). Note that barium paste and barium/meat mixtures are not suitable and oral water-soluble iodine preparations should be used if a perforation is suspected.
- Syringe or stomach tube plus three-way tap.

Restraint
Moderate sedation (to allow positioning); acepromazine has least effect on gut.

Technique
Barium only

1. Administer the required dose of barium liquid by syringe or stomach tube.
2. Roll the patient to coat the gastric mucosa.
3. Take four radiographs: DV, VD, left and right lateral recumbency.
4. Take further radiographs as indicated, e.g. to follow stomach emptying.

Double-contrast gastrogram

1. Stomach tube the patient.
2. Give liquid barium, using the syringe and three-way tap, roll the patient (with the stomach tube still in place) and then distend the stomach with room air.
3. Remove the stomach tube and immediately take four views of the stomach as above.

The second method is preferred if a definite gastric lesion is suspected, but follow-up radiographs of the small intestine may be hard to interpret because of the presence of the air.

Small intestine (barium series)

Indications
Persistent vomiting, haematemesis, abdominal masses, weight loss, malabsorption, intestinal dilatation (usually unrewarding in cases of chronic diarrhoea).

Preparation, equipment and restraint
As for stomach.

Technique
Liquid barium is administered by syringe or stomach tube. Serial lateral and VD radiographs are taken to follow the passage of barium through the small intestine (usually at intervals of 15–60 minutes, plus a 24-hour radiograph) depending on any pathology seen.

Large intestine
Three techniques are used: air only (pneumocolon); barium only (barium enema); and barium and air (double-contrast enema). A pneumocolon will outline soft tissue masses within the colon and the use of barium alone will demonstrate displacement or compression of the colon; but for most purposes a double-contrast enema is indicated, as it yields maximum information about the colonic mucosa.

Indications
Tenesmus, melaena, colitis, identification of certain abdominal masses.

Preparation
Starvation for 24 hours; thorough enema, using tepid water or saline until no faecal matter returns; plain radiographs.

Equipment

- Cuffed rectal catheter or Foley catheter.
- For pneumocolon: three-way tap and large syringe.

- For barium and double-contrast enemas: gravity feed can and hose or a proprietary barium enema bag; barium sulphate liquid diluted 1:1 with warm water.

Restraint
Moderate to deep sedation (to allow positioning) or general anaesthesia.

Technique

Pneumocolon
The rectal catheter is positioned and the colon inflated with room air, using the syringe and three-way tap, until air leaks out around the catheter. Lateral and VD radiographs are taken without removing the catheter.

Barium enema
The rectal catheter is positioned and barium allowed to flow into the colon under gravity, until it just begins to leak out around the catheter (usually 10–20 ml/kg is required). Lateral and VD radiographs are taken without removing the catheter.

Double-contrast enema
The barium technique is followed for initial radiographs. Then, excess barium is allowed to drain out and the colon is reinflated with air. This can be a very messy procedure unless a special barium enema bag is used; when the bag is lowered to the floor the barium drains back down the tube from the colon into the bag. If the bag is then compressed, the air within it will inflate the colon (Figure 20.42). Lateral and VD radiographs are repeated after the introduction of the air.

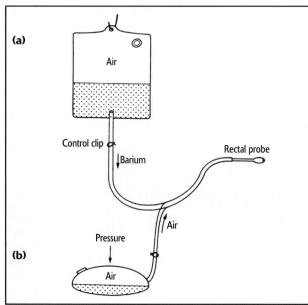

20.42 Barium enema bag. **(a)** In this position, barium flows under gravity into the colon. **(b)** In this position, barium empties from the colon into the bag and then pressure on the bag will distend the colon with air for the double-contrast effect.

Urogenital tract

Kidneys and ureters: intravenous urography (IVU), excretion urography
Contrast radiography of the upper urinary tract involves the intravenous injection of a water-soluble iodine preparation, which is subsequently excreted by, and opacifies, the kidneys and ureters. Two methods are used: rapid injection of a small volume of a very concentrated solution (**bolus intravenous urogram**) and a slow infusion of a large volume of a weaker solution (**infusion intravenous urogram**). The bolus IVU produces excellent opacification of the kidneys. The infusion IVU is preferred for investigation of the ureters, as it produces more ureteric distension by inducing a greater degree of osmotic diuresis.

Indications
Identification of kidney size, shape and position, haematuria, urinary incontinence.

Preparation
Starvation for 24 hours; enema; plain radiographs.

Equipment
- Intravenous catheter (perivascular leakage of contrast medium is irritant).
- *For bolus IVU*: syringe and three-way tap; concentrated contrast medium (300–400 mg iodine/ml) at a dose of up to 850 mg iodine/kg bodyweight, i.e. about 50 ml for a 25 kg dog (if there is poor renal function, the dose may be increased by up to 50% more)
- *For infusion IVU*: drip giving set; weaker contrast medium (150–200 mg iodine/ml) at a dose rate of up to 1200 mg iodine/kg bodyweight, i.e. about 200 ml for a 25 kg dog. Concentrated solutions may be diluted with saline for this study if necessary.

Restraint
General anaesthesia to prevent patient nausea and allow positioning.

Technique

Bolus IVU

1. Warm the contrast medium to body temperature to reduce its viscosity and make it easier to inject.
2. Inject the whole amount as quickly as possible.
3. Take lateral and VD radiographs immediately and at 2, 5, 10 minutes and so on as indicated by the initial pictures.

Infusion IVU
If the patient has urinary incontinence and the position of the ureteric endings is being assessed, a pneumocystogram should be performed first to produce a radiolucent background.

1. Infuse the total dose over 10–15 minutes.
2. Take lateral and VD radiographs once most of the contrast medium has run in.
3. Oblique radiographs are also useful for ureteric endings.

Bladder (cystography)
Direct or retrograde cystography may be performed in three ways: using negative contrast (**pneumocystogram**), positive contrast (**positive contrast cystogram**) or a combination of the two (**double-contrast cystogram**). Pneumocystography is quick and easy but gives poor mucosal detail and will fail to demonstrate small bladder tears, as air leaking out will resemble intestinal gas. Positive contrast cystography is ideal for the detection of bladder ruptures but will mask small lesions and calculi. Double-contrast cystography is usually the method of choice, as it produces excellent mucosal detail and will demonstrate all types of calculi. A positive contrast cystogram will also

be seen following an IVU, if the patient cannot be catheterized for any reason. Excreted contrast should be mixed with urine already present in the bladder by rolling the animal. This type of cystogram is not ideal, as adequate bladder distension cannot be ensured.

Indications

Haematuria, dysuria, urinary incontinence, urinary retention, suspected bladder rupture, identification of the bladder if not visible on the plain radiograph, assessment of prostatic size.

Preparation

Enema, if faeces are present; plain radiographs.

Equipment

- Appropriate urinary catheter
- Syringe and three-way tap
- Dilute water-soluble iodine contrast medium for positive and double-contrast cystogram.

Restraint

Sedation or general anaesthesia to allow catheterization and positioning.

Technique

The bladder is first catheterized and drained completely of urine (obtaining a sterile urine sample if required).

Pneumocystogram

The drained bladder is inflated slowly with room air, using a syringe and three-way tap. The bladder should be inflated until it is felt to be moderately firm by abdominal palpation (usually requires 30–300 ml air, depending on patient size).

Positive contrast cystogram

As for pneumocystogram but using diluted iodine contrast medium instead of air. However, for detection of bladder rupture, a much smaller quantity is required.

Double-contrast cystogram

1. Inject 2–15 ml iodine contrast medium at a concentration of about 150 mg iodine/ml into the empty bladder via the catheter.
2. Palpate the abdomen or roll the patient to coat the bladder mucosa.
3. Inflate with air until the bladder feels turgid.
4. The bladder wall will be lightly coated with positive contrast, and residual contrast will pool in the centre of the bladder shadow, highlighting calculi and other filling defects.

Lateral radiographs are usually more informative, but VD and oblique views may be taken if required.

Urethra: retrograde urethrography (dogs); retrograde vaginourethrography (bitches)

These studies are less frequently performed in cats, but may be carried out using simple cat catheters.

Indications

Haematuria, dysuria, urinary incontinence, urinary retention, prostatic disease, vaginal disease.

Preparation

Enema, if faeces are likely to obscure the urethra on either view; plain radiographs.

Equipment

- Appropriate urinary catheter
- Syringe
- Dilute iodine contrast medium (150 mg iodine/ml) (may be mixed with equal amount of K-Y jelly for studies on male dogs, to increase urethral distension)
- Gentle bowel clamp (for bitches).

Restraint

Sedation (dogs) or general anaesthesia (bitches).

Technique

Retrograde urethrography (males)

1. Insert the urinary catheter into the penile urethra.
2. Occlude the urethral opening manually, to prevent leakage of contrast.
3. Inject 5–15 ml contrast or contrast/K-Y jelly mixture slowly.
4. Release the urethral occlusion and stand back prior to exposure (or make the injection wearing lead mittens and an apron, and ensuring tight collimation to exclude the hands).

Lateral views are most useful and should be taken with the hindlimbs pulled forwards for the ischial arch and backwards for the penile urethra.

Retrograde vaginourethrography (females)

1. Snip off the tip of a Foley catheter, distal to the bulb.
2. Insert the catheter just inside the vulval lips, inflate the bulb and clamp the vulval lips together with the bowel clamp to hold the catheter in place.
3. Carefully inject up to 1 ml iodine contrast medium/kg bodyweight (vaginal rupture has been reported).

Lateral views are most informative, and demonstrate filling of the vagina and urethra.

Spine (myelography)

A narrow gap surrounds the spinal cord as it runs along the vertebral column; this is called the **subarachnoid space** and it contains **cerebrospinal fluid (CSF)**. It may be opacified by the injection of positive contrast medium and will then demonstrate the spinal cord, showing areas of cord swelling (e.g. tumours) or cord compression (e.g. prolapsed intervertebral discs) not evident on plain radiographs. This technique, which is called **myelography**, requires the use of special water-soluble iodine preparations, which have lower osmotic pressures than do the other iodine media and which are therefore less irritant to nervous tissue. The two low osmolar contrast media currently used in veterinary myelography are iohexol and iopamidol.

Two approaches may be made to the subarachnoid space. The one most commonly used in veterinary radiology is the **cisternal puncture**, where the needle is inserted into the cisterna magna – the cranial end of the subarachnoid space just behind the skull. Myelography may also be performed by injection in the lumbar area via a **lumbar puncture**, which is more commonly used in humans. Lumbar myelography involves passing the needle through the spinal cord and injecting into the ventral subarachnoid space. Both techniques involve practice and skill and the patient must be anaesthetized to prevent movement during needle placement or injection.

Indications
Spinal pain, spinal neurological signs (ataxia, paralysis), identification of prolapsed intervertebral discs prior to surgery.

Preparation
Clip relevant area, i.e. caudal to skull or over lumbar spine.

Equipment

- Spinal needle of suitable length, depending on patient size
- Contrast medium, warmed to body temperature to reduce viscosity and ease injection (dose rate 0.25–0.45 ml/kg of 200–350 mg iodine/ml solution – dose administered depends on size of patient and expected site of lesion but no more than a maximum of 15 ml)
- Syringe
- Sample bottles for CSF if required for analysis
- Some means of elevating the head end of the table for cisternal punctures, to aid flow of contrast along the spine.

Restraint
General anaesthesia.

Technique

Cisternal puncture

1. Elevate the table to about 10 degrees tilt with the head at the raised end.
2. Clip and surgically cleanse the injection site.
3. Flex the head to an angle of 90 degrees with neck.
4. Insert the needle carefully into the cisterna magna, between the skull and atlas (Figure 20.43), advancing the needle slowly until CSF drips out of the hub.
5. Collect several millilitres of CSF, then slowly inject warmed contrast medium.
6. Remove the needle and extend the head again.
7. Take several lateral radiographs until either contrast reaches the lesion or the whole spine is shown well. VD and oblique views may also be taken, especially if a lesion is found. Improved filling of the subarachnoid space in the lower neck area can be ensured by obtaining DV rather than VD views of this area. When the animal is on its back for the VD view, this area is furthest from the table and contrast medium runs cranially and caudally away from the area of interest; but with the dog in sternal recumbency, this area is closest to the table and therefore contrast pools here.

Lumbar puncture

1. Clip and surgically cleanse the injection site.
2. Flex the vertebral column by pulling the hindlimbs forwards.
3. Insert the needle carefully (usually at L5–6; as it passes through the cauda equina the animal's hindlimbs and anus will usually twitch slightly. Little or no CSF may appear from this site and if this is the case a small test injection is required to check needle placement.
4. Inject contrast medium.
5. Remove the needle, extend the spine and take radiographs as above.

It is important to keep the head raised during the recovery period, since contrast medium entering the brain may precipitate fits.

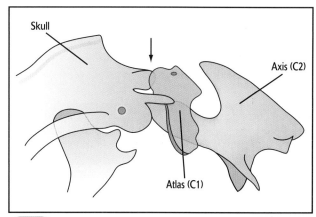

20.43 Myelography: site for cisternal puncture.

Other contrast techniques

Some other contrast techniques occasionally performed in veterinary practice are described briefly.

Angiography

Angiography is the opacification of blood vessels using injected iodinated contrast medium, with a rapid series of radiographic exposures made immediately after injection. This will demonstrate the location and size of arteries (arteriography) or veins (venography), depending on the site of deposition of the contrast medium. Although still used in humans for the investigation of cerebral aneurysms and varicose veins, its applications in veterinary patients are extremely limited, with the exception of portal venography (described below). It has been largely superseded in both medical and veterinary diagnosis by ultrasonography, CT and MRI.

Portal venography

Portal venography is used to diagnose certain types of liver disease (e.g. congenital portosystemic shunts, cirrhosis) by demonstration of the vascular system within the liver parenchyma. Under general anaesthesia a laparotomy is performed and a splenic or mesenteric vein is catheterized. A small quantity of concentrated iodine contrast medium is injected as a bolus and a single radiograph is taken at the end of the injection. The contrast medium enters the liver via the hepatic portal vein and in the normal animal shows branching and tapering portal vessels throughout the liver.

Dacryocystorhinography

Dacryocystorhinography is opacification of the nasolacrimal duct, in order to demonstrate strictures, rupture and communication with cystic maxillary structures. Under general anaesthesia, one of the nasolacrimal puncta in the eyelids is cannulated and a small quantity of warmed, non-ionic iodinated contrast medium is instilled.

Arthrography

Arthrography is the demonstration of a joint space using negative contrast (air), positive contrast (iodine) or double-contrast techniques injected under sterile conditions. The joints most amenable to arthrography in small animals are the shoulder and stifle. General anaesthesia is required as the procedure is uncomfortable. Arthrography will demonstrate joint capsule distension or rupture or defects in the articular cartilage, which is normally radiolucent.

Fistulography

Fistulography is the opacification of sinus tracts and fistulae using water-soluble or oily iodine contrast media. Fistulography will demonstrate the extent and course of these lesions and may outline radiolucent foreign bodies such as pieces of wood.

Other imaging techniques

Diagnostic ultrasonography

Diagnostic ultrasonography is being increasingly used in small animal practice as a complementary imaging tool to radiography. Ultrasound imaging has the advantage that it is painless and safe to both patient and operators and can therefore be used in the conscious patient without the need for sedation or anaesthesia (Figure 20.44). It can differentiate between soft tissue and fluid, which radiography cannot, and it produces a 'real-time' or moving picture, which is invaluable in the assessment of cardiac function and of peristalsis. Its main disadvantage is that it does not penetrate bone or air so it cannot be used for investigations of the skeletal system or lungs. Bone reflects all of the incident ultrasound, resulting in 'acoustic shadows' or radiating black streaks in deeper tissues (Figure 20.45).

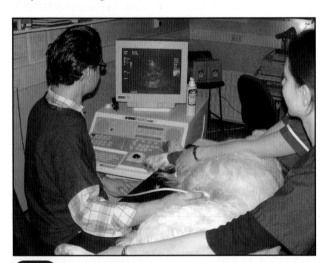

20.44 Ultrasonography of a conscious patient.

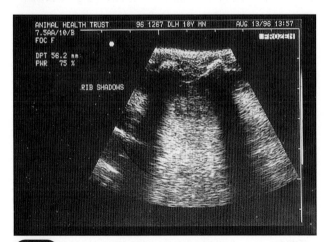

20.45 Acoustic shadows created by ribs.

Ultrasonography is a difficult technique to master since experience is required both to obtain and to interpret the images. However, some simple diagnoses, such as pregnancy diagnoses, may be made even by relatively inexperienced operators.

Principles of ultrasonography

Ultrasound is sound energy at a higher frequency than can be detected by the human ear. In the diagnostic range, the frequencies used range from about 2.5 to 15 megahertz (MHz). Ultrasound of higher frequency produces better image resolution but cannot penetrate so far into the body, and so the highest frequency compatible with the type of study and patient is selected. For most small-animal ultrasonography, a 5 MHz transducer is used. For cats and very small dogs, 7.5 MHz may be preferred; and for very superficial examinations, such as of the eye or tendons, transducers of 10 MHz or higher are needed.

In an ultrasound machine the sound waves are created by the vibrations of special crystals in the probe or transducer that alter their shape when an electrical current is applied to them. This is known as the piezo-electric effect. When the probe is applied to the patient's skin the sound waves are passed through the patient's soft tissues as pressure waves, and at interfaces between organs or between clusters of different cells within an organ a certain percentage of the sound waves are reflected and may return to the transducer. Returning sound waves in turn create a vibration of the tissues and of the crystals in the probe and this is converted back into electrical impulses, which are quickly converted by a computer into an image. The image is basically built of many tiny dots of different brightnesses, depending on the strength of the returning pulses of ultrasound and the location in the body from which they have been reflected. It is a cross-sectional picture of the internal architecture of the tissues under investigation. The basic principle of ultrasound is shown in Figure 20.46.

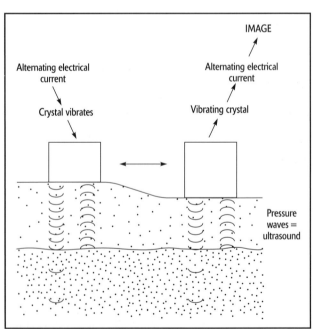

20.46 Diagrammatic representation of the production of ultrasound waves by the transducer and the detection of returning sound waves.

Equipment

Ultrasound equipment consists of one or more transducers, a TV monitor and a control panel (Figure 20.47). There is also likely to be some sort of printer for recording the images.

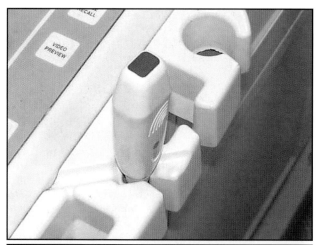

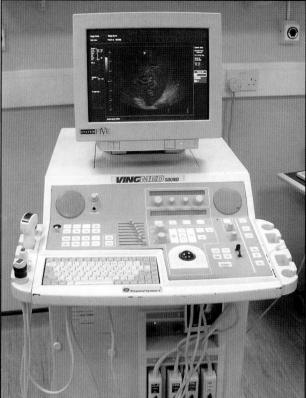

20.47 Ultrasound transducer, TV monitor and control panel.

Ultrasound transducers are of two main types: linear array and sector scanning. In **linear array transducers**, the piezo-electric crystals are arranged in a line and the image is rectangular (Figure 20.48a). Although a wide image of the tissues close to the transducer is obtained, linear array transducers need a long contact area with the patient, which is hard to achieve in small animals (remember that ultrasound does not pass through air). Linear array transducers are mainly used for rectal investigations in large animals. **Sector scanning transducers** are much more suitable for small animal work since the crystals are arranged close together so that only a small area of contact with the patient is required (Figure 20.48b). The ultrasound beam fans out to produce a triangular image that shows as much of the deeper tissues as possible. The image can be altered in depth, brightness and contrast using the ultrasound machine's controls, and measurements can be made on a frozen image.

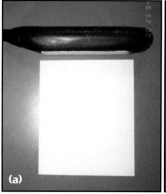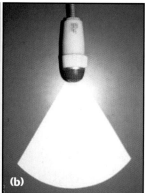

20.48 (a) Linear array transducer and image field.
(b) Sector scanner transducer and image field.

Technique

In dogs and cats the fur must be usually be clipped to allow good contact between the transducer and the skin, since small air bubbles trapped in hair will greatly degrade the image. A special coupling gel is then applied to improve contact further. In long-haired animals, it may be possible simply to part the hair and hold it aside using gel.

Most ultrasound examinations are performed with the animal in lateral or dorsal recumbency, scanning from the ventral surface of the body or through the uppermost body wall. However, **echocardiography** (ultrasonography of the heart) is best performed from beneath through a cut-out in a special tabletop. In lateral recumbency the heart sinks towards the dependent chest wall and therefore the best acoustic window (the least intervening lung) is on the underneath side.

Most ultrasonography performed uses B-mode ('brightness' mode ultrasound), as described above, to create a two-dimensional image of the tissues. Small sound reflections within tissues create a fine, granular pattern to organs, with different organs producing different brightnesses on the image (Figure 20.49). Pathology within an organ can often be recognized as a change in the overall brightness or **echogenicity** of the organ or a mottled appearance disrupting normal architecture (Figure 20.50). Areas of altered echogenicity are said to be **anechoic** (black), **hypoechoic** (dark) or **hyperechoic** (bright). Fluid is usually seen as an anechoic area, because it gives rise to very few ultrasound reflections. Thus, free abdominal fluid can be seen as a black background surrounding abdominal organs (Figure 20.51). One of the main advantages of ultrasound is that it allows examination of the abdominal structures when free fluid renders radiography unhelpful by obscuring the organs.

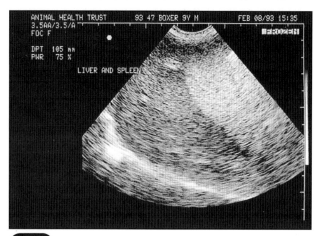

20.49 Ultrasound image of normal liver and spleen.

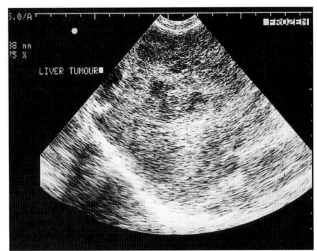

20.50 Ultrasound image of liver tumour in a dog, giving rise to a mottled irregular pattern to the liver.

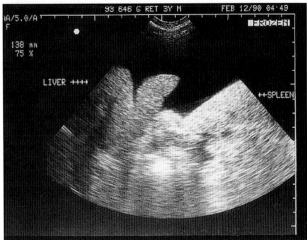

20.51 Ultrasound image of free abdominal fluid, seen as a black area, outlining abdominal organs.

Applications

Polycystic kidney disease

In November 2000 the Feline Advisory Bureau launched an ultrasonographic screening scheme for the detection of polycystic kidney disease (PKD) in cats (see Chapter 5). This follows similar schemes in a number of other countries. PKD is an inherited disease that affects mainly Persian cats, with an incidence of over 50% in the UK. Certain other pedigree breeds, such as the Exotic Shorthair, may also be affected. Although severely affected cats eventually develop renal failure, this is not usually until after their breeding life. Detection of the cysts when they are subclinical means that these cats can be excluded from breeding, which should eventually eradicate the disease. However, a DNA test has also recently been developed.

Biopsy

Ultrasound is increasingly used to assist biopsy or fine needle aspiration of small diseased areas within organs. Since the internal organ architecture and the needle can both be seen, the needle can be guided into the affected area without damaging other structures (Figure 20.52). This technique can often be performed with the patient conscious and avoids the need for surgical biopsy.

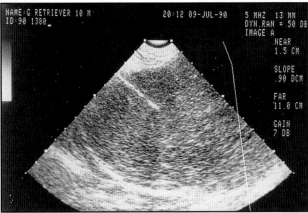

20.52 Fine-needle aspiration of an abdominal mass. The needle is seen as a bright line entering the mass.

Heart motion

A further refinement of ultrasonography is the use of M-mode ('movement' mode) to quantify heart motion. Firstly, a B-mode image is obtained and a cursor (line of dots) is placed on it and moved right or left until it passes through the heart in the required position. At the touch of a button the ultrasound beam produced by the transducer is converted into a thin line that produces a vertical band of dots indicating reflections at tissue interfaces along that line. This is rapidly updated with the movement of the heart and the image is scrolled along a horizontal axis with time. The resultant image shows the degree of heart motion and can be frozen to allow measurements of the heart chambers and walls in systole and diastole. Figure 20.53 shows a combined B-mode and M-mode image of a heart.

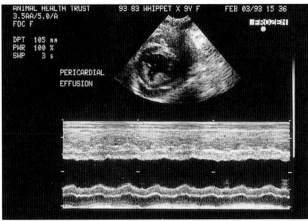

20.53 Ultrasonograms of a dog with a pericardial effusion. Top: B-mode image of heart; the line of dots indicates the position of the fine ultrasound beam. Bottom: M-mode image, with time along the horizontal axis. Blood in the left ventricle and pericardial fluid are seen as black areas on both images.

Doppler ultrasonography

Doppler ultrasonography is the use of ultrasound waves to detect movement, usually blood flow. It is based on the principle that echoes returning from moving reflective surfaces will be of shorter wavelength if the movement is towards the transducer and longer wavelength if it is away. **Spectral Doppler** displays flow quantitatively and graphically against a baseline, whilst **colour flow Doppler** assigns a colour according to speed and direction of flow and this colour mapping is superimposed over a B-mode or M-mode image. Doppler ultrasonography is used mostly in cardiac investigations (echocardiography) but can also be used to show the vascularity of structures, which is helpful prior to biopsy.

Computed tomography (CT scanning)

Principles and equipment

CT involves the production of a highly detailed cross-sectional radiograph of the patient's tissues. The CT scanner is a large piece of apparatus with a central orifice and the X-ray tube head moves quickly around the circumference during the exposure. Radiation emerging from the patient is detected electronically and digitized, producing image information that can be manipulated by computer. The grey scale of the image can be altered to different window widths and levels, emphasizing (for example) bony detail or soft tissue.

Technique

The patient lies on a movable tabletop that is advanced a few millimetres between exposures so that each image shows a different 'slice' of the tissues. Veterinary patients must be anaesthetized for CT scanning because the very high doses of radiation involved preclude manual restraint (Figure 20.54), but conventional anaesthetic and monitoring equipment can be used.

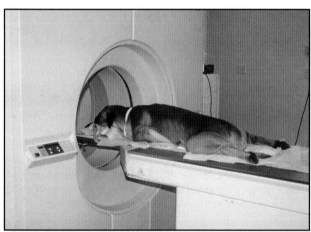

20.54 CT scanner and patient.

With older CT machines, images are always obtained transverse to the patient as it passes through the gantry. Images in other planes must be reformatted, which results in considerable loss of detail. The newer 'spiral' CT scanners are capable of producing images in any plane in very short scan times. Images can also be displayed in three dimensions and with different layers of tissue 'stripped away', allowing surgical planning. Advanced applications such as 'virtual endoscopy' are also possible.

Applications

Although this is essentially a radiographic technique, CT images have much more tissue definition than radiography and can differentiate between different types of soft tissue and between fluid and soft tissue. CT is especially valuable for imaging the skeletal system, as it is very sensitive to areas of osteolysis and new bone formation (Figure 20.55). It is also useful for imaging thoracic and abdominal masses, as it is less susceptible to movement artefacts than is MRI (see below). Iodinated radiographic contrast media can be given intravenously or into the spinal

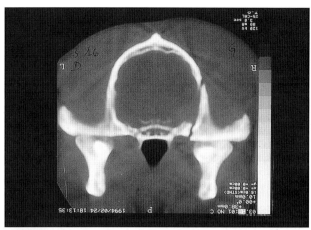

20.55 CT scan of a skull fracture: bone appears white, as in radiography. This image has been processed by the computer to 'flatten' the soft tissues into a single grey shade to give better emphasis to bone.

subarachnoid space to enhance the images further, demonstrating the vascularity of the lesion or damage to the blood–brain barrier and permitting CT-myelography to be performed.

Magnetic resonance imaging (MRI scanning)

Principles and equipment

MRI involves completely different physical principles, combining magnetism and radio energy. The scanner itself is a very powerful magnet, which may be cylindrical in the case of medium- and high-field magnets (Figure 20.56) or open in the case of low-field (weaker) systems. Because MRI does not use ionizing radiation, unlike radiography and CT, it is thought to be completely safe, but veterinary patients must still be anaesthetized to keep them still during the scanning time. This may sometimes be up to an hour or more in complex cases or when using low-field systems, in which scan times are longer. The main danger to patients and handlers lies in the fact that ferrous metal objects taken near the magnet may become dangerous missiles, and serious injuries and even deaths have occurred in medical MRI as a result.

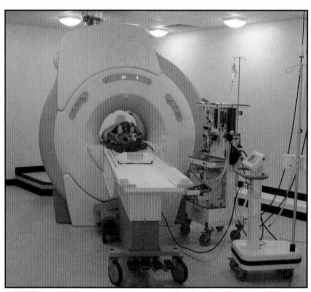

20.56 MRI scanner and anaesthetized patient positioned ready to slide into the bore of the scanner.

The presence of a strong magnetic field means that conventional anaesthetic and monitoring equipment cannot be used. In the case of low-field magnets, placing the anaesthetic machine at a distance from the magnet and using a long circuit may be sufficient to overcome this problem. With higher-field systems, dedicated non-ferrous machines may be required and this of course adds to the expense of MRI. Although total intravenous anaesthesia may be possible, patients with severe disease, especially of the CNS, are often at high risk from anaesthesia, especially if they cannot be monitored adequately.

Technique

During scanning, the patient lies in the magnetic field with the part to be imaged in a radioaerial or RF (radiofrequency) coil. The tissues within the magnet become magnetized, which has an effect on the protons of the hydrogen atoms in the body. The patient is then subjected to a series of radio waves, each lasting for several minutes; these have the effect of disorientating the protons so that they emit tiny radio signals themselves. The emitted signals are detected by the RF coil and are converted to an image by a computer. Unlike CT, in which there is a single image acquisition, with MRI many different types of scan can be performed to show tissues in different ways. For example, using a so-called T1-weighted scan, fluid such as CSF and oedema is dark, whereas with a T2-weighted scan it is bright. Since many more studies are possible than with CT and since each set of image acquisitions takes a number of minutes, overall scan times are much longer than with CT.

Applications

As with CT, the images are cross-sectional slices through the patient's tissues, but can be acquired in any plane and the soft tissue information produced is much greater. Although slightly less sensitive for bony structures and calcification than CT, MRI provides excellent orthopaedic images by showing articular cartilage, joint fluid, subchondral bone and so on. In veterinary work, MRI is used particularly in the diagnosis of brain and spinal conditions in small animals (Figure 20.57) but it can also be used to investigate many other disease processes, such as neoplasia, soft tissue foreign bodies and other space-occupying lesions and inflammation. Intravenous MRI contrast medium is given in many cases. This will show damage to the blood–brain barrier and vascularity of lesions, as with CT, due to 'enhancement' of the tissues absorbing the contrast medium.

The use of MRI, and to a lesser extent CT, has meant that surgery and radiotherapy of brain tumours in cats and dogs can now be performed successfully. The two techniques are also very helpful in planning surgery or radiotherapy for diseases elsewhere in the body, as the full extent of a disease process is often not evident on radiographs. MRI and CT are becoming increasingly used in veterinary diagnostic imaging as referral centres gain access to human scanners (or even obtain their own machines) and as owner expectations and the number of insured animals continue to rise. They are, however, open to misuse if used incorrectly. Appropriate patient selection is required, together with expert acquisition and interpretation of images.

Nuclear medicine (scintigraphy)

Scintigraphy is used mainly in horses for the diagnosis of bony orthopaedic problems. A gamma ray-emitting radioactive substance that will be taken up by the tissue under investigation (usually bone) is injected into the bloodstream under conditions that protect the handler from irradiation. The horse is then returned to an isolation stable. Several hours later the radioactivity will have become concentrated in areas of increased bone turnover, creating 'hot spots' that are emitting more gamma radiation than are the surrounding tissues. The emitted photons can be detected either by a hand-held radioactivity counter or by a large detector known as a gamma camera. A pattern of emitted radioactivity is produced that allows the source of the lameness to be diagnosed. Although the 'image' itself is rather crude, since it reflects metabolism rather than anatomical detail, the technique is very sensitive to early bone changes that cannot be seen with radiography.

Scintigraphy is occasionally used in small animals. Figure 20.58 shows a sedated cat positioned on a gamma camera for scintigraphy of the thyroid gland. Figure 20.59 shows the location of abnormal thyroid tissue in a hyperthyroid cat, allowing surgical planning if thyroidectomy is to be performed.

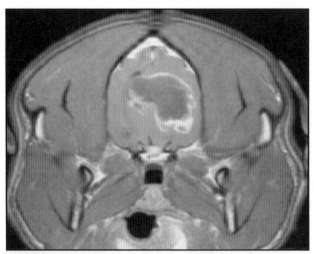

20.57 MRI scan of a brain tumour in an 11-year-old collie cross. The brain is the central light grey area and the tumour is the ring-like bright structure within the brain. Head muscle is dark grey and bones are black (cortical bone) and white (bone marrow). This tumour responded well to radiotherapy.

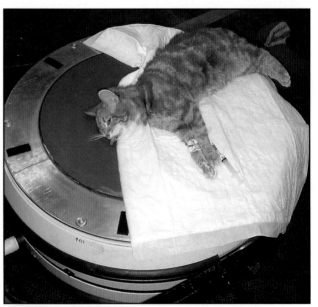

20.58 A sedated cat and gamma camera during scintigraphy.

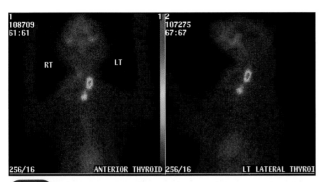

20.59 Scintigrams from a hyperthyroid cat.

Radiography of exotic species

Most of the exotic species seen in general practice are smaller than the more commonly seen cats and dogs. This provides potential problems when performing radiography:

- The smaller size of the species means lower voltages (kVs) are generally used, particularly in small mammals and birds. In chelonians, however, the kV may need to be disproportionately *greater* per kilogram of bodyweight, due to the density of the bony shell.
- Grids are rarely, if ever, used in commonly seen exotic species as few patients are greater than 10 cm in depth. Due to the smaller size of these patients, non-screen films respectively may be more helpful in demonstrating the finer details of their anatomy. These types of film require a greater amperage (mAs) in general. Alternatively rare-earth intensifying screens and so-called 'detail' films (high-definition fine-grain films) are used.
- For most small exotic species, particularly birds, mammals and squamates (snakes and lizards), a radiography unit capable of a range of 40–70 kV with a rapid exposure time of 0.008–0.016 seconds is helpful. The rapid exposure time is important, as many small mammals in particular have rapid respiration rates and therefore longer exposures can lead to blurring of the image produced.

It may also be useful to have a radiography unit that has the facility to alter the focal–film distance, as reducing the distance can allow some magnification of the image produced, which may be of help when imaging very small patients.

Smaller radiographic units, such as human dental machines, are beneficial. They generally operate on a fixed voltage and amperage, the only variable being the exposure time, which may be varied from 0.1 to 3 seconds on modern digital machines. This will allow the fine detail imaging of distal limbs and the head, and, if combined with non-screen dental film, can provide superior imaging to standard veterinary radiography. The possibility of longer exposure times means that patients generally have to be chemically restrained to avoid motion blurring of the image.

Positioning

Small mammals

The usual two views (a lateral and a ventrodorsal or dorsoventral view; Figure 20.60a,b) for small mammals are advisable in order to build up a three-dimensional picture. In addition,

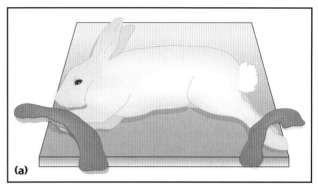

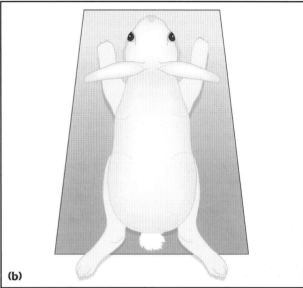

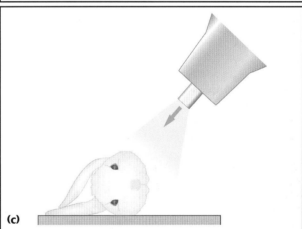

20.60 Rabbit radiographic positioning. **(a)** Right lateral view; the limbs are drawn away from the body. **(b)** Standard dorsoventral whole body view. **(c)** Oblique lateral dental arcade and head view. (Reproduced from the *BSAVA Manual of Rabbit Medicine and Surgery, 2nd edition*)

further specialist views may be useful. For example, in rabbits and chinchillas particularly, where dental disease is a common problem, oblique lateral views (Figure 20.60c) with contrast medium injected into the lacrimal ducts may help to highlight dental and nasolacrimal disease (see Chapter 26).

Rabbits also commonly suffer from otitis media, and dorso-ventral views specifically focusing on the auditary bullae are necessary to confirm presence of disease. Skyline views of the frontal sinuses and craniocaudal views of the skull may also be used where disease is suspected in sinuses or the temporo-mandibular joints.

Birds

As with small mammals, two views are essential and these usually comprise a lateral (generally a right lateral) and a ventrodorsal view (Figure 20.61). With the lateral view, the wings are pulled dorsally away from the body to prevent superimposition. For this reason, it is advisable to anaesthetize the patient to prevent struggling and minimize stress.

These two views are suitable for imaging the body cavity, but they actually result in exactly the same view for the wings, i.e. a ventrodorsal view. To obtain a caudocranial view of the wing, it is necessary to position the patient vertically. This is achieved by holding the anaesthetized and intubated bird head downwards and extending the wing over the radiographic cassette, which can be challenging.

It may also be necessary from time to time to perform skyline views of the skull when examining the sinuses for signs of disease.

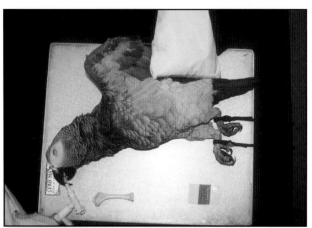

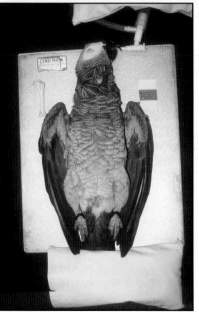

20.61 Grey Parrot positioned for **(a)** lateral and **(b)** ventrodorsal radiography. (Reproduced from the *BSAVA Manual of Psittacine Birds, 2nd edition*. © Nigel Harcourt-Brown)

Reptiles

Reptiles such as chelonians may be immobilized by propping up the centre of the plastron, for example with tin cans or up-turned feeding bowls, so that the legs cannot reach the ground (Figure 20.62). Snakes can be encouraged to enter a clear plastic tube to restrain them for such procedures, but the tube itself will reduce the clarity of the image produced. Lizards, and some snakes, may be placed into a hypotonic immobility by using the vago-vagal response. This is where pressure applied gently to the eyes stimulates the vagal nerve and results in a slowing of respiration, heart rates and a semi-sedative state. Pressure may be maintained by placing cotton-wool balls over the closed eyes and wrapping them in place with bandage material. Fractious animals or dangerous species should be chemically restrained.

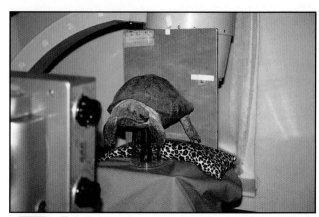

20.62 Tortoises can be propped up by the plastron to keep them immobile during radiography. (Photo courtesy of Mike Jessop)

Due to the absence of a diaphragm in reptiles, the lungs are fully collapsible (unlike birds, where the lungs are relatively rigid in structure). It is therefore advisable to use horizontal beam radiography when performing lateral radiographs. This allows the assessment of the lung fields and viscera in their normal positions without superimposition.

A dorsoventral view is also necessary, to provide a three-dimensional picture, and in chelonians a third view, the craniocaudal view (again using horizontal beam radiography), is helpful. This is because the chelonian lungs sit in the most dorsal part of the carapace. Lateral horizontal beam radiographs will allow the lungs to be examined, but the right and left lung fields are superimposed on each other. The dorsoventral view in chelonians provides little information on the lungs due to their superimposition on the ventrally situated viscera. Therefore to compare left and right lung fields a craniocaudal horizontal beam radiograph (with the X-ray beam focused on the nuchal scute just behind the head) can be performed.

In snakes, it is not advisable to allow the snake to coil up on the cassette, as this distorts the anatomy and makes interpretation difficult. The snake should instead be stretched out and if necessary sequential sections of body should be radiographed. It is helpful to place radiodense markers on the dorsal body wall when performing lateral radiographs, and the lateral body wall when performing dorsoventral radiographs to help with the accurate positioning of any radiographic abnormalities found.

Fish

The fish should be carefully anaesthetized and removed from its water source. Using a perforated plastic bag to do this can minimize the trauma to the skin of the fish. In most cases, a simple lateral radiograph can be performed. A ventrodorsal view is helpful to create a three-dimensional image, but is hampered by the laterally flattened shape of most fish. Foam wedges covered in cling film or other plastic material to prevent waterlogging may be used to prop the fish up.

Endoscopy

Principles and equipment

Endoscopy is the use of optical devices that give visual access to the inside of the body and provide high-quality magnified images of tissues and organ systems (Figures 20.63). Foreign bodies can be removed and tissue samples and biopsies taken, often without the need for open surgery (Figure 20.64). Where surgery is required, the clear magnified image gives greater precision and access to otherwise inaccessible places. Procedures are carried out through natural orifices or tiny incisions (keyhole surgery) resulting in less tissue trauma, reduced intraoperative and postoperative pain, quicker recovery and reduced infection rates. For this reason, these procedures are termed minimally invasive. An increasing number of routine procedures, including bitch spays and cryptorchid testicle removal, are being carried out using these techniques, and this trend is likely to continue as it has in human surgery. Endoscopy can be divided into two broad categories: flexible endoscopy and rigid endoscopy.

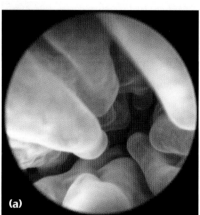

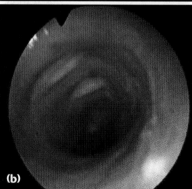

20.63 Endoscopic images of **(a)** normal nasal turbinates and **(b)** normal duodenum in a dog.

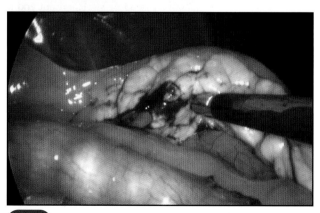

20.64 Laparoscopic biopsy of the pancreas.

Flexible endoscopy

Flexible endoscopes comprise an umbilical cord connected to a light source and suction/irrigation pump, a handpiece and a long flexible insertion tube, the tip of which can be manipulated in two or four directions. These endoscopes are used for examination of the gastrointestinal tract and respiratory tract where they can be directed deep within the body to remove foreign bodies, visualize lesions and take fluid samples or biopsies. Images are observed either through the eyepiece or preferably on a television monitor by means of an attached camera or dedicated video-endoscope. Patients are examined under general anaesthesia and a suitable mouth gag must always be used to prevent inadvertent reflex biting and damage to the endoscope.

Routine positioning for flexible endoscopy is as follows:

- Upper GI (**gastroduodenoscopy**) – left lateral recumbency
- Lower GI (**colonoscopy**) – left lateral recumbency
- Lungs (**tracheobronchoscopy**) – sternal recumbency
- Nose/pharynx (**rhinoscopy**) – sternal recumbency
- Urethra (especially male dogs) (**urethroscopy**) – lateral recumbency.

Rigid endoscopy

Rigid endoscopes are relatively simple steel tubes containing rod lenses, with an eyepiece at one end, and a connection for a light guide cable. They are extremely delicate and require careful handling and care during cleaning. These endoscopes are used for a wide variety of diagnostic and surgical procedures, including:

- **Otoscopy** (examination of the ear)
- **Rhinoscopy** (examination of the nose)
- **Tracheoscopy** (examination of the trachea)
- **Colonoscopy** (examination of the colon)
- **Vaginoscopy** and **urethrocystoscopy** (examination of the urogenital tract and bladder)
- **Laparoscopy** (examination of the abdomen)
- **Thoracoscopy** (examination of the thorax)
- **Arthroscopy** (examination of the joints).

Instrumentation

Smaller endoscopes are placed in a specially designed rigid sheath with instrument and irrigation channels to protect the scope and allow biopsies to be taken in restricted spaces such as the nose, bladder or joints. Grasping forceps or laser fibres can also be passed down the channel, for foreign body removal or surgical resection, respectively. Larger endoscopes are used in the abdomen or thorax through specially designed cannulae, which are inserted through the body wall. A variety of endoscopic instruments may be passed through separate cannulae to perform surgical procedures or take biopsies and tissue samples. A detachable camera clipped to the eyepiece enables procedures to be observed on a television monitor.

Technique

Vaginoscopy and otoscopy may be carried out on conscious patients, but all other procedures require general anaesthesia. Positioning will depend on the site being examined, and the procedure being undertaken:

- Rhinoscopy and cystoscopy – sternal recumbency (some prefer lateral), with nose or abdomen propped up on a rolled-up towel
- Laparoscopy – dorsal recumbency (sometimes dorsolateral)

- Thoracoscopy – dorsal recumbency (sometimes lateral)
- Arthroscopy – usually lateral but depends on the joint being examined.

Rhinoscopy and urethrocystoscopy are best carried out on a wet table as they require considerable amounts of saline flushing. Alternatively a deep tray covered with a wire grid may suffice. It should be noted that laparoscopy requires insufflation of the abdomen with an inert gas (usually carbon dioxide). This increases abdominal pressure on the diaphragm and can restrict respiration, which requires careful monitoring during anaesthesia. It is not unusual for the surgeon to change the position of the patient during laparoscopy in order to allow gravity to move abdominal organs out of the surgical field. For this reason, rigid ties should not be used and movable cradles may be substituted instead. Alternatively an adjustable operating table that can tilt in four directions is ideal.

Further reading

British Veterinary Association (2002) *Guidance notes for the safe use of ionising radiations in veterinary practice.*

Dennis R (1992) Practice tip – choosing an X-ray machine. *In Practice,* **14**, 181–184

Dennis R (1997) Veterinary diagnostic imaging – into a new era. *The Veterinary Nursing Journal,* **12**, 43–52

Dennis R (2003) Advanced imaging: indications for CT and MRI in veterinary patients. *In Practice,* **25**, 243-254

Douglas SW, Herrtage ME and Williamson HD (1987) *Principles of Veterinary Radiography, 4th edn.* Baillière Tindall, London.

Girling SJ (2000) Mammalian imaging and anatomy. In: *BSAVA Manual of Exotic Pets, 4th edn.* (eds A Meredith and SP Redrobe), pp. 1–12. BSAVA Publications, Cheltenham

Girling SJ (2006) Diagnostic imaging. In: *BSAVA Manual of Rabbit Medicine and Surgery, 2nd edn* (eds A Meredith and P Flecknell), pp. 52–61. BSAVA Publications, Gloucester

Krautwald ME, Tellhelm B, Hummel GH, Kostka VM and Kaleta EF (1992) Positioning. In: *Atlas of Radiographic Anatomy and Diagnosis of Cage Birds,* pp. 39–53. Paul Parey Scientific Publishers, Berlin and Hamburg

Lavin LM (2003) *Radiography in Veterinary Technology, 3rd edn.* Saunders, Philadelphia

Latham C (2005) Practical contrast radiography 1. Contrast agents. *In Practice,* **27**, 348–352

Lee R (1995) *Manual of Small Animal Diagnostic Imaging.* BSAVA Publications, Cheltenham

Raiti P (2004) Non-invasive imaging. In: *BSAVA Manual of Reptiles, 2nd edn* (eds SJ Girling and P Raiti), pp. 87–102. BSAVA Publications, Gloucester

Silverman S (1993) Diagnostic imaging of exotic pets. *Veterinary Clinics of North America: Small Animal Practice,* **23**, 1287–1299

Stefanacci JD and Hoefer HL (2005) Radiology and ultrasound. In: *Ferrets, Rabbits and Rodents: Clinical Medicine and Surgery, 2nd edn* (eds KE Quesenberry and JW Carpenter), pp. 395–413. WB Saunders, Philadelphia

Stetter MD (2001) Diagnostic imaging and endoscopy. In: *BSAVA Manual of Fish, 2nd edn* (ed. W Wildgoose), pp. 103–108. BSAVA Publications, Gloucester

Chapter 21

Medical disorders of dogs and cats and their nursing

Susan Howarth, Robyn Gear and Elizabeth Bryan

Learning objectives

After studying this chapter, students should be able to:

- **List the common medical disorders**
- **List the presenting signs, initial treatment and nursing care for a range of common medical conditions**
- **Describe the effects of the pathophysiological states and common pathologies on the animal body**
- **Explain the nurse's role when dealing with a range of medical conditions**
- **Plan the care required by a patient, taking into account the potential and actual problems identified in the assessment process**
- **List the more commonly recognized complementary therapies and their uses**

Upper respiratory tract disease

The upper respiratory tract comprises the nasal cavity, pharynx, larynx and trachea.

Definitions

- **Sinusitis** – inflammation of one or more sinuses
- **Rhinitis** – inflammation of the nasal lining
- **Epistaxis** – bleeding from the nose
- **Laryngitis** – inflammation of the larynx
- **Tracheitis** – inflammation of the trachea

Nasal disease

Clinical signs

- Sneezing
- Snorting
- Facial swelling
- Facial rubbing
- Dyspnoea
- Nasal discharge

Nasal discharge

Nasal discharge can be either bilateral or unilateral, depending on the causal factor. A good indicator as to the causal factor can be the type of discharge:

- Serous
- Mucoid
- Mucopurulent (Figure 21.1)
- Bloody.

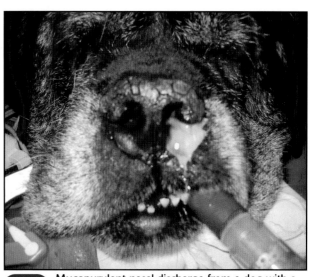

21.1 Mucopurulent nasal discharge from a dog with a nasal tumour.

Causes of nasal discharge (Figure 21.2) include viral, bacterial and fungal infections, allergies, neoplasia and foreign bodies. Trauma, tumours and coagulopathies can cause epistaxis (Figure 21.3).

457

Dog
Distemper
Kennel cough complex
Aspergillus spp.
Foreign bodies, e.g. grass seeds
Neoplasia

Cat
Feline upper respiratory disease
Chlamydophila
Foreign bodies, e.g. blades of grass
Neoplasia
Trauma

Small mammals
Pasteurella multocida in rabbits
Bordetella bronchiseptica in guinea pigs
Lung tumours in guinea pigs and thymic lymphoma in ferrets
Distemper and influenza A virus in ferrets
Mycoplasma spp. and *Streptococcus pneumoniae* in rats and mice
Tooth root abscesses can lead to migration of bacteria into nasal cavity due to the thin layer of bone that separates them
Lung abscessation
Poor husbandry – irritants such as dusty bedding and ammonia from soiled substrate

Birds
Hypovitaminosis A, due to poor diet
Psittacosis (*Chlamydophila psittaci*)
Aspergillus spp.
Mycoplasma spp.
Paramyxovirus, poxvirus, herpesvirus and influenza virus A
Teflon (overheated non-stick frying pans etc) and smoke toxicity
Poor husbandry

Reptiles
Usually lower respiratory disease
Paramyxovirus
Inclusion body disease virus
Gram-negative bacteria (e.g. *Pseudomonas*, *Aeromonas*)
Poor husbandry – low temperatures, inappropriate humidity levels
Chelonid herpesvirus

21.2 Causes of nasal discharge and respiratory disease in various species.

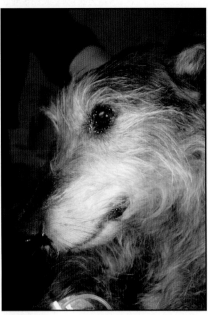

21.3 Epistaxis in a dog with a nasal tumour.

Diagnostics

- History and clinical presentation
- Blood tests: haematology, biochemistry, clotting profile and serology if pathogens suspected
- Rhinoscopy
- Radiography of the nasal chambers and thorax
- Bacterial and fungal culture
- Nasal flush for cytology examination

Treatment

The correct treatment will depend on the causal factor (e.g. supportive treatment for viral infections; antibiotics for primary and secondary infections; antifungal treatment for aspergillosis; removal of foreign bodies; surgery or radio-therapy for neoplasia).

Nursing care

- Isolate and barrier nurse the patient if it is thought to be infectious
- Monitor vital signs
- Keep the patient clean, bathe away discharge and groom as necessary. Prevent excoriation by the use of petroleum jelly
- Encourage the patient to eat by feeding highly palatable, strong-smelling food, warming the food, hand-feeding, etc.

Laryngeal disease

This can include conditions such as **laryngitis**, **laryngeal paralysis**, oedema and trauma. Causes of laryngitis include persistent barking in dogs and respiratory tract infections in dogs and cats.

Clinical signs

- Change in vocal ability (dysphonia)
- Coughing or gagging when attempting to bark or purr
- Exercise intolerance or dyspnoea in the case of laryngeal paralysis. Dogs known as 'roarers' (commonly ageing medium to large breeds)

Treatment

Treatment depends on the cause:

- Severe laryngeal paralysis – surgery often indicated
- Laryngitis – supportive treatment and possibly use of anti-inflammatory drugs and antibiotics
- Cough linctus (not advisable in cats).

Nursing care

- Use a head collar or harness to prevent pressure around the neck
- Provide rest and avoidance of excitement
- Keep cool if patient is becoming hyperthermic
- Administer oxygen if necessary
- Anaesthetize and intubate for severe laryngeal paralysis

Tracheal disease

This can include conditions such as **tracheitis** and **tracheal collapse** and trauma. Clinical signs may include:

- Honking noise (tracheal collapse) – middle-aged obese dogs, especially Yorkshire Terriers
- Dry hacking cough
- Exercise intolerance or dyspnoea in tracheal collapse.

Treatment will depend on the cause.

Nursing care

- Use a head collar or harness to prevent pressure around the neck
- Restrict exercise
- Revise diet if the patient is obese (especially in the case of tracheal collapse)
- Avoid dry, dusty or smoky atmospheres

Lower respiratory tract disease

The lower respiratory tract comprises the bronchi, bronchioles and alveoli.

Definitions

- **Dyspnoea** – difficulty in breathing
- **Apnoea** – cessation of breathing
- **Tachypnoea** – increased breathing rate
- **Orthopnoea** – dyspnoea in lateral recumbency (usually improved in sternal recumbency)

Acute respiratory disease

Acute respiratory disease will occur when any part of normal respiration is interrupted or fails to function adequately. This will lead to the failure of oxygen being transferred to the circulation and of carbon dioxide being eliminated, resulting in hypoxia and hypercarpnia. Causes include:

- Ruptured diaphragm
- Pneumothorax, haemothorax, pyothorax, chylothorax
- Airway obstruction (e.g. foreign body, tracheal collapse)
- Neoplasia
- Infections
- Paraquat poisoning
- Gastric torsion

Clinical signs

- Tachypnoea, orthopnoea, dyspnoea
- Mouth breathing
- Cyanosis
- Tachycardia
- Collapse.

Nursing care

Acute respiratory disease is an immediate life-threatening emergency. When the patient arrives at the surgery the veterinary nurse should inform the veterinary surgeon and begin to set up and administer oxygen therapy. It is vital that the patient should not be stressed, as this will increase the patient's demand for oxygen. The method by which oxygen therapy is given should be chosen carefully to suit the patient (see Chapter 18). Minimal restraint should be used for any procedure to avoid the patient struggling. Tight-fitting collars and leads should be removed or loosened.

The patient may have to be supported in sternal recumbency to allow maximum lung inflation. If the patient is collapsed, the head and neck should be extended and the airways kept as clear as possible, without causing further stress.

Equipment should be prepared in case the patient deteriorates further. This equipment might include:

- Various sizes of endotracheal tube (local anaesthetic spray for cats) and bandage for securing the tube in place
- Oxygen supply and suitable anaesthetic circuit to provide intermittent positive pressure ventilation (IPPV)
- Laryngoscope
- Tracheostomy tube and surgical kit or large-gauge needle
- Thoracocentesis equipment
- 'Crash' box.

The patient should be monitored continually for any changes in its vital signs and the veterinary surgeon should be informed of such changes.

Chronic pulmonary disease

Causes of chronic pulmonary disease (CPD) include:

- Bronchitis
- Pneumonia
- Pulmonary oedema (e.g. in cardiac failure)
- Feline asthma
- Lung worm
- Neoplasia
- Pulmonary haemorrhage.

Clinical signs

- Coughing
- Wheezing
- Tachypnoea
- Exercise intolerance
- Debility

Diagnostics

- Blood tests for haematology and biochemistry
- Thoracic radiographs
- Bronchoscopy
- Faecal analysis for lungworm larvae
- Bronchoalveolar lavage to obtain a sample for culture and cytology

Treatment

- Anti-inflammatory medication – to reduce inflammation
- Bronchodilators – to treat narrowing of the airways (e.g. in the case of feline asthma)
- Mucolytics – to reduce mucous viscosity to aid removal
- Expectorants – to aid removal of secretions
- Antibiotics – for primary or secondary bacterial infections
- Anthelmintics – for lungworm infections
- Antitussives – to suppress coughing if indicated, when coughing is persistent and unproductive

Nursing care

- Monitor vital signs
- Provide rest and avoid stress
- Provide oxygen therapy with or without nebulized medication
- Ensure adequate fluid intake (dyspnoea increases fluid loss)
- Give coupage if indicated (check with veterinary surgeon)

Extrapulmonary disease

Clinical signs

These are all due to the fact that the lungs are unable to inflate adequately as a result of air, fluid, abdominal organs or neoplasia in the thoracic cavity (Figure 21.4).

The signs depend on the severity of the underlying condition but may include:

- Tachypnoea, shallow respiration, orthopnoea, dyspnoea
- Cyanosis
- Severe respiratory distress
- Shock
- Collapse.

Treatment

- Thoracocentesis
- Indwelling chest drain (indicated for pyothorax and chylothorax)
- Specific treatment depending on the cause of the condition (e.g. surgery to repair ruptured diaphragm)

Nursing care

- Monitor vital signs
- Decrease stress and provide a warm quiet environment
- Provide oxygen therapy
- Provide intravenous access and administer fluid therapy under veterinary surgeon's direction
- Set up for and assist with thoracocentesis (see box)

Thoracocentesis procedure

Equipment

- Clippers
- Cotton wool and skin disinfectant
- Local anaesthetic
- Sterile gloves
- Intravenous catheter – suitable size for patient; extension set and three-way tap, suitable size syringe
- Bowl for collection of any fluid
- Sterile sample pots (plain and EDTA)   ▶

Condition	Description	Cause	Other information
Diaphragmatic rupture	Abdominal organs in the thoracic cavity	Rupture of the diaphragm due to blunt trauma (e.g. road traffic accident, being kicked)	Heart can sound muffled, depending on extent of condition Size of rupture can determine how many of abdominal organs are present in chest cavity Patient should be handled carefully as viscera can move around, making the condition worse
Pneumothorax	Accumulation of air in thoracic cavity	Trauma to chest wall either blunt or penetrating (e.g. often seen following road traffic accidents)	Can be classified as **open** (e.g. when thoracic wall is penetrated, air is sucked into thorax from outside) or **closed** (e.g. following rupture to lungs, allowing air to leak from lungs into thoracic cavity) Chest percussion will produce increased resonance
Haemothorax	Accumulation of blood in thoracic cavity	Trauma or disease affecting pulmonary veins, arteries or other blood vessels in chest cavity	Heart can sound muffled depending on the extent of the condition Chest percussion will show decreased resonance in ventral thorax when patient in sternal recumbency
Hydrothorax	Accumulation of fluid (pure or modified transudate) in thoracic cavity	Hypoproteinaemia causing fluid to leak from blood vessels (pure transudate) Congestive heart failure or neoplasia (modified transudate)	Appearance of fluid (pure = clear and colourless; modified = straw coloured, pink, slightly opaque) Laboratory test will reveal: nucleated cell count <7 (1 x 10^9/litre), specific gravity 1.018 or less with pure transudate, protein content <35 g/litre Chest percussion as above
Pyothorax	Accumulation of pus (or exudates) in thoracic cavity	Bacterial infection (pyothorax) Feline infectious peritonitis (wet) Neoplasia	Appearance of fluid – often thick, yellow-brown and foul smelling Laboratory test will reveal: nucleated cell count 5–300 (1 x 10^9/litre), specific gravity >1.018, protein content >30 g/litre Chest percussion as above These patients are often pyrexic
Chylothorax	Accumulation of chyle in thoracic	Trauma or rupture of thoracic duct Congenital abnormalities of thoracic duct	Appearance of fluid – milky, fails to clear when centrifuged Triglyceride levels of the fluid should be tested to confirm that it is chyle Chest percussion as above
Neoplasia	Development of neoplasia involving thymus, mediastinal and sternal lymph nodes	Lymphosarcoma – common in ferrets FeLV infection Cysts	Neoplasia if large enough will interfere with normal lung expansion, but usually it is the pleural effusion generated that produces the clinical signs A non-compressible cranial mediastinum may be present with dull heart and lung sounds on ascultation
Ascites	In avian and reptile patients that do not possess diaphragm, development of ascites places pressure on air sacs (birds) or lungs directly (reptiles), causing dyspnoea	Usual causes of ascites (e.g. congestive heart failure, liver disease etc.)	Radiographically, loss of detail in coelomic cavity; ultrasonography will demonstrate hypoechoic fluid in normally air-filled spaces

21.4 Extrapulmonary disease.

Procedure
1. Place patient in sternal recumbency.
2. Clip thorax over 7th/8th intercostal space.
3. Inject local anaesthetic and wait for it to take effect.
4. Surgically prepare thoracocentesis site.
5. Veterinary surgeon will put on sterile gloves.
6. Hand equipment to surgeon in a sterile manner.
7. Surgeon will hand syringe to nurse.
8. Surgeon will insert catheter into thoracic cavity.
9. Gently withdraw plunger.
10. Once syringe is full, turn the three-way tap and empty of fluid or air.
11. Repeat procedure until no further air or fluid can be aspirated.
12. Repeat on other side of chest if required.
13. Fill sample pots and send for analysis.

Circulatory system disease

Definitions

- **Myocarditis** – inflammation of the muscular walls of the heart
- **Endocarditis** – inflammation of the endocardium (endothelial membrane lining the cavities of the heart), most commonly involving a heart valve
- **Endocardiosis** – chronic fibrosis and thickening of the atrioventricular valves
- **Tachycardia** – rapid heart rate
- **Bradycardia** – slow heart rate
- **Pericarditis** – inflammation of the pericardium
- **Cardiomyopathy** – primary disease of the heart muscle
- **Cardiac tamponade** – compression of the heart due to fluid accumulation in the pericardial sac

Congenital heart disease

Congenital heart disease is present at birth. It represents only 5% of the cases of heart disease seen in practice. Often it is detected at the first vaccination when a heart murmur is auscultated. Clinical signs depend on the severity of the defect and include poor growth and those of heart failure: exercise intolerance, lethargy, dyspnoea and coughing. The diagnosis is made from the history, clinical examination, thoracic radiographs (including contrast studies), echocardiography and ECG. Congenital conditions include, for example: patent ductus arteriosus, valvular defects, septal defects and persistent right aortic arch.

Patent ductus arteriosus (PDA)

This is the most common congenital defect in dogs. In the fetus a vessel (ductus arteriosus) connects the pulmonary artery to the aorta, allowing blood to bypass the lungs. At birth this vessel normally closes but in PDA it fails to do so and blood is shunted from the aorta into the pulmonary artery. This causes left-sided heart failure and ultimately death if not treated.

Clinical signs

- A PDA is usually detected at first vaccination when a loud machinery-type murmur is auscultated
- The patient may be poorly grown, asymptomatic or in heart failure

Treatment
Treatment is via closure of the vessel with either surgery or implantation of a coil (both carried out by cardiac specialists). The prognosis is excellent with treatment.

Aortic and pulmonic stenosis
Stenosis is a narrowing of the aortic or pulmonic valves, obstructing the blood flow leaving the ventricles. This requires the heart muscle to work harder and there is compensatory hypertrophy of the muscle.

Clinical signs

- A heart murmur is auscultated, which may or may not be accompanied by clinical signs
- Patients can present with syncope or signs of heart failure

Treatment
Pulmonic stenosis can be treated with dilation of the area with a balloon (balloon valvuloplasty). Aortic stenosis is treated symptomatically. The narrower the outflow, the worse is the prognosis.

Mitral/tricuspid valve dysplasia
This is a malformation of the mitral or tricuspid valves. Blood regurgitates into the atria, increasing their workload, and they enlarge. This leads to congestion and right- or left-sided heart failure. The condition is less common than PDA or aortic/pulmonary stenosis.

Clinical signs

- A heart murmur is auscultated, which may or may not be accompanied by clinical signs
- Patients can present with heart failure

Treatment
Treatment is symptomatic treatment for heart failure. The prognosis is poor.

Ventricular/atrial septal defects
These defects are known as 'holes in the heart'. A hole connects either the atria or the ventricles. Blood flows through the heart abnormally, leading to heart failure. Ventricular septal defects are the most common congenital defects in cats.

Clinical signs

- A heart murmur may be auscultated
- The patient may be asymptomatic or have congestive heart failure

Treatment
Symptomatic treatment of heart failure. Animals with small defects can live normal lives. The larger the lesion, the more guarded is the prognosis.

Combined defects – tetralogy of Fallot
Some patients can present with a combination of defects. The most common is **tetralogy of Fallot**, which is a combination of a ventricular septal defect, pulmonic stenosis, compensatory right-sided hypertrophy and an overriding aorta. These patients present with cyanosis, as the blood bypasses the lungs. The prognosis is guarded.

Persistent right aortic arch (vascular ring anomaly)

This is a congenital malformation of the major arteries of the heart which traps the oesophagus, obstructing boluses of food from reaching the stomach.

Clinical signs

- Regurgitation and failure to thrive are usually evident when the animal is weaned
- Aspiration pneumonia can be a complication

Treatment

Treatment is surgery to ligate and cut the remnant. If there is permanent oesophageal dysfunction and megaoesophagus, the patient needs to be managed with elevated feeding and monitoring for aspiration pneumonia (see 'Regurgitation'). The prognosis is excellent as long as no permanent damage has been done to the oesophagus.

Acquired heart disease

Endocardial disease

Disease of the heart valves is most commonly due to chronic fibrosis (**endocardiosis**). Endocardiosis is the most frequently encountered heart disease in dogs, but is very rare in cats. The mitral value is most commonly affected, although the tricuspid valve can be affected. It is a progressive condition. Endocardiosis prevents the valves from functioning correctly and blood regurgitates into the atria, increasing their workload, causing congestion and heart failure. Infection of the heart valves (**endocarditis**) is less common.

Clinical signs

Clinical signs of **mitral valve endocardiosis** include a murmur. Other signs are those of left-sided heart failure (see later). Clinical signs of **tricuspid valve endocardiosis** are those of right-sided heart failure (see later).

Clinical signs of **endocarditis** include:

- Pyrexia
- Lethargy
- Shifting lameness
- Anorexia
- Heart murmur.

Diagnostics

A presumptive diagnosis can be made on clinical examination.

- Thoracic radiographs: right lateral and dorsoventral views
- Echocardiography
- ECG
- Blood cultures for endocarditis

Recording an electrocardiogram

This should be carried out with minimal stress to the patient and without sedation.

- The animal is placed in right lateral recumbency and gently restrained.
- ECG pads can be placed on the main pads of the paws. Alligator forceps can be traumatic and painful and should if possible be reserved for emergency situations; they can be attached on the upper part of the leg, where there is some loose skin. ▶

- Good contact is made by using ECG gel or spirit. The latter should not be used if there is a chance that the animal may be defibrillated.
- The electrodes are attached as follows:
    - Red – right forelimb
    - Yellow – left forelimb
    - Green – left hindlimb
    - Black – right hindlimb.
- A standard 6 lead ECG is recorded (leads I, II, III, AVL, AVR, AVF), usually at settings of 10 mV and 25 mm/second.
- The ECG should be labelled with the animal's details, date, settings and leads used.
- Ensure that it is of diagnostic quality, with minimal interference.

The electrode placement can be remembered as 'Red = Right' (both begin with R) and then work in an anti-clockwise direction in the order of traffic lights – yellow, green. Black is placed on the remaining limb, i.e. right hindlimb.

Treatment

- Patients with endocardiosis are treated when heart failure has developed (see 'Heart failure', below)
- Endocarditis is treated with broad-spectrum antibiotics pending blood culture results

Myocardial disease

Cardiomyopathy is the most frequently recognized cardiac condition in cats. It is also seen in large and giant breeds of dog. Cardiomyopathies are diseases of the myocardium associated with cardiac dysfunction.

Hypertrophic cardiomyopathy

Thickening of the heart muscle interferes with relaxation of the heart, preventing normal filling, leading to poor diastolic function, decreases in cardiac output and heart failure.

Clinical signs

Many cases in cats are clinically 'silent', but if congestive heart failure is present, then signs include:

- Dyspnoea, tachypnoea
- Tachycardia
- Heart murmur.

A common complication in cats is **aortic thromboembolism** where a thrombus (blood clot) leaves the heart and lodges in the caudal aorta (most commonly), obstructing blood flow to the hindlimbs. Clinical signs include:

- Acute onset of unilateral/bilateral paresis/paralysis of the hindlimbs
- Lack of arterial pulse in the affected leg(s)
- Pain
- Hindlimb(s) cool to the touch
- Dyspnoea, tachypnoea.

Diagnostics

- Thoracic radiographs: right lateral and dorsoventral views
- Echocardiography
- ECG
- Blood pressure

- Blood tests: T4 (for hyperthyroidism)
- Additional tests if a clot is suspected include blood tests: haematology and biochemistry, clotting profile and abdominal ultrasonography

Treatment

Treatment of hypertrophic cardiomyopathy is aimed at improving cardiac relaxation and slowing the heart rate (e.g. calcium channel blockers and beta blockers). Blood clots are treated with pain relief, antithrombotics and vasodilators.

Dilated cardiomyopathy

This is characterized by dilation of the heart chambers and poor systolic function and heart failure. In dogs, dilated cardiomyopathies are seen most frequently in large breeds and there is a familial predisposition in Dobermann Pinschers, Irish Wolfhounds, Great Danes, Newfoundlands, Boxers and other breeds. The heart enlarges and there is reduced cardiac contractility, decreasing forward flow of blood and causing congestion and heart failure. In cats, the cause may be idiopathic or due to taurine deficiency, though the latter is now rare because of good commercial diets.

Clinical signs

- Apparently acute onset
- Anorexia, weight loss, reduced exercise tolerance, lethargy

- Usually present with signs of left-sided heart failure (coughing, dyspnoea, tachypnoea) and sometimes concomitant right-sided heart failure
- Ascites
- Heart murmur, tachycardia
- Arrhythmias
- Sudden death

Diagnostics

- Thoracic radiographs: right lateral and dorsoventral views
- Echocardiography
- ECG

Treatment

Each patient is assessed and treated based on the severity of the disease but general guidelines are as per management of heart failure (see later).

Arrhythmias

Arrhythmias occur as a result of a disturbance of the electrical activity in the heart. This can be due to primary heart disease, or secondary to another systemic disease. Arrhythmias can be broadly categorized into **bradycardic** (slow) arrhythmias and **tachycardic** (fast) arrhythmias (Figure 21.5). They are further divided according to where the arrhythmia arises.

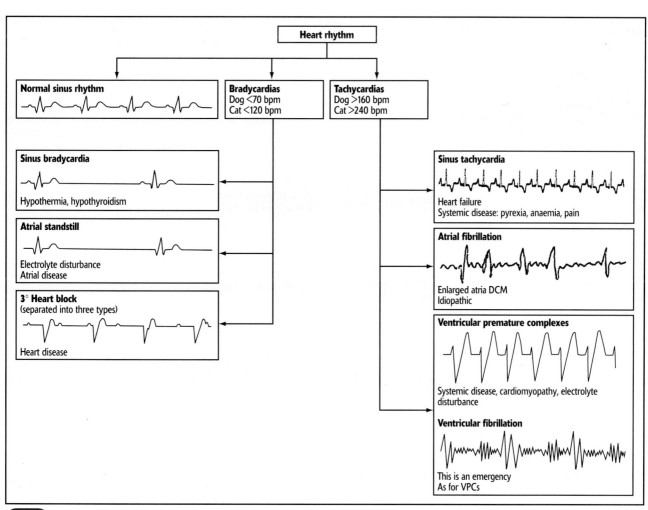

21.5 Arrhythmias.

Clinical signs

- May be asymptomatic
- Collapse
- Exercise intolerance, weakness

Diagnostics

- Blood tests: electrolytes
- ECG to document type of arrhythmia
- Thoracic radiographs, echocardiography for underlying cause

Treatment

Treatment depends on the type of arrhythmia and whether or not the patient is symptomatic. If possible, the underlying cause should be treated. Tachycardia is treated with antiarrhythmic drugs. Bradycardia can be treated with a pacemaker.

Pericardial disease

An effusion accumulates in the pericardial sac and restricts filling of the right side of the heart, leading to right-sided heart failure.

A pericardial effusion may be caused by:

- Haemorrhage (e.g. trauma, neoplasia)
- Transudate (e.g. hypoproteinaemia, neoplasia)
- Exudate (e.g. infection, foreign body).

Clinical signs

- Collapse
- Exercise intolerance
- Pale mucous membranes
- Muffled heart sounds, tachycardia

Diagnostics

- Echocardiography
- Thoracic radiographs: right lateral and dorsoventral views
- ECG

Treatment

Treatment involves relieving the pressure around the heart and removing the fluid via pericardiocentesis; samples should be sent for analysis. Subsequent management will depend on the underlying cause but if pericardial effusion recurs, surgical removal of the pericardium (pericardectomy) is indicated.

Procedure for pericardiocentesis

The following is one of various pericardiocentesis techniques

Equipment
- 60 ml syringe
- Three-way stopcock
- Intravenous fluid extension line
- 16 gauge 3¼-inch or 5-inch over-the-needle catheter
- Sterile gloves
- Lidocaine for local anaesthesia
- Scalpel blade ▶

Technique
This is a sterile procedure. It may be done with the patient standing or in sternal or left lateral recumbency

1. Connect the syringe to the three-way stopcock and intravenous extension tubing.
2. If sedation is required, administer this according to the veterinary surgeon's instructions.
3. The patient should have constant monitoring. Monitor with ECG if available.
4. Surgically prepare the ventral third of the right hemithorax from the 3rd to the 8th intercostal space.
5. The veterinary surgeon will infiltrate the areas with lidocaine, making a small cutaneous incision with the scalpel blade and advancing the catheter. The intravenous extension is attached to the catheter.
6. The assistant will be instructed to aspirate the fluid slowly.
7. During the procedure the catheter may block and the veterinary surgeon will need to reposition it.
8. Ventricular premature complexes may be seen during the procedure. These usually resolve once the procedure is completed. The ECG may need to be monitored intermittently for abnormal rhythms once the procedure is complete.
9. The fluid is usually very bloody. Collect a sterile sample, label it and submit for culture and cytological examination.
10. Measure the PCV of the fluid and compare with venous PCV.
11. Monitor patient's vital signs once the procedure is completed.

Heart failure

Heart failure may be defined as circulatory failure where the heart is unable to maintain an adequate circulation for the needs of the body. The heart has some capacity to compensate for disease. When this is exceeded the heart fails; blood cannot be effectively pumped around the body and congestion occurs. Right-sided heart failure causes systemic venous congestion and ascites. Left-sided heart failure causes congestion in the lungs and pulmonary oedema.

Clinical signs
Some cases will be recognized early on, while others will present with acute decompensation, have severe clinical signs and acute heart failure. These cases require emergency treatment.

Acute heart failure

- Collapse
- Pale mucous membranes
- Slow capillary refill time
- Weak pulse

This is an emergency and requires immediate treatment (see Chapter 18).

Left-sided heart failure

- Pulmonary oedema
- Cough
- Dyspnoea, tachypnoea

- Tachycardia, weak pulses
- Murmurs, dysrhythmias (in many cases)
- Exercise intolerance, fatigue, lethargy
- Cyanosis (rare)

Right-sided heart failure

- Ascites, abdominal distension
- Hepatomegaly, splenomegaly
- Exercise intolerance, fatigue, lethargy
- Pale mucous membranes, tachycardia, weak pulses
- Dyspnoea, tachypnoea, cyanosis
- Murmurs, dysrhythmias (in many cases)

Congestive heart failure

This includes signs of simultaneous failure of both left and right sides, and may occur as a result of myocardial disease or as a sequel to left- or right-sided heart failure. Clinical signs are as for both left- and right-sided heart failure.

Diagnostics

In a patient with heart disease the first indication of failure can be an increased breathing rate and heart rate. Therefore, these need to be monitored at home by the owners.

- Thoracic radiographs: right lateral and dorsoventral views
- Echocardiography
- ECG
- Blood tests: biochemistry, especially urea, creatinine and electrolytes

Treatment

Acute heart failure

- Strict cage rest
- Oxygen supplementation
- Glyceryl trinitrate (applied topically to inside of ear; wear gloves)
- Diuretics
- Catheterize and monitor urine output

Chronic heart failure (left-sided, right-sided, congestive)

- Reduce exercise
- Reduce obesity if present
- Low salt diet (see below)
- Diuretics to relieve ascites, pulmonary oedema
- Cardiac drugs
- Anti-arrhythmic drugs if required

Nursing care

Acute heart failure

- Do not stress
- Provide oxygen
- Provide cage rest
- Keep warm
- Monitor vital signs; continuous ECG monitoring

Chronic cases

- Decrease stress and exercise
- Manage for weight loss if the patient is overweight
- Monitor vital signs

Nutrition

Animals with heart failure can be anorexic; therefore it is important that the diet is palatable. Various formulated diets are available. These have added nutrients and usually increased potassium and magnesium but decreased sodium (salt restriction) (see Chapter 16). As treats are often high in salt, low-salt alternatives need to be used (e.g. formulated treats or a slice of apple or orange). Overweight patients need to be on a weight-control diet.

It should be noted that new cardiac drugs may alter the electrolyte balance of the patient and so these need to be monitored and the diet adjusted as necessary.

Haemopoietic system disease

Definitions

- **Anaemia** – reduced number of red blood cells or reduced quantity of haemoglobin
- **Erythrocytosis** – increased number of red blood cells
- **Leucocytosis** – increased number of white blood cells
- **Leucopenia** – reduced number of white blood cells
- **Thrombocytopenia** – reduction in number of platelets
- **Lymphocytosis** – increase in number of lymphocytes
- **Leukaemias** – distorted proliferation and development of leucocytes and their precursors in the blood and bone marrow

Anaemia

Anaemia is a clinical sign rather than a diagnosis. It may have many causes (Figure 21.6).

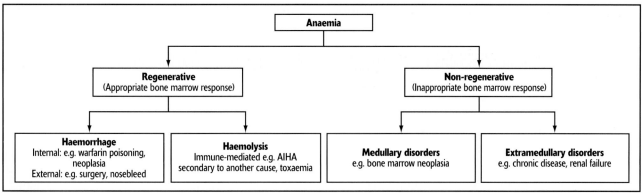

21.6 Types and causes of anaemia.

- In **regenerative** anaemias the bone marrow is capable of making an appropriate response to the anaemia: it increases the production of red blood cells and releases immature red blood cells into the circulation. Regenerative anaemias are distinguished by the presence of reticulocytes in the circulation.
- In **non-regenerative** anaemias the bone marrow is not capable of making an appropriate response to the anaemia: there is no increase in red cell production.

Clinical signs

In acute anaemias the clinical signs can be severe and require emergency treatment. Conversely, mild and chronic anaemias can have very few apparent clinical signs.

- Collapse
- Lethargy
- Inappetence
- Exercise intolerance
- Pale mucous membranes
- Dyspnoea, tachypnoea
- Tachycardia

Diagnostics

- Blood tests: haematology (morphology of the cells is also important, as it can help with determining the cause), including presence of reticulocytes
- Biochemistry
- In-saline agglutination and Coombs' test for autoimmune haemolytic anaemia
- Serology, especially if travel history
- FeLV/FIV tests in cats
- *Mycoplasma* – fresh blood smear needed (see 'Feline infectious anaemia')
- Faecal occult blood (red-meat-free diet for 3 days)
- Non-regenerative anaemias: bone marrow aspiration (see Chapter 17)

Other tests that may be indicated include:

- Coagulation profile
- Radiographs – chest, abdomen
- Ultrasonography – chest, abdomen.

Treatment

The animal may need a blood transfusion (see Chapter 19) if the anaemia is severe or if there are severe clinical signs (Figure 21.7). The underlying cause needs to be treated (e.g. immunosuppresion for immune-mediated disease; chemotherapy for neoplasia; tetracyclines for *Mycoplasma*).

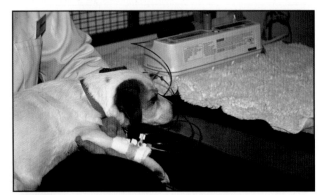

21.7 Blood transfusion in an anaemic dog.

Nursing care

- Monitor vital signs
- Restrict exercise, keep quiet and avoid stress
- Monitor blood transfusion
- Take blood samples to monitor progress

Clotting disorders

The normal blood clotting mechanism (**haemostasis**) is described in Chapter 4a. Clotting defects can result in haemorrhage and thus give rise to anaemia. Clotting disorders may result from primary or secondary defects:

- Primary haemostatic defect:
  - Vessel defect
  - Platelets
    - decreased
    - dysfunction
- Secondary haemostatic defect:
  - Decreased levels of clotting factors
    - decreased production (e.g. liver disease, warfarin toxicity)
    - increased consumption (e.g. disseminated intravascular coagulation).

Clinical signs

A primary abnormality in haemostasis usually leads to haemorrhages in the skin or mucous membranes. These are referred to as **petechial** (pinpoint) or **ecchymotic haemorrhages** (larger; Figure 21.8). An abnormality in clotting factors can lead to bleeding into body cavities such as the pleural or peritoneal space. If the blood loss is severe, the patient will have clinical signs of anaemia. Other clinical signs will be related to the underlying cause and to the physical effect of accumulation of blood (e.g. dyspnoea if there is bleeding in the pleural space).

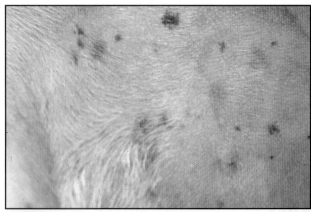

21.8 Ecchymotic haemorrhages in the skin as a result of a primary haemostatic disorder.

Diagnostics

- Haematology and biochemistry
- Clotting profile: prothrombin time, activated partial thromboplastin time
- Activated clotting time
- Buccal mucosal bleeding time (if the above results are normal – assess platelet function)
- von Willebrand factor
- Clotting factor assays
- Platelet function tests
- Fibrin degradation products, D-dimers

Buccal mucosal bleeding time (BMBT)

1. Restrain the patient in lateral recumbency (cats usually require light sedation).
2. Fold back the upper lip and tie a strip of gauze around the maxilla, enough to cause moderate mucosal engorgement.
3. Make an incision on the upper lip by gently holding the buccal mucosal bleeding spring-loaded blade on the lip and firing it.
4. Start the timer.
5. Gently blot away bleeding with filter paper, taking care not to disturb the incision and the formation of the clot.
6. When bleeding ceases, stop the timer.

The normal bleeding time for dogs is less than 4.2 minutes and for cats less than 2.4 minutes.

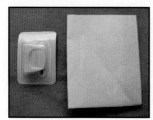

Spring-loaded buccal mucosal bleeding device and filter paper

Treatment

The underlying cause needs to be treated (e.g. immunosuppression for immune-mediated disease; vitamin K for warfarin poisoning). If the bleeding is severe, the patient may require whole blood or plasma to replace clotting factors. Desmopressin can be used to increase von Willebrand factor and can be used prior to surgery in affected Dobermanns.

Nursing care

- Handle gently
- Blood samples should be taken from a peripheral vein to ensure that adequate pressure can be applied to the site
- Avoid intramuscular injections
- Monitor vital signs

Gastrointestinal tract disease

The GI tract comprises the oesophagus, stomach, small intestine, colon and rectum. Dysfunction or disease affecting these organs can lead to regurgitation, vomiting and diarrhoea.

Definitions

- **Dysphagia** – difficulty in swallowing
- **Coprophapia** – eating of faeces
- **Anorexia** – absence of appetite
- **Pica** – depraved appetite (e.g. eating of unusual foodstuff)
- **Inappetence** – reduced appetite
- **Polyphagia** – increased appetite ▶

- **Megaoesophagus** – flaccid dilation of oesophagus
- **Regurgitation** – passive process of returning, usually from oesophagus
- **Vomiting** – active process of expelling stomach contents
- **Diarrhoea** – increased passage of abnormally softer liquid faeces
- **Tenesmus** – straining to pass faeces
- **Dyschezia** – pain on defecation
- **Melaena** – dark tar-like faeces containing digested blood
- **Constipation** – failure to pass faeces of normal frequency or consistency

Regurgitation

It is important to be able to differentiate between regurgitation and vomiting. Regurgitation is a *passive* process: there is no contraction of the abdominal muscles; the head is lowered and undigested food is ejected from the mouth. The severity of the condition can vary from the regurgitation of all solid food to regurgitation of some ingested matter and saliva. Malnutrition and aspiration pneumonia can result, depending on the severity of the condition. If there is any doubt as to the origin of the undigested food matter (i.e. whether it is from the oesophagus or from the stomach) a dipstick can be used to check the pH, as it can sometimes be difficult to determine.

Causes of regurgitation can include:

- Megaoesophagus
- Oesophagitis
- Oesophageal foreign bodies
- Oesophageal strictures
- Persistent right aortic arch.

Diagnostics

- Blood samples for haematology and biochemistry; other specific tests to detect myaesthenia gravis, hypothyroidism and hypoadrenocorticism (Addison's disease)
- Plain and barium swallow radiographs
- Oesophagoscopy

Treatment

The treatment will vary depending on the underlying cause of the problem:

- Medical management to treat any underlying disease that causes megaeosophagus
- Anti-inflammatories and histamine H_2 blockers for oesophagitis
- Surgical removal of oesophageal foreign bodies
- Ballooning for oesophageal strictures
- Surgery for animals with persistent right aortic arch.

Further management can include feeding animals from a height (see Chapter 15). Gravity-assisted feeding can help to control the clinical signs if the problem is not too severe. Keeping the patient's head and forelimbs elevated for 10 minutes after a meal will allow the food to enter the stomach. In other cases liquid food can be fed to pass a stricture, or balls of food may be given for megaoesophagus if some peristaltic activity is present.

Nursing care

- Monitor patient's vital signs and hydration status
- Monitor and record patient's weight
- Observe for regurgitation and record frequency and consistency
- Observe for signs of aspiration pneumonia (coughing, depression, pyrexia)
- Offer food and water from a height
- Groom and clean patient as necessary
- Administer medication and fluid therapy as directed by the veterinary surgeon

Vomiting

Vomiting is an *active* process, where the stomach contents are forcefully ejected out of the mouth by the contraction of the abdominal muscles. It is a common clinical sign of many conditions, as it is a protective mechanism that helps to eliminate toxic substances from the body. Receptors in the brain are triggered by the presence of certain toxins or when normal levels of substances found in the body are exceeded (e.g. urea). Causes of vomiting are shown in Figure 21.9.

Gastrointestinal disease
Dietary indiscretion
Infectious agents: viral (e.g. parvovirus); bacterial (e.g. *Salmonella*); parasitic (e.g. roundworms)
Gastric foreign bodies
Intestinal foreign bodies
Intussusception
Gastrointestinal ulceration
Pyloric stenosis
Gastrointestinal neoplasia
Systemic disease
Uraemia – due to either renal disease or urinary tract obstruction
Hepatic failure
Pyometra
Pancreatitis
Peritonitis
Metabolic/endocrine disorders
Diabetic ketoacidosis
Hypercalcaemia
Hypoadrenocorticism
Drugs/toxins
NSAIDs
Chemotherapy drugs
Heavy metal toxicity
Insecticide toxicity (e.g. organophosphates)
Herbicide toxicity (e.g. chlorates)
Molluscicide toxicity (e.g. metaldehyde)

21.9   Causes of vomiting.

Prior to vomiting the animal may show signs of restlessness, abdominal pain, salivating or licking of the lips. An episode of vomiting may occur many hours after the animal has eaten and the vomitus may contain partially digested food, bile or a mixture of both.

Vomiting can be classified as **acute** or **chronic**, depending on the speed of onset and its duration. Depending on the frequency of vomiting and the volumes involved, there can be a significant loss of water from the body and dehydration if the animal is unable to replace these losses. Electrolytes (sodium, chloride and potassium) are also lost, along with hydrogen ions, and this can result in electrolyte imbalances and metabolic alkalosis (see Chapter 19).

Diagnostics

It can sometimes be difficult to discover the cause of vomiting in a patient. Obtaining a detailed history is an important part of the diagnostic approach. It is equally important that close observations of a patient are made if an animal is hospitalized.

- History
- Clinical examination – abdominal palpation important
- Blood samples for haematology and biochemistry to confirm or rule out systemic disease
- Abdominal radiography and/or ultrasonography
- Barium meal
- Gastroscopy
- Exploratory laparotomy
- Biopsy (via endoscopy or laparotomy)

Assessing the vomiting patient

- **Body condition:** A depressed or lethargic patient is more likely to have systemic disease, dehydration or electrolyte imbalances. Weight loss and general body condition can also provide important information about the cause of vomiting.
- **Age:** Older animals more likely to have neoplasia.
- **Other clinical signs:** Clinical signs such as polyuria and polydipsia can indicate the presence of systemic disease.
- **Vaccination history:** Up-to-date vaccination status can help to rule out some infectious agents.
- **Dietary changes:** Changes in feeding can help to confirm or rule out uncomplicated gastroenteritis. A history of scavenging (or opportunity to scavenge) should also be ascertained.
- **Frequency of vomiting:** Can provide important information about the causal factor. For example, infectious agents such as parvovirus or *Salmonella* are often associated with acute bouts of frequent vomiting.
- **Type of vomit:** Vomit containing blood can indicate ulceration or severe inflammation of the GI tract. Vomition of undigested food long after a meal can suggest gastric motility problems.
- **Faeces:** Lack of faeces can indicate obstruction. Diarrhoea indicates intestinal involvement. Melaena (blackened by digested blood) indicates ulceration and bleeding from the upper GI tract.

Treatment

Uncomplicated **acute** vomiting is managed by starving the patient for 24 hours, whilst providing oral fluid and electrolyte replacement. If the animal responds successfully, an investigation of the cause is often not undertaken. Further symptomatic treatment may also be required.

Treatment for **chronic** vomiting is aimed at treating the underlying disease, controlling the clinical signs and correcting the dehydration. Drug therapy may include:

- Specific drugs acting on the GI tract (see Chapter 9)
- Antibacterial drugs – if cause is bacterial or to prevent secondary bacterial infections if blood is present in the vomit

- Fluid therapy – important to correct dehydration, electrolyte and acid–base imbalances (see Chapter 19)
- Analgesia – to make the patient more comfortable (NSAIDs should be avoided).

Surgery may be indicated for correction of pyloric stenosis, intussusception or removal of foreign bodies and tumours.

Nursing care

- Starve the patient for 24 hours and then feed small frequent meals
- Feed a bland easy-to-digest single-source protein diet
- Keep the patient clean and groom as necessary
- Monitor clinical signs, weight and hydration status and record findings
- Observe and record vomiting type and frequency
- Administer medication and fluid therapy, as directed by the veterinary surgeon
- Isolate and barrier nurse if an infectious agent is suspected (see Chapter 12)

Diarrhoea

Diarrhoea can be classified as either **acute** or **chronic** and can originate from the small intestine, the large intestine or both (Figure 21.10). It results in a loss of water from the body, leading to dehydration, electrolyte imbalances and metabolic acidosis.

Clinical sign	Origin: small intestine	Origin: large intestine
Vomiting	Commonly seen	Occasional
Weight	Loss common	Maintained
Appetite	Often increased	Normal
Faecal volume	Increased	Normal
Faecal type	Watery	Varies with cause
Faecal frequency	3-4 times daily	Up to 10 times daily
Faecal mucus	None	Often present
Blood in faeces	Melaena	Haematochezia
Urgency to pass faeces	Not present	Present; straining on defecation
Flatulence	Minimal	Common

21.10 Clinical signs suggesting the origin of diarrhoea.

Causes

Acute diarrhoea

- Sudden change of diet or scavenging
- Dietary intolerance or hypersensitivity
- Colitis
- Viral infections (e.g. parvovirus, FIV, FeLV)
- Bacterial infections (e.g. *Salmonella, Campylobacter, Escherichia coli*)
- Intestinal parasites (e.g. *Toxocara, Giardia, Cryptosporidium*)
- Intussusception
- Neoplasia
- Foreign bodies

Chronic diarrhoea

- Long-term dietary intolerance or hypersensitivity
- Chronic infections (e.g. *Giardia, Campylobacter*)
- Small intestinal bacterial overgrowth (SIBO)
- Malabsorption (e.g. inflammatory bowel disease (IBD))
- Maldigestion (e.g. exocrine pancreatic insufficiency (EPI))
- Colitis
- Intussusception
- Neoplasia
- Foreign bodies
- Liver disease, due to lack of bile salts being produced
- Endocrine disease (e.g. hyperthyroidism, hypoadrenocorticism)

Colitis
The cause of colitis is not often determined. Many cases of acute colitis are associated with dietary indiscretion, resulting in a secondary bacterial infection. Causes of chronic colitis can include: inappropriate immune response to antigens in the colon (e.g. eosinophilic colitis); infections – *Campylobacter, Salmonella*; neoplasia or polyps; motility disorders and food hypersensitivity reactions. Treatment includes: hypoallergenic diet; change of diet; sulfasalazine – as anti-inflammatory; metronidazole – antibacterial but also has anti-inflammatory effect; corticosteroids – used in cases not responding to other treatment.

Clinical signs

- **Acute** diarrhoea can be mild or severe. In mild cases the animal appears bright and alert with no signs of dehydration. In severe cases the animal is dull, depressed and dehydrated, especially if accompanied by vomiting.
- In **chronic** diarrhoea clinical signs are more commonly weight loss and loss of bodily condition, as the causes result in the animal receiving inadequate nutrition over a period of time.

Diagnostics
A thorough history can provide important information as to the cause of the diarrhoea. Also observation of the frequency and the consistency of the diarrhoea (e.g. steatorrhoea) can indicate exocrine pancreatic insufficiency (EPI).

- Clinical examination
- Routine biochemistry and haematology to rule out systemic disease
- Specific blood tests: trypsin-like immunoreactivity (TLI), folate and cobalamin (B12), to confirm or rule out EPI or bacterial overgrowth
- Faecal analysis – for parasites, undigested food, culture; ELISA test for parvovirus antigen
- Abdominal radiography and/or ultrasonography
- Contrast radiography
- Endoscopy of upper or lower GI tract
- Exploratory laparotomy
- Biopsy (via endoscopy or laparotomy)

Treatment

Acute diarrhoea
In acute cases of diarrhoea, fasting for 24–48 hours is usually sufficient as long as during this period of time the animal is not vomiting, and fluid and electrolytes are supplemented. In severe acute cases, intravenous fluid therapy is indicated to

prevent dehydration and electrolyte imbalance. Fasting for longer periods should be avoided, as the intestine absorbs the majority of its nutrition from the digested food that passes through it. Long periods of starvation can therefore result in reduced functioning capabilities of the intestine.

Treatment of any underlying cause is also important.

When food is reintroduced it should be a bland, easy-to-digest, low-fat and single-source protein diet. This should be fed for a number of days before gradually reintroducing normal food.

Chronic diarrhoea

In cases with chronic diarrhoea, investigation of the underlying cause is important for successful treatment. Treatments can include:

- In cases of hypersensitivity, feeding a novel protein that the animal has never eaten
- Anthelmintics and antiparasitic drugs
- Antibacterials for bacterial overgrowth and to prevent secondary bacterial infections
- Corticosteroids for malabsorption due to inflammatory disease
- Enzyme supplementation in cases with EPI
- Surgery for intussusception, neoplasia and foreign bodies
- Treatment of underlying systemic disease.

Nursing care

- Feed a diet that contains high-quality protein and is low in fat (see Chapter 16)
- Feed small frequent meals
- Keep the patient clean and groom as necessary. It may be necessary to bandage the tail, clip the hair and apply barrier cream to the skin if diarrhoea is severe
- Monitor clinical signs, weight and hydration status and record findings
- Observe and record passing of any diarrhoea
- Allow frequent visits outside to defecate (if not thought to be infectious)
- Administer medication and fluid therapy, according to veterinary surgeon's instructions
- Isolate and barrier nurse if an infectious agent is suspected (see Chapter 12)

Constipation

Constipation is the failure to pass faeces either in normal quantity or at normal frequency, resulting in impaction of the colon and rectum with faecal material. There are many causes of constipation (Figure 21.11). It is seen more commonly in elderly patients taking less exercise.

Clinical signs

- Failure to pass faeces
- Tenesmus
- Passing of very hard faeces (often with fresh blood)
- Vomiting
- Dyschezia (pain on passing faeces)

Diagnostics

- Physical examination/rectal examination
- Radiography
- Proctoscopy

Dietary
Fibre content of diet too low
Eating bones

Colonic
Rectal strictures
Rectal foreign bodies
Rectal tumours
Perineal ruptures
Megacolon (dysautonomia)
Anal sac disease

Orthopaedic
Pelvic fractures causing narrowing of pelvic canal

Other
Dehydration
Neurological dysfunction (Key–Gaskell syndrome; spinal damage)
Prostatic hyperplasia

21.11   Causes of constipation.

Treatment

It is important to find the underlying cause to provide the best treatment, but treatment may include:

- Enemas – various types (use most suitable)
- Changes to diet
- Stool-softening agents (lactulose)
- Bulking agents
- Surgical correction of obstruction.

Nursing care

- Administer enema under veterinary surgeon's instructions
- Administer fluid therapy
- Monitor vital signs
- Keep the patient clean
- Encourage the patient to eat a suitable diet

Hepatic disease

Definitions

- **Hepatitis** – inflammation of the liver
- **Cirrhosis** – a degenerative change, causing fibrosis of the organ, resulting in a loss of functional cells and therefore loss in normal function
- **Ascites** – accumulation of fluid in the abdominal cavity
- **Jaundice** – elevated levels of bilirubin in the tissues and circulation, resulting in a yellowing of the skin and mucous membranes

Causes

Liver disease may be congenital or acquired, and acute or chronic. There are many causes, including:

- **Acute:**
  - Drug-induced (e.g. paracetamol, phenobarbital)
  - Toxins (e.g. bacterial endotoxin, blue-green algae)
  - Bacterial infection (e.g. *Leptospira*, *Salmonella*)
  - Viral infection (e.g. adenovirus I (ICH), canine herpes)

- Parasitosis (e.g. toxoplasmosis)
- Acute pancreatitis
- Surgical hypotension or hypoxia
- Trauma (e.g. bruising or rupture)

- **Chronic:**
  - Drug-induced (e.g. phenobarbital)
  - Neoplasia (e.g. haemangioma, haemangiosarcoma)
  - Metabolic (e.g. diabetes mellitus, hyperadrenocorticism)
  - Copper toxicity (in Bedlington Terrier and West Highland White Terrier)
  - Immune-mediated (e.g. cholangiohepatitis, chronic progressive hepatitis)
  - Congenital (e.g. portosystemic shunts).

Portosystemic shunt

The hepatic portal system enables the products of digestion that are absorbed by the gut to be transported directly to the liver for storage or use. In a normal animal the blood flows:

- From the heart to the capillary beds of the stomach and intestines
- From here to the liver via the hepatic portal vein, where it enters the capillary bed of the liver
- From the liver via the hepatic vein to the posterior vena cava.

With a portosystemic shunt the blood bypasses the liver and deposits blood directly back into the systemic circulation. Shunts can be a developmental abnormality or they can be due to advanced cirrhosis. Congenital shunts can be surgically ligated.

Clinical signs of liver disease

The liver has enormous regenerative capabilities and the clinical signs will not be noticed until 70–80% of the liver cells have been lost due to damage.

Non-specific signs include:

- Vomiting
- Diarrhoea
- Weight loss
- Polydipsia
- Polyuria
- Anorexia.

Specific signs include:

- Anterior abdominal pain
- Jaundice
- Ascites
- Hepatomegaly
- Hepatoencephalopathy
- Pale fatty faeces – due to decreased bile production
- Dark urine – due to bilirubin from red cell breakdown
- Bleeding disorders – due to clotting factor deficiency.

Jaundice (icterus)

Jaundice of the skin and mucous membranes (Figure 21.12) will occur if the capacity of the liver to excrete bilirubin in the bile becomes unbalanced:

- Prehepatic (e.g. excessive haemolysis)
- Intrahepatic (e.g. degenerative liver function
- Posthepatic (e.g. bile flow obstruction).

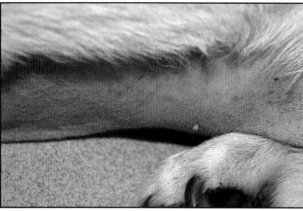

21.12   Jaundice as a result of haemolytic anaemia in a 6-year-old Labrador Retriever.

Hepatic encephalopathy

This occurs when more than 70% of hepatic tissue is lost and neurotoxic substances build up, causing toxaemias and neurological signs. The toxins are mainly from the gastrointestinal tract (e.g. ammonia is a by-product of protein breakdown).

Diagnostics

- Biochemistry:
  - Albumin
  - Globulin
  - Alanine aminotransferase (ALT)
  - Alkaline phosphatase (ALP)
  - Ammonia
- Bile acid stimulation test
- Haematology:
  - Full blood count
  - Coagulation screen
- Radiography – can provide information about the size of the liver
- Ultrasound scan – can give a more useful indication of internal structure of the liver and can identify focal or diffuse lesions
- Liver biopsy – will most likely provide definitive diagnosis, but coagulation screen should be run first
- Paracentesis – can give indication as to cause or nature of the disease
- Urine tests – to include specific gravity, dipsticks and sedimentation

Treatment

- Intravenous fluids (acute cases)
- Antibiotics (to reduce bacterial load)
- Anti-inflammatories
- Water-soluble bile acids
- Lactulose (helps to bind ammonia)
- Special diet (see Chapter 16)
- Vitamin supplement, especially vitamin K

Nursing care

- Isolate and barrier nurse the patient if cause is infectious
- Monitor vital signs
- Administer medication and therapy
- Provide comfort and TLC
- Provide nutritional support (see Chapter 16)

Pancreatic disease

The pancreas is composed of two types of tissue:

- Exocrine – produces digestive enzymes
- Endocrine – produces hormones (insulin, glucagon).

Diseases of the pancreas can be divided into:

- Pancreatitis – acute and chronic
- Exocrine pancreatic insufficiency
- Exocrine tumours.

Pancreatitis

Pancreatitis, inflammation of the pancreas, is caused by self-digestion (**autolysis**) of the pancreas by the digestive enzymes that are stored inside specialized storage pockets. **Acute** pancreatitis is more often seen in dogs, whereas **chronic** pancreatitis is more common in cats.

Acute pancreatitis

This can be life-threatening, as complications such as peritonitis can develop. Causes include:

- Obesity
- High-fat diet
- Pancreatic duct occlusion
- Trauma
- Surgical manipulation.

Clinical signs

- Sudden-onset pyrexia
- Sudden-onset anorexia
- Acute abdominal pain
- Dehydration
- Shock
- Collapse

Diagnostics

- Blood tests (elevated levels of amylase and lipase)
- Radiography
- Ultrasonography

Treatment

- Nothing by mouth (**nil per os**, *NPO*) for 3–5 days, until vomiting has stopped (any food or fluid given orally can stimulate the production of further enzyme release, making the condition worse)
- Intravenous fluid therapy
- Antibiotics
- Analgesics
- Low-fat diet

Nursing care

- Monitor vital signs (this is important, as disease can quickly progress to a life-threatening state)
- Ensure that nothing is given orally
- Keep the patient away from the sight and smell of other patients' food

- Groom and keep the patient clean (it is often necessary to clean the gums and mucous membranes, as the animal is unable to drink oral fluids)
- Administer fluid therapy and other medications, as instructed by the veterinary surgeon
- After clinical signs have resolved, and on the instruction of the veterinary surgeon, introduce small amounts of water and observe the patient's vital signs closely
- If the patient tolerates water, introduce small frequent low-fat meals (see Chapter 16) and observe the patient's vital signs closely

Chronic pancreatitis

This is a low-grade but continual inflammation of the pancreas, leading to functional destruction. The causes include:

- Idiopathic
- Infection
- Cholangiohepatitis (especially in cats)
- Ascending infection (especially in cats)
- Bile duct obstruction (especially in cats)

Clinical signs

- Weight loss
- Reduced appetite
- Abdominal pain

Diagnostics

Diagnostic tests are as for acute pancreatitis, with the addition of testing for trypsin-like immunoreactivity (TLI), folate and B12 levels.

Treatment

- Long-term dietary management (low fat)
- Fluid and electrolyte support
- Enzyme supplementation

Exocrine pancreatic insufficiency (EPI)

This condition is caused by insufficient production of pancreatic enzymes, resulting in maldigestion and malabsorption of food. Pancreatic atrophy occurs. It can be congenital and may be hereditary in German Shepherd Dogs. It can also occur following a severe case of pancreatitis if the cells of the pancreas are damaged. The condition is relatively common in dogs but rare in cats.

Clinical signs

- Diarrhoea
- Steatorrhoea
- Ravenous appetite
- Coprophagia (eating faeces) – due to presence of undigested food
- Weight loss

Diagnostics

- Blood test for haematology and biochemistry, to include trypsin-like immunoreactivity (TLI)
- Faecal analysis for undigested food

Treatment

- Dietary management using a low-fat highly digestible diet is sufficient in some mild cases
- Supplementation of food with pancreatic enzymes – amylase, lipase, and protease; dietary management still required
- Raw ox or pig pancreas obtained following appropriate post-mortem inspection is an inexpensive alternative. Pancreas can be stored frozen for at least 3 months without loss of enzyme activity

Nursing care

- Feed small frequent meals of low-fat diet
- Mix enzyme supplement with food
- Monitor faecal output – colour, consistency and frequency
- Groom and keep the patient clean
- Check and record weight

Renal disease

Definitions

- **Nephritis** – inflammation of the kidney
- **Glomerulonephritis** – inflammation of the glomerulus
- **Pyelonephritis** – inflammation of the kidney and renal pelvis
- **Interstitial nephritis** – inflammation of the renal interstitium

Acute renal failure

Renal failure that occurs suddenly is referred to as **acute renal failure**. It may occur as a consequence of:

- Decreased blood flow to the kidneys (e.g. hypovolaemic shock)
- Direct effect on the cells of the kidneys (e.g. toxins: ethylene glycol toxicity (antifreeze); infectious causes: leptospirosis)
- Post-renal obstruction (e.g. urethal stone causing obstruction, or rupture of the urinary tract)
- Chronic renal failure
- Congestive heart failure.

Clinical signs

- Sudden-onset anorexia, lethargy, depression
- Oliguria and anuria, followed by polyuria
- Vomiting, diarrhoea
- Polydipsia
- Dehydration
- Uraemic breath

Diagnostics

- Blood tests: haematology and biochemistry (urea, creatinine, electrolytes – specifically potassium phosphate)
- Urinalysis: specific gravity, dipstick and sediment examination
- Abdominal radiographs: right lateral and ventrodorsal views
- Abdominal ultrasonography

Treatment

Treatment involves removing the inciting cause and if possible treating the underlying cause. It is usually supportive:

- Intravenous fluid therapy is very important for several reasons: to decrease potassium (which is the initial life-threatening complication); to dilute the built-up waste products; and to rehydrate the animal. It is also the first line in establishing urine output.
- If oliguria persists, drugs such as furosemide, dopamine and mannitol may be administered to improve urine output.
- Antiemetics can be used to manage persistent vomiting.
- Peritoneal dialysis is used to remove nitrogenous waste products when urine output has failed to be re-established with the above treatment.

The condition is often reversible if the patient comes through the acute crisis.

Nursing care

- Administer fluid therapy, as directed by the veterinary surgeon
- Monitor vital signs, respiratory rate and sounds – especially for signs of volume overload
- Monitor urine output. If normal output (1–2 ml/kg/hour) is not re-established, discuss with the veterinary surgeon; a urinary catheter may need to be placed (this needs to be managed aseptically)
- Monitor hydration status
- Monitor bodyweight
- Administer drugs as directed by the veterinary surgeon
- Encourage to eat, and feed an acute renal diet
- Monitor vomiting
- Keep animal clean, grooming and bathing as necessary
- Barrier nurse the patient if an infectious cause is suspected

Chronic renal failure

This slowly progressive loss of renal function over an unidentified period of time results in **azotaemia** (uraemia). The onset of the clinical signs is gradual and may only become noticeable when 75% of the nephrons have already been lost. It is most often seen in animals over 7 years of age (Figure 21.13) but this can depend on the causal factor, as younger animals can be affected.

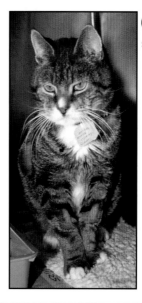

21.13 A 13-year-old cat with chronic renal failure showing poor body condition.

Causes of chronic renal failure include:

- Acute renal failure
- Nephrotoxins
- Pyelonephritis
- Glomerulonephritis
- Ischaemic damage
- Hypercalcaemia
- Congenital/hereditary disease (e.g. polycystic kidney disease)
- Idiopathic.

Clinical signs

- Polyuria/nocturia (as the kidney loses its ability to concentrate the urine)
- Polydipsia
- Uraemia – anorexia, vomiting, lethargy, depression
- Weight loss
- Dehydration
- Oral ulceration and halitosis
- Non-regenerative anaemia (due to lack of erythropoietin production by the kidney)
- Hypertension
- Rubber jaw (renal hyperparathyroidism) – kidneys fail to excrete phosphorus, effectively causing phosphorus levels in blood to become elevated (hyperphosphataemia); parathyroid responds by triggering release of parathormone, resulting in demineralization of calcium from bones to correct imbalance in blood
- Seizures – end-stage of disease

Diagnostics

- Biochemistry – will often reveal high levels of urea, creatinine and phosphorus)
- Hypokalaemia often evident
- Haematology: non-regenerative anaemia
- Urinalysis: lower than normal specific gravity often evident
- Abdominal radiography and/or ultrasonography

Treatment

Chronic renal failure is not reversible. Treatment is aimed at preventing further damage and reducing the workload of the remaining nephrons:

- Treatment of any underlying cause
- Intravenous fluid therapy (allow water to drink, unless vomiting)
- Antiemetics if vomiting
- Electrolyte supplementation, if required due to increased losses
- Dietary management
- ACE inhibitors such as benazepril to help treat hypertension (they also increase blood flow to kidneys)
- Vitamin B supplementation.

Nursing care

- Monitor vital signs and urine output
- Administer fluid therapy and any other medication
- Provide water *ad libitum*
- Take patient outside regularly or keep litter tray clean
- Feed special diet (see Chapter 16)
- Encourage patient to eat if inappetent

If the animal is anorexic it should be offered other more palatable foods; for example, a recovery diet can be used initially until the patient's appetite improves. If the patient does not eat it will become catabolic, as it is metabolizing protein (its own body mass), and by-products of protein metabolism can still contribute to azotaemia. However, in this case the animal will also be losing weight and body condition.

Nephrotic syndrome

This is caused by either immune-mediated damage to the glomerular basement membrane or amyloidosis.

Clinical signs

- Ascites
- Subcutaneous oedema
- Hydrothorax (dyspnoea)
- Weight loss
- Exercise intolerance

May initially be bright until chronic renal failure develops; then additional signs of CRF (see above).

Diagnostics

- Biochemistry – hypoproteinaemia, severe proteinuria
- As for chronic renal failure

Treatment

- Diet – high biological value protein, low phosphate, high B vitamins
- Diuretics
- As for chronic renal failure

Lower urinary tract disease

The lower urinary tract comprises the ureters, bladder and urethra. Disease of these organs results from inflammation, obstruction or dysfunction.

Definitions

- **Cystitis** – inflammation of the urinary bladder
- **Urinary incontinence** – involuntary passing of urine
- **Urinary tenesmus** – straining to pass urine
- **Haematuria** – the presence of blood in the urine
- **Polyuria** – passing of increased volumes of urine
- **Dysuria** – difficulty and pain passing urine
- **Oliguria** – reduced urine production
- **Anuria** – absence of urine production
- **Pollakiuria** – abnormal frequency of urination (used in paediatrics, where it is a benign condition), passing very small amounts of urine

Diagnostic tests

- Blood tests for biochemistry and haematology
- Urinalysis: specific gravity, dipsticks, sedimentation examination, culture and sensitivity (urine for this test must be obtained via cystocentesis)

- Ultrasonography
- Radiography: contrast studies such as pneumocystograms and double-contrast cystograms
- Intravenous excretory urography (IVU)
- Retrograde urethrography
- Histology

Cystitis

Causes of cystitis include:

- Trauma
- Urolithiasis (urinary calculi)
- Primary bacterial infection – often ascending, common in females
- Bacterial infection secondary to other diseases (e.g. diabetes mellitus, hyperadrenocorticism (Cushing's disease), neoplasia, immunosuppressive infections – FIV, FeLV).

Clinical signs

- Pollakiuria (increased frequency of urination)
- Urinary tenesmus
- Haematuria
- Incontinence
- Dysuria
- Polydipsia

Treatment

- Identification and treatment of any underlying cause
- Appropriate antibiotic therapy – bacteria such as *Escherichia coli, Staphylococcus, Streptococcus* and *Pseudomonas* have all been identified as causal agents

Nursing care

- Monitor vital signs
- Ensure that water is freely available
- Take patient outside frequently
- Monitor urine output (note volume and frequency, and whether straining or haematuria is present)
- Administer medications, as directed by veterinary surgeon

Urolithiasis (urinary calculi)

Urinary calculi or uroliths (see Chapter 17) can form within the urinary tract in the renal pelvis, ureters, bladder or urethra. Causes include:

- Urinary tract infection
- High dietary intake of certain minerals
- Systemic disease (e.g. liver disease)
- Genetic predisposition (e.g. high incidence of urate calculi in Dalmatians).

Clinical signs

- Pollakiuria
- Urinary tenesmus
- Haematuria
- Dysuria
- Distended bladder

Treatment

Diet plays a major role in the control and management of some types of urinary calculi (i.e. struvite, urate and cystine) (see Chapter 16). Dietary dissolution of calculi is possible for certain uroliths, but surgical removal is required for calculi such as those composed of calcium oxalate or calcium phosphate. Diet is used to prevent the recurrence of calculi after removal. These diets change the urinary pH, make the urine more dilute, and contain lower dietary levels of the minerals that contribute to calculi formation.

If urinary obstruction occurs, the same steps should be followed as for obstructed feline lower urinary tract disease (see below).

Nursing care

- Monitor vital signs
- Ensure that water is freely available
- Take outside frequently
- Monitor urine output (note volume and frequency, and whether straining or haematuria is present)
- Administer medications as directed by the veterinary surgeon

Urinary incontinence

Urinary incontinence is the involuntary passing of urine. Leakage of urine may be continuous or intermittent and may occur when the animal is recumbent or standing. Causes include:

- Urethral sphincter mechanism incontinence
- Ectopic ureters (congenital; more common in females; ureter often ends in vagina)
- Bladder-neck tumour (transitional cell carcinoma)
- Prostatic disease
- Neurological disease
- Cystitis.

Clinical signs

- Passing of urine when lying down or walking
- Urine around perineum
- Urine scalding of the skin around the perineum

Treatment

Treatment will be specific to the cause, but can include:

- Phenylpropanolamine or oestrogen for sphincter mechanism incontinence
- Surgery for ectopic ureters
- Surgery with or without chemotherapy for tumours
- Castration or delmadinone acetate injections for prostatic hyperplasia
- Antibiotic therapy for cystitis.

Nursing care

- Clip and clean the perineum
- Apply barrier creams to prevent urine scalding
- Administer medication as directed by the veterinary surgeon

Feline lower urinary tract disease (FLUTD)

FLUTD may be obstructive or non-obstructive. In many cases the cause is unclear, but FLUTD is commonly seen in over-weight, young to middle-aged, indoor cats fed on dry food in multi-cat households. It is thought that these cats have a tendency to urinate less frequently than outdoor cats, resulting in stale urine remaining in the bladder for longer periods, which gives rise to increased levels of bacteria in the urine and precipitation of crystals. Stress is also thought to be a contributing factor. Research has found that cats with cystitis have reduced levels of glycosaminoglycan (GAG), a component of the bladder membrane.

FLUTD affects both male and female cats, but male cats tend to be affected by obstructive disease due to the narrow size of the urethra in comparison with females. The distal end of the urethra becomes blocked with calculi or clumps of crystals and mucus (urethral plugs).

Causes of FLUTD include:

- Idiopathic (up to 65% of cases)
- Urethral plugs
- Uroliths
- Bacterial infection.

Clinical signs

Clinical signs for both non-obstructive and obstructive FLUTD are as for cystitis (see above). With obstructive FLUTD these signs may lead to:

- Distress
- Anuria
- Distended bladder
- Renal damage.

Treatment of obstructive FLUTD

Urethral obstruction is a serious life-threatening condition, which requires urgent medical attention.

- Blood tests should be performed to assess the patient's metabolic state (urea and creatinine often elevated due to postrenal azotaemia; potassium levels elevated; analysis of blood gases if available).
- Intravenous fluid therapy should be initiated (a fluid type that does not contain potassium).
- The cat should be anaesthetized.
- Cystocentesis should be performed to empty the bladder or at least alleviate the pressure. A sample can be taken at this time for analysis and culture.
- The blockage can then be dislodged; massage of the penis tip or retrograde flushing is often required to pass a urinary catheter, and the bladder should then be flushed with saline.
- The veterinary surgeon will decide whether or not an indwelling catheter should be left in place, as this can increase the urethral inflammation already present.
- If a urinary catheter is fitted, it should be sutured in place and either plugged or a closed collection system fitted, to prevent ascending infection. The patient should also be fitted with an Elizabethan collar to prevent interference.
- Antibacterial, analgesic and anti-inflammatory drugs are given (avoid NSAIDs in cases with possible renal involvement).

Nursing care of obstructive FLUTD

- Monitor vital signs
- Perform regular blood test as described by the veterinary surgeon to monitor levels
- Administer and maintain fluid therapy
- Monitor urine output and aseptically maintain urinary catheter if in place; apply barrier creams to prevent scalding
- Groom and keep patient clean, especially if fitted with an Elizabethan collar
- Administer any other medications as per veterinary surgeon's instructions
- Encourage eating of a suitable urinary diet; if inappetent, tempt patient with other food initially

Treatment of non-obstructive FLUTD

This usually involves long-term management by the owners at home.

- Dietary management: feeding a diet that has low levels of magnesium and phosphorus. Wet foods are preferable as this increases the urine output. Weight loss is to be encouraged if the cat is overweight.
- Increase water consumption: ensure that the cat always has access to clean water. Cats prefer large shallow bowls. Commercial water fountains are available that provide filtered running water; these are often successful, as cats tend to prefer to drink running water.
- Provide glycosaminoglycan (GAG) supplementation to promote the health of the bladder lining.
- Reduce stress levels; use pheromones or, in severe cases, amitriptyline.
- Make regular biochemistry and urinalysis checks.

Prostatic disease

The prostate can be affected by:

- Benign prostatic hyperplasia (BPH)
- Prostatitis
- Prostatic abscessation
- Prostatic cysts
- Prostatic neoplasia (rare; may occur in young and old dogs).

Clinical signs

- Haematuria
- Dysuria
- Urinary incontinence
- Urinary and faecal tenesmus
- Constipation

Diagnostics

- Ultrasonography
- Radiography
- Urinalysis
- Prostatic massage/flushing/biopsy

Treatment

- BPH is treated with castration or hormone treatment
- Prostatitis is treated as for BPH and with antibiotics
- Surgical intervention is required for cysts and abscessation

Reproductive system disease

Diseases of the reproductive system are discussed in detail in Chapter 25.

Endocrine and metabolic disorders

The hormones manufactured and secreted by various endocrine glands and the functions of those hormones are described in Chapter 4a.

Diabetes mellitus

Diabetes mellitus is caused by the lack of insulin, or a relative lack of insulin. Insulin is required to regulate glucose in the body. In the absence of insulin the animal will become hyperglycaemic. Clinical signs are attributable to this.

In the majority of dogs the condition is caused by immune destruction of the insulin-producing cells in the pancreas. In cats it is generally a result of insulin resistance due to obesity. These cats may produce insulin but the cells do not respond adequately. The cat may only be temporarily diabetic and can sometimes be managed with hypoglycaemic drugs. Insulin resistance can also be seen in entire bitches, and in hyperadrenocorticism (Cushing's disease) and pancreatitis.

If diabetes is left untreated, fats are broken down, leading to a build-up of ketones. These cases quickly become dehydrated, are acidotic and have electrolyte abnormalities. This condition is called **diabetic ketoacidosis (DKA)**.

Clinical signs
The majority of cases present with a history of:

- Polyuria/polydipsia
- Increased appetite (polyphagia) with weight loss.

More serious clinical signs that may indicate that the animal has developed DKA include:

- Vomiting
- Diarrhoea
- Anorexia
- Depression
- Collapse.

Other clinical signs include:

- Cataracts in dogs
- Plantigrade posture in cats.

Diagnostics

- Blood: haematology, biochemistry and fructosamine levels
- Urinalysis: dipstick, especially for presence of glucose and ketones in the urine, culture and sensitivity

Treatment
Treatment involves subcutaneous administration of insulin. There are various types of insulin available.

- **Neutral** or **regular insulin** is short-acting and has a rapid onset of action. It is used to stabilize ketoacidotic diabetics and is the only insulin that can be administered intravenously (it may also be administered intramuscularly or subcutaneously).
- **Lente insulin** has an intermediate duration of action and can be used in long-term stabilization of diabetics. It is administered subcutaneously.
- **Protamine zinc insulin** (PZI) has a long duration of action and can be used in long-term stabilization of diabetics. It is administered subcutaneously.

Patients undergoing anaesthesia should have their glucose measured on the morning of surgery and the insulin given as directed by the veterinary surgeon. Blood glucose levels should be monitored during anaesthesia, and dextrose saline administered intravenously as necessary.

If there is insulin resistance, the underlying cause needs to be treated (e.g. treat hyperadrenocorticism; spay a diabetic bitch).

The 'well' diabetic dog
It is very important that patients follow a routine in their insulin administration, diet and exercise.

- Insulin therapy: intermediate-acting insulin (lente or protamine zinc insulin (PZI)) administered once or twice daily (note that insulin preparations authorized for veterinary use are usually 100 IU/ml or 40 IU/ml)
- Diet: high-fibre, low-carbohydrate – feed twice daily (see Chapter 16)
  - If receiving once-daily insulin, feed once when insulin administered and the second meal 6–8 hours later to coincide with lowest glucose point
  - If receiving twice-daily insulin, meals are given at the time of insulin administration
- Exercise – same time every day.

The 'well' diabetic cat

- Insulin therapy:
  - In non-insulin-dependent diabetes: hypoglycaemic drugs (e.g. glipizide)
  - In insulin-dependent diabetes: intermediate-acting (lente or PZI) once or twice daily as per veterinary surgeon's instructions
- Diet: high-protein, ad libitum (see Chapter 16)
- Exercise – as per usual.

Diabetic ketoacidotic patient
This is a life-threatening condition and needs intensive treatment.

- Fluid therapy needs to be administered to lower the blood glucose, rehydrate the patient and correct acidosis and electrolyte imbalances.
- A short-acting soluble insulin is given intravenously (*note: this is the only insulin that can be administered via this route*), subcutaneously or intramuscularly.
- Glucose and electrolytes need to be monitored frequently and treatment adjusted as directed by the veterinary surgeon.

Long-term monitoring
The diabetic patient is monitored by owner observations (appetite, water consumption, urine output, weight control) and blood tests. The insulin is adjusted on the basis of a combination of these findings.

Blood tests

- Fructosamine: indication of blood glucose control over 2–3 weeks
- Serial blood glucose curves: give indication of how long the insulin is effective for and the time the lowest glucose level occurs. Blood is usually taken every 2 hours over a 24-hour period and the glucose is plotted on a graph. This needs to follow as normal a routine as possible, with minimal stress to the patient, as stress causes hyperglycaemia (this is especially important in cats)
- Urinalysis to monitor for ketones.

Urine glucose monitoring and subsequent adjustment of insulin by the owner is *not* recommended, as urine glucose can be misleading. The presence of glucose in the urine can be a result of overdosing but also of *under*dosing. The reason for the latter is a compensatory mechanism called the Somogyi overswing. An overdose of insulin will make the patient hypoglycaemic; hormones are then released to increase the glucose in the blood; there is a compensatory overswing and the patient becomes hyperglycaemic. Therefore if a patient is found to have an increase in urine glucose prior to the administration of the morning glucose, it is an indication to perform a serial blood glucose curve.

Hypoglycaemia

Hypoglycaemia is a complication that occurs as a result of an insulin overdose. Clinical signs include:

- Lethargy
- Ataxia
- Muscle twitching
- Severe seizures.

It is most likely to occur at the time of peak activity of the insulin. Immediate action must be taken, which may involve feeding, rubbing honey or glucose on the gums, or administering intravenous dextrose (as directed by veterinary surgeon). If left untreated, coma and death will ensue.

Nursing care

Uncomplicated diabetes mellitus

- Assist the veterinary surgeon with diagnostic tests
- Administer insulin, as directed by the veterinary surgeon
- Feed appropriate diet at times requested (see Chapter 16)
- Ensure that water is freely available
- Take the patient outside frequently
- Monitor blood glucose levels
- Monitor urine for glucose and ketones
- Monitor vital signs
- Clean and groom the patient as necessary
- Administer fluid therapy, as directed by the veterinary surgeon
- Administer any other medication

Diabetic ketoacidosis

- Monitor vital signs
- Monitor glucose and electrolyte levels hourly
- Administer intravenous fluid therapy, as directed by veterinary surgeon
- Administer insulin injections, as directed by veterinary surgeon

- Administer intravenous glucose if blood levels fall, as directed by veterinary surgeon
- Supplement intravenous fluids with potassium if blood levels fall, as directed by veterinary surgeon
- Encourage the patient to eat suitable food, or *any* food if anorexic
- Clean and groom as necessary
- Monitor animal's response to treatment

Nutrition

Successful management of a diabetic patient involves an appropriate dietary regime as well as insulin therapy (see Chapter 16). Owner compliance with the dietary regime is essential if an animal is to become stabilized.

Hyperadrenocorticism (HAC) (Cushing's disease)

Hyperadrenocorticism is common in the dog but rare in the cat. It occurs as a result of excessive cortisol in the body. This may be due to excessive administration of steroid or an overproduction of cortisol by the adrenal glands. The latter is a result of either a tumour in the pituitary gland (pituitary-dependent HAC), which overstimulates the adrenal glands to produce cortisol, or a tumour of the adrenal gland (adrenal-dependent HAC). Pituitary-dependent HAC is the most common form.

Clinical signs

- Polyuria/polydipsia
- Polyphagia
- Pot-belly (Figure 21.14)
- Panting
- Bilateral alopecia and skin changes (thin inelastic skin)
- Muscle atrophy and weakness

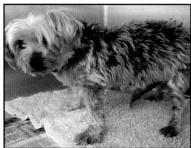

21.14

A dog with hyperadrenocorticism. Note the pot-bellied appearance.

Diagnosis

- Blood tests: haematology and biochemistry
- ACTH stimulation test
- Low-dose dexamethasone suppression test (LDDST)
- High-dose dexamethasone suppression test (HDDST)
- Endogenous ACTH assay
- Abdominal ultrasonography
- Abdominal radiography

The ACTH stimulation and LDDST are confirmatory tests. The HDDST and endogenous ACTH assay are used to discriminate between pituitary-dependent and adrenal-dependent HAC. (See Chapter 17.)

Treatment

Pituitary-dependent HAC is treated medically (trilostane or mitotane). Adrenal tumours can be treated with drugs or by surgical removal.

Nursing care

- Monitor vital and clinical signs
- Assist veterinary surgeon with diagnostic tests
- Observe the patient after blood sampling for haematoma formation and handle carefully for other procedures, as bruising can occur easily in patients with HAC
- Ensure that water is freely available
- Take patient outside frequently
- Clean and groom patient as necessary
- Administer medications, as directed by the veterinary surgeon

Hypoadrenocorticism (Addison's disease)

Hypoadrenocorticism is a reduction in or failure of steroid production by the adrenals. This usually occurs as a result of immune destruction of the adrenal gland, but may also be a consequence of treating *hyper*adrenocorticism. Hypoadrenocorticism causes electrolyte imbalances, hyponatraemia (low sodium), hyperkalaemia (high potassium) and dehydration. The hyperkalaemia can be life threatening and needs to be treated promptly.

Clinical signs

Clinical signs are often initially vague and wax and wane; they include lethargy and inappetence. In the untreated patient this will progress to:

- Anorexia
- Vomiting
- Haemorrhagic diarrhoea
- Hypotension
- Weakness
- Bradycardia
- Collapse.

Diagnostics

- Blood tests: haematology and biochemistry (sodium:potassium ratio)
- ACTH stimulation test (same protocol as for hyperadrenocorticism)
- ECG (Figure 21.15)

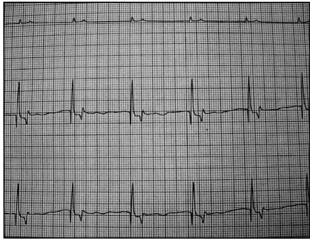

21.15 ECG from a dog presented in an Addisonian crisis. There is bradycardia, and no P waves are evident.

Treatment

An acute crisis is an emergency. Treatment involves fluid therapy at shock rates to reduce the potassium level and rehydrate the patient (see Chapter 19). Intravenous corticosteroids are administered. In the stable patient, glucocorticoids (prednisolone) and mineralocorticoids (fludrocortisone acetate) are administered. Treatment is monitored by observing the sodium:potassium ratio.

Nursing care

- Monitor vital (especially temperature, if patient is in a crisis) and clinical signs
- Assist veterinary surgeon with diagnostic tests
- Administer medication, as directed by the veterinary surgeon
- Administer fluid therapy (high in saline/low potassium) if patient is in a crisis, as directed by the veterinary surgeon
- Encourage patient to eat
- Ensure that water is freely available
- Clean and groom patient as necessary
- Take patient outside frequently

Hyperthyroidism

Patients with hyperthyroidism have an overactive thyroid gland. There is overproduction of thyroxine (T4) that increases the metabolic rate. This is a common condition in the older cat but rare in dogs.

Clinical signs

- Polyphagia with weight loss
- Emaciation
- Aggression and hyperactivity
- Heart murmur and tachycardia
- Polyuria/polydipsia
- Vomiting and diarrhoea

Diagnostics

- Blood tests: haematology and biochemistry, total T4

Treatment

Treatment involves administration of methimazole or radioactive iodine, or thyroidectomy. Success is monitored by measuring T4 levels.

Nursing care

- Monitor vital and clinical signs
- Assist veterinary surgeon with diagnostic tests
- Reduce patient stress as much as possible
- Feed patient a suitable diet
- Ensure that water is freely available
- Clean and groom patient as necessary
- Administer medication, as directed by veterinary surgeon
- Provide postoperative nursing and observation following thyroidectomy
- Follow protocol for nursing patients after radioactive iodine treatment

Hypothyroidism

Patients with hypothyroidism have an underactive thyroid gland. There is decreased production of thyroxine (T4) as a result of atrophy or lymphocytic infiltration of the thyroid gland. This results in a decreased metabolic rate. It is most common in middle-aged dogs and rare in the cat.

Clinical signs

- Lethargy, exercise intolerance
- Obesity
- Bradycardia
- Dermatological abnormalities: alopecia, seborrhoea, hyperpigmentation, pyoderma

Diagnostics

- Blood tests: haematology and biochemistry
- Total T4 and thyrotropin releasing hormone (TRH) assays (thyroid stimulating hormone (TSH) assay preferable, but TSH must be imported into UK with a Special Treatment Authorization (STA))

Treatment

Supplement thyroxine (levothyroxine). Treatment is monitored by measuring T4 levels and improved clinical signs.

Nursing care

- Monitor vital and clinical signs
- Assist veterinary surgeon with diagnostic tests
- Feed patient a suitable diet
- Ensure that water is freely available
- Clean and groom patient as necessary
- Administer medication, as directed by veterinary surgeon

Hypercalcaemia

Calcium is required for many functions in the body. It is regulated in the body by vitamin D, which is ingested and metabolized in the kidneys, and parathormone (PTH) produced in the parathyroid gland (Figure 21.16). Increased vitamin D and PTH will increase the calcium in the body. There are other substances that are able to increase calcium in the body and they are released in certain disease states. In excess, calcium can cause renal failure and death.

Differential diagnoses

- Neoplasia (e.g. lymphoma, Figure 21.17)
- Primary hyperparathyroidism
- Vitamin D toxicity (e.g. some toxic rat baits)
- Renal failure (see 'Chronic renal failure')

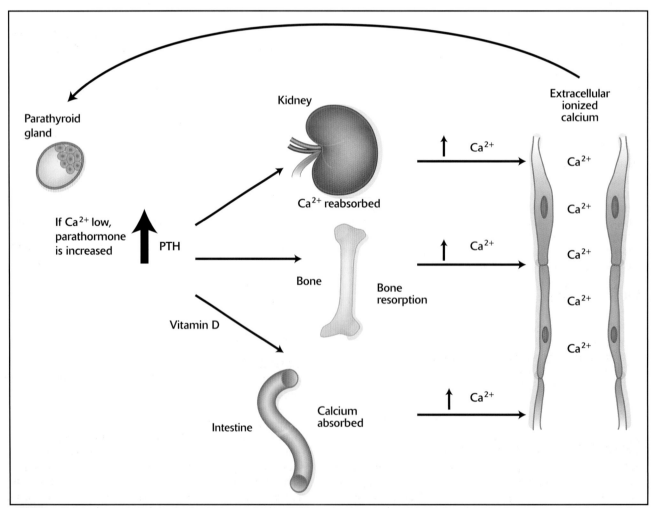

21.16 Calcium regulation in the body. Low calcium: PTH production rises; calcium absorbed by intestine and kidney. High calcium: PTH production decreases; calcium lost in urine and taken up by bones.

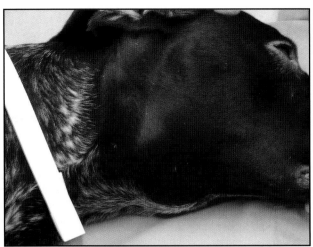

21.17 This dog was presented with hypercalcaemia. It has enlarged submandibular lymph nodes and was diagnosed with lymphoma.

Clinical signs

- Polyuria, polydipsia
- Anorexia, lethargy, weakness
- Vomiting, diarrhoea
- Tremors

Diagnostics

- Blood tests: haematology and biochemistry (total calcium and ionized calcium)
- Urinalysis: specific gravity, dipstick and sediment
- Fine-needle aspiration of a lymph node
- Radiography
- Ultrasonography
- PTH assay and parathyroid-related protein assay

Treatment

Hypercalcaemia should be treated promptly to decrease risk of permanent renal damage. Patients should be placed on intravenous fluids. Once a diagnosis has been made, the underlying cause should be treated (e.g. chemotherapy for lymphoma; parathyroidectomy for primary hyperparathyroidism). After surgery for primary hyperparathyroidism the patient should be monitored for hypocalcaemia. Clinical signs include tremors, seizures and facial rubbing.

Nursing care

- Monitor vital and clinical signs
- Monitor urinary output
- Assist veterinary surgeon with diagnostic tests
- Feed patient a suitable diet
- Ensure that water is freely available
- Clean and groom patient as necessary
- Administer medication, as directed by veterinary surgeon

Diabetes insipidus (DI)

This disease is caused by an impairment in the production of ADH (antidiuretic hormone/vasopressin) or a failure in response. The animal produces large quantities of dilute urine with a compensatory polydipsia. The condition may be referred to as water diabetes. Animals are normally well in all other aspects.

There are two forms of diabetes insipidus:

- **Central DI** – a deficiency in ADH produced by the pituitary, thought to be either congenital or as a result of trauma to the hypothalamus (e.g. tumours, head trauma)
- **Nephrogenic DI** – failure of the collecting tubules in the nephrons to respond to ADH.

Normally ADH controls the water balance within the body by concentrating the urine. If the animal's water intake is decreased, the body will respond by producing more ADH and this will then stimulate the collecting tubules to retain water, preserving the body's water balance.

Clinical signs

- Marked polyuria
- Marked polydipsia
- Vomiting after drinking large amounts
- Weight loss due to poor appetite, due to constant thirst

Diagnostics

- Haematology and biochemistry – normal
- Urinalysis (SG <1.009)
- Water deprivation test
- Trial of ADH

Protocols for water deprivation test and ADH trial

Prior to starting this test, the patient should be well hydrated and have a normal blood urea level. The test should only be performed under close observation.

1. Empty the bladder and measure urine specific gravity (SG).
2. Weigh animal and calculate 5% of its bodyweight.
3. Place animal in a kennel with no access to food or water.
4. Empty bladder every hour, check SG and weigh the animal.
5. Once 5% of the animal's bodyweight has been lost, stop the test.
6. Normal result: SG >1.025. If SG is <1.020, suspect DI.

Once rehydrated, repeat as above but give ADH injection or drops.

- Increased urine SG = central DI
- No change in SG = nephrogenic DI.

Treatment

Central DI

Desmopressin acetate (DDAVP) nasal/eye drops, synthetic vasopressin.

Nephrogenic DI

Chlorothiazide diuretics (hydrosaluric). Although this medication is a diuretic, it can actually reduce the urine output in cases with nephrogenic DI. It works by causing sodium and water to be excreted in the proximal tubules. This leaves less fluid available for the distal tubule to excrete – this is the section affected by nephrogenic DI. It therefore limits the total volume of urine that can be excreted.

Nursing care

- Monitor vital and clinical signs
- Assist veterinary surgeon with diagnostic tests
- Ensure that water is freely available (except during water deprivation test)
- Take patient outside frequently
- Clean and groom patient as necessary
- Administer medication, as directed by veterinary surgeon

Nervous system disease

Definitions

- **Convulsions** – a series of involuntary contractions of the muscles
- **Seizures** – clinical manifestation of a paroxysmal cerebral disorder resulting from a transitory disturbance of brain function due to abnormal electrical activity
- **Epilepsy** – an intracranial disorder that produces recurrent seizures
- **Status epilepticus** – life-threatening series of epileptic spasms without intervals of consciousness
- **Paresis** – weakness of one or more limbs
- **Hemiplegia** – paralysis of one side of the body
- **Paraplegia** – paralysis of the caudal limbs
- **Tetraplegia** – paralysis of all four limbs

Clinical signs of nervous system disease include:

- **Cerebral**:
  - Behaviour changes
  - Ataxia
  - Circling
  - Pacing
  - Seizures
  - Weakness
- **Cerebellar**:
  - Ataxia
  - Tremors
  - Dysmetria
  - Hypermetria
  - Head tilt
  - Nystagmus
- **Spinal**:
  - Abnormal spinal reflexes
  - Weakness
  - Paresis/paralysis
  - Faecal/urinary incontinence.

Seizures

Differential diagnoses

Seizures can result from abnormalities within or outside the brain.

Causes within the brain include:

- Idiopathic epilepsy
- Brain tumours
- Head trauma
- Infections (e.g. canine distemper)
- Congenital abnormalities (e.g. hydrocephalus).

Causes outside the brain include:

- Metabolic (e.g. hypoglycaemia, hypocalcaemia, hepatic encephalopathy, uraemia)
- Toxins (e.g. ethylene glycol (antifreeze)).

Idiopathic epilepsy is more likely to occur in dogs under 3 years of age. Most brain tumours are more common in the older animal.

Clinical signs

Signs can vary from animal to animal, but usually take the form of three phases.

- **Preictal** – just before the fit the animal will usually be asleep or resting; it will then appear restless or anxious.
- **Ictal** – this period describes the actual fit, varying degrees of collapse, clonic and tonic activity. Vocalization, jaw champing, hypersalivation, involuntary urination or defecation may also be present.
- **Postictal** – this is the period following the fit: the animal may be exhausted, disorientated or anxious.

Seizures may be single, multiple (**cluster seizures**) or continuous (**status epilepticus**).

Diagnosis

- Blood test for haematology and biochemistry
- Cerebral spinal fluid (CSF) tap
- Magnetic resonance imaging (MRI scan)
- Computerized tomography (CT scan)
- Electroencephalography (EEG)

Treatment

Any underlying cause should be treated. To control cluster seizures or status epilepticus, initial treatment involves:

- Diazepam initially, can be repeated (intravenously or per rectum) if unsuccessful
- Phenobarbital or propofol infusion
- Status epilepticus should be dealt with as an emergency
- If idiopathic epilepsy is diagnosed, anticonvulsant therapy should be started.

Phenobarbital is used to control seizures; this can also be used in conjunction with potassium bromide.

Nursing care

- Observe and record seizure activity
- Monitor vital signs, especially temperature
- Dim the lighting or partially cover the kennel
- Pad the kennel to prevent trauma
- Keep the room as quiet as possible
- Place and maintain intravenous access
- Administer medication, as directed by the veterinary surgeon
- Administer fluid therapy, as directed by the veterinary surgeon
- Keep airway clear
- Administer oxygen if required
- Cool the patient if hyperthermic

Spinal injuries

Differential diagnoses

- Intervertebral disc disease
- Fibrocartilaginous embolism
- Discospondylitis
- Wobbler syndrome
- Cauda equina syndrome
- Tumour
- Fracture

Clinical signs

- Ataxia
- Paresis of one or more limbs
- Paralysis of one or more limbs (paraplegia, tetraplegia, hemiplegia)
- Urinary or faecal incontinence
- Lack of panniculus reflex
- Lack of tail function

Diagnosis

Neurological assessment

- Localization of pain
- Examination of gait
- Detection of proprioceptive deficits
- Assessment of muscle atrophy/tone
- Assessment of limb, tail, anal and panniculus reflexes
- Assessment of deep pain
- Assessment of bladder function

Other diagnostic tests

- Radiography
- Myelography
- MRI scan
- CSF analysis

Treatment

Surgical correction of some conditions is possible. Other conditions cannot be corrected surgically, or surgical repair is precluded by financial constraints. These patients are then managed by medical treatment, which includes:

- Analgesia
- Restricted or supported exercise (depending on condition)
- Urinary and faecal management – use of catheters and enemas
- Physiotherapy (depending on condition).

Nursing care

- Monitor patient's vital signs
- Assist veterinary surgeon with examination and other diagnostic procedures
- Prevent pressure sores and turn patient frequently
- Avoid excessive movement with spinal fractures
- Assist with emptying bladder and rectum
- Keep patient clean and groom as necessary (this also helps to prevent patient boredom)

- Provide adequate nutrition – make sure that the animal can reach its bowls. Hand feeding or other methods of assisted feeding may be required
- Carry out physiotherapy, as directed by veterinary surgeon
- Administer medication, as directed by veterinary surgeon

Musculoskeletal system disease

Definitions

- **Myositis** – inflammation of a voluntary muscle
- **Tendonitis** – inflammation of a tendon
- **Arthritis** – inflammation of a joint

Bone disease

Rickets

This disease is seen in young growing animals that are fed a diet deficient in vitamin D. The affected animal is unable to absorb calcium from the intestines, leading to reduced bone mineralization around the growth plates. Clinical signs include lameness, bowing of limbs and swollen joints. Radiographic examination shows enlargement of growth plates. Treatment involves feeding an appropriate balanced diet for a young growing dog.

Nursing care

- Feed a balanced diet suitable for a growing puppy
- Administer analgesics as necessary
- Provide soft comfortable bedding

Metaphyseal osteopathy

This is also known as hypertrophic osteodystrophy and Möller Barlow's disease. Metaphyseal osteopathy occurs in young growing dogs, particularly giant breeds. It is associated with abnormal metaphyseal bone formation, usually affecting long bones of the distal limbs. Clinical signs include swollen and painful growth plate regions on all limbs, severe lameness, pyrexia, depression and anorexia. The cause of metaphyseal osteopathy is unknown. Treatment consists of pain relief and feeding an appropriate diet for a young growing dog.

Nursing care

- Feed a balanced diet suitable for a growing puppy
- Administer analgesics as necessary
- Provide soft comfortable bedding
- Ensure urination and defecation are possible

Hypertrophic osteopathy

This is also known as pulmonary osteopathy and Marie's disease. It is associated with a thoracic mass. There is periosteal proliferation, particularly of the metacarpals and metatarsals. There is no joint involvement. Clinical signs includes lameness, bilateral soft tissue swelling of the lower limbs and pain. These changes are usually seen before thoracic signs develop. Treatment depends on the underlying condition but the prognosis is usually poor.

Nursing care

- Monitor vital signs
- Provide soft, comfortable bedding
- Administer analgesics as necessary
- Administer medications as per the veterinary surgeon's instructions

Secondary nutritional hyperparathyroidism

This is caused by a diet grossly deficient in calcium or containing an excess of phosphorus. It is most commonly associated with feeding all-meat diets. Calcium is resorbed from bone, giving rise to lameness, pain, reluctance to stand or walk, and pathological fractures of long bones. Treatment consists of feeding a balanced diet, cage rest to allow fractures to heal, and analgesics.

Nursing care

- Feed a balanced diet
- Administer analgesics as required
- Provide soft comfortable bedding
- Ensure urination and defecation are possible

Osteomyelitis

Osteomyelitis is inflammation, most commonly due to infection, of bone. Clinical signs include pain, swelling, lameness, loss of function, pyrexia, depression and inappetence. A draining sinus tract may develop. Causes include bacterial or fungal infection (the latter is uncommon in the UK) and corrosion of surgical implants. Radiography reveals destruction of existing bone and new bone formation. Treatment includes administration of antibiotics (based on culture and sensitivity results), antifungals and removal of surgical implants or necrotic bone fragments (sequestra) that may be associated with the osteomyelitis.

Nursing care

- Monitor vital signs
- Provide soft, comfortable bedding
- Administer analgesia as necessary
- Administer antibiotics as per the veterinary surgeon's instructions
- Provide postoperative care

Arthritis

Joint disease can be categorized as immune-mediated (e.g. idiopathic polyarthritis, systemic lupus erythematosus, rheumatoid arthritis), inflammatory (infectious or non-infectious) or degenerative (Figure 21.19).

Clinical signs

Patients with arthritis have a variable degree of lameness, pain in the affected joint or joints, and exercise intolerance. A specific clinical sign of degenerative joint disease is that the condition improves with exercise.

- Degenerative:
  - Gradual onset
  - Improvement with exercise
  - Crepitus on extension/flexion
- Immune-mediated:
  - Pyrexia
  - Inappetence
  - Usually multiple joints involved
  - Other signs of systemic disease
- Inflammatory:
  - Joint pain
  - Pyrexia
  - Recent history of surgery or medication

Diagnostics

- Blood tests for haematology, biochemistry, rheumatoid factor and antinuclear antibody
- Radiography
- Joint tap (arthrocentesis) for cytology and culture

Treatment

Treatment is aimed at the underlying cause, or managing the pain associated with degenerative changes:

- Immune-mediated: immunosuppression
- Infectious: antibacterials, pain relief
- Degenerative: pain relief (NSAIDs), diet, glycosaminoglycans.

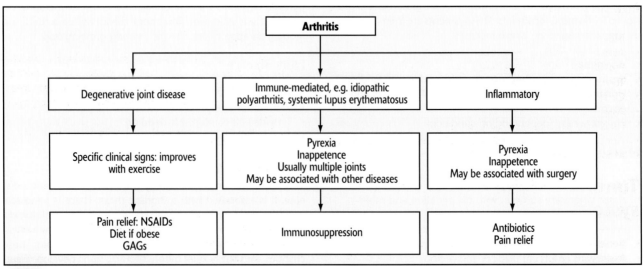

21.19 Classification of arthritis.

Nursing care and nutrition

- Monitor vital signs
- Provide soft, comfortable bedding
- Encourage frequent short walks
- Administer medication, as directed by the veterinary surgeon
- Adjust diet if obese (see Chapter 16)

Muscle disease

Myopathies can be classified as inflammatory and non inflammatory:

- Inflammatory:
  - Infectious (e.g. *Toxoplasma gondii*, *Neospora caninum*)
  - Immune-mediated
- Non-inflammatory:
  - Endocrinopathies (e.g. hyperadrenocorticism, hypothyroidism)
  - Congenital (e.g. 'floppy Labrador')

Clinical signs

- Muscle weakness and loss of function
- Muscle atrophy
- Muscular pain
- Lameness
- Pyrexia, anorexia if inflammatory
- Regurgitation if the oesophageal muscle is affected

Diagnostics

- Haematology, biochemistry
- Electromyography
- Muscle biopsy

Treatment

The underlying cause needs to be treated:

- Infectious – antibacterials
- Immune-mediated – immunosuppression
- Endocrinopathies – treat underlying disease
- Congenital – usually no treatment available

Nursing care

- Monitor vital signs
- Assist walking if required (see Chapter 15)
- Provide soft comfortable bedding
- Turn patient every 4 hours if recumbent
- Carry out physiotherapy (see later)
- Assist feeding if dysphagic
- Feed from a height if regurgitating
- Administer medication, as directed by veterinary surgeon
- Monitor progress

Tumours of the musculoskeletal system

- Bone tumours – most commonly osteosarcoma (malignant) and osteoma (benign); other tumours include fibrosarcomas, haemangiosarcomas and chrondrosarcomas.
- Soft tissue tumours – fibrosarcoma, haemangiosarcomas.

Clinical signs

- **Osteosarcomas** most commonly affect the long bones. Patients may present with only a swelling (Figure 21.20) but these are usually very painful and the patient will be lame and often unable to bear its weight on the affected leg
- **Chondrosarcomas** affect bones such as ribs and the nasal cavity
- **Fibrosarcomas** usually affect the bones of the axial skeleton, including the skull and mandible

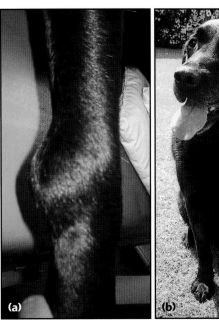

21.20 Bone tumour. **(a)** A swelling on the distal left forelimb of a dog, which was diagnosed as osteosarcoma. **(b)** The dog underwent a course of radiotherapy, as evidenced by the white square.

Diagnostics

- Haematology, biochemistry
- Radiography – local area, thorax (metastasis)
- Ultrasonography – abdomen (metastasis)
- Biopsy

Treatment

Treatment of osteosarcomas involves amputating the affected leg to relieve pain or cure. The best results are achieved by combining this with chemotherapy to slow the development of any metastases. Radiotherapy will also relieve the pain of the tumour.

Soft tissue tumours are best treated by surgical excision.

Nursing care

- Monitor vital signs
- Provide soft comfortable bedding
- Administer analgesia and other medications, as directed by the veterinary surgeon
- Provide postoperative care
- Assist veterinary surgeon with chemotherapy
- Ensure adequate nutrition

Nutrition

- Convalescent diets should be used for patients following surgery and initial chemotherapy
- Specially formulated diets that help to reduce tumour growth may be fed

Diseases of the skin and coat

Definitions

- **Alopecia** – the absence of hair from areas of the skin where it is normally present; can be partial or complete, symmetrical or patchy, diffuse or focal
- **Erythema** – reddening of the skin
- **Pyoderma** – a pyogenic (pus-forming, e.g. infected) condition of the skin
- **Pruritus** – sensation within the skin that provokes the desire to scratch (animal may persistently lick, chew, or rub itself to alleviate the irritation; this can lead to self-trauma)
- **Seborrhoea** – excessive secretion of sebum by the sebaceous glands within the skin, giving the coat and skin an oily appearance

Parasitic and fungal skin disease

These are discussed in Chapters 7 and 8.

Pyoderma

This condition is more common in the dog than the cat and there is usually an underlying cause for its development. The severity of the condition is determined by the depth of the tissue affected (Figure 21.21). *Staphylococcus intermedius* is the most commonly involved bacterium, but other secondary opportunist bacteria such as *Pseudomonas* may also be present.

Feline pyoderma is associated with cat bites. Bacteria such as *Pasteurella, Staphylococcus* and *Fusiformis,* which are routinely found in the cat's mouth, cause cellulitis when bite wounds penetrate deep within the skin. Other clinical signs include pyrexia, anorexia, depression, pain and swelling at the site of the bite wound. This condition is usually successfully treated with antibiotics and drainage of pus from the site of infection.

Allergic skin disease

This is caused by an inappropriate immune response to an antigen, which in cases of allergic skin disease can include many factors. Figure 21.22 outlines the causes, presentation, diagnoses and treatments of various allergic skin diseases.

Tissue depth	Condition	Presentation	Treatment
Surface	Acute moist dermatitis	Often occurs where skin has become damaged due to self-trauma. Can occur anywhere but especially over face, feet and tail base. Erythema often present and area is often moist or crusty due to serum exudates	Treatment of underlying cause (e.g. ear infection). Clip hair from site – patient may require sedation as area can be very painful. Clean area with chlorhexidine. Elizabethan collar to prevent further self-trauma. Topical or systemic antibiotics and anti-inflammatories may be required
	Skin fold dermatitis	Commonly found around lip folds, vulval folds and tail folds. Common in breeds with excessive skin folds	Treat as above. Surgical correction or cosmetic surgery may be required to correct anatomy of skin in severe cases that recur
Superficial	Impetigo	Often known as juvenile pustular dermatitis or puppy pyoderma. Multiple pustules and yellow scabs commonly found along ventral abdomen	Antibacterial shampoo with additional systemic antibiotic and anti-inflammatory therapy if condition extensive
	Folliculitis	Formation of pustules with hair protruding. Sometimes the lesions in ring-like formation, especially ventral abdomen. As a result of underlying disease	Treatment of underlying disease. Appropriate antibiotic medication
Deep	Interdigital pyoderma (pododermatitis)	Often seen in short-haired dogs – paws become painful and swollen and may discharge pus. Area of alopecia seen with ulceration and fistulas in severe cases	Surgical drainage of infected material. Treatment of underlying cause. Long-term antibiotic therapy
	Furunculosis	Often associated with underlying disease such as demodicosis, dermatophytosis or hypothyroidism. Clinical signs include pustules, discharging pus, fistulas, alopecia, pain. Lesions often found on muzzle, flanks and anal regions but can occur anywhere on body	Treatment of any underlying disease. Long-term antibiotic therapy. In severe cases, surgical resection of fistulas may be required if problem recurs

21.21 Classification of pyoderma.

Condition	Cause	Presentation	Diagnosis	Treatment
Urticaria	Induced by drugs, vaccines and insect stings	Sudden development of multiple oedematous swellings or wheals on skin, with hair becoming erect; they are pruritic and can remain for hours or days	Based on clinical signs and accurate history	Removal of cause Treatment with corticosteroids Future avoidance of causal agent
Atopic dermatitis	Large numbers of unknown antigens, including house dust mites, pollens, danders	Usually affects dogs 1–3 years old Intense pruritus and alopecia, especially around eyes, feet, axilla and ventral abdomen Secondary infection common, due to self-trauma Otitis externa and ocular discharges may also be present Cats may present with miliary eczema and eosinophilic granuloma complex	Intradermal skin testing with multiple allergens to determine cause Serum testing for specific antigens	Allergies usually lifelong Depending on causal factors, changes to environment may be required Treatment may include corticosteroids, antihistamines, essential fatty acid supplementation, desensitizing vaccinations
Food hypersensitivity	Causes individual to each animal but can include beef, milk, gluten	Pruritic skin disease and/or gastrointestinal symptoms	Clinical signs and exclusion diet food trial (see Chapter 16)	Avoidance of specific allergens identified by food trial Long-term feeding of novelty diet fed during exclusion trial
Contact dermatitis	Commonly caused by soaps, detergents or chemicals of any kind	Pruritic erythematous lesions mainly on feet, ventral abdomen, neck and face Often secondary bacterial infection due to self-trauma Intolerance generally develops 4–6 weeks after initial exposure	Patch testing: suspected allergen applied to clipped area of skin and kept in contact 48 hours then examined for reaction Contact elimination: hospitalize animal from usual environment to see if clinical signs resolve; suspected items or substances then reintroduced and patient observed for reaction	Avoid contact with identified allergens

21.22   Causes, diagnosis and treatment of allergic skin diseases.

Hormonal alopecia

This is usually associated with one of the following:

- Hypothyroidism
- Hyperadrenocorticism (Cushing's disease)
- Sertoli cell tumour
- Canine ovarian imbalance.

In conjunction with clinical signs of the underlying condition, it usually presents as a bilateral alopecia, often on the flanks. It is usually non-pruritic and the skin is not inflamed. Treatment is based on identifying and treating the underlying cause.

Diseases of the eye

Conditions that affect the eyelids

- **Entropion** – inturning of the upper or lower eyelid, towards the eyeball (often hereditary)
- **Ectropion** – eversion of the lower eyelid, away from the eyeball, with exposure of the conjunctiva; less common than entropion
- **Distichiasis** – extra row of eyelashes behind the normal row; most common hereditary eye abnormality in the dog

All of these abnormalities can result in irritation, inflammation, infection or damage to the cornea and conjunctiva, depending on the severity.

Clinical signs

As well as visible evidence of one of the above conditions, clinical signs may include:

- Blepharospasm
- Squinting
- Increased lacrimation
- Ocular discharge

Treatment

- Anti-inflammatory eyedrops
- Antibacterial eyedrops
- Surgical correction of condition

Conjunctivitis

Inflammation of the conjunctiva can be unilateral or bilateral, depending on the cause.

Causes include bacterial infections (sometimes primary but usually secondary), viral infections (e.g. distemper, herpesvirus) or allergies. It may also be associated with foreign bodies, strong winds, trauma and ectropion.

Clinical signs

- Blepharospasm (constant blinking)
- Increased lacrimation
- Chemosis (oedema and swelling of the conjunctiva)
- Conjunctival hyperaemia
- Ocular discharge ranging from serous to mucopurulent

Treatment

This will vary depending on the causal factor, but may include:

- Surgical correction
- Antibiotic eyedrops
- Anti-inflammatory eyedrops
- Antiviral eyedrops
- Antihistamine eyedrops.

Nursing care

- Prevent patient self-trauma and interference (e.g. Elizabethan collar)
- Bathe eyes to remove any discharge
- Apply medication, following veterinary surgeon's instructions

Keratoconjunctivitis sicca

KCS ('dry eye') is due to a reduction in aqueous tear production from the lacrimal and third eyelid gland. This often results in an overproduction of mucus as an attempt to keep the cornea moist. Most commonly the condition is immune-mediated but it may also be caused by drug toxicity (e.g. sulfasalazine), trauma or surgery (e.g. following removal of the third eyelid gland in dogs with 'cherry eye'). There is considerable variation in the degree of severity.

Clinical signs

- Vascularization, ulceration, opacity of the cornea
- Recurrent conjunctivitis
- Mucoid or mucopurulent discharge on and around the surface of the eye

Diagnostics

A Schirmer tear test (Figure 21.23) will show insufficient tear production. Readings of <10 mm in a minute will confirm the diagnosis, but the test should be repeated for monitoring purposes.

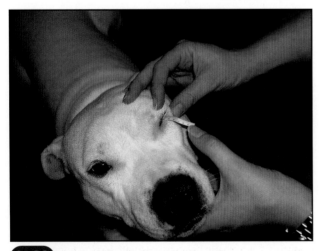

21.23 Schirmer tear test.

Treatment and nursing care

- Tear stimulants, such as ciclosporin or pilocarpine
- Tear substitutes
- Antibiotic drops if infected
- Anti-inflammatory eyedrops
- Good ocular hygiene and frequent cleaning to remove discharge from around the eyes

Corneal ulceration

This common condition can vary in severity depending on depth. Deep ulcers may result in corneal rupture. Causes include:

- Eyelash/eyelid disorders
- Trauma (e.g. cat scratch)
- Keratoconjunctivitis sicca
- Bacteria (primary trauma due to any of the above often allows bacterial overgrowth)
- Melting ulcers – these occur due to bacterial infections (e.g. *Pseudomonas*) resulting in enzymes being released to aid removal of devitalized cells and debris. These enzymes also contribute to the melting of the cornea.

Clinical signs

- Ocular pain
- Ocular discharge
- Blepharospasm
- Increased lacrimation

Diagnostics

- Visual inspection of the cornea
- Fluorescein dye – this dye is taken up by any exposed stroma so that epithelial erosions can be detected

Treatment

This will vary depending on the severity of the ulcer but may include:

- Antibiotic eyedrops
- Analgesia
- Fitting of contact lenses
- Surgical procedures (e.g. debridement of damaged cornea, grid keratotomy, conjunctival grafts).

Nursing care

- Monitor carefully to check for deterioration – infected ulcers can progress rapidly (melting ulcers)
- Prevent patient self-trauma. As well as using correctly fitting Elizabethan collars, prevent the patient from rubbing on cage bars, etc.
- Carefully follow medication regimes

Uveitis

Uveitis is inflammation of the iris, ciliary body and/or choroid. It can be caused by trauma, neoplasia, infection or immune-mediated disease, lens-induced, or associated with corneal insult.

Clinical signs

Clinical signs vary according to duration of the condition, the cause of the inflammation and the extent of the uveal tract involvement. Bilateral uveitis usually indicates systemic involvement. Secondary complications include glaucoma and cataracts.

- Pain
- Blepharospasm
- Miotic pupil
- Red eye
- Photophobia
- Lacrimation
- Reduced intraocular pressure

Diagnostics

Underlying cause must be determined.

- Haematology, biochemistry, specific diagnostic tests (e.g. FeLV, FIV, FIP)
- Serology
- Ophthalmoscopy
- Tonometry
- Fluorescein staining
- Diagnostic imaging

Treatment

- Treat underlying cause
- Topical atropine (contraindicated if glaucoma present)
- Topical corticosteroids (avoid in corneal ulceration, with caution in viral/fungal infections) or topical NSAIDs
- Systemic corticosteroids
- Systemic NSAIDs if systemic corticosteroids contraindicated
- Evaluate response to treatment at regular intervals

Nursing care

- Keep patient away from bright light if has photophobia
- Follow treatment regimes carefully

Glaucoma

This is a condition in which there in an elevation in intraocular pressure due to inadequate drainage of aqueous humour within the globe. This eventually affects the vision and health of the eye, and the condition can be very painful. In acute cases permanent blindness can result if untreated. The condition may be idiopathic: many breeds have a predisposition (including many terrier and spaniel breeds as well as the Great Dane and Flat-coated Retriever). There is a list of breeds that are tested for this condition on the KC/BVA eye testing scheme (see Chapter 5). Other causes include:

- Uveitis
- Cataracts
- Lens luxation
- Neoplasia.

Clinical signs

- Painful red eye(s)
- Corneal oedema
- Swelling of the globe
- Dilated pupil
- Retinal damage

Diagnostics

- Examination of the eye with an ophthalmoscope
- Measuring the intraocular pressure with a tonometer (this is also monitored to check the response to treatment) (Figure 21.24)
- Gonioscopy to measuring the iridocorneal drainage angle

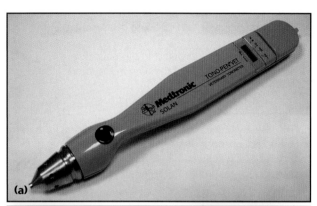
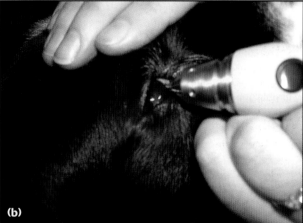

21.24 **(a)** Tonometer. **(b)** Using a tonometer to measure intraocular pressure.

Treatment

- Emergency treatment: intravenous mannitol, to help to draw fluid from the aqueous and vitreous humours and therefore decrease intraocular pressure
- Carbonic anhydrase inhibitors reduce formation of aqueous humour
- Miotics to increase aqueous outflow
- Analgesia
- Surgical treatment in specialist centres

Nursing care

- Prevent patient self-trauma (patient may rub eye when uncomfortable)
- Carefully follow medication regimes

Conditions affecting the lens

These include **cataract formation** and **lens luxation**, both of which require surgical correction (see Chapter 24). Cataract formation is a common finding in dogs with diabetes mellitus. Visual inspection of the eye reveals a clouding of the lens. Poor night vision leading to progressive blindness is the common progression of the disease.

Conditions affecting the retina

Collie eye anomaly

This is a disorder of the deep structures of the eye that affects Collie breeds. It is a congenital disorder and can be detected with an ophthalmoscope in puppies. It can affect the eye in the following ways:

- Choroid hypoplasia – inadequate development of the choroids
- Coloboma – a cleft or defect in the optic disc
- Staphyloma – an area of thinning in the sclera, adjacent to the choroids
- Retinal detachment, with or without haemorrhage.

The severity of the condition varies. In its mildest form there is little effect on sight. In a severe form, total retinal detachment will cause blindness. Affected animals should not be used for breeding.

Progressive retinal atrophy (PRA)

This is a hereditary disease of the eye that causes blindness. The retina is composed of two types of photoreceptor cells: rods and cones. The rods function in dim light and the cones in bright light. A dog affected with PRA begins to have difficulty seeing in dim light and then gradually looses the ability to see in bright light, eventually becoming completely blind. Although most common in dogs, some forms can occur in cats. Age at onset and rate of progression vary. Generalized retinal thinning occurs, manifest as tapetal hyper-reflectivity and attenuation of the superficial retinal vessels. There is no available treatment. Genetic testing is now available to identify carrier animals that are unaffected (see Chapter 5).

Nursing animals with poor vision

If a patient's sight is badly affected, it is important that the patient is aware of the nurse's presence before trying to handle them or apply any medication. Talking to them and stroking should reassure them. Otherwise the patient may be aggressive due to fear. To transport such patients around unfamiliar areas, it is often easier to carry smaller dogs; larger dogs need to be led slowly.

When these animals are nursed as inpatients, food and water bowls should always be located in the same position.

Infectious diseases – canine

Figure 21.25 summarizes information on common canine infectious diseases. Two important features in the care of patients with infectious diseases are barrier nursing and the provision of isolation facilities, which are described in Chapter 12. The subject of vaccination is discussed in principle in Chapter 6.

Disease/ infection	Type of infectious agent	Incubation period	Major organs affected	Main method of transmission	Zoonotic?	Diagnostics	Major nursing needs	Control/ prevention
Canine distemper	Virus	7–21 days	Respiratory, gastrointestinal systems	Inhalation	No	History, clinical signs Blood analysis Post-mortem examination	Fluid therapy Symptomatic	Vaccination Client education
Infectious canine hepatitis	Virus	5–10 days	Liver	Inhalation/ ingestion	No	History, clinical signs Blood analysis	Pain management Fluid therapy	Vaccination Client education
Canine parvovirus	Virus	3–5 days	Gastrointestinal system, bone marrow, heart	Ingestion of faecally contaminated material	No	History, clinical signs CITE faecal test	Fluid therapy Symptomatic Antibiotics	Vaccination Isolation Avoid risk
Leptospirosis	Bacterium	5–7 days	Kidneys, liver	Through mucous membranes and skin abrasions	Yes	History, clinical signs Urinalysis Blood analysis	Antibiotics Fluid therapy	Vaccination Avoid risk
Kennel cough complex	Mixed – bacteria/virus	5–7 days	Respiratory system	Inhalation	No	History, clinical signs	Antibiotics Symptomatic	Vaccination Isolation
Rabies	Virus	1 week to 1+ years, normally 3–8 weeks	Nervous system	Saliva to skin wound	Yes – fatal	History, clinical signs Post-mortem examination	N/A	Stray dog control Vaccination Pet Travel Scheme
Salmonellosis	Bacterium	2–3 days following a stressful experience	Gastrointestinal system	Ingestion of faecally contaminated material	Yes	History, clinical signs Culture	Fluid therapy, +/– antibiotics	Hygiene, disinfection

21.25 Common canine infectious diseases.

Canine distemper

Canine distemper is caused by canine distemper virus, a morbillivirus related to measles virus in humans and rinderpest virus in cattle. Both dogs and ferrets are susceptible. In warm climates the virus persists for 1–2 days in the environment. It is susceptible to routine disinfection.

The disease is most commonly seen in unvaccinated 3–6-month-old puppies. This time coincides with the waning of maternal antibodies (see Chapter 6). In susceptible populations a dog of any age may be affected. Outbreaks occur where there is a high density of dogs, such as rescue centres, housing estates and cities generally.

The virus is shed most commonly in respiratory exudates as well as in urine, faeces, saliva, vomitus and ocular discharges, up to 60–90 days post-infection. The incubation period is 7–21 days and infection is via inhalation. The aerosol droplets, when inhaled, come into contact with the upper respiratory epithelium of the susceptible animal and spread through the body from this point. The respiratory, gastrointestinal and central nervous systems, nose, footpads and conjunctiva can be affected. The severity of the disease depends on the efficacy of the immune response that is mounted and ranges from no clinical signs to death. Secondary bacterial infections can complicate the infection.

Clinical signs (generalized distemper)

- Depression
- Pyrexia
- Anorexia
- Lymphadenopathy
- Conjunctivitis giving ocular discharge (initially serous but rapidly becoming mucopurulent with secondary bacterial infection)
- Rhinitis giving nasal discharge (initially serous but rapidly becoming mucopurulent with secondary bacterial infection)
- Cough (initially dry, may become moist and productive)
- Exudative pneumonia – complicated by a secondary bacterial infection – leading to tachypnoea, dyspnoea
- Vomiting, diarrhoea, dehydration, loss of body condition
- Hyperkeratosis of nose and footpads; footpads become thickened and fissures appear ('hard pad')
- Enamel hypoplasia – permanent damage to tooth enamel in puppies under 6 months old
- Neurological signs (see below)
- Skin rash – pustules, thought to be associated with an immune response (animals that develop rashes often recover)

Neurological signs

Some animals, including those with subclinical infection, can develop neurological signs 2–3 weeks after infection. Clinical signs are usually acute in onset and progressive and are associated with a poor prognosis. Clinical signs depend on the part of the nervous system that is affected and include seizures, paresis/paralysis of one or more limbs, and optic neuritis. Involuntary twitching of muscles (**myoclonus**) may also occur and is said to be a classic sign.

Diagnostics

A presumptive diagnosis is usually based on the history and classical clinical signs in an at-risk patient.

- Blood tests: haematology and biochemistry
- Thoracic radiography: right lateral and ventrodorsal views
- CSF sample
- Specific tests:
  - Epithelial cells with eosinophilic bodies
  - Antibody titre rising at least fourfold
  - Immunofluorescence for virus in lymphoid tissue
  - Detection of antibody in CSF
- Post-mortem examination

Treatment

Prevention is by vaccination. Specific treatment is not available and the patient is treated symptomatically:

- Antitussives for *dry* cough
- Broad-spectrum antibiotics for secondary bacterial infections
- Intravenous fluids for dehydration and electrolyte losses
- Anticonvulsants for seizures
- Antiemetics for vomiting
- Isolation and barrier nursing – of particular importance.

Nursing care

The nursing care of a patient with CDV is centred on managing the symptoms.

- Barrier nurse the patient to prevent transmission
- Monitor vital signs
- Administer medication, as directed by the veterinary surgeon
- Administer and maintain fluid therapy
- Provide general nursing of the symptoms suffered, cleaning of nasal and ocular discharges, and application of petroleum jelly to prevent skin excoriation
- Ensure adequate nutrition of the patient; use of convalescing diets and assisted feeding may be required
- Disinfect the environment
- Provide the owner with advice on vaccination protocols for any other dogs in the household

Infectious canine hepatitis (ICH)

Infectious canine hepatitis is caused by canine adenovirus type I (CAV-1), similar to the CAV-2 adenovirus that causes respiratory disease (see 'Kennel cough complex', below). It is a resistant virus and can survive for days on fomites in the environment. It survives disinfection with various chemicals but is inactivated at temperatures >50°C.

The incubation period is 5–10 days. During the initial infection, virus is shed in all bodily secretions. From around 10 days post-infection, the virus is shed in the urine for at least 6 months. Animals become infected through the oronasal route. The virus localizes in the tonsils and regional lymph nodes before disseminating to other parts of the body and localizing in the liver and vascular endothelial cells. If an appropriate immune response is not made, acute or chronic hepatitis can occur. Immune complexes (antibody and viral antigen complexes) can lodge in the uveal tract and glomerulus and cause a severe uveitis and corneal oedema, or glomerulonephritis.

Dogs younger than 1 year are usually affected, but unvaccinated dogs of any age can be affected. Mortality rate can be high in unweaned puppies. Disease can progress rapidly and the puppies may die within a few hours of developing clinical signs. Infection in older animals is less severe.

Clinical signs

Clinical signs in acute infections may include:

- Pyrexia, depression, anorexia
- Lymphadenopathy
- Vomiting, diarrhoea
- Shock
- Hepatomegaly and anterior abdominal pain
- Jaundice (in a third of cases)
- Petechial haemorrhages
- Corneal oedema (blue eye)
- Neurological signs (in terminal stages)
- Severely affected dogs may die suddenly, without the owner noticing other clinical signs.

In subacute infections, clinical signs include depression, anorexia and mild pyrexia.

Diagnostics

- History and clinical signs
- Blood tests: haematology and biochemistry (especially liver enzymes), clotting profile
- Serological tests – rising antibody titre
- Intranuclear inclusion bodies found within hepatocytes
- Virus isolation from affected organs
- Post-mortem examination

Treatment

Prevention is by vaccination (CAV2 cross-protective). ICH patients are treated symptomatically:

- Intravenous fluids to rehydrate the animal
- Analgesics to control abdominal pain
- Topical steroids should only be used with caution; topical NSAIDs may be preferred.

The corneal changes may remain as a complication leading to permanent visual impairment, but in the majority of cases these are temporary.

Nursing care

- Barrier nurse the patient to prevent transmission
- Monitor vital signs
- Administer medication, as directed by the veterinary surgeon
- Administer and maintain fluid therapy
- Provide general nursing of the symptoms suffered
- Ensure adequate nutrition of the patient; use of convalescing diets and assisted feeding may be required
- Disinfect the environment
- Provide the owner with advice of vaccination protocols for any other dogs in the household, as after recovery dogs can become convalescent carriers for up to 6 months

Canine parvovirus

Canine parvovirus (related to feline panleucopenia virus) is very resistant and can survive in the environment from months to years. It is not killed by normal routine disinfection and a parvocidal disinfectant needs to be used.

It is a common infection and is highly contagious with a high mortality rate. Young puppies are most susceptible between the waning of maternal antibodies and efficacy of a vaccination programme. However, an unvaccinated dog of any age can be affected. Black and tan dogs are at increased risk.

Parvovirus is shed in the faeces. It is spread by direct or indirect contact with infected dogs or their faeces. Infection occurs through ingestion. The incubation period is 3–5 days. The severity of the disease depends on the age, immune/antibody status of the animal, stress and concurrent infections. The virus targets rapidly dividing cells, i.e. the gastrointestinal tract, cardiac tissue and bone marrow. In the gastrointestinal tract there is generalized inflammation, causing the gastrointestinal signs. The virus causes flattening of the villi, which causes malabsorption. Destruction of the bone marrow causes immunosuppression and susceptibility to secondary bacterial infections. In puppies under 4 weeks of age, the myocardium is rapidly dividing and will also be targeted by parvovirus, causing heart failure. The infection is often complicated by secondary bacterial infections.

Clinical signs

- Anorexia, depression, lethargy
- Vomiting and foul-smelling haemorrhagic diarrhoea
- Pyrexia
- Shock, dehydration, hypothermia
- Sudden death

Diagnostics

A presumptive diagnosis is based on history (general and vaccination) and clinical signs.

- Blood tests: haematology (leucopenia) and biochemistry
- Faecal sample: antigen tests – CPV antigen capture CITE test
- Serology
- Post mortem – histopathology

Treatment

Prevention is by vaccination and reducing the exposure of at-risk animals.

Treatment involves:

- Isolation
- Supportive – intravenous fluid therapy to correct dehydration and electrolyte imbalance; whole blood or colloids may be indicated
- Antiemetic if vomiting is intractable
- Nutrition (microenteral nutrition has been shown to decrease the time for which a patient is hospitalized).

Once vomiting has ceased, water can be introduced. If this is kept down, small highly digestible low-fibre low-fat meals need to be offered to the patient. The amounts are gradually increased over the following few days. Sometimes parvovirus causes permanent damage to the gastrointestinal tract and malabsorption may then occur; these patients will need to be maintained on a special diet. Antibiotics are important in treating the secondary bacterial infections.

Nursing care

- Barrier nurse the patient to prevent transmission
- Monitor vital signs
- Administer medication as directed by the veterinary surgeon
- Administer and maintain fluid therapy

- Provide general nursing of the symptoms suffered
- Keep patient clean from vomitus, clip hindquarters, bathe and apply barrier creams to prevent scalding from diarrhoea
- Offer small amount of electrolyte fluid when vomiting stops; then offer small meals as described above
- Disinfect the environment using a suitable parvocide
- Provide the owner with advice on vaccination protocols for any other dogs in the household

Leptospirosis

This is a zoonotic disease. It is important that effective precautions are taken when nursing these cases.

Leptospirosis is caused by the Gram-negative bacterium *Leptospira canicola* or *L. icterohaemorrhagiae*. Other serovars may also be involved. Leptospires can survive in a suitable environment and contaminate water supplies. They are destroyed by desiccation, disinfection and ultraviolet light.

Transmission occurs through contact with infected urine and contaminated water sources, food, soil or bedding. Recovered dogs can excrete organisms, through urine, intermittently for months. Some species of animal can be carriers without exhibiting signs. Rats can be carrier animals of *L. icterohaemorrhagiae* and the source of contamination.

The organism penetrates through mucous membranes or damaged skin, spreads through the body and infects many tissues. The incubation period is approximately 7 days. The extent of damage to organs depends on the serovar. *L. icterohaemorrhagiae* predominantly causes hepatocellular damage, giving rise to hepatitis, whereas *L. canicola* predominantly causes renal dysfunction, leading to an acute interstitial nephritis.

Young animals are usually more severely affected. *L. canicola* infection has a low incidence of clinical disease and is more common in urban areas. *L. icterohaemorrhagiae* causes very severe illness and is more common in rural areas. Peracute cases may die before clinical signs develop. The acute form is the most frequently recognized, as the subacute form often only manifests very mild clinical signs. Mortality rates can be high, with sudden death or rapid deterioration within a few hours.

Clinical signs

- Anorexia, pyrexia, depression, dehydration
- Vomiting, diarrhoea
- Anterior abdominal pain, jaundice, petechiae, bleeding from gum margins (*L. icterohaemorrhagiae*)
- Renal enlargement and pain, polyuria/polydipsia or oliguria (*L. canicola*)

Diagnostics

A presumptive diagnosis is usually made based on history and clinical signs.

- Blood tests: haematology and biochemistry, clotting profile
- Urinalysis: specific gravity, dipstick, sediment and dark field microscopy and culture for leptospires
- Serological testing: demonstration of a fourfold increase in antibody titre
- Post-mortem examination

Treatment

Prevention is through pest control and vaccination.

Antibiotics are used specifically to treat the infection. Penicillins are effective against the bacteraemic state but other antibiotics are required to eliminate the carrier state. Some antibiotics can be nephrotoxic and need to be avoided (e.g. tetracyclines).

Supportive treatment is aimed at restoring fluid and electrolyte balance. If acute renal failure has occurred, urine output needs to be restored. Blood transfusions may be required if the patient is anaemic.

Nursing care

- *This is a zoonotic disease* – care must be taken when nursing
- Barrier nurse the patient to prevent transmission
- Monitor vital signs
- Administer medication, as directed by the veterinary surgeon
- Administer and maintain fluid therapy
- Provide general nursing of the symptoms suffered
- Ensure adequate nutrition of the patient
- Monitor urine output and dispose of urine-soaked bedding carefully
- Disinfect the environment
- Provide the owner with advice on vaccination protocols for any other dogs in the household

Canine contagious respiratory disease ('Kennel cough complex')

A complex of microorganisms can cause the clinical signs of kennel cough. The organisms include canine parainfluenza virus 5 (PI-5), canine herpesvirus, canine reovirus, canine adenovirus 2 (CAV-2), *Bordetella bronchiseptica* and *Mycoplasma*. *B. bronchiseptica* can cause the most severe form of kennel cough when involved in an outbreak. Parainfluenza virus does not last long away from the host. CAV-2, as for CAV-1, is relatively resistant but is susceptible to heat. Quarternary ammonium disinfectants are effective against these viruses. *Bordetella* can be shed for months.

Kennel cough is highly infectious but mortality rate is low. Spread usually occurs in areas of high density by direct dog-to-dog contact, hence the name kennel cough. Transmission occurs through aerosol droplets that localize in the respiratory system and cause a tracheobronchitis. The incubation period is 5–7 days and the clinical signs tend to resolve after 3–7 days. Damage to the respiratory epithelium can predispose to secondary bacterial infections.

Clinical signs

These are usually restricted to a goose-honking cough that is dry and unproductive, and may be associated with retching. Gentle pressure on the trachea will elicit this cough. The animal will remain bright and alert unless the condition is complicated by bronchopneumonia, in which case anorexia, pyrexia, depression, tachypnoea and dyspnoea will be present.

Diagnostics

A presumptive diagnosis is usually made on history and clinical signs.

Treatment

Vaccination is available against *B. bronchiseptica,* CAV-2 and PI-5, the latter as part of combination vaccines including canine distemper virus and canine parvovirus.

The disease is usually self-limiting, but antibiotics can be used to reduce the time of clinical signs and risk of secondary bacterial infections. Antitussives can be used to reduce the persistent cough, but should not be used if there is bronchopneumonia.

Nursing care

*   Barrier nurse the patient (aerosol transmission is an important mode of transmission)
*   Monitor vital signs
*   Administer medication, as directed by the veterinary surgeon
*   Provide general nursing of the symptoms suffered, cleaning of nasal discharge
*   Ensure adequate nutrition of the patient
*   Disinfect the environment
*   Provide the owner with advice on vaccination protocols for any other dogs in the household

Infectious diseases – feline

Common feline infectious diseases are summarized in Figure 21.26.

Feline panleucopenia (feline infectious enteritis, FIE)

Feline panleucopenia is caused by a feline parvovirus and infects domestic and wild cats. It is very similar to the canine parvovirus, with similar properties. It survives for long periods in the environment and is very resistant to heating and routine disinfectants. Parvocidal products are required for disinfection.

The disease is usually seen in unvaccinated kittens living in close proximity (e.g. in rescue shelters). Maternal antibodies protect the kittens in the first 3 months of life.

The virus is shed in faeces, vomit, saliva and urine up to 6 weeks after infection. Transmission occurs via the oral route or transplacentally. Fomites play an important role in transmitting the virus. The incubation period is 2–10 days.

As a parvovirus, feline panleucopenia targets rapidly dividing cells: the lymphoid tissue, bone marrow and intestinal mucosal crypts. Destruction of the lymphoid tissue and bone marrow results in immunosuppression. Damage to the gastrointestinal system leads to gastroenteritis. In the late prenatal and early neonatal stages the lymphoid tissue, bone marrow and central nervous system can be affected. Early *in utero* infection can cause abortion and infertility. The cat recovers when an adequate immune response is mounted.

Damage to the bone marrow (panleucopenia results in low white blood cell counts) and enteritis increase susceptibility to bacterial infections.

Clinical signs

Many cats will have mild or subclinical infection and the disease is unlikely to be recognized. In peracute cases there will be sudden death. In acute cases the clinical signs include:

Disease/ infection	Type of infectious agent	Incubation period	Major organs affected	Transmission	Zoonotic?	Diagnostic methods	Major nursing needs	Control/ prevention
Feline panleucopenia	Virus	2–10 days	Gastrointestinal system Bone marrow	Body excretions	No	History, clinical signs Faecal analysis	Fluid therapy Symptomatic Antibiotics	Vaccination
Feline upper respiratory disease	Virus Bacteria	1–10 days	Upper respiratory tract	Saliva Ocular and nasal discharges	No	History, clinical signs Swabs	Symptomatic Antibiotics for secondary bacterial infections	Vaccination Isolation
Feline leukaemia	Virus	Months/years	Immune system Neoplasia	Saliva	No	Blood analysis	Symptomatic	Vaccination
Feline immuno-deficiency	Virus	Variable – may not show clinical signs for many years	Immune system	Cat bites – saliva	No	Blood analysis	Symptomatic	Restrict cat's movements
Feline infectious peritonitis	Virus	Variable	Severe inflammation of body tissues	Ingestion	No	Combination of history, clinical signs, blood tests, tissue biopsy	Symptomatic	Unknown
Feline infectious anaemia	Bacterium		Red blood cells	Unknown Fighting/fleas?	No	Blood analysis	Antibiotics, immunosuppression Symptomatic	Flea control, cat fight control
Toxoplasmosis	Coccidian	3–10 days	Intestinal tract Systemic	Ingestion faeces, meat	Yes	Tissue biopsy Serology	Antibiotics	

21.26 Common feline infectious diseases.

- Pyrexia, depression, anorexia
- Vomiting
- Diarrhoea (less frequent)
- Dehydration, hypothermia
- CNS signs: ataxia, tremors, incoordination. Cerebellar hypoplasia if fetus infected in second half of pregnancy
- Retinal lesions
- Queens: abortion, infertility.

Diagnostics

A presumptive diagnosis is usually made on history, clinical signs and demonstration of leucopenia on haematology.

- Blood tests: haematology and biochemistry
- CITE test: faecal sample

Treatment

Prevention is by vaccination.

Supportive and symptomatic treatment includes intravenous fluid therapy, antibiotics for secondary bacterial infections and antiemetics for intractable vomiting.

Nursing care

- Barrier nurse the patient to prevent transmission
- Monitor vital signs
- Administer medication, as directed by the veterinary surgeon
- Administer and maintain fluid therapy
- Provide general nursing of the symptoms suffered
- Keep patient clean from vomit and diarrhoea
- Offer small amount of electrolyte fluid when vomiting stops, then offer small meals of a low-fat highly digestible diet
- Advise the owner regarding other cats in the household. As the virus can persist in the environment, advise owners that new cats/kittens are fully vaccinated before entering the household
- Advise owners re disinfection of the environment

Feline upper respiratory disease (FURD, 'cat flu')

FURD is a common syndrome involving several primary infectious agents. It usually causes high morbidity but low mortality. The main infectious agents are:

- Feline herpesvirus type 1 (FHV-1)
- Feline calicivirus (FCV)
- *Bordetella bronchiseptica*
- *Chlamydophila felis.*

FHV-1 and FCV account for 80% of cases.

FURD is a highly infectious disease and the infectious organisms are shed in nasal and ocular discharges and saliva from cats exhibiting clinical signs or from asymptomatic carriers. Aerosolized droplets and contaminated fomites transmit the viruses to susceptible individuals. The virus can remain in the environment for a week following the presence of an infected cat.

Purebred cats, especially Siamese, are prone to a more severe infection. Cats of all ages are susceptible but the disease may be more severe in kittens, elderly cats and immunocompromised cats.

After inhalation, the virus replicates in the local lymph nodes before targeting the epithelial cells of the respiratory tract and conjunctiva. Most cats will become carriers after the clinical signs are no longer evident.

Infectious agents and clinical signs

Feline herpesvirus type 1

FHV-1 survives in the environment for hours only and is killed by routine disinfection. The incubation period is 2–10 days and infection usually lasts for 10–14 days. After infection >80% of animals become carriers, shedding the virus when stressed. Cats remain carriers for life. Severe illness and fatalities can occur in young and old cats. Some cats develop chronic rhinitis or sinusitis ('chronic snufflers').

Clinical signs

- Depression
- Inappetence/anorexia
- Paroxysmal sneezing
- Pyrexia
- Conjunctivitis
- Rhinitis (serous ocular/nasal discharges rapidly become mucopurulent with secondary bacterial infection)
- Salivation
- Dyspnoea and cough if pneumonia develops

Feline calicivirus

The incubation period is 1–7 days and infection usually lasts for 7–14 days. Disease is usually not as severe as with FHV-1. Carriers of FCV shed the virus continuously, some for a short period and some for years.

Clinical signs

- Mild ocular/nasal discharge (becoming mucopurulent with secondary bacterial infection)
- Sneezing
- Inappetence
- Depression
- Pyrexia
- Ulceration of hard and soft palates, tongue and cheeks
- Chronic ulcerative stomatitis and gingivitis in some individuals

Bordetella bronchiseptica

Infection with this bacterium causes mild upper respiratory tract disease in cats. Coughing is less prominent than in infected dogs. Bronchopneumonia may develop and can cause death, especially in kittens. Recovered cats may remain infectious for several months. Infections are more prevalent in multi-cat households, in rescue catteries and in cats in contact with dogs with respiratory disease, suggesting interspecies transmission.

Clinical signs

- Sneezing
- Nasal discharge
- Coughing
- Submandibular lymphadenopathy

Chlamydophila felis

Chlamydophila felis (formerly Chlamydia psittaci var. *felis)* is an intracellular parasite. Strains are species-specific. It is present on the ocular, respiratory, gastrointestinal and genitourinary mucosa of infected cats. The organism is very short lived off the host and transmission is likely to occur through direct contact with infected ocular and nasal discharges. All ages can be affected but kittens the most severely. The incubation period is 4–10 days. Infection may be unapparent to overt. The most common illnesses are acute, chronic and relapsing conjunctivitis. Improvement is normally seen after 2–3 weeks. The organism is responsible for about 30% of conjunctival cases and can cause nasal and lower respiratory infections. Abortions or infertility may also be caused by *Chlamydophila felis* but this remains to be proved clinically.

Clinical signs

- Conjunctivitis, hyperaemia, blepharospasm
- Serous to mucopurulent ocular discharge
- Mild upper respiratory tract disease (less common)

Diagnostics

A presumptive diagnosis is usually made on history and clinical signs.

- Oropharyngeal swab in viral transport medium for isolation of FHV-1 or FCV
- Oropharyngeal or nasal swab in charcoal Amies transport medium for culture of *Bordetella*
- Ocular swab in chlamydial transport medium for detection of *Chlamydophila* antigen

Treatment

Prevention is by vaccination.

Treatment is symptomatic and supportive. Nursing care is particularly important.

- Antibiotics if viral infection complicated by secondary bacterial infection
- Chlamydophilosis: topical or systemic tetracyclines. In multi-cat households the whole cat population should be treated at the same time. Treatment should continue for 2 weeks after clinical signs have abated
- Bordetellosis: antibiotics (tetracyclines, enrofloxacin)
- Intravenous fluid therapy if cat dehydrated and anorexic.

Nursing care

- Barrier nurse the patient (aerosol transmission is an important mode of transmission)
- Monitor vital signs
- Monitor weight and hydration status if the patient is anorexic
- Provide general nursing care, with attention given to cleaning of nasal discharges and grooming
- Provision of a steamy room with added decongestant can help if nasal discharge is severe
- Attention to nutrition is important, as these patients often need assisted feeding due to anorexia
- Administer fluid therapy and medication, as directed by veterinary surgeon
- Advise the owner about contamination, especially in multi-cat households
- Advise the owner regarding vaccination protocols for other cats in the household
- Advise the owner regarding the carrier state of the patient once recovered

Preventive measures in a cattery

- Ensure that all animals are vaccinated before entering the premises
- Cats should not be able to gain access to other cats. Ideally runs should have Perspex walls to provide a sneeze barrier
- Use of disposable feeding bowls to reduce fomite transmission
- Maintain correct disinfection protocols
- Isolate any cats showing symptoms

Feline leukaemia (FeLV infection)

Feline leukaemia virus is a retrovirus. It is host species-specific and affects both domestic and wild cats around the world. It is an important cause of death in young adult cats. It is associated with leukaemia and other lymphoproliferative diseases and non-neoplastic disease.

The virus is shed constantly in saliva; therefore, close contact and mutual grooming are required for spread. Cats in close contact or living in the same household are most likely to become infected. Vertical transmission from dam to offspring via the placenta and milk also occurs. The main source of infection is the persistently viraemic cat who is either a healthy carrier or has FeLV-related disease. Kittens are more susceptible than adults and are more likely to become persistently viraemic.

Although the virus is shed in other bodily fluids (e.g. mucus and faeces), it is unlikely to be spread via this route; it is readily inactivated in the environment. Iatrogenic spread could occur through blood transfusions and contaminated needles or instruments.

After initial oronasal infection the animal may exhibit mild, vague clinical signs of lethargy and inappetence and a corresponding lymphadenopathy. At this point most cats mount an appropriate immune response, recover and do not become carriers. In a minority of cases the cat becomes permanently viraemic. The most important factors that determine whether a cat recovers or is permanently infected are its age at infection and the dose of virus to which it is exposed. Cats with persistent viraemia have a high risk of developing FeLV-related disease.

The diseases caused by FeLV can be divided into two categories: neoplastic and non-neoplastic. Malignancy may be caused by the virus being inserted into the genome and causing changes in the expression of the oncogene, which results in abnormal 'growth' and control of some cell lines. The transformation is usually of lymphoid and myeloid cells, causing lymphoma, leukaemias and myelodysplastic disorders. Anaemias may occur as a result of interference with normal maturation of the red blood cell line in the bone marrow or due to anaemia of chronic disease. Thrombocytopenia and leucopenia are a result of decreased production caused by suppressed or infiltrated bone marrow. The virus also interferes with a normal immune response; therefore these cases are more prone to infections. Circulating immune complexes may cause immune-mediated disease (e.g. glomerulonephritis, polyarthritis). Reproductive disorders include infertility and abortions.

Latent infections may revert to overt viraemia in times of stress, such as pregnancy and glucocorticoid treatment, but this is unusual and latent infection is most likely to be eliminated over time.

The prevalence of FeLV has declined over the years with effective routine testing of kittens in shelters. Vaccination has also helped to decrease prevalence.

Clinical signs

Neoplastic FeLV

Lymphoma can be categorized by the site of origin. FeLV may be associated with some sites, including mediastinal lymphoma. Clinical signs for the latter include:

- Tachypnoea
- Dyspnoea
- Regurgitation
- Horner's syndrome
- Non-specific signs of disease.

Alimentary lymphoma is usually FeLV negative. Clinical signs include:

- Vomiting
- Diarrhoea
- Weight loss
- May only present with anorexia.

Clinical signs for leukaemia include:

- Lethargy
- Bleeding
- Sepsis
- Splenomegaly.

Non-neoplastic FeLV

- Anaemia (see above)
- Platelet abnormalities:
  - Bleeding tendencies (see clotting section)
- Leucocyte abnormalities:
  - Increased incidence of bacterial infections
  - Gingivitis
- Immunosuppression:
  - Increased incidence of infections, e.g. toxoplasmosis, cat flu, gingivitis
- Reproductive disorders:
  - Infertility
  - Abortions.

If kittens are infected *in utero* they often die at an early age of 'fading kitten' syndrome (see Chapter 25). They fail to nurse and become dehydrated and hypothermic within the first 2 weeks of life.

Diagnostics

Before diagnosis in an apparently healthy cat, a definitive test using virus isolation or immunofluorescence is recommended.

- Specific blood tests: FeLV ELISA test
- Other blood tests: haematology for haemopoietic cell lines
- FIV
- Bone marrow cytology
- Fine-needle aspiration/biopsy of lymph nodes
- Radiography and/or ultrasonography

Treatment

Prevention is by vaccination of at-risk cats. Treatment is supportive: although the underlying virus cannot be treated, the secondary disease should be treated as for an FeLV-negative cat. Chemotherapy is appropriate for lymphoma.

Good routine management of disease needs to be maintained to avoid stress to the immune system. For example, good flea and worm control and routine vaccinations need to be continued.

FeLV-positive cats should be removed from multi-cat households if the other cats are found to be negative, using 'test and remove' schemes.

Nursing care

- Barrier nurse the patient
- Monitor vital signs
- Administer medication, as directed by the veterinary surgeon
- Administer and maintain fluid therapy if required
- Provide general nursing of the symptoms suffered
- Ensure adequate nutrition of the patient. Advise the owner *not* to feed raw meat (due to increased risk of infection by *Toxoplasma gondii*)
- Advise the owner regarding preventive vaccination, worming and flea control to protect the patient from contracting other diseases
- Advise the owner to neuter the cat and keep it indoors to prevent transmission to other cats

Feline immunodeficiency (FIV infection)

Feline immunodeficiency virus is a retrovirus. It is related to human immunodeficiency virus (HIV) but is host species-specific, i.e. it only infects cats, both wild and domestic. It is labile and does not survive in the environment.

The virus is transmitted predominantly via bite wounds. The virus is found in large quantities in the saliva. Kittens can also be infected via the placenta and milk. Transmission to other cats in a multi-cat household is infrequent. Intact male cats are at increased risk as they are most likely to roam and fight. The average age of infected cats is around 6 years.

After infection, replication of the virus occurs in the salivary glands and lymphoid tissue. At this point there may be mild and vague clinical signs or infection may be subclinical. An immune response can be mounted that decreases the circulating virus and the cats generally become asymptomatic for a period of time. The virus, however, continues to replicate and over time there is destruction of the cat's immune system. This leaves the cat susceptible to infections and developing various tumours. The brain and kidneys can also be affected, leading to neurological signs and renal failure, respectively.

There are no vaccines for FIV and the virus cannot be eliminated by a normal immune response elicited by infection. The cat will produce antibodies but these are largely ineffective.

Clinical signs

Clinical signs are non-specific. After the initial infection the cats may have mild lethargy, inappetence and pyrexia. In the later stage of infection, clinical signs are associated with opportunistic infections, neoplasia or other syndromes, such as wasting, and include:

- Weight loss, emaciation
- Lethargy
- Inappetence
- Lymphadenopathy
- Pyrexia
- Gingivitis/stomatitis
- Chronic diarrhoea

- Chronic nasal discharge
- Chronic ocular discharge
- Anterior uveitis (directly FIV-related or as a result of toxoplasmosis)
- Chronic renal failure
- Chronic respiratory infection
- Abscesses
- Neurological signs (behaviour changes, seizures, paresis)

Diagnostics

- Blood tests: haematology, biochemistry
- FIV-specific ELISA for antibodies
- Confirmatory tests: virus isolation from the lymphocytes

ELISA-based tests

Some FIV-positive cats produce different antibodies to those detected on the test, leading to a false-negative result. Negative tests should be repeated after 8–12 weeks (anti-FIV antibodies are not produced in the first 8 weeks of infection).

Queens transfer antibodies to their newborn kittens via milk. These maternally derived antibodies (MDA) are then detected when the kittens are tested. FIV is usually only passed on to about one-third of the litter, but all the kittens will have MDA at the time of sampling as they may remain in the kitten's immune system for up to 4 months. Kittens that have been infected with the virus do not usually produce their own antibodies to the virus for a further 2 months. Therefore, to avoid false-positive results, kittens born to FIV-positive queens should not be tested until 6 months old.

Treatment

At this time there is no specific treatment with proven long-term efficacy, although antiviral drugs may be used. Treatment is aimed at the complications of FIV infection, i.e. opportunistic infections and neoplasia. Infections should be treated with appropriate antimicrobials. Dental hygiene is important to reduce stomatitis.

Routine inactivated vaccines can be given to asymptomatic FIV-positive cats living in a high-risk population to reduce the effects of stress that these diseases could have on the cat. Other measures include:

- Routine flea and worming prevention
- Neutering
- Removal of kittens from FIV-positive queens from birth
- Keeping FIV-positive cats indoors and away from FIV-negative cats.

Nursing care

The nursing of a patient with FIV is based on generalized symptomatic care. Symptoms can vary from patient to patient, but in addition to general nursing care the following measures should be taken.

- Administer fluid therapy and other medications, as directed by the veterinary surgeon
- Keep the patient clean and groomed
- Ensure adequate nutrition of the patient
- Advise the owner not to feed raw meat (due to increased risk of infection by *Toxoplasma gondii*)
- Advise the owner regarding preventive vaccination, worming and flea control
- Advise the owner to neuter the cat and keep it indoors to prevent transmission to other cats

Feline infectious peritonitis (FIP)

Feline infectious peritonitis is caused by a coronavirus. Although the incidence is low, the disease is usually fatal. It is a disease of multi-cat households and there is an increased risk in pedigree households. Clinical disease is seen most frequently in cats under 2 years of age, stressed or with concurrent disease.

The virus is shed via the faeces. Cats are usually infected via the oronasal route by direct contact with infected individuals or indirectly through contaminated fomites. Although the virus may survive in the environment, it is readily destroyed by routine disinfection.

Coronavirus infection is common. In the majority of cases the cats are asymptomatic or develop mild signs of diarrhoea and eliminate the virus. Less commonly the virus causes FIP. The reason why these cats develop FIP is not fully understood but it is thought likely to be associated with an inappropriate immune response.

The coronavirus infects macrophages, which are then dispersed around the body via the circulation, targeting the vascular beds of the peritoneum, pleura, eyes, meninges or kidneys. Antibodies produced against the coronavirus form complexes with the antigen that lodge in the vasculature and cause a vasculitis.

- If this occurs in the peritoneum or pleura, it causes protein-rich fluid leakage and accumulation in the cavities. This is referred to as **wet effusive FIP** and is generally seen in cats less than 2 years old.
- The **dry** form of FIP is seen in older cats, often after stress. There is inflammation and development of pyogranulomatous lesions throughout the body, without fluid accumulation.

Both forms are difficult to treat and, as the immune response is not appropriate, the disease is invariably fatal. Therefore the prognosis is poor.

Clinical signs

FIP cats have clinical signs of systemic disease – anorexia, lethargy and depression. The signs may be variable depending on the affected organs.

Wet effusive FIP

- Pleural effusion: dyspnoea and tachypnoea
- Ascites: pot-bellied appearance
- Weight loss

Dry FIP

Common presenting signs include:

- Weight loss
- Inappetence.

Other signs depend on the organs affected:

- Neurological signs
- Eye disease
- GI disease
- Renal disease.

Diagnostics

Diagnosis can be difficult, as the majority of cats are seropositive for coronavirus but do not have FIP. A combination of criteria is therefore used to make a diagnosis of FIP:

- History and clinical signs
- Blood tests: haematology and biochemistry (especially looking for increased globulins)
- Fluid analysis: exudates with increased proteins
- Biopsy of enlarged organs
- Post-mortem examination.

Treatment

The prognosis is poor and treatment is palliative. Corticosteroids may target the inflammation and slow the deterioration of the cat's condition. Supportive treatment involves thoracocentesis to relieve dyspnoea associated with a pleural effusion.

Prevention is aimed at managing the multi-cat households by reducing faecal contamination, keeping cat numbers low, and isolation and early weaning of the kittens.

Nursing care

- Barrier nurse the patient
- Monitor vital signs
- Provide general nursing of symptoms presented
- Provide assisted feeding of the anorexic patient
- Advise the owner regarding other cats in the household

Feline infectious anaemia (FIA)

The organism causing feline infectious anaemia was previously known as *Haemobartonella felis* but it has recently been re-classified as *Mycoplasma felis* and *M. haemominutum*. It is a parasite of feline red blood cells and lives on the cell surface.

The route of transmission is not completely understood. It is potentially spread by cat bites, fleas and blood transfusions. Kittens can be infected transplacentally and via the milk. There is an increased incidence in cats that are FeLV-positive, unvaccinated, roaming or involved in frequent cat fights.

The organism causes damage to the red blood cell surface. This is recognized by the immune system and the red blood cells are destroyed. This results in anaemia, which can be severe, especially if there is a concurrent FeLV infection.

Once infected, there is cyclical parasitaemia resulting in a cyclical anaemia. Some cats will be asymptomatic for infection and others will have severe disease. Infected cats will remain carriers for life.

Clinical signs

Clinical signs may be acute or chronic. The chronic form is the more common. Because cats can adapt their lifestyle they are often very anaemic when first presented.

- Acute:
  - Collapse
  - Dyspnoea
  - Pale mucous membranes
- Chronic:
  - Lethargy, anorexia
  - Tachypnoea, tachycardia
  - Pale mucous membranes
  - Splenic enlargement
  - Enlarged lymph nodes
  - Pyrexia.

Diagnostics

The diagnostic plan is the same as for anaemia:

- Blood tests: haematology (including reticulocytes) and biochemistry (the anaemia is regenerative)

- Fresh blood smears to stain for *Mycoplasma* – Wright–Giemsa stain. The parasites are visible on the surface of the red blood cells. Due to the cyclical nature, multiple smears over time may need to be examined.

Treatment

The infection is treated with doxycycline for 2–3 weeks. As there is an immune component to the red blood cell destruction, the patient is also given immunosuppressive drugs. Supportive care includes blood transfusions for severe anaemia.

Nursing care

- Monitor vital signs
- Administer medication, as directed by veterinary surgeon – especially flea treatment to prevent disease transmission
- Administer fluid therapy with or without blood transfusion, as directed by veterinary surgeon
- Ensure adequate nutrition; assisted feeding may be required
- Reduce environmental stress
- Advise the owner regarding flea control

Toxoplasmosis

This is an important zoonotic disease, especially for pregnant women.

Toxoplasma gondii is an intracellular protozoan parasite (see Chapter 8). It infects all warm-blooded animals but cats are the only species in which the parasite can complete its life cycle (the cat is a definitive host) and the only species that sheds oocysts. The other species act as intermediate hosts.

It is a multisystemic infection. Neurological signs are seen in 10% of affected animals.

Clinical signs

Most infections are subclinical. If infection occurs in a previously uninfected queen during pregnancy, the parasite can multiply in the placenta and spread to the fetuses. Affected kittens may be stillborn or may die before weaning.

Clinical signs depend on the organs affected:

- Pyrexia
- Anorexia
- Lethargy
- Weight loss
- Ophthalmitis (especially uveitis)
- Pneumonia
- Hepatitis
- Myositis
- Pancreatitis
- Myocarditis
- Skin lesions (rare)
- Diarrhoea
- Vomiting
- Muscle hyperaesthesia
- Lameness
- Ascites
- Neurological signs
- Sudden death.

Diagnostics

- Blood tests: haematology and biochemistry
- CSF if neurological signs are present
- Faecal examination
- Serology
- Biopsy

Treatment

Systemic disease should be treated with clindamycin. Corticosteroids are contraindicated.

Nursing care

- *This is a zoonotic disease.* Appropriate care and use of disinfectants are important when handling faeces or cleaning litter trays.
- Administer drugs, as directed by the veterinary surgeon.

Advice for clients on avoiding toxoplasmosis

- Prepare animal food in a separate area, using separate utensils and feeding bowls
- Do not allow pets to lick bowls, utensils or cooking items used by humans
- Empty cat litter trays daily and clean with boiling water and disinfectant
- Regular and prompt cleaning of litter trays will prevent oocysts from sporulating and becoming infectious
- Pregnant women should wear waterproof protective gloves when gardening to avoid contact with buried or decomposed cat faeces, as the oocysts in the environment will have sporulated and become infectious. Hands should be washed thoroughly prior to contact with cups, food, etc.
- Wash all vegetables thoroughly for the same reason
- Cook meat thoroughly
- Cover children's sand pits prevent cats using as litter trays
- Ensure regular worming of cats to prevent infection

Infectious diseases – canine/feline

Rabies

This is a zoonotic disease.

Rabies is caused by a lyssavirus. It is quite labile and does not survive in the environment. Rabies is an important fatal zoonotic disease and is widely spread through the rest of the world except Australasia and Antarctica; the UK is currently rabies-free. Control of stray dogs and rabies vaccinations have been important in reducing the number of rabies cases in pet dog and human populations. Dogs that travel abroad as part of the pet travel scheme are required to be vaccinated against rabies.

Rabies is transmitted directly via saliva in bite wounds or abrasions from infected animals. All warm-blooded animals are variably susceptible to infection. Wild animals can act as a reservoir of infection.

The incubation period can be prolonged, with an average of around 2 months. The length of time to clinical signs is related to the infective dose and the distance the virus has to travel to the central nervous system: after the animal is bitten, the virus replicates locally before spreading up the nerves to the central nervous system. It replicates in the central nervous system before spreading along nerves to other parts of the body and into the salivary glands, where it is secreted in the saliva and capable of infecting another animal. Clinical signs of abnormal behaviour and paralysis are caused by direct damage to the central nervous system. The disease is considered fatal.

Clinical signs

The clinical signs of rabies have classically been divided into two major types: excitative ('furious') and paralytic ('dumb'). However, atypical signs are commonly seen. From the onset of clinical signs in pets, death usually occurs within 2–7 days.

Excitative

These animals become irritable, restless and vicious. They usually develop other neurological signs of incoordination, disorientation and generalized grand mal seizures. Wild animals may be less fearful of humans.

Paralytic

Incoordination is one of the first signs of the paralytic form. The motor neurons are damaged, resulting in hindlimb ataxia progressing to paralysis. Progressive laryngeal and pharyngeal paralysis occurs, giving difficulty in swallowing and profuse salivation and drooling. Facial expression is affected, resulting in drooping eyelids, sagging jaw and squinting. Progressive paralysis ensues, leading to respiratory arrest and death.

The distinction between the two forms is often not clear-cut and both forms progress toward paralysis, coma and death. The paralytic form is very uncommon in cats.

Diagnostics

There are no reliable ante-mortem tests for diagnosis of rabies; therefore, a presumptive diagnosis needs to be based on history and clinical signs. As rabies is a fatal zoonotic disease, suspected cases are euthanased and the diagnosis is made on post-mortem examination of the brain. Rabies is a **notifiable disease**. Suspect cases should be isolated and DEFRA contacted immediately.

Any animal that has potentially been exposed should be handled with great care. Transmission routes should be borne in mind and any abrasions, especially to the hands and face, should be covered. Masks with visors should be worn to avoid infection via mucous membranes.

Treatment

- Dogs are vaccinated in areas where there is a risk of rabies and in those taking part in the Pet Travel Scheme (see DEFRA website)
- Humans are vaccinated if they are deemed at risk (e.g. staff working in quarantine kennels)
- Dogs with clinical signs should be placed in strict isolation and DEFRA contacted immediately. These cases are not treated
- If bitten, the wound should be washed immediately with detergent and then 40–70% alcohol. Medical attention should be sought urgently

Salmonellosis

This is a zoonotic disease.

Salmonellosis is caused by *Salmonella*, of which there are many serotypes. The bacterium is not host species-specific and occurs commonly in the intestinal tract of healthy mammals, birds and reptiles. Under certain circumstances it can cause systemic disease. It can survive for relatively long periods in the environment.

It is shed in the faeces, and transmission occurs through ingestion of faecally contaminated food, water or fomites. The bacteria multiply rapidly in foodstuffs stored at room temperature and in food that is inadequately cooked. Shedding can be intermittent and is usually increased when the animal is stressed. Younger animals are more susceptible to infection and illness. Overcrowding, stress and immunosuppression increase the risk of salmonellosis in dogs and cats.

After ingestion, the bacteria localize in the intestinal epithelium. Acute gastroenteritis is the most common clinical manifestation, but septicaemia can occur and the infection may become established in other tissues (placenta, conjunctiva, joints, meninges). Carrier animals may exhibit GI signs when subject to stress.

Clinical signs

- Anorexia, depression
- Diarrhoea – haemorrhagic in severe cases
- Vomiting, abdominal pain
- Dehydration
- Weight loss
- Pyrexia
- If severely affected and has a bacteraemia, will present in shock
- *In utero* infections result in abortions, stillbirths and the birth of weak puppies

Diagnostics

The diagnosis may be suspected from history and clinical signs.

- Blood tests: haematology/biochemistry are non-specific
- Faecal culture: may be supportive but bear in mind that *Salmonella* can be isolated from healthy individuals

Treatment

- Barrier nursing and isolation
- Antibiotics are only used if the disease is systemic, as they (except fluoroquinolones) may increase risk of shedding once the animal has recovered. The disease is usually self-limiting
- Fluid therapy and other supportive care for acute diarrhoea

Nursing care

- *This is a zoonotic disease* – care must be taken when nursing
- Barrier nurse the patient to prevent transmission
- Monitor vital signs
- Administer medication, as directed by the veterinary surgeon
- Administer and maintain fluid therapy if required
- Provide general nursing of the symptoms suffered
- Ensure adequate nutrition of the patient
- Dispose of faeces carefully
- Advise owner regarding contamination

Campylobacteriosis

This is a zoonotic disease.

The bacterium *Campylobacter* is an opportunistic organism whose role as a primary pathogen is not fully known. *Campylobacter* spp. probably act synergistically with other infections. Spread is through ingestion of undercooked raw food, contaminated water or faeces from infected animals, or via food/water bowls. Clinical infection is more common in animals under 6 months of age.

Clinical signs

- Watery or mucoid diarrhoea
- Faecal tenesmus
- Dullness, inappetence

Diagnostics

- Culture of organisms from fresh (<24h old) faeces, using selective media
- Detection of *Campylobacter* – not always diagnostic on its own because of carrier state

Treatment

- The disease is self-limiting
- Antibiotics may be given to reduce duration and severity of diarrhoea, minimizing risk of infection to humans and other animals
- Fluid therapy

Nursing care

- *This is a zoonotic disease* – care must be taken when nursing
- Barrier nurse the patient to prevent transmission
- Monitor vital signs
- Administer medication, as directed by the veterinary surgeon
- Administer and maintain fluid therapy if required
- Provide general nursing of the symptoms suffered
- Ensure adequate nutrition of the patient
- Dispose of faeces carefully
- Advise owner regarding contamination

Complementary therapies

The use of complementary therapies for the treatment of animals is increasing rapidly in the veterinary profession. A **complementary therapy** is one that is used *in combination with* traditional veterinary treatment, rather than as an alternative to conventional medicine. There are various types of complementary therapy that can be used to aid in the treatment of a range of conditions.

- **Acupuncture** – an ancient form of healing derived from Chinese medicine, involving the insertion of fine needles into specific locations in the body known as 'acupuncture points'
- **Physiotherapy** – therapy using physical or mechanical means such as massage, heat, exercise or electricity in order to relieve pain, regain movement, restore muscle strength and increase weight loss
- **Hydrotherapy** – involves the use of water either internally or externally for the treatment of disease or trauma or for the general maintenance of good health
- **Magnetic therapy** – magnetic products are applied to animals in order to relieve pain and increase mobility
- **Aromatherapy** – treating animals with medicinal remedies that they would once have found in the wild; involves the use of essential oils and plant extracts.

Complementary therapies play an important role in supporting veterinary treatment. Under the direction of a veterinary surgeon, the veterinary nurse can improve the quality and effectiveness of nursing care by employing these therapies. This section will cover the application of the basic techniques of acupuncture, physiotherapy and hydrotherapy.

Acupuncture

The use of acupuncture is becoming more widely accepted in veterinary medicine. It is particularly popular for the management of postoperative and chronic pain. Figure 21.27 shows a range of canine and feline conditions for which treatment has included the use of acupuncture.

System	Canine conditions	Feline conditions
Musculoskeletal	Lameness of unknown origin Hip dysplasia Bruising/sprains Arthritic and rheumatic joints Back pain – spondylosis/spondylitis Cruciate ligament damage	Lameness of unknown origin Cruciate ligament damage Arthritic and rheumatic problems Back pain
Respiratory	Chronic bronchitis Coughing unresponsive to treatment Persistent or periodic kennel cough	Feline asthma Chronic nasal discharges Chronic cat flu Chronic sneezing
Urogenital	Infertility Incontinence in bitches Old-age incontinence Cystitis Ovarian dysfunction	Kidney disease Incontinence Infertility Cystitis
Nervous system	Epilepsy	Epilepsy
Digestive system	Persistent diarrhoea Persistent constipation	Persistent diarrhoea Persistent constipation

21.27 Canine and feline conditions for which treatment has included the use of acupuncture.

Basic principles

Traditional Chinese medicine operates on the principle that the organs of the body interact with each other in order to maintain a balance of good health. This is known as the Yin–Yang Theory and the belief is that when this balance is disturbed the body will suffer from disease. The balance in the body is thought to be maintained by the flow of 'Qi' along energy channels known as meridians that connect all the organs in the body. Acupuncture aims to manipulate the flow of 'Qi' and restore any imbalance by inserting fine needles into specific points on the body.

Acupuncture points can be found all over the body and are located in areas with a rich nerve and blood supply. Each acupuncture point corresponds with an organ system in the body. Following a thorough examination of the animal, the relevant points can be selected for stimulation. The specific effects of acupuncture needling are transferred through stimulation of the peripheral nervous system.

Procedure

The nature of the animal's condition should first be established with a diagnosis by a veterinary surgeon. This is very important, as it is essential to rule out conditions that require surgical treatment. Once a diagnosis has been made, it is safe to proceed with acupuncture.

- Acupuncture is performed by inserting very thin sterile needles into the skin (Figure 21.28).
- The needles used for cats and dogs are generally 2.5 cm in length. The depth of insertion varies between practitioners from superficial to needling of the muscle tissue.
- The needles remain in the patient for as little as 1 minute to a maximum of half an hour. Most commonly the duration of needling is approximately 10–20 minutes.
- The placement of needles causes little or no discomfort and once situated they are painless.
- Once inserted the needles can be gently manipulated with a twisting action in order to stimulate the acupuncture point.
- The number of needles inserted in a treatment session determines the 'dose' of acupuncture. On average four to six needles are used, with this number increasing in chronic cases.
- The dose of acupuncture required for each animal should be recorded for future reference.
- The frequency of treatment sessions is usually once a week, but this is dependent on the severity of the condition.
- A small percentage of animals will object to receiving acupuncture, making it difficult or in some cases impossible to apply the treatment.

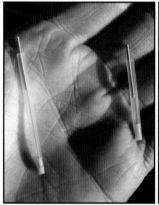
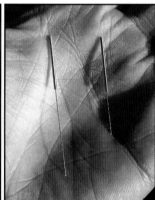
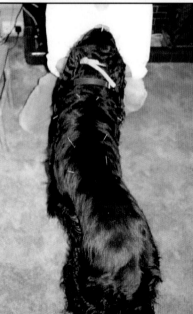

21.28 Acupuncture needles inside and removed from their plastic casings, and in use in a dog. (Courtesy of N Thompson)

⚠ WARNING

Although the insertion of needles is considered to be minor surgery, specialized training and knowledge are essential in order to perform acupuncture safely. The Royal College of Veterinary Surgeons therefore states that 'a Listed veterinary nurse may undertake acupuncture treatment provided that he or she is working under the direction of a veterinary surgeon who is also a qualified acupuncturist'. Veterinary nurses must ensure that they adhere to these guidelines at all times.

Safety

- The use of sterile, disposable needles is recommended.
- The veterinary nurse should ensure that the needles remain sterile when opening the packets for the veterinary surgeon.
- Acupuncture needles should be disposed of in 'sharps' boxes.
- If reusable needles are used, it is essential that they are properly sterilized.

Physiotherapy

Many applications of physiotherapy should only be carried out by a qualified physiotherapist with suitable training, otherwise harm can be caused. A diagnosis is essential before physiotherapy is started.

Knowledge and the effective application of physiotherapy techniques are essential for the veterinary nurse and highly beneficial to the patient. *Physiotherapy must only be performed by the veterinary nurse under the direction of the veterinary surgeon.*

There is a wide variety of musculoskeletal and neurological conditions that can be treated using a range of physiotherapy methods (Figure 21.29). This works in conjunction with traditional veterinary treatment by speeding up the healing process and therefore improving recovery time.

Conditions that will benefit from physiotherapy
Injuries to tendons, ligaments and joints
Muscle atrophy
Chronic inflammation
Reduction of scar tissue
Hip dysplasia
Elbow dysplasia
Osteoarthritis
General pain in back or joints
Paralysis/paresis
Pre/postoperative treatments
Postneurological events (CVA)
Oedema
Excess secretions

Conditions where physiotherapy is contraindicated
Pneumonia
Pleural effusion
Disc prolapse
Serious rupture of soft tissues
Severe developmental problems
Nerve avulsion
Acute inflammation
Fractures
Haemorrhage
Presence of infection or neoplasia

21.29 Conditions in which the use of physiotherapy is beneficial or contraindicated.

Physiotherapy can also be used routinely as a preventive therapy for those with a high level of activity, such as working, racing and competition animals. This helps to reduce the risk of injury and encourages the animal to reach its full physical performance potential.

Physiotherapy is a valuable form of stimulation and enrichment for the hospitalized patient and can help to prevent behavioural problems that may arise due to boredom and frustration.

Aims of physiotherapy

- Increase the flow of blood, thus assisting the healing of damaged tissues and improving circulation in elderly/recumbent patients
- Reduce oedema and chronic inflammation
- Build up physical strength
- Improve mobility and restore normal movement
- Decrease the incidence of muscle spasms
- Relieve pain
- Reduce the length of stay in hospital for the animal following surgery (especially orthopaedic procedures)
- Reduce the build-up of scar tissue

Effleurage

Effleurage is a gentle form of massage that should ideally be performed first before any other physiotherapy techniques are applied. Effleurage massage is directed towards the heart, which improves circulation and promotes the drainage of lymphatic fluid. It is also a useful technique for animals that are reluctant to be manipulated with physiotherapy. Starting with gentle stroking techniques, the animal can become familiar with being touched in this manner, which will enable progression to other methods of physiotherapy.

- The technique is performed using stroking movements, with the palm of the hand progressing from the edge of the area being massaged to the centre.
- A massage session using effleurage should last approximately 10 minutes.
- A nervous or reluctant animal should be initiated with short sessions of 1–2 minutes. The duration can then be increased gradually until the animal is comfortable with the full 10-minute session.

Petrissage

This is a form of massage that involves squeezing, kneading, rolling and compression of the muscles in order to increase circulation. Petrissage aims to warm the tissues in preparation for more intense massage techniques. Other benefits include an increased supply of nutrients and oxygen to the muscle, softening of superficial fascia, decreased muscle tension, and improved mobility by breaking down adhesions in damaged tissues to help repair or prevent injury.

- Petrissage can be performed using the whole palm or simply using the fingertips, and is applied vertically to the muscle tissue.
- The pressure used will vary according to the purpose of the massage and the condition of the tissues being worked.
- Petrissage can be performed for between 10 and 20 minutes, three to four times daily on the hospitalized patient.

Passive exercise

This technique is applied when the animal is unable to move of its own accord (e.g. post fracture, or in the recumbent patient). The aim is to improve balance, strength, coordination and range of motion, and to restore normal function.

- The animal should be positioned in lateral recumbency in a warm, comfortable environment.
- The affected limbs or joints should be flexed and extended in turn through the full range of motion. The limb should be supported.
- It is important that the joints are not overextended.
- Always remember that the manipulation is likely to be painful, therefore the animal should be carefully restrained by a second nurse or muzzled if necessary to prevent any injuries.
- The affected limbs or joints should be manipulated up to ten times in each session, three to four times daily.

Active exercise

With this technique, the animal is encouraged to make the movements itself. The aim is to increase muscle strength and improve proprioception.

- The animal should be supported using a sling or hoist (if not available, towels can be used instead).
- A minimum of two nurses will be required to support a larger dog.
- Ensure that the floor surface is appropriate, i.e. not slippery. A non-slip mat can be placed on the floor if necessary.
- Once the animal is adequately supported in a standing position, the limbs should be placed on the floor.
- The animal should be raised slightly off the floor and lowered gently back down.
- The technique will encourage the animal to bear weight and will therefore help to restore muscle strength and increase awareness of the position of the limbs in relation to the body.
- As the patient progresses and muscle strength increases, supported walking can be encouraged.
- Once this stage has been achieved, the animal can eventually be encouraged to stand and walk on its own.
- Following on from this, obstacles can be placed on the floor for the animal to step over, improving balance and coordination.
- Session length depends on the condition and tolerance of the animal and can vary from as little as 2 minutes up to 10, three to four times daily.

Respiratory physiotherapy

The application of respiratory physiotherapy is beneficial for animals with pulmonary disease and also for recumbent patients. Such animals are likely to suffer from a reduction in lung volume and pooling of pulmonary secretions. The aims of respiratory physiotherapy are to:

- Reduce airway obstruction by improving the clearance of secretions
- Reduce the severity of any infection by clearing infected material
- Maintain optimal respiratory function and exercise tolerance
- Reduce the level of respiratory effort for the animal
- Improve level of comfort for the animal.

Postural drainage

This involves positioning of the patient to allow gravity to assist with the clearance of secretions and to increase lung capacity. Secretions drain from the lungs to the central airway, where they can then be removed by coughing. The cough reflex can be stimulated if necessary by gentle compression of the trachea.

- The animal should be positioned in lateral recumbency, supported using either rolled-up towels or sandbags so that the body is angled downwards, with the head placed lower than the rest of the body.
- Ensure that the lung to be drained is positioned on top.
- The position should be maintained for between 3 and 15 minutes, four to five times daily depending on the patient's condition and tolerance levels.
- Energy can be applied to the chest wall and lung using **percussion**, which is accomplished by rhythmically striking the thorax with cupped hands (**coupage**). This helps to loosen any secretions.
- Session duration and frequency is dependent on the condition and tolerance of the animal but can range from 2 minutes up to 10, three to five times daily.

Standing enables maximum expansion of the lungs, whereas placing the animal in a sitting position will reduce the level of expansion slightly. Lateral recumbency results in the poorest level of lung expansion, which is why it is vital to reposition the recumbent patient regularly. If possible the patient should be encouraged to stand up periodically. It may be necessary to support the patient using towels or a sling in order to achieve this.

Postural drainage is *contraindicated* in:

- Head and neck injuries
- Spinal injuries/surgery
- Surgical/healing wounds
- Rib fractures
- Pregnant animals
- Dyspnoea.

Thermotherapy

Thermotherapy is the use of heat treatment to promote vasodilation, thus increasing the blood supply to the affected area. The application of heat relaxes the muscles and increases flexibility and is effective in reducing muscle spasms, reducing swelling and relieving pain.

- Hot-water bottles, heated pads or infrared lamps can be used to apply heat to the affected area.
- Heat should be applied at a temperature of 40–45°C for between 5 and 30 minutes, up to five times a day.
- Heat therapy can be used for pain relief and prior to therapeutic exercises to increase flexibility of the joint capsule, tendons and ligaments.
- *Care must be taken to ensure that the temperature is correct, so that the heat therapy does not burn the animal.*
- Thermotherapy is contraindicated when there is bleeding at the site of trauma or in patients with peripheral vascular disease or diabetes mellitus.

Cryotherapy

Cryotherapy is the application of cold to an area of the body, which decreases the flow of fluid to the tissues and slows the release of chemicals that cause pain and inflammation. Cold decreases sensation in a localized area by reducing the ability of the nerve endings to conduct impulses.

- A cold compress can be applied to tissues following surgery or trauma.
- The reduced tissue temperature causes vasoconstriction, reducing any swelling, haemorrhage or bruising.
- Ice bags, chemical cold packs, ice cubes wrapped in a cloth or even frozen vegetables can be used as a cold compress.
- It is important to apply a cloth or towel over the area to prevent direct contact with the skin.
- The duration of treatment sessions will vary from 5 to 15 minutes, depending on the condition. If using ice, it is important to move it around the area being treated every 3 minutes to prevent damage to the skin.
- A cold compress can be applied to the affected area several times a day and is most effective in the first 72 hours after the trauma occurred.
- *It is essential not to leave an ice pack on an area of the body for too long, as it can stop the flow of blood. If the injury occurs in an area with little fat or muscle beneath the skin, take the compress off after a maximum of 10 minutes.*
- Cold therapy is contraindicated in patients with open wounds, peripheral vascular disease, diabetes mellitus and ischaemic injuries.

Hydrotherapy

Hydrotherapy is the use of water in any of its three forms (liquid, solid or gas), internally or externally, for the treatment of disease and trauma or for cleansing purposes. The most common form of hydrotherapy is swimming, which is classed as a form of active physiotherapy exercise.

The Canine Hydrotherapy Association has listed the minimum requirements that should be included in any veterinary referral (Figure 21.30). Under the direction of a veterinary surgeon, or with a signed veterinary referral, the veterinary nurse can conduct a programme of controlled exercise in the water for the animal.

- Name and contact details of referring veterinary surgeon
- History of previous veterinary treatment or surgical procedure undertaken or administered in connection with the condition
- Any areas of concern or caution
- Details of current medication
- Signed declaration from referring veterinarian stating that the animal is in a suitable state of health to undertake hydrotherapy
- A record of treatment (see Figure 21.33) must be recorded for all animals and kept on file for a minimum of 12 months following treatment
- A new referral must be obtained every 6 months for longer-term treatments
- Referring veterinary surgery should be updated on animal's progress every ten sessions.

21.30 Minimum requirements that should be included in a veterinary referral for hydrotherapy, as listed by the Canine Hydrotherapy Association.

Swimming is a very effective form of therapy, as movements in water can be performed more easily than in the air medium due to the buoyancy eliminating the effect of gravity. In this weight-free environment the animal is able to exercise the muscles with less stress. However, because of the increased resistance to movement, the muscles are made to work harder in water than in air; therefore a short swim for a dog is comparable to a 5-mile walk. Resistance can be increased with the use of jets that the animal can swim against. Due to the support from the water and specialized hydrotherapy equipment,

hydrotherapy is a very safe form of exercise for the animal, with no risk of damaging joints. For postoperative dogs hydrotherapy removes the weight loading on the affected limb, encouraging the gradual rebuilding of wasted muscle. It also reduces the pain and can accelerate recovery following surgery for a range of conditions (Figure 21.31).

Conditions that will benefit from hydrotherapy

Osteochondritis dissecans (OCD)
Hip dysplasia
Elbow dysplasia
Spinal trauma
Paralysis/paresis
Cruciate ligament injuries
Hip replacement
Patella luxation
Muscle atrophy post fracture
Osteoarthritis
Postoperative muscle restoration
Obesity
Prevention of injury by maintaining optimal condition in racing, working or competition animals

Conditions where hydrotherapy is contraindicated

Presence of infectious disease
Pulmonary disease
Serious instability of the joint
Unstable fractures
Active gastrointestinal disease (vomiting, diarrhoea)
Advanced heart or respiratory problems
Behaviour problems (e.g. aggression)
Uncontrolled epilepsy
Uncontrolled diabetes
Pyrexia
Presence of open wounds
Skin conditions that may be irritated by moisture

21.31 Conditions in which the use of hydrotherapy is beneficial or contraindicated.

Hydrotherapy aims to:

- Restore muscle mass
- Reduce pain
- Increase range of movement
- Assist with weight management
- Improve general fitness
- Improve balance and coordination
- Improve healing
- Reduce oedema.

Procedure

Hydrotherapy can be conducted using a large tub or bath for smaller animals. There may also be access to the increasing number of specially designed hydrotherapy pools for animals, which provide an excellent swimming environment (Figure 21.32). The animal is supported in the water using either an electronic hoist or a manual version that involves a support sling attached to a pole. Buoyancy aids such as life jackets and floats are used, depending on the ability of the patient. The buoyancy aids allow the depth of the animal to be adjusted and ensure that the spine is kept straight while the animal is in the water. The water temperature encourages vasodilation, which improves the flow of oxygen and nutrients to the tissues. Consequently healing time following surgery or trauma is improved.

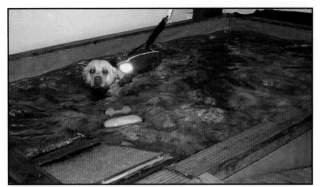

21.32   Hydrotherapy. (Courtesy of Leconfield Kennels.)

- The bath or pool should be clean, safe and conducive to the well-being of the animals undergoing treatment and those operating the pool.
- The temperature of the water should remain between 27 and 32°C. The temperature of spa pools may be higher – up to 40°C.
- To ensure the safety of the animal and the handlers, it is best to have two nurses present when conducting hydrotherapy treatment.
- Ensure that plenty of towels are available and there is a suitable area nearby to dry the animal. A hairdryer may also be used.
- If the patient is hospitalized, ensure that the kennel is clean, warm and dry for the animal to return to.
- Prior to swimming, the temperature, heart rate and respiration rate of the animal should be recorded. If any of these are abnormal, the session should be cancelled.
- The animal should be carefully lifted into the water if using a bath and supported at all times. *Never leave the animal unattended in the water.*
- Entry into a pool should be carefully controlled by walking the animal into the water on a submerged ramp or using an electronic hoist.
- The animal can then swim in the water whilst being supported by the electric hoist or in the harness attached to a pole, which can be controlled by the nurse.
- It may be necessary for one nurse to accompany the animal in the water, particularly if the animal is nervous.
- The length of the session will depend on the condition being treated and on the individual. The first session may be as short as 1 minute following surgery such as a cruciate repair. Usually the initial swim will last 5 minutes, increasing up to a maximum of 30 minutes over time. If the animal appears to be tired or struggling, the session should be ended immediately.

- Frequency of sessions is dependent on the condition being treated, but typically an animal will begin with two sessions per week, reducing to once a week as progress is made.
- Details of each session and the progress made should be recorded (Figure 21.33).

- Name of owner
- Name, breed, sex and age of animal
- Description of condition being treated
- Initial assessment of animal and goals to be targeted
- Date and time of session
- Method of entry into pool
- Duration of swim, including time and power of anti-swim jets if used
- Relevant comments or observations (e.g. range of movement in affected limb)

21.33   Details to be recorded on an animal's treatment record for hydrotherapy.

Acknowledgement

Elizabeth Bryan, author of the section on Complementary therapies, would like to thank Nick Thompson BSc(Hons), BVM&S, VetMFHom, MRCVS, for being a valuable source of information and data.

Further reading

Bowden C and Masters J (2003) *Textbook of Veterinary Medical Nursing*. Butterworth Heinemann, London

Hall EH, Simpson JW and Williams DA (eds) (2005) *BSAVA Manual of Canine and Feline Gastroenterology, 2nd edition*. BSAVA Publications, Gloucester

Klide AM and Kung SH (2002) *Veterinary Acupuncture*. University of Pennsylvania Press, Philadelphia

Millis D, Levine D and Taylor R (2004) *Canine Rehabilitation and Physical Therapy*. WB Saunders, Philadelphia

Mooney CT and Peterson ME (eds) (2004) *BSAVA Manual of Canine and Feline Endocrinology, 3rd edition*. BSAVA Publications, Gloucester

Moore M (ed.) (2000) *Manual of Veterinary Nursing*. BSAVA Publications, Cheltenham

Ramey DW and Rollin BE (2004) *Complementary and Alternative Veterinary Medicine Considered*. Iowa State Press, Ames, Iowa

Ramsey IK and Tennant B (eds) (2001) *BSAVA Manual of Canine and Feline Infectious Diseases*. BSAVA Publications, Gloucester

Chapter 22

Anaesthesia and analgesia

David C. Brodbelt and Simon J. Girling

Learning objectives

After studying this chapter, students should be able to:

- **Describe the necessary steps required to evaluate a patient for general anaesthesia**
- **List the properties of the commonly used premedicants**
- **Discuss a potential analgesia plan to include perioperative analgesia**
- **Describe local anaesthetic techniques**
- **Discuss the administration and maintenance of general anaesthesia, including individual intravenous and inhalational agents**
- **Check the anaesthetic machine prior to anaesthesia and prepare for an anaesthetic**
- **Describe the methods appropriate for the anaesthesia of 'exotic' species**
- **Discuss the potential risks of general anaesthesia**
- **Assist the veterinary surgeon in the event of a cardiopulmonary arrest during anaesthesia**
- **Explain the veterinary nurse's role in anaesthesia and analgesia**

Introduction

Anaesthesia is the reversible production of a state of unconsciousness necessary to perform surgery or undertake diagnostic tests. It relies on the provision of analgesia, muscle relaxation and narcosis/unconsciousness: the 'triad' of anaesthesia. Safe and effective anaesthesia addresses these three components individually and, by using a combination of anaesthetic agents, satisfies these requirements whilst avoiding significant depression of normal physiological function. This is termed 'balanced' anaesthesia, which provides good patient stability and reduces the potential for perioperative complications. It is commonly employed in practice when a patient is premedicated with a sedative and analgesic, providing analgesia during and after surgery, and then maintained with an inhalation agent to provide narcosis.

The veterinary nurse is integrally involved in the provision of anaesthesia and analgesia of the patient presenting for surgery and diagnostic procedures. A solid understanding of each individual patient's requirements and the likely effects of the anaesthetic administered are important aspects of the nurse's duties when involved in an anaesthetic. Careful monitoring of the patient from admission, through the anaesthetic and until discharge is a task often delegated to the nurse by the veterinary surgeon, and the provision of good analgesia is an area in which the veterinary nurse can make a large impact and benefit the patient. In a survey of practitioners' views on analgesia, veterinary surgeons were most often likely to delegate the assessment and administration of analgesics to the veterinary nurse.

Safe anaesthesia requires a good knowledge of the underlying anatomy and physiology of the patient and an appreciation of the pharmacological effects of the anaesthetic given. These subjects are reviewed in Chapters 4 and 9 and other standard texts (see 'Further reading').

Preoperative assessment and preparation

A thorough preoperative examination is essential to identify higher-risk patients and allows appropriate preparation prior to anaesthesia. In those cases that are poor anaesthetic candidates (ASA classes 3–5, see box), particular attention to preparation is required, to minimize the risk of untoward events. Other considerations that affect the degree of preparation include the type of surgery: prolonged or invasive procedures require more preparation than superficial operations. Whether the procedure is elective or an emergency indicates how much preparation is possible. Emergency cases requiring immediate surgery may receive only cursory preparation. Elective procedures may be postponed without compromising the animal.

The American Society of Anesthesiologists (ASA) Risk Assessment

Patients are classified into five categories:

- **Class 1**: Normal, healthy patient
- **Class 2**: Patient with mild to moderate systemic disease
- **Class 3**: Patient with severe systemic disease that is not incapacitating
- **Class 4**: Patient with severe systemic disease that is a constant threat to life
- **Class 5**: Moribund patient not expected to survive 24 hours with or without surgery.

Preoperative examination

The animal's medical condition is primarily determined by taking a good history and performing a comprehensive clinical examination. When necessary, further tests may be required. Those systems of particular concern include nervous, cardiovascular, respiratory, renal and hepatic systems.

History

Much valuable information can be gained from questioning the owner. Questions relating to general health status include recent weight loss, behavioural changes and signs of pain. Information pertaining to cardiovascular and pulmonary function can be gleaned by questioning the owner about the animal's response to exercise, presence of coughing and general demeanour when at rest. Excessive drinking may alert to endocrine, liver and renal problems and may lead to the performance of further tests prior to anaesthesia. Vomiting, diarrhoea and inappetence prior to presentation may also alert the nurse to systemic disease. Reproductive status (neutered/in season) and the presence of discharges (e.g. vaginal discharge) may be relevant. Other background information that may be of value includes:

- Duration of ownership
- Previous medical history
- Previous anaesthetic history
- Vaccination status
- Current medication, including 'over-the-counter' products. The dose, dosing frequency and duration of treatment should be established. Drugs of particular concern are:
  - Antibiotics
  - Glucocorticoids
  - Non-steroidal anti-inflammatory drugs
  - Organophosphorus compounds, flea collars, parasiticides
  - Anticonvulsants
  - Digoxin, beta-blockers, calcium channel blockers and ACE inhibitors
  - Furosemide and other diuretics
  - Endocrine supplements (e.g. thyroxine)
  - Antihistamines
  - Antitussives/bronchodilators
  - Antidepressants (e.g. selegiline).

Physical examination

This concentrates on the organ systems affected principally by anaesthesia.

Central nervous system

Central nervous system status involves particular attention to the patient's state of mind and the presence of depressed function.

Cardiovascular system

Cardiovascular function is assessed with inspection of exercise tolerance, mucous membrane colour and capillary refill time, palpation of peripheral pulse rate and quality, and auscultation of cardiac murmurs and dysrhythmias. Pale mucous membranes suggest hypovolaemia or anaemia, whilst cyanotic membranes indicate poor oxygenation of arterial blood. Cool extremities can be seen during shock and reduced peripheral perfusion. Right-sided cardiovascular dysfunction is associated with pronounced jugular pulses and peripheral oedema.

Practical tip

A good assessment of a dog's cardiovascular fitness for anaesthesia is its response to a short lead-walk. If the animal becomes distressed or dyspnoeic or collapses after minimal exercise, the patient is at a significant risk for anaesthesia, whereas an animal that is unremarkable and remains undistressed should be fit for anaesthesia.

Respiratory system

Examination includes observation of respiratory rate and pattern, auscultation and percussion of the chest. Auscultation of rales and crepitus suggest airway secretion and respiratory disease. Reduced sounds are associated with lung consolidation. Chest percussion with low resonance supports the presence of consolidation, whilst high resonance is consistent with pneumothorax.

Further tests

Haematology and biochemistry

A blood sample should be examined if the history or physical examination raises the suspicion of anaemia, hypoproteinaemia, coagulation disorders, liver or renal pathology. Metabolic and electrolyte disorders, including hypo- and hyperkalaemia, can be detected. Liver function tests and liver enzymes can alert to liver pathology, whilst serum urea and creatinine are useful indicators of renal status. Urinalysis (especially urine specific gravity) is valuable in investigating renal function if particular concern exists.

Radiography and ultrasonography

Animals involved in road traffic accidents, those with neoplastic disease and those with signs of cardiovascular or pulmonary disease should undergo radiographic examination of the thorax and abdomen. Presenting polydipsia and polyuria with or without a vaginal discharge in an unneutered bitch may warrant abdominal radiography to rule out pyometra. Additionally ultrasonography allows thorough investigation of cardiac function and abdominal pathology.

Electrocardiography

Abnormal pulse rhythm requires further investigation. Electrocardiography allows the diagnosis of cardiac arrhythmias and treatment if appropriate.

Significance of clinical findings

Central nervous system disease

Behaviour better indicates an animal's suitability for surgery than age: a tail-wagging, active 15-year-old dog is a better risk than the depressed, small, inactive 8-month-old puppy with a portosystemic shunt. Depression increases patient sensitivity to anaesthetics and may indicate the presence of intracranial pathology (tumours, meningitis), systemic disease (pyrexia, hyperkalaemia, toxaemia) or cardiovascular problems.

Epileptic animals are more sensitive to anaesthetics if anticonvulsant therapy has only recently begun. In time, liver enzyme induction occurs and accelerates the metabolism of some anaesthetics, making the patient more resistant to anaesthetics.

Cardiovascular and respiratory disease

Signs of cardiac and respiratory disease (including exercise intolerance) are always important. When disease is present, the fundamental goal of preparation is to optimize the factors contributing to oxygen delivery to the tissues, i.e. cardiac output, haemoglobin content and pulmonary function.

Cardiac disease is not a contraindication to anaesthesia if the effects on cardiac function and blood flow are appreciated and drugs selected accordingly. In general, 'stress', pain and volume losses are less well tolerated by animals with cardiovascular disease. Drugs used for treating cardiac disease (e.g. digoxin, beta-blockers) may interact with anaesthetics. Cases with congestive heart failure may require cage rest and institution of medical therapy. Pre-existing arrhythmias may require treatment.

Respiratory disease predisposes the animal to hypoxia and hypercapnia. It may contribute to secondary right ventricular changes (cor pulmonale) or polycythaemia. A common form of restrictive respiratory disease is morbid obesity. Restricted airways (e.g. nasal discharge, brachycephalic canine anatomy, collapsing trachea) require careful attention for maintenance of an airway.

Causes of respiratory embarrassment (e.g. pneumothorax, gastric tympany) must be relieved preoperatively. Pleural effusions should be drained preoperatively. Excessive alveolar transudate may be cleared with diuretics, ACE inhibitors and drugs that improve cardiac contractility and function.

Liver and renal disease

Liver disease may prolong anaesthesia, as most drugs administered undergo some hepatic metabolism. Consideration of anaesthetics with least reliance on hepatic function may be appropriate in such circumstances. Secondary problems include coagulation defects, hypoproteinaemia and hypoglycaemia (see below).

Patients with pre-existing **kidney disease** are intolerant of renal hypoperfusion during anaesthesia. Significant cardiovascular depression and reduced kidney perfusion during anaesthesia can cause renal ischaemia and lead to subsequent renal failure. This is a particular concern in geriatric patients already in early chronic renal failure, and can result in acute renal decompensation. Elderly patients (and those in renal failure) should be given fluids during anaesthesia and cardiovascular stability should be maintained.

Unstable blood glucose levels

Diabetes mellitus causes hyperglycaemia with diuresis, fluid loss and ketoacidosis. Severe hypoglycaemia resulting from an insulinoma or liver disease causes considerable neuronal damage if brain glucose supply is curtailed. Glucose levels should be controlled with soluble insulin or dextrose solutions preoperatively.

Hypoalbuminaemia

This can indicate liver or renal disease and has two consequences. First, the albumin-bound fraction of drugs highly bound to plasma proteins (e.g. thiopental) is lowered and so more free drug is available, potentially leading to overdose if a standard dose is administered. Secondly, plasma oncotic pressure may be lowered, promoting oedema and increased diffusion distance for gases in the lung. If severe enough this can result in hypoxia.

Coagulation problems

Clotting failure may be genetic (e.g. von Willebrand's disease in Dobermanns) or may indicate liver failure. Fresh blood products may be required preoperatively.

Electrolyte and pH abnormalities

High potassium levels resulting from hypoadrenocorticism or renal failure must be lowered preoperatively, while low serum potassium should be raised. High potassium levels are lowered with sodium bicarbonate solutions, calcium gluconate, insulin–glucose solutions, or cation-exchange resins. In extreme cases, peritoneal dialysis may be required. Potassium is raised by infusing solutions at rates not greater than 0.5 mmol/kg/h. Extremes of pH are ameliorated by treating the underlying cause.

Hypovolaemia and dehydration

In dehydrated and hypovolaemic animals, tissue perfusion may become compromised during anaesthesia. Animals with chronic fluid loss (e.g. those with chronic vomiting and diarrhoea) may have electrolyte and/or pH disturbances.

Animals with renal failure cannot concentrate urine and become dehydrated if access to water is restricted. Dogs and cats with chronic renal failure, or any disease characterized by polyuria and polydipsia, should not have water withheld preoperatively; if necessary, parenteral fluids may be given.

When reduced, circulating blood volume must be restored preoperatively with appropriate fluids. Oral, intravenous, intraperitoneal, intraosseous or subcutaneous routes may be used, depending on the cause, fluid type and the time available (see Chapter 19).

Anaemia and polycythaemia

Low haemoglobin levels (<8 g/dl) caused by blood loss or renal disease should be resolved before surgery; oxygen flux may become inadequate when compensatory changes (increased cardiac output and modest hyperventilation) are depressed by anaesthetics. In elective cases, low haemoglobin levels may be raised by treating the underlying cause; otherwise blood transfusion therapy, preferably with 'packed' cells, may be required.

High haemoglobin levels can also be deleterious. Haematocrit values in excess of 55% make blood hyperviscous, causing it to 'sludge' in capillaries. They may also indicate that the animal is dehydrated or suffering from chronic hypoxia. High haematocrits in normovolaemic patients can be lowered by the process of normovolaemic haemodilution. This involves the withdrawal of whole blood and simultaneous replacement with plasma or fluids.

Pyrexia

Pyrexia increases metabolic rate; there are rises in the consumption of oxygen and glucose and in the production of carbon dioxide. The cause of pyrexia should be investigated because, while there is little problem anaesthetizing animals with superficial abscesses, there is considerable risk when pyrexia results from endocarditis or meningitis. Pyrexia is treated with antibiotics if the cause is infectious.

Current medication

Pre-existing medical therapy and perioperative medication may affect subsequently administered sedatives and anaesthetics. An understanding of the impact of these concurrent therapies is important to avoid unnecessary side effects. Generally, however, most medications are continued through the perioperative period. Individual considerations include the following.

- **Aminoglycoside antibiotics** (e.g. gentamicin) may potentiate neuromuscular blockade when combined with inhalation anaesthesia, resulting in significant ventilation depression. Further, at high doses these antibiotics can cause renal failure and may be better avoided in patients with pre-existing renal failure.
- **Barbiturates** given to control epilepsy should be maintained perioperatively. Theoretically, enzyme induction may increase anaesthetic requirements, though clinically this is rarely seen.
- **Cardiovascular therapy** including the use of ACE inhibitors, beta-blockers and calcium channel blockers is also best maintained. However, caution should be applied when administering anaesthetic agents and premedicants that decrease blood pressure (i.e. many drugs), and attention to maintenance of cardiovascular function during anaesthesia is particularly important. Digoxin therapy may induce intraoperative arrhythmias, though if cardiovascular function is stable it is best continued.
- **Corticosteroids** administered chronically prior to anaesthesia may inhibit the normal stress response to surgery and parenteral supplementation should be considered.
- **Non-steroidal anti-inflammatory drugs** must be used with caution in the perioperative period because of their effects on renal autoregulation. In general these are best reserved for postoperative therapy.

'Emergency' cases

There are cases where surgical delay is unacceptable:

- Thoracic visceral damage
- Airway obstruction
- Uncontrollable haemorrhage
- Obstetric emergencies in which neonates are at risk.

In emergencies, preparation may be limited to catheterizing a vein, administering fluids and enriching inspired breath with oxygen.

Final details

Before admitting normal animals for surgery, owners must:

- Be informed of the risks and possible outcomes (see Chapter 2)
- Have signed an anaesthetic consent form
- Be asked to withhold food the night before (water can be given).

A full stomach reduces lung volume, limits breathing and predisposes to vomiting; this may result in fatal aspiration pneumonia. If an animal scheduled for surgery has received a large meal, the best option is to delay surgery to allow adequate emptying of the stomach (i.e. at least 6 hours).

Sedation and premedication

Sedatives and tranquillizers can be used on their own to allow minor procedures to be performed or as premedication in preparation for general anaesthesia. Many procedures require restraint only.

Sedation

Effective sedation and chemical restraint require:

- A quiet environment without disturbance of the animal
- Adequate time to allow full effect before handling
- Calm, firm and sensible handling.

Potential cardiovascular and respiratory depression can occur with the use of chemical restraint and a knowledge of the pharmacological effects of the main sedatives is required for their safe use (see also Chapter 9).

Properties of an ideal sedative include:

- Production of stoical indifference to the surroundings
- Recumbency if required
- Analgesia
- No side effects
- The presence of a specific reversal agent.

Sedation is not always safer than general anaesthesia as often no oxygen is supplied, facilities for intermittent positive pressure ventilation are not available and monitoring of the patient is frequently minimal. In debilitated patients that require more than just light sedation, a general anaesthetic with careful monitoring and intraoperative care may be more appropriate than heavy sedation.

Premedication

The objectives of premedication are:

- To calm the patient and reduce anxiety prior to induction of anaesthesia
- To provide sedation
- To aid a 'smooth' induction and recovery
- To reduce induction and maintenance agent requirements
- To provide analgesia
- To reduce associated side effects of the anaesthetic to be given
- To reduce adverse effects of surgery.

Premedication is given before anaesthesia to smooth subsequent events. Long-acting drugs such as acepromazine maleate smooth recovery after induction with barbiturates and other drugs. Similarly, analgesics smooth recovery after painful procedures. In providing 'background' narcosis, premedication and analgesics lower the requirement for maintenance agents and consequently the potential for associated side effects. The premedication given should always be specific to the individual patient and procedure to be undertaken; some patients require greater sedation than others prior to anaesthesia. A good premedication will render the animal calm and tranquil, allowing a smooth, stress-free induction of anaesthesia (Figure 22.1).

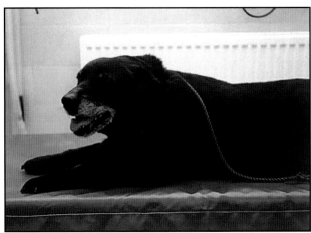

22.1 After light premedication, an elderly Labrador Retriever calmly awaits induction of anaesthesia.

Disadvantages of premedication include the potential for drug interactions and side effects, prolongation of recovery, and the need to allow sufficient time for the drugs to have full effect. Not all animals require premedication, e.g. those already depressed by toxaemia, shock or head trauma. After haemorrhage or in shocked animals, normal doses produce more profound effects.

The route by which preanaesthetic medication is given influences time to peak effect, duration of action and the incidence of side effects (Figure 22.2).

Characteristic	Preferred route of administration
Convenience	s.c. > i.p. > i.m. > i.v.
Pain on injection	i.m. > i.p. + i.v. > s.c.
Restraint needed	i.v. > i.p. > i.m. > s.c.
Animal tolerance	s.c. > i.p. > i.m. > i.v.
Onset of action	i.v. > i.m. > s.c. > i.p.
Duration of action	i.p. + s.c. > i.m. > i.v.
Predictability	i.v. > i.m. > s.c. > i.p.
Relative dose required	i.p. + s.c. > i.m. > i.v.
Technical ease	s.c. > i.m. > i.p. > i.v.

22.2 Comparison of drug administration routes. i.m., intramuscular; i.p., intraperitoneal; i.v., intravenous; s.c., subcutaneous

Phenothiazines – acepromazine maleate

Phenothiazines are antagonists at central dopamine receptors. They are used routinely to premedicate animals prior to anaesthesia. **Acepromazine maleate**, the most commonly used phenothiazine in the UK, is available for small animals as a 2 mg/ml solution and is administered for premedication at doses of 0.01–0.05 mg/kg i.m. or i.v. It remains a popular and useful drug despite important side effects. At normal doses the drug is safe and produces moderate sedation. Increasing the dose above this stated dose range does not increase the degree of sedation but extends the duration of action and increases the severity of adverse reactions. The addition of an opioid potentiates sedation (i.e. neuroleptanalgesia, see below) and can be more effective – with fewer side effects – than an increased dose.

Phenothiazines
Advantages

- Synergism: improve sedative effects of opioids
- Antiarrhythmic: exert antiarrhythmic activity
- Antiemetic: offset the emetic effects of some opioids
- Spasmolytic: reduce discomfort when 'colic' results from gastrointestinal spasm
- Antihistamine: useful with some histamine-releasing opioids

Disadvantages

- Hypotension: this results from vascular smooth muscle relaxation. Problems occur when high doses are used or when normal doses are used in hypotensive or hypovolaemic animals. Acute decompensation and hypotension may result
- Syncope: some breed-lines of Boxers collapse after low doses
- Unpredictability: aggressive dogs are often resistant
- Long-acting: dose-dependent duration of action; clinical sedation lasts 4–6 hours
- Slow onset: peak effect does not occur for 10–20 minutes after intravenous, and for 30-45 minutes after intramuscular, administration
- No analgesia
- Hypothermia: cutaneous vasodilatation and thermoregulatory depression cause heat loss
- Poor muscle relaxation: no relaxant effects but reduced hypertonicity with ketamine
- Penile prolapse may be seen in horses
- Said to reduce threshold to seizures in epileptics

Butyrophenones

These behave like phenothiazines but produce unpredictable results. Hypotension can be a concern at higher doses and they should be avoided in hypovolaemic patients. There are no butyrophenones with market authorization for sole use in small animals, but **fluanisone** and **droperidol** are available combined with opioids. **Hypnorm**, a combination of fentanyl and fluanisone, is licensed for use in rabbits. It is a controlled drug and its use must be recorded in a Controlled Drugs register (see Chapter 2).

Neuroleptanalgesia

Phenothiazines and butyrophenones combined with opioids create a neuroleptanalgesic combination. The two components are synergistic; lower doses of each are needed, which lowers the incidence and severity of side effects. Commercially available mixtures are convenient but effects can be suboptimal:

- Hypnorm (fentanyl 0.315 mg + fluanisone 10 mg/ml).

Neuroleptanalgesics may be 'home-made', with doses and drugs modified to suit the individual case (e.g. acepromazine maleate and buprenorphine). This form of neuroleptanalgesia is commonly used in practice and can provide consistent and effective sedation.

Neuroleptanalgesia
Advantages

- Lower incidence of side effects
- Increased degree of sedation
- Increased predictability
- Stable cardiopulmonary performance

Disadvantages

- Animals remain sensitive to, and are aroused by, certain stimuli (e.g. noise)
- Only opioid antagonism is possible. The neuroleptic is not antagonized and is the longer-acting component
- Behavioural changes are alleged to have occurred after neuroleptanalgesia in dogs

Alpha$_2$ adrenoceptor agonists

Alpha$_2$ adrenoceptor agonists stimulate prejunctional alpha$_2$ receptors within the central nervous system, inhibiting release of noradrenaline, resulting in sedation. They are potent sedatives that provide analgesia, muscle relaxation and anxiolysis. However, they cause significant cardiovascular depression and should be used with caution in debilitated patients. They have specific antagonists and so their effects can be readily reversed.

Xylazine (0.5–1 mg/kg) and **medetomidine** (dog: 5–20 µg/kg; cat: 10–40 µg/kg) are alpha$_2$ adrenoceptor agonists with market authorization in companion animals. Medetomidine is more potent, more specific to the alpha$_2$ receptor and longer acting than xylazine. The lower end of the dose range for these drugs is to be recommended, as increasing doses tend to greater cardiovascular depression. The addition of an opioid (e.g. butorphanol) to the alpha$_2$ agonist increases sedation without increasing cardiopulmonary depression and can produce greater sedation or allow a reduction in the alpha$_2$ agonist dose. The alpha$_2$ agonists can also be used for premedication prior to anaesthesia.

Atipamezole is an alpha$_2$ antagonist and is used to antagonize the effects of medetomidine in companion animals; the antagonist dose is the same volume as agonist injected in dogs and half the volume in cats (50–100 µg/kg i.m.). Its use is desirable because the prolonged effect of medetomidine predisposes to hypothermia, hypostatic lung congestion and prolonged recovery. After painful procedures, antagonism may expose the animal, acutely, to discomfort and appropriate analgesia must be administered.

Alpha$_2$ adrenoceptor agonists
Advantages

- Profound dose-dependent sedation
- Duration of action is also dose-dependent
- Marked drug-sparing effect: doses of induction and maintenance agents are considerably reduced. A greater lag time elapses before effects of induction agents are seen. Circulation time is prolonged, accelerating the uptake of volatile anaesthetics
- Muscle relaxation: relaxant effects offset muscle rigidity seen with ketamine
- Visceral analgesia
- Specific reversal agent

Disadvantages

- Cardiovascular depression: profound cardiovascular effects occur; peripheral vasoconstriction and hypertension initially occur and grey mucous membranes are seen. Severe bradycardia occurs, resulting in reduced cardiac output. Later, centrally mediated hypotension occurs. Anticholinergic pretreatment, which counteracts bradycardia, is controversial; although heart rate is restored, systemic vascular resistance remains elevated, resulting in increased myocardial work. In dogs, xylazine sensitizes the myocardium to adrenaline-induced arrhythmias during halothane anaesthesia
- Respiratory depression: the respiratory rate is reduced, though ventilation is minimally depressed. Arterial oxygenation is maintained. Muscle relaxation of redundant oropharyngeal tissue in brachycephalics may cause respiratory obstruction
- Emesis: vomiting occurs in dogs and cats after xylazine and, to a lesser extent, after medetomidine
- Diuresis: ADH inhibition and insulin suppression contribute to this effect
- Gut motility: this is reduced and barium meal interpretation may be confused
- Thermoregulation: impaired, generally resulting in hypothermia
- Personal risk: data sheet instructs that gloves should be worn when handling medetomidine

Benzodiazepines

Benzodiazepines potentiate the inhibitory activity of the neurotransmitter gamma aminobutyric acid (GABA). They produce anxiolysis, muscle relaxation, sedation, hypnosis and amnesia and have powerful anticonvulsant effects. Paradoxically, intravenous diazepam can cause marked stimulation in non-debilitated dogs. **Diazepam** as its water-insoluble formulation (with propylene glycol as the solvent) causes pain on injection and thrombophlebitis after intravenous injection. It is also available as a water-soluble emulsion which is non-painful on injection. **Midazolam** is water-soluble and also does not cause these problems. It is short-acting; is approximately twice as potent and is more effective after intramuscular injection than is diazepam. Doses of both drugs at 0.1–0.2 mg/kg are routinely used. In debilitated patients, benzodiazepines can be administered intravenously at induction of anaesthesia to reduce the induction agent dose, and hence reduce the latter's cardiopulmonary depressant effects.

Flumazenil is a benzodiazepine antagonist used to treat overdosage in people and accelerate recovery in outpatient anaesthesia. In animals the cost often precludes its use.

Benzodiazepines
Advantages

- Sedation: good sedation can be achieved in the debilitated patient
- Safety: the drugs have high therapeutic indices and minimal cardiopulmonary effects
- Drug-sparing effect: they prolong and enhance effects of other anaesthetics. Anaesthetic doses are lowered and predicted excitement (e.g. recovery after methohexitone) is prevented

- Muscle relaxation: diazepam or midazolam are used with ketamine in cats to provide heavy sedation and eliminate excitation/convulsions and associated muscle hypertonicity of ketamine administration
- Anticonvulsant
- Appetite stimulant in cats

Disadvantages

- Unpredictable: in healthy animals, benzodiazepines often stimulate rather than depress but become increasingly effective as the animal's health status deteriorates
- Formulation: diazepam with propylene glycol as the solvent causes pain on injection and thrombophlebitis

Anticholinergic drugs

The routine use of anticholinergics for anaesthetic premedication is controversial. In previous times, the widespread use of diethyl ether anaesthesia in humans justified this practice; diethyl ether promotes oropharyngeal secretion, bronchosecretion and bronchoconstriction. Modern volatile anaesthetics do not produce excessive secretions and most cause bronchodilatation. In modern practice, anticholinergics are best administered when required. They might be used to:

- Decrease salivation and bronchial secretion
- Treat vagally induced bradycardia
- Block the effects of certain drugs administered (e.g. anticholinesterases).

Atropine crosses the blood–brain barrier and the blood–placental barrier. The former can cause visual disturbances, which can be unsettling, particularly for cats. It is given at 0.02–0.04 mg/kg i.v., i.m. or s.c. **Glycopyrrolate** (dose 0.01–0.02 mg/kg) has a slower onset time, a longer duration of action and a greater antisialogogue effect (i.e. reduces flow of saliva) than atropine. Tachyarrhythmias are said to be less likely and cardiovascular stability is better preserved. Glycopyrrolate does not cross the blood–brain barrier, thus avoiding visual disturbance, and may be a more appropriate agent in the cat.

Anticholinergics
Advantages

- Reduce salivation and bronchial secretions
- Rapidly control intraoperative vagally mediated bradycardia
- Protect against adverse vagal effects of anticholinesterases during antagonism of neuromuscular block

Disadvantages

- Increase heart rate; increase myocardial oxygen consumption
- Increase metabolic rate
- Arrhythmogenic, causing bradyarrhythmias and/or tachyarrhythmias
- Cause gastrointestinal ileus
- Pupil dilatation and visual disturbance

Pain and analgesia

Analgesia is a state of reduced sensibility to pain. Painful stimuli reach the brain in similar ways to other sensations but are amenable to interruption by a greater range of drugs. The perception of pain requires conscious awareness, whilst nociception is the transmission of impulses to lower levels within the central nervous system in response to noxious stimuli. An animal's response to pain depends on the level of the central nervous system to which the pain message ascends (Figure 22.3):

- **Spinal responses** include, for example, reflex limb withdrawal.
- **Medullary responses** include increased heart rate, blood pressure and respiratory rate.
- **Hypothalamic responses** take several forms. The hypothalamus initiates catecholamine release from the adrenal medulla and nerve endings of the sympathetic nervous system. This further increases heart rate and blood pressure. Less obviously, the hypothalamus secretes releasing factors that cause the pituitary gland to release 'stress' hormones such as adrenocorticotropic hormone (ACTH). Other pituitary hormones such as thyroid stimulating hormone (TSH), antidiuretic hormone (ADH) and prolactin (PRL) are also released.
- **Cortical responses** are the most complex: they include activity such as vocalization and voluntary acts such as attempting to escape or to bite at the noxious stimulus.

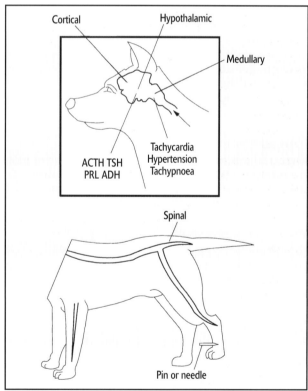

22.3 Responses to pain after peripheral limb stimulation.

The assessment of pain in animals is a subjective process and can be difficult. Recognizing clinical signs associated with pain is invaluable in allowing early treatment (see Chapter 13).

Analgesics

Analgesics interrupt the ascending pain pathway at various levels (Figure 22.4) and suppress the sensation of pain. Some, like the opioids, act at several points along this path. Blocking pain at a number of sites with the use of more than one type of analgesic can produce more effective analgesia; this is termed **balanced analgesia**.

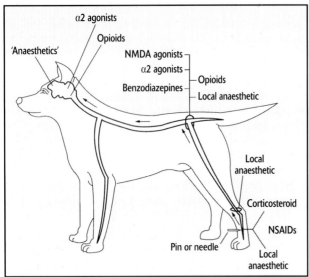

22.4 Location of pain pathways after peripheral limb stimulation and potential targets for analgesia. The arrows show ascending pathways of pain.

Several drug groups suppress pain. These include:

- Alpha$_2$ adrenoceptor agonists
- Dissociative anaesthetics (e.g. ketamine)
- Nitrous oxide
- Glucocorticoids
- Local anaesthetics
- Non-steroidal anti-inflammatory drugs (NSAIDs)
- Opioids.

Peripheral nerve endings

Glucocorticoids and NSAIDs reduce the production of pain-sensitizing chemicals released from damaged tissues that stimulate nerve endings. Topical local anaesthetics block nerve endings.

Peripheral nerves

Local anaesthetics block nerve impulses in peripheral nerves. Local anaesthesia is frequently neglected as a method of pain relief but can produce very effective analgesia. Local anaesthetics are discussed later.

Spinal cord

Pain can be suppressed in the cord by the extradural injection of several drug types:

- **Local anaesthetics** block all nerve fibre types producing anaesthesia, analgesia and muscle relaxation.
- **Opioids** diminish sensitivity to pain but do not eliminate all sensation, proprioception or muscle function. Animals are therefore free from pain but can walk.
- *N*-methyl-D-aspartate (**NMDA**) receptor antagonists and **alpha$_2$ agonists** have analgesic effects at the spinal level but they are less frequently used.

- **Combinations** of drugs that are compatible *in vitro* may be injected in order to take advantage of desirable properties of each (e.g. lidocaine or bupivacaine with morphine).

Brain

Opioids, alpha$_2$ adrenoceptor agonists and general anaesthetics cause analgesia through effects on the brain. Consciousness need not be lost for analgesia to be present.

Pre-emptive analgesia

Administration of analgesic drugs prior to tissue trauma is suggested to reduce postoperative analgesic requirements. This concept is called pre-emptive analgesia. Although work in the human literature remains equivocal, the general consensus is that analgesia given prior to surgery combined with adequate postoperative pain relief is the most effective method of providing analgesia. For example, premedication with the opioid buprenorphine and the NSAID carprofen, followed by a local block prior to surgery and continued with regular dosing of the opioid postoperatively, will provide excellent analgesia and encourage a rapid recovery.

Opioid analgesics

Opioids are often included in premedication:

- To relieve preoperative pain and therefore anxiety
- To contribute to sedation
- To provide analgesia during maintenance and on recovery.

While the properties of individual opioids differ, there are common advantages and disadvantages.

Opioids
Advantages

- Profound drug- and dose-dependent analgesia
- Benign cardiovascular effects: with some exceptions, opioids slow heart rate. In high doses, bradycardia and bradyarrhythmias may occur. Cardiac output is usually maintained
- Anaesthetic-sparing effect: opioids reduce dose requirements of induction and maintenance agents
- Sedation: some opioids produce sedation
- Positive ventilatory effects: by reducing chest-wall pain after thoracotomy or trauma, opioids improve ventilation. This frequently offsets any respiratory depression seen (see below)

Disadvantages

- Dysphoria: in pain-free animals, opioids may stimulate rather than sedate and cause excitation on overdosage (particularly cats). At normal analgesic doses, opioids in pain-free animals do not cause marked stimulation. Stimulation is also unlikely when neuroleptics are given concurrently
- Respiratory depression: this is a greater problem in primates than companion animals, though some respiratory depression can be seen. Intraoperative alfentanil and fentanyl often depress breathing, requiring ventilatory support

▶

- Antitussive effects: opioids suppress the coughing reflex, which may be useful in animals requiring analgesia and prolonged intubation. However, accumulated bronchial secretion may impair respiration
- Gastrointestinal effects: some opioids (e.g. morphine) cause vomiting in dogs. Opioids can induce constipation with prolonged use. With the exception of pethidine, opioids cause increased pressure in the biliary tree; they should be used with caution in pancreatitis and obstructive jaundice
- Urinary retention: epidurally administered opioids cause urinary retention, which may be of significance in cases of pre-existing bladder dysfunction

Individual properties

Opioids have slightly different properties (Figure 22.5) and their use in any situation is governed by several factors.

Drug	Controlled?	Potency	Efficacy	Duration (hours)
Morphine	Yes (Schedule 2)	1	++++	3–4
Pethidine	Yes (Schedule 2)	0.1	+++	1–2
Papaveretum	Yes (Schedule 2)	0.5	++++	3–4
Methadone	Yes (Schedule 2)	1	++++	3–4
Butorphanol	No	1	++	3–4
Buprenorphine	Yes (Schedule 3)	30	+++	6–8

22.5 Comparison of selected features of opioid analgesics.

Potency
Although drugs vary in analgesic potency, this is of little relevance as 'weaker' opioids such as pethidine are given at greater doses. The quality of analgesia is more important. Pure agonists (morphine, fentanyl) should be chosen if severe pain is anticipated.

Pharmacodynamic effect
The central nervous, autonomic, cardiopulmonary and gastrointestinal effects of individual drugs may render them useful or hazardous under different circumstances.

Pharmacokinetic factors
Onset time, duration of action and elimination pathways may be important considerations in choosing specific opioids.

Other factors
Personal preference, cost and controlled drug status may also influence choice.

Drug legislation
Because of their abuse potential, most opioids are controlled drugs (CDs), i.e. their use is controlled by the Misuse of Drugs Act 1971 (see Chapter 9). Controlled drugs are 'scheduled' according to the degree of control applied to their use. Schedule 1 agents (e.g. LSD) are stringently controlled but unused in veterinary practice. Schedule 2 drugs, such as morphine, fentanyl, alfentanil and pethidine, are regulated in terms of:

- Special prescription requirements
- Requisition requirements
- Record keeping: acquisition and prescription must be recorded in a controlled drugs register (CDR)
- Safe custody: Schedule 2 drugs must be kept in a locked receptacle
- Destruction of expired stocks.

Schedule 3 drugs include pentazocine and buprenorphine. These are subject to prescription and requisition requirements but transactions do not have to be recorded in the CDR. With the exception of buprenorphine, they do not have to be kept in a locked receptacle.

Pure agonists (mu-agonists)
Opioids bind to specific opioid receptors in the CNS to produce analgesia. Mu-receptor agonists bind to mu receptors (also termed OP3 receptors) to exert their analgesic effects. This group of analgesics is excellent for treating moderate to severe pain as their action is dose-dependent, with higher doses or repeated doses increasing the analgesic effect.

- **Morphine**: dose 0.1–0.5 mg/kg i.m. (dog), 0.1–0.2 mg/kg (cat). It is the gold-standard analgesic, producing some sedation and lasting approximately 4 hours. However, it can cause vomiting and constipation, and at higher doses morphine can cause excitement in cats. When given intravenously it causes some histamine release.
- **Methadone**: dose as for morphine. It is said to produce less vomiting, sedation, excitement and histamine release compared with morphine and can hence be given intravenously.
- **Papaveretum**: dose 0.2–1.0 mg/kg i.m. It is associated with less vomiting than morphine and greater synergy with acepromazine maleate, producing greater sedation. This is particularly useful for the sedation of vicious dogs.
- **Pethidine**: dose 1–5 mg/kg i.m. It rarely causes vomiting, or excitement in cats, and uniquely is spasmolytic on the intestines. It can be used in cases of pancreatitis and biliary obstruction. It causes histamine release if given intravenously, leading to significant hypotension.
- **Fentanyl**: dose 1–5 μg/kg i.v. Fentanyl is a short-acting opioid, 50 times more potent than morphine, that is more commonly used intraoperatively as an intravenous infusion or as intermittent intravenous boluses when surgical stimulus is particularly severe. Additionally, it is used in cutaneous patches as a continuous controlled release of fentanyl for postoperative analgesia (fentanyl patches). Patches need to be applied 12–24 hours before surgery to provide background postoperative analgesia that can last up to approximately 72 hours in dogs and 104 hours in cats.

Partial agonists/mixed agonist–antagonists
These agents are weak agonists at the mu receptor (partial agonists) or antagonists at the mu receptor and agonists at kappa opioid receptors (mixed agonist–antagonist), giving analgesia of moderate efficacy though variable consistency. They have a bell-shaped dose–response curve, meaning that at higher doses less analgesia may result. This is of significance if the animal is in severe pain, as further doses of these drugs may not adequately treat the pain. As a group they are best reserved for procedures anticipated to result in mild to moderate pain only.

- **Buprenorphine**: dose 10–20 μg/kg, i.m. or i.v. It is a partial agonist and has a relatively slow onset of action (45 minutes) but has a relatively long duration of action (6–8 hours). Tight mu-receptor binding underlies the duration of action and also makes subsequent pure agonists less effective. This is a useful agent for procedures producing mild to moderate pain. The concern about the bell-shaped dose–response curve is less clinically relevant at the doses commonly used in dogs and cats with buprenorphine, and further doses can be safely administered if the patient remains in pain after an initial dose.
- **Butorphanol**: dose 0.1–0.5 mg/kg (cats at lower end of range). It is a mixed agonist–antagonist and provides analgesia of an inconsistent nature, though is reported to be better for visceral than somatic pain. It has antitussant properties and provides good sedation when combined with a sedative.

Antagonists

Opioid antagonists may be beneficial for reversing some aspects of opioid activity. In veterinary medicine, naloxone is occasionally used to reverse sedation and respiratory depression, though analgesia is also reversed. Partial agonists such as buprenorphine can be used to reverse the fentanyl component of Hypnorm to speed recovery without compromising analgesia in exotic species.

Non-steroidal anti-inflammatory drugs (NSAIDs)

NSAIDs act peripherally as a group inhibiting the enzyme cyclo-oxygenase and reduce the level of prostaglandins in the tissues. This reduction in prostaglandins reduces inflammation around the injured tissue. Direct analgesia is also said to occur, though its mechanism is unclear. Preoperative administration of some of the newer agents (carprofen and meloxicam) prior to tissue trauma can reduce tissue inflammation more effectively (i.e. pre-emptive analgesia). However, due to the prostaglandin inhibition, certain side effects can occur:

- **Gastric irritation**: manifest as vomiting, diarrhoea and gastric haemorrhage. Prostaglandins inhibit gastric acid secretion, stimulate mucus production, maintain blood flow to the gastric mucosa and are involved in mucosal repair. Hence reduction in prostaglandins can compromise the gastric mucosa, leading to ulceration.
- **Renal compromise**: prostaglandins modulate renal haemodynamics and are involved in autoregulation of blood flow to the kidneys. They are especially important in states of decreased renal perfusion (e.g. hypotension during anaesthesia) and under such circumstances administration of NSAIDs can lead to renal insufficiency. With the notable exception of carprofen and meloxicam, as a group they are not recommended for preoperative administration.
- **Blood dyscrasias** and **platelet dysfunction**: thromboxane and prostaglandins are involved in induction of aggregation of platelets. Thus NSAIDs prolong bleeding time.

NSAIDs used in veterinary practice include the following:

- **Aspirin**: dose 10–20 mg/kg (dog), 10 mg/kg (cat), orally. The duration of action is 12–24 hours (longer in the cat). Inhibition of platelet aggregation, gastric irritation, aplastic anaemia and hepatoxicity are notable side effects.

- **Paracetamol**: dose 25–30 mg/kg (dog). *Not safe in cats*. The duration of action is 4–6 hours. It inhibits CNS cyclo-oxygenase and is a less effective analgesic than aspirin.
- **Phenylbutazone**: dose 10 mg/kg (dog). Duration of action is 6–12 hours. It produces moderate gastric irritation and sodium and water retention, so caution in renal and cardiac disease.
- **Flunixin**: dose 1 mg/kg (dog); (cats 1 mg/kg, not licensed). It has a 4-hour half-life but is found in tissue exudate for up to 24 hours. It is a good analgesic and antiendotoxic drug. Gastrointestinal toxicity and renal papillary necrosis have been recorded.
- **Ketoprofen**: dose 1–2 mg/kg. It is a potent cyclo-oxygenase inhibitor, additionally inhibits the enzyme lipoxygenase and provides good analgesia.
- **Tolfenamic acid**: dose 4 mg/kg; the half-life is 6.5 hours. Though providing good analgesia, it is associated with greater side effects than some of the 'newer' NSAIDs.
- **Carprofen**: dose 2–4 mg/kg, s.c., i.v. or orally. The duration of action is 12–24 hours. Carprofen produces poor inhibition of cyclo-oxygenase; thus it is prostaglandin sparing. Less renal toxicity and gastric irritation are reported, but it has greater anti-inflammatory potency than phenylbutazone. It is licensed for administration preoperatively prior to tissue trauma.
- **Meloxicam**: dose 0.2 mg/kg s.c. It is licensed for preoperative administration in the dog and cat. It provides good analgesia (18–24 hours after a single dose) and has been used for some time for chronic pain therapy.
- **Firocoxib**: dose 5 mg/kg once daily (dog). It comes as a chewable tablet and is indicated for the relief of pain and inflammation associated with degenerative joint disease in dogs.

Other agents used for analgesia

- **Alpha$_2$ adrenoceptor agonists** provide good analgesia, especially for visceral pain, but these actions are reversed if an antagonist is subsequently administered (e.g. atipamezole). They can be administered epidurally and have been used in combination with local anaesthetics and opioids by this route.
- **Inhalation anaesthetics**, including methoxyflurane and nitrous oxide, provide analgesia (see later).
- **Dissociative anaesthetics** (e.g. ketamine) provide good analgesia for somatic pain. At subanaesthetic doses they can be used to reduce 'wind-up' and hypersensitization of the CNS to painful stimuli.
- The role of **benzodiazepines** as analgesics is controversial, though they have been found to provide analgesia in humans when administered spinally and epidurally.

Supportive therapy

Good patient nursing is essential for postoperative comfort. Bandaging and support of injured areas (e.g. Robert Jones bandage) stabilizes wounds and reduces pain on movement. Warmth, comfortable bedding, an empty bladder, food and water postoperatively and attentive care can significantly improve patient welfare.

Local anaesthesia

Local anaesthetics produce reversible block of nerve impulse conduction. Uses include:

- **Superficial surgery**: some minor procedures may be performed in the conscious animal using local anaesthetics alone (e.g. skin infiltration for wart removal). More invasive procedures may require moderate sedation (e.g. intravenous regional anaesthesia for toe amputation).
- **Adjunct to surgical anaesthesia**: local techniques may be superimposed on light general anaesthesia for major surgery. The local technique usually does not affect cardiopulmonary function, making the combined technique useful in high-risk cases. Animals also recover consciousness rapidly and, importantly, the surgical site remains pain-free.
- **Facilitation of procedures**: topical anaesthetics facilitate intravenous and urethral catheterization, endotracheal intubation and ophthalmic examination.
- **Diagnosis**: local anaesthetics are used to assist lameness diagnosis in horses.
- **Antiarrhythmics**: lidocaine is used to treat certain types of cardiac arrhythmia.

Local anaesthesia

Advantages

- Less equipment required
- Techniques are inexpensive
- Excellent anaesthesia and muscle relaxation
- Consciousness is retained when used alone; there is no loss of protective reflexes
- There is little cardiopulmonary depression; techniques are relatively safe in ill animals
- Some techniques allow titration: the degree, duration and anatomical 'level' of block can be varied

Disadvantages

- Not all procedures can be performed with local anaesthetic techniques
- Some techniques are difficult to perform and subsequent block may be incomplete
- Some techniques are painful to perform; animals may require sedation
- Active animals may require physical or chemical restraint for surgery
- Overdosage and toxicity are possible with some drugs
- Some techniques (e.g. extradural anaesthesia) can produce untoward cardiovascular effects
- Some local anaesthetics have a short duration of action

Mechanism of action

Nerve fibres carrying different sensations (e.g. touch, cold and pain) vary in response to local anaesthetics. Because pain fibres are among the most sensitive, it is possible for local anaesthetics to eliminate pain but allow touch and other sensations to persist. When this occurs, the drug behaves as a local analgesic. If all sensation is lost, the drug is an anaesthetic. Motor fibres are most resistant to local anaesthetics but are usually blocked, resulting in muscle relaxation.

Toxicity

Toxic central nervous system signs (e.g. convulsions or coma) are seen if high levels of local anaesthetic are absorbed. Local anaesthetics can also induce cardiovascular side effects. Lidocaine can be used to control ventricular arrhythmias, but at toxic doses electrical activity is suppressed and cardiac arrest may occur.

Toxicity depends on the route of injection (beware of inadvertent intravenous injection), the total amount injected, the characteristics of the individual agent and whether a vasoconstrictor has been used. Overdosing is avoided by using low concentrations (the minimum dose required to produce effect), by using regional rather than local techniques (where appropriate) and by adding vasoconstrictors to the injected solution.

Pharmacokinetics

Speed of onset

The speed of onset of a local anaesthetic block depends upon the agent diffusing into the nerve cell (usually the axon) where it has its effect. Factors influencing this include the proximity of the injection site to the site of action, the lipid solubility, concentration and volume of the agent used, and the use of potentiating drugs.

Duration of action

The duration of action of a local anaesthetic depends upon the lipid solubility of the agent used, the pH of the tissues, the pharmacological properties of the agent, the blood flow at the site of action and the use of potentiating drugs.

Vasoconstrictors may be added to prolong the duration of block. The most common vasoconstrictor used is **adrenaline**, added to local anaesthetic solutions at 1:100,000 (concentration 0.01 mg/ml). This slows drug absorption from the injection site and prolongs block. Solutions containing adrenaline must not be overused in areas with poor or superficial blood flow; vasoconstriction may cause subsequent tissue ischaemia.

State of tissues

The state of the tissues into which local anaesthetic is injected also has an effect upon the action of the drug. For example, if local anaesthetic is injected into inflamed tissue it will have a reduced action. This is because inflamed tissue is more acidic than normal and so the agent will be more ionized and less able to diffuse through the tissue.

Local anaesthetic drugs

Lidocaine

This is the most commonly used local anaesthetic in veterinary practice. It is available as a gel, a topical cream, a spray or in injectable forms. Injections are usually 1% or 2% solutions with or without adrenaline. The drug has a rapid (less than 5 minutes) onset of action. It spreads rapidly through tissues and produces almost complete block of 50–90 minutes. Adding adrenaline retards absorption (and toxicity) and prolongs the duration of block. Lidocaine can cause tissue irritation after injection. Doses of 1–2 mg/kg are commonly used.

Bupivacaine

This is about four times as potent as lidocaine and so is available in lower concentrations (0.25, 0.5 or 0.75%). It has a slower onset of action (up to 20 minutes) but may last from 4 to 6 hours. It does not irritate tissue but may cause cardiac arrest if inadvertent intravascular injection is made. It is commonly used for epidural analgesia.

Mepivacaine

This drug is favoured for conduction blocks in the equine limb as it is less irritant than lidocaine. Its duration of action is similar to that of lidocaine.

Ropivacaine

This is a homologue of bupivacaine with similar clinical effects but much reduced cardiotoxicity. It is said to have some vasoconstrictive properties and is also commonly used epidurally.

Types of local anaesthesia

A number of different types of block can be performed.

Local block

Desensitization is produced only at or near the site of application. Applications include:

- **Surface or topical**: anaesthetic is applied to skin or mucous membranes to give loss of sensation at the site of application; for example, EMLA cream (lidocaine 2.5% and prilocaine 2.5%) can be applied to the ear margin in rabbits to allow pain-free catheterization of the auricular vein.
- **Intradermal**: anaesthetic is injected into the skin to form a desensitized weal.
- **Infiltration**: a primary injection of local anaesthetic is made at the surgical site, using as small a needle as possible (23–25 gauge). The next injection is made through this site and the process repeated until the surgical area is 'infiltrated' with local anaesthetic. Liberal infiltration must be avoided as overdosage is possible, especially in small animals and birds. Irritant drugs such as lidocaine and those containing vasoconstrictors may interfere with wound healing.
- **Intrasynovial**: local anaesthetics injected into painful joints and synovial sheaths relieve pain but the effects are not long-acting.

Regional block

Anaesthetic is used to produce desensitization remote from the site of injection.

- **Perineural**: this involves drug injection in proximity to identifiable nerves, as opposed to nerve endings. The technique requires knowledge of topographical anatomy. Injection is made using sterile needles and syringes. Common blocks include the intercostal nerve block, where the intercostal nerves are blocked behind each rib. This is particularly valuable after thoracotomy (e.g. with bupivacaine). This relieves postoperative chest-wall pain, allowing adequate ventilation. Additionally, desensitization of the distal forelimb below the elbow can be achieved by performing a brachial plexus block, blocking the nerves of the brachial plexus medial to the scapula.
- **Intravenous regional anaesthesia (IVRA)**: this is used for surgical procedures on limb extremities (e.g. digit removal). The limb is first exsanguinated using an Esmarch's bandage, which is then left in place as a tourniquet. Local anaesthetic (e.g. 2–5 ml lidocaine

without adrenaline) is then injected into any vein distal to the tourniquet. Surgery may begin after 15 minutes. Anaesthesia persists until the tourniquet is removed.
- **Spinal and epidural block**: anaesthetic is injected within the bony confines of the spinal canal (see below).

Epidural anaesthesia

In this method, drug is injected into the space between the dura mater (the thick fibrous outermost covering of the spinal cord) and the periosteum lining the spinal canal. Here, the drug blocks the nerves as they leave the cord. A large spinal needle is used and usually injection is made into the L7–S1 interspace. The technique is useful for pain relief and muscle relaxation during pelvic-limb orthopaedic procedures in dogs, and less commonly in cats. In current practice, the technique is usually performed on anaesthetized animals. Lidocaine or bupivacaine combined with an opioid (e.g. preservative-free morphine) are commonly used. The main advantage of epidural opioids is prolonged and profound analgesia.

Spinal anaesthesia

This technique is rarely used in clinical veterinary anaesthesia. It involves a midline injection at the L5–L6 interspace or, at a higher level, into the CSF-filled subarachnoid space below the dura and arachnoid mater. Lower doses produce the same effects as extradural injection, but there is a slightly greater risk of overdosage.

Injectable anaesthesia

General anaesthesia can be induced and maintained with injectable anaesthetics. The intramuscular and intravenous routes are most often used but occasionally, particularly in small mammals, the intraperitoneal or subcutaneous routes may be used. Recently, maintenance of anaesthesia via the intravenous route has received more interest. Total intravenous anaesthesia (TIVA) can provide a good alternative to gaseous anaesthesia, providing good cardiovascular stability without the potential pollution hazards of the inhalation agents (see later). Whichever route is used, the provision of a patent airway and a supply of oxygen are always to be recommended. If the intravenous route is to be used the placement of an intravenous catheter is recommended, particularly for prolonged and complicated procedures (Figure 22.6).

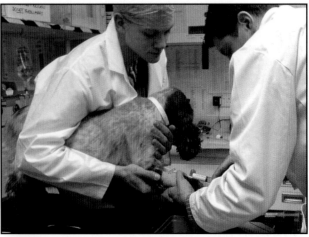

22.6 Intravenous induction of anaesthesia after intravenous catheter placement.

Injectable anaesthetics

Advantages

- Convenient; simple to inject
- Inexpensive – less equipment needed
- Intravenous injection usually causes a rapid loss of consciousness
- No airway irritation
- No explosion/pollution hazard
- Rapid recovery after a single dose
- Some drugs can be antagonized
- Endotracheal intubation not always necessary
- Rapid deepening of anaesthesia possible
- Respiratory function does not influence drug behaviour

Disadvantages

- Stressful restraint may be required
- Technical skill is required for intravenous injection and catheterization
- Myositis and pain may result from injection
- Perivascular injection may cause irritation with certain drugs
- Effects may be slow to be reversed; for drugs without antagonists, recovery depends on cardiovascular, hepatic and renal function
- Anaesthesia is readily deepened, but not lightened
- Dose-range requirements are wide
- Self-administration is a potential hazard with some drugs
- Repeated doses may cause drug accumulation and prolonged recovery
- Injectable drugs have varying side effects
- Airway protection and supply of oxygen are often neglected

Pharmacology

The brain has a rich blood supply and receives a high concentration of drug shortly after intravenous injection. When a critical brain concentration is exceeded, unconsciousness occurs. In time, organs less well perfused than the brain (such as skeletal muscle) begin to take up drug. Plasma levels fall and this creates a diffusion gradient which promotes movement of drug from brain to plasma. Consciousness returns when brain drug levels fall below a critical level. The duration of action of most modern injectable anaesthetics depends on 'redistribution' of drug from brain to less well perfused tissues; this depends on factors including cardiac output and the mass of tissues available for redistribution of drug.

Most anaesthetics are metabolized in the liver by conversion from lipid to water-soluble molecules. These forms are more easily excreted in bile (appearing later in faeces) or urine. Only very small amounts are excreted unchanged in bile and urine as lipid-soluble drug. The duration of action of drugs that are rapidly metabolized by the liver (e.g. propofol and methohexitone) depends on a combination of redistribution and metabolism.

Practical tip

Label all drugs. This will avoid dangerous mistakes.

Barbiturates

Barbiturates like thiopental, methohexital and pentobarbital cause unconsciousness but have poor analgesic properties. Muscle relaxation is usually adequate during anaesthesia.

Thiopental

Thiopental (formerly known as thiopentone) is available as a powder and requires reconstitution with water. In solution it is highly alkaline (pH of 10.8) and irritant if injected perivascularly. It is highly protein-bound (80–85%) and slowly metabolized in the liver, relying primarily on redistribution away from the brain for recovery after administration. Solutions of various strengths may be made. A 1% solution contains 1 g (or 1000 mg) in 100 ml. A 1% solution, therefore, contains 10 mg/ml and a 2.5% solution of thiopental contains 25 mg drug/ml. It is reconstituted by adding 100 ml water to 2.5 g of powder.

Thiopental is a useful anaesthetic agent for short-duration procedures or for induction prior to maintenance with inhalation agents. Doses of 10 mg/kg i.v. are used following premedication. Incremental doses should be avoided as they prolong recovery and contribute to 'hangover'.

Mild cardiovascular depression is seen, with hypotension, reduced cardiac output and tachycardia reported. Cardiac dysrhythmias may be seen. Dose-dependent respiratory depression occurs transiently. Thiopental reduces cerebral blood flow and intracranial pressure and is useful in patients with increased intracranial pressure (e.g. some brain tumours).

The drug is safe in high-risk cases provided that the factors which increase patient sensitivity are known (many of these apply to drugs other than thiopental). Doses are reduced in hypoalbuminaemia, acidaemia, hypovolaemia, congestive heart failure, azotaemia, toxaemia and obesity. Doses are also reduced when diazepam is injected immediately before or afterwards.

Special precautions

Thiopental causes prolonged recoveries in sight-hounds (e.g. Whippet, Greyhound, Saluki) after otherwise uneventful anaesthesia. The drug should not be used if there is difficulty achieving venous access.

Practical tip

Concurrent administration of a benzodiazepine will significantly reduce the induction agent dose and help to smooth anaesthetic induction and endotracheal intubation. This is particularly valuable in high-risk cases.

Methohexital

Methohexital is available as a dry powder and is reconstituted to produce a 1% solution. Being twice as potent as thiopental, its dose is halved to 5 mg/kg. Onset time is similar but its duration of action is shorter; extensive and rapid hepatic metabolism occurs in addition to redistribution. It also is alkaline in solution (pH of 11) but is less irritant when injected outside a vein and is similarly protein bound compared with thiopental.

Cardiovascular and respiratory depression are similar to that of thiopental. Recoveries are not always smooth, especially when preanaesthetic medication is withheld. Good premedication prior to methohexital induction of anaesthesia is recommended. The drug has been favoured in sight-hounds because it produces rapid recoveries.

Pentobarbital

This once useful drug has been superseded by newer agents except, perhaps, in laboratory animal anaesthesia. Following injection, its onset of action is relatively slow (related to delay in crossing the blood–brain barrier) and recoveries are prolonged. It is only moderately protein-bound (approximately 40%). In companion animal practice it is used as an anticonvulsant and for humane destruction.

Steroid anaesthetics – Saffan

Saffan is a mixture of alfaxalone (9 mg/kg) and alfadolone (3 mg/kg); the former is the major active component. Induction doses of 3–6 mg/kg i.v. are routinely used in the cat. Doses are always expressed in milligrams of total steroid. The drug has been favoured for some time in cats as it has a high therapeutic index with a wide safety margin. It produces only mild cardiovascular and respiratory depression at clinical doses, with transient hypotension similar to that of thiopental.

The two steroids are insoluble in water and the formulation contains Cremophor EL (polyethoxylated castor oil). *This agent causes histamine release in dogs and cannot be used safely in this species.* In cats, it causes only mild anaphylactoid reactions with swelling of the pinnae and paws. Very infrequently cases of fatal pulmonary oedema have been seen. Because Saffan contains no bacteriostatic agent, open ampoules must be discarded. Saffan is only weakly protein-bound (approximately 50%).

The intravenous route is preferred because effects are less predictable after intramuscular injection. The solution is viscous but non-irritant. The subcutaneous route is unsuitable as the rate of drug metabolism over absorption is high and so anaesthetic levels are not achieved.

A formulation of alfaxalone without alfadolone (Alfaxan, Jurox Pty) is authorized for use in cats and dogs in Australia, New Zealand and South Africa; authorization in the UK is under review.

Dissociative anaesthetics – ketamine

Ketamine is described as a dissociative anaesthetic, producing a unique state of anaesthesia. Protective airway reflexes are maintained, the eyes remain open and the pupils are dilated. Cranial nerve reflexes are less depressed than with other agents, although it cannot be assumed that these will remain entirely protected.

It is presented in an aqueous solution (pH of 3–3.5). It can be given by intravenous, intramuscular, subcutaneous or intraperitoneal injection and is also active when given sublingually. Intramuscular injection is painful, though injection volumes are low because the drug is available as a 100 mg/ml solution. Doses of 2–5 mg/kg i.v. or 5–10 mg/kg i.m. are frequently used.

Heart rate is increased and blood pressure is normally maintained. Breathing is modestly reduced, but at higher doses an apneustic pattern can be seen in which the breath is held after inspiration. Salivation increases. Spontaneous muscle movement unrelated to surgery is a disconcerting feature of ketamine anaesthesia but can be suppressed by concurrently administered drugs. Ketamine is considered to provide good somatic analgesia. Its use to reduce 'wind-up' and central sensitization to pain has been described.

Poor muscle relaxation is provided and for this reason it is usually given with or after another agent such as an alpha₂ agonist or a benzodiazepine. Convulsions are seen in dogs when it is used alone, and its use in this species can only be recommended when combined with a sedative/tranquilliser.

Phenols – propofol

This water-insoluble phenol derivative (2,6-di-isopropylphenol) forms a characteristic milky-white solution when solubilized in an egg–phosphatidyl–soybean oil emulsion. The solution must not be frozen, though cooling is said to reduce the low incidence of pain on intravenous injection. Perivascular injection does not cause irritation. The solution contains no bacteriostat and so opened ampoules must be discarded.

The drug produces dose-dependent levels of unconsciousness after intravenous injection. Good muscle relaxation is seen. Dogs require 4–6 mg/kg i.v., whilst cats require higher doses (6–8 mg/kg i.v.) for anaesthesia. The drug is also longer-acting in these species, with induction doses lasting up to 20 minutes. Being rapidly metabolized it is a useful agent for total intravenous anaesthesia (TIVA). Maintenance of anaesthesia can be achieved by infusing it at rates of 0.3–0.5 mg/kg/min.

Cardiovascular and respiratory depression are comparable to those induced by thiopental but are generally of longer duration. Similarly it reduces cerebral blood flow and can be used in patients with raised intracranial pressure. Occasionally, twitching and spontaneous muscle activity occurs with propofol anaesthesia and excited recoveries have been described. Repeated anaesthesia with propofol in cats (30 minutes daily for 3–7 days) has been associated with red blood cell damage (Heinz body production), prolonged recoveries and anorexia and should be used cautiously if multiple anaesthetics are considered in cats.

Propofol has some advantages over thiopental:

* Recovery is rapid and free from hangover when a single dose is given. This makes it useful in sight-hounds.
* Non-cumulative: maintenance of anaesthesia with top-up injections or by infusion results in less risk of prolonged recoveries.
* Non-irritant when administered perivascularly.

Combinations and neuroleptanalgesia

Minor surgical procedures may be performed using neuroleptanalgesia, benzodiazepine/ketamine and alpha₂ agonist/ketamine mixtures.

Ketamine mixtures

Several drugs are used with ketamine to reduce muscle hypertonicity. These include acepromazine maleate, diazepam, midazolam, xylazine and medetomidine. Some of these also have anticonvulsant effects and render the combinations safe for use in dogs. However, some combinations have adverse physiological effects such as inducing hypoventilation and arrhythmias.

Intravenous catheterization
Advantages

* Reduces risk of extravascular injection, ensures full doses are given and prevents tissue damage with irritant drugs
* Provides rapid intravenous access for emergency drugs
* Allows fluids to be given rapidly
* Allows rapid 'deepening' of anaesthesia with injectable anaesthetics

▶

Disadvantages

- Vein damage: poor catheterization technique may damage the vein and preclude further access. This occurs when haematoma or thrombosis forms
- Sepsis: in immunosuppressed animals (e.g. diabetics) poor surgical preparation and management of catheters lead to phlebitis
- More severe conditions such as bacteraemia may follow

Technique

Adequate physical and/or chemical restraint is a prerequisite. The site must receive surgical preparation. A small skin incision over the vein may facilitate catheter placement in animals with thick skin (e.g. male cats). The catheter is introduced through the skin and directed proximally along the line of the vein. When blood is seen to flow back down the catheter, it is advanced a small distance further, to ensure presence of both catheter and stylet within the vein. The catheter is then gently advanced off the stylet whilst stabilizing the latter. An obturator or three-way tap is attached to the catheter, the catheter is flushed with heparinized saline and then it is secured to the skin with tape or superglue. Catheters should be bandaged to protect them from the patient when not under direct observation.

Inhalation anaesthesia

Inhalation, volatile or 'gaseous' anaesthesia refers to the inhalation of anaesthetic vapours or gases delivered into the respiratory tract. Inhalation agents are commonly used to maintain anaesthesia, but they can also be used to induce anaesthesia.

Inhaled anaesthetics commonly used in animals include halothane, isoflurane and nitrous oxide (N_2O). Other agents used include methoxyflurane, enflurane, ether and more recently sevoflurane and desflurane. Oxygen (O_2) and N_2O are known as carrier gases because they 'carry' the volatile anaesthetics.

Inhalation anaesthetics
Advantages

- Recovery depends on respiratory function and is normally rapid and predictable
- The depth of anaesthesia is readily controlled
- Single dose rate; minimum alveolar concentration (MAC) is similar in most species
- Concurrent oxygen delivery; volatile agents are usually 'carried' in oxygen
- Volatile agent activity is independent of hepatic and renal function
- Continued administration does not necessarily cause prolonged recoveries
- Surgery may be prolonged without complication
- Inhalation drugs have broadly similar effects
- The airway is usually protected

▶

Disadvantages

- Induction and recovery may be delayed by inadequate ventilation or lung pathology
- A considerable range of equipment is required; some items are expensive
- Intubation is usually necessary
- Knowledge of breathing systems and anaesthetic machines is required
- Hazards associated with compressed gas
- Fire and explosion risks with some agents
- Possible personnel health risk associated with exposure to volatile agents

Pharmacokinetics

The behaviour of inhalation anaesthetics can be predicted and compared if two important features are known. These are the blood/gas solubility coefficient and the minimum alveolar concentration.

Blood/gas solubility coefficient

This value describes the solubility of agents in blood. Drugs with low solubility produce rapid induction and recovery rates, and changes in the level of anaesthesia on changing vaporizer settings are more rapid. Values for modern anaesthetics (starting with the most insoluble) are:

- Desflurane: 0.42
- N_2O: 0.47
- Sevoflurane: 0.60
- Isoflurane: 1.39
- Enflurane: 1.8
- Halothane: 2.4
- Methoxyflurane: 12.0

Hence the use of isoflurane, which is more insoluble than halothane, would be expected to result in a faster induction of anaesthesia, change in depth and recovery.

Minimum alveolar concentration (MAC)

MAC of anaesthetics is the alveolar concentration that prevents responses occurring to a specified stimulus (e.g. skin incision) in 50% of patients. It is a measure of potency. Agents with low values have the greatest potency; low inspired concentrations are required for surgery. Many factors alter MAC, the most important being other drugs given during anaesthesia; for instance, N_2O, analgesics and preanaesthetic medication all reduce MAC of the inhalation agents. Although the MAC of an anaesthetic is similar across species, there are some species differences. Value ranges (starting with most potent) are as follows:

- Methoxyflurane: 0.23%
- Halothane: 0.8–1.1%
- Isoflurane: 1.3–1.6%
- Enflurane: 2.2%
- Sevoflurane: 2.2–2.6%
- Desflurane: 7.2–9.8%
- N_2O: 188–220%

Critical tension

Volatile anaesthetics produce anaesthesia when a critical tension is exceeded in the central nervous system (CNS). This tension is achieved by movement of drug molecules down a series of tension gradients, beginning at the anaesthetic machine and ending at the site of action within the CNS. At equilibrium, the tension of drug in the brain mirrors that in arterial blood, which in turn depends on that in the alveoli. Therefore, factors influencing alveolar tensions ultimately determine brain tensions.

Alveolar drug levels depend on those factors that affect delivery to, and removal from, the lung. Factors increasing alveolar delivery include alveolar ventilation rate and the inspired gas concentration. When these are high, induction of anaesthesia is rapid. Removal of anaesthetic from the alveolus depends on blood solubility of the gas, cardiac output and alveolar–venous anaesthetic gradient. Alveolar tensions rise rapidly (and induction is rapid) when cardiac output is low (e.g. in haemorrhagic shock), when insoluble agents (e.g. isoflurane) are used and when the pulmonary venous tension of anaesthetic is high.

Principles of recovery

Recovery from anaesthesia relies on principles similar to those of induction in the process of removing inhaled agent from the CNS. An added consideration is the presence of a poorly perfused fat-soluble compartment (i.e. adipose tissue). During a prolonged period of anaesthesia, a significant uptake of volatile agent into this compartment can occur and this can affect recovery, as release of the inhalation agent from this tissue to the blood will result. Highly fat-soluble agents will produce a greater effect than poorly fat-soluble inhalation agents, as more agent will have partitioned within this fatty compartment. Metabolism of the anaesthetic may also play a role in recovery from certain anaesthetics, particularly for drugs undergoing significant hepatic metabolism (e.g. halothane, methoxyflurane).

Individual inhalation agents

Halothane

Currently one of the most common volatile anaesthetics in veterinary anaesthesia in the UK, this halogenated hydrocarbon is a sweet-smelling, clear liquid which decomposes in ultraviolet light (and so is stored in amber bottles) and contains an antioxidant (0.01% thymol). It readily evaporates, producing a maximum concentration of 32%. For this reason it must be used from a calibrated vaporizer, or dangerously high levels of anaesthetic could be delivered to the patient. Halothane is a fast-acting anaesthetic. Up to 12–25% of absorbed halothane is metabolized to bromide ions, trifluoroacetate and chloride by the liver. Halothane affects physiological function of the patient as described below.

CNS effects

Halothane is a potent anaesthetic. Concentrations of 1.0–3.0% may be needed for induction but adequate surgical conditions are obtained with inspired concentrations of 0.75–2.0%. Muscle relaxation is modest but analgesia is poor; adrenergic responses occur until deep levels of anaesthesia are reached.

Cardiopulmonary system effects

Halothane lowers blood pressure by depressing cardiac contractility and reducing cardiac output. Heart rate remains unchanged. Halothane produces minimal reduction in systemic vascular resistance, though it causes vasodilatation in capillary beds of the brain, uterus and skin. As a halogenated hydrocarbon, the drug 'sensitizes' the myocardium to adrenaline, predisposing the heart to arrhythmias under conditions of high circulating catecholamines (e.g. when stressed).

Halothane depresses ventilation in a dose-dependent manner, causing decreased tidal volume and decreased respiratory rate. It depresses ventilation to a lesser extent than other volatile anaesthetics with the exception of diethyl ether. It is non-irritant to respiratory mucosa and well tolerated for mask induction.

Other effects

In people, halothane-associated hepatitis occurs with repeated halothane anaesthetics. The cause is not fully understood, but seems related to preoperative enzyme induction caused by smoking and alcohol consumption, as well as intraoperative hypoxia. The condition has not been conclusively demonstrated to occur in animals during surgical anaesthesia.

Halothane lowers body temperature by inhibiting thermoregulatory mechanisms and producing cutaneous vasodilatation.

Special precautions

Halothane triggers malignant hyperthermia in sensitive pigs and this genetically determined condition also occurs in humans. It has occurred in dogs, horses and cats but is rare.

Isoflurane

Isoflurane is an isomer of enflurane and a more recently developed volatile agent. Although it is a halogenated ether, it has an unpleasant pungent smell. Its saturated vapour pressure is similar to halothane and the same (cleaned) precision vaporizer may be used for its administration. At room temperature, the maximum concentration possible is 31.5%. It is more expensive than halothane, but this difference in cost is reduced when isoflurane is delivered via a rebreathing anaesthetic system.

Isoflurane has a low blood/gas solubility coefficient and so inductions and recoveries are rapid, the latter even after prolonged administration. At induction, inspired concentrations of 2–3% are needed. Because it has a higher MAC value than halothane, higher inspired concentrations are needed to maintain anaesthesia (1.5–2.5%).

CNS effects

It is a potent anaesthetic, providing narcosis and muscle relaxation. Recoveries are rapid but may be associated with transient excitatory effects, especially after painful surgery. It decreases cerebral vascular resistance and cerebral metabolic rate, with an increase in cerebral blood flow, though to a lesser degree than halothane.

Cardiopulmonary system effects

Isoflurane causes dose-dependent hypotension despite non-dose-dependent increases in heart rate. At 1.0 to 1.5 times MAC, cardiac output is maintained whilst systemic vascular resistance is reduced. Isoflurane does not sensitize the heart to catecholamine-induced arrhythmias. Isoflurane is a potent respiratory depressant, depressing ventilation to a greater extent than halothane. Because of its pungent odour it is poorly tolerated for mask inductions.

Sevoflurane

Popular in human anaesthesia in Japan and veterinary anaesthesia in North America, sevoflurane is now licensed for use in dogs in the UK. Sevoflurane has a low blood/gas partition coefficient resulting in rapid inductions and recoveries. It has a pleasant, non-irritant odour. It is only moderately metabolized (approximately 3%) and the potential for hepatotoxicity is low. It is unstable in the presence of soda lime and degrades, producing toxic metabolites (i.e. compound A) that have been shown to produce renal pathology in rats. Clinically this effect on kidneys has not been reported in small animals.

CNS effects

It is a potent anaesthetic, providing narcosis and muscle relaxation. It decreases cerebral vascular resistance and cerebral metabolic rate, but the resultant increase in cerebral blood flow is less than that seen with isoflurane.

Cardiopulmonary system effects

Cardiopulmonary effects are similar to those of isoflurane. Sevoflurane causes dose-dependent hypotension, primarily via reduction in systemic vascular resistance, though it does cause some myocardial depression. It does not sensitize the heart to catecholamine-induced arrhythmias. Sevoflurane causes dose-dependent respiratory depression, but because it is a non-irritant gas it is well tolerated for mask inductions.

Enflurane

Enflurane, a halogenated ether with a fruity smell, has never gained popularity in veterinary anaesthesia despite some useful features. Chemically it is very stable and contains no preservative. Because it is highly volatile, with a saturated vapour pressure (SVP) of 171.8 at 20°C, the maximum concentration achievable is 22% (at that temperature) and so the use of an 'Enfluratec' is advisable.

In humans, deep enflurane anaesthesia causes seizure-type electroencephalographic (EEG) activity which is exacerbated by hypercapnia. Involuntary muscle twitches are seen during anaesthesia and recovery in animals. Enflurane depresses blood pressure to a similar extent as isoflurane. Heart rate is increased in a dose-dependent manner. Cardiac output is reduced. It is the most potent respiratory depressant, decreasing rate and depth. Enflurane produces excellent muscle relaxation and markedly potentiates neuromuscular blockers.

Desflurane

This is a relatively new agent. Its blood/gas partition coefficient (0.42) is similar to that of nitrous oxide, so it is very insoluble and is associated with very rapid induction and recovery. It requires a special temperature-controlled, pressurized vaporizer and is expensive, though use in a closed circle system makes it more cost effective. It undergoes minimal metabolism (0.2%) and hence its potential for toxicity is low.

Cardiopulmonary properties are similar to those of isoflurane, with dose-dependent vasodilatation and only moderate myocardial depression seen, though sympathetic tone is maintained. Respiratory depression also occurs to a similar degree as with isoflurane, and it is irritant to the respiratory system at higher concentrations, though it is said to be well tolerated by animals for mask induction. Its use in veterinary anaesthesia is at present mainly experimental, but it may become licensed for use in animals in the future.

Methoxyflurane

This fruity-smelling halogenated ether is the most potent volatile anaesthetic. It is non-reactive but decomposes slowly when exposed to soda lime and ultraviolet light and so it contains butylated hydroxytoluene. Methoxyflurane evaporates poorly; no more than 3% can be delivered at room temperature. It has high blood/gas (12.0) and rubber/gas (630) solubility coefficients, making induction and recovery very slow. This precludes its use in large animals.

It is a potent anaesthetic with good muscle relaxant and analgesic properties. Cardiac output is reduced in a dose-dependent manner, causing hypotension. Heart rate tends to be slow. It causes more respiratory depression than halothane. In humans, prolonged methoxyflurane anaesthesia causes renal tubular destruction, polyuria and dehydration lasting several days after administration. This is partly due to fluoride and oxalate ions generated from hepatic methoxyflurane metabolism. In dogs, acute renal failure has occurred when flunixin has been given perioperatively and it is not currently used in clinical practice.

Ether

Rarely used now in veterinary anaesthesia, this is a pungent irritant vapour. Oxygen–ether mixtures are explosive. It is less potent than halothane, but produces sympathetic stimulation providing cardiovascular support. Ether does not sensitize the heart to catecholamine-induced arrhythmias. It has some analgesic activity.

Nitrous oxide (N₂O)

Nitrous oxide is an odourless, relatively inert gas that is non-flammable but supports combustion. Its MAC is greater than 100% in animals and so it cannot be used as a sole anaesthetic agent. Nitrous oxide is combined with oxygen as a carrier gas. It must not be used at concentrations greater than 80% as this lowers O_2 below normal levels. Usually no more than 66% is delivered.

The percentage of gas mixtures is calculated on a flow ratio basis. For example, a 50% O_2/N_2O mixture is produced when O_2 and N_2O flows are the same (e.g. 3 litres of O_2/min and 3 litres of N_2O/min). Commonly, 66% or 2:1 N_2O/O_2 mixtures are used. These are produced when N_2O flow is exactly twice that of O_2.

Anaesthetic 'sparing' effect

Nitrous oxide is less potent in animals than in humans but does lower the concentration of volatile agent required to produce a given level of anaesthesia. For example, 66% N_2O reduces halothane requirements by about 25%. Because N_2O has minimal effects on cardiac output and ventilation, its inclusion preserves cardiopulmonary performance.

Second gas effect

During induction with N_2O and a volatile agent, the rapid uptake of N_2O from alveoli causes the alveolar concentration of the volatile agent, or second gas, to rise. This accelerates uptake of the second gas and speeds the rate of induction of anaesthesia.

Gas-filled viscus

Because N_2O is 35 times more soluble in blood than nitrogen, N_2O diffuses into gas-filled spaces faster than nitrogen is reabsorbed during denitrogenation of the body. Hence it can accumulate in gas-filled spaces, e.g. the dilated stomach of dogs with gastric dilatation–volvulus complex or the pleural space of animals with a closed pneumothorax. Nitrous oxide compromises the animal by enlarging or increasing the pressure within such spaces and reducing the space for lung ventilation.

Cardiopulmonary effects

Nitrous oxide has a very modest stimulant effect on cardiac output and blood pressure. It has no effect on ventilation; when it is added to volatile agents, ventilation remains unchanged even though anaesthesia deepens.

Hypoxia

Whenever N_2O is used, the O_2 content of inspired gas is lowered; this increases the possibility of hypoxia arising from other causes like hypoventilation. When used in a rebreathing system after the initial stabilization period, uptake of N_2O from the circuit declines and can build up within the circuit if low flow anaesthesia is being performed. For this reason N_2O should be used with caution in circle or to-and-fro systems, and preferably only if inspired O_2 concentration is measured or a pulse oximeter is used. Nitrous oxide should not be used in animals whose arterial O_2 tensions are lowered by disease or where a gas-filled viscus is present.

Diffusion hypoxia

When N_2O delivery is ended, its direction of diffusion reverses – from blood into the alveolar space. The volume evolved in the first few minutes after termination may dilute alveolar O_2. If alveolar O_2 levels are low because the animal is breathing air, not 100% O_2, 'diffusion hypoxia' may occur. Therefore on ending N_2O administration, animals should receive 100% O_2 for at least 5 minutes.

Pollution

Nitrous oxide is relatively odourless and high atmospheric levels are difficult to detect. There is some evidence that N_2O causes toxic effects, including bone-marrow depression after chronic low-level exposure. It is not absorbed by activated charcoal and so 'canister' scavenging is useless.

Oxygen

Oxygen is an odourless reactive gas that allows combustion and, in the presence of organic material and activation energy (i.e. sparks or naked flames), explosions. The gas is given whenever the normal delivery of atmospheric oxygen to active tissue is threatened. This includes anaesthesia (even that produced with injectable agents). Pure oxygen (100%) is usually given to animals that are anaemic, have pulmonary pathology or are hypoventilating. During inhalation anaesthesia, 100% oxygen may be used as the 'carrier gas' but it is frequently diluted to 50% or 33% concentrations by nitrous oxide. Oxygen is also supplied during recovery until the animal is capable of maintaining haemoglobin saturation with room air (21% O_2).

Techniques

Endotracheal intubation

When animals are rendered unconscious by injectable or inhalation drugs, protective airway reflexes are lost. Endotracheal intubation is an important means of ensuring a patent airway and preventing aspiration of fluids and regurgitated food. The equipment and its care are described later (in the section on 'Other anaesthetic equipment').

Tube selection

Ideally, the tube should extend from the incisor table to a point level with the spine of the scapula. Provided that the cuff lies beyond the glottis, the airway will be secure. Surplus dead-space is minimized by cutting off the projecting tube. The maximum tube diameter appropriate to the patient minimizes resistance to air flow.

Intubation

The jaws must be relaxed and laryngeal reflexes suppressed before intubation is attempted. Laryngeal reflexes persist in cats to relatively 'deep' levels of anaesthesia, and laryngospasm is not uncommon following tactile stimulation of the glottis. In this species, laryngeal reflexes may be depressed with topical lidocaine administered as an aerosol.

Laryngoscopy is useful during intubation in cats, in dogs with pigmented oral mucosae or in those with surplus soft tissue in the upper airway.

Endotracheal intubation
Advantages

- Airway protection from saliva and gastric contents: if cuffed tubes are not available an oropharyngeal pack (layers of moistened gauze laid in a horseshoe pattern over the tube and 'packed') may suffice. This is important during dental and oral surgery
- Allows positive pressure ventilation: a leak-proof cuff allows lung inflation without gas escape
- Reduces waste-gas pollution
- Reduces anatomical dead-space

Disadvantages

- Resistance: cuffs limit the size of tube that can be introduced atraumatically. Small internal diameters critically increase resistance to breathing
- Kinking or occlusion: overinflated cuffs may compress the underlying tube. Severe occipito-atlantal flexion (e.g. during cisternal puncture) may cause tubes (especially red-rubber types) to kink. If tubes are inadequately cleaned, dried secretions accumulate within the lumen
- Traumatic laryngitis: poor intubation technique or the use of oversized tubes may physically damage the larynx and/or trachea, causing post-operative respiratory embarrassment
- Chemical/ischaemic tracheitis: if tubes are inadequately rinsed or irritant sterilants are used, the tracheal mucosa may be irritated. For this reason, tubes must be adequately aired after ethylene oxide sterilization. Overinflated cuffs left *in situ* for prolonged periods may produce an ischaemic tracheitis and cause postoperative coughing
- Apparatus dead-space: correctly sized endotracheal tubes reduce anatomical dead-space. However, overlong tubes extending beyond the incisor table constitute apparatus dead-space, which should be minimized
- Endobronchial intubation: excessive advancement of the endotracheal tube down the airway may result in endobronchial intubation. In these circumstances, one lung receives no ventilation and blood deoxygenation may occur
- Interference: conventionally placed (orotracheal) tubes interfere with some types of oral surgery. In such cases pharyngotracheal or tracheostomy placement may be required. In some species nasotracheal intubation is practised

Mask inductions

Masks are used to provide oxygen in comatose or recovering animals, or for the delivery of volatile anaesthetics when intubation is not performed. Induction of anaesthesia using masks is a useful technique in high-risk cases because animals receive oxygen during induction; if crises develop, switching the vaporizer off may prove life-saving.

Induction by mask
Advantages

- Do not damage the airway
- Produce smooth inductions when patients are depressed or heavily sedated

Disadvantages

- Mask inductions are resisted and cause inelegant inductions in poorly sedated animals
- Masks increase mechanical dead-space. They do not necessarily add to air-flow resistance but, because the airway is not clear, turbulence or obstruction can occur
- Ventilation is possible with tightly applied gas-tight masks. Even so, some gas inevitably enters the stomach, which inflates and limits diaphragmatic movement
- Atmospheric pollution is greater with masks. This is reduced by using close-fitting face-masks

Chamber inductions

This technique is useful in laboratory animals and can be used in cats and small dogs. Sedation or depression should be present, otherwise inductions may be violent. Pollution is a problem when the chamber is opened. High inspired oxygen levels are present when consciousness is lost; indeed, the chamber usefully serves as an oxygen cage for neonates or small animals.

Equipment

Anaesthetic equipment centres on the administration of inhalational anaesthetics. Modern techniques require an anaesthetic machine and an anaesthetic breathing system or 'circuit'. The main components include:

- Oxygen source
- Vaporizer/source of anaesthetic gas
- Breathing system.

Anaesthetic breathing systems

The anaesthetic system takes the fresh gas from the common gas outlet of the anaesthetic machine and delivers it to the patient. The functions of the system include:

- Removal of exhaled carbon dioxide (CO_2)
- Supply of oxygen (O_2)
- Supply of anaesthetic gases
- Allowing performance of intermittent positive pressure ventilation (IPPV).

System classification varies throughout the world and can be confusing. A simple basis of classification depends on whether expired carbon dioxide is flushed from the system by high gas flow (non-rebreathing system) or removed by chemical reaction (e.g. with soda lime; rebreathing system).

Rebreathing systems

Rebreathing systems (circle and to-and-fro) remove CO_2 from expired gas by chemically absorbing it. Expired breath, in comparison with inspired gas, is low in O_2 and anaesthetic but contains more CO_2 and water vapour and is warm. In rebreathing systems, expired gas passes through soda lime (absorbent), which removes CO_2. Warm, moist gas is then reinspired and so rebreathing systems conserve heat and moisture. Fresh gas flow requirements are based on the O_2 consumption of the patient. Because this value is low (Figure 22.7), rebreathing systems are very efficient.

Species	Respiratory rate (breaths/min)	Tidal volume (ml/kg)	Minute volume (ml/kg/min)	Oxygen consumption (ml/kg/min)
Dogs >30 kg <30 kg	15–20 20–30	12–15 16–20	150–250 200–300	5.8 6.2
Cats	20–30	7–9	180–380	7.3

22.7 Respiratory variables in companion animals.

Carbon dioxide absorbent
The two main absorbents that absorb CO_2 are soda lime and barium lime, based on the metallic base used.

Soda lime consists of granules of:

- 80% calcium hydroxide ($Ca(OH)_2$) ('lime')
- 4% sodium hydroxide (NaOH) ('soda')
- 14–20% water.

Barium lime consists of granules of:

- 80% calcium hydroxide ($Ca(OH)_2$)
- 20% barium hydroxide ($Ba(OH)_2$) (octahydrate).

Carbon dioxide reacts chemically with the absorbent to produce carbonates, changes the pH of the absorbent and produces heat in the process. As absorbent reacts with CO_2 and becomes exhausted, pH indicators change colour. Changes depend on the dyes used. Common absorbents turn from pink to white or green to purple. The container label describes the colour change that its contents undergo and should be consulted.

When soda lime granules are 'spent', they lose their soapy, soft texture and fail to become warm when exposed to CO_2. Spent soda lime should be replaced, as it will no longer absorb CO_2. If left overnight the surface of the spent granules can return to pink; however, the granules are still exhausted and should be replaced.

The absorbent is contained in canisters with contents of approximately 50% granules and 50% air space. Efficient absorption requires an air-space volume in excess of tidal volume and so the minimum 'working' canister size is two times the tidal volume of the patient, though generally greater volumes than this are used.

Soda lime is irritant (alkali); gloves should be worn when refilling canisters and the dust should not be inhaled or allowed to contact the eyes. Soda lime reacts with trichloroethylene (a once popular volatile agent) to produce phosgene and other toxic gases and should not be used in rebreathing systems. It also reacts with sevoflurane, producing 'compound A'. Detrimental effects of compound A have been demonstrated on kidneys in rats but not in other companion animals or in humans.

'Closed' and 'low-flow'
Rebreathing systems are used in one of two ways. In 'closed' systems, gas inflow precisely replaces anaesthetic and O_2 taken up by the patient. Approximately 5–10 ml O_2/kg/minute

is required. Under these conditions the pressure relief valve is closed. When the system is run in a 'low-flow' fashion, oxygen delivery is in excess of basal requirements (above 10 ml/kg/min) with surplus gas leaking through the open pressure-relief valve. This is the easiest system to operate and therefore the most commonly used in practice.

Nitrous oxide

Once a rebreathing circuit has reached equilibrium the addition of further N_2O can result in its accumulation within the inspired gas, as O_2 continues to be withdrawn from the inspired gas by the patient and CO_2 is removed by the absorbent. At low flow rates and during long operations this can result in dangerously low oxygen levels developing in the inspired gas, and hypoxia of the patient can result. This problem can be avoided at higher gas flow rates, i.e. > 30 ml O_2/kg/min (and the same of N_2O). A 1:1 ratio of $N_2O:O_2$ is recommended if N_2O is to be used. In general this gas is best used in rebreathing systems only if inspired O_2 content, arterial O_2 saturation or arterial blood gas analysis can be performed.

Denitrogenation

When connected to breathing systems at the onset of anaesthesia, patients expire considerable volumes of nitrogen (which is present in normal air but not in anaesthetic gas mixtures). This may lower circuit O_2 to hypoxic levels unless purged through the pressure-relief valve (denitrogenation). This is achieved by using high flow rates for the first 10–15 minutes of anaesthesia.

Rebreathing systems
Advantages

- Low gas flow requirements
- Low volatile agent consumption rate
- 'Closed' or 'low-flow' options
- Expired moisture and heat conserved
- Ventilation can be altered (spontaneous to controlled) without changing system performance
- Low explosion risk (when explosive gases are used)
- Less pollution

Disadvantages

- Greater resistance to breathing
- Nitrous oxide must be used cautiously in rebreathing systems
- Some versions expensive to purchase
- Regular absorbent replacement required
- Inspired gas content undetermined
- Denitrogenation required
- Slow to change level of anaesthesia
- Cumbersome

Circle system

Circle systems are becoming increasingly popular in the UK and modern small-animal circles can be used in patients weighing > 5–10 kg. The circle system has valves causing unidirectional gas movement. With one-way flow of gas around the circle, absorption of CO_2 from the soda lime canister is very efficient. The main components of the circuit are shown in Figure 22.8.

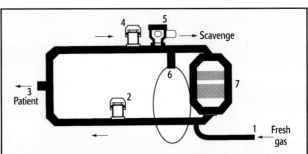

- *Fresh gas inflow (1).* This pipe connects the circuit with the common-gas outlet on the anaesthetic machine.
- *Unidirectional valves (2 and 4).* These are light transparent discs resting on knife-edge valve seats, enclosed within a transparent dome. Units should be easy to disassemble for drying and cleaning.
- *'Y' connector (3).* This connects inspiratory and expiratory limbs with endotracheal tube connectors or masks.
- *Adjustable pressure limiting (APL) valve (5).* This is opened to release surplus gas from 'low-flow' systems, during denitrogenation, and closed when lung inflation is imposed. APL valves should be shrouded for attachment to scavenging hoses.
- *Reservoir bag (6).* This allows IPPV; its volume should be 3–6 times the animal's tidal volume. Large bags increase circuit volume, make respiratory movement less obvious and are harder to squeeze. Inadequately sized bags collapse during large breaths and overdistend during expiration.
- *Absorbent canister (7).* Canisters for circle systems may have two compartments. When absorbent in one becomes exhausted, it is discarded; after refilling, the canister is replaced in the reverse direction. This allows optimal use of absorbent.
- *Hoses.* These are corrugated to prevent kinking.

22.8 Circle breathing system.

Circle system
Advantages

- High gas efficiency
- Mechanical dead-space remains unchanged with use (unlike to-and-fro system)
- Bronchiolitis unlikely (unlike to-and-fro system)
- Less circuit inertia than to-and-fro system
- Ventilation readily controlled

Disadvantages

- Some models expensive
- Complex, cumbersome and difficult to sterilize
- High resistance to breathing for animals less than 5–10 kg
- Unidirectional gas flow dependent on functioning one-way valves

To-and-fro (Waters' canister) system

In this system (Figure 22.9) gas oscillates over absorbent in the Waters' canister. The patient breathes in gas from the fresh gas outlet and recycled (CO_2 free) gas that has passed through the soda lime canister. Gas is then exhaled through the soda lime canister where CO_2 is removed and excess gas is vented out of the expiratory valve. Canisters are designed for either vertical or horizontal use; only the latter are used with companion animals.

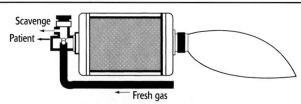

• *Fresh gas inflow.* This is situated adjacent to the endotracheal tube connector, allowing dialled concentrations of anaesthetic to be preferentially inspired and therefore giving greater control over anaesthesia.

• *Filter.* A metal gauze screen should be sited at the patient end of the canister to limit inhalation of alkaline dust.

• *Scavenging shroud.* Scavenging waste gas from a to-and-fro system relies on a suitable shroud on the adjustable pressure limiting valve.

• *Canister.* Transparent canisters allow absorbent colour and filling adequacy to be checked. Canisters in horizontal to-and-fro systems must be filled to capacity, otherwise the expired gas will 'channel', i.e. take the low resistance path over the absorbent, retaining CO_2.

22.9 To-and-fro breathing system.

To-and-fro system
Advantages

• High gas efficiency
• Bidirectional gas flow improves CO_2 scrubbing efficiency
• Greater heat conservation (hyperthermia is possible on warm days)
• Lower resistance to breathing than with circle systems (no valves and lower overall circuit length)
• Low circuit volume
• Denitrogenation achieved rapidly
• Rapid changes in gas concentration
• Simple, robust construction
• Readily sterilized
• Inexpensive

Disadvantages

• Valve position is inconvenient for positive pressure ventilation
• Mechanical dead-space increases during surgery as absorbent is exhausted
• 'Channelling' occurs if the canister is not adequately filled
• Bronchiolitis; aspiration of alkaline dust from canister may cause chemical injury
• Considerable drag
• The system has some inertia and is inconvenient during head surgery

Non-rebreathing systems

Non-rebreathing systems rely on high fresh gas flow rates, based on multiples of minute volume, to flush expired CO_2 from the circuit so that it cannot be rebreathed at the next breath. **Minute volume** is respiratory rate multiplied by tidal volume and can be calculated on a weight basis (see Figure 22.7). Individual circuits have different fresh gas requirements based on the multiple of the minute volume required to prevent rebreathing of CO_2. This multiple of minute volume is called the **circuit factor**. Circuit factors will be described for individual systems.

Non-rebreathing systems
Advantages

• Low resistance; ideal for small animals and birds
• Simple construction
• Inexpensive to purchase
• Soda lime not required
• Inspired gas content similar to that 'dialled' at anaesthetic machine
• Denitrogenation not required
• Circuit concentration of anaesthetic can be changed rapidly, allowing more precise control over patient's level of unconsciousness

Disadvantages

• High carrier gas flow requirements
• High volatile agent consumption rate
• Expired moisture and heat usually lost
• Ventilatory modes affect system performance for some circuits
• Different types of non-rebreathing circuits behave differently and have different flow requirements

The Magill system

The Magill system (Mapleson A) consists of a reservoir bag and a corrugated hose that ends at an expiratory APL valve (Figure 22.10). On inspiration, fresh gas is drawn down the corrugated hose to the patient. On expiration, exhaled gas is pushed back towards the reservoir bag and fresh gas outlet, and when the pressure in the reservoir bag exceeds the pressure to open the expiratory valve, subsequently exhaled gas goes out of the APL valve.

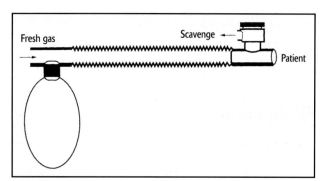

22.10 Magill breathing system.

The first component of the exhaled gas (dead-space gas) has only been in contact with non-gaseous exchanging tissues (e.g. trachea, primary bronchi) and is CO_2-free gas. This gas passes back up the corrugated hosing. The second component of exhaled gas comes from deep within the lungs and is CO_2-rich (alveolar gas). This CO_2-rich gas is vented out of the expiratory valve. Hence during spontaneous ventilation the Magill circuit is an efficient system as it conserves the CO_2-free dead-space gas. Fresh gas flow rates equal to or greater than patient minute volume (1 to 1.5 times minute ventilation, approximately 200 ml/kg/min) are required. When N_2O is used, its flow rate is included within this value. For example, a 15 kg dog with a minute volume of 3 litres receives an inspired concentration of 66% N_2O with flows of O_2 at 1 l/min and N_2O at 2 l/min (fresh gas flow rate 3 l/min).

During IPPV the ability of the circuit to conserve dead-space gas is lost and higher fresh gas flow rates are required to prevent rebreathing of CO_2. The late inspired gas (fresh gas) is vented through the expiratory valve and the late expired gas (alveolar gas) is reintroduced into the lungs during inspirations rather than expelled through the valve. For longer periods of IPPV this circuit is not recommended.

Magill system
Advantages

- Efficient general-purpose circuit
- Readily maintained and sterilized
- Inexpensive

Disadvantages

- Expiratory valve resistance precludes its use in animals weighing less than 10 kg
- Valve location is inconvenient for scavenging and during head and neck surgery
- Not good for prolonged IPPV

The Lack breathing system
The inconvenient valve location in the Magill system is overcome by adding an expiratory limb ending with the APL valve distant to the patient in the Lack system (also classified as Mapleson A). In the coaxial Lack system (Figure 22.11), a reservoir bag connects to an outer inspiratory limb; this surrounds an inner expiratory tube which ends at the expiratory APL valve. Fresh gas flow rates are equivalent to those of the Magill.

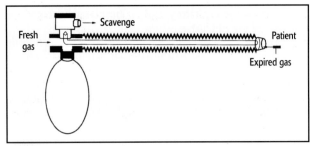

22.11 Coaxial Lack breathing system.

Problems of coaxial geometry (inner tube disconnection, fracture or kinking of the inner limb) are avoided when the inspiratory and expiratory limbs are placed in a parallel configuration in the parallel Lack system (Figure 22.12). This system also behaves like the Magill system and has the same fresh gas flow rate requirements.

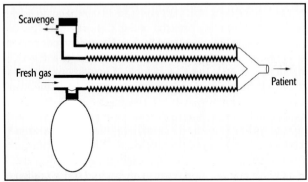

22.12 Parallel Lack breathing system.

A mini-Lack is also available in the UK. It has the same configuration as the parallel Lack breathing system but with a low-resistance APL valve. It has the same fresh gas flow requirements as for the Lack and can be used in cats and small dogs.

Lack system
Advantages

- Lightweight and exerts marginally less drag than Magill system
- Valve position facilitates surgery on the head and scavenging
- Length of system (1.5 m) allows anaesthetic machine positioning away from surgery
- Can be used in lieu of the Magill system

Disadvantages

- In coaxial versions the inner hose can become disconnected, causing considerable rebreathing
- The system is stiffer and inconvenient to use in very small animals
- Because the Lack system behaves like the Magill, it should not be used for prolonged IPPV

Ayre's T-piece
The Ayre's T-piece (Mapleson E system) (Figure 22.13) is ideal for small patients weighing under 10 kg as it has no expiratory valve and low expiratory resistance. Gas is inspired from the fresh gas outlet and the expiratory limb (hose). On expiration all expired gas (dead-space and alveolar gas) is exhaled down the expiratory limb, where it is vented via a shrouded scavenging port. Hence it is less efficient than the Magill system as dead-space gas is not conserved. Gas flows for T-piece systems of approximately 2 to 2.5 times the minute volume are required (approximately 500 ml/kg/min). Nitrous oxide is included at 66% of these levels.

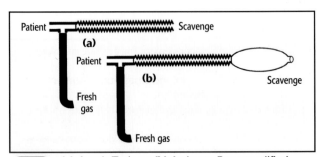

22.13 **(a)** Ayre's T-piece; **(b)** Jackson–Rees modified Ayre's T-piece.

The addition of the reservoir bag (Ayre's T-piece with Jackson–Rees modification or Mapleson F system) allows easy IPPV via occlusion of the bag outflow followed by gentle manual compression of the reservoir bag. Gas flow rates remain unchanged during IPPV. The bag also allows observation of respiratory movements.

A further modification of the Ayre's T piece with Jackson–Rees modification has become available on the veterinary market. The addition of a low-resistance APL valve to the expiratory limb after the reservoir bag allows easier controlled ventilation and scavenging of exhaled gas. This system functions as a modified Bain system.

Ayre's T-piece
Advantages

- Minimal apparatus dead-space and resistance, therefore ideal for cats, small dogs, neonates and birds
- Simple, inexpensive and easy to sterilize
- Bag facilitates IPPV and bag movement acts as a useful respiratory monitor
- Good for IPPV
- The system is scavenged with appropriate connectors

Disadvantages

- Fresh gas flow rates are high for larger patients
- With scavenging shrouds the expiratory connections can twist, obstructing expiratory outflow

The modified Bain system

The modified Bain system (Mapleson D system) is a coaxial (tube within a tube) T-piece with an inner inspiratory limb surrounded by an outer expiratory hose (Figure 22.14). The expiratory limb ends in a reservoir bag and expiratory APL valve.

It functions like a T-piece and as such requires similar fresh gas flow rates. The presence of an expiratory valve precludes its use in patients weighing less than 10 kg. It is a useful circuit for IPPV as circuit characteristics remain constant under spontaneous and controlled respiration.

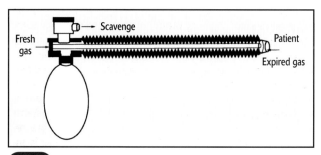

22.14 Modified Bain breathing system.

Bain system
Advantages

- Inexpensive
- Low drag and mechanical dead-space
- Good for IPPV
- Length of the system (1.8 m) allows anaesthetic machine to be positioned away from surgery, improving access
- Easily maintained and sterilized

Disadvantages

- Too much resistance for patients under 10 kg
- High fresh gas flows in larger patients
- Rebreathing problems can result from inner limb disconnection

The Humphrey ADE

The Humphrey ADE is a hybrid system that functions in spontaneous ventilation as a parallel Lack breathing system (Mapleson A), and in controlled ventilation as a T-piece (Mapleson D or E). The system consists of parallel inspiratory and expiratory hoses mounted on a 'Humphrey' block with a reservoir bag and an APL valve. There is a lever switch within the Humphrey block controlling the direction of gas flow within the block, determining the configuration of the system. In the 'A' mode during spontaneous ventilation, with the lever switch up, it functions as a Mapleson A or parallel Lack. With the switch of the lever down, it is converted from the 'A' mode to the 'D/E' mode for controlled ventilation (T-piece, Mapleson D or E) and can be attached to a ventilator. Additionally, the Humphrey ADE has been adapted to include the option of a carbon dioxide absorber and function as a circle system.

Anaesthetic machines

The functions of an anaesthetic machine (Figure 22.15) are to produce and deliver safe concentrations of anaesthetic vapour and to provide a means of supplying oxygen and imposing IPPV during apnoea or cardiopulmonary arrest. It also often

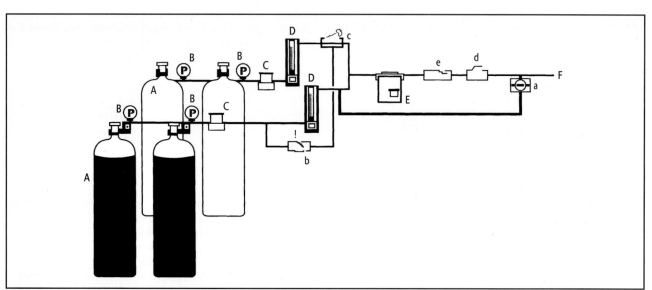

22.15 The anaesthetic machine begins at a carrier gas source (A), passes through a pressure gauge (B), a pressure regulator (C) and flowmeter assembly (D), and ends at the common gas outlet (F), where the anaesthetic breathing system attaches. Vaporizers (E) are usually positioned downstream from the flowmeter assembly. Other features include emergency oxygen valves (a), low oxygen alarms (b), nitrous oxide cut-out devices (c), over-pressure valves (d) and emergency air-intake valves (e).

provides storage for monitoring and other anaesthetic equipment. Understanding the function of anaesthetic machines is needed for the safe administration of volatile anaesthetics and oxygen and for machine maintenance; this prolongs the life of equipment, limits pollution and reduces the risk of equipment failure.

Gas supply

Cylinders are metal containers designed to withstand the pressure of compressed gases. Their size determines the volume of gas contained (in litres) and this is described by letters from AA (very small) to J (large). The volume of oxygen in filled cylinders at room temperature is shown in Figure 22.16.

Cylinder size	Content (litres)
E	680
F	1340
G	3400
J	6800

22.16 Oxygen cylinder sizes and contents.

Gas cylinders colour-coding in the UK

- **Oxygen** cylinders are black with white shoulders.
- **Nitrous oxide** cylinders are blue.
- **Carbon dioxide** cylinders are grey.
- Old machines may have a facility for **cyclopropane**, which is delivered in orange cylinders.

Cylinders are opened by anticlockwise rotation of the spindle. Before attachment to the cylinder yoke, the protective cellophane sleeve is removed from the cylinder valve. Once connected in the hanger yokes, spindles should be opened slowly two full turns, as partially restricted valves may reduce flow when the cylinder pressure falls.

Low-volume 'E' or 'F' cylinders attached to hanger yokes on the machine suit most practices. Machines usually hold two cylinders of O_2 and two of N_2O. The cylinder valve face has holes that correspond with pins sited within the hanger yoke. The pin-and-hole pattern constitutes the 'pin-indexing' system and ensures that N_2O or CO_2 cylinders cannot be connected to the O_2 yoke.

Vertically standing banks of three to five 'J' or 'G' size cylinders are used in busy practices. Two banks for each gas (O_2 and N_2O) are preferable, with one being 'in use' and the other 'in reserve'. Gas flows to the operating room through pipes in the wall. These end in wall-mounted Schrader-type sockets, which receive probes from the anaesthetic machine. Pipes are colour-coded and the probes size-coded so that lines cannot be accidentally crossed.

Pressure/contents gauge

The pressure gauge (see Figure 22.15) is indispensable for oxygen, because it indicates the gas volume in the cylinder. A cylinder at half its full cylinder pressure will be half full.

The N_2O pressure gauge is less useful; the full N_2O cylinder contains liquid and gas and the gauge measures the pressure of gaseous N_2O in equilibrium with liquid. This remains constant until all liquid evaporates, after which pressure falls rapidly. Gas volume in N_2O cylinders is found by weighing the bottle and applying the following formula:

litres N_2O present =
(net weight (g) – tare weight (g)) x 22.4/44

Net weight is the weight of the cylinder and its contents. Cylinder tare weight is stamped on the cylinder neck and represents the weight of the empty cylinder.

Pressure-reducing valves or regulators

These valves (see Figure 22.15) produce constant 'downstream' pressure (and therefore flow) as cylinder pressure falls with use. Without them, the cylinder valve would need incremental opening to maintain constant flow. They are sited immediately downstream from the hanger yoke, and in modern machines they may be incorporated in the yoke.

Flowmeters

Flowmeters (see Figure 22.15) control and measure the rate of gas passing through them. The units are litres per minute (l/min). A freely moving 'float' (either a ball or a bobbin) is supported in a transparent tapered tube by an ascending flow of gas. The flow rate is etched on the tube and read from the top of a bobbin or the equator of a sphere. The greater the flow, the higher the indicator rises in the glass tube. Flowmeters become inaccurate if dirt or non-vertical positioning makes the float rub against the tube. Flowmeters are calibrated for one gas only and so oxygen flowmeters do not accurately indicate the flow of nitrous oxide. Because of this, flowmeter control knobs are often colour-coded. Flowmeter control knobs must not be over-tightened.

Vaporizers

Vaporizers (see Figure 22.15) dilute the saturated vapour of volatile anaesthetics to yield a range of useful concentrations of vaporized inhalation agent. Concentrations leaving the vaporizer depend on:

- Temperature
- Surface area
- Gas flow
- Volatility of the anaesthetic.

As anaesthetic liquid vaporizes, the remaining liquid cools and the delivered anaesthetic concentration falls. With increased flow rates, the delivered concentration tends to decrease. Hence, ensuring a constant output is not always easy. A number of compensating devices can be employed to maintain output:

- **Heat source** (or heat sink) – surrounds the liquid anaesthetic to prevent rapid cooling. Heat is transferred from this source to buffer the drop in chamber temperature associated with vaporization.
- **Flow-splitting valve** – varies the proportion of carrier gas that passes through or bypasses the vaporizing chamber, allowing control of the percentage of anaesthetic vapour delivered.
- **Temperature compensating mechanism** – compensates for fall in vaporizing temperature and subsequent fall in vapour concentration. Two methods are commonly employed:
  - A bimetallic strip of two dissimilar metals, placed back to back, bends in proportion to a given change in temperature. When placed in the flow of the anaesthetic fresh gas it can alter the flow through the vaporizing chamber (increasing or decreasing the amount of anaesthetic vaporized) and compensate for a change in anaesthetic vapour pressure caused by a change in temperature.

- Alternatively, an ether-filled bellows attached to a flow-splitting valve, which expands or contracts in relation to temperature, performs a similar function of compensating for variation in vapour concentration with changes in temperature.
- **Wicks and baffles** – increase the surface area of vaporization, maximizing vaporization of the inhalation agent.

Draw-over vaporizers

Early vaporizers relied on the patient's respiratory efforts to 'draw' carrier gas (often air) over the liquid anaesthetic. They offer relatively little resistance to flow but are subject to large variations in inspiratory flow, being dependent on the ventilation characteristics of the patient. Compensation for changes in temperature is rarely employed. Consequently, their output is frequently variable and they cannot be reliably calibrated.

They are more commonly used when placed within the anaesthetic circuit, i.e. within a circle system. In this position they are termed **in-circuit vaporizers (VICs)**. Anaesthetic machines such as the Stephens' machine and the Komezaroff machine incorporate VICs, and work in small animals has demonstrated that they can safely be used. However, caution must be exercised when IPPV is initiated, as dangerously high concentrations of anaesthetic gas can be delivered. Some models still in use include:

- **Goldman halothane** vaporizer – simple, small, inexpensive. It is neither temperature nor flow compensated.
- **Oxford miniature** vaporizer – used primarily with portable anaesthetic equipment. It is not temperature compensated, though has a heat sink (a sealed water/antifreeze compartment). It can be drained of one anaesthetic and refilled with another and detachable scales of approximate vapour percentage delivered are supplied.
- **EMO** (Epstein, Macintosh, Oxford) vaporizer – used for ether delivery. It has a water-filled compartment as a heat sink.

Plenum vaporizers

Plenum vaporizers are designed for use with constant flow of carrier gas and offer greater resistance to flow. Hence they are positioned out of the breathing circuit, i.e. they are **out-of-circuit vaporizers (VOCs)**. They are mostly calibrated vaporizers with compensatory devices for variations in temperature and flow and are those most commonly used in veterinary practice. Earlier models include uncalibrated types but these are infrequently seen today.

- **Uncalibrated vaporizers** – the **Boyle's bottle** is simple, inexpensive and easily maintained. It does not have any temperature compensation, though it does have a cowl that can be lowered towards and below the liquid anaesthetic surface to increase vapour uptake for a given control lever position. However, output concentrations are not guaranteed and they 'drift' despite constant control settings. With age, the sealing washer (usually cork or rubber) becomes brittle and allows leakage of anaesthetic vapour. The cork stopper placed in the filling orifice is normally retained with a metal chain and often the metal anchor of the chain passes through the cork. If the chain breaks, the cork can act as a sparking plug; if someone charged with static electricity touches the cork–metal top, an explosion may result.

- **Calibrated vaporizers** – temperature and flow compensation are incorporated as well as a heat sink into these vaporizers. Anaesthetic concentration from calibrated vaporizers is similar to that 'dialled' on the spindle, provided that the gas flow through the vaporizer and the temperature of liquid anaesthetic are within ranges specific for the model. In Mark III 'Tecs (Ohmeda), output is constant between 18 and 35°C. Dialled and delivered concentrations are similar at flows between 0.2 and 15 l/min. In the earlier 'Tec 2, vapour output is reliable from above 2–4 l/min fresh gas flow. Lower flows, as used in low-flow anaesthesia, produce delivered concentration different from that displayed on the dial. They come with a performance chart that indicates the delivered vapour concentration for a given dial setting and flow rate. Though obsolete, they are still seen in veterinary practice.

Vaporizers are agent-specific. Filling with the wrong anaesthetic is prevented by keyed filling ports. These accept a key-ended tube that only attaches to the corresponding anaesthetic bottle. Used properly, the system also assists pollution control, because vaporizer filling occurs without spillage.

Back bar

Flowmeters and vaporizers may be joined by tapered connectors and attached to a back bar, producing a series of semi-permanent fixtures. The 'Selectatec SM' manifold allows rapid attachment or removal of 'Tec 3 and 'Tec 4 vaporizers, facilitating vaporizer removal for refilling out of theatre, servicing and rewarming. In accommodating up to three vaporizers, a range of volatile agents may be available.

Common gas outlet

This connects the anaesthetic machine to breathing system connectors, ventilators or O_2 supply devices (Figure 22.15).

O_2 flush

Also known as the bypass or purge valve (see Figure 22.15), this receives O_2 from the cylinder and bypasses the vaporizer. Activation produces high flows of pure O_2 to the common gas outlet. The device is used to provide oxygen in emergency situations. It is used to flush anaesthetic from breathing systems before patient disconnection, thus lowering pollution.

Nitrous oxide cut-out devices

These devices (see Figure 22.15) curtail N_2O flow and sound an alarm when oxygen runs out. They are invaluable if N_2O is used, but some older anaesthetic machines do not have them.

Over-pressure valve

High pressures downstream from the common gas outlet open this valve and sound an alarm (see Figure 22.15). The device is useful for leak-testing breathing systems; the valve's presence is confirmed by occluding the common gas outlet while pressing the oxygen bypass valve.

Emergency air intake valve

When gas flow from the machine accidentally ceases, the patient's inspiratory effort opens an emergency valve (see Figure 22.15) that allows room air to enter the breathing system. The valve's opening action is accompanied by a 'whistling' sound. This valve is tested by attaching a pipe to the common gas outlet and applying suction; when sufficient vacuum is present, the valve opens and a whistle is heard.

Checking the anaesthetic machine before use

The anaesthetic machine should receive a major check at the beginning of each working day and a minor check between cases.

Major checking procedure

1. Ensure that flow control valves (at the flowmeter) are 'off'.
2. Ensure that cylinders are closed and fit securely on the hanger yoke.
3. Press the O_2 flush valve until no gas flow is apparent from the common gas outlet.
4. Check that flowmeters and pressure gauges read '0'.
5. Open the O_2 cylinder valve slowly (anticlockwise) and observe the registered pressure. On machines that carry two O_2 cylinders, test the 'full' or reserve cylinder first.
6. Open the O_2 flowmeter control valve to 2–4 l/min to ensure smooth function.
7. Whilst this is flowing, repeat the procedure for the 'full' N_2O cylinder and open the flowmeter to 2–4 l/min. Close the tested O_2 cylinder. As the O_2 runs out, the low-oxygen alarm should sound and the N_2O cut-off device should trigger, with both bobbins dropping to zero flow.
8. The 'full' N_2O cylinder is closed.
9. Repeat the test for the 'in use' O_2 and N_2O cylinders.
10. Replace bottles that have little remaining gas.
11. Open the 'in use' O_2 and N_2O cylinders.
12. Ensure that the vaporizer is full, with the filling port tightly closed, that spindle operation is smooth, and that the connection hoses (if appropriate) are connected to the vaporizer.
13. Check over-pressure and emergency air-intake valves.

The testing of machines that receive a service supply from banked cylinders requires additional steps. These machines should have an emergency oxygen cylinder attached to the machine and this should be tested with the vaporizer as above. The back-up cylinder is then turned off. The piped sources of oxygen and nitrous oxide are then connected to the machine and checked with a 'tug' test – a sharp pull at the connection – to ensure they are correctly attached. The O_2 and N_2O flowmeters are opened to check adequate flow and then turned off ready for the anaesthetic.

'Shutting down' the anaesthetic machine

When all surgery is finished, the content status of all cylinders is checked and empty cylinders are removed. If piped gases are present, the Schrader probes are removed from the wall sockets and the pipes neatly coiled. The N_2O and O_2 cylinder valves are closed. The N_2O and O_2 flowmeters are opened to a flow of 2 l/min and closed once the flow indicator has fallen to '0'. The O_2 flush valve is activated until no pressure registers on the pressure gauge. Machine surfaces are wiped down.

Pollution control systems

Exposure to anaesthetic gases has been associated with the development of malignancies, neuropathy, bone marrow toxicity, a higher incidence of abortions and infertility in theatre personnel and congenital abnormalities in their offspring. Although many of the studies reporting these effects have been criticised for weaknesses in methodology, the risk of chronic exposure remains a serious concern to veterinary staff. Under COSHH (Control of Substances Hazardous to Health) Regulations (see Chapter 1) the employer has a duty to assess the risk of exposure to anaesthetic gases to employees and take the appropriate measures to protect their health. The Health and Safety Executive has proposed the following occupational exposure standards (OES) based on an 8-hour time-weighted average (TWA), i.e. the average level of anaesthetic gas in the environment if measured over an 8-hour period:

- Nitrous oxide: 100 ppm
- Halothane: 10 ppm
- Enflurane: 50 ppm
- Isoflurane: 50 ppm
- Ether 400 ppm.

For shorter periods of operation, as more commonly seen in veterinary practice, it is suggested that short-term exposure should not exceed three times this average environmental inhalant limit. The use of scavenging systems combined with careful anaesthetic techniques can reduce pollution by up to 90% and ensure an environment safely below these OES levels. Scavenging systems include both passive and active methods. Generally, active methods are more efficient, though in some circumstances passive methods are adequate.

Passive scavenging

This relies on the patient's respiratory efforts to void the waste gases via a wide-bore (22 mm) tube to the outside of the building. To be effective the exit must be protected from significant air currents such that excessive sub-atmospheric or positive pressure could be generated within the tube and affect function. Further scavenging to the roof level would produce a back pressure due to the heavier gases pooling in the tube. Generally, a tube length of no more than 2.6 m is acceptable.

A variation of this method is the active charcoal absorber that chemically absorbs hydrocarbon inhalation anaesthetics. It collects gas via a short tube from the scavenging shroud of the breathing circuit and removes the inhaled anaesthetic. However, it does not absorb nitrous oxide, and confirming that it is not exhausted can only be performed by weighing the absorber. It also adds further resistance to the passive system.

Active–passive scavenging

Similar to the passive system, a wide-bore tube scavenges exhaled gas from the expiratory valve of the circuit, but passes the gas to a forced ventilation system rather than outside. It is important to ensure that this ventilation system does not dump the gas in another workplace or recirculate the gas.

Active scavenging

This is the preferred method and the most likely to meet COSHH standards. It consists of three main components:

- **Transfer system** – consists of a tube and connector (usually 30 mm) attached to the expiratory port of the circuit.
- **Receiving system** – functions as an air break, preventing excessive positive or negative pressure reaching the breathing system. Often it consists of a simple open-ended reservoir system, allowing venting of excess positive pressure or uptake of atmospheric gas if excess negative pressure develops. Alternatively a reservoir bag and safety valve can be used.

- **Disposal system to the exterior** – delivers the gas to the outside of the building and includes an active suction method. Frequently this consists of a fan unit or a pump system.

Safety procedures

Good anaesthetic technique is also important to ensure minimal exposure to waste gases. Recommended procedures include the following.

- Check the anaesthetic machine and circuit for leaks.
- Turn on the scavenging system and connect it to the breathing circuit prior to anaesthesia.
- Intubate the patient with an appropriate-sized cuffed endotracheal tube and inflate the cuff.
- Avoid the use of face masks when possible.
- Turn on the anaesthetic gases (other than oxygen) only after the patient is connected to the circuit.
- Avoid disconnecting the patient during anaesthesia.
- Flush the circuit with oxygen for 30 seconds prior to disconnection at the end of procedure and empty the remaining gas in the reservoir bag into the scavenging system.
- Fill the vaporizers at the end of the day in a well ventilated area.
- Service all equipment annually.
- Monitor theatre pollution annually.

Other anaesthetic equipment

Other equipment required for anaesthesia includes endotracheal tubes, masks, laryngoscopes and suction devices. Proper use and care of these pieces of equipment is invaluable in ensuring safe anaesthesia.

Endotracheal tubes

These connect the patient to the anaesthetic breathing system. Most patterns have cuffs at the distal (patient) end which, when filled with air, produce a gas-tight seal. Construction materials confer different properties on the tube. Red rubber tubes have poor resistance to kinking and conform poorly to airway contours. Tubes made of polyvinyl chloride (PVC) are the softest and least irritating to the tracheal mucosa; they have little tendency to kink and they mould to the curve of the airway at body temperature.

Care, maintenance and storage depend on the material of construction. Red rubber tubes are deteriorated by oil and petroleum-based lubricants. After cleaning and sterilization, tubes should be dried thoroughly and stored in a cool, dry environment. They should not be exposed to direct sunlight.

Before use, the tubes should be checked for patency and the cuffs' ability to hold pressure should be established. The tube connector should be tight and fit snugly with the chosen breathing system. The tube should be an appropriate length and a range of tube diameters should be made available.

After use, the tubes should be rinsed in running water and left to soak in detergent solution. Later they should be scrubbed inside and out to remove residual mucus. Rinsing must be thorough to remove detergent.

Sterilizing procedures depend on the material. Red rubber tubes are deteriorated by heat sterilization but can be autoclaved for 10 to 20 times. Alternatively they can be disinfected with chlorhexidine solutions. Polysiloxane tubes can also be autoclaved. While most PVC tubes are designed for single use only, they may be safely reused after cleaning and sterilizing. Ethylene oxide must be used cautiously and adequate aeration allowed afterwards (at least 48 hours). Gamma-irradiated single-use items and PVC tubes should not be sterilized with ethylene oxide.

Masks

These are used for administering oxygen and for volatile anaesthetics when an endotracheal tube is not present. Patterns made of malleable rubber can be shaped to fit the animal's face and minimize apparatus dead-space. Others are made of rigid plastic with a perforated rubber diaphragm; they have high dead-space and so require greater gas flows. However, for birds and laboratory animal species they can be constructed from syringe cases and latex gloves. Customized equipment should have minimum dead-space; it should not confer resistance to respiration; and it should allow the animal to be seen.

Care, maintenance and storage considerations for masks are the same as those for endotracheal tubes. Masks can be sterilized by soaking in a 0.2% chlorhexidine solution.

Laryngoscopes

Laryngoscopes consist of a handle and a blade and are available in several patterns and sizes. They serve to depress the base of the tongue during intubation; in so doing, they evert the epiglottis. A bulb at the tip of the blade illuminates the oropharynx. Ideally, the bulb should only illuminate when the blade is 'fixed' in the working position.

Before use, it is important to ensure that the bulb is firmly positioned and that the batteries are charged. After use, blades should be wiped clean with a swab soaked in alcohol. Laryngoscopes must not be immersed in water.

Suction devices

Connected either to a central vacuum pipeline or to a portable pump unit, these devices allow suction of body secretions and are particularly relevant to anaesthesia. They are probably the most important piece of resuscitation equipment and are used to clear mucus, blood and other debris from the pharynx, trachea and main bronchi. Suction is also used to clear the surgical site of blood, and allow gastrointestinal drainage, wound drainage and pleural drainage. The devices consist of three essential components:

- Source of vacuum
- Reservoir or collection vessel
- Suction tubing.

The **vacuum source** can be via a central vacuum pipeline or a portable unit. An appropriate-sized **collection vessel** is one that is large enough to collect the aspirated material but not too large or cumbersome. The interface between the collection vessel and the rest of the unit must be kept clean and free from damage to ensure adequate suction function.

Addition optional features include:

- Cut-off valve – to prevent aspirated liquid entering the pump
- Bacterial filter – to prevent contamination of the room with aspirated bacteria
- Vacuum control valve – to allow adjustment of the degree of vacuum applied
- Vacuum gauge – to indicate the degree of suction
- Foam prevention – foam may cause closure of the cut-off valve or contaminate the filter or pump
- Stop valve – to occlude the suction tubing and allow build-up of vacuum
- Two collection vessels – to allow continuous operation when one vessel is full or non-functional and to provide overflow when the first vessel is full.

Muscle relaxants

Several types of drug produce muscle relaxation, including general anaesthetics. When absolute relaxation is required, however, neuromuscular blocker agents ('muscle relaxants') are used because they are the most effective and predictable. These drugs, derived from poisons used with blow-darts by indigenous South Americans, act on nicotinic receptors at the neuromuscular junction of skeletal muscle. They have no direct effect on smooth or cardiac muscle.

Neuromuscular blocking drugs do not cross the blood–brain barrier and so do not alter consciousness. However, they eliminate some of the obvious signs of inadequate anaesthesia – movement, ocular position and cranial nerve reflexes – so that monitoring the level of anaesthesia becomes more complicated. Because the animal cannot respond normally to inadequate anaesthesia, the anaesthetist must ensure that the animal is unconscious.

The respiratory muscles (external intercostals and diaphragm) are blocked by relaxants and so ventilation stops. Therefore a means of supporting ventilation must be available, e.g. a cuffed endotracheal tube and a suitable breathing system. There are two types of relaxant based on their mechanism of action: depolarizing and non-depolarizing drugs.

Depolarizing drugs

Succinylcholine has a rapid onset time (seconds) and is short-acting (3–5 minutes) in horses, pigs, cats and humans. It is used to facilitate endotracheal intubation in humans, and less commonly in pigs and cats, or during induction of anaesthesia in horses.

Non-depolarizing drugs

Many types of non-depolarizing drug have been used in veterinary practice and some have more or less fallen out of use.

- D-**Tubocurarine** is seldom used these days because injection causes histamine release in dogs, resulting in vasodilatation, hypotension, tachycardia and bronchial spasm.
- **Gallamine** became unpopular because of tachycardia and hypertension after injection. Prolonged relaxation occurs with animals in renal failure.
- **Alcuronium**, a long-acting relaxant, is only occasionally used nowadays.
- **Pancuronium** has an intermediate onset and long duration of action (more than 30 minutes), causes modest tachycardia after injection, but remains a useful agent.
- **Vecuronium**, a popular drug, derived from pancuronium, has an intermediate duration of action (20–30 minutes). It has little cumulative effect after repeated doses and little, if any, cardiovascular effect.
- **Atracurium** is another popular relaxant because of its intermediate duration of action and rapid onset time. It is spontaneously degraded (Hofmann degradation) and so the agent is favoured in animals with diseased elimination pathways (liver and kidneys).

Indications for neuromuscular blockade

High-risk cases
Neuromuscular blockers reduce anaesthetic requirements and so cardiopulmonary function is preserved. Positive pressure ventilation must be imposed.

Thoracic surgery and diaphragmatic hernia repair
For thoracic surgery and repair of diaphragmatic hernias, positive pressure ventilation is required. Positive pressure ventilation can be imposed without neuromuscular blockade; however, in paralysed animals, reduced rigidity in the thoracic cage (ribs and diaphragm) means that lower inflation pressures can be used, producing less cardiovascular compromise. Anaesthesia is frequently smoother.

Oesophageal foreign body removal
Oesophageal foreign body removal in dogs is facilitated by neuromuscular blockade, as a significant component of oesophageal musculature is skeletal in the dog. Relaxed oesophageal musculature allows retrieval of relatively large objects without the need for thoracotomy.

Laparotomies
During laparotomy, neuromuscular blockers reduce the amount of traction required to produce exposure, causing less tissue trauma on the wound margins with less postoperative inflammation and pain.

Microsurgery
Intraocular and neurological surgery (which is frequently performed under microscopy) requires guaranteed immobility.

Inefficient ventilatory pattern
Joint surgery and other procedures occasionally cause bizarre breathing patterns that are inefficient in terms of gas exchange. In these, relaxants allow positive pressure ventilation to be imposed without the animal 'fighting the ventilator'.

Monitoring blockade
The degree of relaxation is measured using a peripheral nerve stimulator. Clinical signs must be used when stimulators are unavailable. Because diaphragmatic and respiratory muscles are relatively resistant to neuromuscular blockers, the first sign of a waning block is diaphragmatic 'twitching'.

Neuromuscular blockers paralyse facial skeletal muscle and eliminate normal reflexes; after paralysis, the eyelids are open and the eye is central. There are no corneal or palpebral reflexes. In animals that are paralysed but not unconscious, there may be increased jaw tone and mydriasis, lacrimation, salivation, tachycardia and hypertension. When these signs are present, anaesthesia must be deepened by increasing the vaporizer setting or, by injecting intravenous anaesthetic.

Antagonism
Non-depolarizing neuromuscular blockers can be antagonized using a combination of anticholinesterase and antimuscarinic drugs, commonly either edrophonium or neostigmine with atropine or glycopyrrolate.

Monitoring

Monitoring anaesthesia is an important aspect of safe anaesthesia and is commonly performed by the veterinary nurse. Close attention to the patient allows rapid intervention if the patient becomes too light, too deep or physiologically compromised. Good monitoring and rapid correction of developing problems will prevent minor disturbances from becoming major complications.

The goals of monitoring are to provide an appropriate depth of anaesthesia for the procedure required, whilst maintaining normal physiological function of the patient. Central nervous system function is assessed to maintain depth of anaesthesia, whilst cardiovascular and respiratory function are the main systems monitored to ensure normal body function. In addition, close attention to body temperature is required. In performing good monitoring, regular and continuous observation of the patient is required. The maintenance of detailed written records of each anaesthetic is to be recommended; it will focus the anaesthetist on patient monitoring, allow identification of developing trends and provide a legal record of the anaesthetic.

Monitoring central nervous system function

Monitoring CNS function during anaesthesia is a major component of assessing 'depth' of anaesthesia. Depression of cranial nerve reflexes gives valuable information on this. Additionally, changes in cardiopulmonary parameters during anaesthesia give further indirect information on patient depth. Under normal circumstances, the 'deeper' the level of anaesthesia, the greater is the cardiopulmonary depression. Hence, to provide adequate conditions for performing the procedure requested whilst preserving patient physiological function, anaesthesia is generally maintained at a relatively 'light' level.

Stages in anaesthesia

For convenience, the 'depth' of anaesthesia has been categorized into four stages (though this is somewhat arbitrary, because it is based on observations in humans anaesthetized with ether). Stages I and II are unpleasant for the patient and hazardous for the anaesthetist. An elegant induction passes through these stages rapidly. This is achieved by adequate preanaesthetic sedative medication and sufficient anaesthetic for induction.

Stage I: stage of voluntary excitement

This begins with induction and lasts until unconsciousness is present. The animal resists induction, shows signs of apprehension and fear but later becomes disorientated. Pulse and respiratory rates are elevated, but breath-holding may occur if irritant or pungent vapours are given. The pupils are dilated. Skeletal muscle activity may be marked and hyper-reflexia may be present.

Stage II: stage of involuntary excitement

This lasts from the onset of unconsciousness until rhythmic breathing is present. All cranial nerve reflexes are present and may be hyperactive. Initially the eye is wide open and the pupil dilated. Later, eyes begin to rotate to a ventromedial position. Responses to toe withdrawal reflexes are brisk. Breathing is irregular but later becomes regular.

Stage III: surgical anaesthesia

This is subdivided into three planes:

- **Plane 1**. Respiration is regular and deep. Spontaneous limb movement is absent but pinch reflexes are brisk. Nystagmus, the lateral oscillation of the eyeball, if present, slows and stops by the end of Plane 1. Eyeball position in

the orbit is ventromedial; opening the eye reveals mainly sclera. The third eyelid moves part way across the corneal surface. Palpebral reflexes begin to slow but the corneal reflex is brisk. Cardiovascular function is only slightly depressed. This plane is suitable for abscess lancing and superficial surgery such as skin suturing and cutaneous tumour removal.
- **Plane 2**. Eye position is ventromedial and the eyelids may be partially separated. The palpebral reflex is sluggish or absent although corneal reflexes persist. The conjunctival surface is moist and the pupil constricted. Muscle relaxation is more apparent. The pedal reflex becomes sluggish and ultimately is lost. Tidal volume is decreased; respiratory rate may be increased or decreased. The heart rate and blood pressure may be modestly reduced. This plane is adequate for most surgery except some laparotomy and thoracotomy.
- **Plane 3**. The eyeball becomes central and the eyelids begin to open. The pupillary diameter increases. The pedal reflex is lost and abdominal muscles are relaxed. Heart rate and blood pressure are lowered. This plane is adequate for all procedures.

Stage IV: overdosage

This is characterized by progressive respiratory failure. The pulse may be rapid or very slow and becomes impalpable. The eye becomes central, the eyelids open, the pupils are maximally dilated and the corneal surface is dry. Capillary refill time becomes prolonged. Accessory respiratory muscle activity, indicated by twitching in the throat, represents agonal gasping. This may superficially mimic inadequate anaesthesia.

Indicators of 'depth' of anaesthesia

Cranial nerve reflexes as indicators

- **Palpebral reflex** – a 'blink' occurs when the medial canthus of the eye is stroked with a finger. If the test is repeated too frequently, the reflex becomes sluggish.
- **Corneal reflex** – 'blinking' also occurs when the cornea is gently touched with a moistened cotton bud. This is not a very sensitive test as during clinical anaesthesia it should always be present.
- **Eye position** – during increasing depth of anaesthesia the globe first rocks ventromedially within the orbit and then returns to a more central position with increasing depth.
- **Pupillary diameter** – with increasing depth of anaesthesia the pupil dilates.
- **Jaw tone** – tension in the jaws indicates light levels of anaesthesia.
- **Tongue curl** – during 'light' anaesthesia, the tongue curls when the jaws are opened.
- **Lacrimation** – the eye becomes dry at deep levels of anaesthesia.
- **Salivation** – profuse salivation indicates inadequate anaesthesia.

During surgical anaesthesia the eye will be rotated ventromedially (Figure 22.17) or be just beginning to rotate back dorsally, with a weak or absent palpebral reflex and a constricted pupil.

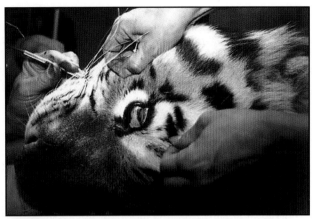

22.17 Siberian tiger with eye rotated ventromedially during anaesthesia for dental surgery.

Respiratory signs

The rate, depth and pattern of respiration are altered by the level of anaesthesia and the degree of surgical stimulation. Increasing respiratory rate often suggests 'light' anaesthesia but can also be seen when the patient is too deeply anaesthetized, so should be used in conjunction with other signs.

Cardiovascular signs

Heart rate, blood pressure and capillary refill time are influenced by the interaction between anaesthetic depth and surgical stimulation. Increasing depth of inhalational anaesthesia is often associated with a dose-dependent decrease in blood pressure with or without a fall in heart rate.

Musculoskeletal tone and withdrawal responses

Light anaesthesia is associated with greater skeletal muscle tone and limb withdrawal reflexes. However, these reflexes are generally lost during clinical anaesthesia.

Drug concentrations

The end-tidal inhalation agent concentration can give an indication of the approximate level of anaesthesia when compared with the specific agent's MAC (minimum alveolar concentration). Individual patient variation will occur and the required end-tidal concentration will depend on what concurrent drugs have been administered, but generally approximately 1–1.5 times MAC is required for surgical anaesthesia. Alternatively, the infusion rate of a total intravenous anaesthetic will give an indication of the likely depth of the patient.

Electroencephalogram (EEG)

The EEG is a recording of the thalamocortical activity of the brain and potentially can be used to assess anaesthetic depth. A number of parameters can be measured but the ones more commonly recorded include the spectral edge frequency, the median frequency and the bispectral analysis (BIS). The first two have enjoyed limited success and only the latter, the BIS, has shown much potential for clinical anaesthetic monitoring. None of these are currently routinely recorded in animals.

Monitoring cardiovascular function

Assessing cardiovascular variables continuously provides information on the depth of anaesthesia, on the effects of surgery (e.g. haemorrhage, inadequate anaesthesia, untoward reflexes) and on cardiovascular function itself. The primary goal is to ensure adequacy of tissue perfusion. In practice there is no single parameter that indicates perfusion absolutely, but rather the veterinary nurse must assess cardiovascular function on the basis of a number of signs. Monitoring of heart rate and pulse characteristics is combined with assessment of the mucous membranes, blood pressure and other parameters to form an overall picture of the state of the cardiovascular system of the patient. The regular direct assessment of peripheral pulse character, strength and rate should form the central component of cardiovascular monitoring around which other aspects and electronic monitoring can be added.

Pulse characteristics, heart rate and rhythm

Pulse quality

The pulse strength gives useful information as to the adequacy of the peripheral circulation. The palpated pulse is the difference between systolic and diastolic arterial blood pressure (i.e. pulse pressure) and though not a direct indicator of blood pressure, it generally gives reliable information as to changes in blood pressure and cardiovascular function. A weak pulse is usually associated with hypotension, often due to myocardial depression during anaesthesia, and an increasingly weak pulse suggests that cardiovascular depression is increasing.

Heart rate

The absolute rate is important as very high and low heart rates are undesirable. Equally changes in the rate give information as to the depth of the patient and cardiovascular stability of the patient. For example, tachycardia may be seen during very light anaesthesia due to sympathetic stimulation, or during periods of hypotension following blood loss, or during excessively 'deep' anaesthesia and severe cardiovascular depression. The rate is drug dependent (e.g. bradycardia with alpha$_2$ agonists) and so a knowledge of what drugs have been administered is important.

Heart rhythm

The heart rhythm gives an indication as to the presence of arrhythmias. A difference in recorded heart and pulse rates is called a **pulse deficit** and usually indicates the presence of a significant arrhythmia. Characterization of such a deficit requires the recording of an ECG (see below).

Palpation of the apex beat is useful in very small companion animals and laboratory animals, or when hypotension makes peripheral pulses impalpable. It gives information on heart rate and rhythm but not pulse strength. Similarly cardiac auscultation allows assessment of heart rate and rhythm but not pulse quality. While heart sounds may be heard with standard (precordial) stethoscopes, these tend to fall off even when adhesive tape is used. Oesophageal stethoscopes are less prone to displacement.

Heart rate monitors detect ECG signal and produce an audible beep or digital read out. This provides limited information as it only indicates the presence of electrical activity and not cardiac output. Such monitors will continue to register a 'beat' long after output from the heart and a palpable pulse have been lost. The ECG and pulse oximeter can also be used as heart rate monitors (see below).

Mucous membranes and capillary refill time

The general appearance of the mucous membranes can provide valuable indications as to the state of the cardiovascular system (see Chapter 13). Ideally they should be pink, indicating good tissue oxygenation, but bright pink suggests hypercapnia. Pale, grey or dry mucous membranes are indicative of poor peripheral perfusion. White can indicate anaemia, peripheral vasoconstriction, or hypovolaemia.

The capillary refill time indicates adequacy of peripheral perfusion. Generally the refill time should be between 1 and 2 seconds. A time of greater than 2 seconds is associated with poor perfusion. It is not absolute, as the refill time may be adequate in some situations of impaired venous return and poor arterial perfusion: capillaries can refill from engorged veins as well as arteries.

Arterial blood pressure

Arterial blood pressure gives information about adequacy of the cardiovascular system. It is not a direct monitor of cardiac output but, in the presence of myocardial depressant anaesthetic agents, it is a useful indirect indicator. Arterial blood pressure (ABP) is related to cardiac output (CO), right atrial pressure (RAP) and total peripheral resistance (TPR) by the following equation:

$$ABP - RAP = CO \times TPR$$

Most anaesthetics decrease cardiac output and total peripheral resistance (right atrial pressure remains minimally affected). The degree of inhalant-induced hypotension is dose-dependent, hence blood pressure is a useful indicator of cardiovascular depression as well as depth of anaesthesia. An exception occurs where vasoconstrictors have been given, producing hypertension without increased CO. This is seen after the administration of an alpha$_2$ agonist. In general, during anaesthesia the aim is to maintain mean ABP above 70–80 mmHg.

Direct measurement of blood pressure is the gold standard allowing continuous recording of blood pressure even at low pressures. A catheter is aseptically placed in an accessible artery (e.g. dorsal pedal, femoral, middle auricular arteries). It is connected via a heparin saline column to an anaeroid manometer or to a strain-gauge pressure transducer. The anaeroid manometer is cheap but only indicates mean ABP. The electronic pressure transducer provides systolic and diastolic pressures as well and a pulse waveform, but is expensive. Arterial catheters allow blood gas analysis and are particularly valuable in high-risk patients.

Indirect methods are based on the use of a cuff applied around a limb or tail and a method of detecting the peripheral pulse distal to or under the cuff. Cuff width should be about 40% of limb circumference. Wider cuffs transmit pressure more efficiently and underestimate pressure, whilst narrow cuffs overestimate it. The following two methods are commonly used.

Oscillometric method

The occluding cuff also senses pulsation. The cuff is inflated above systolic blood pressure and no blood flows past it. As the cuff is deflated, blood starts to pulse through it; the cuff senses this oscillation. Return of pulsation occurs at systolic ABP. Maximum oscillation corresponds to mean ABP. This method indicates systolic, mean and diastolic pressures and gives a heart rate. It is automated and reasonably accurate in dogs, but less reliable in hypotensive states and cats, and is moderately expensive.

Doppler flow detection

A Doppler ultrasound flow detector placed over a peripheral artery senses blood moving in the artery and produces an audible sound for each pulse. A cuff is applied proximal to the

sensor on the limb or tail. The cuff is inflated above systolic blood pressure, above which the audible sound is abolished, and then the cuff is deflated until the audible pulsation returns. The pressure in the cuff at this time-point gives systolic ABP. It is simple and cheap, works well in dogs and cats, is reliable in hypotensive states, and is probably the most appropriate method for general practice (Figure 22.18).

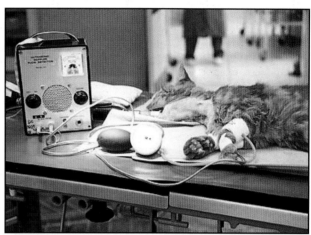

22.18 Doppler flow detector blood pressure monitor used in a cat.

Central venous pressure

Often neglected, central venous pressure (CVP) reflects filling of right heart and provides a valuable indicator of the circulating blood volume. A catheter is introduced into the jugular vein and advanced to the anterior vena cava. The zero point is the pressure of the right atrium or level of the sternal manubrium. It is a useful inexpensive indicator of response to fluid therapy. A change is as important as the actual value, indicating response to therapy, and as long as it is within the normal range the risk of overinfusion of fluids is minimal. Normal values are between 0 and 7 cm H_2O in the dog and cat.

Electrocardiography

An electrocardiogram (ECG) describes the electrical activity of the heart. Changes in rhythm can be associated with systemic abnormalities (hypoxia, electrolyte disturbance) and cardiac pathology. It is not indicative of cardiac output or mechanical activity of the heart and electrical activity can remain normal minutes after onset of cardiac arrest.

Monitoring respiratory function

Assessment of respiratory function is as important as monitoring cardiovascular function in ensuring the well-being of the patient during anaesthesia and centres on ensuring adequate ventilation and oxygenation of blood. The veterinary nurse should be continuously observing the respiratory rate and pattern of the animal as well as the extent of reservoir bag inflation and deflation during each breath. In addition, there are a number of electronic monitors that can add valuable information to the assessment of ventilation.

Respiration rate, depth and pattern

The rate of respiration gives some information about adequacy of ventilation and depth of anaesthesia. Though only a crude indicator, it alerts to problems when the rate is very slow (**bradypnoea**) or very fast (**tachypnoea**). When combined with the assessment of depth of ventilation, a better assessment of ventilation (and depth of anaesthesia) can be made. Observing chest excursion or reservoir bag movement can give a good idea of the adequacy of ventilation for the size of the animal. In addition, mechanical and electronic monitors can be used that record the **minute volume** (i.e. volume of gas inspired per minute) of the patient. An example of a mechanical minute volume recorder is Wright's respirometer.

The pattern of respiration can also provide valuable information. Irregular ventilation can indicate pathology; for example, Cheyne–Stokes breathing or gasping suggests dangerously 'deep' anaesthesia. Certain drugs are associated with irregular respiratory patterns; for example, ketamine anaesthesia in the cat produces an apneustic pattern with periods of apnoea interspersed with regular bursts of a number of breaths. Very shallow rapid breathing can be seen during inappropriately light planes of anaesthesia.

Pulse oximetry

Pulse oximetry is a non-invasive method of measuring arterial oxygen saturation and gives valuable information about gas exchange and arterial oxygenation. It rapidly responds to falling arterial oxygen saturation and can be life saving in situations such as during airway obstruction and hypoxia. It does not allow accurate assessment of adequacy of ventilation as it does not tell the clinician anything about arterial carbon dioxide, which is what mammals primarily regulate their ventilation to. A patient on 100% O_2 during anaesthesia can easily have an arterial O_2 saturation of $> 95\%$ even when it is underventilating. However, if ventilation became so reduced as to produce hypoxia, the pulse oximeter would then display a reduced O_2 saturation. Primarily it alerts to hypoxaemia and is particularly valuable when the patient is just being disconnected from the oxygen at the end of a procedure. During this early period of recovery, rapid detection of hypoxia and compromised ventilation can allow early correction of ventilatory problems (e.g. during respiratory obstruction), preventing the development of serious complications and cardiopulmonary arrest (Figure 22.19).

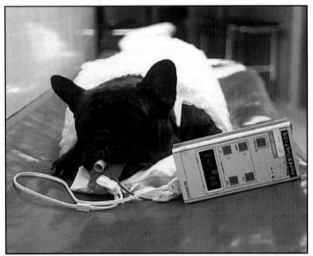

22.19 Pulse oximeter being used postoperatively after airway surgery.

The pulse oximeter can be placed anywhere on the patient where there is an area of non-pigmented skin where light can easily be transmitted through tissue. Common sites where it is applied include the tongue, ear pinna, mammary teat and the vulva.

Capnography

Capnography is based on the measurement of exhaled carbon dioxide (end-tidal CO_2) and provides valuable information on respiratory as well as cardiovascular function. Usually it is measured from gas withdrawn from a small tube placed between the circuit and the endotracheal tube. End-tidal CO_2 approximates to alveolar and arterial CO_2 and so gives an excellent indicator of ventilatory adequacy: if the end-tidal CO_2 level is high, it suggests that ventilation is inadequate as the body is not blowing off sufficient CO_2, whereas a low level suggests overventilation.

The end-tidal CO_2 level is also related to how much CO_2 is produced in the tissues and how effectively it is delivered to the lungs. Thus a very high end-tidal CO_2 level is seen with malignant hyperthermia due to massively elevated levels of CO_2 production by the tissues (especially muscles). Further, if the heart's ability to pump blood is compromised (e.g. very deep anaesthesia or onset of cardiac arrest), the amount of CO_2-rich blood (venous blood) delivered to the lungs and exhaled will be reduced. In this situation, although blood CO_2 is high, the measured end-tidal CO_2 will be low.

Capnography is becoming cheaper and increasingly popular in practice. It is a valuable non-invasive monitor to aid patient assessment.

Blood gas analysis

Blood gas analysis of a blood sample withdrawn from an artery allows the definitive assessment of respiratory gas exchange. The blood gas analyser measures the partial pressure of CO_2 (pCO_2) and O_2 (pO_2) in the sample and pH. It allows the assessment of adequacy of ventilation (pCO_2), arterial oxygenation (pO_2) and acid/base status (pH) of the patient.

Blood gas machines are expensive and require regular maintenance. Presently they are found primarily in referral institutions.

Monitoring temperature

General anaesthesia interferes with the animal's ability to regulate temperature and the patient may become hypothermic or hyperthermic. Hypothermia is most commonly seen during anaesthesia. It delays recovery, increases morbidity and at very low temperatures can result in mortality. Though often overlooked during anaesthesia, it is important to monitor temperature perioperatively. Particular attention should be given to monitoring temperature of very small patients, young and old animals and during prolonged periods of anaesthesia.

Mercury thermometers are the most commonly used thermometers but they need to be removed to be read. During anaesthesia thermistors or thermocouples are more useful, as they allow a continuous record of temperature.

Central body temperature ('core' temperature) is the most informative during anaesthesia. It can be estimated by measuring temperature in the thoracic oesophagus or at the tympanic membrane. Rectal temperature is less accurate but still an acceptable alternative. In addition, peripheral temperature can be measured at the skin. The difference between 'core' and peripheral temperature gives an indication of the state of peripheral tissue perfusion. During shock the core–peripheral gradient is elevated; this is commonly seen in the shocked animal that presents with cold paws and distal limbs.

General monitoring of the patient

Other monitoring activities performed during the anaesthetic period include the following:

- **Urine output:** Catheterizing the urinary bladder and measuring the collected urine enable estimation of urine output. This is a simple and valuable method of assessing kidney function. A value in excess of 1 ml/kg/h is held to represent adequate renal perfusion, and therefore vital organ perfusion
- **Fluid administration:** If fluids are being given, the administration rates should be checked periodically. If a catheter is in place but fluids are not given, it should be flushed with heparin–saline regularly
- **Surgery:** The veterinary nurse should be aware of what surgical activity is occurring throughout anaesthesia. Haemorrhage must be continuously assessed. Liaison with the veterinary surgeon is vital during complicated surgery (e.g. thoracotomy)
- **The breathing system:** The system must be continuously monitored for behaviour, disconnection, soda lime exhaustion, valve action etc. The pilot balloon of the endotracheal tube must be periodically checked to ensure that the cuff remains gas-tight
- **Gas flows and vaporizer settings:** Flowmeters may 'drift' with time and should be constantly checked. Vaporizer fluid levels, settings and temperature should also be monitored. Cylinder contents must be assessed continuously.

Special anaesthesia

Occasionally, animals with severe physiological disturbances present for procedures requiring general anaesthesia. Each procedure carries its own individual risks; however, the anaesthetic approach should be similar. Careful preoperative assessment and stabilization (where possible) are required. Anaesthesia should be smooth, with minimal disruption of physiological function, and careful attention should be given to the recovery period.

General considerations

Preoperative assessment

Careful patient evaluation is important (see the beginning of this chapter). Consideration of cardiovascular, respiratory, liver and renal function and concurrent therapy should be given.

Preoperative stabilization

Aspects include fluid therapy and electrolyte and acid–base stabilization, oxygen therapy for hypoxaemia and blood product administration for anaemia, clotting defects and protein deficits. Also analgesia, antibiosis and specific procedures may be required, e.g. stomach decompression in gastric dilatation–volvulus (GDV).

General anaesthesia

The high-risk patient is less able to tolerate physiological disturbance. Hence it is important to maintain normal physiological status especially cardiovascular, respiratory and thermoregulatory function. Pre-oxygenation with a face mask prior to induction of anaesthesia can be beneficial.

Anaesthetic agents have a more profound effect in the debilitated animal. It is important to reduce drug doses, use drugs that depress cardiopulmonary function less and give induction agents slowly to effect. Careful monitoring is important to be alert to dangers and allow rapid correction of problems.

Recovery

Careful attention into the recovery period is often neglected. Monitoring should be continued with fluid therapy, rewarming and analgesia when appropriate.

Anaesthesia of the neonate

Neonates are defined as immature animals under 12 weeks of age. Significant differences exist from the mature animal. Overestimation of neonate size often leads to overdose; and immature body systems make them more sensitive to anaesthetics and less able to accommodate alterations in their normal function. An understanding of these differences is necessary for safe anaesthetic management.

Physiological considerations

Respiratory system

Oxygen consumption is two to three times that of the adult; minute ventilation is about three times that of the adult; there is a greater risk of airway obstruction; and alveolar collapse is more likely. All these factors predispose the neonate to hypoxia during anaesthesia. Careful IPPV may be appropriate but excessive pressure can cause damage. Neonates aged 4–14 weeks can be allowed to ventilate spontaneously.

Cardiovascular system

The myocardium is less contractile, the baroreceptors are immature, and there is a predominance of parasympathetic nervous system activity. Haemoglobin concentrations are lower and the red blood cells have a shorter life span. Thus neonates are less able to increase force of contraction to meet changes in demand; increases in cardiac output are heart-rate dependent. Hence hypotension is a particular problem and neonates are less able to cope with blood loss.

Hepatorenal function

Enzyme systems are immature or absent. Hypoglycaemia is likely. Renal function is immature, thus there is poor renal concentrating function and reduced ability to tolerate dehydration. Maximum preparatory starvation of 2–3 hours is suggested. Intraoperative fluids, preferably including glucose (e.g. dextrose–saline), should be given.

Thermoregulation

Neonates have immature thermoregulatory control, with reduced shivering ability and reliance on non-shivering thermogenesis. There is a large ratio of surface area to volume and less subcutaneous fat. Hence neonates are prone to hypothermia.

Pharmacokinetics

Low albumin and a larger percentage of body water, lower body fat and reduced hepatorenal function affect the pharmacology of drugs used. In general the dose of parenteral drugs needs to be reduced in the neonate.

Anaesthesia

The addition of an anticholinergic to maintain heart rate and reduce respiratory secretion is recommended in young neonates. Sedatives should be used sparingly

- Benzodiazepines are useful, though often sedation is poor.
- Below 10 weeks, acepromazine maleate is best avoided.
- Alpha$_2$ adrenoceptor agonists are potent sedatives and best avoided.
- Analgesics such as opioids are useful, though may have a prolonged action; a reduced dose is recommended.

Induction of anaesthesia can be achieved by injectable or inhaled methods. The latter is generally more stressful, but in young neonates can be a valuable technique. With less body fat and reduced metabolic function, prolonged recoveries are likely in the neonate after barbiturate anaesthesia.

- Propofol produces smooth induction of anaesthesia and a relatively rapid recovery and may be preferred.
- Dissociative agents (e.g. ketamine) can be used.
- Saffan can be used in cats but a prolonged recovery may be seen.

Maintenance with inhalation anaesthesia is recommended for all but the shortest procedures. Isoflurane, with its lower blood gas solubility than halothane, less reliance on metabolism in the liver, and less myocardial depression, is preferred over halothane. Caution is required with endotracheal intubation; the larynx is more susceptible to trauma and small narrow tubes are more liable to obstruction. Preservation of body temperature is important and these patients should be well insulated and actively warmed during anaesthesia. During recovery, attention should be given to body temperature to encourage a rapid return to consciousness.

Anaesthesia of the aged patent

As for the neonate, ageing affects physiological function and anaesthesia. Age results in a reduced capacity for adaptation and reduced functional reserves of organ systems. Though not a disease itself, it is frequently accompanied by systemic disease.

General considerations

- **Central nervous system:** There are generally reduced requirements for anaesthetics.
- **Respiratory system:** Reduced tidal volume and efficiency of gas exchange increase the risk of hypoxia.
- **Cardiovascular changes:** The maximum heart rate falls with age and the response to stress/catecholamines is reduced. Geriatric (senior) animals are poorly tolerant of volume depletion.
- **Hepatorenal function:** Renally excreted drugs are more slowly eliminated. Renal tubular function is reduced, the renin–angiotensin system less responsive and kidneys are less tolerant of hypotension. The older patient may be in chronic renal failure and prolonged periods of reduced renal perfusion (e.g. during hypotensive anaesthesia) may further damage the kidneys, resulting in acute renal failure. Hepatic clearance decreases with decreasing liver mass.
- **Thermoregulation:** Geriatric animals are prone to hypothermia.
- **Pharmacokinetic considerations:** Contracted blood volume increases plasma concentration of intravenous agents. Protein binding is reduced, due to reduced albumen in plasma. Highly protein-bound drugs are more active.

Anaesthesia
There is no one ideal protocol and all drugs should be administered slowly to effect. Heavy premedication should be avoided, as it can significantly compromise the patient and prolong recovery. Caution should be exercised with alpha$_2$ adrenoceptor agonists, as they are potent sedatives, causing significant depression of cardiovascular function. Benzodiazepines are valuable and can produce good sedation, particularly in combination with an opioid, in the older patient. A rapid smooth induction and calm recovery are preferred. Barbiturates may be associated with a prolonged recovery in patients with significant liver pathology. Propofol ensures a good rapid recovery and Saffan appears acceptable in cats. Inhalation anaesthesia with isoflurane provides a more rapid recovery than halothane.

The shorter the procedures are, the better. Attention to heat loss and fluid therapy are important. Intraoperative fluid therapy is important to maintain renal perfusion and kidney function. Monitoring arterial blood pressure is particularly valuable in ensuring preservation of renal autoregulation and perfusion.

Anaesthesia for caesarean operation

Anaesthesia for caesarean operation is often an emergency without time for extensive preparation. Both dam and fetal viability are important considerations.

General considerations

Maternal physiology
Pregnancy alters maternal physiology:

- **Central nervous system** – increased sensitivity to inhalation agents occurs.
- **Respiratory system** – increased alveolar ventilation, reduced functional residual capacity due to anterior displacement of the diaphragm and increased oxygen consumption are seen. Hence there is increased inhalation agent uptake but also the dam is prone to developing hypoxia and hypercapnia.
- **Cardiovascular system** – aortocaval compression (compression of the large vessels by the gravid uterus) can occur in dorsal recumbency, compromising venous return from the hindquarters. Increased blood volume (30%), reduced haematocrit and plasma proteins, increased cardiac output (30–50%) and reduced total peripheral resistance occur. There are reduced cardiac reserves and relative anaemia. Thus the dam is less tolerant of cardiovascular compromise.
- **Gastrointestinal system** – increased gastric acidity, cranial displacement of stomach by the uterus and altered tone in the lower oesophageal sphincter make the dam more prone to regurgitation, vomiting and aspiration pneumonia.

Uteroplacental circulation and fetal viability
Preservation of blood flow to the fetus is essential to prevent hypoxia and acidosis of the fetus developing prior to removal from the placenta. Reduced uterine blood flow reduces placental perfusion and induces fetal hypoxia. This is particularly seen with shock and hypovolaemia, dehydration, and after administration of drugs such as oxytocin and ergotamine. Stress and release of catecholamines can vasoconstrict the uterine blood vessels and reduce blood flow to the fetus.

Fetal tissues

The umbilical vein delivers drugs derived from the maternal circulation to the fetal liver and the ductus venosus. The fetal circulation attempts to protect vital tissues from exposure to sudden high concentrations of drugs. However, most drugs administered to the dam are transferred rapidly across the placenta and, even when diluted, may depress the fetus or neonate.

Preoperative preparation

This includes clipping (if it is not stressful to the patient), as it will reduce anaesthesia time. Preoperative fluid therapy is indicated if the patient is shocked. Starvation is rarely possible. Positioning in off-dorsal recumbency reduces aortacaval compression.

Anaesthesia

The goals of anaesthesia are the provision of a smooth induction and maintenance of anaesthesia with a rapid recovery of the dam to consciousness to allow nursing, and delivery of viable alert neonates ready to feed. Minimal sedation is preferred. Induction of anaesthesia should be smooth, with rapid endotracheal intubation. Barbiturates inhibit fetal respiration, which may be significant if delivered soon after induction. Recovery of the dam and neonate may be delayed. Propofol gives a rapid and smooth induction and recovery and is recommended. Saffan in cats causes minimal respiratory depression, and is also adequate. Ketamine produces minimal fetal depression but may result in disorientated kittens. Inhalation induction is potentially stressful; if used, intubation must be rapid.

For maintenance of anaesthesia, inhalation anaesthesia is recommended, and isoflurane is preferred over halothane for a more rapid recovery. A light plane of anaesthesia should minimize dose-dependent cardiorespiratory depression and reduce the potential for fetal hypoxia. It is important to maintain blood pressure to protect the fetal circulation, and intraoperative fluid therapy can be valuable. Postoperative pain relief should be administered.

Neonate resuscitation requires adequate help:

- Clean mucus from the upper airways.
- Administer oxygen if required.
- Stimulate the skin.
- Prevent cooling.
- Aim to get the neonate feeding as soon as possible.

Anaesthesia in pyometra

The bitch with pyometritis often presents dull and depressed. Closed pyometritis, in which the mucopurulent discharge accumulates in the uterus, can be life-threatening. Presurgical stabilization is important, but complete stabilization is often impossible prior to removal of the septic focus.

General considerations

- **Shock:** This is a major concern. Hypovolaemia develops via fluid loss to the uterus combined with losses via vomiting and polyuria. Toxaemia can induce septic shock.
- **Renal disease:** Pre-renal uraemia due to hypovolaemia, glomerular disease associated with antibody–antigen complexes and tubular disease due to toxins and immune complexes all interfere with the ability to concentrate urine. Concurrent renal disease of the old bitch may be present.
- **Acid–base and electrolyte disorders:** Metabolic acidosis is common with sodium and potassium loss.

- **Bone marrow suppression and clotting disorders:** Reduced erythrocyte and platelet production occurs. Anaemia is common. Clotting disorders may occur.
- **Liver disorders:** Hepatocellular damage develops due to intrahepatic cholestasis and bile pigment retention. Damage can also be secondary to endotoxaemia, dehydration and shock.
- **Arrhythmias:** Arrhythmias may be present, induced by toxins.

Preoperative preparation

Fluid therapy is essential to restore circulating blood volume, protect renal function, and correct electrolyte and acid–base disorders. Potassium may need to be supplemented. Broad-spectrum antibiosis should be commenced. Platelet-rich plasma, whole blood or red blood cells may be required if there is thrombocytopenia, low plasma proteins, clotting disorders or anaemia.

Anaesthesia

Premedication should cause minimal depression. Sedation is often unnecessary, though benzodiazepines may be beneficial to reduce the induction agent dose required. Analgesia is recommended (e.g. morphine or buprenorphine) to reduce intraoperative and postoperative pain. Induction of anaesthesia should be smooth with minimal cardiopulmonary depression. Most injectable anaesthetics cause cardiovascular depression and should be administered at a reduced dose. Maintenance with inhalation anaesthesia with isoflurane over halothane is preferred. Attention to monitoring and intraoperative fluid therapy are important. Postoperatively, fluid therapy may be required as well as further analgesia with opioids.

Anaesthesia in gastric dilatation–volvulus (GDV)

GDV is an acute emergency of the large dog with a high incidence of mortality (12–43%). Complete stabilization prior to surgery is often impossible, but a significant degree of stabilization dramatically reduces complications and mortality.

General considerations

- **Respiratory compromise:** Ventilation is compromised by the dilated stomach. Endotoxic mediators can disrupt ventilation/perfusion balance, compromising gas exchange in the lungs. Pulmonary oedema can occur.
- **Cardiovascular disturbances:** Compression of the caudal vena cava and portal veins, and pooling of blood in splanchnic, renal and capillary beds, reduces venous return and cardiac output. Cellular hypoxia and metabolic acidosis result. Circulating catecholamines, release of myocardial depressant factor and endotoxin, myocardial hypoxia and ischaemia, metabolic acidosis and electrolyte disturbances all predispose to arrhythmias and myocardial depression.
- **Endotoxaemia:** Ischaemic injury to the gut compromises the mucosal barrier, with increased absorption of endotoxin. Liver clearance of endotoxin is reduced. Shock can ensue with disseminated intravascular coagulation and multiple organ failure.
- **Gastric and splenic damage:** Increased intraluminal pressure and reduced gastric perfusion result in gastric ischaemia. Mucosal compromise allows leakage of plasma proteins, resulting in hypoproteinaemia and oedema. Gastric torsion may compromise perfusion of the spleen, inducing ischaemic damage.

Preoperative preparation

Treatment for shock is essential prior to anaesthesia. Aggressive intravenous fluid therapy to restore circulating blood volume is required. Crystalloids, e.g. lactated Ringer's (up to 90 ml/kg/h), can be used alone or combined with colloids and hypertonic saline (7.5% 4 ml/kg). Positive inotropes (e.g. dopamine or dobutamine) for hypotension unresponsive to fluids may be required. Correction of acidosis and electrolyte disturbances (especially hyperkalaemia) is necessary. The administration of steroids or NSAIDs remains controversial.

Gastric decompression with an orogastric tube with gastric lavage can dramatically improve cardiopulmonary function. Alternatively, percutaneous trocar placement (18 gauge needle) or a gastrotomy may be required. Oxygen therapy should be given if the patient is hypoxic. Antibiosis is appropriate as the mucosal barrier may be compromised. Antacids (e.g. ranitidine or cimetidine) have been suggested and control of cardiac arrhythmias may be necessary.

Anaesthesia

Premedication is rarely required. Minimal cardiovascular depression is essential during induction of anaesthesia. Arrhythmias are likely. An intravenous opioid/benzodiazepine combination is good (e.g. fentanyl 1–2 µg/kg and diazepam 0.1–0.2 mg/kg). Alternatively, a benzodiazepine followed by a reduced dose of propofol given slowly may be acceptable. Maintenance of anaesthesia with isoflurane is preferred; it is less arrhythmogenic and causes less cardiovascular depression than halothane. Nitrous oxide should be avoided until the stomach is decompressed, as it partitions into gas-filled bodies. Careful monitoring is essential and fluid therapy should be continued.

During recovery, complications are frequent. Monitoring is important. Fluid therapy for shock should be continued. Arrhythmias in the postoperative period are common and may require therapy. Anaemia may result from significant blood loss. Reperfusion injury may occur after derotation of the stomach. Bowel mucosal ischaemia occurs due to gastric torsion and compromise to stomach blood supply. Oxygen free radicals and superoxide ions are produced and can be released to the blood when the volvulus is corrected, resulting in further shock.

Small mammals

Relevant anatomy and physiology

Gastrointestinal tract

The majority of species considered here are small herbivores and so have enlarged GI tracts and comparatively small thoracic cavities. This has importance when considering anaesthesia, as hypoventilation and hypoxia may easily occur.

Respiratory tract

Respiratory tract infections and lung consolidation are relatively common in many small herbivores, particularly rats and rabbits. This may further compromise oxygenation and the safety of anaesthesia.

The majority of small herbivores have very narrow openings to their oral cavities and their epiglottis is situated caudally. In addition, the majority are nasal breathers and the epiglottis is therefore positioned dorsal to the soft palate. This makes intubation difficult. The exception is the ferret, which has a large gape and a very easily accessible epiglottis for intubation.

Body size

Many of these species are very small and so have a large body surface area to weight ratio. This allows often excessive heat loss during anaesthesia, and dehydration from the drying effect of anaesthetic gases. Fluid therapy and external heat sources are therefore necessary.

Preanaesthetic preparation

As with other species, a thorough examination prior to anaesthesia is important. Particular care should be taken to observe any signs of respiratory disease, such as the nasal discharge and matted fur of the forepaws seen in rabbit snuffles (a respiratory tract infection due to *Pasteurella multocida* that is frequently accompanied by lung disease).

Fasting is not necessary in most small herbivores such as rabbits, which have a very tight cardiac sphincter and therefore do not vomit. Food should be withheld immediately prior to anaesthesia in species such as guinea pigs to allow emptying of the oral cavity. Ferrets should be starved for a short while, usually 4 hours, as they can vomit, but longer starving may be detrimental and cause hypoglycaemia due to their high metabolic rates.

Weight measurement is vitally important when using injectable medications, as a miscalculation of 4–5 g in a rodent weighing 50 g can lead to a 10% under- or overdosage of medication.

Preanaesthetic medications

- **Atropine** at 0.05 mg/kg 30 minutes before anaesthesia is useful in some species (such as the guinea pig) where excessive salivation and lacrimation occur when using isoflurane. Atropine is not so useful in rabbits, as around 60% have a serum atropinesterase that breaks down atropine before it has a chance to work. **Glycopyrrolate** functions in a similar manner but is not affected by the atropinesterase and may be used instead at doses of 0.01 mg/kg s.c.
- **Acepromazine maleate** can be used at doses of 0.2 mg/kg in ferrets, 0.5 mg/kg in rabbits and 0.5–1 mg/kg in rats, mice, hamsters, chinchillas and guinea pigs. In general it is a very safe premedicant even in debilitated animals, though should be used with caution in hypotensive patients. It is advisable that acepromazine maleate is not used in gerbils, as it reduces the seizure threshold and many gerbils suffer from hereditary epilepsy.
- **Diazepam** is useful as a premedicant in some species. In rodents doses of 3 mg/kg can be used, even in gerbils. In rabbits the benefits are somewhat outweighed by the larger volumes required, and intramuscular injection with the oil-based formulation may be painful. Water-soluble emulsion versions can be given intravenously.
- **Fentanyl/fluanisone** combination (Hypnorm) may be used at varying doses as either a premedicant, a sedative, or as part of an injectable full anaesthesia. As a premedicant, doses of 0.1 ml/kg for rabbits, 0.08 ml/kg for rats or 0.2 ml/kg for guinea pigs (one-fifth the recommended sedation doses) can produce sufficient sedation to prevent breath-holding and allow gaseous induction. These doses are given intramuscularly 15–20 minutes before induction. Hypnorm is irritant and large doses in one spot may cause postoperative lameness. It can be reversed after the operation with butorphanol at 0.2 mg/kg i.v., or buprenorphine at 0.05 mg/kg.

- **Medetomidine** may be combined with ketamine (see section below) or used on its own. For example, in ferrets a dose of 0.1 mg/kg has been suggested as a premedication dosage.

Fluid therapy

Fluid therapy is vitally important. In most species, lactated Ringer's solution is adequate. Maintenance doses are higher than for cats and dogs. with levels of 80–100 ml/kg/day being advised for most small mammals. In cases of mild dehydration or for routine perianaesthetic fluid therapy, subcutaneous administration is acceptable. In cases of moderate to severe dehydration, intraperitoneal, intravenous or intraosseous fluids are advisable.

- Intraperitoneal fluids are given ventrally into the abdominal cavity with the patient in dorsal recumbency.
- Intravenous fluids may be given by the lateral ear vein or the cephalic or saphenous veins in the rabbit, the cephalic or saphenous veins in ferrets, guinea pigs and chinchillas, and the lateral tail veins in rats and mice.
- Intraosseous fluids may be administered where there is severe dehydration and venous access is not possible. These are usually given via the proximal femur in the trochanteric fossa between the hip joint and the greater trochanter of the femur. Sedation and analgesia are often needed to insert the hypodermic or spinal needle, but the advantages are direct venous support via the medullary cavity of the bone, and the ability to attach a drip set and syringe driver to administer a continuous infusion of fluids.

Local anaesthesia

The use of EMLA cream (a lidocaine/prilocaine topical anaesthetic cream) applied to the skin surface prior to placement of intravenous catheters is extremely useful, particularly in rabbits. To avoid laryngospasm, lidocaine spray should be used when intubating small mammals.

Induction of anaesthesia: injectable agents

Propofol

This has some limited usage in small mammals. It may be used in ferrets at 10 mg/kg after the use of a premedicant such as acepromazine maleate (0.2 mg/kg), or at 1–3 mg/kg after the use of a premedicant such as medetomidine (0.08–0.1 mg/kg). Its use is limited in rabbits and hystricomorphs (because of the ensusing apnoea) and in the smaller rodents (because it needs to be given intravenously).

Ketamine combinations

Rabbits

Ketamine is used at a dose of 20–35 mg/kg in conjunction with medetomidine at 0.3–0.5 mg/kg or with xylazine at 5 mg/kg. Lower doses are used for debilitated animals. The advantages are a quick and stress-free anaesthesia, but the vasoconstrictive effects of medetomidine make detection of hypoxia difficult. Respiratory depression during longer procedures may become a problem and intubation is often advised. A triple combination of ketamine, medetomidine and butorphanol may also be used safely in rabbits. Doses of 0.2 mg/kg medetomidine plus 10 mg/kg ketamine and 0.5 mg/kg butorphanol may be given subcutaneously to induce anaesthesia. Medetomidine may be reversed using atipamezole at 1 mg/kg.

Rats and mice

In rats, ketamine can be used at 90 mg/kg in conjunction with xylazine at 5 mg/kg, i.m. or i.p. In mice and hamsters it is used at 100–150 mg/kg in conjunction with xylazine at 5 mg/kg. These combinations provide about 30 minutes of anaesthesia. In gerbils the dose of xylazine may be reduced to 2–3 mg/kg as they appear to be more sensitive to the hypovolaemic effects of the alpha$_2$ agonist drugs, with ketamine doses at 50 mg/kg. Ketamine may also be used at doses of 90–100 mg/kg in combination with medetomidine at doses of 0.5 mg/kg.

Chinchillas and guinea pigs

In guinea pigs, ketamine at 40 mg/kg may be used in conjunction with xylazine at 2 mg/kg to produce a light plane of anaesthesia. Ketamine at 40 mg/kg may also be used with medetomidine at 0.5 mg/kg in guinea pigs. In chinchillas, ketamine at 30 mg/kg can be used with medetomidine at 0.3 mg/kg. Reversal with atipamezole at 1 mg/kg may be performed. Anaesthesia may be improved after premedication with acepromazine maleate at 0.25 mg/kg.

An alternative combination for chinchillas is ketamine at 40 mg/kg with acepromazine maleate at 0.5 mg/kg. Induction with these drugs takes 5–10 minutes and typically lasts for 45–60 minutes, but recovery may take 2–5 hours for the non-reversible acepromazine maleate combination. Reducing the dose of ketamine and using the reversible alpha$_2$ antagonists may be beneficial, but should be weighed against the greater hypotensive effects of the alpha$_2$ agonist drugs.

Ferrets

Ketamine has been used alone for chemical restraint in the ferret at doses of 10–20 mg/kg but, as with cats and dogs, the muscle relaxation is poor and salivation occurs. Ketamine at 10–30 mg/kg may be combined with xylazine at 1–2 mg/kg, preferably giving the xylazine 5–10 minutes prior to the ketamine. Ketamine at 5 mg/kg may be combined with medetomidine at 0.08 mg/kg, and this may be reversed with half the volume in millilitres (2.5 times the dose in milligrams) of atipamezole.

Hypnorm

Hypnorm is a neuroleptanalgesic combination of fentanyl (a full opioid agonist) and fluanisone. The fentanyl portion may be reversed in all cases with the partial opioid agonist buprenorphine at 0.05 mg/kg or butorphanol at 0.5 mg/kg, or with the full antagonist naloxone at 0.1 mg/kg. Unlike buprenorphine and butorphanol, naloxone does not have any analgesic effect.

Rabbits

Hypnorm may be used as sedation only, on its own at a dose of 0.5 ml/kg i.m. This produces sedation and immobilization for 30–60 minutes, but its analgesic effect due to the opioid derivative fentanyl will persist for some time after.

To provide anaesthetic depth, fentanyl/fluanisone may be combined with diazepam (0.3 ml Hypnorm to 2 mg diazepam/kg) i.p. or i.v. (but in separate syringes as they do not mix), or with midazolam (0.3 ml Hypnorm to 2 mg midazolam/kg) i.m. or i.p. in the same syringe. Alternatively, first the Hypnorm may be given intramuscularly and then 15 minutes later the midazolam may be given intravenously into the lateral ear vein. These two combinations provide good analgesia and muscle relaxation, with a duration of anaesthesia of 20–40 minutes.

Fentanyl/fluanisone combinations are well tolerated in most rabbits, but they can produce respiratory depression and hypoxia, which can lead to cardiac arrhythmias and even arrest.

Rats and mice

Hypnorm may be used as sedation only, on its own at a dose of 0.01 ml/30 g bodyweight in mice and 0.4 ml/kg in rats. This produces sedation and immobilization for 30–60 minutes.

For anaesthesia, it may be combined with diazepam (mice: Hypnorm at 0.01 ml/30 g with diazepam at 5 mg/kg i.p.; rats: Hypnorm 0.3 ml/kg with diazepam 2.5 mg/kg i.p.) where the diazepam and Hypnorm are given in separate syringes as they do not mix. Alternatively, Hypnorm may be combined with midazolam, with which it is miscible. In this combination, for rodents the recommendation is that each drug is mixed with an equal volume of sterile water first and then mixed together. Of this stock solution, mice receive 10 ml/kg and rats 2.7 ml/kg as a single intraperitoneal injection. These two combinations provide anaesthesia for a period of 20–40 minutes.

Chinchillas and guinea pigs

Hypnorm may be used for sedation only, on its own at a dose of 1 ml/kg i.m. Alternatively it may be combined with diazepam (Hypnorm at 1 ml/kg and diazepam at 2.5 mg/kg) in separate syringes and given intraperitoneally, or it may be combined with midazolam by making the stock solution as described above for rats and mice, and then administering this solution at 8 ml/kg i.p.

Induction of anaesthesia: gaseous agents

Sevoflurane

Sevoflurane is well accepted by all small mammals and stimulates much less breath-holding in species such as rabbits and less lacrimation in species such as guinea pigs when compared with isoflurane. Induction without a premedication may be performed using 4–5% sevoflurane in 100% oxygen, then turning the sevoflurane down to 2–3% once a stable anaesthetic plane has been achieved.

Isoflurane

Isoflurane is less well tolerated than sevoflurane, though it is currently the only licensed gaseous anaesthetic for small mammals. When it is used to induce anaesthesia, a premedicant should be used wherever possible to prevent breath-holding. It is best to provide 100% oxygen with no isoflurane at first, via face mask or induction chamber, for a couple of minutes. The isoflurane may then be carefully increased to 0.5% and the patient observed for 2 minutes further to ensure that it continues to breathe regularly. If everything is stable, the isoflurane flow is increased by 0.5% increments until surgical anaesthesia is achieved at 1.5–2%. If breath-holding develops, the isoflurane is dropped by 0.5% until breathing resumes.

Maintenance of anaesthesia

Gaseous anaesthesia

Isoflurane is becoming the most widely used gaseous anaesthetic for maintenance and induction. Usually premedication with an analgesic is used, as isoflurane's analgesic effects are minimal. It is well tolerated in the liver-compromised patient as < 0.3% of the gas is metabolized hepatically, the rest merely being exhaled for recovery to occur. Recovery is therefore rapid.

Induction levels vary between 2.5 and 4% and maintenance is usually 1.5–2.5% if adequate analgesia is given as a premedicant. Breath-holding still occurs, but the practice of supplying 100% oxygen to the patient for 2 minutes prior to anaesthetic administration helps to minimize hypoxia. The isoflurane is gradually introduced initially at 0.5% for 2 minutes; then if breathing is regular, this is increased to 1% for 2 minutes and so on until surgical anaesthesia is reached. This usually allows a smooth induction.

Intubation

Ferrets may be intubated easily using the same technique as for cats. All other small mammals routinely anaesthetized are more difficult to intubate, as the epiglottis can rarely be visualized.

Rabbits may be intubated without the use of a laryngoscope by first sedating them, placing them in sternal recumbency and then lifting the head and inserting the endotracheal tube midline and gently feeding it caudally until a swallowing reflex or cough is elicited, indicating that the end of the tube is over the epiglottis (Figure 22.20). The tube may then be advanced into the trachea. Alternatively the rabbit may be turned on its dorsum and a 0 blade Wisconsin laryngoscope used to locate the epiglottis to intubate it visually.

Other small mammals are often maintained on close-fitting face masks due to the inaccessible nature of their epiglottis and trachea.

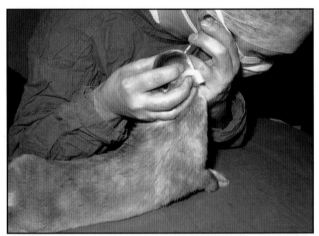

22.20   'Blind' intubation in a rabbit. (Reproduced from *BSAVA Manual of Rabbit Medicine and Surgery, 2nd edition*)

Anaesthetic circuits

Most small mammals weigh < 2 kg and many < 150 g. Low volumes of dead-space are essential, and whilst Ayre's T-piece circuits may be used for the larger rabbits and ferrets, the small species should have mini-Bain system.

Positioning

Care should be taken when placing species such as rabbits and guinea pigs in dorsal recumbency, as the large weight of the ingesta and gut can press on the diaphragm and restrict breathing. Slightly tilting the table or raising the cranial end of the animal when in this position can ease the situation.

Monitoring

Temperature

Regular rectal temperature readings should be taken to ensure that any hypothermia is corrected quickly. Most small mammals have rectal temperatures between 38 and 39°C. Temperature may be maintained using radiant heat mats, hot-water bottles or blown hot-air systems. Care should be taken to avoid thermal burns and hyperthermia.

Cardiovascular and respiratory systems

Doppler probes may be used on peripheral vessels, such as the lateral ear vein (rabbits), saphenous or metatarsal veins (rabbits, guinea pigs, chinchillas and ferrets) or lateral tail veins (rats and mice), to assess pulse strength and rate. Electrocardiography may also be relatively easily employed using modern machines that can cope with heart rates above 300 beats per minute.

Pulse oximeters may be used to assess pulse and oxygen saturation of the blood, but care should be taken to use those that can cope with the higher heart rates, as not all will read pulses above 250 bpm. The medial ear artery is an excellent site for this in the anaesthetized rabbit. Alternatively the probe may be placed under the base of the tail ventrally.

Capnography and breath monitors may be placed between the anaesthetic circuit and the ET adaptor when animals are intubated. Due to the difficulties discussed in intubating other smaller species, their use is often restricted to rabbits and ferrets.

Depth of anaesthesia

Eye position cannot be used in small mammals to assess the depth of anaesthesia. Instead the anaesthetist must rely on other reflexes, such as toe withdrawal reflex or pain sensation reflexes, and the corneal reflexes, as well as the respiration depth and rate to assess depth of anaesthesia. Generally, most small mammals should have lost the toe withdrawal reflex when they have entered the surgical plane of anaesthesia. The exception is the rabbit, which should have lost the toe withdrawal reflex in its hindlimbs but should still have a slight withdrawal response in its forelimbs when pinched firmly. If the latter is lost, the rabbit is starting to become too deeply anaesthetized and should be lightened.

If respiration becomes lighter in depth or erratic, it may suggest that the patient is too light or too deep. A positive toe withdrawal reflex at this stage indicates that the plane is too light, a negative one that the patient is too deep and part or full reversal of the anaesthetic should occur.

Resuscitation

If it is possible to intubate the patient, this should be performed and IPPV started. If not, a tight-fitting face mask may be used and the animal bagged via this in combination with caudal thoracic/cranial abdominal massage. As most small mammals breathe by diaphragmatic movement rather than by chest wall movement, alternate compression and relaxation of the cranial abdomen/caudal thorax wall will have more effect upon respiration via the diaphragm than massage of the chest alone. Doxapram at 0.5 mg/kg either orally or i.m. may be used to stimulate respiration centrally.

If the animal has been intubated, endotracheal administration of adrenaline at 0.1 mg/kg may be used if cardiac arrest has occurred.

Analgesia

Figures 22.21 to 22.23 outline common analgesics used in small mammals.

Drug	Dose rate	Frequency of dosing
Buprenorphine	0.01–0.05 mg/kg s.c., i.m., i.v.	q6–12h
Butorphanol	0.1–0.5 mg/kg s.c., i.m., i.v.	q2–4h
Carprofen	2.2 mg/kg s.c., oral	q24h
Ketoprofen	1 mg/kg i.m., s.c.	q12–24h (< 2 days)
Meloxicam	0.3 mg/kg oral	q24h
Pethidine	10 mg/kg s.c., i.m.	q2–3h

22.21 Analgesics used in rabbits.

Drug	Dose rate	Frequency of dosing
Buprenorphine	0.01–0.03 mg/kg s.c., i.m., i.v.	q8–12h
Butorphanol	0.05–0.5 mg/kg s.c., i.m., i.v.	q6–8h
Carprofen	1–2 mg/kg s.c., oral	q12–24h
Flunixin	0.3–0.5 mg/kg i.m., i.v.	q12–24h (no more than 3 days)
Ketoprofen	1 mg/kg i.m., s.c.	q24h (no more than 5 days)
Meloxicam	0.2 mg/kg oral, s.c.	q24h
Morphine	0.5–5 mg/kg s.c., i.m.	q2–6h

22.22 Analgesics used in ferrets.

Drug	Rats	Mice	Gerbil	Hamster	Guinea pigs	Chinchillas and Degus	Hedgehogs	Sugar gliders
Buprenorphine	0.02–0.5 s.c. q6–12h	0.05–2.5 s.c. q6–12h	0.1–0.2 s.c. q8h	0.5 s.c. q8h	0.05 s.c. q8–12h	0.05 s.c. q8–12h	0.01 s.c. q6–8h	0.01 s.c. q6–8h
Butorphanol	1–5 s.c. q2–4h	1–5 s.c. q2–4h	1–5 s.c. q2–4h	1–5 s.c. q2–4h	2 s.c. q2–4h	0.2 s.c., i.m. q4h	0.1–0.4 s.c., i.m. q6–8h	0.2–0.5 i.m. q6–8h
Carprofen	5 s.c., oral q24h	5 s.c., oral q24h	1–4 oral, s.c. q24h	1–4 oral, s.c. q24h	1–4 oral, s.c. q24h	1–4 oral, s.c. q24h	1 oral, s.c. q12–24h	1 oral, s.c. q12–24h
Flunixin	2.5 s.c. q12–24h	2.5 s.c. q12–24h	2.5 s.c. q12–24h	2.5 s.c. q12–24h	2.5–5 s.c. q6–12h	2.5 s.c. q12–24h	0.1–0.3 s.c., i.m. once	0.1 s.c., i.m. once
Ketoprofen	1–2 s.c. q12–24h	1 s.c. q24h	1 s.c. q24h	1 s.c. q24h	1 s.c. q24h	1 s.c. q24h	1 s.c. q24h	1 s.c. q24h
Meloxicam	0.2–0.5 oral, s.c. q24h	0.1–0.2 oral, s.c. q24h	0.1–0.2 oral, s.c. q24h	0.1–0.2 oral, s.c. q24h	0.1–0.2 oral, s.c. q24h	0.1–0.2 oral, s.c. q24h	0.2 oral, s.c. q24h	0.2 oral, s.c. q24h
Morphine	2–5 s.c., i.m. q4h	2–5 s.c. q4h	2–5 s.c. q4h	2–5 s.c. q4h	2–5 s.c. q4h	2–5 s.c. q4h	2 s.c. q4h	2 s.c. q4h

22.23 Analgesics used in other small mammals. All doses are in mg/kg.

Birds

Relevant anatomy and physiology

The avian patient has a number of variations on the basic respiratory system.

Vestigial larynx

The bird does have a glottis, but there are no vocal cords or epiglottis to worry about on intubation. All of the sounds a bird makes come from an area known as the syrinx, which lies at the bifurcation of the trachea into the bronchi.

Trachea

Birds have complete cartilaginous rings to the trachea. This means that there is no 'give' to the trachea and so inflatable cuffs on endotracheal tubes should not be inflated, as this will cause pressure necrosis to the lining of the trachea. In some cases, such as flushing the crop or stomach of the bird, it may be necessary to inflate the cuff in order to prevent inhalation pneumonia, and extreme care must be taken.

Lungs

The lungs of birds are relatively rigid structures, attached to the underside of the thoracic vertebrae. To allow air to move back and forth, the bird has a series of thin-membrane air sacs that act as inflatable/deflatable balloons for inspiration and expiration. Inspiration is initiated by the outward movement of the ribcage and downward movement of the sternum, which increases the volume of the body cavity (coelom) and creates a relative negative pressure. Air moves through the lungs (where gaseous exchange occurs) and into the inflating caudal air sacs. When the bird breathes out, the air in the caudal air sacs moves back into the lungs through a series of one-way valves where more oxygen exchange can occur. The next inspiration allows the air in the lungs to continue its journey cranially and move on into the cranial air sacs. The cranial air sacs then empty their contents on the second expiration. Birds therefore extract oxygen from air during inspiration and expiration and the whole respiratory cycle occurs over two inspirations and two expirations. This has applications when dealing with avian anaesthesia, as surgery may be performed on the upper respiratory tract and the patient anaesthetized by placing an ET tube into a caudal air sac by making a hole in the body wall over the bird's flank (see below).

Preanaesthetic preparation

Every patient should be clinically examined to ensure that they are safe to anaesthetize. This may also include a preanaesthetic blood test to check liver and kidney function and erythrocyte and leucocyte levels. Veins used for venepuncture include the right jugular, basilic and medial metatarsal veins.

Birds have a very high metabolic rate and so prolonged fasting for many of them is not advisable. Some period of fasting is useful to allow emptying of the crop and proximal GI tract to prevent passive reflux of ingesta during anaesthesia. Most birds are fasted between 1 and 3 hours before anaesthesia, depending on body size. Smaller species have shorter fasting periods. Many birds weighing more than 300 g may have longer fasting periods; for example, some of the larger birds of prey should be fasted for 12–24 hours.

Local anaesthesia

Minor procedures may be performed under local anaesthesia after sedation/tranquillization with parenteral drugs such as midazolam (see below). These include repair of small skin wounds, replacement of cloacal prolapse and removal of haemorrhaging blood feathers.

The drug of choice is lidocaine with adrenaline. It is advisable to dilute the standard solution (2%) at 1 part to 3 parts sterile water to create a 0.5% solution, particularly if dealing with species weighing less than 150 g. Even then, smaller birds should be given doses no greater than 0.1–0.15 ml of the 0.5% solution per 100 g bodyweight.

Preanaesthetic medications

These are used infrequently in birds.

- **Atropine** and **glycopyrrolate** are rarely used, as they create unacceptably high heart rates and thickening of the mucus in the airways, leading to endotracheal tube blockage.
- Benzodiazepines such as **diazepam** and **midazolam** have been used as premedicants in waterfowl, as these species are prone to apnoea when gaseous anaesthesia is being induced by face mask. Midazolam is more potent and doses of 0.1–0.5 mg/kg i.m. have been suggested.

Fluid therapy

Fluid therapy is probably the most important preanaesthetic medication, to ensure adequate hydration and cardiovascular support. Fluid levels of 10 ml/kg/h for the first 2 hours and then 5–8 ml/kg/h thereafter during anaesthesia are advised. Lactated Ringer's solution warmed to 40–42°C given via the right jugular, basilic or medial metatarsal vein is advised.

Blood transfusion

If blood loss occurs that is greater than 30% of the total blood volume, a blood transfusion or use of a blood replacer such as Oxyglobin should be considered. Other indicators for blood transfusion include a total protein level less than 25 g/l. Blood donors should be of the same species (e.g. African Grey parrot to African Grey parrot).

Induction of anaesthesia: injectable agents

Propofol

This has to be administered intravenously or intraosseously (the latter needs to be administered via a non-pneumonized bone such as the tibiotarsus; see Chapter 4b). The drug produces profound apnoea and is rarely used in birds.

Ketamine and ketamine combinations

Used alone at doses of 20–50 mg/kg, ketamine produces inadequate anaesthesia and recoveries are often traumatic, with the patient flapping excessively. Recovery may be prolonged, with ensuing hypothermia and hypoglycaemia.

It is therefore advisable, if using ketamine, to give lower dosages and combine it with an alpha$_2$ agonist such as xylazine. Ketamine at 20 mg/kg with xylazine at 4 mg/kg gives 1–2 hours anaesthesia, or ketamine at 5–10 mg/kg with xylazine at 1–2.2 mg/kg is useful for minor procedures, but this combination should be avoided in pigeons, doves and all wading birds.

The alpha$_2$ agonist medetomidine may also be used. Doses of ketamine may be reduced to 5 mg/kg with medetomidine at 60–85 µg/kg, but higher doses of medetomidine at 100–150 mg/kg with ketamine at 10 mg/kg may be required for full surgical anaesthesia in owls and waterfowl. Medetomidine may be reversed by using the same volume of atipamezole, thus speeding recovery.

Ketamine may also be used at 30–40 mg/kg in combination with diazepam at 1–1.5 mg/kg.

All of the above combinations are administered intramuscularly, usually in the breast/pectoral muscles.

Induction of anaesthesia: gaseous agents

The recommended gaseous agents for induction of anaesthesia are isoflurane or sevoflurane in 100% oxygen. Nitrous oxide is not used in birds. Halothane, due to its arrhythmogenic properties and its metabolism by the liver (most avian patients that are presented as sick will have some hepatic function impairment), is not advised as an anaesthetic agent in birds.

Anaesthesia may be induced via face mask with gentle towel restraint of the patient, or in the case of very small birds via induction chamber. Induction with isoflurane is usually at the level of 3–4% (vaporizer setting) in 100% oxygen. This can be turned down to 1.5–2% once a stable plane of anaesthesia has been induced. Induction with sevoflurane is usually at the level of 4–5% in 100% oxygen. This can be turned down to 2–3% once a stable plane of anaesthesia has been induced.

Maintenance of anaesthesia

For any prolonged procedures, or where the patient is particularly fragile or sick, the maintenance agents of choice are either isoflurane or sevoflurane in 100% oxygen. Isoflurane and sevoflurane are minimally metabolized inside the body, have very low solubility levels and so are readily removed from the blood and the body via exhaled air. This leads to rapid recoveries and minimal postanaesthetic side effects.

Intubation

The patient's airway should be intubated with an endotracheal tube. This is easily done as the glottis is readily visible at the base of the tongue. A snug-fitting tube, pre-sprayed with lidocaine spray, is inserted. Tubes without cuffs are preferable for reasons mentioned above. Once intubated, the patient may then be maintained easily and IPPV may be instituted as required.

Anaesthetic circuits

Anaesthetic circuits should have minimal dead-space, due to the generally small size of the patient. Modified Bain systems are useful as are Ayre's T-pieces.

Positioning

Avian patients should be preferably positioned on their side or sternum to minimize the pressure of the internal organs on the air sacs and lungs. If the patient has to be placed in dorsal recumbency, IPPV should be considered, as apnoea after anaesthetic induction is common.

Intermittent positive pressure ventilation (IPPV)

If the respiratory rate becomes depressed for more than 15–20 seconds, respiratory assistance in the form of IPPV should be instituted. The anaesthetic circuit and the depth of anaesthesia should be checked to ensure that the patient is not too deep. If all is stable, IPPV is started. This may be in the simple form of manual ventilation of the patient 10–15 times a minute if apnoeic. The aim is to allow a gentle rise and fall of the body wall by approximately 30–50%. Use of the cardiorespiratory stimulant doxapram at 5–10 mg/kg orally or i.m. should also be considered.

If performing a lot of bird anaesthetics, it is often preferable to use a mechanical ventilator. These may be set to create a pressure of 10–15 cm water (7–11 mmHg). The frequency of respiration may also be set, as above. Certain anaesthetics are known to be respiratory depressants, such as xylazine, and isoflurane in African Grey parrots.

Air sac intubation

In the event of an upper respiratory tract obstruction, or where surgery is to be performed on the upper respiratory tract, an ET tube may be inserted into a caudal body air sac via the lateral body wall to introduce oxygen and anaesthetic gases for anaesthesia.

The bird is placed in right lateral recumbency and the left leg is pulled caudally. A small skin incision is made caudal to the last rib and just cranial to the left thigh on the flank. A pair of haemostats is used to dissect bluntly through the thin body wall muscles and into the body cavity and the caudal air sacs. A shortened piece of ET tube, or a specific air sac tube, can be placed and sutured to the skin. An adaptor allows connection to the anaesthetic circuit (Figure 22.24). Usually IPPV is required to maintain anaesthesia via an air sac tube, as birds frequently become apnoeic.

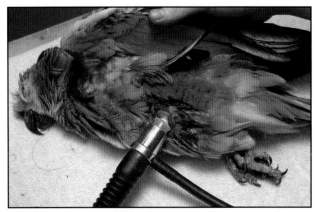

22.24 Air sac intubation in a parrot. (Reproduced from *BSAVA Manual of Psittacine Birds, 2nd edition*)

Monitoring the patient

Temperature

Hypothermia is common in anaesthetized birds, due to the cooling nature of gaseous anaesthesia and the small size of the patient. The use of an electronic measuring device (avian body temperature is normally around 41–42°C) with the probe placed into the bird's cloaca is advisable.

To maintain temperature, the use of warmed intravenous fluids and of radiant heat mats, hot-water bottles or hot-air devices (e.g. the Bair Hugger) should be considered, taking care not to induce thermal burns.

Cardiovascular and respiratory systems

Heart rate may be determined directly via a stethoscope externally, or an oesophageal stethoscope. An ECG trace may also be performed, the leads being attached as for cats and dogs, except that the forelimb leads are attached to the relevant wings at the level of the wing web/propatagium (the web that stretches from the shoulder to the carpus across the elbow joint cranially). Alligator forceps are often too traumatic; instead 25 gauge hypodermic needles may be placed through the skin at the relevant sites, and the alligator forceps attached to the projecting needle. The avian ECG differs from the mammalian in that the majority of species have a small R wave and a large S wave. This makes the trace look as if it is inverted, as the main deflection of the QRS complex is a negative one.

Doppler probes may be used to monitor blood flow through peripheral vessels such as the brachial vein over the ventral upper wing, or the medial metatarsal vein over the medial aspect of the lower leg (tarsometatarsus).

Pulse oximetry may also be used to monitor the patient, but many pulse oximeters have difficulty coping with the high heart rates of birds. The probe is usually used inserted into the cloaca.

Respiratory flow monitors and capnography may be used when the patient is intubated. An end-tidal carbon dioxide level of 30–45 mmHg has been shown to indicate adequate ventilation in the African Grey parrot.

Depth of anaesthesia

During the initial stages of anaesthesia the respiratory rate, as with cats and dogs, will be shallow and erratic. The patient will be lethargic and have drooping eyelids, a lowered head and ruffled feathers. As the depth increases, palpebral, corneal, pedal and cere reflexes will remain, but all voluntary movement ceases.

As depth of anaesthesia increases further, the respiration rate becomes regular, depth of breathing is increased and corneal and pedal reflexes are slow but the palpebral reflex disappears. This is the level at which most surgery is performed. As anaesthesia is allowed to progress, respiratory rate and tidal volume will continue to decrease, until (if allowed) respiratory arrest will occur. Just before apnoea, the corneal reflex will disappear.

Resuscitation

With gaseous anaesthetics such as isoflurane and sevoflurane, respiratory arrest generally precedes cardiac arrest, allowing some time to reduce anaesthesia and start mechanical ventilation. The ABC of emergency medicine applies to birds as for cats and dogs (see below). Therefore intubation should be performed wherever possible initially to facilitate resuscitation. The drug doxapram at 5–10 mg/kg orally or i.m. can aid with stimulation of the cardiac and respiratory centres in the CNS.

Where intubation is not possible, the bird should be placed in right lateral recumbency and the uppermost (left) wing grasped by the carpus and drawn vertically. By extending and flexing the wing from this point, the forces are transferred to the body wall and ribcage, causing increasing and decreasing of the body cavity size and thus allowing inspiration and expiration.

If cardiac arrest occurs, manual rhythmical palpation of the caudal sternum will compress the heart and act as cardiac massage. This may be combined with doxapram and the use of adrenaline administered via the ET tube at a dose of 0.1 mg/kg. If bradycardia is detected prior to arrest, atropine at 0.01–0.02 mg/kg i.v. should be administered.

Analgesia

Local anaesthesia has been mentioned above. Systemic analgesics such as the non-steroidal anti-inflammatory drugs (NSAIDs) meloxicam and carprofen may be used with care, as may the opioids buprenorphine and butorphanol (Figure 22.25). Limited studies in avian patients suggest that they predominantly have kappa rather than mu opioid receptors in their CNS, leading to the suggestion that butorphanol is the better opioid analgesic. NSAIDs should be avoided, or used with caution, where pre-existing GI ulceration or renal disease is present.

Drug	Dose rate	Frequency of dosing
Butorphanol	1–4 mg/kg s.c., i.m. 0.02–0.04 mg/kg i.v.	q6–8h
Buprenorphine	0.02–0.06mg/kg s.c., i.m.	q8–12h
Meloxicam	0.1–0.2 mg/kg s.c., i.m., oral	q24h
Carprofen	2–4 mg/kg s.c., oral	q24h

22.25   Analgesics used in birds.

Reptiles

Relevant anatomy and physiology

Vestigial larynx

Reptiles have a glottis, but there are no vocal cords or epiglottis to worry about on intubation.

Trachea

Chelonians have complete cartilaginous rings to the trachea. This means that there is no 'give' to the trachea and so inflatable cuffs on endotracheal tubes should not be inflated in chelonians, as this will cause pressure necrosis to the lining of the trachea. Snakes and lizards have C-shaped rings of cartilage, as for mammals, and so gentle inflation may be performed.

Lungs

The lungs of snakes are elongated, and the left lung of many may be absent or vestigial. The right lung of many snakes often ends in an air sac. In chelonians and lizards there are two lungs, which are largely elastic in nature.

There is no true diaphragm in reptiles. The lungs are inflated by the outward movement of the ribcage in the case of lizards and snakes. In chelonians, the outward movement of the head and limbs from the shell increases the body cavity volume and so creates a negative pressure to draw air into the elastic lungs. Pulling the head and limbs back in again applies positive pressure, which allows expiration.

Respiratory stimulus

The stimulus for respiration in reptiles is a low pO_2 rather than a high pCO_2 as is seen in mammals (see Chapter 4b). Thus if anaesthesia involves 100% oxygen via IPPV, this must be reduced to allow voluntary respiration to occur.

It should be noted that some chelonians can survive with little or no inhaled oxygen for up to 24 hours, or more, making induction of anaesthesia via face mask almost impossible.

Preanaesthetic preparation

Routine clinical examinations should be made, and any hint of respiratory disease should be investigated further with radiographs, lung washes and blood samples. Blood may be drawn from the jugular or dorsal tail veins in chelonians, the ventral tail veins in lizards and the ventral tail vein or by cardiac puncture in snakes.

Fasting is advised in snakes: 24 hours in smaller species and up to 1 week for giant species such as an adult Burmese python. The idea is to ensure an empty stomach and minimal ingesta that may cause a bacterial population explosion or result in regurgitation and aspiration pneumonia. In small insectivorous lizards (e.g. leopard geckos) live prey should be withheld for 24 hours prior to anaesthesia to ensure that any prey consumed is truly dead and not still within the stomach. Chelonians rarely if ever regurgitate and so generally do not need to be fasted.

Preanaesthetic medications

These are rarely used in reptiles. **Acepromazine maleate** at 0.1–0.5 mg/kg i.m or **midazolam** at 2 mg/kg i.m. may aid in the control of a fractious animal and allow a smoother recovery, but they also markedly prolong anaesthesia and so are generally avoided.

Fluid therapy

This is necessary, as reptiles, like birds, excrete uric acid as their main waste product of protein metabolism (the so-called urates or whites produced in the droppings). Uric acid is insoluble; therefore if dehydration occurs, and consequently excretion of uric acid by the kidneys does not occur, the levels build up inside the body and can precipitate deposits of uric acid on internal organs (so-called visceral gout) or in the joints (articular gout). Fluids used include lactated Ringer's solution, and mixtures of mammalian isotonic fluids with sterile water as there is some suggestion that isotonicity is lower in reptiles than in mammals (0.8% for reptiles versus 0.9% for mammals). Maximum doses of fluids have been recommended as 20–25 ml/kg/day and may be given by a number of routes.

Oral fluids may be used where the gastrointestinal tract is functioning and if only mild dehydration occurs. The oral route is not useful if the patient requires an anaesthetic, so for reptiles with mild dehydration subcutaneous fluids are used (over the ribcage in lizards, over the lateral body wall in snakes and over the thigh region in chelonians). More dehydrated reptiles may have intracoelomic fluids (the equivalent of intraperitoneal fluids in mammals). In snakes, the caudal third of the body is used, the needle just popped through the body wall, two rows of scales up from the ventrum on the lateral body wall. In lizards, the same technique as for mammals is used, with the reptile being turned head down, in dorsal recumbency and the needle inserted in the right lower quadrant of the body wall ventrally. In chelonians, a slightly longer needle (25 mm) is used and placed just cranial to each hindleg to access the coelomic cavity (the cavity is known as the coelom as there are no divisions into thorax and abdomen).

Local anaesthesia

This may be used for minor procedures such as skin biopsy techniques and cloacal prolapse replacement.

Induction of anaesthesia: injectable agents

These are useful due to the breath-holding capabilities of many reptiles, which makes gaseous induction difficult or stressful.

Propofol

This is one of the agents of choice in many reptiles. It may be administered intravenously via any of the veins used for venepuncture, or intraosseously. Dosages of 10–15 mg/kg are generally used.

Ketamine

Ketamine's effects depend on species and dose. Doses of 22–44 mg/kg i.m. have been suggested for sedation, with doses of 55–80 mg/kg being required for anaesthesia. Effects occur within 10–30 minutes but can take up to 4 days to wear off at the higher doses. Ketamine is excreted by the kidneys, so should be given via the cranial half of the body to avoid the renal portal system and immediate excretion before effect and dosages should be reduced where known renal damage exists.

Alfaxalone/alfadolone (Saffan)

This can allow intubation within 3–5 minutes after intravenous administration at 6–9 mg/kg. Given intramuscularly, induction is longer (25–40 minutes) and the dosages used must be higher (9–15 mg/kg). Recovery is quicker than with ketamine, but still may take 4 hours or more.

Succinylcholine

This is a neuromuscular blocking agent (see 'Muscle relaxants') and produces immobilization without analgesia. It should therefore never be used on its own where surgery or any technique likely to cause pain is going to be performed. It is useful in giant chelonians at doses of 0.5–1 mg/kg i.m. and allows rapid intubation and conversion to gaseous anaesthesia. Respiration usually continues voluntarily at these doses, but the anaesthetist should be aware that blockade of the respiratory muscles can also occur and so IPPV may need to be performed and should always be available.

Induction of anaesthesia: gaseous agents

It is possible to induce anaesthesia using sevoflurane or isoflurane in 100% oxygen in many snakes and lizards. Due to breath-holding problems, chelonians are not good candidates for gaseous anaesthetic induction. Snakes and lizards may be induced in anaesthetic chambers or via face masks. Snakes are often easily induced by encouraging them to crawl into a clear tube attached to the anaesthetic circuit.

Maintenance of anaesthesia

Injectable agents

Anaesthesia may be maintained with injectable agents.

- **Ketamine** may be combined with:
  - Midazolam (ketamine 40 mg/kg with midazolam 2 mg/kg) in turtles
  - Xylazine (xylazine 1 mg/kg, given 20 minutes before ketamine 20 mg/kg) in crocodiles/alligators
  - Medetomidine (ketamine 50 mg/kg with medetomidine 100 μg/kg) in snakes.
- **Propofol** may be topped up intravenously or intraosseously at 1 mg/kg/min. Apnoea is common and so intubation, IPPV and maintenance on 100% oxygen are advised.
- **Alfaxalone/alfadolone** may be used for surgery at 6–9 mg/kg i.v. and is particularly useful in chelonians.

Gaseous agents

The anaesthetic of choice is isoflurane in 100% oxygen. Levels of 1–2% (vaporizer setting) will generally maintain anaesthesia after injectable induction, or levels of 3–4% may be used to mask down snakes and lizards. Induction of anaesthesia by gaseous means is not easy in chelonians. Sevoflurane may also be safely used, at higher levels of 2–3% for maintenance and 5–6% for induction. Reptiles generally need to be intubated to maintain anaesthesia, due to the likelihood of apnoea and the need for intermittent positive pressure ventilation (IPPV).

Intubation

In **snakes** the glottis sits rostrally on the floor of the mouth just caudal to the tongue sheath (Figure 22.26) and is easily seen in an open mouth. Intubation may be performed consciously if

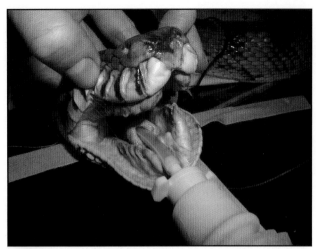

22.26 A snake intubated for gaseous general anaesthesia. (Reproduced from *BSAVA Manual of Reptiles, 2nd edition*)

necessary, as reptiles do not have a cough reflex. The mouth is opened with a wooden or plastic tongue depressor and the endotracheal tube is inserted during inspiration. Alternatively, an induction agent may be given and then intubation attempted.

In **chelonians** the glottis sits slightly more caudally at the base of the tongue. The trachea is very short and the ET tube should be inserted only a few centimetres, otherwise there is a risk that one or other bronchus will be intubated, leading to only one lung receiving the anaesthetic. As mentioned, an induction agent such as ketamine or propofol is advised for chelonians prior to intubation, due to their ability to breath-hold and difficulty in extracting the head from the shell.

Lizards vary depending on the species of lizard involved, most having just a glottis guarding the entrance to the trachea, but some species possess vocal folds (notably some species of gecko). Some may be intubated when conscious, but most are better induced with an injectable method, or gaseous induction by face mask. Some species may be too small for intubation.

Anaesthetic circuits

For species weighing less than 5 kg, a non-rebreathing system with oxygen flow at twice the minute volume (which approximates to 300–500 ml/kg/min for most species) is suggested. The Ayre's T-pieces and modified Bain systems are commonly used.

Positioning

Many chelonians are placed in dorsal recumbency for intracoelomic surgery (surgery entering the body compartment known as the coelom), as already mentioned. Other groups of reptiles may also be placed in this position for similar techniques. The use of foam wedges or positional polystyrene-filled vacuum bags is essential to maintain stability.

This also applies to snakes, as they become extremely flaccid during surgery, and in order to provide stability they may be strapped to a long board, or wedged in place with foam/vacuum bags. The use of IPPV and the need to keep the body wall of non-chelonian species free of constraint is necessary.

IPPV

If intubation is performed when the animal is fully conscious, anaesthesia may be induced (even in breath-holding species) by using positive pressure ventilation, in a matter of 5–10 minutes. This does have some advantages, as the avoidance of injectable induction agents leads to rapid postoperative recovery.

Many species require positive pressure ventilation during the course of an anaesthetic. Chelonians, for example, are frequently placed in dorsal recumbency during intracoelomic surgery. As they have no diaphragm and the lungs are situated dorsally, the weight of the digestive contents pressing on the lungs will reduce inspiration and slowly lead to hypoxia. This is in addition to the fact that most inspiratory effort is induced by movement of the chelonian's limbs, which should be immobile during anaesthesia. If a neuromuscular blocking agent such as succinylcholine has been used, positive pressure ventilation may be needed as respiratory muscle paralysis may occur.

The aims of IPPV lie in inflating the lungs with oxygen/anaesthetic mixture, just enough for an adequately oxygenated state to be maintained and for the animal to remain anaesthetized. To this end it is sufficient to ventilate most reptiles two to six times a minute and no more, and with 10–15 cm water (7–11 mmHg) pressure levels. As with birds, a ventilator unit makes life much easier, but with experience manual ventilation of the patient with enough pressure to just inflate the lungs and no more can be achieved. A rough guide is to inflate the first two-fifths of the reptile's body at each cycle.

Monitoring the patient

Temperature

Digital temperature gauges with probes that may be inserted into the reptile's cloaca should be used to ensure that the reptile stays within or close to its preferred body temperature (PBT). Heat may be provided by radiant heat mats, hot-water bottles and hot-air systems, as for birds.

Cardiovascular and respiratory systems

Monitoring the heart rate and rhythm can be extremely difficult with a conventional stethoscope, due to the reptile's rough scales interfering with sound transmission and due to the three-chambered heart, which reduces the clarity of the heartbeat. Some of this can be overcome by placing a damp towel over the area to be auscultated, so deadening the sound of the scales, but in many cases the best solution is to use a Doppler probe (see 'Monitoring cardiovascular function', above). This is an ultrasound probe unit attached to a microphone which responds to fluid movement such as blood flow, converting it to sound. Pulse oximetry may also be used to assess blood saturation with oxygen. The flat probe may be placed alongside the tongue of the reptile when anaesthetized, or into the cloaca. A drop of >5% saturation indicates mild hypoxia and >10% is classified as an emergency requiring increased ventilation.

Apnoea alert monitors may also be used, but as many reptiles require IPPV, these may be of limited use.

Depth of anaesthesia

Light anaesthesia is highlighted by slow movements of the reptile and the retention of the positive righting reflex (a reptile will flip back on to its feet after being inverted) and, in snakes, the tongue withdrawal reflex. The reptile still responds to noxious stimuli.

In deepening anaesthesia the righting reflex and vent tone are absent and in snakes the tongue reflex is absent. In chelonians and lizards the palpebral reflex is much reduced. Subsequently, with increasing depth of anaesthesia there is no response to noxious stimuli. The tongue reflex in snakes is absent, as is the Bauchstreich reflex (the contraction of the ventral muscles when a finger is run along the ventrum of the snake).

Resuscitation

The ABC determined for small mammal medicine should be used in reptiles. Ensuring a clear airway is best achieved by intubation. As reptiles do not have a diaphragm, there is no cough reflex and so even conscious but collapsed patients may be intubated with minimal distress. IPPV is required, to maintain breathing. It should be remembered that the stimulus to breathe in reptiles is a lowered partial pressure of oxygen (pO_2) in the airways/blood rather than an increased partial pressure of carbon dioxide (pCO_2) and so IPPV with 100% oxygen (though often necessary) will prevent stimulation for inspiration. Therefore pauses should be made in the IPPV to allow the oxygen levels to drop slightly to see if the reptile will breathe for itself. Pulse oximetry may be used to assess adequacy of oxygenation.

Should cardiac arrest occur, use of adrenaline via the ET tube is advised with chest massage in lizards and snakes. The heart is located high in the chest, inside the pectoral girdle in lizards such as iguanas and agamids. In monitor lizards, the heart is located more caudally towards the end of the ribcage and in snakes the heart is generally located at the caudal end of the first third of the snake. In chelonians, the heart is generally located caudal to the neck and so is difficult to access for cardiac massage. Instead, movement of the head and neck and movement of the forelimbs into and out of the shell may be used. This is also useful for attempting artificial respiration in chelonians, mimicking the conscious method of inspiration and expiration.

Drugs that may be of help include doxapram at 5–10 mg/kg orally or i.m. to stimulate respiration, or adrenaline at 0.1 mg/kg should cardiac arrest occur.

Analgesia

Figure 22.27 outlines some of the more commonly used analgesics in reptile medicine. Care should be taken with the NSAID family where dehydration or renal disease is suspected.

Drug	Dose rate	Frequency of dosing
Butorphanol	0.4 mg/kg s.c., i.m.	q6–8h
Buprenorphine	0.01 mg/kg s.c., i.m.	q8–12h
Meloxicam	0.1–0.2 mg/kg s.c., i.m., oral	q24h
Carprofen	2–4 mg/kg s.c., oral	q24h (first day higher dose, then decrease)

22.27 Analgesics used in reptiles.

Amphibians

Relevant anatomy and physiology

Some amphibian species, such as the anurans (frogs and toads) possess lungs; others, such as the axlotl, possess external gills. Many can breathe/exchange oxygen across their skin surface.

Preanaesthetic preparation

All amphibians are carnivorous and should be fasted for 12–24 hours prior to anaesthesia.

General anaesthesia

MS-222

MS-222 is commonly used to anaesthetize anurans. It is used at a concentration of 100–500 mg/l and may be syringed on to the skin. To reverse the process, fresh, dechlorinated water without MS-222 can be trickled over the skin. Induction with MS-222 results in loss of the righting reflex and pinch reflexes when surgical anaesthesia is achieved. In the course of the induction the skin of the ventrum of many anurans will redden markedly.

Ketamine

Ketamine may be used at 50–100 mg/kg i.m. to provide deep sedation, but its recovery time is prolonged.

Other agents

A preparation of clove oil has also been used, chiefly in anurans at 0.3 ml/l (approximately 310 mg/l) and seems to be safe.

Analgesia

Opioids have been safely used in amphibians. Examples include fentanyl at 0.5 mg/kg s.c., butorphanol at 0.2–0.4 mg/kg i.m. and buprenorphine at 38 mg/kg in leopard frogs.

Fish

Local anaesthesia

Lidocaine with adrenaline may be employed when taking skin biopsies or removing small masses. It is preferable to combine this with sedation/anaesthesia to minimize stress. Local infiltration of the 2% stock solution previously diluted 1 part solution with 10 parts sterile water for injection to avoid overdosage is advised.

Induction and maintenance of anaesthesia

Topical/in-water agents

MS-222

MS-222 may be added to the water as a stock solution of 80–100 mg/l. This is generally safe for most fish such as Koi carp, but where an unfamiliar species is being anaesthetized a 20 mg/l solution should be used first and then gradually added to reach 100 mg/l.

Initially the fish becomes slightly more active, flashing its gills and fins. This slows as the anaesthetic takes effect. Eventually the fish stops actively swimming and remains motionless in the water. When a surgical plane of anaesthesia has been reached, the fish loses its righting reflex, i.e. it becomes unable to stay upright and turns belly upwards in the water. At this point it may be removed from the water, placed on a water-soaked towel and its upper eye covered from the light to reduce stimulation.

To reverse the process, fresh dechlorinated water without MS-222 can be trickled over the gills, or the fish may be placed in a tank of fresh non-medicated water and gently moved through the water by hand to allow the water to pass over the gills.

Benzocaine

This may be used at a concentration of 25–50 mg/l. Benzocaine needs to be dissolved first in acetone and is acidic in nature and needs to be mixed with a buffering agent.

Lidocaine

This has been used at 100 mg/l in carp as an in-water anaesthetic.

Isoflurane

It is possible to bubble isoflurane through the water to induce anaesthesia, but its low solubility makes induction lengthy.

Injectable agents

Medetomidine and ketamine

These have been used as an injectable anaesthetic in goldfish. The combination is administered intramuscularly into the tail base, avoiding the lateral line, at doses of 1–2 mg ketamine/kg and 50–100 µg medetomidine/kg. The medetomidine may be reversed using the same volume of atipamezole.

Anaesthetic circuits

A simple water pump may be used to pump tank water with the in-water medication MS-222 via a pipe into the mouth of the anaesthetized fish. The anaesthetic solution then flows over the gills and the flow rate may be adjusted to maintain the correct depth of anaesthesia.

Positioning

Lateral recumbency is usually sufficient for growth removals, gill sampling and skin biopsies. Occasionally when intracoelomic (fish have no lungs or diaphragm and so the body cavity, as with birds and reptiles, is referred to as a coelomic cavity) surgery is required, the fish may be placed in dorsal recumbency with foam wedges.

Monitoring

Cardiovascular system

Doppler probes may be used to monitor blood flow through the primitive heart, which is generally located between the pectoral fins, immediately caudal to the lower jaw ventrally.

Depth of anaesthesia

This is assessed by the use of pinch reflexes and the lack of response. There may be the occasional gill movement, but no flapping of the body or eye movements.

Resuscitation

The fish is moved through clean, well oxygenated water.

Analgesia

Butorphanol at 0.05–0.1 mg/kg intramuscularly has been used for analgesia, and doses as high as 0.4 mg/kg have been safely used in Koi carp.

Invertebrates

Local anaesthesia

Local infiltration of diluted lidocaine may be used to amputate limbs in spiders. However, generally this is combined with a general anaesthetic to reduce stress and pain. As with the other animals listed above, the 2% lidocaine solution is best diluted 1 part with 10 parts sterile water for injection prior to use, to reduce the chances of overdosage.

General anaesthesia

Injectable agents

These are rarely used in invertebrates.

Gaseous agents

Isoflurane or sevoflurane may be used via an induction chamber to successfully anaesthetize many invertebrates, such as arachnids (spiders and scorpions), stick insects and giant millipedes.

Carbon dioxide will also render many insects unconscious but it provides no analgesia.

Topical agents

Aquatic species of invertebrate may be anaesthetized with MS-222 at 100 mg/l.

Accidents and emergencies

Accidents are frequently avoidable problems, affecting patients or personnel and sometimes involving equipment. Problems may be of minor consequence individually, but collectively they may create emergencies. Emergencies are crises that require rapid responses, as they quickly lead to cardiopulmonary arrest. The most common complications involve respiratory and cardiovascular compromise, body temperature abnormalities and delayed return to consciousness. Problems can develop at all stages of anaesthesia, from premedication through to recovery. An understanding of the nature of common complications is important if they are to be avoided. When accidents do occur, rapid and effective therapy is essential if permanent disability or death is to be avoided.

Definitions

- **Apnoea**: the arrest of breathing
- **Hypoventilation**: reduced alveolar ventilation
- **Tachypnoea**: rapid respiration
- **Bradypnoea**: slow respiration
- **Hypoxia**: reduced oxygen in the body tissues
- **Hypoxaemia**: reduced oxygen in the blood
- **Hypercapnia**: excess of carbon dioxide in lungs or blood
- **Tachycardia**: rapid heart rate
- **Bradycardia**: slow heart rate
- **Arrhythmia**: irregular heart rhythm
- **Hypotension**: low arterial blood pressure
- **Haemorrhage**: bleeding
- **Hypothermia**: low body temperature.

Respiratory complications

Compromise to ventilation is a significant concern during anaesthesia when the patient is unable to protect its own airway and normal regulation of ventilation is depressed. Apnoea is a particular emergency: severe hypoxia and hypercapnia rapidly cause cardiac arrest. Hypoventilation is less of an acute emergency but if severe may lead to cardiopulmonary arrest also. The circumstances in which apnoea can occur are:

- An acute event that prevents breathing (e.g. pneumothorax, upper airway obstruction, anaesthetic overdose)
- As a sign of cardiac arrest
- As the end result of progressive hypoventilation.

Signs of apnoea include absence of breathing or irregular gasping with twitching neck muscles and spasmodic diaphragm contractions. In conscious animals the neck is extended, the mouth is wide open, the eyes are staring and the pupils are dilated. Mucous membranes are blue or dirty grey. In anaesthetized animals, only ineffectual breathing attempts, discoloured mucous membranes and signs of overdosage may be present.

There are three main causes of hypoventilation and apnoea (Figure 22.28) and elements of all three are usually present during surgery:

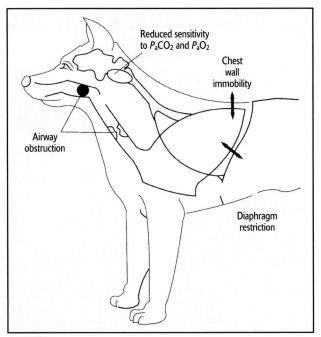

22.28 Causes of apnoea and hypoventilation.

- Failure of the brain to respond to elevated blood carbon dioxide or reduced blood oxygen levels
- Airway obstruction (partial or complete)
- Chest-wall fixation and lung collapse.

Failure of the brain to respond to blood carbon dioxide and oxygen levels

This occurs:

- In severe head trauma
- When intracranial pressure is raised (e.g. by tumours or by inflammatory processes)
- In anaesthetic overdose
- In severe hypothermia.

The most common cause of hypoventilation is profound anaesthesia, which reduces medullary sensitivity to carbon dioxide and abolishes chemoreceptor stimulation by hypoxia. The deeper the level of anaesthesia, the greater is the degree of respiratory depression. Hypoventilation under anaesthesia is exacerbated by hypothermia. High doses of opioids may induce respiratory depression.

Transient apnoea is common after induction of anaesthesia with propofol and thiopental. While spontaneous respiration resumes in the course of time, lung inflations should be imposed intermittently until regular ventilation returns.

Reduced alveolar ventilation results from reduced tidal volume and/or reduced respiratory rate. Conversely, very high respiratory rates with low tidal volumes (tachypnoea) also cause hypoventilation, because inspired gas does not reach the alveoli effectively.

Airway obstruction

Airway obstruction in the non-intubated animal contributes to hypoventilation because it causes turbulent gas flow, which increases resistance to breathing. Partial or total obstruction is indicated by inspiratory snoring noises and/or paradoxical thoracic wall movement during inspiration (the abdomen moves outwards whilst the chest wall moves inwards). The airway may become obstructed in several ways, as follows.

Soft-tissue obstruction
This is likely in brachycephalic breeds when sedatives or anaesthetics depress reflex control of oropharyngeal and nasopharyngeal muscles. Sedated brachycephalics must be observed closely and endotracheal intubation performed once consciousness is lost. During recovery, the return of gag reflexes indicates the need for extubation. Thereafter, surveillance must continue because obstruction remains possible.

It must be appreciated that oxygen by mask is ineffective during obstruction. Endotracheal intubation, transtracheal oxygen or tracheotomy may be required until the obstruction is relieved. During recovery, sustained airway protective reflexes should be restored rapidly in cases at risk of obstruction by using drugs with little residual effect, or by administering an antagonist.

Blood and debris
Obstruction also results from mycotic or neoplastic lesions, or from blood clots after nasal and dental surgery. After surgery involving the oropharynx, nasopharynx or any part of the upper airway, surgical debris must be cleared before the animal recovers and is extubated.

Vomiting/regurgitation
This may occur during induction or postoperatively. Rarely, passive regurgitation occurs during surgery. When there is regurgitation, the animal must be positioned head-down. If it remains conscious, its mouth is gagged and the oropharynx cleared of material. Initially, dry swabs held with towel forceps or haemostats will suffice. Later, moistened swabs may be needed. If consciousness is lost, cursory pharyngeal lavage must be followed by endotracheal intubation and positive pressure ventilation with oxygen. Suction and lavage are then performed.

Fluid–pulmonary oedema
A froth-filled airway indicates pulmonary oedema, which results from end-stage left-sided heart failure or, rarely, after use of Saffan in cats. Endobronchial suction should be performed, but the prognosis is poor.

Bronchospasm
Severe bronchospasm (status asthmaticus) is fortunately a rare cause of airway obstruction in companion animals but in theory could occur in response to histamine-releasing drugs, e.g. high doses of pethidine or morphine given intravenously. The administration of adrenaline, beta$_2$ agonists and steroids may be required.

Endotracheal tube complications
The presence of endotracheal tubes does not guarantee a patent airway. Overinflated cuffs may cause the lumen to collapse, or extreme neck positions may cause kinking. Lightly anaesthetized animals may bite the tube and close the lumen. Cats have particularly sensitive larynxes and are prone to spasm if poor intubation technique is used. Desensitization of the larynx with local anaesthetic prior to intubation is required in this species. Oesophageal intubation is possible and may result in premature awakening or respiratory compromise.

Chest-wall fixation and lung collapse
Breathing ceases when the chest wall and diaphragm are immobilized or when the lungs are prevented from expanding. In pneumothorax, the lungs are collapsed by thoracic expansion with gas accumulation in the pleural space, resulting in hypoventilation. Similarly, fluid accumulation in the pleural space, in patients with pleural effusions, can compromise ventilation.

Some breathing systems have expiratory valves. If these are inadvertently left closed, there is a rapid build-up in circuit pressure, preventing expiration and causing rapid death. In very small animals, breathing may be suppressed when the chest wall is 'stiffened' by heavy drapes, when surgeons rest heavy instruments on the chest, or when the chest wall is covered by adipose tissue. Breathing is also inhibited by restrictive postoperative bandages and by pain after road traffic accidents or thoracotomy.

Treatment of apnoea or hypoventilation

If the cause of apnoea or hypoventilation is in doubt, the trachea is intubated and a breathing system is connected. The level of anaesthesia is assessed. Anaesthetic administration is ended if cranial nerve signs indicate overdosage.

The lungs are then inflated at a rate of 8–15 breaths per minute. If this is possible without high pressure being needed, the cause is probably upper airway obstruction or central nervous depression. If the lungs feel 'stiff', there is probably pneumothorax, pleural effusion or bronchospasm. If the animal does not breathe after 5 minutes or so, imposed hyperventilation may have caused hypocapnia. In this case the respiratory rate should be reduced.

Opioid antagonists (naloxone) or analeptics (doxapram) may be considered as a last resort. Doxapram stimulates respiration and elevates consciousness but its use is futile when respiratory embarrassment is caused by chest-wall fixation or airway obstruction. Its effects are short-lived and so the drug is only useful for 'buying time'.

Cardiovascular complications

Cardiovascular complications are a major concern during anaesthesia. Most drugs depress cardiovascular function, often in a dose-dependent manner. This, combined with pre-existing pathology, makes such complications relatively common. Alterations in heart rate and rhythm, vascular tone and myocardial contractility can all occur.

Tachycardia and bradycardia

Changes in heart rate are important because they can affect the adequacy of the heart to pump out blood to the organs, they can increase the workload of the heart (especially tachycardia) and they can predispose to serious arrhythmias. Further they may indicate serious underlying pathology or inappropriate depth of anaesthesia. The causes and treatment of these two conditions are given in Figure 22.29.

Arrhythmias

Irregularities in heart rhythm may reduce cardiac output and cause hypotension. Without treatment some rhythms may deteriorate into more dangerous forms associated with cardiac arrest (e.g. ventricular fibrillation).

Causes

Arrhythmias are caused by inadequate anaesthesia or overdosage, electrolyte and blood-gas abnormalities, certain surgical procedures and pre-existing heart disease. Certain medical conditions, such as GDV complex, are associated with ventricular arrhythmias.

Treatment

This depends primarily on diagnosis with electrocardiography and treatment with antiarrhythmic drugs. Often, ensuring an adequate level of anaesthesia and ventilation restores normal rhythm.

Cause	Treatment
Tachycardia	
Inadequate anaesthesia	Increase vaporizer setting or give intravenous anaesthetic/analgesic
Hypoxia	Ventilate with 100% oxygen, end nitrous oxide administration (if used)
Hypercapnia	Ventilate, reduce anaesthetic depth
Hypotension	Begin fluid infusion at rapid rate, reduce anaesthetic depth, administer inotropes
Hyperthermia	Cool body surfaces, administer cool IV fluids
Drugs	Reversal not generally required
Bradycardia	
Anaesthetic overdose	Reduce vaporizer setting and ventilate. Administer reversal agent (if available)
Terminal hypoxia	Stop anaesthetic and ventilate with 100% oxygen. Initiate CPR
Hyperkalaemia	Instigate fluid therapy, give sodium bicarbonate and or glucose and insulin
Vagal activity	Check surgeon's activity. If this is related to bradycardia then temporarily suspend surgery and give atropine or glycopyrrolate
Drugs	Alpha$_2$ agonists and high doses of opioids produce bradycardia. Anti-muscarinic drugs offset the effects of opioids, but their use with alpha$_2$ agonists is controversial. Reducing the depth of anaesthesia may increase heart rates reduced by drugs
Hypothermia	Rewarm, and end surgery as soon as possible. Reduce vaporizer setting and ventilate

22.29 Treating tachycardia and bradycardia.

Hypotension

Prolonged hypotension diminishes perfusion in splanchnic and renal vasculature, ultimately causing tissue damage. When hypotension is severe or prolonged, fatal myocardial and cerebral damage occurs.

Causes

Low blood pressure results from several factors. Inadequate cardiac output and reduced systemic vascular resistance cause hypotension. Cardiac output falls because of either extremes of heart rate or inadequate stroke volume. The latter results from poor contractility (e.g. anaesthetic overdose) or reduced preload (hypovolaemia). Alternatively, hypotension can occur from reduced systemic vascular resistance, e.g. when high doses of acepromazine maleate are given.

Treatment

If the animal is 'deep', anaesthetic depth should be reduced and intravenous fluids should be infused rapidly until improvement is seen. If no improvement occurs, inotropes (e.g. dobutamine) may be needed.

Haemorrhage

Blood loss during surgery causes hypotension and ultimately haemorrhagic or hypovolaemic shock. Obvious signs of shed blood at the surgical site combined with tachycardia, pallor and a weak pulse should raise the suspicion of significant haemorrhage. Loss can be estimated by weighing swabs: 1 ml blood weighs 1.3 g. The volume of shed blood can be quantified by deducting the weight of dry swabs from those soaked in blood.

Lost blood is replaced with blood, plasma expanders or electrolyte solutions. If blood is used, the volume required equals the volume lost. For blood losses of up to 20% of circulating volume, electrolyte solutions such as Hartmann's can be infused on a 3:1 basis (3 ml fluids are given for each 1 ml of blood lost).

Thermoregulatory complications

Both hypothermia and hyperthermia are seen during anaesthesia. Anaesthetics depress the body's ability to regulate temperature and occasionally can upregulate metabolism, inducing hyperthermia (e.g. malignant hyperthermia). Hypothermia, however, is most common under anaesthesia and results from a number of factors:

- Hypothalamic thermoregulation is impaired by anaesthetics.
- Skin blood vessels vasodilate.
- Skeletal muscle activity ceases.
- Shivering is inhibited during surgical anaesthesia.
- Visceral surfaces are exposed.
- Inspired gases are cold and dry.

Animals most at risk are those with high ratios of surface area to volume (e.g. neonates, birds and small mammals) and those with underdeveloped or impaired thermoregulatory reflexes (the very young and old).

There are important adverse effects of hypothermia:

- Alveolar ventilation is reduced.
- Heart rate and cardiac output are reduced.
- Haemoglobin binds oxygen more strongly.
- Erythrocytes become stickier; blood viscosity increases.
- During recovery, shivering elevates oxygen consumption and plasma catecholamines.

Consequences

Primarily prolonged recovery is seen. This results from reduced elimination of volatile agents, reduced redistribution and retarded metabolism of injectable drugs and may become a self-reinforcing cycle. In human anaesthesia there is evidence that perioperative hypothermia predisposes to increased morbidity and wound complications. If hypothermia is very severe, cardiac arrest may result. Ventricular fibrillation is likely when body temperature falls below 28°C.

Prevention

Prevention of hypothermia is better than treatment and can be addressed in a number of ways.

Physical factors

- Increase operating room temperature.
- Do not lay animals on cold, uninsulated surfaces.
- Do not expose to draughts.
- Insulate animals with aluminium foil or bubble wrap.
- Use heated blankets, hot-air blankets (Bair huggers), insulated hot-water bottles and radiant heat lamps.

Anaesthetic factors

- Favour the use of short-acting anaesthetics.
- Avoid deep planes of anaesthesia.
- Provide adequate but not excessive ventilation.
- Use rebreathing systems where appropriate.
- Use warm intravenous fluids.

Surgical factors

- During surgical preparation of high-risk animals, do not unnecessarily wet the animal, clip excessively or use volatile preparations such as alcohol.
- Minimize surgical time.
- Exposed visceral surfaces must be moistened with warm irrigation fluids. Non-surgical areas must not be allowed to get wet. Incision size must be as small as possible. Viscera should be replaced in body cavities as soon as examination or surgery is completed.

Treatment

Postoperatively, the animal should be thoroughly dried using towels and hair dryers. Topical heat may then be applied using hot-air blankets, judicious use of 40 W light bulbs, radiant infrared lamps or insulated hot-water bottles. Small mammals may be placed in an incubator. If these methods fail, warm-water gastric or rectal lavage may be performed.

Delayed return to consciousness

Prolonged recovery is occasionally seen. Inappropriate depth of anaesthesia, the use of drugs with prolonged durations of action and individual patient sensitivity all contribute to this problem. Acepromazine maleate may cause slow recoveries in certain breeds of dog and in dogs with diminished liver function. Multiple doses of barbiturates may also delay recovery, particularly in sight-hounds. Drug retention may result from inadequate perfusion or failure of the liver or kidney. Hypothermia causes retarded expiration of volatile agents and the redistribution and reduction of metabolism of injectable agents.

The fundamental approach to prolonged recovery is based on maintaining organ physiological function, providing good nursing (e.g. raising temperature, preventing dependent sore) and creating a diffusion gradient from the drug's site of action to the organ of elimination. Monitoring of the patient should be approached as for the anaesthetized patient. Maintenance of cardiovascular and respiratory function in these cases is vital. Haemodynamic support with intravenous fluids (with or without the use of positive inotropes) may be required. For patients with prolonged periods of unconsciousness, urinary catheterization and measurement of urine output is valuable. This gives a simple yet excellent indicator of renal perfusion and function and, indirectly, cardiovascular performance. If the patient is hypoxic, oxygen supplementation is necessary; and if hypoventilating, positive pressure ventilation may be required. Rewarming and maintenance of body temperature are also important. Persistent drug activity can be countered if the suspect agent has an antagonist (Figure 22.30).

Agonist	Antagonist
Opioids	Naloxone, nalbuphine
Benzodiazepines	Flumazenil
Alpha$_2$ agonist	Atipamezole

22.30 Agonists and antagonists.

Miscellaneous accidents

Accidents during recovery

Poor attention to recovering animals contributes to postoperative mortality. Problems are probably more likely at this time because attention relaxes, the perceived high-risk periods of induction and maintenance having passed. Responsibilities during recovery (Figure 22.31) include the following:

- Monitoring vital signs and keeping records
- Keeping animals calm and dry, and surgical sites and orifices clean
- Attending to wounds and preventing interference
- Providing postoperative medication
- Monitoring fluid and energy balance
- Reporting recovery problems.

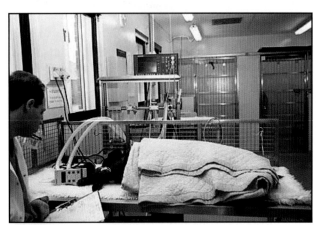

22.31 Careful postoperative monitoring following laryngeal surgery.

Excitation
Bad recoveries characterized by excitation, hyperaesthesia, vocalization, exaggerated responsiveness and excessive activity may result from pain, emergence, pharmacological phenomena and epilepsy/convulsion.

Pain
Pain responds to analgesic administration.

Emergence
Some animals recover after non-painful surgery as if in pain. Disconcerting signs are normally short-lived. The incidence is higher with certain drugs (e.g. Saffan) but may be reduced if sedative premedications are used and recovery occurs in a quiet environment.

Convulsions/epilepsy
Postoperative convulsions traditionally followed myelographic investigation with certain contrast media. Epileptic patients may be at increased risk of postoperative seizures.

Hypoxia
Although extubation must be performed when gagging, 'bucking' and other cranial nerve reflexes are restored, it is not wise to assume that oxygen delivery may be safely discontinued. Hypothermia, residual anaesthetic drug activity and lung changes may combine to diminish blood oxygenation, while shivering and pain increase oxygen consumption. Oxygen (100%) should be delivered until animals can maintain satisfactory oxygenation on room air. If extubation is necessary before this time, oxygen should be given by mask, intranasal catheter, tracheostomy tube or transtracheal catheter.

Oxygen must be given for at least 5 minutes after the discontinuation of N_2O in order to avoid diffusion hypoxia. Animals incapable of maintaining sternal recumbency should be repositioned every 2–4 hours to prevent hypostatic congestion of the lungs.

Discharge
Animals must not be discharged before full recovery from anaesthesia and surgery. The client must also be forewarned of other anaesthetic and surgery-related complications such as haemorrhage.

Extravascular injections
Extravascular injection of irritant drugs such as thiopental results in tissue sloughs. These are painful, take a long time to heal and leave unsightly blemishes. The risk of this is minimized by:

- Effective patient restraint (physical or chemical) before injection
- Venous catheterization
- Using dilute solutions of drug (e.g. 1.25% for thiopental) in animals with poorly accessible veins.

If extravascular injection does occur, the deposition is enthusiastically diluted with sterile saline or water. Large volumes may be safely injected under the skin and massaged. Later a record should be made of the accident.

Burns
Burns occur if excess heat is applied to cold animals. This is more likely when skin blood flow is reduced, as in shock, because poorly perfused skin conducts heat less effectively.

Decubital ulcers
These sores appear when bony prominences remain in prolonged contact with hard surfaces. They are prevented by adequate bedding and frequent turning of the patient.

Hypostatic congestion
Capillaries in the dependent (lowermost) lung fill with blood and alveoli partially collapse when recoveries are prolonged and cardiac output is low. Both changes result in hypoxia. Prevention is based on frequent (2-hourly) turning.

Equipment-based accidents

Cylinders
Cylinders contain gas at high pressure (nearly 1935 psi or 13,300 kPa) and will explode if mistreated. They must not be dropped or placed in a position where they might fall or become damaged. They should not be exposed to high temperatures (including direct sunlight). They must be stored in dry conditions away from flammable materials.

When a full oxygen cylinder is exposed to elevated temperatures caused, for example, by naked flames, the pressure within it rises and may exceed the test pressure. Eventually the bottle bursts and releases oxygen, which fuels further conflagration.

Explosions and fires
Explosions require a source of fuel (usually carbon-based), oxygen and activation energy (a spark or a naked flame). Once initiated, heat released from the reaction provides further activation energy and the reaction proliferates. Explosions are more likely when fuel–oxygen rather than fuel–air mixtures are present.

For these reasons, 'sticking' valves or apparatus involved with pressurized oxygen must never be lubricated or sealed with carbon-based or petroleum-based lubricants. In the past, cyclopropane and diethyl ether were commonly used for anaesthesia. They lost popularity because of their flammability and explosive properties, and their redundancy was accelerated by the introduction of thermocautery and electrical monitoring devices in the operating room. Surgical alcohol remains a possible source of fire and explosion.

Risks of fire and explosion are minimized by keeping the three 'components' separate:

- Inflammable agents must not be used when heat, sparks (from static electricity or electrical apparatus) or naked flames are present
- If thermocautery is required, cyclopropane and ether must be avoided
- Naked flames, carbon-based fuels and dust must be minimized.

If fires or explosions occur, the emergency services must be informed that supplies of inflammable material and compressed oxygen are within the vicinity of the accident.

Accidents to personnel

Bites and scratches
These are minimized by suitable physical and chemical restraint techniques, by equipment and by commonsense precautions. Fingers should not be placed within the mouth of an ungagged, unconscious animal, especially during endotracheal intubation. Owners should not normally be allowed to restrain animals, in case they are injected accidentally or bitten.

When an accident occurs, the appropriate report form must be completed (see Chapter 1). The injured person should report to hospital for examination and tetanus immunization. If known, details of the animal's condition should be supplied.

Self-administration of drugs
There is risk associated with self-administration of all drugs. In particular, there is risk with sedatives, especially alpha$_2$ adrenoceptor agonists; toxicity has not yet been reported in humans, though the potential is great. Absorption of these drugs across oral mucous membranes is rapid and so placing of needle-caps in mouths is especially hazardous. Ketamine has been inadvertently self-administered, with ensuing toxic signs.

Whenever drug-based accidents occur, the data sheet or NOAH Compendium should be taken to the emergency room with the injured person. Self-administration can be avoided by taking sensible precautions:

- Ensure that the animal is adequately restrained
- Do not resheath needles but dispose of them immediately after use
- Do not carry syringes and needles in pockets
- Do not place syringe caps in the mouth
- The needle used for drug withdrawal from the vial should be discarded and a new needle used for injection
- Wear gloves
- Do not pressurize the vial
- Have eye and skin washes available.

If a drug splashes on to the skin or into the eye, the site must be thoroughly irrigated with copious amounts of fresh water. If injection occurs, or if toxic signs follow splashing accidents, medical advice must be sought.

Cardiopulmonary arrest

Cardiopulmonary arrest occurs when cardiopulmonary function fails. Failure to initiate effective cardiopulmonary–cerebral resuscitation (CPCR) under these circumstances leads rapidly to death. Sometimes CPCR is not appropriate: it is futile when animals with 'terminal' conditions arrest. Factors predisposing to arrest can develop rapidly (acute arrests) or more slowly (chronic arrests). 'Acute' arrests result from single devastating events occurring in otherwise normal cases (e.g. thiopental overdose). 'Chronic' arrests result when many derangements develop slowly and remain unnoticed until the cumulative effect is catastrophic. The latter are probably more common in veterinary practice and indicate that close monitoring and rapid treatment of even mildly deteriorating conditions are important. The axiom 'prevention is better than cure' is most important in the context of CPCR.

Causes of arrest

- Myocardial hypoxia (e.g. tachycardia, bradycardia, hypotension, myocardial disease)
- Toxins (e.g. toxaemia, azotaemia, anaesthetic overdose)
- pH extremes (e.g. hypoventilation, shock, diabetic ketoacidosis)
- Electrolyte changes (e.g. hyperkalaemia, hypocalcaemia, hypokalaemia)
- Temperature extremes.

Clinical signs

- Blood at surgical site becomes dark and clots easily.
- Bleeding stops.
- Either 'gasping' ventilation or apnoea is seen (the former resembling 'light' anaesthesia).
- Mucous membranes may become dirty grey, blue or white.
- Capillary refill time becomes prolonged (more than 2 seconds).
- Heart sounds are not audible.
- No palpable pulse.
- Central eye position.
- Pupils dilate.
- Dry cornea.
- Cranial nerve reflexes are lost.
- Generalized muscle relaxation.
- Arrhythmias. Those normally associated with arrest include ventricular fibrillation and asystole. However, in electromechanical dissociation there is a near-normal ECG while mechanical cardiac activity is lost. This is a common cause of arrest in dogs.

Treatment
When these clinical signs are recognized, assistance must be summoned immediately. Simultaneously, preparations are made for CPCR (see Chapter 18), the elements of which are remembered with the mnemonic:

- Airway
- Breathing
- Circulation
- Drugs
- Electrical defibrillation
- Follow-up.

Before these begin, the animal is laid in right lateral recumbency, positioned against a hard surface and, if possible, in a slight head-down position.

Practical tip
Rehearse CPCR so that when an emergency occurs everybody knows what to do.

Airway
Effective CPCR requires an appropriately positioned, cuffed patent endotracheal tube of suitable size. Alternatively, a tracheotomy may be performed or a catheter may be passed to the level of the tracheal bifurcation to allow oxygen insufflation.

Breathing
Positive pressure ventilation with oxygen-enriched gas must be imposed. This can be done using any of the following:

- An anaesthetic machine and appropriate breathing system flushed with 100% oxygen
- Self-inflating resuscitation bags (e.g. Ambu resuscitator) which connect to endotracheal tubes and allow manual lung inflation with either air (20% oxygen) or 100% oxygen
- Expired air (containing 16% oxygen).

The lungs are inflated using sufficient volume to produce visibly supranormal chest-wall excursions. The lungs are reinflated immediately expiration is ended, but must be allowed to deflate to the normal end-expiratory position. In single-handed resuscitation attempts, two or three large lung inflations should be delivered for every 15 chest-wall compressions.

The femoral pulse, mucous membrane colour and heart sounds should be checked within 30 seconds of beginning ventilation. Thereafter they should be monitored continuously, if assistance is available, or at half-minute intervals. Ventilation alone may restore the pulse but in most cases circulatory support will be required.

Circulation
When the heart stops, cardiac output must be supported by either compressing the rib cage (external cardiac compression) or directly squeezing the surgically exposed heart (internal cardiac compression). Cardiac output produced by either method depends on adequate venous return. This is enhanced by rapid fluid infusion, posture, abdominal compression and adrenaline.

External cardiac compression
There are two forms of external cardiac compression: the 'cardiac pump' method and the 'thoracic pump' method.

The **cardiac pump** method is most suitable for cats, dogs weighing less than 20 kg, or those with narrow chests (e.g. whippets). The chest wall is compressed in the ventral third of the thorax between the 3rd and 6th rib. This is facilitated if the animal is positioned on a hard surface in right lateral recumbency. For very small dogs, cats and puppies, the heart is massaged by compressing the ribs between thumb and forefinger. The compression rate is 80–100 per minute.

The **thoracic pump** method is suitable for larger dogs weighing over 20 kg or lighter dogs with 'barrel' chests (e.g. bulldogs). The rib cage is compressed at the widest point – the junction of the dorsal and middle thirds of the 6th to 7th rib –

at 60–120 times per minute. If possible, compressions should be made during peak lung inflation. The efficiency of this second technique is increased by three manoeuvres:

- **Abdominal binding.** Applying tight bandages to the hindlimbs and then the abdomen directs blood flow (generated by external cardiac compression) towards the head.
- **Abdominal counterpulsation** (interposed abdominal compression). The abdomen is manually compressed during the diastolic or relaxation phase of chest compression to increase coronary perfusion and assist venous return.
- **Synchronous lung inflation/chest wall compression.** Cardiac output increases when the chest is compressed.

Because ventilation and cardiac compression must never be suspended, abdominal binding and counterpulsation require the presence of a third resuscitator.

The advantages of external cardiac compression are:

- Reasonably effective in certain patients
- Requires little preparation
- Rapidly applied
- Few hazards
- Can be performed by lay staff.

The disadvantage is that it is ineffective in some circumstances.

Internal cardiac compression
Internal cardiac compression requires a thoracotomy and direct manual compression of the heart. It is more effective than external cardiac compression and is recommended if the latter is ineffective at generating a palpable pulse within 2–3 minutes of onset of cardiac arrest. Internal cardiac massage allows visualization of the beating heart and intracardiac drug administration. However, it does require a surgical approach to the thorax and often practitioners are reluctant to perform it or they attempt internal massage too late after onset of arrest.

To perform internal thoracotomy a rapid clip of the 3rd to 6th intercostal space on the left side may be needed in long-haired dogs. The appropriate site can be identified by flexing the forelimb so that the olecranon transects the costochondral junction; this point overlies the 5th intercostal space. However, time must not be wasted in surgical preparation. A bold skin incision is made from dorsal to the sternum to ventral to the transverse process of the thoracic vertebrae at intercostal space 5. Scissors are used to cut through the intercostal muscles and the ribs are spread with rib retractors. The heart is then manually compressed.

Signs of effective CPCR
Early signs

- Palpation of pulse during cardiac compression
- Constriction of the pupils
- Ventromedial relocation of the eye
- Improvement of mucous membrane colour
- ECG changes
- Restoration of a trace on the capnograph when ventilating, indicating that CO_2 is being returned to the lungs from the tissues, to be blown off in the lungs

▶

Later signs

- Lacrimation
- Return of cranial nerve reflexes (e.g. blinking, gagging and coughing)
- Return of spontaneous respiratory activity (diaphragmatic twitches and irregular breathing appear at first)
- Then return of regular deep breathing (this is a good prognostic sign)
- Return of special senses: response to sound
- Return of other central nervous function: vocalization righting reflexes, purposeful movement

If early signs of successful CPCR are not seen within 2 minutes, resuscitative drugs and electrical defibrillation (D and E of the mnemonic) can be used, or an emergency thoracotomy and internal cardiac compression can be undertaken.

Drugs

In cases unresponsive to ventilation and cardiac massage or where a definite diagnosis of an arrhythmia has been made, drug therapy is instituted. The use of a central vein (e.g. jugular vein) is to be recommended, as peripheral vein drainage back to the heart is often reduced in these patients. Alternatively, intratracheal drug administration can be used. Commonly used drugs and their doses are included in Figure 22.32.

Drug	Route	Indication	Dose
Adrenaline	i.v., i.t.	Asystole, atropine-resistant bradycardia myocardial depression	0.1–0.2 mg/kg
Atropine	i.v., i.t.	Vagal bradycardias, asystole	0.02–0.04 mg/kg
Bicarbonate	i.v.	Metabolic acidosis	Approx. 1 mEq/kg
Calcium	i.v.	Hyperkalaemia, hypocalcaemia myocardial depression	10 mg/kg
Dobutamine	i.v.	Hypotension	1–5 µg/kg/min
Dopamine	i.v.	Hypotension, renal failure	1–10 µg/kg/min
Electrical defibrillation		Ventricular fibrillation	0.1–0.5 J/kg (internal) 1–5 J/kg (external)
Lidocaine	i.v., i.t.	Ventricular tachycardia	2–4 mg/kg (dog) 40–80 mg/kg (cat)
Dexamethasone	i.v.	Post-resuscitation	1–2 mg/kg

22.32 Drug doses for cardiopulmonary resuscitation. i.v., intravenous. i.t., intratracheal.

Electrical defibrillation

If ventricular fibrillation has occurred, early electrical defibrillation is advised (see Chapter 18). A fully charged and readily available defibrillator is required.

Follow-up

If the patient has been successfully resuscitated, careful postoperative intensive care will be required. Maintenance of cardiovascular function may be necessary. Fluid therapy is usually continued into the recovery period and inotropes may be given if blood pressure is not maintained. Attention to renal output is important and some patients may need diuretic therapy in addition to fluid therapy. Those patients inadequately ventilating may require ventilatory support (with or without sedation) into the recovery period. Maintenance of body temperature is often required with the use of methods including heated blankets, heat lamps and warm intravenous fluids. Postoperative attention to neurological status is also often required. Treatment of seizures and brain oedema may be necessary.

Too much practice at resuscitation is not necessarily a good thing, as it suggests more accidents are happening than would be liked. However, the veterinary nurse can prepare for such eventualities and can significantly improve the chances for successful resuscitation. A fully stocked and maintained resuscitation box with in-date drugs can be invaluable. Contents of a resuscitation box are described in Figure 22.33.

Drugs
Adrenaline
Atropine
Lidocaine
Isoprenaline
Dopamine
Dobutamine
Propranolol
Furosemide
Mannitol
Methyl prednisolone
Procainamide
Calcium gluconate
Sodium bicarbonate
Edrophonium or neostigmine
Verapamil
Doxapram
Naloxone
Atipamezole

Equipment
Needles and syringes
Urinary catheters for intratracheal drug administration
Emergency surgical pack
Self-inflating resuscitator bag
Defibrillator
Internal and external paddles
Intravenous catheters
Endotracheal tubes

22.33 Drugs and equipment required for cardiopulmonary resuscitation.

Acknowledgements

The author (DB) is indebted to Mr RE Clutton, the author of this chapter in a previous edition, from which information and some diagrams have been drawn, and to Dr PM Taylor for permission to use information from her University of Cambridge Undergraduate Veterinary Anaesthesia lecture notes.

Further reading

Bennet RA (1998) Reptile anaesthesia. In: *Reptile Medicine and Surgery* (ed. D Mader), pp. 241–247. WB Saunders, Philadelphia

Beynon P, Forbes NA and Harcourt-Brown N (1996) Formulary. In: *BSAVA Manual of Psittacine Birds*, pp. 228–234. BSAVA Publications, Cheltenham

Coles B (1997) *Avian Medicine and Surgery*. Blackwell Publishing, Oxford

Davey A, Moyle JTB and Ward CS (1994) *Ward's Anaesthetic Equipment, 3rd edn*. WB Saunders, London

Edling TM (2005) Anaesthesia and analgesia. In: *BSAVA Manual of Psittacine Birds, 2nd edn* (eds N Harcourt-Brown and J Chitty), pp. 87–96. BSAVA Publications, Gloucester

Girling S (2002) *Veterinary Nursing of Exotic Pets*. Blackwell Publishing, Oxford

Hall LW, Clarke KW and Trim C (2000) *Veterinary Anaesthesia, 10th edn*. Baillière Tindall, London

Hall LW and Taylor PM (1994) *Anaesthesia of the Cat*. Baillière Tindall, London

Harms CA and Lewbart GA (2000) Surgery in fish. *Veterinary Clinics of North America: Exotic Animal Practice*, **3**, 759–774

Mason DE (1997) Anaesthesia, analgesia and sedation for small mammals. In: *Ferrets, Rabbits and Rodents: Clinical Medicine and Surgery* (eds EV Hillyer and KE Quesenberry), pp. 389–391. WB Saunders, Philadelphia

Meredith A and Redrobe S (eds) (2002) *BSAVA Manual of Exotic Pets, 4th edn*. BSAVA Publications, Cheltenham

Page CD (1993) Current reptilian anaesthesia procedures. In: *Zoo and Wildlife Medicine: Current Therapy 3* (ed. M Fowler), pp. 140–143. WB Saunders, Philadelphia

Seymour C and Gleed R (1999) *BSAVA Manual of Small Animal Anaesthesia and Analgesia*. BSAVA Publications, Cheltenham

Thurmon JC, Tranquilli WJ and Benson GJ (1996) *Veterinary Anesthesia, 3rd edn*. Williams & Wilkins, Baltimore

Chapter 23

Theatre practice

Dawn McHugh

Learning objectives

After studying this chapter, students should be able to:

- Explain the principles of surgical asepsis
- Describe the role of the veterinary nurse in the establishment and maintenance of asepsis in the operating theatre
- Describe the different methods of sterilization available and discuss their suitability and use for a range of surgical instruments and equipment used in veterinary surgery
- Describe the care and maintenance of surgical instruments/packs and equipment
- Recognize a range of surgical instruments used in all types of veterinary surgery
- Describe the preparation of a patient for surgery, intraoperative and immediate postoperative care of a patient
- Explain the roles of a veterinary nurse in the operating theatre as both a scrubbed and a circulating nurse
- Describe the ideal properties of suture materials and discuss the advantages and disadvantages of different types
- Recognize different suture patterns commonly used in veterinary surgery

Definitions

- **Sepsis** – the presence of pathogens or their toxic products in the blood or tissues of the patient; more commonly known as infection
- **Asepsis** – freedom from infection, i.e. exclusion of microorganisms and spores
- **Antisepsis** – prevention of sepsis by destruction or inhibition of microorganisms using an agent that may be safely applied to living tissue
- **Sterilization** – the destruction of all microorganisms and spores
- **Disinfection** – the removal of microorganisms but not necessarily spores
- **Disinfectant** – an agent that destroys microorganisms, generally chemical agents applied to inanimate objects (see Chapter 12)

Factors influencing the development of infection

Infection of a clean surgical wound is always a matter of great concern. It is far better to prevent infection than to try to treat it. The use of antibiotics should not be relied upon to protect patients from the consequences of poor asepsis.

It has been established that most surgical wound infections occur at the time of surgery, not during the postoperative period. Poor aseptic technique will undoubtedly affect the success of any surgery and in the long term the success and reputation of the practice. Strict theatre discipline is essential if high standards are to be maintained. There has to be a specific protocol that is adhered to rigidly and that everyone involved with surgery respects. This will include correct theatre attire, scrubbing-up procedures, patient preparations, draping techniques, sterilization, organization of surgical lists, cleaning protocol and conduct during surgery.

Introduction

The veterinary nurse is usually given the responsibility for running the operating theatre. This involves: maintenance of hygiene in the theatre; care and maintenance of instruments and equipment; preparation of theatre, the patient and the surgical team; and assistance as both scrubbed and circulating nurse.

The most important factor in successful theatre practice is the establishment and maintenance of a good aseptic technique, i.e. all the steps taken to prevent contact with microorganisms.

Sources of contamination in the operating theatre include the operating room, equipment, personnel and the patient.

Operating room and environment

Many microorganisms are airborne and any movement within the operating theatre will disperse them. Good ventilation is necessary as hot, humid conditions are a great threat to asepsis. Clean procedures should be performed first because microorganisms from contaminated sites will remain in the air. The operating room itself must be easily cleaned and should contain as little furniture and shelving as possible.

Equipment and instruments

All equipment and instruments used in the operative site must be sterile. There must be a new set of instruments for each operation.

Personnel

The more people present in theatre, the greater is the likelihood of infection. All theatre personnel should wear theatre clothing, caps, masks, scrub suits and antistatic footwear. These are only worn in the designated theatre area. In addition, those who are in the surgical team should prepare their hands aseptically and wear sterile gowns and gloves.

The patient

The patient is probably the greatest source of contamination, especially as animals are covered in hair. The source of microorganisms may be endogenous or exogenous:

- **Endogenous** – those that originate from within the body of the patient
- **Exogenous** – those that are found on the outside, i.e. the skin and coat. This term is also used with reference to environmental sources of microorganisms (e.g. air, equipment).

It does not necessarily follow that introduction of microorganisms will result in an infected wound. Microorganisms can and will enter any wound that has been exposed to air, but whether infection follows depends on several variable factors.

Factors that influence wound infection

- **Virulence** (disease-producing ability) of the organism and **resistance** of the patient (see Chapter 6)
- **Duration of surgery** – bacterial contamination increases the longer the wound is open (infection rate doubles for every hour of operative time)
- **Surgical technique** – excessive trauma to tissues and damage to vascular supply may increase the likelihood of infection
- **Impaired host resistance** – may increase the risk of infection if it is due to drugs, nutrition or underlying disease
- **Contamination of the wound** – surgical wounds are classified with respect to their potential for contamination and infection (see also Chapter 24):
  - **Clean** – where there is no break in asepsis. The respiratory, gastrointestinal and urinary tracts are not entered and there is no break in aseptic technique ▶
  - **Clean-contaminated** – where a contaminated area is entered but without spillage or spread of contamination (i.e. ingesta, urine, mucus). Minor break in asepsis
  - **Contaminated** – where there is spillage from a viscus or severe inflammation is encountered, but no infection present. Open fresh traumatic wounds
  - **Dirty** – infected where there is pus present or viscus perforation spilling pus or intestinal contents. Traumatic wound containing devitalized tissue or foreign bodies.

Sterilization

All instruments, drapes, gowns and equipment should be washed thoroughly prior to sterilization, as the presence of protein (e.g. blood) and grease will impede or prevent the sterilization process. Most will also require drying and all items should be inspected for damage and wear prior to packing for sterilization.

Sterilization can be divided into: heat sterilization and cold sterilization (Figure 23.1).

Heat sterilization
Autoclave (steam under pressure):   • Vertical   • Horizontal   • Vacuum-assisted   Dry heat: • Hot-air oven   • High-vacuum oven   • Convection oven

Cold sterilization
Ethylene oxide   Commercial solutions: • Chemical   • Alcohol-based   Gamma irradiation

23.1 Heat and cold sterilization.

Heat sterilization

Steam under pressure (autoclave systems)

Steam under pressure is the most widely used and efficient method of sterilization. It is also the most economical, although the initial outlay may be large. Items that may be sterilized in the autoclave include:

- Instruments
- Drapes
- Gowns
- Swabs
- Most rubber articles
- Glassware
- Some plastic goods.

Heat-sensitive items that may be damaged in the autoclave include fibreoptic equipment, lenses and plastics (especially those designed to be disposable, such as catheters).

The three main types of autoclave are the vertical pressure cooker, the horizontal or vertical downward displacement autoclave and the vacuum-assisted autoclave.

Vertical pressure cooker

This very simple machine operates by boiling water in a closed container, like a household pressure cooker. It usually has an air vent at the top, which is closed once the air has been evacuated and pressure (15 psi) is allowed to build up. As the air vent is at the top, the main disadvantage of this type of autoclave is the danger that some air will be trapped underneath the steam. The temperature in this area will be lower and sterility cannot be guaranteed. It is also manually operated and there is room for human error in the sterilizing cycle.

Horizontal or vertical downward displacement autoclave

This type is larger and usually fully automatic. It uses an electrically operated boiler that is incorporated in the autoclave as a source of steam. Air is driven out more efficiently by downward displacement. There is an air outlet at the bottom and a steam outlet at the top.

Most of these machines are designed for loose instrument sterilization only, rather than packs, as they have insufficient penetrating ability and drying cycles: packs may seem to be dry but they remain damp, allowing entry of microorganisms during the storage period.

There is usually a choice of programmes on this type of autoclave with temperatures of 112, 121, 126 or 134°C.

Vacuum-assisted autoclave (porous load)

This type of autoclave works on the same principle as the other two but uses a high-vacuum pump to evacuate air rapidly from the chamber at the beginning of the cycle. Steam penetration after evacuation is almost instantaneous and sterilization occurs very quickly. A second vacuum cycle rapidly withdraws moisture after sterilization and dries the load. It is suitable for all types of instruments, drapes and equipment and there is a choice of cycles using different temperatures and pressures.

Vacuum-assisted autoclaves are fully automatic, with failsafe mechanisms (usually warning lights and alarms) that indicate whether the load is non-sterile or has been sterilized effectively. They are generally much larger and more sophisticated than other types and are invariably connected to a central boiler to supply steam. The cost of purchase and maintenance are higher, but the machine's efficiency and reliability in sterilization far outweigh those of the smaller types.

Principles of sterilization using steam under pressure

Although autoclaves vary in size and type, the basic principle of function remains the same. When water boils at 100°C some bacteria, spores and viruses are resistant to heat, and remain unchanged even if exposed to such a temperature for a long time. By increasing the pressure, the temperature of the steam is raised and resistant microorganisms and spores will be killed by coagulation of cell proteins. It is the increased temperature, not the increased pressure, that leads to this destruction of microorganisms. The higher the temperature, the shorter is the time needed to achieve sterilization (Figure 23.2).

Temperature (°C)	Pressure (psi)	Pressure (kg/cm²)	Time (minutes)
121	15	1.2	15
126	20	1.4	10
134	30	2	3½

23.2 Autoclave temperature, pressure and time combinations.

The autoclaving process

The central sterilizing chamber of the autoclave is surrounded by a steam jacket. The pressure in the jacket is raised (depending on the cycle). Steam then enters the chamber and as it does so air is displaced downwards, because steam is lighter. When all the air is evacuated, exhaust vents are closed and steam continues to enter until the desired pressure is reached. The more sophisticated types of autoclave have a vacuum prior to introduction of steam to displace air from materials to be sterilized. If any air remains in the chamber the temperature will be lower than steam at that pressure and sterility cannot be guaranteed.

Once the air has been evacuated, steam that has entered the chamber begins to condense on the colder surfaces in the chamber, i.e. instruments etc. The steam produces heat, which penetrates to the innermost layer of the pack. The moisture increases the penetrability of the heat. After the given amount of time the steam is exhausted. As the temperature drops, the pressure returns to normal. In vacuum-assisted autoclaves the instruments are then heat dried, with filtered air replacing the exhausted steam. On modern machines the door cannot be opened until the end of this stage.

Effective sterilization also depends on correct loading of packs into the autoclave. There should be adequate space between them to allow steam to circulate freely. Care should be taken to avoid overloading and blocking of the inlet and exhaust valves. Before packing for sterilization, instruments must be free of grease and protein material to allow effective penetration of steam.

Maintenance of the autoclave

All types of autoclave should be serviced by a qualified engineer to ensure that they remain in good working order and remain electrically safe. Vacuum-assisted autoclaves with a separate boiler should be serviced every 3 months to comply with Health and Safety regulations. Thermocouple testing is recommended at least annually to ensure that effective sterilization is taking place.

Monitoring efficacy of sterilization in the autoclave

- **Chemical indicator strips** (TST Strips) show colour changes when the correct temperature, pressure and time have been reached. A strip is placed inside each pack. It is important that the appropriate strip is used for each different pressure/time/temperature cycle, otherwise a false result may be given.
- **Browne's tubes** work on the same principle, i.e. a colour change. Small glass tubes are partly filled with an orange-brown liquid that changes to green when certain temperatures have been maintained for a required period of time. Tubes are available that change at 121, 126 or 134°C. It is essential to ensure that the correct type of tube is selected for any particular temperature cycle. Browne's tubes are also available for hot-air ovens.
- **Bowie–Dick indicator tape** is commonly used to seal instrument and drape packs. It is a beige-coloured tape impregnated with chemical stripes that change to dark brown when a certain temperature is reached (121°C). As with ethylene oxide indicator tape, it is not reliable as an indicator of sterility as it does not ensure that the temperature was maintained for the required time.
- **Spore tests** are strips of paper impregnated with dried spores (usually *Bacillus stearothermophilus*). A strip is included in the load; on completion of the cycle it is placed in the culture medium provided and incubated at

the appropriate temperature for up to 72 hours. If the sterilization process has been successful, the spores will be killed and there will be no growth.

Spore systems are more accurate than chemical indicators but the delay in obtaining results is a major disadvantage. A combination of both systems is recommended: chemical indicators should be included in each pack and spore strips should be used at regular intervals.

Vacuum-assisted autoclaves will usually have visible **temperature and pressure gauges** on the front. Some systems have a **paper recording chart** that indicates the efficiency of sterilization.

Thermocouples (electrical leads with temperature-sensitive tips) are placed in various parts of the sterilizing chamber with the leads passed out through an aperture to a recording device outside. The temperature within the chamber can be constantly recorded throughout a cycle to check that required temperatures are achieved and held for the specified time.

Dry heat

Dry heat kills microorganisms by causing oxidative destruction of bacterial protoplasm. Microorganisms are much more resistant to dry heat than when heated in the presence of moisture and so higher temperatures are required (150–180°C). Dry heat below 140°C cannot destroy bacterial spores in less than 4–5 hours.

The range of equipment sterilized in this way is restricted: fabrics, rubber goods and plastic cannot withstand these high, dry temperatures and are easily damaged.

There are certain items for which dry heat sterilization is the method of choice. These include glass syringes, cutting instruments, ophthalmic instruments, drill bits, glassware, powders and oils.

Hot-air ovens

These are heated by electrical elements (Figure 23.3). They are usually small but are economical in terms of purchase and running costs. They have been largely superseded by the autoclave, which is more efficient and suitable for most types of material.

Item	Temperature (°C)	Time (min)
Glassware	180	60
Non-cutting instruments Powders, oils	160	120
Sharp-cutting instruments	150	180

23.3 Temperature and time ratios recommended for hot-air ovens.

A long cooling period is needed before the items may be used. The door should be fitted with a safety device to prevent it being opened before the oven is cool. It is important to ensure that the oven is not overloaded and that items are placed so that air can flow freely.

Spore strip tests and Browne's tubes are available that are designed specifically for testing sterility in hot-air ovens.

Moist heat (boiling)

Boiling is no longer considered as a method of sterilization. It cannot be guaranteed to kill all microorganisms and spores, because the maximum temperature of 100°C is insufficient to kill resistant spores.

Cold sterilization

Ethylene oxide

Ethylene oxide is a highly penetrative and effective method of sterilization. However, concerns have been expressed about its use in veterinary practice as it is toxic, irritant to tissue and a very inflammable gas. Its use is currently permitted and the danger to operators should be negligible as long as the manufacturer's recommendations are followed. COSHH Regulations may make its use impractical in some veterinary practices.

Ethylene oxide inactivates the DNA of the cells, thereby preventing cell reproduction. The technique is effective against vegetative bacteria, fungi, viruses and spores. Several factors influence the ability of ethylene oxide to destroy microorganisms, including temperature, pressure, concentration, humidity and time of exposure. As the temperature increases, the ability of ethylene oxide to penetrate increases and the duration of the cycle shortens. The only system available in the UK operates at room temperature for a period of 12 hours.

Use of the ethylene oxide sterilizer

The sterilizer consists of a plastic container fitted with a ventilation system to prevent gas entering the work area. It should be located in a clean, well ventilated area (e.g. fume cupboard) away from work areas. The temperature of the room must be at least 20°C during the cycle.

Individually packed items to be sterilized are placed in a polythene liner bag. The plastic bag is a gas diffusion membrane of known permeability whose function is to contain the gas given off by the ampoule and to release it at a controlled rate during the sterilization cycle. A gas ampoule containing the ethylene oxide liquid surrounded by a plastic shield is placed within the liner bag. Excess air is then pressed out before the mouth of the bag is closed. A flexible plastic purge tube protrudes into the sterilization unit. The end of this purge tube is placed in the mouth of the liner bag and, using a plastic locking bag tie, the neck of the liner bag is sealed around the purge tube. The top of the glass vial is snapped from outside the liner bag to release the sterilant gas. The door to the sterilizer unit is closed and locked, the ventilator switch is turned on and the items are left for 12 hours (the sterilization process is frequently performed overnight). At the end of the 12-hour period, the unit is unlocked, the liner bag is untied and a purge pump is switched on to aerate the chamber. The door may be opened after 2 hours and the load removed.

The latest model of the Anprolene ethylene oxide sterilizer has a 'cycle start' button, which is pressed when the glass vial is snapped. This then automatically begins a 2-hour purge at the end of sterilization. A green light indicates the end of that period and when the unit may be opened.

Preparation of materials for sterilization

Ethylene oxide is effective for the sterilization of many different types of equipment but its use is limited by the size of the container, the duration of the cycle and concerns about toxicity. Its use therefore tends to be restricted to items that are damaged by heat:

- Fibreoptic equipment
- Plastic catheters, trays, etc.
- Anaesthetic tubing, etc.
- Plastic syringes
- Optical instruments
- High-speed drills/burs
- Battery-operated drills.

Many commercially available products are now sterilized by this method, e.g. syringes, synthetic absorbable suture materials and catheters. Equipment made of polyvinylchloride (PVC) should not be sterilized by this method as the material may react with the gas.

Materials to be sterilized by ethylene oxide must be cleaned and dried. Water on instruments at the time of exposure may react with the gas and reduce its effectiveness.

Occlusive bungs, caps or stylets must be removed from instruments so that gas can penetrate freely. Syringes should be packaged disassembled.

Ethylene oxide penetrates materials more readily than steam and so a wider variety of packaging materials may be used when preparing items for sterilization and storage. However, nylon film designed for autoclaving should not be used, as it has been shown that there is poor penetration by ethylene oxide.

Testing efficiency of sterilization
To indicate exposure to ethylene oxide, blue/green **indicator tape** (resembling Bowie–Dick tape in design) with yellow stripes that turn red following prolonged exposure to the gas may be used. It does not guarantee sterility as it gives no indication that exposure was for the correct length of time. In fact the colour change will occur after a fairly short period of time.

Indicator stickers provided by the manufacturer have a yellow dot that turns blue following prolonged exposure to ethylene oxide. These are useful but not 100% reliable as sterility indicators, as the colour change will occur following prolonged exposure to light. It is recommended that the box containing the roll of stickers is kept in a drawer or cupboard to prevent this change occurring before use.

Dosemeter strips that undergo a colour change when exposed to ethylene oxide for the correct time may be placed in the centre of a pack or load to test the penetration efficiency.

Spore strips placed into a load are added to a culture medium on completion of the cycle and are incubated for 72 hours. This is a useful test of the efficiency of the system but is obviously not suitable as an immediate indicator of sterility.

Commercially produced solutions
There are a number of chemical disinfectant solutions produced commercially. Some are ready for use, others require dilution (usually with purified water) prior to use.

Until recently a solution containing glutaraldehyde was the most widely used product for chemical disinfection. Although it is still readily available, COSHH regulations may prevent its use in veterinary (and medical) practice.

Chemical solutions
This method should really only be considered as a means of disinfection, though some manufacturers guarantee sterilization following prolonged immersion (usually 24 hours).

It remains a useful method for surgical equipment that may not be sterilized by any other means. It has gained particular popularity for the disinfection of endoscopic and arthroscopy equipment. There are several proprietary brands available.

Care should be taken to use the specific concentrations and immersion time stipulated by the manufacturer. Before immersion, check with the manufacturer that the equipment will not be damaged by wet disinfection. The chemical solution and the article to be disinfected should be placed in a tray or bowl, preferably with a lid to prevent evaporation and contamination by airborne microorganisms. Following immersion in chemical solutions, instruments should be rinsed in sterile water

and dried before use. Chemical solutions should be discarded after use and a fresh solution made up each time.

Alcohol-based solutions
A variety of these have been used, such as ethyl alcohol and isopropyl alcohol. They work by denaturation and coagulation of proteins.

Irradiation
This type of sterilization uses a form of gamma-irradiation and can only be carried out under controlled conditions. Many pre-packaged items are sterilized by this method, including suture materials and surgical gloves.

Packing supplies for sterilization
Various materials and containers are available for packing supplies for sterilization, each having advantages and disadvantages. Choice will depend on several factors:

* The packaging material must be resistant to damage when handled and not damage the equipment to be sterilized.
* Steam or gas must be able to penetrate the wrapping for sterilization to occur and must be easily exhausted from the pack once sterilization is complete.
* Microorganisms must not be able to penetrate from the outer surface of the wrap to the inner.

Other factors include:

* Size of autoclave/gas sterilizer
* Cost
* Personal preference
* Time taken to achieve sterility.

Materials and containers

Nylon film
Nylon film designed specifically for use in the autoclave is available in a variety of sizes. It has the advantages of being reusable and transparent so that items can be easily seen. Its main disadvantage is that it becomes brittle after repeated use, resulting in development of tiny unseen holes and therefore contamination of the pack. It may also be difficult to remove sterile items from packs without contaminating them on the edges of the bag. The packs are often sealed using Bowie–Dick tape.

Seal-and-peel pouches
Disposable bags, consisting of a paper back and clear plasticized front with a fold-over seal, are available in a wide variety of sizes. They may be used with ethylene oxide or the autoclave. The risk of contamination during opening is small. Double wrapping decreases the risk of damage to the instrument during storage or when opening the pack. They are most suitable for individual instruments.

Paper
Paper-based sheets are used for packing instruments. The most suitable type consists of a crepe-like paper that is slightly elastic, conforming and water-repellent. It is therefore ideal as an outer layer for packs. Although it is intended to be disposable, it is frequently reused. It is available in large sheets that can be cut to the appropriate size.

Textile

Textile sheets, usually linen or a cotton/polyester combination, are used to wrap surgical equipment for sterilization. They are conforming, strong and reusable but have the major disadvantage of being permeable to moisture. Usually a double layer of linen is covered by a waterproof paper-based wrap for surgical packs.

Drums

Metal drums with steam vents in the side, which are closed after sterilization, can be used for instruments, gowns and drapes. Their main disadvantage is that they are frequently multi-use and so there is a degree of environmental contamination each time the lid is opened. There is also a risk of contamination of items touching the edge or outside of the drum when they are removed. Initial outlay is relatively high but they will last for years.

Boxes and cartons

A variety of cardboard boxes and cartons are available for use in the autoclave. They are useful for gown or drape packs and for specialized kits (e.g. orthopaedic kits). They are relatively inexpensive and may be reused.

Care and sterilization of equipment

Gowns and drapes

After use, surgical gowns and drapes should be washed, dried and inspected for damage. Gowns should then be folded correctly so that the outside surface of the gown is on the inside (Figure 23.4). This is so that the surgical team can put on gowns in an aseptic fashion (described later). Plain drapes may be folded concertina style (Figure 23.5) or so that two corners are on the top surface (Figure 23.6). Fenestrated drapes are usually folded concertina style.

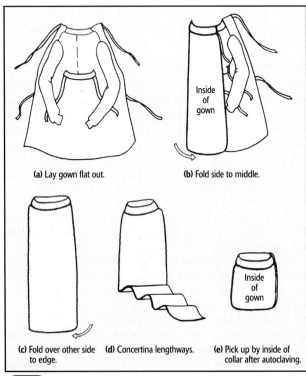

(a) Lay gown flat out. (b) Fold side to middle.

(c) Fold over other side to edge. (d) Concertina lengthways. (e) Pick up by inside of collar after autoclaving.

23.4 Folding a gown.

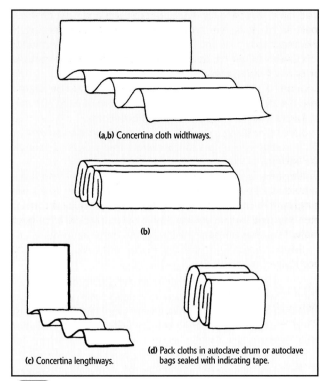

(a,b) Concertina cloth widthways.

(b)

(c) Concertina lengthways. (d) Pack cloths in autoclave drum or autoclave bags sealed with indicating tape.

23.5 Folding surgical drapes.

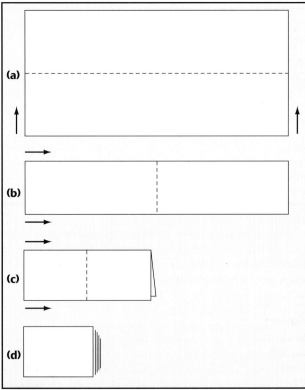

(a) (b) (c) (d)

23.6 Folding a plain drape, corner to corner. **(a)** The drape is folded in half widthways, and then **(b–d)** folded in half lengthways three times, so that there are two corners at the top.

Both gowns and drapes may be sterilized by ethylene oxide but this method is often uneconomical in a large practice, owing to the small size of the sterilizer, duration of the cycle (12 hours) and the airing time (24 hours). Autoclaving is a quicker, more efficient method but it is essential that the machine has a porous load cycle to ensure complete penetration and drying of the load. A hot-air oven is unsuitable as it will lead to charring of the material.

Gowns and drapes may be sterilized in drums, boxes, bags or packs. A handtowel is usually placed with the gown when packing for sterilization. Drapes are sometimes incorporated into the instrument pack.

Disposable sterile gowns and drapes are now widely used and are to be recommended (see later).

Swabs

Swabs may be purchased sterile or non-sterile. Each pack should have a consistent number which is known to all surgery staff (usually packs of five). Swabs may be incorporated into the instrument pack, supplied in drums or packed individually in packets.

Swabs should be sterilized in the same way as gowns and drapes.

Urinary catheters

Although designed for single use, most urinary catheters may be re-sterilized once. The exception to this is the Foley catheter, which will usually be unfit for reuse. After use, catheters should be washed, rinsed and then dried. They should be packed, without coiling if possible, in appropriate bags.

Many brands of catheter may be sterilized by autoclaving but some will be damaged by heat. Ethylene oxide can be successfully used for all types of catheter. It is essential to ensure that they are aired for the recommended time before use.

Syringes

Plastic syringes are designed to be disposable. To ensure sterility after storage they must be packed individually. It is therefore rarely economical to re-sterilize small syringes but it may be profitable to resterilize 30 and 50 ml syringes. They should be disassembled, washed thoroughly and dried prior to sterilization.

Most plastic syringes can be autoclaved safely but some brands will be damaged. Ethylene oxide may be used effectively to sterilize syringes. The plungers should be removed from the barrel prior to this. Glass syringes may be sterilized using a hot-air oven, autoclave or ethylene oxide.

Liquids

It is usual to purchase liquids presterilized, though more sophisticated autoclaves have a cycle for the sterilization of fluids. The risk of breakage of glass bottles is high and it is probably more economical to purchase fluids that have been commercially prepared.

Power tools

Air drills, saws and mechanical burrs are usually autoclavable but individual manufacturer's instructions should always be followed. Autoclaving can in some cases lead to jamming of the motor. Ethylene oxide can be used for all air-driven tools. Battery drills frequently have a plastic casing that would melt in an autoclave but they can be sterilized by using ethylene oxide.

Storage after sterilization

There should be a separate area for storage of sterile packs. It should be dust free, dry and well ventilated. Ideally all packs should be kept in closed cupboards. They should be handled as little as possible to minimize risk of damage, and packed loosely on shelves so that bags are not damaged. The length of time for which packs may be safely stored after sterilization

is the subject of much debate, with recommendations varying from a few weeks to 6 months. A sealed pack should remain sterile for a limitless period but it may become contaminated by excessive handling, resulting in damage to the pack, or moisture. It is therefore recommended that unused packs should be repacked and resterilized after 6–8 weeks.

The operating theatre suite

The design and layout of the operating theatre will rarely be within the control of the veterinary nurse. It is important, however, to have some knowledge of ideal requirements and desirable features in order to appreciate differing standards or aseptic techniques and to try to make the best of existing facilities. The layout of rooms within the theatre suite is important for the sake of asepsis. There should be a one-way traffic system, so that the surgical team and sterile supplies enter through one door and unscrubbed personnel enter and leave through a separate doorway.

The operating theatre suite should ideally consist of:

- Operating theatre
- Anaesthetic preparation area
- Area for washing and sterilizing equipment
- Sterile storage area
- Scrubbing-up area
- Changing rooms
- Recovery room

The operating theatre

Many practices have just one operating theatre, which is used for all surgery. Larger hospitals may have theatres that are used specifically for particular types of surgery, such as orthopaedic work, general surgery and 'dirty' surgery (e.g. dental work).

The size of the theatre will depend on the purpose for which it is intended. If it is to be used for simple routine surgery, it can be quite compact; if it is to be used for orthopaedic surgery, a large amount of surgical equipment may be needed. If the theatre is too small, working conditions will be compromised and it may be difficult to maintain a high standard of asepsis. It has to be large enough to accommodate the patient, anaesthetic equipment, surgical instrument trolley, other equipment and personnel.

There are several other requirements that are essential, or at least desirable, as follows.

Basic design and materials
The operating theatre should be an end room, not a thoroughfare to other rooms.

It must be easily cleaned. Walls and floors must be made of impervious non-staining materials; floors should be non-slip and hard wearing. Walls and ceiling should be painted with a light-coloured 'waterproof' paint. The corners and edges of all walls should be coved to facilitate easy cleaning.

Ceramic tiles are often used on walls in operating theatres. These are hard wearing and easy to keep clean, but crevices between the tiles may be difficult to keep clean and may harbour dust and bacteria. The use of drains should be avoided where possible but should not pose a problem if maintained properly.

Lighting and electricity

Good lighting is essential. Advantage should be taken of natural daylight. Ideally lighting should be concealed within the ceiling with additional side lights on the wall and an overhead theatre light.

There should be a good supply of electric sockets (in waterproof casing), preferably recessed into the wall.

Heating and air-conditioning

Heating is an important consideration, since anaesthetized animals are unable to control their own body temperature. The ambient temperature should be between 15 and 20°C. Fan heaters cause air and dust movement and should be avoided. Modern wall-mounted radiators are the most realistic method of heating. Panel heating within the walls is ideal, but expensive.

A system of air-conditioning and ventilation is necessary, and may become mandatory under COSHH Regulations.

Doors and windows

The rooms should have double swing doors, which should normally be kept closed.

There should be no clear-glass window to the outside, as this will be distracting. Windows should not open, as this will be a threat to asepsis.

Operating table

The operating table should be adjustable to facilitate positioning of the patient and to suit the height of the surgeon. The base of the table may be static or maintained on wheels for easy moving. There is usually a hydraulically operated pump to adjust the height, and some electrically operated pumps are also available.

Other equipment

There should be as little shelving and furniture as possible as it will harbour dust. All equipment, including the operating table, must be easily cleaned.

An X-ray viewer, preferably flush with the wall, is an important fixture in the operating theatres.

An air supply for power tools may be needed. This should ideally be piped into the theatre from cylinders housed outside the theatre. Anaesthetic gases can be delivered in the same way. A scavenging system for anaesthetic waste gas will also be necessary (see Chapter 1). A wall clock is needed for anaesthetic monitoring and timing of surgery.

A dry-wipe board is useful for recording details such as swab numbers, suture details, blood loss etc.

Anaesthetic preparation area

There should be a separate area where the induction of anaesthesia and other preoperative procedures (e.g. clipping, catheterization of the bladder and preparation of the surgical site) can be carried out. It should lead directly into the operating theatre.

Area for washing and sterilizing equipment

There needs to be a room where dirty instruments are washed, packed and sterilized. It should be situated close to the operating theatre but away from the sterile storage area. It should include a washing machine and tumble drier (specifically for theatre wear, gowns and drapes), sterilization facilities and possibly an ultrasonic instrument cleaner.

Sterile storage area

Sterile supplies should be stored in closed cupboards away from the instrument washing area, but adjacent to theatre. Instrument trolleys can be laid out here prior to surgery. Entry should be directly into the theatre.

Scrubbing-up area

There should be a separate scrub room within the theatre suite, but outside the theatre itself. This should lead directly into the sterile preparation area and theatre. Swing doors, which can be foot operated, should separate the rooms.

Changing rooms

Changing rooms for personnel should be situated at the entrance to theatre. It is useful to have a red line delineating the sterile area and appropriate notices displayed to indicate these areas. Footwear for use in theatre should be placed at the entrance to theatre beyond the red line. This barrier should be adhered to at all times to ensure a high level of asepsis.

Recovery room

A room where the patient can recover following surgery may be situated near the operating theatre suite. It should be quiet and warm and should contain essential equipment to deal with any postoperative emergencies that might occur.

Maintenance and cleaning of the operating theatre

A routine cleaning programme in the operating area is essential if a high standard of asepsis is to be maintained.

Routine cleaning of the operating theatre

- **At the beginning of each day:**
  - All the surfaces, furniture and equipment in the theatre suite should be damp-dusted, using a dilute solution of disinfectant (a dry duster would simply move dust around the room)
- **Between cases:**
  - The operating table should be wiped clean
- **At the end of the day:**
  - The floors in all rooms of the theatre suite should be vacuumed to remove debris and loose hair
  - They should then be either wet-vacuumed or washed using disinfectant
  - All waste material should be removed
  - Surfaces, equipment, lights and scrub sinks should all be washed down with disinfectant
- **Once a week** there should be a more thorough cleaning session:
  - All equipment is removed from the room and the floors and walls are scrubbed
  - A disinfectant with detergent properties that will remove organic matter and that is active against a wide range of bacteria, including *Pseudomonas* spp., should be used ▶

- After removing any excess solution, allow the disinfectant to dry on the surface rather than rinsing it off, for longer residual activity
- All equipment should be meticulously wiped over

Cleaning equipment

Cleaning utensils should be designated specifically for use in the theatre suite. They should be rinsed and allowed to dry after use. Buckets should always be emptied and rinsed out. All utensils should be stored away from the sterile area.

Autoclavable mops are available and should be used whenever possible. Failing this, cloths and mop heads should be washed daily in a washing machine.

Cleaning checks

A selection of swabs for bacterial culture should be taken from a variety of sites in the operating theatre from time to time to ensure efficacy of the cleaning regime and to alert staff to any potential problems. There should be no growth of bacteria from sterilized equipment and most other sites (e.g. sinks, operating tables, trolleys, drains, positioning aids, surfaces, lights).

Preparation of the surgical team

Theatre attire

If good surgical asepsis is to be achieved, all those involved in the surgery should change from their ordinary clothes into correct theatre attire before entering the operating theatre suite.

Theatre wear, which should be worn only within the theatre suite, usually consists of a simple two-piece **scrub suit**. A clean suit should be worn each day, or it should be changed more frequently if it becomes soiled.

Theatre **footwear** should be antistatic and traditionally has consisted of white clogs or wellingtons. These have the advantage of being easy to clean. Canvas shoes are sometimes worn but have the disadvantage of being difficult to clean on a daily basis and should be covered by waterproof overshoes. All footwear should be wiped over with a disinfectant at the end of the day; plastic or rubber footwear can be more thoroughly cleaned in a washing machine. Plastic overshoes are available that fit over normal shoes, but they are not recommended since they wear through in a very short time.

To accommodate longer hairstyles and beards, various styles of **headwear** are available. These are usually disposable and paper-based.

The purpose of **masks** is to filter expired air from the nose and mouth and to prevent transmission of microorganisms from the surgical team to patient. Masks are effective filters for relatively short periods only and so should ideally be changed between operations.

Scrubbing up

Preoperative scrubbing up is a systematic washing and scrubbing of the hands, arms and elbows, which is performed by all members of the surgical team before each operation. As it is not possible to sterilize the skin, the aim of the scrubbing-up routine is to destroy as many microorganisms from the surface of the arms and hands as possible, prior to donning a sterile surgical gown and gloves. Many different scrub routines have been described and no single technique is necessarily better than another. It is recommended that one of the tried and tested regimes is adopted and adhered to strictly. The scrubbing procedure should take between 5 and 10 minutes: the clock should be checked at the start of the first stage and again at the start of the final stage, to ensure that the procedure has not been rushed.

Example of a scrub routine

1. Remove watch and jewellery.
2. Fingernails should be cut short and any nail varnish removed.
3. Adjust the water supply (which should be elbow or foot operated) to a suitable temperature and flow. Once the scrubbing-up routine has started, the hands should not touch the taps, sink or scrub dispenser. If they are inadvertently touched, the last stage of the procedure should be repeated.
4. Wash the hands thoroughly using a plain soap. At this stage, clean the nails using a nail pick.
5. Once the hands have been washed, wash the arms up to and including the elbows. Always keep the hands higher than the elbows so that water drains down towards the unscrubbed upper arms rather than the other way round (which would lead to recontamination). The purpose of this stage of the procedure is to remove organic matter and grease from the skin.
6. Rinse the hands and then the arms by allowing water to wash away the soap from the hands towards the elbows.
7. Repeat this procedure using a surgical scrub solution, e.g. povidone–iodine or chlorhexidine (see below). Use only sufficient water to produce a lather, as bactericidal properties of the scrub solution are dependent on contact time with the skin. Excessive amounts of water will rinse away the scrub solution before it has achieved its aim.
8. Rinse off the scrub solution, as in stage (6).
9. Take a sterile scrubbing brush and systematically scrub the hands. Scrub the palms of the hand, wrist and four surfaces of each finger and thumb (back, front and both sides) and the nails. Either rinse the brush and use it on the other hand or discard it and take a second brush. It is not recommended that the backs of the hands and arms are scrubbed as this may lead to excoriation, which predisposes to infection.
10. The final stage is a repeat of stage (7). Wash the hands and arms in surgical scrub but this time the scrubbing process is not extended to include the elbow, so that there is no danger that a previously unscrubbed area is touched.
11. Rinse the hands and arms as before.
12. Take a sterile handtowel, holding it at arm's length. Use a different quarter to dry each hand and each arm. Then discard the handtowel.

Surgical scrub solutions

The ideal properties of a surgical scrub solution are:

- Wide spectrum of antimicrobial activity
- Ability to decrease microbial count quickly
- Quick application
- Long residual lethal effect against microorganisms
- Remains active and effective in the presence of organic matter

- Safe to use without skin irritation or sensitization
- Economical
- Practical for veterinary use.

Examples of commonly used agents are given in Figure 23.7.

Putting on a surgical gown

There are two different types of gown: back-tie and side-tie. The technique for putting on the gown is similar for both, with slight variation (Figure 23.8).

Agent	Properties
Povidone–iodine	Iodine combined with a detergent Broad-spectrum antimicrobial activity (bactericidal, viricidal and fungicidal) May cause severe skin reactions and irritation in some individuals Efficacy impaired by organic matter
Chlorhexidine	Effective against many bacteria (including *Escherichia coli* and *Pseudomonas* spp.) Viricidal, fungicidal and sporicidal properties Effective level of activity in presence of organic material Longer residual activity than povidone–iodine Relatively low toxicity to tissue
Triclosan	Newer agent, claimed to be antibacterial against both Gram-positive and Gram-negative bacteria

23.7 Commonly used surgical scrub solutions.

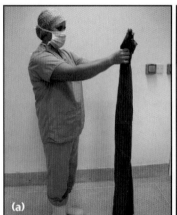

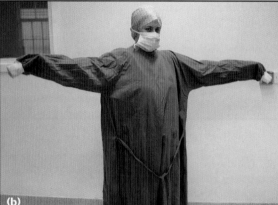

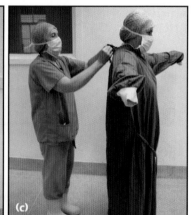

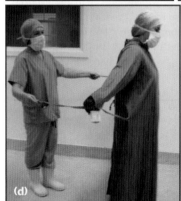

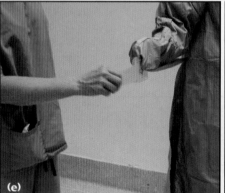

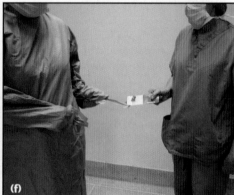

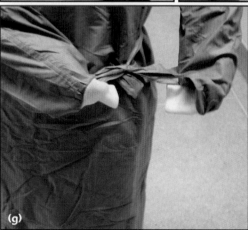

23.8 Putting on a sterile gown. **(a)** The sterile gown (folded inside out) is taken from its sterile pack, held at the shoulders and allowed to fall open. **(b)** One hand is slipped into each sleeve. No attempt should be made to try to pull the sleeves over the shoulder or to readjust the gown, as this will lead to contamination of the hands or outside of the gown. **(c)** An unscrubbed assistant should pull the back of the gown over the shoulders (touching only the inside surface of the gown) and secure the ties at the back. **(d)** With the hands retained within the sleeves, the waist ties should be picked up and held out to the sides. In the case of a **back-tying** gown, the unscrubbed assistant will then take the ends of the waist ties and secure them at the back. The back of the gown is now no longer sterile and must not come into contact with sterile equipment, drapes and gowns. **(e)** In the case of a **side-tying** gown, the unscrubbed assistant takes hold of the paper tape on the longer waist tape and takes the tie around the back to the opposite side. **(f)** The scrubbed person then pulls the tape, so that the paper tape comes away. **(g)** The gown is tied at the waist by the scrubbed person. This type of gown provides an all-round sterile field.

Putting on surgical gloves

Three methods are available: closed gloving, open gloving and the plunge method.

Closed gloving

The hands are kept inside the sleeves while gloving takes place. This technique has the advantage that it minimizes the chances of contaminating the gloves, since the outside of the gloves do not contact the skin.

Closed gloving procedure

1. Hands remain within the sleeves of the gown. The glove packet is turned so that the fingers point towards the body. (The right glove will now be on the left and *vice versa*.)
2. The glove is picked up at the rim of the cuff of the glove.
3. The hand is turned over so that the glove lies on the palm surface with fingers of the glove still pointing towards the body.
4. The rim is picked up with the opposite hand.
5. It is then pulled over the fingers and over the dorsal surface of the wrist.
6. The glove is then pulled on as the fingers are pushed forwards.

Open gloving

The hands are extended out of the sleeves while gowning. This technique has the disadvantage that the gloves are relatively easily contaminated by skin contact.

Open gloving procedure

1. The glove pack is opened by an assistant.
2. With the left hand, the right glove is picked up by the turned-down cuff, holding only the inner surface of the glove.
3. The glove is pulled on to the right hand. Do not unfold the cuff at this stage.
4. The gloved fingers of the right hand are placed under the cuff of the left glove and pulled on to the left hand, holding only the outer surface of this glove.
5. The rim of the left glove is hooked over the thumb whilst the cuff of the gown is adjusted.
6. The cuff of the left glove is pulled over the cuff of the gown using the fingers of the right hand.
7. Repeat for the right hand.

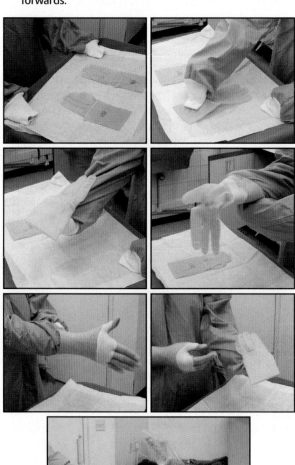

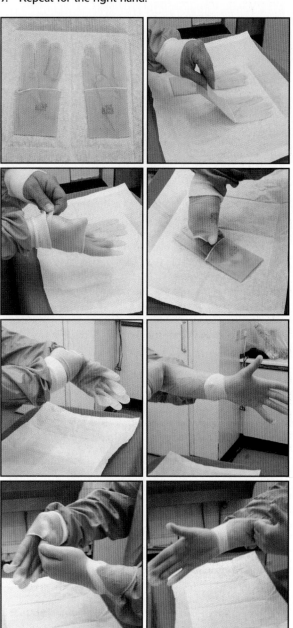

Plunge method

With this method (Figure 23.9) the sterile glove is held open by a scrubbed assistant and the hand is inserted. There is a risk of contaminating both personnel involved. This technique is not commonly employed in veterinary operating theatres.

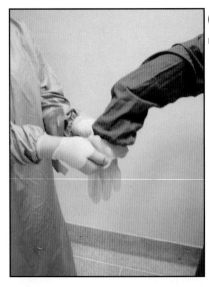

23.9 The plunge method of gloving.

Preoperative preparation of the patient

Surgical cases may be categorized as follows:

- **Elective** and **non-urgent** – the patient is usually healthy and often young (e.g. ovariohysterectomy, castration, corrective osteotomy)
- **Necessary** or **urgent** – not immediately life-threatening but requiring prompt attention (fracture repair, airway, gastrointestinal surgery)
- **Emergency surgery** – life-threatening conditions (e.g. abdominal crisis), often traumatic (e.g. chest injury).

The time between admission and surgery will depend on various factors. In the simplest elective procedures, the patient is admitted on the morning of surgery and returns home later that day. Preoperative preparations in these cases are minimal. In others there may be a delay before surgery is performed. Reasons for this may include:

- **Investigative procedures**, e.g. diagnostic tests, radiographic and ultrasonographic studies
- **Fluid therapy or transfusion** – to improve the patient's physiological status before surgery
- **Presence of other injuries** that require treatment before surgery may be undertaken (e.g. thoracic trauma associated with a limb fracture)
- To allow **reduction of swelling/debridement** of wounds – bandaging of fracture site, application of wound dressings etc.
- **Stabilization** of patient with concurrent metabolic disturbance (e.g. diabetes mellitus, renal disease, hyperadrenocorticism).

Admission of the patient

- All relevant details must be recorded on the case records.
- Check the reason for admission.
- Where relevant, identify the site (draw a diagram if necessary).
- Ensure that the owner understands what is to be done and how the patient will look when discharged (e.g. it will have a clipped area and may be wearing a bandage, cast, Elizabethan collar).
- Ensure that the patient is in good general health or that symptoms have not changed since last seen by a veterinary surgeon.
- Always ensure that there is a contact telephone number and that an anaesthetic consent form is signed.
- The patient should then be weighed.
- It is sensible at this stage to fit a plastic identicollar containing the patient's name/number, weight and reason for admission, to minimize the risk of mistakes occurring.

Preoperative procedures

Withholding food

Food is usually withheld for 12 hours prior to surgery. This is primarily to prevent regurgitation of food under general anaesthesia or during recovery. A full stomach could also interfere with the surgical procedure in very young animals, very old animals and those with metabolic disorders, but prolonged withholding of food may be contraindicated. It is preferable for such cases to be placed as early as possible on the surgical list and then fed promptly afterwards to minimize metabolic disturbances and potential problems in the postoperative period.

Clipping

Clipping the surgical site is necessary for most procedures (except intraoral). It may be carried out before anaesthesia or under general anaesthesia (Figure 23.10)

	Advantages	**Disadvantages**
Under general anaesthesia	Often takes less time Fewer people required to restrain animal Desirable with fractious animals or painful/inaccessible sites	Decreases asepsis: small loose hairs are extremely difficult to remove even with a vacuum cleaner Increases anaesthetic time
Pre-anaesthesia	Shorter anaesthetic time Improves asepsis: loose hairs generally shed before surgery Can give initial skin preparation Improves operating theatre efficiency (more operations can be performed)	Patient may be uncooperative Requires two or more people Clipping more than 12 hours before surgery may increase skin bacteria

23.10 Advantages and disadvantages of clipping.

Considerations for preoperative clipping

- Clip a large area around the surgical site. Ensure that the clipping is neat (this is what the owner will notice)
- Ensure that clipper blades are in good order. Tears in the skin will cause irritation, which may encourage postoperative licking and scratching at the site, which will predispose to infection of the site
- When clipping around a wound, K-Y jelly placed in the wound and on the coat at the edges of the wound will help to prevent hair entering the wound
- Clean the clipper blades in between cases. It may be necessary to sterilize them after clipping contaminated sites (e.g. abscesses)
- Clipping should be performed away from the operating theatre, to minimize contamination by hair
- Do not allow clipper blades to become too hot during use, as this may cause inflammation or excoriation that is not apparent until the postoperative period. Have a second pair of blades ready so that they can be swapped during procedures
- Some surgeons advocate shaving of the skin after clipping but this may lead to severe excoriation of the skin, which encourages postoperative licking, scratching and soreness

Bathing

Ideally all patients should be bathed before surgery to decrease the risk of contamination, but this is not always feasible. It should be considered in elective orthopaedic procedures such as total hip replacement.

Administration of an enema

For some surgery (e.g. rectal/colonic) it is desirable to give an evacuant enema prior to surgery (see Chapter 15). A soap-and-water enema is simplest. The patient may need bathing afterwards to remove faecal contaminants from the skin.

Preparation immediately before surgery

Some form of premedicant drug is usually given by either intramuscular or subcutaneous injection, 15 minutes to 1 hour before induction of anaesthesia. Antibiotic drugs are often given at the same time as the premedicant drugs, to ensure effective antibiotic blood levels at the time of surgery. Eyedrops are often applied immediately prior to ophthalmic surgery. Catheterization of the bladder may be required, for the following reasons:

- Monitoring of urine output during and after surgery
- Minimizing risk of soiling during surgery
- Facilitating access to abdominal organs
- Preventing risk of bladder perforation or rupture during surgery.

Other possible preparations include:

- Purse-string suture around anus to prevent contamination by faecal material during surgery in the perianal region (the nurse should ensure that it is removed at the end of surgery)
- Application of Esmarch's rubber bandage and tourniquet for a bloodless operating field during surgery on distal limbs
- Introduction of a throat pack to prevent aspiration of blood, mucus etc. during oral or nasal surgery (usually a dampened conforming bandage is used for this purpose)

- Covering of any additional wounds not associated with the surgery, to prevent risk of further contamination
- Application of a foot bandage to cover any unclipped areas where surgery involves a limb.

Preparation of the skin

The skin and coat are two of the greatest sources of wound contamination, as it is not possible to remove all bacteria from the skin. The aim is to reduce significantly the number present without damaging the skin itself. Skin bacteria include species of *Staphylococcus*, *Bacillus* and occasionally *Streptococcus*.

As antiseptic and detergent properties are required in skin-cleansing agents, surgical scrub solutions such as chlorhexidine and povidone–iodine are ideal. An antiseptic solution (which may be water or alcohol-based) is then usually applied to give residual bacterial activity.

Initial skin preparation should be done in the preparation room. There are several different techniques that are used commonly.

Skin preparation technique

1. Surgical gloves should be worn to prevent contamination of the patient's skin from the nurse's hands. It is not necessary for the gloves to be sterile during the initial preparation.
2. Using lint-free swabs, wash the site using a surgical scrub solution and a little warm water, beginning at the proposed incision site and working outwards. Once the edges of the clipped area are reached, discard the swab and take a new one.
3. Continue this procedure until the area is clean, i.e. there is no discoloration on a white swab.
4. A small amount of a 70% alcohol solution can then be sprayed over the site to remove any remaining detergent. It should not be used on open wounds or mucous membranes. Avoid over-wetting the patient.
5. Move the patient into theatre and position for surgery. For limb surgery, a tape is applied over the foot and attached to a drip stand to allow preparation around all sides of the limb.
6. As the site is likely to have been contaminated to some extent in the transition to the theatre, the skin is given another wash in the manner previously described. This time, however, sterile gloves, water and swabs are used.
7. The final stage of preparation is carried out by the scrubbed surgical team with an antiseptic solution using sterile swabs on sterile Rampley sponge-holding forceps, which are then discarded.

Care should be taken to avoid soaking the coat, as this will increase the risk of 'strike-through' from the drapes and may make the patient hypothermic.

Preparation of eyes and mucous membranes

The solutions commonly used for preparation of the skin are likely to be irritant and cause damage to mucous membranes and in particular the eye. Dilute solutions of povidone–iodine (0.1–0.2%) are commonly used to irrigate the eye and may also be used on oral and other mucous membranes. Chlorhexidine solutions are shown to be more irritant to the surface of the cornea. Alcohol-based solutions should not be used on this sensitive tissue.

Some surgeons do not advocate clipping around the eye for intraocular surgery but use adhesive drapes to protect the eye from the hair and skin. Others prefer to clip a minimal amount of hair around the eye. Application of petroleum or K-Y jelly to the hair prior to clipping with a narrow fine blade will help to prevent hair being introduced into the eye. The skin around the eye is extremely thin and sensitive, and so it is important that the clippers are in good order and great care is taken when clipping. The eye should then be irrigated several times with physiological saline before irrigating with a povidone–iodine solution, as described. The skin should also be prepared with the povidone–iodine solution.

Positioning the patient for surgery

Most surgeons have individual preferences with regard to positioning of the patient for surgery, but there are some standard positions for specific operations. The veterinary nurse needs to be familiar with positioning for different surgical techniques and individual variations. When there is any doubt, the nurse should check well in advance of surgery.

Some operating tables have adjustable sides and tilting facilities that assist in positioning the patient. If not, the use of additional restraining aids such as troughs, sandbags and tapes will be necessary. Care should be taken to avoid placing heavy sandbags over the limbs or tying tapes tightly, which may occlude blood supply to the area.

Draping the patient

The reason for draping the patient is to maintain asepsis by preventing contamination of the surgical site from the hair and the immediate environment. Drapes must therefore cover the entire patient and operating table, leaving only the surgical site exposed. Drapes may be disposable or reusable. The relative advantages of each type are shown in Figure 23.11.

	Advantages	Disadvantages
Disposable	Labour saving Less laundry Presterilized Usually very water repellent Always in perfect condition	Expensive Cheaper brands can be less conforming Large stock needed
Reusable drapes	Cheaper	Porous – all fluids leak through leading to a break in asepsis Time-consuming – washing and folding Danger of threads detaching and gaining access to wounds After repeated use quality becomes poor

23.11 Advantages and disadvantages of disposable and reusable drapes.

Disposable drapes

These are usually paper-based. Most are designed for the human surgical market but many are suitable for veterinary use. They are usually water-resilient and may be purchased presterilized. Cheaper varieties tend to be non-conforming and may tear easily, but many commercial brands of disposable drapes are of high quality, and their use is recommended. Good disposable drapes tend to be more conformable than cotton drapes and the high water resistance helps to prevent bacterial strikethrough. They also help maintain body temperature during surgery.

Reusable drapes

These are usually linen or cotton/polyester mixes. They may be custom-made to suit practice needs.

Draping systems

Plain drapes

Four rectangular drapes are used to create a 'window' (**fenestration**) for the surgical site (Figure 23.12). The fenestration created can be of any size. The first drape should be placed between the surgeon and the nearest side of the table. Then a drape is placed over the opposite side of the patient (i.e. furthest from the surgeon). Drapes are then placed over both ends. They are then secured in place using towel clips.

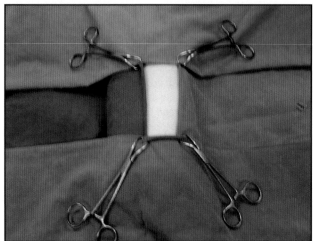

23.12 Draping the surgical site. Plain drapes are first placed longitudinally on both sides of the operating table. More drapes are then placed over each end and secured by towel clips.

Fenestrated drapes

Fenestrated drapes achieve the same effect as the plain drapes in leaving a surgery window, but the window is already formed in a single ready-made drape. Fenestrated drapes can be large enough to cover the entire animal and table top. A selection of different-sized fenestrations are needed to cater for all the different surgical sites.

Adhesive 'barrier' drapes

Sterile clear adhesive plastic sheets are sometimes placed over the surgical site. Standard drapes are then applied in the usual way. The skin incision is made through the adhesive material.

Draping limbs

There are various ways of draping limbs for surgery (Figure 23.13). The surgeon's individual preference will govern the choice of method. Commonly, the lower limb is tied to a drip stand, using tape. A sterile drape is placed on the tabletop underneath the limb. Then either a sterile drape or stockinette is secured to the lower limb and the suspending tape is cut. The surgical site is then draped in a routine fashion.

Sub-draping

Additional towels are sometimes used to protect the incision site from contamination. They are applied to each side of the incision by towel clips. The towel is then folded back over the towel clips.

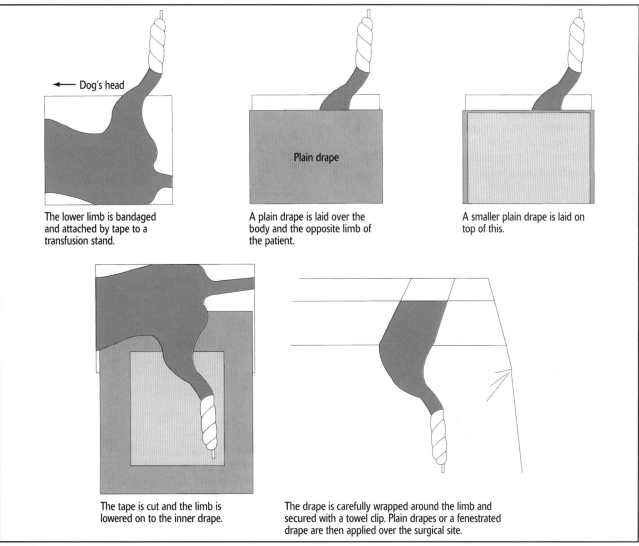

◄— Dog's head

The lower limb is bandaged and attached by tape to a transfusion stand.

A plain drape is laid over the body and the opposite limb of the patient.

Plain drape

A smaller plain drape is laid on top of this.

The tape is cut and the limb is lowered on to the inner drape.

The drape is carefully wrapped around the limb and secured with a towel clip. Plain drapes or a fenestrated drape are then applied over the surgical site.

23.13 Draping a limb for surgery.

Surgical assistance

The theatre nurse has two main roles: as scrubbed nurse, and as circulating nurse.

Duties of a circulating nurse

- Helping to prepare theatre, instruments and equipment for surgery
- Tying the surgical team into gowns
- Helping to position the patient on the table
- Preparation of the surgical site
- Connecting the apparatus (diathermy, suction, airlines etc.)
- Opening packs of sutures/instruments etc.
- Counting swabs, sutures etc. with the scrubbed nurse
- Being in theatre at all times when surgery is in progress
- Assisting the anaesthetist
- Preparing postoperative dressings
- Helping to move the patient to recovery
- Helping to clear theatre at the end of surgery

Duties of a scrubbed nurse

- Preparing the instrument trolley
- Assisting in draping the patient and connecting equipment (e.g. suction)
- Passing instruments, swabs etc. to the surgeon
- Assisting with surgery: retracting tissue, cutting sutures etc.
- Being responsible for all equipment, swabs, sutures, needles etc.
- Keeping instrument trolley tidy

Scrubbed nurse

The role of the scrubbed nurse is an extremely important one and requires rigid adherence to a set of rules. It is very easy to make mistakes if corners are cut or changes made. Knowledge of the procedure to be performed is important so that the needs of the surgeon can be anticipated.

- It is essential to know exactly what instruments and equipment are on the trolley at the start and throughout surgery.

- All swabs, sutures, needles etc. must be counted before surgery begins and again before the wound is closed, to prevent any items being accidentally left within a wound cavity.
- The nurse should watch the operation carefully in order to anticipate the surgeon's needs.
- Instruments should be passed to the surgeon so that they are ready to be used, i.e. not upside down.
- Instruments should be returned to the same place on the trolley each time so that the nurse knows exactly where they are. They should not be left around the surgical site, because they are likely to fall on the floor and because they will not be immediately to hand when needed.
- Instruments should be wiped over with a dry swab when they are returned to the trolley.
- Only one swab should be given to the surgeon at any time and the nurse must keep a constant check on the number of swabs used.
- Swabs should be applied firmly to a bleeding site, without wiping across the tissue, which may both damage the tissue and disturb a clot.
- All tissues should be handled gently to avoid trauma. Viscera in particular should be handled very carefully.
- One of the nurse's roles may be to irrigate the tissues with warmed saline to prevent desiccation, particularly during long operations.
- On completion of surgery the nurse should ensure that all instruments, needles and swabs are returned to the trolley and that needles, blades and glassware are disposed of safely.

General rules for maintenance of asepsis

- Correct theatre attire should be worn at all times
- There should be a minimum number of people present and movement should be kept to a minimum
- There should be a new set of sterile instruments for each operation, even when dealing with a contaminated site
- Plan to perform 'clean' operations first, i.e. orthopaedic operations (especially when implants are used), and to carry out contaminated surgery last (e.g. aural and oral).
- Wherever possible there should be a room for 'dirty' procedures
- An efficient sterilization programme should be adopted
- The theatre should be maintained at an ambient temperature and the ventilation must be good. Hot, humid conditions will encourage the growth of pathogens, in particular *Pseudomonas* spp
- Wherever possible, the patient should be clipped and bathed before it is taken to theatre.
- The surgical team must ensure that they do not touch any non-sterile surfaces during surgery. Any break in asepsis must be reported and rectified
- No contaminated instruments or equipment should be returned to the sterile trolley
- A record book of all operations should be kept, so that if any sepsis problems arise the cause can be detected
- A strict cleaning protocol must be maintained
- Written standards of procedures for maintaining asepsis in the theatre should be prepared

Preparing an instrument trolley

Instrument trolleys should be prepared immediately prior to use. The longer that the instruments are exposed to air, the greater is the chance of contamination from the environment or personnel. If there is a delay once the trolley has been laid out, a sterile drape should be placed over the top. Trolleys can be laid up by hand by a scrubbed nurse or by using sterile Cheatle forceps. The top of the metal instrument trolley will not be sterile and it is important to cover this with a water-proof sterile drape first, to prevent bacterial strike-through from the trolley if it becomes wet.

Instrument sets may be packed in trays complete with drapes, swabs, blades, etc. In these cases the outer wrappings of the set can be unfolded to cover the base of the trolley.

Where instruments are taken from multi-use containers the trolley should be covered by a waterproof drape followed by two layers of linen cloth. Swabs, drapes and instruments are then added.

Hazards in the operating theatre

The avoidance of accidents to patients and staff in the operating theatre is of the utmost importance. The Health and Safety at Work etc. Act and the COSHH regulations (see Chapter 1) are designed to ensure safety in the workplace, including the operating theatre.

Equipment

With the increasing use of new and sophisticated equipment, the risk of accidents has also increased. It is very important that all nursing staff are instructed in the use and maintenance of all new equipment. It is also important that all equipment is serviced regularly and tested for electrical safety to minimize risks.

Pollution from anaesthetic gases and chemicals

All staff should be aware of the dangers associated with inhaling anaesthetic gases. An anaesthetic gas-scavenging system must be fitted or absorptive filters used to minimize exposure to gases.

In the operating theatre, nursing staff will be exposed to various chemicals. Protective clothing, masks and gloves should be worn where appropriate.

Care of the patient during surgery

It is important to remember that underneath the drapes is a live patient. Care must be taken by the surgical team to avoid leaning on the animal's chest, which may compromise breathing in a small patient. Careful positioning of towel clips is important to avoid delicate structures such as the eye, which cannot be seen once drapes have been placed. Attention should be paid to the conservation of heat, especially in the small or very young. The use of heated water beds, insulation (e.g. bubble-wrap) and warmed intravenous and irrigation fluids should be encouraged. Direct heat (e.g. hot-water bottles) should be avoided during both surgery and recovery periods, as the unconscious animal cannot move away if this is too hot. Serious burns can occur, which will not become apparent until the postoperative period. Careful positioning of the animal on the table is also important, to avoid post-operative complications.

Immediate postoperative care

Recovery from anaesthesia
The patient should not be left unattended until it is conscious. The endotracheal tube is usually removed just before the cough reflex returns. The animal should be watched closely to ensure that an adequate airway is maintained once the tube has been removed, especially in brachycephalic breeds or following airway surgery. Cats should be observed closely for any signs of laryngospasm following endotracheal tube removal. A source of oxygen and a means of ventilation should be available during this time in case any problems arise. Colour of the mucous membranes and the presence or absence of respiratory noise and effort will be indicators of effective ventilation by the animal. The ability to maintain body temperature is lost under anaesthesia and so steps should be taken to prevent hypothermia.

Haemorrhage
During recovery the patient should be observed for signs of external haemorrhage (which is usually obvious) or internal haemorrhage (signs of shock).

Recognition of pain
It is important to be able to recognize when an animal is in pain. The nurse should obtain instructions from the veterinary surgeon regarding postoperative analgesia.

Application of dressings or casts
Many orthopaedic and some soft-tissue cases will require postoperative bandages or casts. This should be done before the animal regains consciousness. Care should be taken not to apply these too tightly (especially head and ear dressings).

Comfort
- Make sure that the animal has comfortable bedding, especially orthopaedic patients.
- Turn the animal regularly if it is disinclined or unable to do so by itself.
- Give opportunities for the animal to urinate, or empty the bladder manually if necessary.
- Do not forget to offer food and drink if this is allowed, especially in young and old patients.

Instrumentation

The cost of good-quality surgical instruments is extremely high but they will last for years if handled correctly, whereas cheaper instruments of poor quality will require early replacement.

- **Stainless steel** is the material of choice for most surgical instruments. It combines high resistance to corrosion with great strength and it has an attractive surface finish.
- **Tungsten carbide** inserts are often added to the tips of stainless steel instruments that are used for cutting or gripping, such as scissors and needle-holders. They are very hard and resistant to wear but tend to be expensive. Instruments with tungsten carbide inserts are often identified by their gold-coloured handles.
- **Chromium-plated carbon steel** surgical instruments are commonly used in veterinary practice because they are lower in price. However, they will rust, pit and blister when in contact with chemicals and saline and they tend to blunt quickly.

Care and maintenance of surgical instruments
Surgical instruments should be handled carefully at all times. They should not be dropped into trays and sinks or on to trolleys. Special care should be taken of sharp edges and pointed instruments.

Care of new instruments
Most new instruments are supplied dry without lubrication. Before use, therefore, it is recommended that they are washed and dried carefully and their moving parts lubricated with a proprietary instrument lubricant.

Cleaning after use
To comply with Health and Safety legislation, the veterinary nurse must wear protective clothing (i.e. a plastic apron and rubber gloves) when dealing with surgical instruments.

- Sharp items such as needles, glass vials and scalpel blades should be safely disposed of (see Chapter 1) before removing other disposable items such as suture packets and swabs from the instrument trolley.
- Any specialized or delicate equipment should be separated from the general instruments and cleaned separately.
- Large instruments, such as some orthopaedic instruments, should be washed separately from general instruments as they may cause damage to them or be damaged themselves.

Instruments should be cleaned as soon as possible on completion of surgery to prevent blood, tissue debris or saline drying on them, as this will lead to pitting of the surface and subsequent corrosion. Initial soaking or rinsing in cold water is highly effective for this. Hot water should not be used, as it causes coagulation of proteins (e.g. blood). Alternatively, instruments may be soaked in a chemical cleaning solution specifically manufactured for instrument cleaning.

Where indicated, instruments should be dismantled and ratchets or joints opened before immersion.

Instruments should then be cleaned under cool or warm running water, using a hand brush with fairly stiff bristles. Particular attention should be paid to joints, ratchets, serrations etc. Abrasive chemical agents should never be used as they may damage the surface of the instrument. Ordinary soap should also be avoided, as it causes an insoluble alkali film to form on the surface, thus trapping bacteria and protecting them from sterilization.

After washing, instruments should be rinsed thoroughly – preferably in distilled or deionized water – and then dried prior to packing, as water collecting in trapped areas may lead to corrosion.

After cleaning, each instrument should be inspected for distortion, misalignment, sharpness and incorrect assembly. Pivot movements, joints and ratchets should also be checked for correct function.

Ultrasonic cleaners
Bench-top ultrasonic cleaners suitable for veterinary use are readily available and are relatively inexpensive. They are extremely effective at removing debris from areas inaccessible to

brushes (e.g. box joints). They work by the production of sinusoidal energy waves with a vibration frequency in excess of 20,000 vibrations per second. This produces minute bubbles within the cleaning solution. These form on the surface of instruments. As the bubbles implode, energy is released and breaks the bonds that hold debris on the surface.

Following an initial rinsing or soaking in cold water to remove excess blood and debris, the instruments are placed in the wire mesh basket of the ultrasonic cleaner. The unit is filled approximately half full with water to which a specific ultrasonic cleaning detergent has been added. The basket is placed in the solution, the lid replaced and the unit switched on. Usually a period of approximately 15 minutes is sufficient. On completion of the cycle, the basket is removed and the instruments are rinsed individually under running water. They are then dried, as already described.

Lubrication

Lubrication of instruments on a regular basis is recommended, particularly after using an ultrasonic cleaner. It is important to use lubricants which are recommended by the manufacturer. Mineral oils and grease must be avoided as they leave a film on the surface under which bacterial spores may be trapped, preventing adequate penetration during sterilization. Antimicrobial water-soluble lubricants (instrument milk) are available: instruments are dipped into the solution for a short period and then removed and allowed to dry. They do not need to be rinsed.

Sharpening

- Scissors that become blunt should be returned to the manufacturer for sharpening.
- Drill bits may be resharpened but replacement will give a more reliable instrument.
- Oscillating saw blades become worn and blunt and will require replacement.

Cleaning compressed air machines

Compressed air machines should never be immersed in water or put in ultrasonic cleaners. The machine should have detachable parts (drills, saw blades, etc.) which can be cleaned in a standard fashion as already described. The main handpiece should be detached from the air hose and cleaned according to the manufacturer's recommendations.

For metal air drills and oscillating saws it is usually possible to wash the outside of the body of the handset under running tap water, taking care to avoid water getting into the air hose attachment and internal mechanism of the handpiece. With more delicate air- or battery-powered tools where this is not recommended, cleaning will usually involve wiping over the instrument thoroughly with a disinfectant cleaning solution, paying particular attention to triggers and couplings. Use of a small brush such as a nailbrush may be necessary to remove debris. The air hose should be wiped over with a damp cloth in a similar fashion and at the same time inspected to check that there is no damage to the outer sheath. The handpiece and hose attachments should be lubricated according to manufacturer's instructions. The machine should then be reassembled, attached to the air supply and run for approximately 30 seconds to allow oil to circulate and ensure patency of the equipment prior to packing and resterilization.

General surgical instruments

There is a wide variety of different surgical instruments available. It is not expected that the veterinary nurse should be familiar with them all but a broad knowledge of general instruments can be gained by reference to manuals and catalogues to learn the names and appearance of the more common ones.

Scalpel

The scalpel is the best instrument for dividing tissue with minimal trauma. Usually scalpel handles with interchangeable disposable blades are used (Figure 23.14). A size 3 handle is commonly used for small animal surgery with blade sizes 10, 11, 12 and 15. A size 4 handle is used for large animal surgery with blade sizes 20, 21 and 22. The primary advantage of disposable blades is consistent sharpness. A scalpel with a blade and handle as a disposable package is available, as is a small, rounded (Beaver) handle with smaller disposable blades which has gained popularity with ophthalmic surgeons.

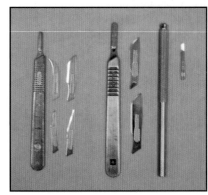

23.14 Scalpel handles and blades. From left to right: size 3 handle and sizes 10, 11, 12 and 15 blades; size 4 handle and sizes 21 and 20 blades; Beaver handle with one blade.

Dissecting forceps

These are commonly referred to as thumb forceps (Figure 23.15) and are designed to hold tissue. They have a spring action and the jaws are opposed by holding the metal blades together. They may have plain or toothed ends. Generally, forceps with plain ends are used for handling delicate tissues such as viscera, whilst toothed forceps are used for denser tissues. Dissecting forceps should be held like a pencil.

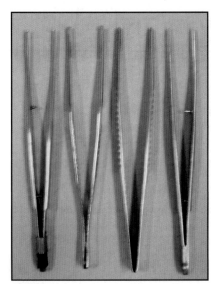

23.15 Dissecting forceps. From left to right: fine-toothed; heavy-duty toothed; plain broad dressing forceps; fine plain forceps.

Scissors

Operating scissors are available in various lengths and shapes (Figure 23.16). Mayo dissecting scissors are commonly used for routine surgery; the finer, long-handled Metzenbaum scissors tend to be used for more delicate work. Special suture scissors (e.g. Carless scissors) should be used for cutting

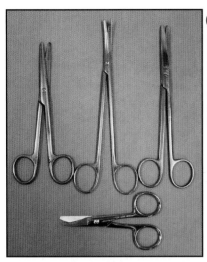

23.16 Surgical scissors. Clockwise from top left: Mayo; Metzenbaum; Carless suture-cutting; Payne's suture removal scissors.

sutures to prevent unnecessary blunting of dissecting scissors. For removal of sutures, Payne's scissors are used. These are small and curved with the cutting surface of one blade hollowed out to fit under the suture easily. Scissors should be held with the ring finger and thumb inserted in the ring of the scissor and the index finger placed on the shaft to guide the scissors.

Haemostatic or artery forceps

Artery forceps (Figure 23.17) are designed to clamp blood vessels and thus stop bleeding. They come in several different lengths and shapes. Most have transverse striations to facilitate holding tissue. There are many different patterns of artery forceps. Some of those commonly used include the Spencer Wells, Dunhill, Crile's, Cairn's and Kelly. Mosquito forceps are very small artery forceps for finer blood vessels, the most common type being the Halstead forceps. Like scissors, artery forceps should be held with the ring finger and thumb, using the index finger to steady the forceps.

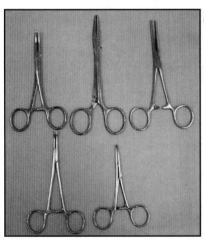

23.17 Artery forceps. Clockwise from top left: Dunhill; Spencer Wells; Kocher's; Crile's; Halstead.

Bowel clamps

These are designed to clamp bowel in an atraumatic manner. Several different types are available but the most common type used in veterinary surgery is the Doyen's bowel clamp (Figure 23.18).

Sponge-holding forceps

These are designed to hold sponges or swabs for skin preparation prior to surgery (Figure 23.18).

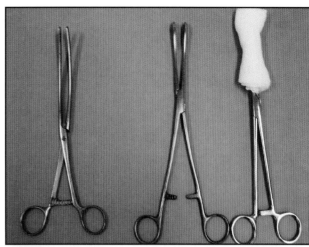

23.18 (Left) Doyen's bowel clamps. (Middle and right) Rampley's sponge-holding forceps.

Tissue forceps

Allis tissue forceps and Babcock's forceps are the most commonly used types of tissue forceps (Figure 23.19). They are designed to grasp tissue with minimal trauma but neither type should be used to grasp and hold viscera, for which more specialized forceps such as Duvall's should be used.

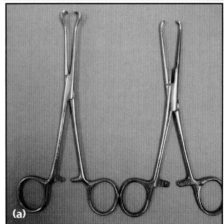
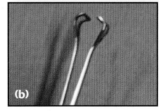
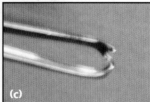

23.19 Tissue forceps. **(a)** (Left) Babcock's; (right) Allis. **(b)** Close-up of Babcock tip. **(c)** Close-up of Allis tip.

Towel clips

Towel clips (Figure 23.20) are used to attach drapes to the patient (see Figure 23.12) and to attach instruments to the operating site. Backhaus and Mayo forceps have a ringed handle and curved, pointed, tongue-like tips. Gray's cross-action forceps, commonly used in veterinary surgery, have a strong spring-clip attachment.

Needle-holders

Needle-holders (Figure 23.21) are forceps that are specifically designed for holding suture needles during suturing and for knot tying.

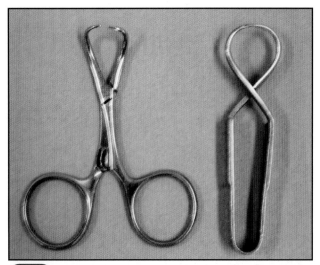

23.20 Towel clips. (Left) Backhaus; (right) Gray's.

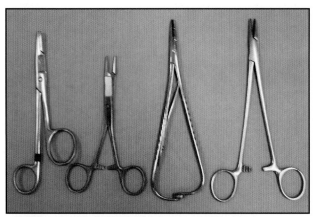

23.21 Needle-holders. From left to right: Gillies; Olsen–Hegar; McPhail's; Mayo–Hegar.

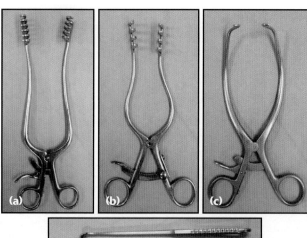

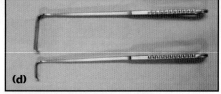

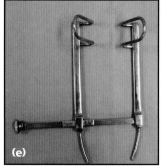

23.22 Retractors: (a) Travers; (b) Weitlander; (c) Gelpi; (d) Langenbeck; (e) Gossett.

- **Gillies** needle-holders are very commonly used in veterinary surgery. They have a scissor action as well for cutting the suture ends. Their major disadvantage is that they have no ratchet, and so the needle has to be held in place by gripping the blades tightly.
- **Olsen–Hegar** needle-holders also have a cutting edge but have the advantage of a ratchet to hold the needle securely in place. The disadvantage of the scissor edge is that the suture material may be inadvertently cut.
- **McPhail's** needle-holders traditionally have copper inserts in the tips, but those with tungsten carbide inserts are of superior quality. The handles have a spring ratchet so that by squeezing them together the jaws open and release the needle.
- **Mayo–Hegar** needle-holders resemble a pair of long-handled artery forceps. They have a ratchet but no scissor action. This is one of the most popular types of needle-holder.

Retractors

Retractors (Figure 23.22) are used to facilitate exposure of the operating field. They may be hand held or self-retaining. Hand-held retractors include Langenbeck, Senn and Czerny. Muscle and joint retractors include Gelpi, West's and Travers. Examples of abdominal wall retractors are Gossett and Balfour; and Finochietto retractors are used for the chest.

Orthopaedic instruments

See also Chapter 24.

Osteotomes, chisels and gouges

These are used to cut or shape bone or cartilage. They are available in a wide variety of sizes. The cutting edge of the osteotome is tapered on both sides, whereas the chisel is tapered on one side only (Figure 23.23). The gouge has a U-shaped edge to remove larger pieces of cartilage or soft bone.

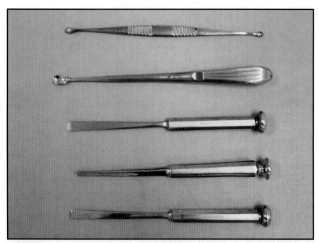

23.23 Some basic orthopaedic instruments. From top to bottom: Volkmann's scoop; curette; chisel; gouge; osteotome.

Curettes

Curettes have an oval-shaped cup (Figure 23.23). They scoop the surface of dense tissue to remove loose or degenerate tissue (e.g. cartilage flaps, necrotic bone). The cup has a sharp cutting edge and is available in various sizes.

Periosteal elevators

Periosteal elevators (Figure 23.24) are used to lift periosteum and soft tissue from the surface of bone.

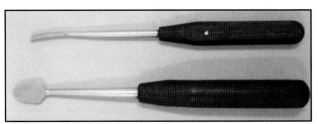

23.24 Small curved and large straight periosteal elevators.

Bone-holding forceps

Bone-holding forceps (Figure 23.25) are designed to grip bone fragments during reduction and alignment in fracture repair.

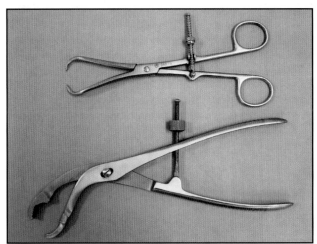

23.25 Bone-holding forceps. Top: Reduction forceps; (bottom) Verbrugge.

Bone cutters and rongeurs

Bone rongeurs (Figure 23.26) are used to cut out small pieces of dense tissue such as bone or cartilage. Bone cutters (Figure 23.26) are designed to cut larger pieces of bone.

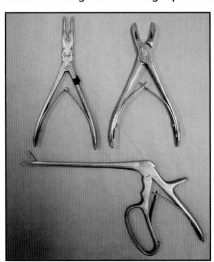

23.26 Clockwise from top left: bone rongeurs; Liston's bone-cutting forceps; arthroscopic rongeurs.

Bone rasps

Bone rasps may be used to remove sharp edges following arthroplasty procedures.

Retractors

Standard retractors are commonly used in orthopaedic surgery. In addition, hand-held Hohmann retractors (Figure 23.27) are often used for retracting muscle, tendons and ligaments.

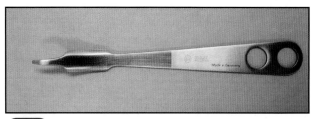

23.27 Hohmann retractor.

Drills, saws and burs

Hand, battery and air drills (Figure 23.28) are commonly used in orthopaedic surgery. Hand drills are useful around delicate structures and when only minimal drilling is required but for most major surgery a battery-operated or air drill should be a prerequisite. These allow more speed and precision than hand drills. Battery drills tend to be slower and more cumbersome than most of the compact air drills available but they are suitable for most veterinary procedures and are less expensive. They should be recharged after each use.

Oscillating saws and mechanical burs are either air or electrically driven. Great care should be taken when connecting attachments and during use. The power supply should not be applied until the couplings are assembled.

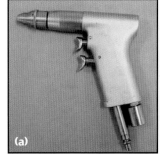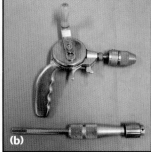

23.28 Orthopaedic drills: **(a)** air drill; **(b)** hand drill and Jacob's chuck.

Wire forceps

Various wire-cutting and twisting forceps are available for applying cerclage wires and for stabilizing bones with wire.

Gigli wire and handles

These are used in osteotomy techniques to saw through bone with a cheese-wire effect.

Instrumentation for fracture repair

The instruments required for fracture repair depend on the technique that is to be used. Materials used to repair fractures internally include Steinmann pins, orthopaedic wire, bone plates, screws and external fixator apparatus (Figures 23.29 and 23.30; see also Chapter 24).

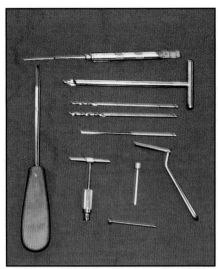

23.29
ASIF (Association for the Study of Internal Fixation) instruments for internal fixation.

Screw dia. (mm)	Drill (mm) Gliding hole	Drill (mm) (Pilot hole)	Tap (mm)
5.5	5.5	4.0	5.5
4.5	4.5	3.2	4.5
3.5	3.5	2.5	3.5
2.7	2.7	2.0	2.7
2.0	2.0	1.5	2.0

23.30 Drill and bone tap combinations for ASIF screws commonly used in veterinary surgery.

Packing a surgical set

Instrument sets are often packed together with swabs, drapes, suction tubing, etc. They are usually wrapped so that, when unfolded, the layers of wrapping will cover the base of the instrument trolley. A metal or plastic tray is lined with a towel or linen sheet. The instruments should then be laid out in a specific order. This is generally the order in which they are likely to be used (Figure 23.31). Swabs, drapes etc. are then added. A water-resistant paper wrap is laid over the top of the trolley, followed by two layers of linen sheet. The tray is placed on this and the pack is then wrapped (Figure 23.32). The set is secured with Bowie–Dick tape and tied with string. It should be labelled and dated prior to sterilization. Sharp or pointed instruments can be protected by application of autoclavable plastic tips.

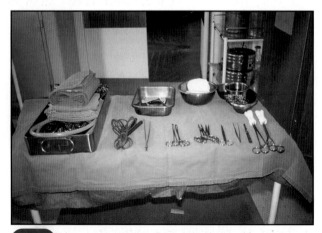

23.31 Instruments laid out ready for use.

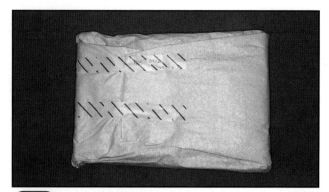

23.32 A wrapped instrument set.

Instrument sets

Instrument sets are made up to suit individual requirements and they vary from one veterinary practice to another. Some practices have sets for specific procedures (e.g. bitch spay set). Others have a standard instrument set that is used for all operations, to which other instruments will be added depending on the procedure. Often a smaller set will be available for minor procedures such as a cat spay. It is important that each of the standard instrument sets should contain the same number and type so that the surgical team always know what instruments they will have and so that it is easy to check that all are present at the end of the procedure. Instrument sets can be colour-coded by application of a piece of instrument identification adhesive tape. Figures 23.33 to 23.36 list suggested contents for various instrument sets required for soft tissue, orthopaedic and ophthalmic surgery, but these are only guidelines. Dental instruments are described in Chapter 26.

Standard instrument set	No. of pairs
Scalpel handle no. 3	1
Dissecting forceps – rat-toothed fine rat-toothed heavy duty fine plain	1 1 1
Mayo scissors – straight	1
Metzenbaum scissors	1
Artery forceps	10
Mosquito forceps	5
Allis tissue forceps	4
Suture scissors	1
Needle-holders	1
Langenbeck retractors	2
Gelpi retractor	1
Probe	1
Backhaus towel-holding forceps	10
Gallipot	1
Receiver	1
Suture tray	1
Suction tubing and tip	1
Electrocautery and handle	1
Swabs (X-ray detectable)	10
Scalpel blades sizes 10 and 15	2

23.33 Standard instrument set.

Abdominal surgery

Self-retaining retractors; Doyen's bowel clamps; long dissecting forceps; long artery forceps (e.g. Roberts); towels to pack abdomen

Thoracic surgery

Rib cutters; Finochietto rib retractors; periosteal elevator; chest drain; suture wire; oscillating saw if sternotomy approach; lobectomy clamps; long-handled artery forceps (e.g. Roberts); rib raspatory

 23.34 Additional instruments required for abdominal and thoracic surgery.

General

Osteotome; Gigli wire and handles; chisel; periosteal elevator; curette; hand drill; gouge; mallet; Hohmann retractor; putti rasp; hacksaw; Lister's bone cutting forceps; bone rongeurs

Power tools

Battery drill; air drill; mechanical burr; oscillating saw

Implants

Stainless steel wire; intramedullary pins; Kirschner wires; rush pins; staples; screws; plates

Bone pinning

Jacob's chuck and key; pin cutters;Steinmann pin

Wire fixation

Stainless steel wire; wire-holding forceps; wire-cutting forceps

Bone staples

Bone staples; staple introducer; staple remover

External fixator

Steinmann pins; Kirschner Ehmer rods; Kirschner Ehmer nuts; pin cutter; drill or Jacob's chuck

Bone plating or screw fixation

Venables/Sherman bone plates; Sherman screws; drill bit; air/hand drill; depth gauge; screw driver; plate bender

ASIF technique

(Association for the Study of Internal Fixation)

Dynamic compression plates and screws; bone drills: standard and overdrill; bone tap and handle; drill guide – neutral and loaded; tap sleeve; drill insert; depth gauge; countersink; screwdriver; plate bender or irons

 23.35 Additional instruments required for orthopaedic surgery.

No. 3 scalpel handle
Scalpel blade sizes 11, 15 or Beaver handle and blades
Fine dissecting forceps
Fine scissors
Corneal scissors
Capsule forceps
Vectis
Iris repositor
Castroviejo needle-holders
Eyelid speculum
Irrigating cannula
Distichiasis forceps

23.36 Additional instruments required for ophthalmic surgery.

Packing and sterilization of orthopaedic implants

Orthopaedic implants made of stainless steel or titanium may be sterilized by autoclaving or using ethylene oxide. They may be packed and stored in various ways, from individual packs for each plate, pin, screw or wire to complete sets. Choice will depend on individual preference, facilities and throughput of cases. The ends of Steinmann pins and Kirschner wires (K-wires) should be protected by plastic instrument tips. All packs or items should be labelled clearly with name, size, length, diameter, etc. as relevant.

Suction apparatus

A suction unit in the operating theatre is important for several reasons. It may be used for: aspiration of the oropharynx and nasopharynx during or after surgery; thoracocentesis following surgery; or for suction of fluids and blood during the surgical procedure. Various suction machines are available and a size suitable for individual requirements should be chosen. It is sensible to choose a unit with two bottles (Figure 23.37) so that there is always a spare when one bottle becomes full.

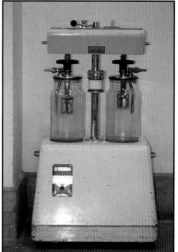 **23.37** Suction apparatus with two bottles.

Diathermy

Diathermy is a useful method of coagulation of blood vessels or cutting of tissues during surgery by means of high-frequency alternating electrical current, which produces heat within the tissues at the point of application.

The advantages of diathermy are that it:

• Allows rapid control of haemorrhage and minimizes blood loss (particularly important in very small patients, where even small amounts of blood loss may be life threatening)
• Allows clear visualization of surgical field
• Helps to minimize surgery time
• Reduces amount of foreign material in the form of ligatures that need to be left in the surgical site.

The nature of the waveform of the applied current used in diathermy can vary the effect from cutting to coagulation:

• Continuous waveforms are employed for cutting tissue.
• Interrupted waveforms are used for pure coagulation.

Diathermy unit

There are several different types of diathermy machine available for surgical use. Most units require the patient to be 'earthed' or 'grounded'. A ground or earth wire transfers the electrical current to a harmless place such as the ground. This 'earth' wire usually takes the form of a plate that is placed under the patient and is connected to the diathermy unit by a cable. If the patient is not sufficiently earthed, the electricity will pass along the line of least resistance, which may be the patient or the surgeon. This may lead to serious burning or electric shock to the patient or surgeon. The earth plate may be disposable or reusable. To provide a good contact between the plate and the patient some form of coupling gel (e.g. obstetric lubricant) spread on the earth plate is usually necessary in animals, since they are covered in hair. A diathermy probe or pair of forceps or scissors is attached to one end of an insulated diathermy lead. The other end of the lead attaches to the diathermy unit. The lead and forceps must be sterilized for use during surgery. The current is usually activated by depression of a foot pedal connected to the machine. Coagulation is achieved by applying the probe or forceps directly to the bleeding vessel or by touching the artery forceps clamping the vessel. Alcohol and other flammable materials should not be used with diathermy, because of the risk of fire.

Care of the diathermy unit

After use the diathermy earth plate, if of the reusable type, should be washed to remove coupling gel, hair, blood etc. The cable and lead should be washed, inspected for patency and resterilized. The unit should be serviced and maintained by a qualified engineer.

Cryosurgery

Cryosurgery is a technique used to destroy living tissue by the controlled application of extreme cold. The aim is to kill cells in a diseased target while producing minimal damage to normal surrounding tissue.

By the application of a refrigerant (usually liquid nitrogen) to the tissues, the temperature is reduced so that intracellular and extracellular water begins to freeze, with the formation of ice crystals. This eventually leads to cell denaturation and death. A rapid freeze followed by a slow thaw is recommended and usually 2–3 freeze–thaw cycles are necessary to achieve maximal effect. It is usually possible to approach a local hospital or research facility to obtain small amounts of the refrigerant as required.

Precautions

Liquid nitrogen is a harmful substance. To comply with COSHH regulations (see Chapter 1), a standard operating procedure (SOP) should be employed to prevent possible accidents when handling the substance. All persons involved in using liquid nitrogen should be trained and aware of the SOP.

- Liquid nitrogen should be transported only in containers provided by the supplier of the liquid nitrogen or manufacturer of the cryosurgical equipment. These are insulated metal vessels of varying sizes.
- Wear protective eye goggles, apron and insulated gloves when handling the refrigerant and equipment.
- Avoid splashing liquid nitrogen on clothes, floors and equipment as it will splash and disperse over a wide area.
- Avoid skin contact with refrigerant and probes whilst in use.
- Take care when filling cryosurgical unit. A metal funnel should be used to pour liquid nitrogen from the reservoir vessel into the unit.

Cryosurgical units

In veterinary practice small thermos-sized units are normally used. These are easy to handle and manipulate. The liquid nitrogen may be applied via a probe that adheres to the tissue surface or from a more diffuse pulsating spray.

Care of equipment following use

Once the probe or spray attachment has thawed, it should be washed using an instrument disinfectant. Any remaining liquid nitrogen should be poured back into the reservoir vessel. Probes may be autoclaved if desired.

Preparation of the patient

- Clip hair around the site to allow effective contact of the liquid nitrogen with the lesion.
- The site should have a basic skin preparation with a surgical scrub solution.
- Protect surrounding healthy tissue with insulation (e.g. polystyrene pieces). This is particularly important when using a spray around delicate structures such as the eye.

Postoperative care following cryosurgery

Initially there may be erythema and oedema, which should be monitored carefully in the immediate postoperative period. A slough will then follow, which may be moist. This should be cleaned once or twice a day. If there is any discharge, it is a good idea to apply petroleum jelly to the skin around the lesion to prevent excoriation.

Owners should be warned beforehand that following cryosurgery the affected area may be unsightly and there may be a copious foul-smelling discharge. They should also be told that the skin may become unpigmented, resulting in formation of white hair.

Endoscopes

There are two types of fibreoptic endoscopes in common use in veterinary practice (see also Chapter 20):

- **Flexible** – used for diagnostic examination of body tracts (e.g. upper respiratory tract, bronchi, urinary tract, oesophagus, stomach, rectum and colon)
- **Rigid** – used for diagnostic evaluation of trachea and bronchi, oesophagus, nasal cavities. Used for evaluation of joints (arthroscopy) and abdominal cavity (laparoscopy).

In small-animal practice the flexible endoscope is more commonly used. Many instruments are obtained second-hand from the medical field. Whilst this is an excellent source of good-quality inexpensive endoscopes, caution should be employed when purchasing such instruments as it may prove difficult to obtain spare parts for older models when repairs are necessary.

The fragile fibreoptic bundles contained within the endoscope are easily damaged by twisting and bending. The more fibres that are damaged, the less light will be transmitted. A second-hand instrument will almost certainly have some damaged fibres. A separate light source is needed to provide illumination. This may be purchased with the endoscope or separately. Relatively inexpensive portable light sources are readily available. These will usually incorporate an air pump for insufflation and a water bottle for flushing and washing the lens during use.

Video-endoscopes

Arthroscopy and laparoscopy are performed more extensively in equine practice, but are becoming more common in small-animal practice. A video camera may be attached to the endoscope so that a remote and enlarged image is produced on a TV monitor. These video-endoscopes are expensive and require careful maintenance by a qualified engineer.

Care of endoscopes

Endoscopes should be cleaned as soon as possible after use, otherwise blood, mucus, etc. will become dried on and may block the air and fluid channels

Flexible endoscopes

All modern flexible endoscopes are designed so that the whole instrument can be immersed to allow thorough cleaning. In most older endoscopes, although the tubing is immersible, the handset is not and the internal mechanism will be irreparably damaged if it is soaked. It is very important therefore to follow the manufacturer's recommendations with regard to cleaning.

Cleaning a flexible endoscope

1. With immersible endoscopes a leak test should be performed after use to ensure that it is safe to soak the instrument when cleaning. A leak test kit and instructions will usually be provided by the manufacturer at the time of purchase. If there is evidence of fluid leakage within the endoscope, it should *not* be immersed but should be sent for repair immediately, otherwise the instrument may be permanently damaged. If the leak test is satisfactory, the endoscope may be safely immersed.
2. The outer surface of the endoscope is then wiped over with an instrument disinfectant. At this stage the instrument should be inspected for external damage.
3. The biopsy channel should be flushed with the disinfectant solution and then a flexible wire brush introduced to clean the channel. It should then be flushed again.
4. The endoscope is attached to its power source and the distal tip of the endoscope is placed in disinfectant solution. Fluid is aspirated by depression of the suction button. This should then be flushed with distilled water.
5. The water and air buttons should be pressed to blow all water out of the system.
6. If the flush channel is blocked, the tip of the endoscope should be gently brushed with a soft toothbrush to try to dislodge debris from this tiny orifice.
7. Thorough drying of the endoscope is recommended. The instrument should ideally be hung up so that the tubing can hang straight down to allow drainage of any remaining fluid.
8. Once dry, the endoscope may be packed in its case or preferably hung in a cabinet so that the cable may remain straight.

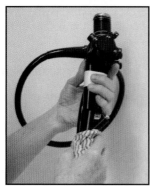 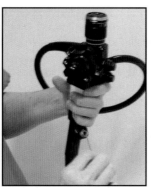

Flexible endoscopes may be safely sterilized with ethylene oxide if desired. This is to be recommended, especially when they are used frequently or where there is a risk of infection.

It is important to coil the fibreoptic cable in large loops when packing the sterilizer unit, to prevent risk of damaging the light fibres in the endoscope.

Rigid endoscopes

Rigid endoscopes are as easily damaged as flexible ones and they must be handled with care. Sterilization by ethylene oxide is recommended, but where several procedures are to be performed in one day it will only be possible to use cold chemical disinfection.

Suture materials

The ideal suture material should:

- Be suitable for use in any situation
- Be readily available and inexpensive
- Be readily sterilized by steam or ethylene oxide
- Show high initial tensile strength, combined with small-diameter material
- Have a good knot security (it should tie easily, with no tendency to slip or loosen, and the knot should hold securely without fraying)
- Produce minimal tissue reaction – it should be inert (i.e. not cause pain or swelling or delay healing), non-allergenic, non-carcinogenic and non-electrolytic
- Show good handling characteristics (it should be easy to handle when wet or dry and pass through tissue without friction or cutting)
- Not create an environment for bacterial growth, i.e. not show capillarity or wicking of fluids (ideally monofilament)
- Be absorbed after its function has been served.

No single suture material in the wide range available possesses all of these ideal characteristics. Selection tends to depend on the surgeon's teaching and preferences. Figure 23.38 explains the terms used to describe the characteristics of suture materials.

Term	Meaning
Tensile strength	The breaking strength per unit area of tissue
Knot security	Related to the surface frictional characteristics of the material Every suture is weakest where it is tied. Often the strongest sutures have the poorest knot security
Tissue reaction	The response of the tissue to the suture material involved
Tissue drag	The degree of frictional force developed as the material is pulled through the tissue
Capillarity	The extent to which tissue fluid is attracted along the suture material. Materials with high capillarity act as a wick and encourage fluids to move along them. Such materials should not be used in the presence of sepsis
Memory	The tendency of the material to return to its original shape. A material with high memory tends to unkink during knot tying, i.e. knot security is poor with materials possessing high memory

23.38 Characteristics of suture materials.   *continues* ▶

Term	Meaning
Chatter	The lack of smoothness as a throw of a knot is tightened down
Stiffness and elongation	The less force required to stretch a suture, the more it will elongate before it ruptures
Sterilization characteristics	The ability of the material to undergo sterilization without deteriorating. Autoclaving is satisfactory for the nylon materials. Repeated autoclaving will, however, weaken them. The natural products and synthetic absorbable materials should not be steam sterilised. Ethylene oxide sterilization is safe for all sutures provided the packs are sufficiently aerated

23.38   *continued*   Characteristics of suture materials.

Classification of sutures

Suture materials are either absorbable or non-absorbable. They may be further classified as natural or synthetic, and as mono-filament or multifilament (Figure 23.39; see also Chapter 24).

	Natural fibres	Synthetic
Absorbable	**Multifilament:** Catgut (plain/chromic)	**Monofilament:** Polydioxanone [PDS II] [a] Polyglyconate [Maxon] Polyglecaprone 25 [Monocryl]
		Multifilament: Polyglactin 910 [Vicryl] [a] Polyglycolic acid [Dexon] [b]
Non-absorbable	**Multifilament:** Silk Linen [Supramid]	**Monofilament:** Polyamide [Ethilon] [a] Polypropylene [Prolene] [a] Polybutylester [Novafil] [b] Polyethylene [Dermalene] [a] Stainless steel
		Multifilament: Braided polyamide [Nuralon] [a] Polyester [Mersilene] [a] Coated polyester [Ethibond]

23.39   Examples of absorbable and non-absorbable suture materials. [a] Ethicon; [b] Davis & Geck Ltd.

Absorbable sutures

These materials are degraded within the tissues and lose their tensile strength by 60 days. Natural fibres (catgut) are removed by phagocytosis, which tends to produce some degree of tissue reaction. The synthetic absorbable materials are hydrolysed and tend to produce minimal tissue reaction. In general, absorbable suture materials are used when closing internal tissue layers or organs that do not require long-term support.

Catgut

Catgut was made from the submucosa of sheep small intestine or the serosa of cattle intestines. 'Plain catgut' is untreated; 'chromic catgut' is tanned with chromic salts to slow its absorption, increase its strength and decrease the tissue reaction. For many years chromic and plain catgut have been used in both human and veterinary surgery. However, following an EU ruling they have been withdrawn from manufacture and sale in the United Kingdom.

Polyglactin 910

This material is a copolymer of lactide and glycolide and is absorbed by hydrolysis. It is available in dyed and undyed preparations, the latter causing less tissue reaction; it is coated to improve its handling characteristics and it is braided.

- Polyglactin 910 has a higher initial tensile strength than catgut.
- It loses 50% of its strength in 14 days and is totally absorbed in 60–90 days.
- There is considerable tissue drag and careful placement of knots is necessary.

Polyglycolic acid

This is an inert, non-antigenic, non-pyrogenic polyester made from hydroxyacetic acid and it is braided. It is absorbed by hydrolysis; the hydrolysed breakdown products have been found to be bacteriostatic experimentally, therefore its use has been advocated in infected sites.

- Polyglycolic acid loses approximately 30% of its strength in 7 days and 80% in 14 days.
- Tissue drag is considerable even in the coated formulation.
- It has poor knot security.

Polydioxanone

This is a monofilament absorbable suture that is absorbed by hydrolysis.

- Polydioxanone loses only 30% of its strength in 2 weeks and is minimally absorbed at 90 days.
- Tissue reaction is minimal.
- As it is monofilament, tissue drag is reduced.
- It is ideal in infected sites and where an absorbable material is required for a long period of time.
- Its main disadvantage is its springiness.

Polyglyconate

This synthetic monofilament absorbable suture is very similar to polydioxanone. It is slightly less springy and therefore easier to handle than polydioxanone.

Polyglecaprone 25

This new synthetic monofilament absorbable suture is similar to both polydioxanone and polyglyconate, but duration of tensile strength is shorter. It is broken down by hydrolysis.

- Polyglecaprone 25 is less springy than polydioxanone and polyglyconate.
- Tissue reaction is minimal.
- Tissue drag is minimal.
- Its main disadvantage is that at 14 days only 30% original strength maintained.

Non-absorbable sutures

These maintain their strength for longer than 60 days. The material is neither hydrolysed nor phagocytosed: it becomes encapsulated within fibrous tissue. Non-absorbable sutures are used where prolonged mechanical support is required. The main indications for use are:

- In skin closure, where sutures are generally removed after 10 days
- Within slow-healing tissues.

Silk

This is available as braided or twisted strands. It is obtained from threads spun by the silkworm larvae. It may be coated with silicone or wax to minimize the capillarity, which may promote infection.

Silk has good handling characteristics, excellent knot security and good tensile strength. It is relatively inexpensive. Its main uses include cardiovascular and thoracic surgery and it can be used on genital mucosa and adjacent to eyes. It should not be used in infected sites, oral mucosa or hollow organs, where it may act as a nidus for infection.

Linen

This is twisted from long strands of flax. It is easily sterilized, handles well and has excellent knot security. It does show capillary properties, however, and has been shown to contribute to sinus formation. It has been largely superseded since the advent of the synthetic absorbable materials.

Polypropylene

This is an inert, non-absorbable monofilament material. It has high tensile strength but tends to stretch and will snap if crushed by needle-holders. The knot security is varied and a bulky knot may be formed. It is very springy but shows little tissue drag. It becomes encapsulated in a thin fibrous covering.

Polyamide

This may be either monofilament or braided. The monofilament form causes little tissue reaction, has little tissue drag and is non-capillary. Its handling characteristics are not good and knot security can be poor. It loses approximately 15% of its tensile strength each year. It can be used on fascia and muscle, but the buried ends can be irritant in serous or synovial cavities. The braided form is usually sheathed in an attempt to decrease capillarity, but its use as a buried suture is not recommended. It shows more tissue drag than the monofilament variety, although it handles better.

Polyesters

Various braided polyesters are available. They are easy to handle and retain their tensile strength well. Some are coated with silicone, Teflon or polybutylate to reduce tissue drag. They tend to have poor knot-tying quality and some have shown signs of capillarity.

Stainless steel

This is available in monofilament or braided varieties. It is very strong, inert and non-capillary. It is relatively difficult to handle as the wire lacks elasticity and knots may be difficult to tie, but knot security is good. It is useful in slow-healing tissues such as bone, tendon and joint capsules, and in contaminated sites. It has become less popular in recent years as newer materials have become available.

Alternatives to sutures

Staples

Metal clips or staples for use in skin and other tissues have gained popularity in the field of veterinary surgery over the last few years. Staples designed for skin closure are packed in a gun-like applicator for rapid insertion. These instruments are intended to be disposable, but they may be safely sterilized by ethylene oxide.

The main advantage of staples is speed of insertion. They are inert and well tolerated. Reusable staple-removing forceps are available to remove metal skin staples.

Stapling machines have also been designed for gastrointestinal anastomosis. Although designed for the human market, they are suitable for veterinary applications and are gaining popularity. They may permit resection of areas of bowel that are inaccessible to routine suturing, particularly in the equine abdomen. Their major disadvantage is cost, but their ease of use and the shortened surgery time have much to recommend them.

Metal clips are also available for use as ligatures. They come in various sizes with reusable applicators. They are simple and quick to use.

Tissue glue

There are cyanoacrylate monomers that polymerize on contact with moisture in the wound. They have been found useful by some surgeons.

Adhesive tapes

Designed for use in humans, these have been of limited use in animals as they do not adhere well to moist skin.

Suture selection

The veterinary surgeon will normally select the suture material (see Chapter 24) but the veterinary nurse should have some idea of which materials may be used in different tissues (Figure 23.40) and the sizes that will be required (Figure 23.41).

Tissue	Suture materials
Skin	Monofilament nylon or polypropylene Metal staples Avoid materials with capillary action
Subcutis	Fine synthetic absorbable material with minimal tissue reaction, e.g. polydioxanone, polyglactin, polyglycolic acid
Muscle	Synthetic absorbable, non-absorbable, e.g. nylon
Fascia	Synthetic non-absorbable if prolonged suture strength required
Hollow viscus	Synthetic absorbable or polypropylene In bladder: monofilament synthetic
Tendon	Nylon, polypropylene, stainless steel
Blood vessels	Polypropylene: least thrombogenic is silk
Eyes	Synthetic absorbable, e.g. polyglactin, polydioxanone
Nerves	Nylon or polypropylene: minimal tissue reaction

23.40 Suture materials suitable for different tissues.

Metric	USP	Metric	USP
0.2	10/0	3	2/0
0.3	9/0	3.5	0
0.4	8/0	4	1
0.5	7/0	5	2
0.7	6/0	6	3 and 4
1	5/0	7	5
1.5	4/0	8	6
2	3/0		

23.41 Sizes of suture materials.

Packaging of suture materials

Most suture materials are purchased in presterilized individual packets. This guarantees a sterile suture (unless the packet is damaged) and a needle in perfect condition where one is attached. The only disadvantage is that of cost. Synthetic absorbable suture materials are only available packaged in this way.

Some suture materials are provided on a reel in surgical spirit, where the suture material is pulled off and a length cut as needed. This is a much less reliable way of storing suture materials and should be avoided for internal use.

Suture materials can also be purchased as lengths, which are then threaded on to resterilizable needles. This causes more tissue trauma, due to drag through the tissues where the suture material is doubled over through the eye of the needle. The needle is also more likely to become blunt.

Multi-use cassettes are still used in veterinary practice for packaging catgut (not UK), nylon and stainless steel sutures. The disadvantage of these is the likelihood of contamination of cassettes during use – they often become damaged. It is also easy to contaminate the material as it is cut from the reel and transferred to the instrument trolley. Their use is to be discouraged.

Suture needles

Suture needles are designed to pass through tissue easily. They must be sharp enough to penetrate tissues with minimal resistance, rigid enough to prevent excessive bending and yet flexible enough to bend before breaking. They should be made from corrosion-resistant stainless steel.

Swaged needles

Swaged or atraumatic needles are attached to the suture material, i.e. they do not require threading. The advantage of this is that a needle in perfect condition is available with each strand and tissue trauma is minimized by the passage of material and needle of a comparative size. All of the prepacked suture materials are available with a variety of different needle shapes and sizes.

Eyed needles

This type of needle requires threading. The primary indication for its use is economy of suitable material or use of speciality needles (e.g. for large-animal work). The disadvantages are increased tissue trauma due to the eye size, loss of sharpness of the needle tip, and bending and corrosion following repeated use. The needle shape refers to both the longitudinal shape of the shaft and the cross-sectional shape.

Longitudinal shape

Of the great variety of different sizes and shapes that are available, some of those used in veterinary surgery are shown in Figure 23.42.

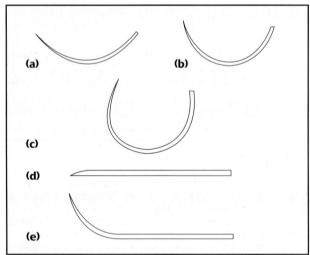

23.42 Suture needle shapes: **(a)** $^3/_8$ circle; **(b)** $^1/_2$ circle; **(c)** $^5/_8$ circle; **(d)** straight; **(e)** $^1/_2$ curved.

Cross-sectional shape

Round-bodied

These are designed to separate tissue fibres rather than cut them, and are used for soft tissue or in situations where easy splitting of tissue fibres is possible.

Modified point

The **taper-cut** needle has a cutting tip on the point of the needle and a round body. This provides increased penetration of the needle without increased tissue trauma.

The **trocar-point** needle has a strong cutting head and a robust round body. This is useful in dense tissue.

Cutting needles

These are required wherever dense or tough tissue needs to be sutured. The cross-sectional appearance of the needle is usually a triangular cutting edge, which extends at least halfway along the shaft. The **reverse cutting needle** has the cutting edge on the outside of the needle curvature to improve strength and resistance to bending.

Micropoint needles

These are very fine needles with a sharp cutting edge. They are designed for ophthalmic surgery and microsurgery.

Selection of needles

The use of swaged needles is to be encouraged – their advantages far outweigh those of eyed needles. Other needles should be as close as possible in diameter to that of the suture. A large needle tract invites bacteria and foreign substances to enter the wound, thus delaying healing. The needle should be of the appropriate shape and size to enable the veterinary surgeon to close the wound accurately and precisely.

The smaller and deeper the wound, the greater the curve should be. Straight needles are designed to be hand held and tend to be used in the skin. Half-curved cutting needles have been commonly used in veterinary surgery but have little to recommend their use.

The tissue type will determine the necessary point of the needle. Generally speaking:

- Round-bodied needles are used for viscera, subcutaneous and friable tissue
- Taper-tip needles are used for easily penetrated tissue, i.e. for denser tissue
- Cutting needles are generally used in the skin.

Suture patterns

Veterinary nurses maintained on the list held by the RCVS are now legally allowed to perform minor acts of surgery, including the suturing of wounds. It is important that they should be familiar with basic suturing techniques. The veterinary surgeon should give practical instruction and reference should be made to surgical technique textbooks.

Suture patterns may be interrupted or closed, and may be further classified as apposing, everting or inverting.

- **Apposing** sutures bring the tissues in direct apposition.
- **Everting** sutures tend to turn the edges of the wound outwards.
- **Inverting** sutures turn the tissue inwards (e.g. towards the lumen of a viscus).

Surgical knots

A surgical knot has three main components:

- The **loop** is the part of the suture material within the opposed or ligated tissue.
- The **knot** is composed of a number of throws, each throw being the linking of two strands of tissue around each other.
- The **ears** are the cut ends of the suture that prevent the knot coming untied.

Knots can be tied by hand or by an instrument. Hand ties may be single or two-handed.

The basic surgical knot is the **reef knot** or **square knot**. A **surgeon's knot** has an initial double throw instead of a single throw. This reduces the risk of the first throw loosening before the second throw is placed.

Hand-tying helps to prevent slippage of the first throw, since tension can be kept on both ends of the suture throughout the procedure. However, it tends to be wasteful on suture material.

The knots of skin sutures should be pulled to one side of the incision and the suture loop should be loose. Sutures that are too tight compromise the vascular supply, enhance infection and delay healing. They are also uncomfortable and encourage the patient to interfere with the wound.

Suture material should not be crushed in the jaws of needle-holders. When tying knots, only the end of the suture material should be grasped. Needle-holders should not be clamped on to the eye of swaged needles, as this will cause damage or breakage of the needle.

Interrupted sutures

The main advantage of the interrupted suture is its ability to maintain strength and tissue apposition if part of the suture line fails. Each suture is individually tied and cut distal to the knot. Its main disadvantage is the amount of suture material used and left within the tissue and the time required to suture.

Continuous sutures

These are neither knotted nor cut, except at each end of the suture line. The advantages of the continuous suture line are ease of application, use of minimal amount of suture material and ease of removal. The main disadvantage is that slippage of either the beginning or end knot is likely to cause failure of the entire suture line.

Common suture patterns

Common suture patterns used in the skin, in muscle and fascia, and in hollow organ closure are listed in Figure 23.43. Skin sutures (Figure 23.44) should be placed at least 5 mm from the skin edge and be placed squarely across the wound. The skin should be handled gently with fine rat-toothed forceps. The wound edges should be apposed or slightly everted with no gaping or overlapping.

In skin	In muscle and fascia	In hollow organ closure
Simple interrupted	Simple interrupted	Simple interrupted
Simple continuous	Simple continuous	Parker–Kerr
Ford interlocking	Ford interlocking	Purse-string
Interrupted vertical mattress	Cruciate mattress	Connell
	Horizontal mattress	Cushing
Interrupted horizontal mattress	Vertical mattress	Lembert
	Mayo mattress	Gambee
Cruciate mattress		Halstead

23.43 Common suture patterns.

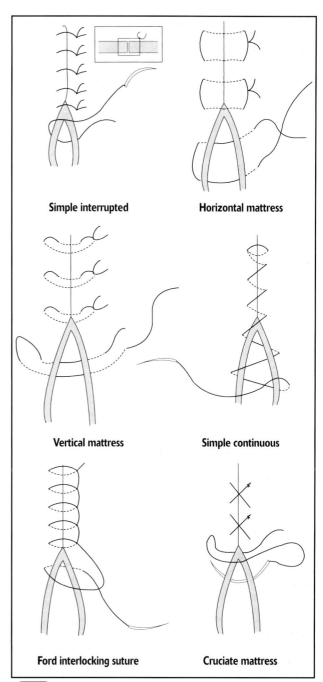

Simple interrupted — Horizontal mattress

Vertical mattress — Simple continuous

Ford interlocking suture — Cruciate mattress

23.44 Common suture patterns used in the skin.

Further reading

College of Animal Welfare (1997) *Veterinary Surgical Instruments*. Butterworth-Heinemann, Oxford

Garden C (1999) The surgical environment and instrumentation. In: *BSAVA Manual of Veterinary Nursing*, Moore M (ed.), pp. 163–176). BSAVA Publications, Cheltenham

Knecht CD, Allen AR, Williams DJ and Johnson JH (1987) *Fundamental Techniques in Veterinary Surgery, 3rd edn*. WB Saunders, Philadelphia

McCurnin DM (1990) *Clinical Textbook for Veterinary Technicians, 2nd edn*. WB Saunders, Philadelphia

Slatter D (2003) *Textbook of Small Animal Surgery*. WB Saunders, Philadelphia

Tracey D (2000) *Small Animal Surgical Nursing*. Mosby, St Louis

Williams D and Niles J (2005) *BSAVA Manual of Canine and Feline Abdominal Surgery*. BSAVA Publications, Gloucester

Chapter 24

Surgical nursing

Davina Anderson and Jenny Smith

<table>
<tr><td colspan="2">

Learning objectives

After studying this chapter, students should be able to:

- **List the common surgical conditions encountered in the dog and cat**
- **Understand the common terms used to describe surgical conditions**
- **Describe the basic physiology and treatments of surgical diseases**
- **Describe the physical signs of normal and delayed healing of tissues and wounds**
- **Discuss the common complications and nursing requirements of surgical diseases**
- **Provide information to the owner on the postoperative nursing care required for surgical diseases**

</td></tr>
</table>

Introduction

This chapter discusses the recognition of surgical diseases, surgical procedures, management and nursing of the postoperative patient, and the stages of normal and abnormal healing. In order to understand this subject a basic knowledge of terminology is required; accurate communication between nursing staff and veterinary surgeons, and reliable record-keeping, can only be accomplished if correct terminology is used. Many terms used in the description of surgical diseases or procedures are created by the combination of two or more components. A knowledge of how these terms are created allows a new term to be understood without extensive learning by rote. The first part of the word usually describes the relevant anatomical area or structure whilst the suffix describes the nature of the procedure. For example, cystotomy, cystostomy and cystectomy all describe surgical procedures on the bladder (Figure 24.1).

Terminology	Meaning
General terms	
Prognosis	The prognosis is an indication of whether the animal is likely to survive the procedure – or at least how long the disease is likely to be controlled. For example a poor prognosis suggests that the animal will die fairly soon despite treatment, whereas an excellent prognosis suggests that the disease may be cured
Postoperative morbidity	This refers to the degree of complications that the animal may be expected to suffer after the surgery. High morbidity would suggest that an animal will need a lot of nursing care (e.g. paraplegics), whereas low morbidity suggests that the animal is expected to make a rapid and full recovery
Emergency surgery	Surgery that is performed immediately as a life-saving procedure despite increased anaesthetic and recovery risks in the ill patient
Elective surgery	Surgery that is planned and can be performed at a time convenient to the veterinary surgeon or owner
Stay sutures	These are long lengths of suture material temporarily placed in tissue so as to hold the tissue without causing bruising during surgery. Usually, the ends are held together with artery forceps, which are used as 'handles' to manipulate the tissue
Temporary openings	The suffix **-otomy** denotes a procedure for cutting open or dividing tissue during surgery. The tissue is then repaired to allow it to heal normally

Laparotomy or coeliotomy	A temporary opening into the abdomen. These are the standard terms of abdominal surgery. These terms can be further defined by identifying the site of the incision:
	    midline (linea alba)
	    paramedian (slightly to one side of the midline)
	    parapreputial (to one side of the prepuce)
	    paracostal (caudal and parallel to the last rib)

24.1 Surgical terminology.

continues ▶

Terminology	Meaning
Temporary openings	
Rhinotomy	A temporary opening into the nasal cavity
Tracheotomy	A temporary opening into the trachea
Thoracotomy	A temporary opening into the thorax
Gastrotomy	A temporary opening into the stomach
Enterotomy	A temporary opening into the intestine
Nephrotomy	A temporary opening into the kidney
Urethrotomy	A temporary opening into the urethra
Cystotomy	A temporary opening into the bladder
Hysterotomy	A temporary opening into the uterus (e.g. a caesarean)
Arthrotomy	A temporary opening into a joint space
Osteotomy	A temporary division of a bone
Myotomy	A temporary division of a muscle
Tenotomy	A temporary division of a tendon
Maintained openings	The suffix **-ostomy** denotes the creation of an opening or stoma ('mouth') which communicates with the outside through the skin. Usually a device is used to keep the stoma open, and then this is removed when the opening is allowed to close. Permanent stoma are sutured to the skin and allowed to heal open
Pharyngostomy	An opening in the pharynx, to allow feeding via a tube, or placement of an endotracheal tube bypassing the mouth
Tracheostomy	An opening in the trachea, to allow the animal to breathe when there is an obstruction in the larynx or pharynx, or when it is important not to have the endotracheal tube in the mouth during surgery. The opening may be maintained temporarily via a special tracheostomy tube, or it can be a permanent airway
Gastrostomy	An opening in the stomach to allow decompression or feeding bypassing the oesophagus, via a tube
Jejunostomy	An opening in the jejunum, to allow feeding bypassing the stomach and duodenum via a special feeding tube
Urethrostomy	A permanent opening in the urethra, to allow urination when there is an obstruction or stricture in the urethra distally
Cystostomy	An opening in the bladder, to divert urine from the urethra, via a drain
Removal of structures	The suffix **-ectomy** denotes the surgical removal of all or part of a structure. Where part of a structure is removed, the remaining part must be sutured back together. The point at which the tissue is rejoined is called the anastomosis
Tonsillectomy	Removal of the tonsils
Lung lobectomy	Removal of a lung lobe
Gastrectomy	Removal of part of the stomach
Pancreatectomy	Removal of part of the pancreas
Cholecystectomy	Removal of the gall bladder
Enterectomy	Removal of a length of intestine
Colectomy	Removal of part or all of the colon
Nephrectomy	Removal of a kidney
Cystectomy	Removal of part of the bladder wall
Mastectomy	Removal of some or all of the mammary glands
Orchidectomy	Removal of the testes
Ovariohysterectomy	Removal of the ovaries and uterus (spay)
Splenectomy	Removal of part or all of the spleen
Ostectomy	Removal of a section of bone

24.1 *continued* Surgical terminology.

Physiology of surgical nursing

Inflammation

Inflammation may be a normal physiological response to injury or irritant, or part of a pathological process causing disease. An inflammatory response will be present as part of the healing process, but then persist for longer than expected if disease develops. For example, the redness and swelling of the inflammation seen along the line of a surgical incision over the first 2–3 days post surgery are normal. If the animal licks at the sutures or the surgical incision becomes infected, the inflammation will persist and then would be considered part of a pathological response to continued injury.

The classical signs of inflammation are:

- Redness
- Swelling
- Heat
- Pain
- Loss of normal function of the tissue.

These signs of inflammation have been recognized for 2000 years. The redness, heat and swelling are due to an increase in the blood flow to the tissue. Swelling occurs as white blood cells and protein-rich fluid leave the blood vessels and accumulate in the tissue. Pain is due to stimulation of the nerve endings in the tissue as a response to the increased pressure because of the swelling, as well as inflammatory mediators and toxins released by the cells in the area. This fluid is known as **inflammatory exudate** and is an important part of the inflammatory process.

Inflammatory exudate serves a number of functions:

- Dilution of irritant substances in the tissues
- Delivery of immune cells to the tissues
- Delivery of immunoglobulins and other immune-response substances
- Delivery of fibrinogen into the area to help with 'walling off' of the inflamed site
- Initiation of the response to injury and start of the healing process.

However, the inflammatory response can also lead to loss of function either due to destruction of the tissue (e.g. destruction of cartilage in erosive arthritis) or just due to muscle spasm and pain.

Acute inflammation

Acute inflammation is the immediate and rapid response to injury (Figure 24.2). In ideal circumstances where the injury is self-limiting, the inflammation should settle down very quickly, i.e. within 2–3 days.

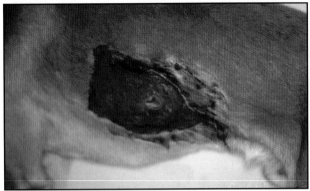

24.2   An acute avulsion of the skin on the flank of a Lurcher. The skin edges are painful and inflamed and there is serous ooze wetting the fur at the edges of the wound. This is a classic example of the very acute inflammatory phase of a wound.

There can be systemic signs of acute inflammation, including:

- Fever
- Increased pulse rate
- Increased circulating white blood cells, particularly polymorphonuclear leucocytes (PMNs).

In most circumstances, the acute inflammation resolves quickly once the injury is repaired or the initiating factor is eliminated. However, where inflammation persists, it may become chronic, and pathological (Figure 24.3). The acute inflammation seen in response to injury is a key stage in the development of normal healing.

Outcome	Notes
Resolution	No significant tissue injury
Healing	Tissues are slowly regenerated or repaired
Abscessation	An accumulation of pus which persists in a walled off cavity
Degeneration	Damaged cells degenerate and are not repaired
Mineralization	Calcified deposits are laid down in soft tissues in response to chronic inflammation
Necrosis	Cell death occurs and the affected tissue is sloughed. Particularly seen in the skin or intestinal epithelium in response to severe inflammation
Gangrene	Cell death is associated with loss of the local blood supply and putrefaction of the tissues by anaerobic bacteria

24.3   Outcome of inflammation in tissues.

Chronic inflammation

Chronic inflammation refers to the fact that the inflammatory response has gone on for longer than expected – possibly weeks or months. These changes in the tissue may become irreversible and affect the normal function of the tissue permanently. The main difference in the tissue is that, instead of PMNs, a mononuclear cell population is seen together with proliferation of fibroblasts. There are three common situations where the inflammation persists and chronic inflammation results:

- Persistent low-grade infections (e.g. intracellular organisms or fungi)
- Prolonged exposure to foreign material (e.g. suture material)
- Autoimmune diseases (in these the inciting cause is the animal's own tissues and treatment aims to reduce the inflammatory response rather than remove the cause).

Inflammation of specific tissues

In different tissues, the same basic processes occur, with production of fluid, swelling, oedema, increased blood supply and sometimes increased pain. For example, inflammation of the pancreas (pancreatitis) results in oedema and reddening of the pancreas with severe cranial abdominal pain. Peritonitis has been likened to an 'internal burn' as the peritoneum may become bright red, and produce large amounts of abdominal fluid.

Definitions: Inflammation of tissues

The suffix -itis indicates inflammation and or infection of that tissue. This may be chronic (long term) or acute (sudden in onset)

- **Adenitis** – Inflammation of a gland
- **Arthritis** – Inflammation of a joint
- **Colitis** – Inflammation of the colon – often referred to as 'irritable bowel'
- **Conjunctivitis** – Inflammation of the conjunctiva of the eye
- **Cystitis** – Inflammation of the bladder
- **Dermatitis** – Inflammation of the skin. Specific terms may be used to describe the nature of the inflammation, e.g. pyoderma – an infected inflammation of the skin
- **Enteritis** – Inflammation of the small intestines (i.e. diarrhoea)
- **Gastritis** – Inflammation of the stomach (i.e. vomiting). Symptoms of vomiting and diarrhoea may be referred to as gastroenteritis
- **Gingivitis** – Inflammation of the oral gingiva
- **Hepatitis** – Inflammation of the liver
- **Metritis** – Inflammation of the uterine lining. Pyometra denotes a concurrent infection of the inflamed uterus
- **Nephritis** – Inflammation of the kidney, often called pyelonephritis to denote infection in the kidney
- **Neuritis** – Inflammation of a nerve or nerve roots
- **Orchitis** – Inflammation of the testes
- **Otitis** – Inflammation of the ear. This may be the external ear canal (otitis externa) or the middle (otitis media) or inner ear (otitis interna)
- **Pancreatitis** – Inflammation of the pancreas
- **Peritonitis** – Inflammation of the abdominal lining
- **Pleuritis** – Inflammation of the thoracic lining
- **Pneumonia** – Inflammation of the lungs
- **Rhinitis** – Inflammation of the nasal cavity
- **Tracheitis** – Inflammation of the trachea
- **Urethritis** – Inflammation of the urethra
- **Uveitis** – Inflammation of the iris of the eye
- **Vaginitis** – Inflammation of the vagina

Treatment of acute inflammation

The aims of treatment of inflammation are to remove the inciting cause and to prevent the development of chronic inflammation or long-term disease.

Removal of the inciting cause may be as simple as **lavage** (washing away) of debris or chemicals, or treatment of a bacterial infection with antibiotics. In the early stages, inflammation can sometimes be reduced by using cold compresses to reduce blood flow and thereby reduce swelling. Rapid treatment of burns (within 20 minutes) with cold water can reduce the extent of the injury by dissipating the heat and reducing the inflammatory response around the edge of the burn.

Sometimes it is necessary to limit the inflammatory response and drugs can be used. Drugs can reduce the inflammation and often have a secondary analgesic effect due to reduced stimulation of nerve endings and reduction of swelling. The commonly used drugs are corticosteroids and non-steroidal anti-inflammatories (NSAIDs). These two groups of drugs have potential toxic side effects; they should never be used together and are only used under the direction of a veterinary surgeon. If ongoing inflammation is caused by infection, topical antiseptics or systemic antibiotics may be used to kill the bacteria.

Fluid accumulation

Fluid can accumulate in tissues or in body spaces as part of a pathological process or as a response to injury and often is part of the inflammatory response. Analysis of the fluid is necessary in order to make a diagnosis of the disease process causing the fluid to accumulate.

Body fluid accumulations

- **Exudate** is the term used to describe inflammatory fluid that contains white blood cells and proteinaceous debris.
- **Blood** may accumulate in body cavities after organ haemorrhage or in tissue planes.
- **Serosanguineous exudate** is fluid that has the appearance of blood, but on analysis has a lower packed cell volume (PCV) than blood, and other inflammatory cells predominate.
- **Transudate** is fluid that has shifted across semi-permeable membranes and is largely acellular. It may accumulate due to loss of osmotic pressure (proteins in the circulating blood) or increased venous pressure.
- **Modified transudate**. When a transudate has been in the body cavity for a while, it causes irritation in its own right and some cells start to move into the transudate as part of the inflammatory response.
- **Physiological fluid in an inappropriate space** (e.g. urine, bile, chyle, saliva). The body produces some fluids that should always travel out through lined ducts. If there is a leak in the system, large volumes of these fluids may be identified in inappropriate spaces, such as free urine or bile in the abdomen.

Fluid-filled masses

Fluid-filled masses are often identified as part of investigation of disease, and they are differentiated according to the type of fluid within.

Seroma

Seromas are probably the commonest type of fluid-filled mass encountered in surgical nursing. A seroma is usually an accumulation of inflammatory exudate within the tissue underneath a surgical site. Some surgeries result in loss of normal tissue structure (**dead space**) and the spaces fill with fluid rapidly after the surgery. If measures are not taken to prevent this, the fluid may take a long time to resolve or may even need drainage.

Haematoma

This is the term used for a 'blood blister', where a blood vessel bursts due to trauma or surgery and the blood accumulates in the surrounding tissues. It is important to differentiate between a haematoma due to direct trauma (or surgery) and a haematoma due to clotting defect or vessel wall abnormality.

Abscess

An abscess is an accumulation of inflammatory exudate that is full of dead and dying white cells (pus) in response to severe irritation or infection. It is usually walled off with a fibrous reaction (see below).

Physiological fluid leak

Sometimes normal body fluids can leak into tissue planes and get walled off by the inflammatory response to form a persistent fluid-filled mass. A good example of this is the **salivary mucocele**, where saliva leaks from the salivary duct and forms a fluctuant subcutaneous mass.

Abscesses and cellulitis

Abscesses and cellulitis are very common presentations of acute inflammatory disease in veterinary practice. When pyogenic organisms locate in a solid tissue, they cause cell death and a strong inflammatory response. This leads to the formation of pus. If this is not localized, it may distribute diffusely throughout the tissue and is known as **cellulitis**.

Abscesses are nearly always secondary to bacterial infection, and the pus is full of bacteria and dead bacteria inside white blood cells. However, an abscess can also be sterile when there are no bacteria involved but there is an accumulation of dead and dying cells and tissues within a fibrous capsule.

Within an abscess, there are often several stages of inflammation going on at the same time, with pus in the centre, an acute inflammatory response around this with PMNs reacting to the toxins produced in the pus and, on the outside, a chronic inflammatory response with mononuclear cells and fibroblasts laying down a fibrous capsule. Sometimes the toxins produced by the abscess are not contained and they cause a **toxaemia**, which makes the animal systemically ill. The toxaemia can be life threatening, causing pain, fever, vomiting, shock or even heart or kidney failure. Once the pus is discharged from the abscess, the systemic signs resolve and recovery is usually very rapid.

Abscesses that occur superficially (e.g. cat bite abscesses in the skin; Figure 24.4) often rupture spontaneously, releasing the pus through a hole in the overlying skin. Some abscesses occur internally (e.g. prostate, liver or peritoneal). If these abscesses rupture and release the pus generally throughout the abdomen, the consequences could be fatal.

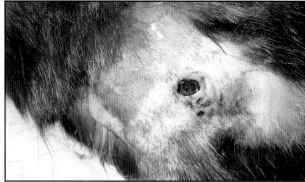

24.4 Cat bite abscess. This abscess over the gluteal region has ruptured, releasing the pus. It has been clipped and cleaned and will now heal by second intention.

Treatment

Cellulitis is too diffuse to be treated except with systemic antibiotics, analgesics and anti-inflammatories, but abscesses can often be drained and this provides immediate relief from symptoms. Once the abscess is drained, the cavity collapses and the fibrous tissue granulates in and the hole heals over rapidly. If the diagnosis is not certain, a small needle and syringe can be used to aspirate some fluid from the abscess for analysis prior to treatment. Treatment of abscesses is most effective if done under general anaesthetic, but at the very least, sedation and analgesics should be administered prior to treatment, as abscesses can be extremely painful.

- **Hot compresses** can be applied to very superficial abscesses. The principle is to soften the overlying skin and encourage rupture of the abscess through the surface. The use of poultices containing boric acid is not to be recommended, as they irritate the surrounding skin.
- **Surgical drainage** is a much quicker and more reliable way of treating abscesses. A hole is made in the skin at the most superficial point of the abscess, using a scalpel blade. The pus is allowed to drain and the cavity is lavaged with sterile fluids. The drainage hole should be encouraged to stay open for a few days, either by using a drain (see later) or by daily bathing with lavage of the cavity.
- **Resection** of abscesses. Very deep abscesses or internal abscesses are not suitable for treatment by simple lancing. Deep abscesses may be dissected out around the fibrous capsule and removed in one piece. Internal abscesses may be either resected (e.g. a lung lobe abscess) or they may be suctioned out under sterile conditions and the omentum used as a natural drain (e.g. prostatic abscesses).
- **Rabbits** are a special case as they can get recurrent abscesses in the submandibular and cheek area. These are filled with a particularly thick type of pus that is very difficult to drain and remove. It is important to open up the abscess adequately in order to allow treatments for some days afterwards. Compounds that debride the inside of the cavity, such as hydrogels or debriding solutions, are often used to continue the cleaning process inside the cavity while it granulates. Sometimes the abscess is related to tooth root disease and this must also be treated in order to prevent recurrence. In some cases, there are multiple abscesses and it may be necessary to resect them.

Wound healing

Generally, acute inflammation of tissue is followed by healing. There are some basic processes that are common to all tissues:

- Removal of dead and foreign material
- Clearance of the inflammatory response
- Regeneration of lost tissue components if possible
- Replacement of lost tissue components by connective tissue.

The different outcomes of the healing process depend on the type of tissue and the degree of damage. There may be resolution, regeneration or organization.

Resolution

Where there is no tissue destruction and the inflammatory process is very mild (e.g. a superficial graze), the tissue can return to its original state prior to the injury.

Regeneration

The damaged tissue is completely replaced by proliferation of the remaining cells. This depends on the type of tissue, as regeneration can only occur if the lost cells can be replaced and if the connective tissue and vascular supply are still intact. In this context, cells are classified into three basic groups:

- **Labile cells** can divide and proliferate throughout life. They are highly capable of regeneration (e.g. epithelial cells, blood cells and lymphoid tissue)
- **Stable cells** do not normally divide, but can do so in response to certain stimuli, and may divide following injury to the tissue (e.g. cells in the liver, kidney, endocrine glands, bone and fibrous tissue)
- **Permanent cells** only divide during fetal growth and are incapable of regeneration (e.g neurons, cardiac muscle cells and, to some extent, skeletal muscle cells).

Organization

Where the cells cannot repair the damage by regeneration, the tissue heals by the formation of **scar tissue**, which is organized fibrous tissue with a large number of collagen fibres. Often this means that the tissue will lose its normal function, or be more susceptible to recurrent damage (e.g. scar tissue in skin) (see later).

Most tissues heal by a combination of these processes, with some parts capable of regeneration and others forming scar tissue. Skin is a good example of tissue that heals in the dermis by the formation of scar tissue (organization) and by regeneration in the epidermis.

Normal wound healing in skin

The normal process of healing follows a predictable pattern that can be used to determine the progress of any healing tissue. There is always overlap between the phases as they progress from one predominant cell type to another, and they are not distinct.

Inflammatory phase

After injury, there is an initial inflammatory phase triggered by activation of the platelets and fibrin in the blood clot, which in turn attracts neutrophils to the damaged tissue. The neutrophils will clear up bacteria, necrotic tissue and foreign material. They also release inflammatory mediators that attract macrophages into the tissue. Once the macrophages arrive, the final debridement process begins and the tissue starts to proliferate to repair the damage. The wound will look exudative, swollen and red during this phase (Figure 24.5).

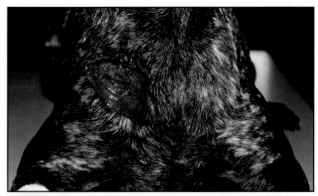

24.5 Gunshot wound across a dog's shoulder. The wound is peracute; there is tissue loss and inflammation and healing processes have not started yet.

Proliferative phase

The proliferative phase is triggered by the macrophages and involves fibroblasts that lay down the matrix of the tissue, endothelial cells that lay down new blood vessels and epithelial cells that migrate over the top of the wound to reconstitute the epidermis (**epithelialization**). This phase is the most crucial part of wound healing, as it demonstrates that it is progressing normally. The classic appearance of this phase is the development of **granulation tissue** (Figure 24.6). Granulation tissue is bright red, very vascular and has a granular surface due to the capillary loops growing into the tissue. It is highly resistant to infection and is a sign that the wound is clear of bacterial infection. During the formation of granulation tissue, the wound starts to contract and this process alone can close a wound by up to 30% of its area. Gradually, the granulation tissue is replaced by collagen fibres and scar tissue is laid down.

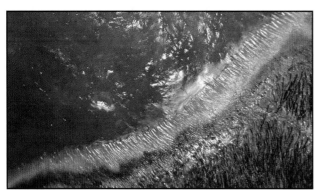

24.6 Close-up of a wound edge, showing healthy granulation tissue with an advancing epithelial edge.

Remodelling phase
Once the proliferation and repair of the tissue is complete, the scar will remodel and strengthen over a period of days to weeks as the hair regrows and the fibroblasts rearrange the matrix of the tissue according to the tensions during normal function.

In a clean surgical wound in skin, the inflammatory phase should only last 24–48 hours, then a thin layer of granulation tissue develops between the edges of the surgical wound. By the time the sutures are removed at 7–10 days, the remodelling phase is well under way.

In larger skin wounds, the inflammatory phase may last longer due to infection or foreign material and the granulation tissue may not start to develop until at least 3–5 days. Depending on how large the wound is, the proliferative phase (granulation, contraction and re-epithelialization) may take days to weeks to be completed.

Normal wound healing in other tissues
All tissues follow the same basic healing pattern as skin, with inflammatory, proliferative and remodelling phases.

Tendon and muscle injuries are often associated with trauma and other tissues may be simultaneously damaged, prolonging the healing process. The basic pattern is as for skin, but the remodelling phase is much more important as tendons and muscles have to retain function as well as strength. **Muscle** should heal quickly but may have to be immobilized to allow development of strength in the scar. **Tendons** take a very long time to develop strength; they have to be supported and only gradually reintroduced to weight bearing, otherwise they may stretch or rupture.

The **gastrointestinal, urinary and reproductive tract** tissues heal more rapidly than skin, with the fibrin clot helping to seal the wound initially, but the main support comes from the sutures for the first 3 days. The epithelium can regenerate and starts to close the wound almost immediately, with fibroblast proliferation giving the wound strength by 3–4 days after

wounding. The urinary bladder heals the fastest and the colon the slowest. Normal healing in the gut depends on good nutrition and a good blood supply. Nutrition for the surgical wound comes from the lumen and feeding the patient will also stimulate blood supply to the gut and accelerate healing. This simple concept emphasizes the importance of postoperative nursing and feeding of the patient.

Factors that affect normal wound healing
Normal wound healing in companion animals is fairly efficient. Most wounds are delayed in healing either because the animal has another undiagnosed disease or because the management of the patient is poor (Figure 24.7). Sometimes treatments affect the rate of healing and these may have to be modified until the wound is healed.

Factors affecting healing	Clinical examples
Systemic diseases	Hypothyroidism, hyperadrenocorticism (Cushing's disease), protein-losing disease, renal or hepatic disease, diabetes mellitus, malnutrition, cachexia, cancer, severe cardiovascular disease
Wound management	Choice of wound dressing (primary layer), bandage technique, inadequate bandage protection, infrequent dressing changes, patient interference with the wound
Surgical factors	Prolonged anaesthetic time, wound infection, overly tight sutures, tension on the suture line, choice of suture material, poor surgical techniques, contamination of instrumentation or surgical site during surgery, inadequate closure or drainage of dead space. Foreign material left in the wound, including suture material may delay healing by increasing the inflammatory response
Therapy	Corticosteroids, antimetabolite chemotherapeutic drugs, radiotherapy

24.7 Causes of delayed wound healing.

Inflammation: a summary
- Inflammatory processes may be a normal part of the healing process but they can also be part of the pathology.
- Prolonged inflammation is usually a sign that the healing process is delayed.
- Responses to inflammation can aid in the diagnosis of the disease process.
- Some tissues can heal by regeneration, but others may have to heal by the formation of scar tissue.

Wounds

Classification of wounds
Wounds may be classified according to aetiology, depth of skin loss, contamination or infection, extent of soft tissue or bony involvement, duration since wounding and site. For example: 'An abrasive, full-thickness, infected injury to the distal hindlimb with shear and fracture of the lateral metatarsal bone and loss of ligaments' (Figure 24.8). It is important to know how the wound was incurred in order to determine the extent of the injuries and the expected progression of the wound. Some types of injury affect the way in which the tissues heal and their susceptibility to infection.

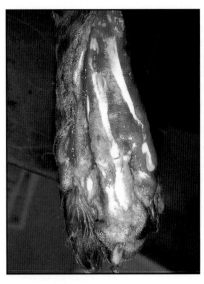

24.8 Traumatic wound on the distal limb as a result of a road traffic accident. The foot has been sheared, losing the skin and some soft tissue and damaging the collateral ligaments and metatarsal bones. (Photograph courtesy of John Houlton)

Aetiology

There are 10 basic groups of wounds classified by cause:

- Surgical (incisional)
- Surgical wound dehiscence
- Laceration
- Puncture
- Abrasion/shear
- Degloving/ischaemic/skin slough (avulsion)
- Burns – chemical, cold and heat, electrical
- Ballistic/gunshot
- Crush injury
- Chronic fistulae/sinuses.

These general groups are distinguished by the degree of tissue trauma, contamination and associated injuries. Identifying the cause of injury helps in determining appropriate wound management and also the expected healing time. Wounds that are heavily contaminated or with large amounts of tissue loss will have longer inflammatory phases and longer healing times. The category also helps to indicate the type and degree of contamination of the wound.

Degree of contamination

The only truly clean wound is a surgical wound; all other types of wound can be considered contaminated or infected. The optimal time for treatment of an open wound is within the first 6 hours. This is known as the 'golden period' and the wound is considered as contaminated, but not infected:

- 0–6 hours – little bacterial multiplication: contaminated
- 6–12 hours – bacteria beginning to divide: early infection
- Over 12 hours – bacterial invasion of tissues: (infection) established.

Surgical procedures are also classified according to infection and contamination (see later).

Viability and vascular supply to the tissue

Wounds may also be more susceptible to infection if there is associated tissue damage. Tissue that is devitalized (or necrotic) due to laceration or compression of blood vessels is more likely to become infected. Surgical wounds are more at risk of infection if a tourniquet has been used, and cardiovascular disease may also delay healing due to poor blood supply to the limbs. Shock can result in vasoconstriction and if this circulation is not

regained there may be reduced blood supply (and therefore increased risk of delayed healing or infection) to wounds in any area of the body.

Different types of tissue have a greater or lesser ability to resist infection. Well vascularized areas of skin have good bacterial defences; they should heal well and resist infection. Tissue may become devitalized due to poor surgical technique or desiccation during surgical debridement, which then increases the risk of infection or delayed healing.

Foreign material

All foreign material has to be removed before the wound will be able to heal, but the immune system can cope better with less irritant particles, such as sand, than with clay soil particles or organic debris.

Healing of wounds (closure)

Primary closure (first intention healing)

Wounds that are closed surgically heal rapidly with a very short healing phase, because there is little foreign material or bacteria (see also Chapter 15).

Delayed primary closure

Some wounds that are contaminated are best cleaned and managed as an open wound for 1–3 days in order to ensure that there is no residual infection. These wounds are then closed surgically once the earliest signs of granulation tissue formation are seen.

Secondary closure

Wounds that are heavily contaminated, or where the surrounding skin is thought to be damaged, may be managed as an open wound for several days until it is possible to close the wound surgically. These wounds will have well established granulation tissue filling the wound and it may be necessary to excise some of the granulation tissue in order to close the wound.

Second intention healing

In some instances, it is not possible or it is unnecessary to close the wound surgically and it is dressed and bandaged until the wound heals. In these cases, the wound heals by granulation (Figure 24.9), epithelialization and contraction (see also Chapter 15). Large wounds may take weeks or months to close in

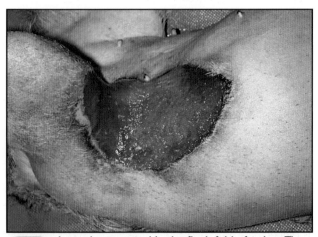

24.9 Large burn wound in the flank fold of a dog. The wound is healing by second intention and has filled in with granulation tissue. The edges of the wound are beginning to epithelialize but there is little evidence yet of contraction.

this way and during this time the wound has to be regularly rebandaged. It is often more cost-effective and better for the patient to attempt secondary closure using a reconstructive technique than continue with second intention healing.

Management of primary closure wounds

This group of wounds covers all surgical incisions that are sutured, and will be the commonest wound management area that veterinary nurses have to provide advice on. Prevention of complications associated with surgical wounds relies on meticulous management in four main areas:

- Preoperative preparation of the patient
- Systemic or local wound factors that may affect wound healing (see above)
- Surgical technique and wound closure (see later)
- Postoperative management.

Preoperative management of the patient

The general principle behind preoperative management is that the patient should be as healthy as possible at the time of the surgery in order to reduce postoperative risks. Therefore elective procedures may be delayed if, on the day of admission, the animal has another incidental condition (e.g. diarrhoea). Patients that have concurrent injuries should be stabilized as much as possible prior to surgery, particularly if a long operation is necessary. However, longer stays in hospital before operations also increase the risk of wound infection and breakdown. The specific reasons for this are not known, but it is probably due to increased stress during hospitalization and the colonization of the patient's skin with microorganisms other than its normal skin commensals.

Skin preparation and patient preparation are important in reducing the bacterial load and therefore also the risk of postsurgical inflammation and infection.

Prior to surgery, the number of microorganisms on the skin should be reduced as much as possible. Very dirty animals (e.g. farm dogs) may benefit from a general bath with non-medicated soap to remove dust and dirt that might contaminate the wound (as well as the operating theatre). With 'normal' levels of contamination, bathing makes no difference unless antiseptic solutions such as 4% w/v chlorhexidine are used. Generally, it is not necessary to bathe preoperatively; standard skin preparation at the time of surgery is adequate.

Clean wounds do not generally become infected postoperatively. The risks of infection can be determined by classifying the type of surgery and using an appropriate antibiotic protocol perioperatively (see later).

Hair removal

Ideally the hair is removed prior to anaesthesia after the premedication has been administered, so as not to prolong anaesthetic time. This also allows for loose hairs to fall off prior to skin preparation. The clipping should always be done outside theatre so that the contaminated hair can be removed from the vicinity of the surgery. Depilatories and shaving have been shown to increase wound infection rates and so clipping is the recommended technique for the removal of hair. Coarse hair is clipped with a No. 10 blade first and all clips are completed with a No. 40 blade. The blade is held gently against the skin and run in the opposite direction to the lie of the hair. Lubricants and coolants are applied regularly to prevent overheating of the blade and it is important to ensure that the blade is

sharp and has no missing teeth. Poor technique results in nicks in the skin, dermatitis and increased risk of postsurgical wound infection. A vacuum cleaner is often used to remove the loose hair from the patient and the table.

A minimum of 15 cm on either side of the proposed incision site should be clipped. For reconstructive procedures, the whole side of the animal may need to be clipped. For surgery on the limbs, the whole circumference and up to or beyond the adjacent joint should be clipped.

Small mammals have much thinner skin than dogs and cats, and extra care must be taken during hair removal (Figure 24.10). Although a No. 40 clipper blade is often used, variable high-speed clippers specifically designed for animals with fine hair are much better. These clippers make hair removal easier and cause less accidental cutting and burning of the skin.

Preparation of avian skin requires feathers to be plucked rather than clipped, in order to ensure regrowth of the feather.

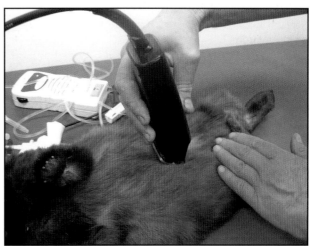

24.10 Rabbit fur should be clipped with very fine clippers to ensure that the underlying skin is not torn. The skin is gently held steady with the free hand.

Skin preparation

The patient's skin can never be made completely sterile. The aim of preoperative preparation is to reduce the bacterial count without damaging the skin's natural barriers to infection. Firstly, a surgical scrub solution is used that has antiseptic and detergent properties to degrease and kill bacteria on the skin surface. Secondly, a surgical antiseptic solution is applied to leave some residual activity to kill bacteria that may migrate out of the hair follicles or sebaceous glands during the surgery. For procedures that require particularly high standards of surgical asepsis for prolonged periods (e.g. specialist orthopaedic surgery), an adhesive impermeable transparent drape may be applied after the skin has been prepared. The surgeon then incises through the drape, which remains stuck to the edges of the skin incision, thereby protecting the surgical site from contamination during the operation.

Postoperative management of surgical wounds

When an animal is discharged, the owner should be given instructions for wound care, potential problems and when to seek advice. It is a good idea to explain the procedure that has been performed and to show the owner the wound before the animal goes home. Some surgeries will give specific instructions such as limited exercise, special diet, care of a bandage or physiotherapy. It is advisable for the owner to be given written instructions on postoperative care so that there can be no misunderstanding at a later date if there is a complication associated with poor home care.

Immediate perioperative care

At the end of the surgery, blood stains and clots should be gently wiped away using sterile fluid such as saline. Wetting of the surgical incision should be avoided if possible. Agents such as hydrogen peroxide solutions may be used to help to clean the fur, but should not be used on the peri-surgical skin as it may cause a dermatitis.

The main principles of managing a clean surgical wound are:

- Dressing the wound
- Observation of the wound and patient
- Prevention of self-mutilation
- Suture removal.

Dressing surgical wounds

Surgical wounds (Figure 24.11) are dressed if necessary for various reasons:

- To protect the wound from contamination or trauma
- To protect the wound from self-mutilation
- To absorb exudate from the wound
- To limit movement of the wound to reduce pain, or tension on the sutures
- To limit swelling of the surgical site.

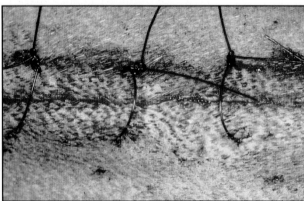

24.11   Close-up of a fresh surgical wound. The skin edges are gently apposed by the sutures and a thin line of blood clot is just visible. The edges of the wound are slightly swollen by the early inflammatory response. This swelling should be resolved by 2 days post surgery if the wound is healing well.

Some surgical wounds do not require a dressing. Simple dressings consist of a non-adherent primary layer with a thin absorbent pad held in place by an adhesive tape. After 24 hours, this dressing can be removed as the wound will have formed a fibrin seal that is resistant to bacterial contamination. A commercial example of this kind of dressing is Primapore (Smith & Nephew) which has a strip of non-adherent dressing with an adhesive edge to hold it to the skin. Spray-on dressings can also be used to seal the wound in the first 24 hours with a waterproof and gas-permeable polymer layer.

In some cases, additional padding is required and a thick cover of absorbent material such as cotton wool or gamgee may be used, which is held in place by tertiary dressings. Pressure bandages (e.g. Robert Jones) should always have substantial padding to prevent focal pressure points. All bandages should be replaced 24 hours after surgery to prevent the development of pressure injuries secondary to swelling under the dressing.

Wounds that are expected to exude heavily may need to be dressed more than once daily in order to ensure that the absorptive capacity of the dressing is not exceeded and the healthy tissues are kept dry and clean.

Monitoring of postsurgical wounds

Veterinary nurses are well placed to detect early signs of wound complications by careful observation of the surgical wound. If a dressing has been placed on the wound it may not be possible to observe the wound directly, but the skin surrounding the wound and the dressing itself can be observed.

The factors to pay particular attention to are:

- **Exudate** – note the amount, colour and type (serous or purulent). If exudate continues to leak through a dressing, the dressing must be changed to observe the wound.
- **Erythema** (reddening) – note whether this is limited to the vicinity of the sutures or whether it extends further. Has the erythematous area increased or decreased in size since the surgery?
- **Oedema** – note how severe the oedema is and whether it is increasing or reducing.
- **Haematoma** – note how severe the haematoma is and whether it is increasing or reducing.
- **Pain** – note the severity of the pain (a subjective score of 1–10 is sometimes helpful) and whether the pain is continuous, intermittent, only present when the wound is handled, or if there is no pain.
- **Odour** – Note if there is a foul odour from the wound.

In addition to monitoring the wound, good postsurgical wound care also involves monitoring the patient for any signs of systemic illness that may be associated with wound complications. Both subjective and objective assessments should be performed:

- **Subjective assessment** – note whether the animal is bright, alert and responsive or whether there has been a change in demeanour since before the surgery. Also note progressive changes in demeanour throughout the postoperative recovery phase.
- **Objective assessment** – daily monitoring of temperature, pulse and respiration rates, a note of appetite, defecation and urination should constitute the minimum daily assessment of hospitalized patients in the postoperative phase. In some cases, a more detailed clinical examination including other factors such as water intake, neurological reflexes or blood parameters may be necessary.

Prevention of self-mutilation

Self-mutilation at the surgical incision often leads to wound dehiscence. Some tendency to lick the wound postoperatively is seen in almost all animals, but persistent licking or chewing at the wound may be an indicator of wound complications. Animals may also lick or chew at the wound because of concern at the foreign material on the skin (the sutures) or due to generalized skin disease causing pruritus.

Dressings will help to reduce self-mutilation, but a determined animal or young animal will soon destroy most bandages. Bitter sprays are available to protect either the bandage or the surgical site, but they are not as effective as preventing access to the wound altogether. The Elizabethan collar (see Chapter 15) is one of the most useful and commonly employed devices to prevent self-mutilation. These aids are available as opaque or clear plastic and are placed around the neck secured by a collar or harness. They must be large enough to prevent the nose from reaching over the edge of the collar and accessing the wound. Scratching with the hind feet can be prevented using well padded bandages on the feet, and other devices available include neck braces or body braces that prevent the animal turning round to reach the wound. Basket muzzles are helpful in preventing animals from destroying bandages, but they must be carefully fitted to ensure that the animal can pant and drink water through the muzzle. Owners should be warned that other pets may interfere with the wound by grooming or playing.

Exotic species may require some ingenuity to prevent them interfering with sutures. One alternative is to use subcuticular sutures so that there are no skin sutures to irritate the fine skin. Elizabethan collars may be made out of light card or plastic and splints can be made out of syringe cases or ice-lolly sticks. Care should be taken to ensure that the collar does not irritate the skin around the neck. Some species (e.g. rabbits) may 'freeze' on application of an Elizabethan collar and refuse to eat or drink. As it is important that herbivores eat as soon as possible after surgery, an 'anti-scratch' collar may be more appropriate in these situations.

It may be difficult to protect a laparotomy wound in cavies or rodents where the surgical site is in constant contact with the floor. These animals should be housed separately until the wound is healed and the bedding changed to a non-powdery source, such as shredded paper. The bedding must be completely changed daily to ensure minimal contamination of the wound with urine or faeces.

Removal of sutures

Sutures approximate the wound edges and this allows rapid first intention healing with minimal scarring. Sutures are removed as soon as the skin is healed and in most cases this will be in 7–10 days. Healing may be quicker in some young animals, whereas in older animals the sutures may be left in for a few extra days. Subcuticular sutures may be used to appose the skin edges, using absorbable suture material where the surgeon does not wish to use skin sutures. In these cases, the wound should still be checked 7–10 days later to ensure that the wound has healed normally.

If the wound has healed, the sutures should be easy to remove and *should not be a painful procedure*. As the swelling resolves, the sutures become slightly loose and the tag can be lifted up with fingers or forceps, allowing a scissor blade to be slipped underneath, and the length entering the skin is cut, without needing to touch the skin surface. The suture then slides out of the skin. Skin staples require a special device for removal.

Reptiles are a special case, in that the sutures may remain in place until the next ecdysis (moult), as then the epidermis is more active and healing may be considered complete.

Complications of surgical wounds

The main complication of surgical wounds is **dehiscence** (the breakdown of a wound along all or part of its length) (Figure 24.12). Factors that increase the risk of wound dehiscence are:

- Poor postoperative care of the wound
- Infection of the wound
- Seroma formation or haematoma
- Poor preoperative preparation of the patient
- Poor surgical technique
- Poor suture technique or inappropriate suture materials
- Decreased blood supply to the wound
- Poor general health of the patient.

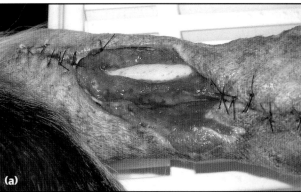

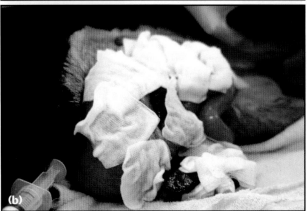

24.12 Surgical wound dehiscence. **(a)** A wound, sutured on the limb of a dog, that has been under too much tension. The central part of the wound has broken open and is now granulating slowly over the exposed bone. The edges of the sutured part are still inflamed. **(b)** A much more serious consequence of wound dehiscence in a bitch spay, where the midline repair has broken down and the abdominal contents (covered here by sterile swabs) have fallen out.

Infection is by far the commonest cause of dehiscence and may be a result of either the poor postoperative care or the surgical preparation and technique.

Other complications of wound healing include sinus formation, fistula and incisional hernia.

Sinus formation

This is a late infective complication. It is usually a small blind-ending tract lined with granulation tissue leading to an abscess cavity. Sinuses in surgical wounds are often focused around suture material or other foreign material inadvertently left in the wound at the time of surgery. Suture sinuses are often seen surrounding skin sutures if they are left in place for too long. They resolve on removal of the foreign material.

Fistula

This is an abnormal tract that forms between two epithelialized surfaces, or connects an epithelial surface to the skin. It can be a complication of wound healing, for example in anal or oronasal surgery. Occasionally it is seen as a congenital abnormality (e.g. rectovaginal fistula). Fistulae have to be surgically repaired.

Incisional hernia

This is a late complication of abdominal surgery where there is dehiscence of the incision in the muscle layers, while the skin repair remains intact. Abdominal contents may herniate out and lie in the space between the muscles or under the skin. It should be repaired as a matter of urgency in case the skin ruptures and the abdominal contents become contaminated.

Management of contaminated or infected wounds

Initial assessment

First aid measures are important in the initial assessment of the injury:

- Take brief details on the duration and site of the injury.
- Assess bleeding and determine whether arterial or venous.
- Arrest bleeding using a bandage or tourniquet if necessary.
- Cover the wound with a sterile dressing to prevent further contamination in the hospital.
- Assess the animal's general state of health; look for signs of shock.
- Assess the animal for other life-threatening injuries.
- Provide antibiotic cover and analgesia, as directed by a veterinary surgeon, and treat for shock if necessary.
- Take a more detailed full history from the owner.

The history helps to determine the origin of the wound and the likely concurrent injuries. It will also determine whether the wound is classified as infected or contaminated.

Principles of management

The first stage is decontamination as far as possible, given the state of the wound and the condition of the patient. This also means prevention of further contamination in the hospital or by the animal. The second stage is debridement of necrotic or devitalised tissue and removal of any foreign debris. The final result should be control of infection and establishment of a healthy wound bed enabling closure of the skin deficit.

One of the important first steps is to clip and clean the surrounding undamaged skin (Figure 24.13). This not only helps to clean the wound, but also helps to assess the extent of the wound and viability of the skin. Ideally, the wound should be protected from further contamination, and it may be closed using towel clips or a continuous suture. This is not always possible and so most wounds are packed with sterile swabs or filled with a water-soluble jelly (e.g. K-Y1, Johnson & Johnson) during clipping and cleaning. The jelly can then be washed away with any hair or dirt from the adjacent skin later on. The clipper blades must be properly disinfected and without chips that might cause dermatitis on nearby skin. Hair at the edges may be trimmed with scissors wetted with saline or dipped in mineral oil. Thorough and wide removal of hair is important in keeping the wound clean during the next phases of management.

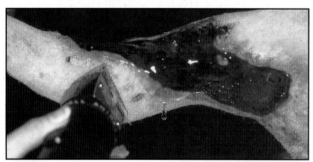

24.13 The skin surrounding a wound should be carefully clipped, using a covering such as K-Y jelly in the wound to protect it from contamination with hair clippings.

Lavage of wounds

The principles of wound lavage are to wash debris out of the wound, to dilute the bacteria, and not to cause any further damage. It is therefore important to use large volumes of fluids and also not to lavage too vigorously. This may be achieved by using a 20 ml syringe with an 18 gauge needle or catheter attached to a giving set on a bag of fluids (Figure 24.14).

Gross contamination or necrotic tissue may be washed away with gentle tap-water lavage using a hand shower. After this, the wound should be treated in a sterile manner to prevent further contamination.

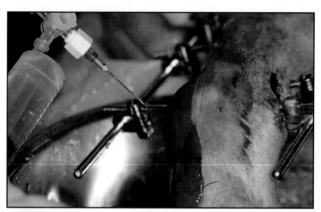

24.14 Once the surrounding skin has been clipped and cleaned, the wound itself can be irrigated or lavaged using sterile isotonic fluids (such as 0.9% saline). A 20 ml syringe is attached to a giving set and a three-way tap is used to fill the syringe with fluids from the fluid bag. The fluid is then sprayed on to the wound using an 18 gauge needle, as shown here. The procedure is repeated until the wound is completely clean.

Not all solutions are suitable for wound lavage; substances added to a lavage solution may damage the host cells and delay healing (Figure 24.15). Although it is tempting to use antiseptic solutions for infected wounds, they do not stay in the wound for long and may delay wound healing. In general it is best just to use large volumes of sterile isotonic fluids to lavage wounds (see box). If antiseptic solutions are used, it is important to use the solution, rather than the surgical scrub, as the latter contains detergents that can irritate the wound.

Solution	Concentration	Indications
Sterile saline	0.9%	Any wound – no tissue damage; no antibacterial action other than dilution
Lactated Ringer's solution	As supplied	As above
Chlorhexidine (Hibitane 4%)	0.5%	Contaminated or infected wounds – *Staphylococcus aureus* often resistant. Toxic to fibroblasts. Residual activity good
Povidone–iodine (Pevidine solution: BK)	1%	Contaminated or infected wounds. Inactivated by debris, pus or blood. Broad spectrum, poor residual activity. Toxic to host cells
Hypochlorite (Dakin's solution)	0.125%	Toxic to cells. Irritant for 4–5 days after use *Not recommended*
Hydrogen peroxide	1–3%	No bactericidal activity. Very toxic to all cell types *Not recommended*
Cetrimide/ chlorhexidine (Savlon)		Very toxic to cells. Irritant *Not recommended*

24.15 Suitability of solutions for wound lavage.

Wound lavage procedure

1. Select at least a 1000 ml bag of sterile isotonic fluids.
2. Attach a giving set with a three-way tap on the end.
3. Attach a 20 ml syringe and an 18 gauge needle or catheter to the three-way tap.
4. Lavage the wound over a bowl or tray to catch the fluid, using the 20 ml syringe to spray the wound surface.
5. Keep refilling the syringe from the fluid bag until all the fluids have been used to clean the wound or the wound fluid runs clear.
6. Carefully dry the healthy skin adjacent to the wound and cover the wound with sterile dressings.

Debridement of wounds

Debridement is the next crucial step in wound management. It involves removal of all infected, necrotic or contaminated tissue from the wound. This may be done in three ways:

- Surgical debridement
- Primary layer dressings
- Enzymatic debridement.

Antiseptics or antibiotics should not be a substitute for good surgical debridement. Debridement is the single most important step in the management of a wound and is often performed inadequately.

Surgical debridement

This is the best way to remove grossly contaminated tissue. The wound should be draped and prepared as for surgery and a scalpel is used to cut away necrotic or dirty tissue. The instruments, gloves and drapes may be exchanged for sterile ones as the debridement progresses and the wound becomes cleaner. Surgical exploration of the wound also enables visualization of local anatomical structures and determination of the extent of the wound.

Debridement dressings

These are used in the initial stages until it is clear that there is no residual infection or necrotic material. Debridement dressings should not be left on the wound for more than 24 hours and in some instances may need changes twice daily. There are three main dressing types available for debridement (see section on primary layer bandaging):

- Adherent dressings
- Hydrogels
- Hydrocolloids.

Other techniques

Commercial enzyme preparations can be applied to the wound to break down and allow removal of necrotic debris, but they are stopped once the granulation tissue is established.

Maggots have been used to debride wounds, allowing rapid establishment of healthy granulation tissue. Sterile maggots are produced commercially and are available at the correct larval stage for clinical use. They must be removed from the wound before they start to invade healthy tissue.

MRSA

Methicillin-resistant *Staphylococcus aureus* (MRSA) has been called the hospital 'superbug' by the Press. Newspaper reports of the disastrous consequences of this infection post surgery have frightened healthcare professionals, patients and clients.

In veterinary care, the incidence of this infection has increased over the last few years and there have been a number of reports of MRSA causing clinical problems, particularly in orthopaedic cases.

MRSA is often found in the upper respiratory tract of healthy people and is a unique strain of *S. aureus* with a particular sensitivity pattern that makes it difficult to treat. Currently, most veterinary cases probably arise from MRSA acquired from the owner *or veterinary staff.* One study showed that hospital staff were two or three times more likely to carry MRSA and this suggests that pets belonging to people who work in hospitals may be more at risk of carrying MRSA.

When MRSA is identified during a routine culture test, it does not necessarily mean that the infection is untreatable. In many cases there is documented sensitivity to potentiated sulphonamides and human carriers can be treated with intranasal mupirocin. However, there is considerable evidence for MRSA protection in biofilm on orthopaedic implants or permanent suture materials and resolution of the infection usually relies on removal of these implants. Even then, there is still a risk of septicaemia and death in cases that have not been dealt with early enough.

Currently the sample is tested *in vitro* against a number of antibiotics, one of which is oxacillin, and resistance to this suggests a phenotype consistent with an MRSA. Some of the isolates will show sensitivity *in vitro* to other beta-lactam antibiotics, but it is important to be aware that this will not be the case *in vivo*.

Simple hygiene will make a big difference to transmission of MRSA to patients. This includes regular hand washing, alcohol rubs and wearing gloves as often as possible. However, recent evidence suggests that MRSA and other nosocomial organisms can be protected from disinfectants in live amoebae, thus avoiding the standard techniques for decontamination. Disposable gloves to handle any patient thought to be at risk, or for changing dressings and cleaning wounds, should be considered standard policy. Some larger veterinary hospitals have considered screening staff for MRSA carrier status, but with employment rights this policy would have to be introduced with informed consent and members of staff could not be required to cooperate. Regular monitoring of culture results in practice, accurate theatre records and staff records will enable a rapid response in anticipating or monitoring outbreaks of MRSA infection.

Management of secondary closure wounds

Principles of wound dressings

Wound dressings are usually applied to the wound in three layers: the primary, secondary and tertiary layers. The general construction of the dressing depends on the location of the wound and the function of the dressing. Knowledge of the normal process of wound healing enables the veterinary nurse to choose the appropriate dressing at different stages of healing.

Wound dressing functions include:

- Absorption of exudate
- Analgesia
- Protection of the wound
- Prevention of infection
- Promotion of wound healing.

Both the owner and the nursing staff should closely monitor all dressings for signs of complications. Poorly managed dressings will cause delayed wound healing and may cause further damage; dressings that have been applied too tightly to the limb can cause damage ranging from areas of skin loss to loss of the whole limb, or even death.

Reasons to remove the dressing

- Persistent chewing at the dressing
- Foul smell from the dressing
- Soiling or wetting of the dressing while on a walk or with urine
- 'Strike-through' of exudate from the wound to the outside of the dressing
- Slippage of the dressing from its original placement.

Written instructions should always be given to owners if an animal is discharged with a dressing in place.

Primary layer

The primary layer is the material that is placed in contact with the wound itself. The principle behind the primary layer is that it should at least do no harm to the wound and, at best, should improve the rate of healing of the wound. Current thinking on wound management is that optimal healing occurs in a 'moist' environment. Dressings are therefore designed to provide a controlled environment that is not too 'wet' nor too 'dry'.

There are numerous products available and it is important to realize that there is no perfect wound dressing. By understanding the way in which the different classes of dressings work, the veterinary nurse should be better equipped to use these dressings appropriately (see Chapter 15).

The functions of the primary layer will include some or all of the following at different stages:

- Debridement of necrotic tissue (this may require rehydration, lysis of fibrin attachments and physical removal from the wound)
- Absorption of fluid away from wound (if fluid is allowed to remain on the wound surface, it can macerate the tissues or provide a reservoir for infection)
- Stimulation of granulation tissue (some dressings actively promote and speed up the formation of granulation tissue)
- Promotion of epithelialization (epithelialization can only occur across healthy granulation tissue and is faster in a moist warm environment)
- Allowing contraction or controlled contraction of the wound.

Categories of primary layer dressings

Wound dressings can be described according to their basic characteristics. Some dressings may fall into more than one of the following categories, or dressings may be designed so that they have more than one general function:

- Adherent or non-adherent
- Absorbent or non-absorbent
- Passive, interactive or bioactive (passive: having no action on the wound; interactive: responding to the wound environment in some way; bioactive: having a biological effect on the wound)
- Occlusive, semi-occlusive or non-occlusive (this refers to the degree of the dressing's permeability to gas or vapour).

Adherent and non-adherent dressings

Saline-soaked gauze swabs are often used as passive adherent dressings in the early stages of wound management for debridement of necrotic tissue. These are cheap to apply and very effective, but they may be painful to remove and can damage healthy tissue. They are often referred to as wet-to-dry dressings.

Passive non-adherent dressings are typically used over surgical wounds, skin grafts or granulation tissue. Perforated polyurethane membrane and paraffin gauze are common examples. These do not interact with the wound in any way, but prevent the secondary layers from sticking to the wound.

Absorbent dressings

Sometimes, the secondary layer of the dressing is used to absorb exudate, but some primary layer dressings are specifically designed to absorb fluid and prevent it accumulating at the wound surface, causing maceration of the tissues.

Foam dressings usually have a semi-permeable membrane backing that allows absorption of fluid and some controlled evaporation, so that the wound environment remains moist without being too wet. These passive dressings can be useful for exudative granulating wounds, as they allow epithelialization in a moist environment.

Wounds that are producing copious amounts of fluid can be dressed with ordinary disposable baby nappies. These can be weighed to calculate how much fluid the animal is losing and to document improvement as the fluid exudate decreases.

Complex dressings

Alginate dressings are bioactive and interactive. They are sheets of a protein derived from seaweed and release sodium or calcium when in contact with body fluids. This results in the stimulation of haemostasis and inflammation. They are used to stimulate the formation of granulation tissue and for haemostasis in low-level bleeding. Once they are wet, they form a gel that keeps the surface of the wound moist. The disadvantage is that sometimes they cause the formation of excessive granulation tissue.

Hydrogel dressings are interactive, consisting of insoluble hydrophilic polymers. They are provided either as a sheet with a semi-permeable backing or as a gel. The hydrogel can rehydrate necrotic tissue, absorb exudate and reduce oedema. Where it is in gel form, a second primary layer must be put over the gel to prevent it from drying out and often the foam dressings are used for this purpose. It is useful where parts of the wound are granulating well and other parts require further debridement, as the gel will not harm healthy granulation tissue. The disadvantages are that the debridement process is very slow, and the combination of dressings may be expensive.

Hydrocolloids are bioactive and interactive suspensions of polymers in an adhesive matrix. They are usually provided as a sheet with an occlusive backing that prevents dehydration of the wound. They can both rehydrate and debride necrotic wounds and will stimulate the formation of granulation tissue. Because they are adhesive, they may prevent contraction of the granulating wound by sticking to the edges and sometimes cause exuberant granulation tissue. They should not be used for infected wounds and they need to be changed regularly, so may be expensive.

Topical wound treatments

- **Aloe vera** ointment actively stimulates the development of granulation tissue, but only if very pure products are used.

- **Silver sulfadiazine** ointment (Flamazine, Smith & Nephew) is a topical broad-spectrum antibiotic, with prolonged activity, and is the agent of choice for prevention of sepsis from burns.
- **Zinc bacitracin** ointments may enhance epithelialization.
- **Malic, benzoic and salicylic acid solution** (Dermisol, Smithkline Beecham) has a very low pH and is a debriding agent; it is toxic to granulation tissue and should not be left in the wound.
- **Nanocrystalline silver** is used for infected wounds and is particularly useful in management of infections that are resistant to commonly used antibiotics. It also decreases the use of antibiotics and reduces the risk of multi-drug resistance.

Secondary bandage layer

The secondary layer of a dressing is used either to hold the primary layer in place, to provide padding to the wound underneath, to absorb exudate or to distribute the pressure of the bandage evenly. The secondary layer is most commonly an **orthopaedic wool**, which is available as rolls of viscose or polyester fleece in different widths. The bandage is applied evenly in a spiral with overlapping layers of 50% of the width of the material. If the bandage is required to distribute pressure (see Robert Jones bandage), more substantial materials such as rolls of cotton wool are used. For heavy levels of exudate, cotton wadding such as gamgee may be incorporated into the secondary layer. The secondary layer is then stabilized using a conforming stretch bandage. This layer is again applied evenly with 50% overlap of width, only slightly compressing the wool layer underneath. It is important not to overstretch the bandage during application, particularly over narrow points in the limb, as pressure points may arise.

Tertiary bandage layer

The tertiary layer is primarily to protect the main functional layers of the bandage from soiling or mutilation by the animal. This outer layer is usually an elastic cohesive or adhesive bandage, applied in a spiral with 50% overlap of width. It is important that this layer is applied with even pressure, as the layers cannot slide over one another to relieve pressure points when the animal moves around in the bandage. At the top of the bandage, this layer must not extend over the top of the secondary layer padding as it will cause chafing of the skin. Finally, adhesive bandages should not be used to stick the bandage to the bare skin or fur as an attempt to help keep the bandage in place. The bottom of the bandage may be covered with an elastic adhesive bandage to increase wear. In order to keep the bottom of the bandage dry, empty intravenous fluid bags or commercially available canvas boots may be used to protect a foot temporarily, but they should not be left on permanently.

Reconstructive surgery

General principles

Major reconstructive procedures are used when there is inadequate skin or other tissue available to close the deficit created by the surgery or trauma. Usually the surgical procedure is planned in advance, so that the patient can be prepared and positioned appropriately. The general principles behind reconstructive surgery include the following.

- The patient should be haemodynamically stable prior to surgery.
- The patient should be prepared for a long period of anaesthesia.
- A very wide area of skin should be clipped and surgically prepared to allow for moving skin around into the wound.
- The skin must be handled gently to prevent bruising that might damage its blood supply.

Reconstructive procedures require good wound management in advance of the surgical procedure. Often the success of the surgery relies on the elimination of infection and foreign or necrotic material prior to surgery.

When an incision is made in the skin, or a skin deficit occurs after trauma, the elastic recoil of the skin makes the edges gape apart. When the skin edges are advanced to close the large wound, there may be too much tension on the edges, causing delayed healing or dehiscence. The skin of the dog and cat generally is extremely mobile and can be manipulated to close skin deficits, but by taking into consideration the tension lines prior to surgery, sometimes the problems associated with the recoil of the skin edges can be avoided.

Suturing skin

Sutures are used to appose the tissues together so that they heal more quickly (see Chapter 23). Sutures in the skin should appose the tissues and not cause eversion or inversion of the skin edges. Generally:

- **Absorbable** sutures are used in deep tissues where they are not accessible for removal.
- **Non-absorbable** sutures, which cause less tissue reaction, are used in the skin and then removed about 7–10 days after the surgery.

Sutures should not be placed too tightly, particularly in the skin, which swells slightly in the first 2–3 days after surgery. Tight sutures may either tear out as the skin swells, or cause itchiness, which encourages the animal to interfere with them. Finally, sutures that are placed too tightly may also constrict the vessels at the wound edge and delay wound healing.

Strategies to combat tension may be employed in most simple wounds, either as a single procedure or in combination:

- **Subcuticular** sutures are used to hold the dermis together so that the skin sutures do not have to be too tight.
- **Walking** sutures can advance skin towards the centre of the wound, taking the tension off the main incision line.
- **Vertical mattress** sutures can also be used as tension-relieving sutures to take the pressure off the incision line for a few days and then they are removed before the incision sutures.

Suture materials

There are many different types of suture material, all developed to perform different tasks in different surgical situations. They are divided into two main groups: natural and synthetic. Within these categories, suture materials may be either **braided** or **monofilament**, and either absorbable or non-absorbable (see Chapter 23).

Sizes

Suture materials are manufactured in different sizes (see Chapter 23). The **metric** gauge is the actual suture diameter in millimetres multiplied by 10. However, suture sizes are often referred to by the United States Pharmacopeia (**USP**) sizing, which has a different figure for the same suture; for example, 2 metric is the same gauge as 3/0 USP.

Packaging

Suture can be purchased in individual sterile packets, with a needle attached to the end of the material by a method known as **swaging**. This is ideal: it is known to be reliably sterile, the needle sharp and the material undamaged.

Selection criteria

When choosing a suture material, the following points need to be considered:

- *How secure is the knot?* Monofilament materials have high memory (i.e. they are very springy) and therefore the knots are less secure than braided materials.
- *How strong is the material?* Often braided materials are stronger than monofilament materials of an equivalent size.
- *How long does the material last in the tissues?* This may depend on the mechanism by which the suture material is broken down in specific tissues, but some materials (e.g. polydioxanone) are designed to be long lasting.
- *How much drag is there when the material is drawn through tissues?* Generally, the braided materials drag through the tissues more than monofilament and are more likely to cause damage.

Tissues treat all suture materials as foreign material and mount an inflammatory response. Therefore it is a good surgical principle to use the minimum of suture material possible to achieve closure of the wound, and to use the smallest gauge of suture material that will be strong enough.

Generally, the natural materials cause much more inflammation and are less reliable than the synthetic materials.

Primary closure of large skin deficits

Large skin defects may not be amenable to simple closure and special reconstructive surgical techniques have to be used. These often involve moving flaps of skin around and it is important that the blood vessels supplying the flap are carefully protected from damage during the surgery. Very fine rat-toothed forceps, stay sutures or specialist skin hooks may be used to handle the skin. The vessels should also be prevented from going into spasm during the surgery; hypotension, hypothermia, shock, dehydration and pain will all decrease blood flow to the skin and risk damage to the skin flap. These cases need very careful peri- and postoperative nursing:

- Clip and prepare very wide areas of skin surrounding the surgical site.
- Protect the drapes from 'strike-through' that might compromise aseptic technique.
- Watch for hypothermia and dehydration during surgery.
- Count the swabs and estimate blood loss.
- Provide soft bedding, good postoperative analgesia and close observation to improve circulation to the skin.

Some oncological surgeries will entail removal of part of the abdominal or thoracic wall. In these cases, a synthetic mesh made of absorbable or non-absorbable material may be used to close the defect. These meshes are expensive and can result in the development of sinus tracts if aseptic technique is not good enough.

Random skin flaps

Incisions are made running away from the skin defect to create a flap of skin that is then undermined so that it can be advanced to cover the defect. These flaps rely on the network of blood vessels in the dermis to supply the skin edges at the end of the flap. They have to have a wide base to ensure that enough vessels run into the flap to keep it alive, and can only be moved into adjacent areas as far as the tension will allow.

Axial pattern skin flaps

These are specialist skin flaps that are defined and named by the specific artery and vein supplying that area of skin. The skin is elevated according to anatomical landmarks and the artery and vein are identified underneath. The flap of skin can then be moved as far as the vessels will allow. This flap is very reliable as it has a well defined blood supply and can be used over wounds that have poor blood supply.

Free skin grafts

Skin grafts are pieces of skin removed from a donor site and then sutured in place on to a wound (Figure 24.16). They are usually used for wounds on the limbs that are difficult to repair using skin flaps. The skin graft is very susceptible to failure, as it has to rely on the wound bed for nutrition from the first day and has no independent blood supply. If the blood supply fails to grow into the skin graft within 3–4 days, the graft will fail.

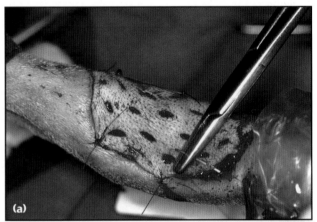
(a)

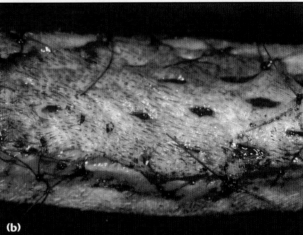
(b)

24.16 A free skin graft. **(a)** Graft in the process of being applied to the wound; sutures are being placed to secure it. The graft has been punctured with stab incisions so that fluid cannot accumulate under it during healing. **(b)** The same graft 7 days later: the hair is just beginning to grow, the stab incisions have almost healed over and the graft has healed on to the wound bed.

Skin grafts may be harvested as split-thickness grafts, which include only the epidermis and superficial dermis, or as full-thickness skin grafts (FTSGs), which include the whole of the epidermis and dermis. In animals, full-thickness pieces of skin are usually used, as this also transfers the hair follicles and so the final result is more cosmetic and hard wearing.

If it is difficult to harvest a large piece of skin from the flank, punch grafts or stamp or strip grafts may be taken and embedded into the wound, allowing the surface to re-epithelialize by growing out from the islands of little skin grafts.

- **Punch grafts** are usually taken with a skin biopsy punch and pushed into little holes in the granulation tissue.
- **Stamp or strip grafts** are small squares or strips of skin laid on to the granulation tissue with gaps between the grafts. These tend to have very sparse hair regrowth between the grafts and are quite fragile.

Usually FTSGs are **meshed** by making little stab incisions in the skin (Figure 24.16) to allow it to conform better to the surface of the wound and also to allow drainage of fluid out from underneath the graft.

Management of free skin grafts

- A well padded bandage (Robert Jones) must be kept on for the first 5–7 days to immobilize the limb.
- Bandage changes must be done carefully so that the graft does not move.
- Aseptic wound management is required, to prevent infection.
- A non-adherent primary dressing layer is essential.

Postoperatively, grafts are dressed with a non-adherent dressing such as paraffin gauze or silicone mesh and heavily bandaged (e.g. with a Robert Jones bandage) to prevent movement of the graft site. The dressing is changed as infrequently as possible, in order to minimize disruption of the fragile process of graft healing over the first 7 days.

Free skin grafts may fail due to inadequate preparation of the wound bed (e.g. chronic avascular granulation tissue), infection of the graft, failure to immobilize the graft or adherence of the primary dressing to the graft. They may also fail if serum or haemorrhage accumulates underneath the graft and lifts it off the wound surface so that the blood vessels cannot grow into the graft quickly enough.

Complications associated with reconstructive surgery

Many reconstructive procedures are long surgeries with large areas of tissue exposed for some time. Patients may dehydrate and become hypotensive more rapidly than expected and also become hypothermic, resulting in longer recovery times and poor skin circulation. If the surgical technique is poor, these skin flaps have a high risk of failure. If the circulation fails in the skin flap, it rapidly becomes ischaemic and over the first 3–4 days is cold to the touch, finally becoming hard and blackened as the skin dies.

Drains

Drains are used where there is a need to perform repeated lavage of a space, where there is a need for repeated aspiration of fluid (or air) from a space, or where the surgeon wants to prevent the accumulation of fluid in a space (e.g. seroma).

Passive *versus* active drains

Passive drains rely on gravity and capillary action, whereas active drains have a suction apparatus on one end – either intermittent or continuous.

Passive drains

The commonest passive drain is the **Penrose drain**, which is a soft latex tube (Figure 24.17) usually placed in the dead space created at surgery to allow drainage of fluid after surgery. One end of the drain is anchored in the wound with an absorbable suture and the other is anchored at the skin. The end of the drain should always exit through a separate skin incision site to the surgical incision so that it does not interfere with wound healing. As it relies on gravity, the drain should exit at the lowest possible point. To increase drainage, a larger drain or several drains may be placed (drainage volume depends on surface area for the capillary action).

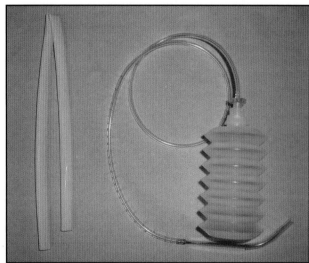

24.17 Drains can be used postoperatively to drain dead space and prevent seroma formation after reconstruction. **Penrose drains (left)** are soft latex tubes that allow fluid to drain out of the space along the surface of the drain (passive drainage). A dressing should be applied to protect the drain from contamination and to collect the fluid. An **active drain (right)** is a rigid tube in the wound with a device that exerts constant gentle negative pressure (suction). Active drains often have a sharp curved needle-like device on the end of the tube in order to place the drain through the skin. This 'needle' is then cut off and disposed of.

Active drains

Active drains usually have rigid walls and may have a radio-paque marker down the side so that their position can be checked. The most common is the **thoracic drain**, where a drain is placed through the skin, under a skin tunnel and then between the ribs into the thorax. The end of the drain is closed securely with clamps and bungs. The drain may be used to aspirate air or fluid out of the chest or to introduce treatment into the chest cavity (e.g. in pyothorax). The drain can be attached to a syringe for intermittent suction or to a suction device that continuously drains the chest. These drains have to be very carefully bandaged in, as the animal could die if it chewed the end of the tube and the chest communicated directly with the outside.

Active drains are also used underneath surgical wounds, attached to suction devices that are little vacuum tubes. The continuous gentle suction applied to the dead space is a very effective way of preventing the formation of a seroma.

Closed *versus* open drains

The thoracic drain is always a closed drain and the system is sealed from the outside.

- Active drains are closed, as they collect the fluid in a reservoir bottle or tube.
- Passive drains will always be open, as they allow the fluids to drip out on to the patient or the floor.

When a passive drain is used, there is a potential risk of bacterial contamination of the wound as bacteria may migrate up the sides and lumen of the tube. In addition, there is increased nursing involved in keeping the skin clean and dry underneath the wound and preventing the fur from becoming matted with exudate. The skin may be protected by using either a thin layer of barrier cream under the end of the drain or a commercial synthetic spray that makes a breathable but waterproof barrier on the skin to help to prevent maceration, e.g. Cavilon (3M, Arnolds). Where possible the drain should be bandaged in place with a sterile dressing to absorb the fluid from the end of the drain. This has to be changed regularly to ensure that the skin does not become macerated.

Active drains still have some risk of bacterial contamination, as there will be some migration of bacteria up the sides of the tube, but the risk is smaller, particularly as they can often be bandaged into place using antiseptic ointments and sterile dressings.

Care and management of drains

All drains should be handled in an aseptic manner, and the animal treated with broad-spectrum antibiotics until the drains are removed. The animal must be prevented from interfering with the drain; and the drain must be protected from the animal's urine or faeces. For removal, the skin suture is cut and then the drain is pulled out quickly, with light pressure over the hole to help it to seal. Thoracic drains should have a purse-string suture pre-placed in the skin ready to close the skin on removal. With most other drains, the hole is allowed to granulate over after removal.

Wounds: a summary

- Wounds heal in a predictable manner, which can be manipulated by the veterinary surgeon or veterinary nurse to accelerate – or delay – the recovery of the animal.
- Classification of wounds is important in order to make a rational plan of approach to management of a case.
- Wounds allowed to heal by second intention should be assessed closely at each bandage change in order to determine what stage of healing the tissues have reached and to apply the appropriate dressing.
- Reconstructive surgery is the technique of choice where possible.

Fracture management

A fracture is a complete or incomplete break of bone continuity, with or without displacement of the resulting fragments.

Initial assessment and management

It is essential that the patient is adequately restrained before being examined or treated with first aid. However placid an animal is under normal circumstances, it will often attempt to bite when in a lot of pain. A muzzle is often required.

Fractures may be accompanied by other injuries and some of these can be life threatening. More often than not, the fracture is of lesser priority and its repair (depending on its nature) can be left for several days until the patient is in a stable condition. It is important to prioritize these injuries and deal with the most life-threatening first (see Chapter 18). Once these issues have been managed, a full and careful examination can be carried out by the veterinary surgeon, analgesics administered and the limb temporarily supported with splints and bandages. When the veterinary surgeon has established that there is a fracture, two orthogonal radiographic views must be taken in order to make a specific diagnosis.

Fracture healing

Indirect fracture healing

This process was previously called secondary healing. Local events immediately after fracture are the same as in other tissues: haemorrhage, formation of a clot, and acute inflammation. The clot is gradually replaced by granulation tissue and blood vessels grow into the organizing clot from periosteal blood vessels and blood vessels in the medullary canal of the bone. Fibrous tissue is produced by fibroblasts in the organizing clot around the fracture and forms a cuff around the bone ends. This fibrous tissue is important: it stabilizes the fracture and allows cartilage to develop. This large cuff of stabilizing tissue is known as **callus**, which is composed of fibrous tissue, cartilage and immature bone and which envelops the ends of the bone.

The cartilage is slowly replaced by bone in endochondral fashion. Cells called **chondroclasts** resorb cartilage and new bone is formed when **osteoblasts** line the surfaces and secrete a mineralized matrix. As this process progresses, the callus gradually contains more cartilage and bone and less fibrous tissue. As the callus becomes stiffer, the fracture becomes more stable until eventually the callus rigidly unites the bone ends and this is the point of **clinical union**. Callus is not always helpful; sometimes the callus formed may be disorganized and excessive and can interfere with the normal movements of muscle and tendons.

There is then a long remodelling phase where the callus is replaced by mature bone. **Osteoclasts** are responsible for bone resorption in the remodelling phase; they remove the mineral part of the callus and degrade the collagenous and non-collagenous proteins. Simultaneously, mature bone is laid down by osteoblasts, thus recreating the original bony structure.

Haversian remodelling is a process of bone resorption and formation within the cortex and is the final step in restoration of the normal compact bone structure. The surface of the cortices is smoothed out and the bone's strength restored in response to normal weight bearing.

Direct fracture healing

Direct fracture healing (previously called primary healing) occurs when the bone edges are so close together that callus formation does not occur and the bone forms without the interim stage of fibrous tissue and cartilage. In cases where callus formation is detrimental to the return of function (e.g. joint surfaces), direct fracture healing is preferable and this usually requires surgical intervention as soon as possible after the trauma. The fragments must be held in rigid anatomical alignment (i.e. with plates, screws or wires, or a combination), and this allows Haversian systems to cross a minute fracture gap and repair the cortical bone directly with little or no callus formation.

Rate of fracture healing

Provided that there are no complications, clinical union is usually achieved in 12–16 weeks in adult dogs and cats. Remodelling may continue for many months, or even years, after clinical union has occurred. The rate of fracture healing is assessed by clinical examination to detect the increase in rigidity and the firm swelling associated with union by callus formation. Radiographs are taken to assess the degree of callus formation and the extent of mineralization within the callus. Many factors influence the rate at which fractures heal and it is important to be aware of these when contemplating fracture repair.

- Fractures in immature animals heal more quickly than in adult animals.
- Fractures in geriatric animals heal more slowly.
- Fractures in debilitated animals heal more slowly. Debilitation may be due to poor nutrition or systemic illness such as hormonal disorder or kidney failure.
- Osteomyelitis interferes with healing and is one of the most common causes of poor fracture healing after surgical repair. Healing can progress normally once the infection is overcome.
- Fractures of cancellous bone heal more quickly than fractures in cortical bone.
- Fractures in bones that have a good blood supply heal more quickly than those in areas with a poor blood supply. For example, the pelvis and scapula are covered by large muscle masses which have a good blood supply and these bones heal well. The distal one-third of the radius and ulna has little muscle cover and a poor blood supply, therefore fractures at this site heal poorly, especially in very small breeds of dog.
- Oblique fractures heal more quickly than transverse fractures, because there is a larger area of contact to promote tissue regrowth.
- Poor reduction or fixation of a fracture will result in a slow rate of healing.
- Movement of the fracture site delays or prevents healing.

Complications of fracture healing

- **Non-union** – complete failure of the fractured ends of the bone to unite.
- **Delayed union** – fracture healing progresses slowly. Clinical union is not achieved within the expected time.
- **Malunion** – fracture heals in an abnormal position. Untreated fractures and those not treated properly often heal in an abnormal position.
- **Shortened limb** – limb shortening occurs if there is healing with inadequate reduction of overriding fracture fragments. Limb function may be severely compromised.
- **Osteomyelitis** – inflammation of the bone. Bacterial osteomyelitis is commonly caused by inadequate asepsis during surgery. It is more likely to occur if there is also damage to the local blood supply. This is recognized by heat, pain and swelling of the affected part, systemic illness, inappetence and fever.
- **Fracture disease** – a syndrome of muscle wastage and inability to flex joints in a limb after fracture repair. One or more joints in the affected limb may be held rigid due to scar formation within the joints or within muscles surrounding the fracture site. Fracture disease is more common after fixation by external coaptation or when there is inadequate reduction. ▶

- **Sequestrum** – a necrotic piece of bone not incorporated successfully in the fracture repair.
- **Implant failure** – this can occur through poor choice of implants or technique, stress applied through the implant caused by overactive behaviour of the patient, or failure of the implant itself. This will result in a sudden deterioration, with instability and pain returning at the fracture site.

Classification of fractures

Modern classification of fractures provides information for both treatment and prognosis: the bone involved, type of displacement, direction of the fracture line and the number and type of fragments.

Open *versus* closed fractures

- A **closed** fracture describes a fracture with no break in the skin.
- An **open** fracture has a wound that has penetrated the skin and the fracture ends are open to the outside environment. This type carries a bigger risk of infection and is often contaminated (e.g. a road traffic accident where the limb has been dragged along the road).

Anatomical description

- **Articular** – involving the joint
- **Diaphyseal** – a fracture in the midshaft or diaphysis of the bone
- **Metaphyseal** – a fracture of the area between the midshaft and the end of a long bone (epiphysis)
- **Physeal** – a fracture through the growth plate of an immature animal
- **Epiphyseal** – a fracture of the epiphysis
- **Condylar** – a fracture of the epiphysis when condyles are involved, e.g. the distal humerus or femur. Other common sites of fractures include the pelvis, the mandibles and the ribs

Type of displacement

- **Greenstick** – an incomplete (i.e. only one cortex) fracture of a bone of an immature animal
- **Fissure** – a fine crack, which may displace during surgery or when stressed
- **Depressed** – especially fractures of the skull, where fragments may be pushed into the underlying cavity
- **Compression** – often refers to fracture of a vertebral body where a compressive force has resulted in the shortening of a vertebra by a crushing effect
- **Impacted** – cortical fragments forced into cancellous bone
- **Avulsion** – a fracture in which a bony prominence has been torn away from the rest of the bone, usually by the pull of a muscle (e.g. fracture of the olecranon or avulsion of the tibial crest)

Direction of fracture line

- **Transverse** – fracture line is at 90 degrees to the axis of the bone
- **Oblique** – fracture line is at an angle of at least 30 degrees
- **Spiral** – fracture line curves around the bone
- **Longitudinal, Y or T** – refers to the appearance of the fracture lines on the bone

Number or types of fracture

- **Simple** – one fracture line, creating two fragments
- **Comminuted** – more than one fracture line, creating more than two fragments
- **Wedge** – a multifragmented fracture with some contact between the main fragments after reduction
- **Segmental** – one or more large complete fragments of the shaft of a long bone
- **Irregular** – a diaphyseal fracture with no specific pattern
- **Multiple** – more than one fracture in the same or different bones

Other classifications

Some fractures are further classified to provide more detail about the appearance. Epiphyseal or growth plate fractures are classified by the Salter–Harris system, ranging from Type I to Type VI. Accessory carpal bone and central tarsal bone fractures are important fractures in racing Greyhounds and are each classified Type I to Type V.

Diagnosis of fractures

Clinical signs

Owners may have witnessed what happened to their pet and can give the veterinary surgeon vital information. A good clinical history may then give a good indication of the nature of the injuries.

The first signs, as with any injury, can be attributed to acute inflammation. The major clinical signs seen with fractures are:

- Pain localized to the affected bone
- Local swelling and heat
- Bruising at the fracture site leading to discoloration of the overlying soft tissues
- Marked loss of function (i.e. very lame or non-weight-bearing)
- Visible or palpable deformity of the affected bone
- Abnormal mobility at the fracture site
- Crepitus when the injured part is moved.

Radiography

General anaesthesia is usually necessary to obtain good quality radiographs (see Chapter 20). At least two views are essential to enable the veterinary surgeon to make a proper diagnosis and a plan for repair. Radiographs of the normal contralateral limb are useful in planning reconstruction of a severe fracture, e.g. comminuted or multiple fractures. Although it may be obvious that a limb is fractured, a good-quality radiograph will confirm details such as hairline fractures, small fissures and chips, or alterations in bone density, which could affect the treatment plan.

Principles of fracture repair

The primary aim of fracture fixation is to restore the functional anatomy of the fractured bone. This is achieved by:

- Restoring the continuity of the bone
- Restoring the length of the bone
- Restoring the functional shape of the bone
- Maintaining essential soft tissue function.

Essential soft tissues include the blood vessels supplying the bone, muscles acting on the bone and the nerves supplying the muscles. Any techniques for fracture repair must be sympathetic to these tissues because without them there is no chance of restoring function to the injured limb. Many techniques exist for successfully restoring bone continuity, length and shape. The same basic principles apply to all the techniques:

- **Reduction** – the fracture fragments should be brought together in the correct anatomical alignment. This may be done 'closed', by traction and manipulation of the limb, or 'open', by performing surgery at which time the fracture is visualized and the individual fragments are manipulated back into position.
- **Fixation** – the fragments should be immobilized in the correct alignment until clinical union occurs. The fragments may also be compressed together to narrow the fracture gap.
- **Blood supply** – the blood supply to the bone fragments must be preserved. Fractures will only heal if there is an adequate blood supply.

Stabilization of fractures

After reduction of a fracture, the bones must be held in position until healing occurs. Indications for immobilization at the fracture site are:

- To relieve pain
- To prevent displacement of the fragment (loss of reduction)
- To prevent movement that might cause delayed union or non-union.

In some cases, such as greenstick fractures and some pelvic fractures, immobilization may be unnecessary and simple restriction of activity will suffice.

Fixation techniques

Fracture fixation techniques are broadly classified into three groups:

- External coaptation, using casts or splints
- Internal fixation, using pins, plates, screws and other devices
- External–internal fixation using 'external fixators'.

There are a number of ways to repair fractures and there are a number of factors to be taken into account before deciding on the technique for repair:

- Classification of the fracture
- Age of the patient
- Size of the patient
- Temperament of patient
- Presence of any underlying disease
- Cost to owner
- Expectations of owner (e.g. working animal versus pet).

For example, a young dog's fractures will heal more quickly than an older dog's, and a fracture in a small breed, such as a Chihuahua, presents different problems than the same fracture in a Great Dane.

External coaptation

The aim of external coaptation is to limit motion at a fracture site by immobilizing the joints above and below the fracture. If the joints above and below the fracture cannot be immobilized, external coaptation is not suitable.

External coaptation techniques

Advantages

- Technically simpler than some internal fixation techniques
- Economical
- Non-invasive

Disadvantages

- They have limited applications. For example, casts are most useful for fractures below the stifle in the hindlimb and below the elbow in the forelimb
- They do not provide sufficient stability for many fractures, particularly comminuted or severely oblique fractures
- They are at risk of causing decubital ulcers
- Slower healing of fracture and greater callus formation
- They restrict activity of joints and muscles in the limb and are therefore prone to causing fracture disease

Methods of external coaptation fall into three main groups: casts, splints and extension splints.

Types of fracture suitable for casting

Relatively stable fractures are ideal: greenstick fractures or simple oblique or spiral fractures that are stable after manual reduction. Where one bone is fractured close to an intact bone that provides a splint-like mechanism, a cast can be used (e.g. a fractured radius with an intact ulna). Casts are also used for postoperative support of arthrodeses, internal fixations or tendon repair.

Casting material should:

- Be conformable and easy to apply
- Reach maximum strength quickly.

The ideal finished cast should be:

- Hard wearing
- Radiolucent (to enable monitoring of fracture healing without removal of the cast)
- Strong and lightweight but not too bulky
- Easy to remove
- Water resistant, but 'breathable'
- Economical.

There are various types of casting materials available:

- **Polypropylene impregnated with resin** (e.g. Dynacast Optima, Smith & Nephew) is easy to apply, radiolucent, strong, lightweight and hard wearing.
- **Fibreglass impregnated with resin** (e.g. Vetcast Plus, 3M) is easy to apply, strong and lightweight but less hard wearing than a polypropylene cast. It causes slightly reduced radiographic detail. Some newer products can be immersed in water and then dried with a hairdryer.
- **Thermoplastic polymer mesh** (e.g. Hexcelite, Hexcel UK) and **thermoplastic sheets** (e.g. Turbocast, Transthermo Systems) are easy to apply, radiolucent (though the mesh creates a distracting pattern on the radiograph) and hard wearing. They are expensive to purchase but can be reused, making them more economical.
- **Plaster of Paris** is cheap and conformable but messy to apply. It makes a heavy, bulky and weak cast, is slow to reach maximum strength and loses strength when in contact with water. It is radio-opaque and has to be removed to monitor fracture healing.

Application of a cast

The casting material must be applied in close proximity to the bone to be able to give good support to the fracture. There is a fine line between using too much padding and too little. Too much will allow the fractured ends to move within the cast or cause the cast to slip. Too little can lead to decubital ulcers. The cast must contain at least one joint above the fracture and one below, and prevent weight bearing across the fracture.

Applying a cast

The manufacturer's instructions should be followed closely. Collect all the materials needed before applying the cast.

Equipment

- Gloves
- Stockinette
- Synthetic cast padding, such as Soffban (Smith & Nephew)
- Enough rolls of casting material of appropriate size
- A bowl of water at the temperature recommended by the manufacturer.

Technique

1. Open or surgical wounds are covered with non-adherent dressing.
2. Stockinette is rolled up the limb, taking care to prevent any creases.
3. Cast padding is carefully and evenly wound on to the limb with 50% overlap at each turn, paying special attention to any bony prominence. Do not overpad these parts; instead use ring 'donuts'. Donuts can be made by cutting holes in small pads made out of cast padding; these are usually placed on the accessory carpal bone and olecranon of the forelimb or the calcaneus of the hindlimb. This prevents pressure ulceration on these structures
4. One roll of casting material is prepared by immersing it in the bowl of water and squeezing several times to allow the water to penetrate into the roll.
5. Excess water is squeezed out and the roll of casting material is applied to the limb in the same manner as the padding but with even tension. The casting material starts to set within minutes (depending on the type used), therefore it is important to work quickly.
6. Each roll is wetted individually just before application. Depending on the type of casting material used and the size of the patient, usually 2–3 layers are applied with 4–6 layers for larger dogs.
7. The pads and nails of the middle two toes are left exposed at the bottom of the cast.
8. A 1–2 cm length of padding is left exposed at the top and bottom of the cast.
9. Once the cast has hardened the stockinette and padding at each end are turned down over the edge of the cast and secured with tape.
10. A cast can be made stronger by applying splints made out of several lengths of casting material laid longitudinally down the compression side of the cast.

Splints

Zimmer and gutter splints can be used as a fixation technique in some fractures, particularly those occurring below the carpus or hock in cats and small dogs. Splints can also be made from casting material (except plaster of Paris). A cast is applied as before, and then an oscillating saw is used to cut the length of the cast on the medial and lateral sides. The limb is dressed and bandaged appropriately and the two halves of the cast are reapplied to the limb and secured with an adhesive bandage.

Postoperative care of casts and splints

Owners should be given *written* instructions of how to look after the cast and what to look out for if things start to go wrong.

- When the patient is taken outside, the bottom of the cast should be covered with a plastic bag (old drip bags are useful for this) and secured with tape – never elastic bands, as these may easily be forgotten and cause problems later on.
- Casts may have to be reapplied if the animal chews extensively or damages the cast. Growing animals will need a new cast every week to allow normal growth of the limb.
- Give medication as prescribed.
- Check cast daily and any of the following signs should be reported to the veterinary surgeon immediately:
  - Swelling of the limb or toes
  - Chafing at the edges of the cast
  - Staining of the cast with a discharge
  - A foul smell coming from the cast
  - Slipping of the cast from its original position
  - Chewing or other signs of discomfort
  - Collapse or bending of the cast (especially plaster of Paris)
  - General illness – depression, lethargy, lack of appetite.

Complications of casts

- Limb swelling – if the cast is too tight, it restricts the lymphatic and venous drainage, which results in oedema of the lower limb. This is usually seen within 1 hour of applying the cast and needs urgent attention.
- Decubital ulcers – usually seen if the cast is poorly padded or is slightly loose and sliding on the skin.
- Cast loosening – if the cast was put on when the limb was swollen, the cast may loosen once the swelling subsides.
- Prolonged immobilization of the limb may cause any of the following complications:
  - Joint stiffness and fibrosis
  - Cartilage degeneration
  - Muscle atrophy
  - Osteoporosis of disuse.
- Joint laxity – rapidly growing young large-breed dogs are particularly at risk.
- Delayed union, malunion and non-union may be seen with poor case selection, poor cast selection, poor casting technique or frequent reapplication of the cast and movement of the fracture site.
- Refracture on removal of the cast – provided that the limb had good callus formation (clinical union) on the radiograph at the time of cast removal, this should not happen.

Removal of the cast

Generally limbs remain in a cast for 4–6 weeks. Radiographs are taken to establish the degree of healing and callus formation. The patient should be sedated or anaesthetized. An oscillating saw is the most suitable tool for removing casts. Two cuts are made in the cast, with the line of cut carefully chosen to avoid bony prominences. The saw should never come into contact with the skin. The saw moves in an arc of 5–6 degrees and only cuts the solid casting material; the padding underneath catches on the blade and is not cut. The oscillating blade can become hot while cutting the cast and the saw should be rotated to use a cooler part of the blade. The padding underneath can then be removed with scissors. Plaster shears can also be used: they are inserted at the distal end of the cast and the cut is advanced proximally in small regular steps.

Internal fixation

Internal fixation uses pins, plates, screws and wire to repair fractures.

Internal fixation

Advantages

- Suitable for fractures in any bone
- Versatile and can handle the full range of fracture types
- Allows accurate reduction and rigid fixation
- Allows the limb to return to full function early, encouraging fracture healing and minimizing the risk of fracture disease.

Disadvantages

- Technique is relatively expensive and time-consuming.
- Some internal fixation techniques are technically demanding.
- There is capital expenditure on the equipment.
- The risks of surgery (wound healing problems, infection) are inherently greater in an open reduction and fixation than in closed reduction and fixation.
- Open fractures with extensive soft tissue injury may not be suitable.

Implants and techniques used in internal fixation

Intramedullary pins

These are called Steinmann pins; they are stainless steel rods with a sharp trocar point at each end, and it is possible to have one end threaded. They come in different widths ranging from 1.6 to 8 mm in diameter and are placed into the medulla of the bone that is fractured. They are inserted with a Jacobs chuck or power drill.

- *Advantages:* cheap to purchase, quick to use, require minimal surgical exposure, easier to implant and remove than bone plates.
- *Disadvantages:* less stable fixation, slower return to function, secondary bone union (i.e. slower healing), more aftercare required, not suitable for unstable fractures.

Postoperative management of intramedullary pins

- Two radiographic views are required to assess repair.
- Provide clients with written instructions outlining convalescent period and dates for follow-up examinations.
- Give medication (analgesics and possibly antibiotics) as directed.
- Exercise restrictions: lead-exercise only to allow patient to urinate and defecate. Cats should be restricted to a cage or a section of a room. ▶

- Avoid stairs and prevent animal jumping on or off furniture.
- Sutures are usually removed after 10 days.
- At the first check, evaluate for limb function and assess joints adjacent to the fracture for range of motion. The point where the pin emerges from bone is examined for swelling or evidence of pin migration. There should be regular checks to monitor bone healing and watch for pin migration.
- The pin is usually removed under anaesthetic once clinical union is achieved.

Interlocking nails

These are solid rods of 4, 4.7, 6 or 8 mm in diameter, with holes through which screws are inserted. The nails are placed in the medulla and the screws fix the rod within the bone. Diaphyseal fractures are suitable for this method of repair and it gives a more reliable fixation than an intramedullary pin. It requires expensive equipment and technical expertise to insert. Equipment and implants are available in the UK but they are mostly used in specialist referral centres.

Arthrodesis and Kirschner wires

These are smaller pins with diameters of 0.9 to 2 mm. Arthrodesis wires have trocar points at each end, and K-wires (Kirschner wires) have a flattened bayonet point at one end and trocar point at the other. These pins can be used as intramedullary pins in very small bones, as an aid in stabilizing a fragment while primary fixation is taking place or to create a tension-band wire. They are also used in various types of fractures in small dogs and cats but not for midshaft fractures of long bones.

Cerclage wire

This is malleable monofilament stainless steel wire. It is often used to supplement the use of intramedullary pins, external skeletal fixators and bone plates. It compresses large fragments by encircling the bone and the fragment and then is twisted with wire twisters, pliers or special tighteners. It is also used to create a tension-band wire (see below).

Tension-band wire

This is used to fix an avulsed fracture. It uses two different directional forces to create compression of the fracture. A K-wire or pin is placed into the fragment and main bone and a wire is placed in a figure-of-eight pattern around the end of the pin. It is anchored through a predrilled hole to a solid part of the bone on the opposite side to the ligament or muscle that pulled off the fragment.

Venables and Sherman plates

A Venables plate is a rectangular bone plate with round holes. The number of holes varies from four to eight. The plate is secured to the bone, bridging the fracture with Sherman self-tapping screws. A Sherman plate is similar to the Venables plate but narrows between the holes, making it lighter but not as strong. Sherman screws are also used to attach this plate to the bone. Self-tapping screws (Sherman) differ from tapped screws by their slotted heads and two notches at the tip of the screw. They are available in two widths (7/64 and 9/64) and various different lengths.

After the plate has been contoured (bent to fit the bone), it is held in position with bone-holding forceps. Each hole is drilled with the correct-size drill bit to include both near and far cortices. The hole is then measured with a depth gauge and the

correct length screw is selected. The screw is driven into the hole with a screwdriver. These screws cut their own thread as they are screwed into the hole. (For this reason they cannot be taken out and replaced in the same hole, because they would strip the thread as it was replaced and not be secure.) Screws are not inserted into holes that cross the fracture line; these holes are best left empty or a lag screw (see later) can be inserted prior to placing the plate.

ASIF/AO systems

ASIF stands for the Association for the Study of Internal Fixation and is used in North America to name the patent and copyright of the system of orthopaedic equipment used for internal fixation. The European designation for the same equipment is AO, which stands for Arbeitsgemeinschaft für Osteosynthsefragen.

There is a wide variety of different plates and equipment for repairing every conceivable type of fracture. The most commonly used plate in veterinary practice is the **dynamic compression plate (DCP)**. It is a strong plate with oval holes. These are available in different widths named by the size of screw they take and the length or number of holes. A 2.0 mm plate takes 2.0 mm screws; a 2.7 mm plate takes 2.7 mm screws; 3.5 mm and 4.5 mm plates come in narrow or broad widths and take 3.5 and 4.5 mm screws, respectively.

The DCP can serve various functions depending on how it is appplied to the fractured bone. It can be used as a compression plate, as a neutralization plate, or as a buttress plate. A compression plate is used in simple transverse diaphyseal fractures to compress the ends of the bone together. A neutralization plate is used in oblique, spiral and comminuted fractures where compression is not possible, and the fracture has been reconstructed with wires or screws but the repair needs additional support. A buttress plate is used to help to stabilize the fracture site and to bridge a fracture that is not reconstructable. The defect at the fracture site is usually filled with a cancellous bone graft.

Pre-tapped screws (AO type)

These screws are identified by the hexagonal head, which needs a special type of screwdriver to be able to place them. They are available in different widths and lengths, and some larger screws are cortical or cancellous. Figure 24.18 is a guide to the sizes and drill bits to use.

Size of screw (mm)	Drill bit for core (mm)	Drill bit for gliding hole (mm)	Tap (mm)
1.5[a]	1.1	1.5	1.5
2.0[a]	1.5	2.0	2.0
2.7[a]	2.0	2.7	2.7
3.5[a]	2.5	3.5	3.5
4.0[b]	2.0	4.0	4.0
4.5[a]	3.2	4.5	4.5
6.5[b]	3.2	6.5	6.5

24.18 Sizes of AO-type screws and corresponding drill bits. [a] Cortical; [b] cancellous.

Technique

A drill bit is selected to drill a hole the size of the core of the screw; for example, if a 3.5 mm cortical screw is to be used, a 2.5 mm drill bit will be selected. The hole is then measured with the depth gauge and the correct length of screw is selected. The hole is then 'tapped' to create a thread for the screw. A **tap** is a special device designed to cut the thread in the bone. It is especially important to use the correct tap for the screw being inserted. The tap designed for the 4.0 mm cancellous screw cannot be used for the 3.5 mm cortical screw even though both screws are of similar widths, because the thread has a different pitch. The screw is finally driven into the hole using the hexagonal-head screwdriver.

Lag screw technique

A lag screw is not a type of screw but a technique. It is used to stabilize and compress fragments in a fracture. The fracture is reduced and held in place using bone-holding forceps. A hole the same width as the screw (the gliding hole) is drilled in the fragment, and the far cortex is then drilled with a drill bit the same size as the core of the screw. The far cortex is tapped, but the near cortex (in the fragment) is not. When the screw is driven into the hole, it does not grip the fragment but just grips the far cortex; this has the effect of compressing the fragment into place.

Postoperative care after internal fixation

- Two radiographic views are required to assess the repair immediately postoperatively.
- Analgesia and nursing during recovery aim to enable a smooth and peaceful recovery of consciousness.
- Early recovery of appetite and adequate nutrition is important.
- Long anaesthetic times and blood loss during reconstruction of the fracture may necessitate continuation of intravenous fluids into the recovery period.
- Assisted walking may be necessary to allow the animal an opportunity to urinate and defecate while limiting the use of the fractured limb.
- Daily monitoring of temperature, pulse and respiratory rates is required during hospitalization.
- Give medication and analgesia as directed in the days following the surgery.
- Sutures are usually removed after 10 days.
- Clients should be provided with written instructions outlining the convalescent period and dates for follow-up examinations and re-radiography. These should be on a regular basis as directed by the veterinary surgeon. The owners should be instructed on how to recognize possible complications and how to seek veterinary advice if these occur.
- Exercise restrictions: cage rest is outdated with modern methods of rigid immobilization. It is considered to be beneficial to fracture healing and well-being of the patient to give short controlled bouts of lead-exercise: 10–15 minutes (on a lead) a couple of times a day for the first 3–4 weeks is usually sufficient. Swimming is also of great benefit once any wounds have healed, but must be controlled in the early stages of healing to prevent overenthusiastic movements.

Complications associated with internal fixation

The most common complications are osteomyelitis and infection associated with the implants, and implant failure. Both are often due to poor technique or poor choice of implants. In some cases, the postoperative care in the home environment is not sufficiently rigorous to protect the implants from failure.

External skeletal fixation (ESF)

External skeletal fixation stabilizes fractures using pins that are inserted through a small stab incision in the skin and then into the bone. They usually travel through both cortices and are then fixed on the outside of the limb with bars and clamps or acrylic resin. Different types of frame can be made according to the requirements of the fracture. A simple frame would consist of one bar and three or four pins exiting from the bone. A more complex frame could consist of multiple pins and three or more bars in three different planes.

Pins come in different sizes (1.6 mm, 2 mm, 3 mm and 4 mm). Pins may be smooth with a trocar end or have threaded ends. End-threaded pins have either a **negative thread**, where the thread is cut out of the pin and the overall diameter of the pin remains the same, or a **positive thread**, where a thread is wound on to the pin and the overall diameter of the pin is slightly larger. Pins are also available with a positive thread in the middle of the pin rather than at the end. The advantage of a threaded pin is that it is less likely to loosen or be pulled out than a smooth pin. Pins are placed in both cortices of the bone but do not necessarily exit both sides. The centrally threaded pins are designed to exit both sides of the limb. Clamps and bars are available to fit each size of pin.

External skeletal fixation

Advantages

- Minimal instrumentation required
- Clamps and bars reusable
- Minimal disruption of soft tissues
- Minimal foreign body at fracture site
- Open wound management easy
- Easy to combine with other implants
- Rigidity and alignment easily adjustable
- Assessment of fracture healing easy
- Easy to remove.

Disadvantages

- Soft tissue problems possible
- Application technique requires practice
- Premature pin loosening common
- Difficult to apply to proximal limb
- Can be difficult to obtain good radiographs of the limb.

Types of fracture suitable for external fixation

- Long bone fractures
- Comminuted fractures
- Open and infected fractures
- Delayed unions and non-union
- Mandibular fractures.

APEF system

The acrylic pin external fixator (APEF) system uses corrugated tubing which is filled with polymethylmethacrylate, a type of bone cement. All the pins are placed in the bone and the corrugated tubing is fixed to the ends of the pins. The cement is mixed and poured into the tubing. The tubing is then held in alignment until the cement has hardened. The hardening process is a chemical reaction between the liquid and powder components and intense heat is generated. It is important to protect the soft tissues (and fingers) from this heat. Heat can also be conducted down the pins and cause necrosis of the bone. Sterile swabs soaked in cool sterile saline can be placed on the tissues to help to protect them; saline can also be dribbled from a syringe on to the pins. The cement takes up to 10 minutes to set. Mandibular fractures are particularly suitable for this system; the acrylic can be formed around the pins and the shape of the jaw into a 'bumper bar'.

Bone grafts

Bone grafts can be harvested from either cortical or cancellous bone. They are used to supplement fracture repair and accelerate healing across a wide fracture gap during reconstruction. The term **autograft** refers to bone taken from a site and used elsewhere in the same dog. An **allograft** refers to bone taken from one patient and transferred into another patient of the same species.

Cortical bone grafts consist of a whole segment of solid bone or else chips of cortical bone either in a fracture or taken from a non-essential site. These bone grafts are very robust and can even be taken from a different dog for use in limb salvage, though this is a very specialized technique. It takes a long time for the cortical graft to become fully incorporated in the repair.

Cancellous bone is harvested from inside the medulla of long bones and the commonest sites used are the proximal humerus or the ilium. A drill is used to make a hole in the cortical bone and the cancellous bone is scraped out from the inside of the bone using a curette. Cancellous bone is very sensitive as it contains live cells. It should be handled in a sterile manner and stored in a blood-soaked swab on the trolley until used. Cancellous bone grafts are an essential part of the repair of complex fractures as they contribute cells and growth factors involved in bone healing.

Postoperative care of external fixators

- Open wounds should be treated and dressed appropriately.
- The limb should have a compressive bandage applied for 2–3 days (changed daily) to minimize swelling. This bandage should go between the limb and the bars/acrylic and in between the pins, and should include the toes.
- The ends of the pins protruding from the clamps or tubing should be covered with self-adhesive tape to prevent damage to furniture and owners.
- Air should be allowed to circulate between the skin and pins.
- Cats should be confined to cage rest.
- Exercise should be limited to lead-exercise only, taking care to avoid fences or other objects that are likely to catch the frame.
- Owners should be told to expect a small amount of scab formation at the site of the pin. This is normal and does not need cleaning on a daily basis. However, excess exudate does need to be cleaned and should be seen by the veterinary surgeon.
- Generally external fixators are well tolerated by the patient but an Elizabethan collar can be put on to prevent the patient interfering with the frame.
- Written instructions should be given to the owner regarding medication, postoperative checks and radiographs.

Complications of external fixation

- Swelling of the soft tissues impinging on the clamps or acrylic bars
- Excessive exudate from the pin site caused by movement of the skin and soft tissues
- Loosening of pins, but in some cases individual pins can be removed without losing the stability of the frame.

Luxations and subluxations

A **luxation** (also called a dislocation) is a displacement of articular surfaces from the normal position within a joint. The joint surfaces no longer touch each other. A **subluxation** is a partial dislocation of the joint surfaces.

Luxations and subluxations may be classified into two types: congenital and acquired.

- **Congenital** luxations or subluxations are anatomical abnormalities present at birth, which may or may not be inherited. The most common congenital luxation is that of the patella. In most cases a surgical procedure can replace the patella in its normal position, but some congenital luxations are so severe that they cannot be corrected. Some small dogs and cats may be able to cope with the permanently luxated joint, but in larger breeds severe congenital luxation may cause great disability.
- **Acquired** luxations and subluxations result from some form of trauma, such as a road traffic accident. The ligaments keeping the joint in its normal position are damaged and the joint is forced out of alignment. Acquired luxations most commonly occur in the hip and elbow joints. Also affected but less commonly are phalangeal joints, the hock and shoulder joints.

First aid treatment for dislocations should follow that for fractures as presenting signs and trauma are often similar.

Clinical signs and diagnosis

The signs shown by the patient can mimic those of a fracture and it can be difficult to differentiate between them. Pain, deformity, loss of motion, non-weight bearing and crepitus are common signs to both. Sometimes typical stance positions are characteristic of an animal with a dislocation. Radiography is essential to confirm the diagnosis and also the presence or absence of other conditions, e.g. small fractures.

Treatment

Treatment of luxations requires the return of the joint to its normal anatomical position and repair of the damaged ligaments. Like fracture reduction, reduction of luxations may be achieved in several ways:

- **Closed reduction** is reduction of the joint by manipulation of the limb. This is the method that should be attempted first. Closed reduction should be attempted as soon as possible after injury, as the longer the delay the less chance there is of successful reduction of the joint. Most joints are impossible to reduce under sedation, causing unnecessary pain and suffering to the patient, and reduction should be carried out under general anaesthetic. The joint should be re-radiographed afterwards to check that the reduction has been successful.
- **Open reduction** involves a surgical approach to the joint: the luxated bones are visualized and manipulated back into the joint. Some form of stabilization technique is usually required.

Postoperative care

Postoperative care is similar after both open and closed reductions except that open luxations require the added precautions taken following surgery. The main postoperative aim is to avoid forces that could cause a recurrence of the luxation.

Once the joint is reduced, it must be immobilized. After a hip dislocation the hindlimb is supported in an Ehmer sling; after a shoulder dislocation the forelimb can be supported in a Velpeau sling. The slings are kept on for 5–7 days. Exercise should be restricted for 3–4 weeks and then slowly increased.

Complications

- Re-luxation is the most common complication, especially if activity is not sufficiently restricted or if there is other pathology in the joint, such as a fracture.
- Joint infection is a risk, especially if an open reduction has been performed.
- There may be injury to surrounding soft tissues, associated either with the original trauma or with the reduction of the joint. These injuries may not be obvious at first. They include damage to nerves in the region of the joint.

Oncological surgery

Oncology is the study of cancer and its related diseases. A **neoplasm**, or tumour, is an abnormal uncontrolled growth of cells that develop faster than the surrounding normal tissues. Most tumours arise as the animal ages and typically they are found in dogs or cats over 8–10 years of age. However, there are some very aggressive tumours that occur in dogs or cats as young as a few months old. Some breeds are specifically susceptible to certain tumours and may develop more than one tumour at the same time (e.g. Boxers, mast cell tumours; Flat-Coated Retrievers, sarcomas). Many owners will be very concerned about the possibility that their animal has cancer, and they must be reassured that many tumours are benign and, if removed completely, will not grow again.

Neoplasia

Neoplasia is extremely common in small-animal practice and all unexplained lumps on an animal should be investigated with the possibility of neoplasia in mind.

Tumours cause problems in a number of ways:

- The physical mass of the tumour presses on other structures and causes pain or loss of function (e.g. pressing on the pharynx and preventing swallowing).
- A rapidly growing tumour may use up energy resources and cause the animal to feel unwell and depressed.
- Cytokines released by the tumour can cause distant physiological effects (see 'Paraneoplastic syndromes', below).
- The tumour may spread to other vital organs (e.g. heart, kidney, liver, lungs) and invade the tissues, causing loss of function and resulting in clinical signs.

Tumours may arise from any body tissue and the name of the neoplasm is derived from its tissue of origin. Very aggressive tumours may lose all their identifying characteristics because they are growing so fast, and in these cases it may not be possible for the pathologist to identify the tissue of origin. It is important to know the tissue of origin, because this enables the veterinary surgeon to predict how the tumour will behave and also to decide what treatment is most appropriate.

The terminology used in oncology is very specific and often describes both the type of tumour and how it behaves. Neoplasms may be benign or malignant and this description indicates whether or not the tumour is likely to spread to other organs or tissues in the animal and result in its death.

Benign tumours

Benign tumours usually grow quite slowly and are discrete and encapsulated. They are often freely mobile relative to neighbouring tissues.

- **Lipoma** – a benign tumour of adipose (fat) cells, very common in the subcutaneous tissues of older overweight animals
- **Papilloma** – a benign wart-like tumour of epithelial cells, most often seen on the skin of cats and dogs (e.g. at the lip margins, eyelid and ear) but they also occur in the bladder and rectum
- **Melanoma** – a benign pigmented skin tumour of melanocytes; some melanomas, however, are highly malignant, particularly if they arise in the mucous membranes of the mouth
- **Fibroma** – a benign tumour of fibrous tissue, present as firm superficial tumours of the skin, and may be difficult to differentiate from other more malignant skin tumours
- **Adenoma** – a benign tumour of glandular tissue, may be quite common in older dogs (e.g. anal adenoma).

Malignant tumours

Malignant tumours may grow quickly or slowly. They may not have a definite capsule and may be closely attached to neighbouring tissue. Some malignant tumours will spread (**metastasize**) very readily to other organs such as the lungs, liver, spleen and bones. Metastasis may occur via various routes:

- In the circulation after invasion of blood vessels
- In the lymphatic system to the draining lymph node and beyond
- By direct contact of tumour cells with neighbouring organs by direct invasion (**extension**) or by exfoliation of tumour cells into a cavity such as the abdomen (**transplantation**).

Malignant tumours are also classified according to the tissue from which they arise:

- **Carcinoma** is a malignant tumour arising from epithelial cells:
  - **Squamous cell carcinoma** arises from squamous epithelium such as the oral cavity
  - **Transitional cell carcinoma** arises from the transitional epithelium characteristic of the bladder epithelium.
- **Adenocarcinoma** is a malignant tumour of glandular tissue in epithelia.
- **Sarcoma** is a malignant tumour arising from mesenchymal tissues (mainly connective tissues):
  - **Lymphosarcoma** is a tumour of the lymphoid tissues, common in dogs, and may be seen in association with feline leukaemia virus in cats.
  - **Fibrosarcoma** arises from fibroblasts, and may be found in any connective tissue.
  - **Osteosarcoma** is a malignant tumour of osteoblasts and is usually in the limb bones. In the dog, these tumours are commonly found in the distal radius or ulna, proximal humerus, distal femur or proximal tibia.

When the tumour is examined histopathologically, it can be further graded to determine its degree of malignancy by assessing its rate of proliferation and degree of differentiation of the cells.

Preparation for oncological surgery

Many forms of neoplasia are amenable to surgery. In order to plan treatment and advise the owner, a specific diagnosis of the type of tumour is necessary. This entails taking a sample from the tumour and submitting it for histopathology. Benign tumours may be completely cured by excisional surgery and a number of treatments are available for malignant tumours that will extend the lifespan of the animal while maintaining its quality of life.

Many animals are older and will require some investigation to establish whether there is evidence of other disease before the surgery is carried out. The animal should also be radiographed or scanned to check whether the neoplasia has spread to other sites. All animals should have a right and left lateral chest X-ray taken to check for metastases. Finally, many patients may be cachexic, malnourished or suffering from paraneoplastic disease that makes them increased surgical risks. Attention to nutrition, planning for postsurgical care and nursing are important for successful oncological surgery.

Paraneoplastic disease

Tumours can cause other signs of illness apart from the physical effects of the mass itself. Some tumours secrete biologically active hormones that may cause generalized non-specific ill-health, or they may cause well defined syndromes of disease. Sometimes the paraneoplastic syndrome is more acutely life-threatening than the tumour itself. For example:

- Anal adenocarcinoma and lymphosarcoma can cause hypercalcaemia, which causes polydypsia, polyuria and renal failure.
- Insulinomas secrete active insulin, which causes episodes of acute hypoglycaemia.
- Mast-cell tumours can secrete histamine, causing generalized or local acute inflammatory responses.
- Thyroid adenomas secrete excess thyroxine, causing tachycardia, weight loss and hyperactivity.

Tumours can also cause pyrexias, cachexia and generalized poor nutrition due to other substances released into the circulation.

Biopsy

Fine-needle aspiration

This is the commonest and most useful method of obtaining tissue for diagnosis of tumours. It is also used to assess draining lymph nodes for evidence of metastasis. A fine-gauge hypodermic needle is inserted into the tumour to aspirate a few cells for cytological analysis (see Chapter 17). Sometimes ultrasound guidance is used to direct needles into intra-abdominal or intrathoracic tumours.

Bone marrow biopsy

Aspirates are also used to sample bone marrow, using a special bone marrow biopsy needle. Usually the sample is taken from the wing of the ilium under sedation with local anaesthesia, or general anaesthesia. The overlying skin is prepared as for surgery and a small skin incision is made over the bone. The bone marrow biopsy needle is driven through the cortex of the bone with the stylet in place. Once in the medullary cavity, the stylet is removed and a syringe is used to aspirate bone marrow. The samples are dripped on to slides tilted at 60 degrees to the vertical so that they run down the slide, forming a smear. These are air dried and submitted for cytology.

Needle core biopsy

A small cylinder of tissue is obtained using a specialized instrument such as a Tru-Cut needle. There is a central notched obturator, with an outer sleeve or cannula with an attached handle. General anaesthesia, or local anaesthesia of the overlying skin, is necessary. A stab incision is made in the skin to allow the loaded instrument to be introduced through the soft tissues, and ultrasound guidance may be used to direct the instrument into the centre of the tumour. Once the obturator is in the tumour, the sleeve is pushed sharply over the notch in the obturator, cutting out a tiny cylinder of tissue. The closed instrument is withdrawn and a hypodermic needle is used gently to dislodge the sample from the opened obturator.

Other biopsy methods

- **Punch biopsy** samples are taken from superficial lesions in the skin, using small circular cutters. The biopsy site may be closed using a single interrupted suture.
- **Trephine biopsy** samples are taken from bony tumours, using a trephine or a Jamshidi needle. A core of bone/tumour a few millimetres in diameter is obtained and pushed out of the trephine or needle using a stylet.
- **Incisional biopsy** is used for tumours that are big enough to remove a piece of tissue from without affecting the ultimate surgical treatment. Usually a wedge of tissue is taken from a part of the tumour that appears to be actively growing and then the wedge is repaired with sutures. This is the most reliable way to obtain a diagnosis.
- **Excisional biopsy** is usually used for small tumours that are easy to remove with a margin of normal tissue, particularly if they are suspected to be benign. It involves the complete removal of the tumour at the first surgery.

Principles of oncological surgery

The mainstay of any cancer therapy is to maintain the animal's quality of life. Side effects of treatment must be balanced by the clinical improvement – or cure. Most tumours are treated with surgical excision, and usually the aim is to remove the entire tumour. Sometimes it is the mass of the tumour that is causing the animal discomfort and in these cases **debulking** surgery may be used to remove as much of the tumour as possible, in order to improve the animal's quality of life until the mass regrows.

Well encapsulated benign tumours may be cured by simple excision of the tumour. However, many tumours require a **surgical margin** around the tumour in order to ensure that the tumour is entirely removed (Figure 24.19). Fibrosarcomas are a good example of tumours that are very invasive and require very wide margins of excision in order to attempt to cure the tumour. This may in turn require complex reconstructive surgery to repair the defect made where the tumour was removed. Intraoperative techniques may be used to reduce the risk of spreading the tumour into normal tissues; for example, the surgeon may change gloves, instruments or drapes prior to closure.

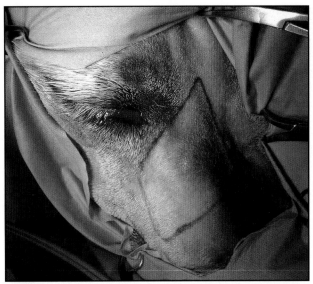

24.19 Skin tumours need to be removed with a margin of unaffected tissue, to ensure that the whole tumour is removed. Here a small mast cell tumour is to be removed with a margin of 2–3 cm. The surgeon has drawn the lines of incision on the skin with a sterile marker.

In some areas, a 'clean' surgical margin may not be possible and further types of therapy for the cancer may be indicated after the surgery. Some tumours are so malignant that post-operative chemotherapy or radiotherapy may be suggested even if the tumour appears to have been completely removed.

Palliative surgery may be used to remove a tumour to improve the animal's quality of life even though it does not alter the prognosis.

Submission of tissue for histopathology

All tissue removed from an animal should be submitted for histopathology or stored in formalin in case of recurrence.

Ideally all tissue removed from the animal should be submitted to the pathologist with a detailed history, in order to maximize the information available with which to analyse the tumour. Large tumours may be difficult to submit by post and representative samples may have to be taken from the mass; the main bulk of the tumour should be kept until the pathologist's report is complete in case more tissue is requested. Very bony samples have to be decalcified prior to cutting and this may result in a delay of up to 3 weeks before the report is received by the veterinary practice.

Where the tumour is malignant or locally invasive, the pathologist should be requested to assess the margins of the tumour in order to determine whether excision has been complete. Sometimes the surgeon may orientate the tumour by placing a marker suture at the cranial/caudal ends, or the edges of the mass can be painted with different colours of Indian ink, which are allowed to dry before fixation.

Fixation

Tissue should be fixed in 10% neutral buffered formalin in a volume ratio of 1 part specimen to 10 parts of formalin solution. Tissue thicker than 1 cm may need to be incised to allow more rapid access of the formalin to the deeper parts of the tissue so that adequate fixation occurs. Once the tissue has been fixed for 2–3 days, it can be posted with a 1:1 ratio of tissue to formalin. Formalin is carcinogenic and health and safety regulations must be observed during handling of the solution and preparing packages for posting (see Chapter 1).

Other treatments

- **Cryosurgery** is where tumour tissue is destroyed by freeze–thaw cycles that cause the cells to rupture due to ice crystal formation. This is not very selective and normal cells are also killed.
- **Chemotherapy** is the use of cytotoxic drugs to kill tumour cells selectively; it is only used for specific tumour types.
- **Radiotherapy** is used in specialist centres to kill dividing tumour cells.
- **Hyperthermia** is a specialist technique that uses local application of heat via needles introduced into the tumour to try to kill the dividing tumour cells.
- **Photodynamic therapy** is a specialist technique using photosensitizing chemicals and light to kill tumour cells.

Often treatments may be combined with surgery. Adjunctive therapy in the form of analgesics, antibiotics, anti-inflammatories, specialist nutritional requirements and nursing management may be an important part of managing these patients.

Postoperative management and advice

Ongoing nursing and monitoring of cancer patients is often necessary. Radiographs may be repeated at 4–6-month intervals to check for the development of metastases.

Oncological surgery carries with it the stigma of the dreaded word 'cancer' and many owners will continue to be concerned about the outcome long after the surgical wound has healed. Some animals have a very good quality of life for a considerable period of time even if the treatment has not been curative, and owners may need reassurance that the animal is not suffering. Some tumours carry a poor prognosis, despite surgery, and owners may need extra time and advice on how to observe their animal for recurrence and quality of life. It can be very distressing for owners to think that the animal will die from the condition and be waiting for it to happen, and all staff should be aware of the condition. Discussion about what to look for and how they might want to manage the final euthanasia may be best carried out before the animal is terminally ill.

Surgery and diseases of body systems

This section covers the main surgical diseases in the different body systems, and outlines the surgery and nursing implications of disease or potential surgical complications.

Nearly all surgical procedures are carried out under general anaesthetic and much of the postoperative nursing involves monitoring of the recovery from anaesthesia, and assessment and provision of analgesia. However, some surgical procedures also require postoperative monitoring for specific complications such as haemorrhage, infection, suture dehiscence or respiratory difficulties.

Surgical intervention in different areas of the body can be classified in terms of their potential for infection (Figure 24.20). Areas that can be prepared for aseptic surgery pose a different risk from those that are clearly infected and impossible to make aseptic.

Category	Classification	Definition	Examples of surgical procedures
I	Clean surgery	A surgical wound made under aseptic conditions that does not enter any contaminated viscus, and where there is no break in sterile technique	Neutering Uncomplicated hernias
II	Clean–contaminated surgery	A surgical wound made under aseptic conditions that enters the oropharynx, respiratory, alimentary or urogenital tracts, but where there is no other source of contamination	Lung lobectomy Gastrotomy Tracheotomy
III	Contaminated surgery	There is a major spill of contaminated material at surgery, or a break in sterile technique, or entry into a viscus with a high bacterial load (e.g. colon or rectum)	Abdominal surgery where gut contents spilled accidentally Oral surgery Wounds <4 hours old Lower bowel surgery
IV	Infected surgery	The surgical site is known to be already infected	Aural surgery Abscesses Old wounds Removal of necrotic tissue

24.20 Surgical classifications.

These classifications of surgical procedures enable the surgical team to assess the risk of postoperative infection and treat appropriately. For example, category I does not require postoperative antibiotics; and category IV may be treated with antibiotics both before, during and after surgery. The most effective way to use antibiotics during surgery is to give an intravenous preparation before the first incision. Antibiotics given after the surgery has been completed will make no difference to the incidence of infection.

Reducing risk of infection

During surgery, the risks of infection can also be reduced by other means:

- Thorough lavage of contaminated tissue using sterile fluids
- Surgeon changing gloves or re-scrubbing after handling infected or contaminated tissue, prior to closing the unaffected tissue
- Changing instruments for fresh sterile ones
- Discarding suture material if used in contaminated areas and supplying fresh material for closure of clean areas
- Covering drapes with fresh sterile drapes prior to closure

These techniques are commonly used after surgery on the gastrointestinal tract.

The eye

Ophthalmic surgery is one of the most meticulous areas of small animal surgery, where preparation, technique and postoperative care can have an enormous impact on outcome. General anaesthesia is required for all but the most minor procedures. Specialized instruments, theatre equipment and facilities for magnification may be necessary for some ophthalmic surgery.

General principles and preparation for eye surgery

The conjunctival sac is filled with a gel or lubricant and the fur is clipped very carefully from a small area surrounding the eye. The first stage is to clean gross contamination or exudate off the eye and eyelids using gauze swabs soaked in sterile saline. Skin preparation is completed using diluted povidone–iodine solution (note that surgical scrub solutions are not used in eye preparation) in preference to chlorhexidine solutions. The corneal and conjunctival surfaces should then be irrigated with sterile balanced salt solutions or saline and a drop of broad-spectrum antibiotic solution may be instilled on to the surface prior to surgery. Alcohol solutions should not be used near the eye surface. During surgery, Lacri-Lube (Allergan) may be used to keep the eye lubricated while the eyelids are held open for the surgery.

Postoperatively, the eye is usually protected using an Elizabethan collar, and sometimes it is necessary to bandage the front paws. Bandages are difficult to keep secure over the eye and they limit postoperative monitoring and treatments.

Inflammation of the eye in the postoperative phase is often detrimental, particularly where specialist surgery has been performed on structures within the eye. In this regard ocular surgery is unusual, as corticosteroids may be used in the postoperative phase to reduce inflammation despite the delay in wound healing. Postoperative treatments may include topical ointments or drops for administration of antibiotics, steroids or cycloplegics (to reduce pupil spasm). In general, ointments can be applied less frequently than drops and may be easier for the owner to administer.

Analgesia is important and will make administration of treatments easier. Owners may need special advice and instruction on how to administer treatments safely.

Surgical conditions of the cornea and conjunctiva

Conjunctivitis
This is inflammation of the conjunctival membrane characterized by reddening of the conjunctiva. Usually the animal also shows increased tear production and overflow (**epiphora**). If the eye is very sore, the animal may hold the eyelids closed and be very reluctant to allow examination of the eye (**blepharospasm**). It is not a surgical disease in its own right, but is often a symptom of other conditions in the eye. In cats and rabbits it can be a primary infection.

Keratitis and ulceration
Keratitis is inflammation of the cornea, which may be accompanied by ulceration. The inflamed cornea has a cloudy appearance due to the oedema. Using the dye fluorescein in the eye allows ulceration to be visualized, and is important in diagnosis and monitoring of the healing of the ulcer. Where ointments containing corticosteroids are to be used to treat the keratitis, it is extremely important to ensure that no ulceration is present as the corticosteroid will prevent the ulcer from healing.

Ulcers may be secondary to penetration of the conjunctiva by a foreign body or due to keratitis or exposure of the surface of the eye and drying out of the conjunctiva. Severe ulcers may cause erosion of the cornea and ultimately result in rupture of the eye.

Ulcers are treated using techniques to protect the surface of the eye while the ulcer heals by second intention. Small ulcers may be treated with removal of the initiating cause and antibiotic ointment. Large ulcers may require surgical treatment. Traditionally, the third eyelid used to be sutured across the front of the eye to cover the ulcer. However, newer techniques such as conjunctival flaps and corneal contact lenses provide better visualization of the ulcer to monitor healing and make it easier to apply treatments.

Keratitis can also be caused by the instillation of irritant chemicals on to the surface of the eye. This may be accidental, malicious or iatrogenic, and requires emergency treatment to prevent permanent scarring to the cornea. The eye should be irrigated with copious amounts of water or sterile saline to wash out as much of the chemical as possible. The eye should then be closely monitored for ulceration and treated appropriately.

Foreign bodies

Presentation with acute severe conjunctivitis may indicate the presence of a foreign body such as a grass seed trapped behind the eyelids. Careful examination of the inner surfaces of both eyelids and the third eyelid is necessary to identify and remove the foreign material. In calm animals, it may be possible to do this after application of local anaesthetic drops, but many animals will require sedation or general anaesthesia, as it can be very painful. After removal, the eye should be checked for ulceration.

Surgical conditions of the eyelids

Entropion

This is inversion of the eyelid margin such that the eyelashes rub on the cornea (Figure 24.21). There is often secondary conjunctivitis and keratitis. Entropion is treated by surgery to return the eyelid margin to its normal position.

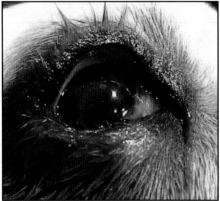

24.21 Entropion (shown here on the lower eyelid) is seen when the eyelid turns inwards and the eyelashes contact the conjunctival surface of the cornea causing constant irritation. (Photograph courtesy of David Williams)

Ectropion

This is eversion of the eyelid margin. In most cases ectropion does not require surgical intervention, but in some dogs it prevents normal lubrication of the eye and gives rise to a chronic exposure keratitis. Certain breeds of dog may have both ectropion and entropion at different points along the eyelid margin.

Distichiasis

This is the most common of a group of disorders characterized by abnormal growth of hairs at the eyelid margin so that the hairs rub the surface of the cornea. In many cases the hairs do not cause a clinical problem, but in some cases they cause a chronic keratitis requiring treatment. There are several surgical treatments described to remove the offending hairs and the follicle permanently.

Tumours

Tumours on the margin of the eyelid are very common in older dogs. They cause irritation by rubbing on the surface of the cornea and some are malignant. They are treated by excising a wedge of the eyelid margin containing the tumour.

Surgical conditions of the globe

Eyeball prolapse

Complete prolapse of the eyeball out of its socket (**proptosis** of the globe) can occur, particularly in brachycephalic dogs. First aid treatment is important if there is to be any chance of saving the eye. The eye must be kept moist using K-Y jelly (Johnson & Johnson) or Lacri-Lube (Allergan), supported by sterile saline-soaked swabs. Definitive surgery to replace the eye in the socket must be carried out as soon as possible.

Lens luxation

The lens is usually held in place by ligaments behind the pupil. If these fail, it can luxate either into the anterior chamber of the eye or caudally. This is usually a spontaneous event, often in terrier breeds, but can also be seen as a result of trauma. It requires emergency treatment to remove the lens, as the condition will lead to the development of glaucoma and blindness.

Glaucoma

This is an acute elevation in the pressure within the eye which can result in permanent blindness within 24 hours if not treated. There are several causes of glaucoma, but the commonest are anterior uveitis and lens luxation. The eye is extremely painful, the sclera engorged and the pupil is usually dilated. Emergency medical treatment includes analgesia and intravenous hypertonic fluids (mannitol) to try to draw fluid out of the eye. Surgical treatments are available in specialist centres.

Cataracts

A cataract is the opacification of the fibres or capsule of the lens of the eye, ultimately resulting in blindness. It should be distinguished from ageing changes in the lens that result in an apparent blue colour of the lens, but through which the animal can still see. Cataracts may be a primary disease or secondary to other conditions such as diabetes mellitus. They may be left untreated or they can be surgically removed by specialist ophthalmic surgeons. Removal of the lens enables the animal to recognize objects and people, as the lens is not as important in focusing as it is in humans. This restores quality of life to the older animal.

Ocular trauma

The eye may be penetrated by foreign bodies or lacerated by claws or teeth during fights with other animals. All these conditions may potentially result in loss of the eye and should be examined and treated as an emergency.

Retina

Most retinal diseases are not amenable to surgery, but the retina is an important site of disease in the eye. Of particular importance is a group of inherited diseases of the retina known as **progressive retinal atrophy** which are known to occur in certain breeds (see Chapter 5).

Skin

Skin biopsy

Skin biopsy is indicated for diagnosis of skin disease. Minimal preparation of the skin surface should be performed in order not to disrupt the surface cells that may aid the pathologist in making a diagnosis. The sample is taken using either a skin biopsy punch or just with a scalpel blade. Several samples should be taken from representative sites and the incisions closed with simple interrupted sutures. In severely diseased skin, there may be delayed wound healing.

Skin tumours

Skin masses should ideally be identified histologically prior to removal. The best way to identify the tumour is using fine-needle aspiration biopsy (see oncological section, above). Surgery should be performed in the normal aseptic way and the skin closed with sutures. It is important to be aware that some small skin tumours may require tissue margins in three dimensions and therefore some fat and muscle may need to be removed along with the overlying skin.

Surgical management of local pyoderma

Some chronic local skin infections are related to long-term skin disease such as atopy (allergic skin disease) and are then exacerbated by the animal's anatomical skin folds. If the skin folds are not due to obesity, then it may be appropriate to resect the skin folds in order to prevent the recurrence of painful pyoderma. The common examples are vulval folds, screwtail folds and lip folds. Certain breeds, such as the brachycephalics and spaniels, are more likely to suffer from these conditions. Patients with allergic skin disease are most likely to interfere with their sutures as they are always itchy.

Urine/faecal scalding and decubital ulcers

Recumbent or incontinent patients are prone to soiling with urine or faeces and it is a failure of nursing management which then results in the development of decubital ulcers (pressure sores) or 'scald' (dermatitis). The skin and fur must be kept clean and dry at all times. In some cases, this may involve several baths per day or clipping away fur to enable exposure of the skin so that it can be checked easily. Traditional treatments are to protect the skin with a thin layer of Vaseline or similar oil-based cream, so that the urine does not irritate the skin surface. However, this does not allow the skin to breathe and although the creams will prevent the skin from becoming worse, they will not help to treat any dermatitis. Commercial spray-on products are available (e.g. Cavilon™) that provide a semi-permeable membrane under which the skin can heal while it is protected from the urine/faeces. The skin can also be covered with self-adhesive semi-permeable membranes.

Decubital ulcers (Figure 24.22) are much easier to avoid than to cure. Padded bedding will help to prevent the development of pressure points in recumbent, obese or bony patients, and the use of 'Vetbed' material or incontinence pads will help to keep the skin dry, by wicking moisture away from

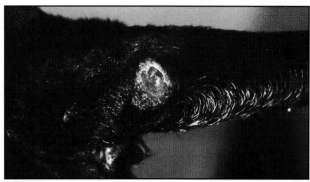

24.22 Decubital ulcers are commonly a sign of poor patient care, but occasionally they are seen in dogs with medical conditions that predispose them to decubital ulcers. They are usually on pressure points where the bone is near the surface, such as the elbows or iliac crests. They often appear very round and have a variable depth of tissue loss. Sometimes they are so deep that the underlying bone becomes infected.

the surface. Paralysed patients should be turned every 2–4 hours and all pressure points protected. Physiotherapy will encourage the blood supply to the skin and reduce the risk.

Anal sacs

The anal sacs are situated on either side of the anus and contain anal glands which produce a creamy coloured pungent exudate. The sacs are normally emptied on top of the faeces at the time of each defecation, and should not swell up or cause irritation. If anal sacs become impacted they fill with fluid, which then becomes secondarily infected, or they can eventually rupture and spill irritant infected contents into the tissues around the anus. This is often the case with animals with chronic **anal furunculosis**, which is a deep-seated infection with sinus tracts in the skin around the anus and under the tail. It is very painful and usually associated with colitis, dietary intolerance and autoimmune disease.

The classic clinical sign of anal gland irritation is persistent chewing at the rump or tail and rubbing the perineum on the ground, particularly after defecation. Anal gland disease may be secondary to a number of non-surgical diseases such as flea allergic dermatitis, atopy, obesity or diarrhoea. In some cases, it is necessary to remove chronically diseased anal sacs to prevent recurrence of infection.

Interdigital disease

Interdigital disease may be part of generalized skin disease, but some breeds are particularly predisposed to development of interdigital cysts or interdigital foreign bodies such as grass seeds. Dogs with long fur between the toes are particularly at risk of grass seeds becoming embedded in the thin interdigital skin. This causes painful swellings or abscesses. Sometimes it is possible to identify the end of the grass seed in the swelling and it is removed with forceps. If the seed has migrated into the leg, the sinus tract must be surgically explored. Surgical exploration is often easier if done with a tourniquet on the leg during the surgery. During the summer and autumn months, owners should be advised to check between and under the toes daily, or else keep the fur trimmed very short.

Aural surgery

The most common conditions of the ear are usually related to generalized skin disease. Recurrent shaking of the head and scratching at the ears can result in an aural haematoma, and persistent dermatitis may result in otitis externa.

Aural haematoma

This is the most common injury of the pinna. It is secondary to self-induced trauma and there is nearly always underlying otitis externa. A blood vessel bursts, usually on the underside of the pinna, and forms a large haematoma (Figure 24.23). This is painful and, if not treated, will cause the pinna to scar in a deformed shrivelled shape. Generally a haematoma is treated surgically. The haematoma is drained and cleaned out, allowing the skin to flatten again against the cartilage. Recurrence is prevented by suturing the skin to the cartilage to close the dead space, with the knots tied on the outer surface of the pinna. Buttons, quills or X-ray film have all been used to help to flatten the skin and prevent the sutures from pulling out.

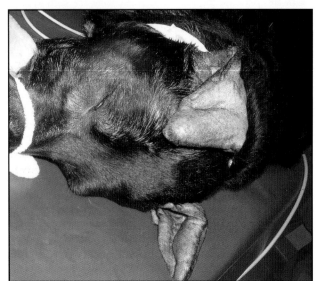

24.23 An aural haematoma forms when a blood vessel bursts and bleeds into the subcutaneous space between the skin and cartilage of the underside of the pinna. Often the pinna is heavy and painful, and drainage of the haematoma provides considerable relief. It is important to treat the underlying ear disease. This dog has been prepared for surgical drainage of bilateral aural haematomas, and the pinnae have been clipped.

Postoperatively it is important to treat any underlying skin or ear disease and to prevent the patient from scratching at the ear again. This is achieved either with an Elizabethan collar or with a figure-of-eight head bandage.

Otitis externa

Otitis externa (Figure 24.24) is very common in both dogs and cats. There are many causes and these have to be investigated prior to treatment:

- Foreign bodies in the ear canal (e.g. grass seeds)
- Ear mites (*Otodectes*)
- As an extension of generalized skin disease (e.g. atopy)
- Poor ear conformation, especially in the floppy-eared breeds or very hairy breeds
- Polyps or tumours
- Bacterial or yeast infection of the ears (this is usually secondary to one of the above).

Animals usually present with head shaking, scratching at the ears, aural pain and there may be bleeding or discharge out of the ear canals.

It may be necessary to clean the ears with saline before they can be examined. They are often extremely painful and this procedure should be done with analgesia or under anaesthetic.

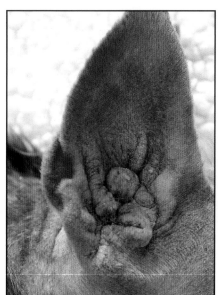

24.24 Chronic otitis externa. The external ear canal is completely obliterated with chronic greyish proliferative tissue. At this stage, it is not possible to salvage the ear by controlling the underlying skin disease and surgery would be recommended.

Tumours in the ear, or where cases of otitis externa have become very severe, are treated surgically:

- **Lateral wall resection**: the lateral wall of the vertical canal is removed so as to open up the ear to the air and allow better drainage and access for cleaning. This is only suitable for ears that have no disease on the medial wall of the vertical canal or in the horizontal canal.
- **Vertical canal ablation**: the vertical canal is completely removed and the horizontal canal opening is sutured to the skin. This is only for ears where the disease is confined to the vertical canal.
- **Total ear canal ablation**: this procedure is most commonly used and is usually for severe long-term otitis externa. Often the infection has ruptured the tympanic membrane and there is otitis media too. The middle ear (**tympanic bulla**) is accessed at the time of surgery by enlarging the bony opening (**bulla osteotomy**) and the middle ear is scraped and lavaged clean. The whole of the vertical and horizontal ear canal are removed and the tissue and skin sutured closed over the top. This procedure is more challenging than the others but often is the only solution as it removes all the diseased tissue.

Ear surgery is regarded as infected and antibiotics are usually given both before, during and after the surgery. Ear infections are often longstanding and opportunistic pathogens such as *Psuedomonas* or *Proteus* establish. They are difficult to treat as they are often resistant to most of the antibiotics commonly used. A foul-smelling greenish discharge may be an indication of these pathogens and a swab should be submitted for culture and sensitivity testing.

Postoperatively, the patients need analgesia, and the ear must be protected from self-inflicted injury. An Elizabethan collar may be used, or a head bandage, or the pinnae may be bandaged together to stop them flapping against the wound. There is often a discharge of blood or exudate from the wound for several days and this must be gently cleaned away using sterile saline. The sutures may have to stay in slightly longer than usual, but small areas of dehiscence are allowed to heal by second intention.

Otitis media

In the dog this is often an extension of otitis externa, but in the cat it may occur as a primary disease as an ascending infection via the eustachian tube. Access to the middle ear is either via a total ear canal ablation as described above if there is external disease or via a ventral approach (ventral bulla osteotomy). The animal is placed in dorsal recumbency and the dissection made directly over the tympanic bulla. A small drill is then used to make a hole in the bulla to allow drainage and lavage.

Otitis interna

Inflammation of the inner ear structures causes loss of balance, vomiting, head tilts, nystagmus and disorientation (vestibular syndrome). If this is secondary to severe middle ear disease, surgical management of the middle ear disease may be necessary to resolve the otitis interna.

Mammary tumours

Mammary neoplasia is the commonest tumour in the bitch, and the second most common tumour in all dogs. It is less common in the cat, but it is seen in breeding queens (particularly Siamese) or cats that have been treated for oestrus suppression or skin disease using megestrol acetate.

In bitches the most commonly affected glands are the two caudal pairs, while in queens the cranial glands are most often affected. About 50% of mammary tumours in the bitch are benign, but in cases with multiple masses they may all be different tumour types (Figure 24.25). In cats, over 80% of mammary masses are malignant and carcinomas tend to be particularly aggressive, most having metastasized by the time of presentation.

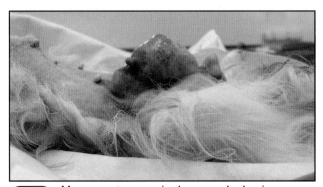

24.25 Mammary tumours in dogs may be benign or malignant and can grow to considerable size by the time the owner presents the animal for treatment. (Photograph courtesy of Pierre Barreau.)

Fine-needle aspirate biopsies are rarely helpful except to differentiate mammary tumours from mastitis or hypertrophy. The type of tumour is rarely confirmed prior to surgery, as it does not change the management of the disease.

Surgery is the treatment of choice for mammary tumours. In the bitch the type of surgery has little effect on the survival time and radical surgery is generally unnecessary, as many tumours are benign. Surgery involves removing either just the affected gland (**mammectomy**), or that gland and an adjacent gland (**local mastectomy**) or all the glands on the affected side (**radical mastectomy** or 'mammary strip'). In the cat, the tumours are often aggressive and radical surgery is more important.

All mammary gland surgery is prone to dehiscence and ideally a drain should be used and postoperative antibiotic therapy. To reduce the risk of wound complications, surgery on both sides simultaneously is usually avoided.

Although in humans there are many other treatments used alongside surgery for mammary tumours, in dogs and cats there are currently no other treatments that are known to make a difference to survival after removal of malignant mammary tumours.

Gastrointestinal tract

Many diseases affecting the GI tract have serious adverse effects on the fluid and electrolyte status of the patient. These deficits should be identified and stabilized prior to anaesthesia and surgery. Long periods of anorexia or vomiting and diarrhoea will cause the animal to be dehydrated and in a negative energy balance and therefore a poor candidate for surgery. Steps must be taken to replenish nutritional deficits and to maintain nutrition to minimize the effects of surgery on the patient. This may mean placement of feeding tubes prior to or during the surgical procedure to help with nursing the patient postoperatively. For example, an anorexic cat is likely to recover much more quickly if feeding tubes are placed at the time of surgery than if hand feeding or 'tempting' food is relied upon in the early postoperative stages.

Oral surgery

Oral tumours

These are generally seen in older dogs and cats. Tumours may arise on any structure of the oropharynx (tongue, gingiva, lips, palate, tonsils, etc.), and the prognosis depends very much upon both the site of the tumour and the type of tumour. As owners generally do not inspect their pet's mouth regularly, these tumours may be large before they are presented for treatment. The first sign of a tumour may be halitosis, loss or displacement of teeth or facial swelling, and the tumour may only be identified at the time of dental examination by the veterinary surgeon.

Surgical resection carries the best prognosis for all oral tumours in the dog and cat. Where tumours are on the mandible or maxilla (Figure 24.26), bone and teeth may have to be removed along with the tumour in order to get adequate margins. The defect is then closed using flaps of mucosa from the lips and sutured with absorbable suture material. Postoperative nursing focuses on analgesia and ensuring that the patient can eat and drink easily. Food should be soft and formed, but not dry or abrasive (which might tear the sutures) or too sloppy (which might seep between the sutures). Tumours of the tonsils or palate often carry a worse prognosis, particularly in cats.

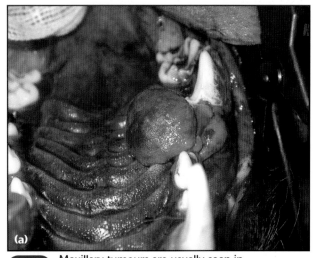

24.26 Maxillary tumours are usually seen in middle-aged to older dogs. **(a)** This dog has a tumour centred between premolar 3 and the carnassial tooth. The tumour must be removed with a margin of at least one uninvolved tooth on each side as well as the oral mucosa and underlying bone.

continues ▶

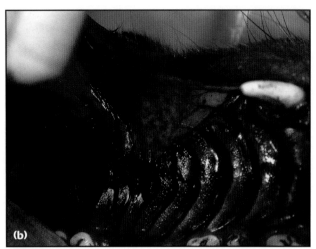

24.26 *continued* Maxillary tumours are usually seen in middle-aged to older dogs. **(b)** The maxilla after the tumour has been removed along with all of the dental arcade up to the incisor. The defect has been repaired with a flap of mucosa from the lip.

Oronasal fistulae

These may be secondary to trauma, dental extraction or tumour resection. All fistulae should be repaired surgically, to prevent food material impacting in the nasal cavity and causing a rhinitis. Preoperative preparation involves using saline and then dilute chlorhexidine or povidone–iodine solution to flush out debris accumulated in the cavity and nasal passages. Postoperatively, the defect should heal rapidly and may be kept clean with gentle oral lavage using chlorhexidine solutions.

Cleft palate

Puppies should always be checked for cleft palate at the time of birth, but it can also be traumatic in origin. Some clefts are simply repaired using advancement flaps; others require more advanced techniques, depending on the degree of involvement of the soft and hard palate. Protection of the suture line in the mouth is difficult and restriction of food intake or use of feeding tubes is counterproductive. The animal should be given soft formed food that will not get stuck in the suture line and is easy to swallow.

Foreign bodies and penetrating injuries

Foreign bodies such as sticks, bones, fish hooks or grass seeds may lodge in the soft tissues of the mouth and pharynx. All cause pain associated with the mouth, difficulty in swallowing and drooling.

The mouth can be opened in the conscious animal by using ropes behind the canine teeth of the upper and lower jaws, but the examination will be more effective under general anaesthesia. Penetrating injuries of the oesophagus and pharynx caused by sticks thrown for dogs by the owners can be potentially life threatening and should be surgically explored as an emergency.

Oesophageal surgery

Oesophageal foreign bodies

Partial obstruction of the oesophagus with bones is common in terrier breeds and results in regurgitation of food and sometimes fluids. In cases where there is complete obstruction, dehydration is extremely rapid and hypovolaemia may be life threatening. These cases are always emergencies. The foreign body is usually retrieved by extraction via the mouth through a rigid endoscope, but occasionally bones may have to be pushed down into the stomach. Digestible foreign bodies (such as bones) are not removed from the stomach but plastic toys or balls have to be removed via a gastrotomy. Postoperatively, the patient is treated with drugs to reduce gastric acidity in case of gastric reflux, which will exacerbate oesophagitis. The oesophagus is also assessed for tears and inflammation, using the endoscope. Small tears or bruising may be treated with nil by mouth and food and water via a gastrostomy tube for 3–5 days. Severe full-thickness tears may have to be explored via a thoracotomy to prevent development of sepsis, and the prognosis may be poor.

Oesophageal stricture

This condition may arise as a result of trauma secondary to an oesophageal foreign body, but is also known to arise as a consequence of general anaesthesia. The animal presents 2–4 weeks after the initiating cause with a history of regurgitating all solid food. It is difficult to treat successfully. Therapy relies on stretching the stricture endoscopically and using steroid therapy to reduce the rate of recurrence of scar tissue. Animals may manage on a liquidized diet.

Gastric surgery

Foreign body

The cardinal sign of a gastric foreign body is persistent or intermittent vomiting. Diagnosis may be confirmed by radiography, contrast radiography or gastroscopy. Some foreign bodies may be retrieved endoscopically, but many will require surgical removal. The stomach is accessed via a cranial midline laparotomy and pulled out of the abdomen as far as possible. The rest of the abdominal organs are packed off with sterile moist towels or swabs to protect them from contamination. The incision is usually made in an avascular area of the body of the stomach. The whole stomach should be inspected for other foreign bodies and mucosal damage, prior to closure with a synthetic absorbable suture material.

Pyloric obstruction

This can be caused by a foreign body, but more often it is because of pyloric thickening, due either to hypertrophy of the muscle or to neoplasia. These diseases are often known as **gastric outflow diseases**, and congenital forms are more common in specific breeds such as brachycephalic dogs or Siamese cats. Once the diagnosis is confirmed, surgery is performed to either widen the pylorus (**pyloroplasty**) or to remove the pylorus altogether (**pyloric resection**).

Immediately postoperatively, small amounts of water are made available to the patient and then small quantities of a liquidized low-fat diet are offered 24 hours later. It is important to stimulate normal gastric motility without inducing vomiting, and some cases may have a gastrostomy tube placed at the time of surgery to help to decompress the stomach postoperatively for a few days.

Gastric dilatation–volvulus

This is a peracute rapidly fatal syndrome resulting from accumulation of food and gas in the stomach. The stomach dilates initially and this precipitates rotation of the stomach around its axis, resulting in occlusion of the oesophagus and the venous drainage. Severe hypovolaemic and toxic shock starts during the dilatation phase and escalates once rotation occurs. If not treated promptly, death results from the shock, gastric wall necrosis, ventricular dysrhythmias and disseminated intravascular coagulation (DIC). The specific aetiology is poorly understood, but usually the dogs are deep chested, often middle to older aged, and the condition may be associated with a nervous temperament. Preoperatively, nursing involves aggressive management of the shock and attempts to deflate the stomach either by passage of a stomach tube or by percutaneous needle gastrostomy (see Chapter 18).

Confirmation of rotation of the stomach is obtained with a right lateral abdominal radiograph (Figure 24.27) and indicates that surgical derotation is necessary.

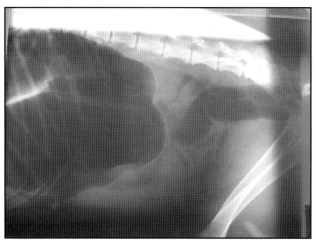

24.27 Right lateral abdominal radiograph of a dog with gastric dilatation–volvulus. The stomach can be seen hugely dilated with air and there is a characteristic fold of tissue crossing the dilated stomach, which indicates torsion.

Gastric dilatation–volvulus

1. Treat for shock with rapid administration of large volumes of intravenous fluids
2. Intravenous antibiotics
3. Decompression of the stomach via passage of a stomach tube
4. Right lateral radiograph to confirm volvulus
5. ECG – treat if necessary for ventricular dysrhythmias
6. Surgery for decompression, derotation and assessment of stomach wall viability.

Usually a gastrostomy tube is placed at the time of surgery to allow decompression of the stomach if there is reduced gastric motility postoperatively, and the tube may be used for feeding if the animal is moribund. In order to prevent recurrence of the rotation, a gastropexy may be carried out where the pylorus is anchored to the body wall with sutures, but this does not prevent the recurrence of dilatation. Postoperative nursing continues treatment of fluid and electrolyte losses and in particular monitoring and treating ventricular dysrhythmias.

Gastric neoplasia
Gastric neoplasms are often aggressive and may be very advanced before diagnosis. Clinical signs include haematemesis, weight loss and gastric pain. Some neoplasms can be resected if they are on the greater curvature of the stomach.

Tube gastrostomy
This is a useful tool for nutritional support (see Chapter 16) or decompression of the stomach. The tube is anchored in the stomach and exits through the body wall, where it is sutured to the skin and bandaged in place. The tube can be placed without surgery, using an endoscope to push the end of the tube through the skin (percutaneous endoscopic gastrostomy tube or PEG tube) or it is placed via a laparotomy. A mushroom-tipped catheter is usually used, although a Foley catheter may also be substituted (Figure 24.28). It is important to protect the tube from mutilation by the animal, particularly if the tube was placed endoscopically, as it is less secure in the stomach wall than if sutured. Tubes are removed by pushing a probe into the end of the mushroom tip to straighten out the tip and allow it to be pulled through the abdominal wall. They should not be removed too early (< 3 days) before a seal has formed around the hole in the gastric wall. The resultant wound in the body wall may leak gastric contents for 1–2 days, but is kept clean with skin antiseptics and allowed to granulate closed.

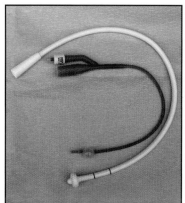

24.28 Depezzer (mushroom-tipped) and Foley catheters. These catheters can be used in situations where they need to be self-retaining (e.g. as a tube gastrostomy). To remove it, the Depezzer has to have the tip cut off, or straightened out. The Foley is removed by removing the fluid in the bulb.

Small intestine
Surgery on the small intestine (duodenum, jejunum and ileum) is common in small-animal practice. The intestines are lifted out of the abdomen during surgery so that other organs are not contaminated if gut contents spill (Figure 24.29). They should be kept moist using sterile saline-soaked swabs or towels, but this will mean that waterproof surgical drapes are necessary. Heat loss is rapid when the intestines are removed from the abdomen and it is necessary to provide a heating pad or warmed fluids.

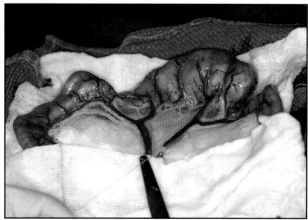

24.29 Intestinal surgery in a cat to remove a tumour in the small intestine (enterectomy). Note how the affected segment of intestine has been exteriorized from the abdomen and packed off with sterile swabs. The drapes underneath are also waterproof.

Biopsy

Intestinal biopsy is usually indicated when investigations of gastrointestinal signs such as persistent or recurrent vomiting or diarrhoea have been unrewarding. It is not possible to sample the jejunum or ileum via endoscopy and these have to be accessed via a laparotomy. Animals presented for intestinal biopsy may be poor candidates for surgery. Healing may be delayed due to hypoproteinaemia or cachexia. Small samples of intestine are taken from several sites all the way down the gastrointestinal tract and submitted in separate containers, each labelled with the site of the sample. All the biopsy sites are sutured closed and wrapped with omentum.

Postoperatively, the animal is encouraged to eat and drink as soon as possible in order to encourage rapid healing of the biopsy sites.

Enterotomy: foreign body removal

Foreign bodies in the cat small intestine are often linear, i.e. they are string, wool or thread-and-needle. The material may be lodged behind the back of the tongue or trapped at the pylorus and travel all the way down the GI tract into the small intestine. Smooth muscle contraction of the gut wall then concertinas the gut up the linear material and eventually either blocks the lumen or cuts through the wall of the intestine. Dogs more commonly ingest balls or plastic toys, which pass to a point along the jejunum and then become lodged.

Sometimes the foreign body can be palpated through the abdominal wall, but often radiography is necessary to make the diagnosis. The animal is stabilized and the foreign body removed via a laparotomy.

Usually the foreign body can be removed via a scalpel incision in the gut wall and then the hole is closed with synthetic absorbable sutures. Sometimes the gut is very inflamed and appears necrotic, in which case an enterectomy may be necessary.

Enterectomy

Enterectomy is indicated where the gut is necrotic or there is a tumour in the wall. A section of the gut is removed and then the ends are sutured together to form an **anastomosis**. The affected section of gut is separated off, using Doyen bowel clamps or just an assistant's fingers to prevent leakage from the remaining bowel, and then cut with a scalpel to remove it. Once it is removed, the cut ends are held close together while the surgeon sutures the edges, using synthetic absorbable suture material. Often the anastomosis is then wrapped in omentum to help to seal the surgical site. Postoperatively, healing is enhanced if the animal is encouraged to eat as soon as possible.

Intussusception

In this condition the small intestine invaginates into itself (like a telescope closing up). It is very rare in the cat, but usually seen in young dogs, often secondary to an episode of diarrhoea. The invaginated portion of intestine is called the **intussusceptum** and the outer part is the **intussuscipiens**. The blood supply to the intussusceptum is compromised and it often becomes necrotic. Symptoms are similar to those for intestinal obstruction and the diagnosis is usually made by radiography. Surgery to reduce the intussusception is necessary and if the intussusceptum is necrotic it is resected. Sometimes the disease recurs and the intestines may be sutured to each other (**enteropexy**) to prevent this.

Volvulus

Mesenteric volvulus is rarely reported in the dog and cat, though it is relatively common in horses. In all species it is rapidly fatal, due to endotoxic and hypovolaemic shock secondary to death of most of the small intestine.

Large intestine

Surgery of the large intestine carries greater risk than higher up the GI tract as there is an increased bacterial load and a slower rate of healing. Enemas near the time of surgery are detrimental to surgical asepsis as the slurry is more likely to spill and contaminate the abdomen. Preoperative oral antibiotics with anaerobic activity may help to reduce the bacterial load, but perioperative antibiotics are essential and should be continued postoperatively. Hospital feeding should be careful not to induce a dietary enteritis, i.e. easily digested protein sources may be better than high-protein diets, which may cause a nutritional diarrhoea. Often constipation or tenesmus is a sign of the disease and dietary fibre supplements and faecal modifiers, such as Isogel or Peridale (GSL), are used to increase faecal mass and increase peristalsis. Paraffin pastes or liquids are less suitable as they only lubricate the faeces and do not alter the water content or soften impacted faeces.

Biopsy

Biopsy samples of the rectum and distal colon can be taken using rigid proctoscopy, but these are only of partial thickness. Full-thickness samples are taken via laparotomy, and carry an increased risk compared with small-intestinal biopsy. Strict aseptic technique, packing off the uncontaminated viscera and thorough lavage of the abdomen at the end of the procedure are important.

Colectomy

Removal of the colon is most often indicated for the treatment of chronic constipation in cats. Cats present with multiple episodes of complete obstipation requiring enemas and evacuation each time. Eventually, the episodes become more frequent and the colon loses all function. It is important to check that the cat does not have an obstruction to defecation in the pelvic canal by rectal examination and radiography of the pelvis. Surgery involves careful identification and ligation of the vessels supplying the colon, and resection and reanastomosis of the colon ends. In animals that are severely affected, the ileocaecocolic valve may need to be removed as well. The animal is prepared for surgery with antibiotics, but an enema is not performed as it is easier to prevent contamination of the abdomen during surgery if the faeces are dry and hard and can be removed within the colon.

These animals are often inappetent postoperatively and early nutritional support is important to healing in the colon. Dehiscence of the anastomosis is often fatal.

Rectal polyps/tumours

Rectal polyps (**papillomas**) cause faecal tenesmus, bleeding and discomfort and are often treated initially as a colitis. Removal of the polyps is indicated because they are a premalignant change of the rectal mucosa. They can be removed by using a 'pull out' technique, where the rectum is everted through the anus to allow removal of the polyp (Figure 24.30). The defect should be sutured using monofilament absorbable material, and postoperative care is directed at reducing postoperative straining using analgesics, anti-inflammatories, local anaesthetic gel and dietary fibre. Where the tumour is identified as malignant or has invasive characteristics, a wider excision is carried out to remove the full thickness of the rectal wall.

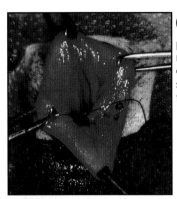

24.30 An intraoperative view of a rectal pull-out procedure to remove a rectal polyp. The everted rectal mucosa is stabilized using Allis tissue forceps.

Rectal prolapse

This is eversion of the wall of the rectum through the anus. It is usually secondary to chronic straining and may be associated with a rectal tumour. Successful management requires treatment of the primary disease as well as reduction of the prolapse itself. The prolapse should be protected from self-mutilation and kept moist and lubricated, using lidocaine gel. Once the rectum is reduced, it is maintained using a loose temporary purse-string suture around the anus. This may have to be loosened intermittently to allow defecation. Dietary faecal modifiers should be given to make the faeces soft and bulky.

Imperforate anus

This is a congenital condition where the anus fails to unite with the rectum, thus creating complete obstruction to the normal passage of faeces from the moment of birth. Sometimes it is possible to correct surgically.

Peritoneum

The peritoneum is the lining of the abdominal cavity and functions to help with healing of the intestinal tract and to protect it from infection if it becomes contaminated. Peritonitis occurs if there is contamination or irritation that results in an inflammatory response. Peritonitis can be due to surgical contamination, urine leakage from the bladder, intestinal content leakage due to perforation of any part of the GI tract, penetrating abdominal injury or leakage from the biliary or pancreatic systems. Initially, if there is no infection, peritonitis develops in response to the irritant nature of the fluid (e.g. urine or bile) and clinical signs may take a few days to develop. However, if the fluid is septic, or where there is leakage from the GI tract, the peritoneum becomes infected and this rapidly leads to severe illness, with septicaemia, shock and cardiovascular collapse within a few hours.

It is important for nurses to recognize peritonitis as part of postoperative monitoring of a patient, particularly after surgery on the GI tract. An animal may show some, or all, of the following clinical signs:

- Pyrexia
- Anorexia
- Depression
- Tachycardia
- Vomiting
- Ascites
- Abdominal pain.

The mainstay of treatment is to explore the abdomen surgically and find the source of contamination. In mild cases, or where there is no infection, thorough lavage of the abdomen may be sufficient. Where there is infection, the abdomen is best treated with open peritoneal drainage.

Abdominal lavage

Abdominal lavage involves pouring large volumes of warmed sterile isotonic fluids into the abdomen via a laparotomy and using suction to remove them until they come out clear. It is important to remove all the contaminated fluid to be effective and waterproof surgical drapes should be used.

1. Give thorough abdominal lavage using sterile isotonic fluids (Hartmann's or saline) at body temperature.
2. Repeat lavage until the fluids come out clear.
3. All lavage fluid must be removed from the abdomen, as remaining fluid reduces the ability of the immune system to clear remaining bacteria.
4. Use omentum to cover any potential sites of leakage.
5. Change the surgeon's gloves and instruments. Re-drape with sterile drapes over the top of the contaminated drapes (preferably with waterproof drapes).
6. Give a second dose of intravenous antibiotics. Do not use topical antibiotics or antiseptics in the abdomen.

Open peritoneal drainage

Open peritoneal drainage is a technique whereby the abdomen is not fully closed after the lavage and is dressed with sterile dressings and a thick absorbent bandage (or disposable nappies). This dressing is changed using sterile technique 2–3 times per day while the infection drains from the abdomen. At each dressing change, the abdomen may be lavaged again through the open wound. Nursing of these patients is very complex and involves close monitoring of blood albumin and electrolyte levels, hydration and care of the bandage.

Respiratory tract

Respiratory distress is potentially life threatening in any species and the veterinary nurse must be able to recognize respiratory difficulties quickly in order to respond with potentially life-saving first aid.

Respiratory difficulty arises from inadequate oxygen delivery to the tissues, which causes hypoxia. There are a number of ways this can come about:

- Obstruction to the passage of air into the respiratory tract (e.g. laryngeal paralysis, tracheal collapse, foreign body)
- Inefficient oxygen exchange at the air–tissue interface (e.g. pulmonary oedema, pneumonia)
- Inadequate blood supply to the alveoli, despite normal delivery of gases (ventilation perfusion mismatch) (e.g. pulmonary thromboembolism, right-sided heart failure)
- Inadequate oxygen-carrying capacity (e.g. severe anaemia, carbon monoxide poisoning)
- Inadequate blood delivery to the tissues (e.g. hypovolaemia, circulatory collapse).

The clinical signs of respiratory distress will develop from an initial increase in respiratory rate and effort to visible cyanosis of the mucous membranes, loss of consciousness and death:

- Increased respiratory rate at rest
- Increased respiratory effort (there may be visible 'heaving' of the ribs)
- Exercise intolerance
- Open-mouth breathing (particularly cats)
- Cyanosis of the tongue and gingiva
- Collapse.

First aid treatment is essential even for only mildly affected patients (see Chapter 18). Animals that show any signs of respiratory difficulty may suddenly decompensate when they are stressed during examination, and become profoundly hypoxic.

Respiratory distress

- Do not stress
- Keep patient away from other animals
- Monitor continuously
- Provide oxygen supplementation
- Sedate if necessary
- Keep the patient cool (this prevents panting and improves ventilation)
- Be prepared for emergency tracheostomy, CPR or endotracheal intubation for ventilation

Nasal disease

The dog and cat have different patterns of nasal disease, with the cat being predominantly affected by infectious agents causing acute or chronic rhinitis. Diagnosis of nasal disease can be very challenging and relies mainly on radiography, rhinoscopy, biopsy and in some cases MRI or CT scanning.

Rhinoscopy and biopsy

Rhinoscopy is used to visualize the nasal turbinates in order to take biopsies or look for a foreign body. Ideally a small rigid endoscope is used, but sometimes an auroscope is used or a small flexible endoscope to look behind the soft palate at the choanae.

Biopsy of the nose in most instances relies on radiographic diagnosis of a lesion and then taking a blind sample using biopsy forceps measured against the radiograph. In some cases, the sample may be taken using the rhinoscope to guide the biopsy forceps. Biopsy of inflamed turbinates causes profuse bleeding, and the pharynx must be packed. Usually pressure over the external nares is sufficient to arrest bleeding, but in severe cases adrenaline diluted to 1:100,000 may be sprayed up the nares to assist vasoconstriction of superficial vessels. Success in biopsy of nasal tumours often results in little haemorrhage.

Rhinotomy

Occasionally, it is necessary to open the nasal cavity to take biopsies, remove foreign bodies or remove a benign tumour. This is done via an incision on the bridge of the nose and the nasal cavity is accessed through the nasal bones. Postoperative complications can include emphysema of the head and neck due to air leaking out through the rhinotomy incision.

Nasal aspergillosis

This is a fungal infection of the nasal cavity usually seen in younger dolichocephalic breeds of dog. It causes a purulent nasal discharge and often causes epistaxis, which can be very severe. Diagnosis is made sometimes on biopsy or rhinoscopy, but it is more usually diagnosed with a blood test for the aspergillus antibodies. Treatment usually involves flushing the nasal cavity with an antifungal agent via tubes implanted through the frontal sinus. The flushing has to be done in the conscious animal so that there is no risk of the dog aspirating the drug into the lungs.

Nasal neoplasia

Nasal tumours tend to affect older dolichocephalic dogs and are most often carcinomas. In the cat, the Siamese may be more at risk and adenocarcinoma is the most common diagnosis, but lymphoma is also seen. The diagnosis is made by radiography and biopsy of the abnormal region seen on the radiograph. Surgical treatment is not usually an option and nasal tumours are treated with a course of radiotherapy.

Stenotic nares (BAOS)

Brachycephalic airway obstruction syndrome (BAOS) affects brachycephalic breeds with deformed airways, resulting in difficulty with breathing. The commonest breeds affected are Bulldog, Pekingese and Pug; occasionally Persian cats may be affected. The animal presents with noisy breathing, which results from a combination of obstructions to the upper airway:

- Stenotic nares
- Overlong soft palate
- Tonsillar hypertrophy
- Pharyngeal hypertrophy.

Some dogs may also have a collapsed larynx and a narrow trachea.

Severely affected animals may have exercise intolerance and episodes of cyanosis and syncope. Animals may present as an emergency in hot weather, when they may be suffering from heat stroke, dehydration, cyanosis and severe stress. Nursing requires oxygen supplementation, cooling, sedation and if necessary an emergency tracheostomy.

Surgical treatment depends on the most severely affected part of the airway: the stenotic nares can be widened and the tonsils and part of the soft palate resected to improve upper airway flow.

Laryngeal surgery

Surgery on the larynx is a complex procedure and can potentially result in severe difficulty during recovery due to mucosal swelling. The animal must be closely observed for signs of respiratory distress and facilities should be available for oxygen supplementation or emergency tracheostomy if necessary.

Laryngeal paralysis

This typically occurs in the older medium-sized breeds of dog. It is rarely seen in the cat. The disease results from paralysis of the recurrent laryngeal nerve, which means that the dog cannot abduct its arytenoid cartilages to open the airway on inspiration. The clinical signs range from increased noise on breathing when excited, panting on exercising, to cyanosis and collapse. These dogs often present in the summer when they are panting more to lose heat and the paralysed larynx becomes oedematous and swollen, thereby further reducing airflow. They may collapse and be brought into the practice cyanotic and struggling to breathe. In hot weather they may also have heat stroke.

In an acute situation, the animal may have to be anaesthetized so that the airway can be intubated and oxygen administered. Prior to recovery, the appropriate surgery is to 'tie back' the arytenoid cartilage so that it no longer obstructs the airway. If this is not possible, then it would be necessary to place a tracheostomy tube to bypass the larynx and allow the dog to breathe until surgery is possible.

Some breeds of dog are predisposed to laryngeal collapse, which is not amenable to laryngeal tieback and is treated with a permanent tracheostomy. The diagnosis is made on laryngoscopy. These dogs sometimes respond to weight loss and medical management.

Laryngeal tumours

These are rare, but also cause respiratory obstruction. Complete resection of the larynx is not very successful and there is little treatment possible, unless the tumour is sensitive to chemotherapy.

Trachea

The trachea is a rigid cartilaginous structure that prevents collapse of the airway when the animal creates negative pressure on inspiration.

Collapsing trachea

This is most often seen in toy or miniature breeds of dog, most notably the Yorkshire Terrier. The tracheal rings are not rigid, and when the dog is excited, or exercising, the trachea flattens and causes a harsh honking cough. Severely affected dogs may become cyanotic during coughing episodes, or even syncopal. Some dogs respond to medical management of weight loss, anti-inflammatories, antitussives and use of a harness rather than a collar. Dogs that are severely affected may require surgery to place rings around the outside of the trachea to provide a rigid support for the airway. There are other techniques that place the support on the inside of the trachea. The surgery is very complex and the postoperative period very risky, as the surgery can make the tracheal irritation worse.

Avulsion of the trachea

Typically this is seen in the cat after a road traffic accident. The trachea is torn apart usually quite distal within the thorax. The cat may initially appear normal, but becomes tachypnoeic over the first few days after the accident and may develop emphysema over the neck and shoulders. Surgical repair is urgent and involves a thoracotomy to re-anastomose the ends of the trachea. The surgery is technically difficult and the anaesthetic complicated by the fact that the cat requires IPPV during the surgery through a sterile endotracheal tube placed by the surgeon through the incision into the distal trachea. Postoperatively, a chest drain is placed to monitor for pneumothorax and the cat is closely monitored for signs of leakage from the anastomosis.

Tracheostomy

This may be temporary or permanent. It may be used for administration of anaesthetic gases during oral surgery or as a means of bypassing an obstructed upper airway. Most often it is used as a life-saving procedure in an emergency situation to bypass an obstructed upper airway.

Usually the airway is not completely blocked and administration of oxygen with a face mask provides some relief while the animal is prepared for tracheostomy. However, where the animal is unconscious or severely cyanotic, the veterinary nurse should be prepared to perform the tracheostomy using only local anaesthetic or no anaesthetic and no surgical preparation if the animal is likely to die with any delay. If airway obstruction is anticipated (e.g. after surgery on the upper airway), the ventral aspect of the neck may be prepared in readiness for an emergency tracheostomy. Tracheostomy tubes are illustrated in Figure 24.31.

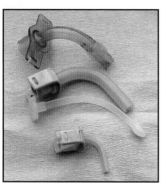

24.31 There are different types of tracheostomy tubes but all have a curved tube that enters through the skin into the trachea. The middle tube shown here also has a trochar that fits inside the tube. They are available in different sizes to accommodate different sizes of animal.

Emergency tracheostomy

1. Make sure that the oxygen delivery tube will fit the tracheostomy tube.
2. Clip and surgically prepare the ventral aspect of the neck.
3. Have a sterile surgical kit ready, together with the appropriate-sized tracheostomy tube, and suture material to open up the tracheal incision.
4. Suction may be necessary for the lower airway.
5. Prepare for postoperative monitoring.

Management of a tracheostomy tube

- Constant monitoring for at least the first 12–24 hours
- Regular suction of the tracheostomy tube every hour
- Humidification of the trachea by instilling 5–10 ml sterile saline into the tube every hour
- Changing the tracheostomy tube for a fresh sterile one every 2–6 hours, depending on the quantity of exudate.

Emergency airway

If an animal is very close to death and the materials are not immediately available, oxygen can be administered via a wide-gauge hypodermic needle or catheter pushed quickly through the ventral midline of the neck between the tracheal rings. This can then be used to administer oxygen via a narrow tube or urinary catheter.

Tracheal foreign body or neoplasia

Rarely an animal presents with obstruction of the trachea. If this is a foreign body, it may be removed under anaesthesia using endoscopic forceps. Small tumours can be removed by resection of some of the tracheal rings and re-anastomosing the trachea.

Lungs

Principles of thoracotomy

The thorax can be approached either by entering the cavity between the ribs (lateral or **intercostal thoracotomy**) or by splitting the sternum and approaching the thorax from the ventral aspect (sternal thoracotomy or **sternotomy**). If more access is required, a rib can be resected.

Intercostal thoracotomy is the commonest approach and allows the surgeon access to the lungs, heart, oesophagus and pleural cavity on one side only. The advantage of a sternotomy is that both sides of the chest can be explored at the same procedure. Sternotomy in large dogs requires the facilities to saw through the sternum. During the thoracotomy, the animal must be on IPPV continuously, and it should be monitored for heat loss and dehydration.

Following thoracotomy, great care is taken to close the incision with an airtight seal. A chest drain is used to remove the pleural air during closure and also postoperatively to monitor air or fluid leaks within the chest (Figure 24.32). A sterile drain is placed through a skin tunnel between the ribs and the other end is linked to a water seal, which allows continual aspiration of air, or it may be occluded and drained intermittently (see 'Drains', above).

Analgesia is very important after thoracotomy. It is also important to get large dogs up and moving around as soon as possible to reduce the risk of thromboembolism.

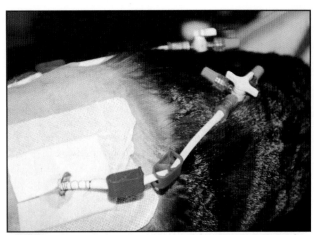

24.32 Chest drains placed in a cat for the treatment of pneumothorax. The drains are secured to the skin with a Chinese finger-trap suture. The drains should be further stabilized by a dressing and monitored continuously, as interference could be fatal. (Courtesy of C. Sturgeon)

Lung lobectomy

Lung lobes are removed via an intercostal thoracotomy as this gives the best access to the arteries, veins and bronchus. The vessels and bronchus may be ligated and oversewn manually or a lung lobectomy stapling device can be used to perform the procedure in one step. After the lung lobe has been removed, the bronchus is checked for air leaks by filling the chest with warm sterile saline, inflating the lungs, and looking for bubbles.

Pyothorax

This is an infection of the pleura in the thoracic cavity. It is commonly seen in cats probably secondary to cat bites, and in dogs probably due to migrating grass seeds. The animal presents with difficulty in breathing, due to large volumes of pus in the thoracic cavity. Mostly these cases are treated by placing thoracic drains in both sides of the chest and draining and lavaging the chest twice daily with sterile fluids and antibiotics. Persistent cases may require a thoracotomy to open up the chest cavity and debride infected tissue or look for the foreign body.

Cardiovascular system

Heart

Persistent ductus arteriosus (PDA)

This occurs when the ductus arteriosus fails to close at birth, and blood bypasses the lungs and left side of the heart, travelling from the pulmonary artery directly into the aorta. It creates a characteristic **heart murmur** that should be easily detected at the first vaccination check. If the condition is left untreated, the dog will eventually die from heart failure. The treatment is surgery via a left lateral thoracotomy to tie off the PDA. Alternatively, coils can be placed inside the PDA to occlude it.

Vascular ring anomaly

Congenital defects of the heart and great vessels sometimes occur and result in entrapment of the oesophagus between the ligamentum arteriosum (the remnants of the closed ductus arteriosum) and the other vessels. The commonest is a **persistent right aortic arch** (PRAA) when the aorta is found on the right side instead of the left and the ductus crosses the oesophagus and makes a constriction that prevents the normal passage of food on swallowing. The treatment is ligation and separation of the ductus from the surface of the oesophagus via a left-sided thoracotomy.

Arteries and veins

Vascular access: 'cut-down'

Intravenous treatments are usually given via an intravenous catheter placed in the cephalic vein. In patients that are very collapsed, dehydrated or in severe shock it can be very difficult to identify the superficial veins in order to place the catheter. If it is not possible to place a jugular catheter, a 'cut-down' technique may be used instead to access a vein. The area over the vein is clipped and prepared surgically and a tourniquet is placed above the vein to increase visibility. An incision is made directly over the vein, and careful dissection down through the tissue planes is used to identify the vessel. The catheter is then placed routinely, flushed with heparin–saline and usually sutured in place. The skin is sutured over the surgical site and the wound is dressed.

Aortic thromboembolism

This is a serious emergency condition, usually seen in the cat, when a blood clot (**embolism**) breaks off and travels down the aorta to block the iliac arteries at the end of the aorta. This completely blocks the blood flow to one or both hindlimbs. The hindlimbs are cold, stiff and very painful and there is no palpable femoral pulse. Occasionally the condition is responsive to medical management; and surgical removal of the thromboembolism has been reported, but is only rarely successful. The condition is usually secondary to heart disease and the prognosis is poor.

Emergency vessel occlusion

Vessels may be lacerated or ruptured during the course of surgery or as a result of severe trauma. If the event occurs during surgery, small arteries (< 2 mm) and veins (< 4 mm) can be sealed using electrodiathermy, or may stop bleeding with a few minutes of direct pressure. Large vessels are ligated or double ligated, using absorbable synthetic suture material with good knot security. There are also commercial staples available to seal arteries and veins during surgery.

Traumatic haemorrhage may have to be stemmed prior to identifying the specific vessel. If the bleeding is clearly arterial (pumping), surgical exploration and ligation of the artery is a priority. However, the bleeding may be profuse and non-specific. Initially direct hand-held pressure on the wound using a sterile pack of absorbent material may be sufficient to slow the bleeding. If the bleeding continues to be profuse, other options are a tourniquet above the site of bleeding on a limb, application of a very heavily padded bandage or immediate surgical exploration under anaesthesia. It is very important to time the duration of a tourniquet to prevent ischaemic necrosis. It is also important to remove the bandage as soon as possible, otherwise high pressure underneath the bandage may result in the same effect. Weighing the material used to absorb the blood before and after use will help in estimating blood loss.

Major arteries may be repaired if necessary and blood flow can be temporarily stopped during the repair using bulldog clips or a Rommel tourniquet. Very fine-gauge polypropylene suture material is usually used to repair arteries or veins, as it causes very little tissue reaction.

Endocrine system

Thyroid gland

Thyroidectomy (dog)
In the dog, thyroidectomy is usually carried out as treatment for thyroid carcinoma. Small tumours may be easy to remove, but they can be very vascular and may be attached to vital structures in the neck.

Thyroidectomy (cat)
Hyperthyroidism is a common condition of the older cat due to a thyroid adenoma (a benign tumour) which secretes excess thyroid hormone. It results typically in restlessness, weight loss, polyphagia and tachycardia. Some cats may also have concurrent kidney disease and heart failure. The thyroid gland may be palpated in the neck, or it may be diagnosed from a blood sample. Initially, the cat is usually stabilized using an orally administered antithyroid drug (carbimazole), but ultimately surgery to remove the affected thyroid gland or glands is a curative treatment. The main risk associated with surgery is damage to the parathyroid glands, which are closely attached to the cranial end of the thyroid gland. This results in loss of control of calcium metabolism, and hypocalcaemia develops in the first 2–3 days after surgery. If the damage is severe, the cat may need calcium supplementation intravenously and then orally for weeks until the parathyroid glands recover.

Adrenal glands
The adrenal glands in the dog and cat are sometimes removed as a treatment for hyperadrenocorticism (Cushing's disease) or phaeochromocytoma, where the adrenal gland is the primary source of the problem. Surgery involves deep dissection in the region of the dorsal abdominal vena cava, and there can be severe haemorrhage. The patient may have delayed wound healing due to the medical condition and should be closely monitored for wound dehiscence. Sudden hormonal changes in the postoperative period can also destabilize a patient and they should be closely monitored for electrolyte abnormalities, hypotension and vomiting/diarrhoea. Adrenal tumours are common in ferrets and often removed successfully.

Pancreas
The pancreas is a lobulated gland that is closely associated with the stomach and duodenum. The commonest disease is a sterile inflammation (pancreatitis), which causes severe abdominal pain and vomiting. This is not a surgical disease and surgical exploration will make the symptoms worse. Other conditions include pancreatic abscesses, damage due to abdominal trauma and pancreatic tumours.

Pancreatectomy
Abscesses and tumours may be removed by a partial pancreatectomy. If the lesion is in the body of the pancreas or involves the blood supply to the duodenum, it is generally considered inoperable. The commonest tumour of the pancreas is an **insulinoma**, which is a tumour that secretes excess insulin and causes hypoglycaemia. After the surgery, the animal has to be carefully managed to ensure that acute pancreatitis does not occur. No food or water is given by mouth for the first 48 hours, and hydration is maintained with intravenous fluids and electrolytes. Monitoring of the glucose levels is critical in postoperative management of insulinoma patients and they may need a glucose drip. When the animal is fed, it should initially be given small quantities of a low-fat diet.

Pancreatic biopsy
In some patients with chronic low-grade pancreatitis, it is difficult to diagnose the disease without biopsy. Ideally, this is performed via laparoscopy ('key-hole' surgery) to reduce the risk of a flare-up of the disease. Otherwise, a small piece of pancreas is removed via laparotomy and the patient is managed as above.

Liver
Liver disease can potentially result in a number of medical conditions that would adversely affect the success of surgery. Many patients may have low levels of albumin vitamin K and increased susceptibility to sedatives or anaesthetic drugs. Animals with suspected liver disease should always have blood-clotting times tested prior to surgery, and they may need a transfusion of fresh-frozen plasma. The liver also has remarkable powers of regeneration and can compensate for removal or damage to liver lobes.

Biopsy
The purpose of performing a liver biopsy is to achieve a specific diagnosis. It can be done either by laparoscopy or via a laparotomy incision. Usually, just a small piece of the edge of a liver lobe is removed, and normal clotting stops the bleeding spontaneously. Occasionally a Tru-Cut needle may be used with ultrasound guidance to obtain the sample.

Lobectomy
A whole liver lobe may need to be removed if it is diseased or damaged. The blood supply to the liver may be temporarily shut off using a small tourniquet during the surgery. Postoperatively, the animal must be monitored closely for haemorrhage into the abdominal cavity as this is the commonest complication of the surgery.

Portosystemic shunts
A portosystemic shunt (PSS) is a congenital or acquired vascular anomaly that redirects blood flow in the portal vein so that it bypasses the liver. The clinical signs include poor growth, abnormal behaviour a few hours after feeding (**hepatic encephalopathy**), seizures, urate calculi in the urinary tract and hypoglycaemia. The disease is usually diagnosed with blood tests and ultrasound scans of the liver. More detailed investigations such as a **portovenogram** (contrast material injected into a mesenteric vein) or contrast fluoroscopy may be necessary.

- Small breeds of dog are most commonly affected with **congenital shunts** that are usually single large vessels draining into the abdominal vena cava (**extrahepatic shunts**).
- Large breeds of dog are usually affected with **intrahepatic shunts**.
- **Acquired shunts** are seen in older dogs or cats and are related to the development of veins that bypass the liver secondary to chronic liver disease that obstructs the normal flow of blood in the portal vein.

Only congenital PSS is treated surgically. The patient is usually stabilized with medical management first and then the shunt is tied off with silk via a laparotomy, in one or more surgical procedures. Some referral centres use constrictor devices to occlude the shunt slowly, allowing the liver more time to adapt to the increased blood flow. Postoperative complications include abdominal pain, hypoglycaemia, diarrhoea, vomiting, hypotension, hypothermia, prolonged recovery time due to poor metabolism of anaesthetic drugs, seizures and shock.

Cholecystectomy

Cholangitis or **cholecystitis** (infection or inflammation of the biliary ducts and gall bladder) and **cholelithiasis** (stones in the gall bladder) may be treated by removal of the gall bladder. The surgery is carried out through a cranial midline laparotomy and the gall bladder is ligated and removed. The bile continues to drain into the duodenum through the bile duct, the only difference being that it does not collect in the gall bladder between meals. Postoperatively the animal should be treated with antibiotics, but abdominal drains are not necessary.

Spleen

The spleen is a large vascular organ in the abdomen on the left side next to the stomach. Although removal of the spleen in humans can result in the development of septicaemia, this has not been reported in dogs and cats and total splenectomy is not usually associated with any long-term problems.

Splenectomy

Indications for removal of the spleen include neoplasia, splenic torsion, trauma and haemorrhage. Haemangiosarcoma is the most common primary tumour of the spleen and some tumours will be metastases from elsewhere. Up to half of splenic tumours may be benign or even just haematomas, and so splenectomy can carry a good prognosis.

Sometimes patients present with acute haemorrhage from the spleen and splenectomy is performed as an emergency procedure. More often, the bleeding is intermittent and the spleen is removed as an elective procedure to prevent a haemorrhagic crisis. If the haemorrhage has been severe, the animal may require a blood transfusion prior to surgery; if the haemorrhage is due to trauma and not neoplasia, an **autotransfusion** of blood can be carried out. At the time of the laparotomy, the blood is suctioned via sterile apparatus out of the abdomen, mixed with the appropriate volume of anticoagulant, filtered and transfused into a peripheral vein. If there is any likelihood of neoplastic disease, autotransfusion should not be carried out.

Splenectomy may be performed using conventional surgical instruments and technique (Figure 24.33a) or using a stapler (Figure 24.33b).

The most common postoperative complication is haemorrhage as a result of displacement of a ligature in the abdomen. The patient needs to be closely monitored for signs of intra-abdominal bleeding.

Urinary tract

All surgery on the urinary tract runs the potential risk of acute renal failure if kidney function is affected and urine production stops postoperatively. Urine production should be maintained at a minimum of 2 ml/kg/hour using intravenous fluid therapy during the postoperative period. Urine needs to be collected and measured in order to calculate these figures, and diuretics or other treatments given if urine output is inadequate. Blood samples can also be analysed for urea, creatinine and electrolyte (potassium) levels, which also indicate renal function.

Kidney

The kidneys are **retroperitoneal**, which means that they lie outside the peritoneal cavity of the abdomen. They receive 25% of total cardiac output and are one of the vital organs of the body. Surgical handling or trauma that might disrupt the blood supply or cause the artery to spasm could potentially be life threatening.

Ureteronephrectomy

A kidney may be removed if there is severe trauma, neoplasia, **hydronephrosis** (enlargement of the kidney secondary to back pressure from the bladder), or severe **pyelonephritis** (infection). It is essential to be sure that the other kidney is functioning normally prior to this procedure, otherwise the animal may go into postoperative renal failure. The kidney is removed together with its ureter, which is traced all the way down to the bladder, and the arteries and veins are ligated. Postoperatively, intravenous fluids should be maintained until normal urine flow has been monitored and recorded.

Nephrotomy

Calculi can occasionally form in the kidney. These are very painful and result in severe secondary infections of the kidney, which may cause permanent damage. They are removed by a nephrotomy into the renal pelvis, when the calculus is removed and the incision repaired. Postoperative intravenous fluid therapy is important to ensure good urine production, along with close monitoring of blood urea and creatinine to check for evidence of urine leakage.

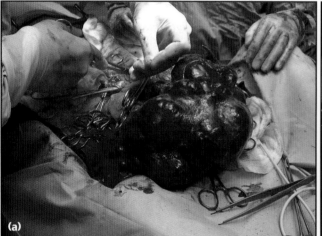
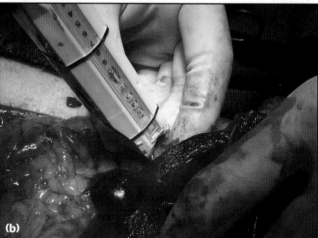

24.33 Splenectomy. **(a)** A splenectomy being carried out using conventional surgical technique, with hand-tied sutures and artery forceps for haemostasis. **(b)** A splenectomy being carried out using an LDS stapler. This is much faster but the LDS stapler is expensive.

Renal biopsy

Biopsy of the kidney can be performed, but this is only done after extensive investigation of the renal disease, as it carries considerable risks of haemorrhage and damage to renal function. Ideally, the sample is taken through a surgical incision, but sometimes it is done percutaneously using a Tru-Cut needle with ultrasound guidance. Postoperatively, pressure is used to stop bleeding and urine output is monitored with intravenous fluids and urinalysis.

Ureter

The ureters travel in the retroperitoneal space from the kidney to the bladder. They can be imaged using intravenous excretory urography or ultrasound examination, but are not seen on plain radiographs.

Avulsion of the ureter

Rarely, the ureter may be torn secondary to abdominal trauma. This causes urine leakage into the retroperitoneal space, causing cellulitis with electrolyte abnormalities. In some cases the damage can be repaired surgically, but often ureteronephrectomy is necessary. It is important to stabilize the animal with respect to renal and electrolyte parameters prior to anaesthesia.

Ectopic ureters

This is a congenital condition where one or both ureters implant distal to the bladder so that urine flows directly into the urethra. This results in a constant urinary incontinence, usually in a young dog. Golden Retrievers, Poodles and Labradors are most commonly affected. The condition is diagnosed using excretory urography and ultrasonography. The ureters are often enlarged and abnormal due to ascending infections. In some cases, the ascending infection results in severe pyelonephritis and a ureteronephrectomy is carried out. Where the ureter and kidney are healthy, it is possible to reimplant the ureter surgically into the bladder. Surgery on the ureter can result in spasm that causes the kidney to stop producing urine on that side for up to 48 hours. Ideally, therefore, if both ureters need surgery, one side should be done at a time. As in renal surgery, urine production is carefully monitored postoperatively. In some cases, the incontinence may persist due to other bladder abnormalities.

Ureteric entrapment

The ureters run down to the bladder and in the female pass the uterine body and cervix. At this position they are at risk of entrapment in the ligature during routine ovariohysterectomy. This is life threatening, particularly if both ureters are involved. If the ligature is removed within 7 days, little damage is done to the kidney and it should completely recover.

Bladder

Surgery on the bladder is common in veterinary practice. The bladder lies in the caudal abdomen and can be accessed via a midline laparotomy. The bladder should be emptied prior to surgery, either using a catheter via the urethra or using a small-gauge needle and syringe at surgery. The bladder wall is delicate and prone to oedema and bruising with rough handling, so it is usually held during surgery using stay sutures or fine forceps. Urine continues to collect in the bladder during surgery, so it is important to protect the other abdominal organs from contamination with the urine during cystotomy.

Cystotomy and cystectomy

The commonest indications for cystotomy are to remove calculi (stones) or tumours. Usually, the incision in the bladder wall is made in the ventral aspect and more stay sutures may be placed lateral to the incision to help to open up the bladder for inspection. Sometimes the calculi are located well down the bladder neck and it may be necessary to place a urethral catheter and flush them into the bladder with sterile saline. For removal of neoplasms, the full thickness of the bladder wall is cut away with a margin around the tumour, and the bladder reconstructed. The incision is closed in two layers using a synthetic absorbable suture material. Postoperatively, the animal should be given the opportunity to empty the bladder as frequently as possible and monitored for normal urination and evidence of urine leakage (uraemia, hypothermia, abdominal pain) for 3–4 days.

Bladder rupture

This occurs either secondary to blunt abdominal trauma or because prolonged urethral obstruction is causing severe back pressure and accumulation of urine. Occasionally bladder rupture occurs when attempts are made to express the bladder manually in paralysed patients. The condition may be diagnosed from the history, absence of urine in the bladder or using diagnostic imaging. The immediate concern is the uroperitoneum and the metabolic consequences of the absorption of urine from the peritoneum. There may be uraemia, electrolyte imbalances, dehydration and shock, which may have to be treated prior to surgery. At surgery, the abdomen should be lavaged with sterile saline to remove urine and contaminants, and the bladder is repaired. Postoperatively, blood urea levels and urine production should be closely monitored.

Tube cystostomy (urinary diversion)

This is the placement of a drain through the abdominal wall in order to drain the bladder, bypassing the urethra. This may be used as a temporary measure prior to urethral surgery or after bladder or urethral surgery to divert urine flow. It can also be used for diversion of urine in patients with urethral obstruction due to tumours, or paralysis of the bladder. A Foley catheter is drawn into the abdomen through a stab incision lateral to the midline (Figure 24.34). The tip is placed into the bladder, the balloon inflated with sterile saline and the catheter secured with sutures and omentum. The catheter is then secured to the outside of the body wall with sutures or zinc oxide butterfly tapes. In the hospital, this should be attached to a closed

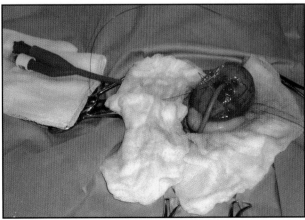

24.34 An intraoperative view of a bladder exteriorized for placement of a cystostomy tube using a Foley catheter.

urine collection system to prevent the risk of ascending infections. In long-term use, the bladder is emptied at least four times daily by removing a bung from the end and attaching a syringe. When the drain is removed, the tip should be submitted for culture and then appropriate antibiotics used to treat any associated infection. Use of antibiotics while the drain is in place will not prevent infection and only increases the likelihood of resistant strains developing.

Urethra

Surgery on the urethra is most often done secondary to damage caused by calculi. Preoperatively, the systemic consequences of urethral obstruction may need to be addressed prior to anaesthesia and often a urinary catheter is passed before surgery to make identification of the urethra easier.

Urethral obstruction

Blockage of the urethra in any species results in accumulation of urine in the bladder which if not relieved causes back pressure on the kidneys and then bladder rupture. The urine spills into the abdomen and causes uraemia and death. The clinical signs may be severe abdominal pain with persistent straining to urinate.

Animals straining to urinate should be checked as an emergency to assess the bladder.

The cat is usually more severely affected than the dog, which may have only partial obstruction.

The urethra in the female is short and wide and unlikely to obstruct except secondary to neoplastic growth. In the male dog and cat the urethra is narrower, particularly at the tip in the male cat and at the level of the os penis in the male dog. This anatomical characteristic makes it prone to obstruction by urinary calculi. The type of stone that blocks the urethra depends on the disease and it should always be submitted for analysis in order to determine the most appropriate prophylactic treatment for the future.

Male cats also develop obstruction of the urethra secondary to feline lower urinary tract disease (FLUTD) and in these cases, the obstruction is not always due to a calculus, but can be a mucoid plug.

The priority is to stabilize the animal with intravenous fluids and to decompress the bladder. If a urinary catheter cannot be passed, then it may be necessary to empty the bladder by cystocentesis. Once the pressure is reduced, it may then be possible to pass a catheter or to flush the urolith or plug back into the bladder with sterile saline (**retropulsion**). If it is not possible to remove the calculus in this way, urethrotomy is necessary.

Cystocentesis

1. Sedation is only necessary in very fractious animals, but analgesia should be provided.
2. The distended bladder is identified as a hard mass in the caudal abdomen.
3. A small area of skin on the ventrolateral abdomen directly over the bladder is clipped and surgically prepared.
4. A 20 gauge needle of the appropriate length for the size of animal is selected and attached to a 20 ml syringe via a three-way tap.
5. Sterile gloves are put on or a short hand scrub is performed.
6. The bladder is gently held still with one hand and the needle is introduced into the bladder through the prepared area of skin. ▶

7. The urine is drawn off and the three-way tap is used to expel the urine into a bowl. This is repeated until the bladder feels empty.
8. The volume of urine is recorded.

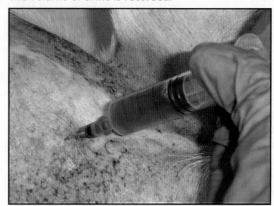

(Photo courtesy of S Chandler)

Urethrostomy

In some circumstances, either the cause of the urethral obstruction cannot be treated (e.g. calcium oxalate crystals) or the tip of the urethra is so damaged that it is prone to recurrent obstruction. In these cases, it may be necessary to create a new opening for urination through a wider part of the urethra. In the dog this is done at the level of the scrotum. In an intact male dog, castration and scrotal ablation are performed and then an incision into the urethra at that level is sutured to the skin edges (**scrotal urethrostomy**). In the male cat, the penis is amputated and the urethra is opened out and sutured to the skin edges (**perineal urethrostomy**). A urinary catheter should not be placed after surgery, and it is extremely important that the animal does not lick at the site at any stage during the healing process. Initially, there may be considerable bleeding associated with urination and it may be easier to hospitalize the patient until this has reduced. Nursing involves keeping the site clean and free of urine or blood, and preventing urine scald until the animal learns how to reposition during urination.

Urethral rupture

The urethra is exposed to damage in the male dog as it runs down the perineum and inguinal area, and in all animals as it runs through the pelvic canal. The most common cause of rupture is trauma to the pelvic area and it is often seen secondary to pelvic fractures. The urine leaks out of the urethra and can cause severe inflammation of the pelvic tissues. Reabsorption of the urine then causes changes in the blood biochemistry such as uraemia and hyperkalaemia, which cause systemic illness. If the tear is small, the urethra may be treated with placement of a soft silicone indwelling urinary catheter, allowing it to heal by second intention. Larger tears or complete ruptures (avulsion) should be repaired surgically once the animal has been stabilized for the anaesthetic. Urine is then diverted through a cystostomy tube until the site is healed.

Urethral neoplasia

This is more common in the bitch than the dog and is occasionally seen in the cat. It usually presents with acute obstruction to urination, though there may be a history of cystitis. Surgery can be performed to try to remove the urethra and reconstruct it using part of the vagina, but the prognosis is very poor.

Urinary incontinence

Incontinence is most common in the bitch. It has to be investigated in order to determine the primary cause or causes:

- Ectopic ureters
- Pelvic bladder
- Short bladder neck
- Urinary tract infection
- Urinary sphincter mechanism incompetence (USMI).

The only condition that has to be treated surgically is ectopic ureters. The other conditions often present in a slightly older bitch, or in the young bitch after spaying. They may respond to medical management, but occasionally surgery is necessary to try to reposition the bladder neck to increase the pressure around the sphincter, and thereby increase the holding capacity of the bladder and reduce incontinence. This is specialist surgery. Postoperative care involves carefully monitoring for urinary tract infections and ensuring that there is no retention of urine.

Incontinence in the male dog is usually secondary to prostatic disease. Castration may make the incontinence worse and it is very difficult to treat successfully either with drugs or with surgery.

Reproductive system

Testes

The testes are the reproductive organ producing spermatozoa in male animals. They should normally descend after birth into the scrotum and remain externally located.

Elective castration (orchidectomy)

Castration may be carried out for therapeutic reasons (treatment of orchitis, perineal hernia, anal adenoma, testicular tumours or prostatitis), social reasons or as part of a neutering programme. Occasionally, castration is recommended to control behavioural abnormalities or difficulties such as roaming, excessive libido or aggression. Castration in the tomcat is usually carried out to prevent territorial spraying.

Castration in the cat is usually carried out via an incision in the scrotum; the testis is pulled out gently and then either ligated with suture material or the vas deferens and vascular bundle are tied in a knot to secure haemostasis. The vascular bundle is released into the scrotum and the procedure repeated on the other side. The cat is observed postoperatively for signs of haemorrhage, and then discharged with instructions for a litter tray to be used with shredded newspaper for 2–3 days. The wounds in the scrotum are not sutured, but allowed to heal by second intention.

Castration in the dog can be carried out either through a pre-scrotal midline incision or via scrotal ablation. **Pre-scrotal castration** involves pushing the testes forwards into the single incision and then the arteries and veins are ligated before removal of each testis. The skin incision is sutured closed, and the scrotum is left in place. **Scrotal ablation** involves removal of the scrotum and then the testes are removed with ligation as described above directly through the scrotal area. The skin is sutured closed. Pre-scrotal castration is quicker but leaves an unsightly scrotal sac behind and risks seroma or haematoma formation in the scrotum. Scrotal ablation takes longer, but has fewer complications associated with the healing of the surgical site.

Postoperatively, it is important that the owner is warned not to let the dog lick the sutures and that the dog is monitored for signs of ventral abdominal or scrotal swelling or bruising that might indicate ligature slippage.

Retained testes (cryptorchidism)

Failure of one or both testes to descend is an inherited condition (see Chapter 25). It is more common in small-breed dogs, and is very rare in the cat. Both the retained testis and the descended testis are at risk of the development of neoplasia and they should be removed. Owners should be encouraged not to breed from affected animals.

The retained testis may be found at any point from the kidney down through the inguinal canal to just above the scrotal sac. The path is carefully explored surgically to locate the testicle, which is then removed in the standard way. The removed testis should be submitted for analysis to confirm that the correct tissue was removed.

Testicular neoplasia

These tumours are relatively common and are usually seen in older dogs. There are three main tumour types:

- Sertoli cell tumour (SCT)
- Seminoma (SEM)
- Interstitial cell tumour (ICT).

Sertoli cell tumours are more likely to metastasize than the other types to the lymph nodes, lung or liver. Sometimes SCT or SEM can cause a paraneoplastic syndrome associated with the production of hormones. Usually a feminization syndrome is seen that causes hair loss, **gynaecomastia** (enlarged mammary glands), prostatitis, atrophy of the unaffected testis and a pendulous prepuce, and the dog may become attractive to other male dogs. More severely affected dogs may also have bone marrow suppression, causing changes such as anaemia. Treatment with castration should carry a good prognosis.

Prostate

The prostate gland completely regresses after castration and should not develop disease later in life. Uncastrated dogs may develop prostatic disease secondary to the influence of the hormone testosterone. Symptoms may include infertility, impotence, incontinence, dysuria, haematuria, caudal abdominal pain and faecal tenesmus. The prostate can be examined by caudal palpation of the abdomen or rectal examination. Ultrasonography and radiography are also useful. Samples of the prostate gland can be taken by needle aspirates through the abdomen, alongside the rectum or via a urinary catheter. Ejaculation samples will also give some information about the fluid that the prostate is secreting.

Benign prostatic hyperplasia (BPH)

This occurs in the older male dog, when the prostate becomes acutely enlarged and very painful. It may be secondarily infected. Castration may be indicated to prevent recurrence. Anti-testosterone drugs can also be used (delmadinone acetate).

Prostatic cysts and abscesses

If BPH persists the prostate may develop cysts or abscesses, which can become enormous. Prostatic abscesses may be life threatening, presenting with toxaemia and systemic disease similar to pyometra in the bitch. Cysts and abscesses should be operated on before they rupture and cause peritonitis. The approach is through a midline laparotomy; the abscess or cyst is drained and lavaged with sterile fluids until clean, and then packed with omentum before routine closure.

Prostatic neoplasia

Cancer can develop in the prostate gland of older dogs, whether castrated or entire. The gland is very painful and has similar signs to other prostatic diseases. Prostatic carcinoma rapidly spreads to the adjacent lymph nodes and sometimes the vertebral bodies. The prognosis is poor. Prostatectomy is unsuccessful at achieving a cure and results in complete urinary incontinence.

Penis

Amputation

Penile amputation is indicated where there is severe trauma to the penis or if there is neoplastic disease. The penis is extremely vascular and the procedure should be done under a tourniquet. Usually the whole of the os penis is removed and the urethra is reconstructed at the end of the inguinal part of the penis.

Mucosal eversion

Occasionally, hypersexed dogs may present with mucosal eversion of the tip of the urethra on the end of the penis. The mucosa is very vascular and bleeds because of the trauma. Castration may help, but usually the mucosa has to be resected from the end of the penis. Again it helps to use a tourniquet during surgery and then absorbable fine-gauge suture material is used to resuture the mucosa at the end of the urethra. Postoperatively there may be some bleeding, and wadding may be used inside the prepuce to help to provide gentle pressure to stop this.

Ovaries and uterus

Elective ovariohysterectomy (spay)

In the UK, female companion animals are usually neutered (removal of the uterus and ovaries) to prevent unwanted litters and prevent oestrous activity. Bitches are also neutered to decrease the risk of development of mammary tumours; the best effect of this is seen if the bitch is neutered before the first season. Bitches, rabbits and ferrets are also neutered to prevent the development of pyometra (uterine infection) later in life.

The ovaries are identified and the arteries tied off before cutting the ovarian ligament. Then a ligature is placed around the uterine stump as close to the cervix as possible, to tie off the uterine arteries, before removal of the whole of the genital tract. The most important part of the procedure is to ensure that the ovaries are removed intact and no remnants are left behind that might secrete hormones. In some countries, only the ovaries are removed (**ovariectomy**); this is a shorter procedure and there is no documented increased risk of uterine disease. Bitches and exotic pets are usually operated on from the midline, but in the UK cats are usually operated on from the left flank approach lying in lateral recumbency. There is some suggestion that spaying increases the likelihood of urinary incontinence in some breeds of dog, but this is not certain and is only likely if there is already an underlying bladder abnormality.

Postoperative analgesia and observation are important. The wound should be observed for signs of bleeding or bruising, and the recovery monitored. Any postoperative spay patient that has a prolonged recovery from anaesthesia should be assessed for the possibility of intra-abdominal haemorrhage. Pale mucous membranes, generalized weakness, a rapid thready pulse, hypothermia, or bleeding from the laparotomy wound or vagina are all symptoms that should be investigated. Postoperative instructions relate to wound care and restricted activity to prevent dehiscence of the abdominal repair.

Pyometra

This is the accumulation of pus in the uterus (Figure 24.35), which may be infected or sterile. It occurs most commonly in middle- to older-aged animals that have never had a litter. It is potentially life threatening and often presents as an emergency. Affected animals may be depressed and polydipsic and may have a history of abnormal or more frequent oestrus. They may have a fever and often vomit. If the cervix is open (**open pyometra**), there is a vaginal discharge and they may be less ill than when the cervix is closed (**closed pyometra**) and all the pus is retained in the uterus.

The animal may be in severe toxaemic shock and will often require intensive fluid therapy before being fit for anaesthesia. Ovariohysterectomy is needed as a life-saving procedure as soon as the animal is stable enough for surgery. Intensive nursing is required in the postoperative phase to ensure that recovery from the toxaemia and renal function are complete after the removal of the infected uterus. Fluid therapy should continue until renal function and urine output are normal.

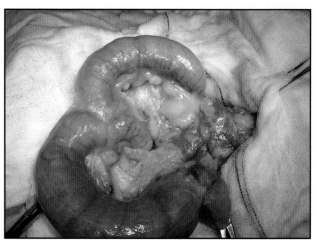

24.35 Intraoperative view of a pyometra. The uterus is grossly swollen and very vascular.

Caesarean operation

This is necessary when a bitch or queen presents with dystocia (see Chapter 25). The caesarean may be necessary if the animal is not able to progress with normal birth (e.g. hypocalcaemia, uterine inertia) and is not responding to medical management, or sometimes the fetus becomes stuck or dies in the birth canal and caesarean operation is carried out to save the remaining litter.

Any attempts to assist the animal to deliver the fetuses per vagina must be carried out under strict aseptic conditions to reduce the risk of post-delivery infections. Generally, the decision is made based on the possibility of live offspring and the duration of the labour so far.

Usually caesarean operation is carried out under general anaesthetic, but epidural anaesthesia is the technique of choice where the facilities are available. Preparation for the caesarean operation focuses around the provision of enough personnel to resuscitate the puppies or kittens (see Chapter 18). Most veterinary surgeons use a midline approach to the abdomen, despite the possibility of interference with the sutures by the young. Preparation of the abdomen for aseptic surgery must be thorough, but the use of antiseptics that might cause dermatitis around the mammary glands should be avoided. The incision is closed routinely, though some surgeons may use a subcuticular closure so as not to have skin sutures in the region where the offspring will be suckling.

Postoperative care involves close monitoring of the recovery from anaesthesia, and prevention of hypothermia. Regular postoperative checks are necessary to ensure that the dam is suckling and caring for the litter, despite the stress of hospitalization and surgery. Many cases will be discharged to their home environment as soon as possible after recovery and monitored with home visits. It is particularly important that the owner is given advice on postoperative nutrition of the dam and that frequent small meals are offered in the early stages postoperatively. Often these patients will develop a transient diarrhoea due to hormonal influences as well as eating placentae. The litter and bedding must be kept as clean as possible to prevent postoperative sepsis.

In some circumstances, an ovariohysterectomy will be performed at the same time as the caesarean operation. This is not ideal but is sometimes indicated where there is uterine rupture or risk of recurrent unwanted pregnancy (e.g. in 'stray' animals).

Neoplasia

Older animals may develop tumours of the ovaries or uterus. These can be very aggressive, but some are benign. Ovariohysterectomy is indicated.

Vagina

The vagina is usually only affected by disease in the entire bitch or queen. It rarely causes problems after neutering.

Hyperplasia

Vaginal hyperplasia is seen most often in brachycephalic breeds. The vaginal mucosa has an exaggerated hyperplastic response to the oestrogens secreted during oestrus, and excessive folds of vaginal mucosa protrude through the vulva. It often has the appearance of a tumour, but it regresses at the end of oestrus. The exposed mucosa must be kept clean and lubricated with K-Y1 jelly. Treatment to prevent recurrence is by ovariohysterectomy.

Prolapse

Vaginal prolapse is less common than hyperplasia, but occurs in the same breeds. Mild prolapses may not require treatment other than protection of the exposed mucosa. Spontaneous regression should occur during the dioestrous period.

Neoplasia

Neoplasia of the vulva and vagina is seen occasionally. Most large fibrous tumours identified in the wall of the vagina are leiomyomas, and are infiltrative hard nodules usually in the dorsal vaginal wall. The tumours are removed using an episiotomy to access the vaginal lumen from the perineum, and the bitch is also neutered. The urethra should be catheterized during surgery, so that the urethral orifice can be identified during the resection. Neoplasms of the vulva tend to be more aggressive carcinomas or mast-cell tumours and require complex surgery for removal and reconstruction.

Hernias and ruptures

- A **hernia** is an abnormal protrusion of an organ or organs through a physiological opening in the lining of the cavity in which it is normally enclosed.
- A **rupture** is a pathological tear in the lining of the cavity through which enclosed organs may protrude.

Most hernias and ruptures affect the abdominal cavity, but a few occur elsewhere. An example outside the abdomen includes herniation of the occipital or temporal lobes of the brain under the bony tentorium cerebelli as a complication of space-occupying lesions of the cranium.

The openings through which a hernia may occur are either a normal opening that has enlarged to allow organs through (e.g. inguinal canal), or an opening that should have closed during normal development (e.g. umbilicus). Hernias and ruptures share some characteristics in terms of the risks associated with the protrusion of viscera; however, as hernias are physiological, they are usually lined by an outpouching of the cavity lining (e.g. the peritoneum). Ruptures are not lined and the cavity lining is ruptured along with the body wall.

Hernias and ruptures are further described by the following terms:

- **Reducible** – the contents of the hernia or rupture can be replaced in the original anatomical location by gentle pressure on the swelling to push the viscera back through the defect itself
- **Irreducible** or **incarcerated** – the contents of the hernia or rupture cannot be replaced, usually because of the formation of adhesions in chronic cases
- **Strangulated** – the contents of a hernia or rupture can become devitalized due to entrapment of the blood vessels passing through the defect. Strangulation is life threatening and a serious emergency.

Umbilical hernia

This is a congenital condition where the umbilicus fails to close over properly and so fat and abdominal contents protrude through under the skin. Small hernias are of no consequence as they usually do not increase in size as the puppy grows. Large hernias should be repaired, due to the risk of incarceration of small intestine or other abdominal organs.

Inguinal hernia

Herniation occurs through the inguinal canal, which is a physiological opening in the muscle of the caudal abdominal wall. It is more common in females than males, particularly in elderly overweight small-breed dogs. In the bitch a swelling may be seen in the groin extending towards the vulva. The hernia may contain fat in the broad ligament, uterus, intestines or bladder. If the bitch is pregnant, the gravid uterus can become strangulated. In male dogs, fat or intestine may herniate into the scrotal sac and can become strangulated because of the small opening.

The hernia should be scanned or X-rayed to determine what structures are in the hernia. The owner should be warned about the possibility of strangulation. All hernias should be surgically corrected and the inguinal canal narrowed to prevent recurrence. Ideally the animal should also be neutered.

Perineal hernia

Perineal hernia occurs almost exclusively in older male dogs. It is associated with degeneration of the muscles of the pelvic diaphragm (coccygeus and levator ani). Affected dogs have difficulty defecating and have an obvious swelling on one or both sides of the anus (Figure 24.36). The swelling is associated with impaction of faeces in the rectum as well as herniated abdominal contents. An important complication of perineal hernia is retroflexion and incarceration of the bladder and prostate. This can result in acute urethral obstruction and is an emergency.

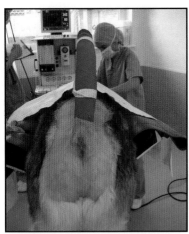

24.36 A bilateral perineal hernia. The perineal area is swollen with herniated contents of the caudal abdomen. Faeces are sometimes impacted in the caudal rectum, contributing to the perineal swelling. Rectal examination confirms the absence of the pelvic diaphragm.

There are a number of surgical techniques described for hernia repair that involve apposing the remains of the atrophied muscles using a monofilament long-lasting suture material (e.g. PDS or polypropylene). Some techniques also involve transferring muscle flaps to help support the hernia repair and these techniques are usually more successful. All dogs are castrated to help to prevent recurrence.

Pre- and postoperative nursing
Preoperatively, the animal should be assessed for bladder position and the possibility that the bladder could be retroflexed into the hernia, obstructing the urethra. If there is doubt, the hernia may be radiographed or the urethra catheterized in order to empty the bladder. Sometimes the bladder has to be emptied by cystocentesis before it can be catheterized or reduced. The surgical site is considered contaminated and peri- and postoperative antibiotic cover is required. Before the surgical preparation, the rectal sacculation is manually emptied of faeces and a purse-string suture is placed to prevent faecal material contaminating the surgical site during surgery. Enemas are not used as they may result in a loose slurry that could easily spill into the surgical site. Postoperatively, the purse-string is removed and faecal modifiers (Sterculia, Isogel) are given in the food to prevent straining against the hernia repair and also to improve rectal function. Bilateral hernia repairs sometimes develop rectal prolapse, which requires a loose purse-string suture around the anus for a few days until the anus regains normal tone.

Diaphragmatic hernia
Diaphragmatic rupture is most commonly associated with trauma such as a road traffic accident, causing a sudden increase in abdominal pressure when the glottis is closed. The diaphragm tears either around the edge (**circumferential**) or across from the centre to the edge (**radial**). The loss of a functional diaphragm makes breathing more difficult and this is coupled with herniation of abdominal contents such as intestine, liver, spleen or stomach into the pleural space. The trauma may also have caused **pulmonary contusion** (bruising of the lungs) which adds to the animal's respiratory distress. Some cases are missed at the time of the original trauma and may present months later with dyspnoea when more abdominal contents herniate through into the chest.

Congenital defects in the diaphragm are also seen, the commonest of which is the pericardial–peritoneal diaphragmatic hernia. In this condition, the ventral portion of the diaphragm is absent and abdominal contents herniate into the mediastinum (not the pleural space). Often the animal also has a large umbilical hernia.

All diaphragmatic hernias are repaired surgically. Congenital defects are repaired as elective procedures, but ruptures may need to be operated on as an emergency if the stomach is in the chest and it begins to dilate. Ideally the animal should be stabilized after the accident to improve the anaesthetic risk, but in some cases the dyspnoea is so severe that immediate surgery is necessary. The tear is sutured closed using long-lasting absorbable suture material. Chronic cases may be difficult to reduce, due to adhesions to the pleura; also, due to contraction of the abdominal muscles, the abdomen may be difficult to close once all the abdominal contents are returned. A chest drain may be necessary, particularly in chronic cases where there may be a pleural effusion.

Pre- and postoperative nursing
Preoperative nursing focuses on provision of supplementary oxygen, reducing stress on handling, analgesia and treatment of shock. The nurse should be prepared to provide IPPV during the anaesthesia and to monitor for sudden changes in blood pressure when the abdominal viscera are moved back into the abdomen. A catheter may be used to aspirate air out of the thorax as the rupture is closed, or a chest drain may be used. Postoperatively, the animal should be watched carefully for signs of discomfort associated with increased abdominal pressure and evidence of continuing difficulty with oxygenation due to pulmonary contusions. Some cats may be inappetent after surgery, due to liver damage.

Prepubic tendon or abdominal wall rupture
This condition is usually seen as a consequence of abdominal wall trauma, most commonly a road accident, but also due to a blunt blow such as a kick. There may be other injuries associated with the trauma. Usually there is an extensive area of severe bruising over the rupture and the associated subcutaneous swelling.

The rupture is repaired surgically using long-lasting absorbable materials such as PDS. Very macerated muscle tissue may not repair easily and a synthetic mesh might be necessary to replace devitalized muscle. Where the prepubic attachment is ruptured, wire sutures may be used to reattach the ventral abdominal wall to the pubic bone.

Pre- and postoperative nursing
The animal should be stabilized and given analgesia prior to surgical repair. If the bladder is in the rupture, urine production should be closely monitored or the animal catheterized to ensure that the bladder neck is not entrapped. Analgesia is important as the abdominal wall is often very bruised. Anti-inflammatories may help with resolution of bruising, as well as padded bedding and cage rest. Faecal modifiers should be given to assist with defecation so that the animal does not strain and put pressure on the abdominal repair. Animals that require a mesh implant should be closely monitored for signs of infection or sinus tracts associated with the implant. Postoperative exercise is restricted and the animal should be prevented from jumping up or stretching the abdomen.

Musculoskeletal system

Tendon and muscle repair
Tendon and muscle damage are usually secondary to trauma, unless a myotomy or tenotomy has been performed as part of a surgical approach to a joint.

Muscle damage is usually repaired as soon as possible after injury, using absorbable monofilament material. Trauma to muscle often results in very macerated fragile tissue and it can be difficult to reappose successfully. Normal healthy muscle heals quickly after a myotomy as it has a good blood supply.

Tendons heal very slowly and have to be supported to ensure that they do not stretch and lose function. Orthopaedic implants may be used to protect the tendon until it has fully repaired and remodelled.

Limb amputation

Amputation is an unfortunate but not infrequent surgical procedure in all of the companion animals. It is a very difficult concept for many owners to come to terms with and they may need special counselling and advice. Most animals cope with amputation much better than the owner will expect (Figure 24.37) and some may even be walking and running within hours of anaesthetic recovery.

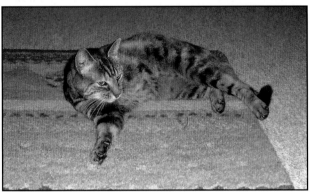

24.37 Animals frequently tolerate limb amputation remarkably well, as long as the remaining three limbs are free of any other orthopaedic or neurological disease. This cat has had her left forelimb amputated yet lives a full and normal life.

Amputation may be recommended for the following reasons:

- Curative removal of a benign tumour (e.g. haemangiopericytoma)
- Palliative removal of a malignant but very painful tumour (e.g. osteosarcoma)
- Injury to the distal limb that is beyond repair (e.g. shear injury)
- Nerve root avulsion resulting in permanent paralysis of the limb
- Economic reasons, if the complex fracture or soft tissue injury is too expensive for repair.

The most important aspect of assessment of a patient for amputation is establishing that the other three limbs are fit and free of arthritic or other disease. On admission it is very important to check and state on the consent form exactly which limb should be amputated. Obese patients or very large breeds may not be suitable candidates for amputation as they will have difficulty shifting the centre of gravity over to the remaining legs and may be less agile.

Postoperative nursing

Postoperative nursing is important to help these patients to their feet as soon as possible so that they can quickly adapt to a new gait. Walking must be assisted if the floor is slippery or else rubber mats may be laid down to give the animal confidence. Surgery may be prolonged and there can be considerable blood loss from the cut muscle ends if diathermy is not available, so intravenous fluids are important to ensure a rapid recovery. Prevention of seroma formation at the site of the amputation can be achieved by bandaging or use of a drain.

Arthrotomy

Some surgical conditions of the joints require surgery inside the joint itself (arthrotomy). The commonest indications for joint surgery in the dog and cat are dislocations, ligamentous injuries (in particular, cruciate ligament rupture), **osteochondrosis** (abnormal development of cartilage in the joint), penetrating wounds of the joint and fractures involving the joint surface. The elbow, stifle and hip are the most commonly affected joints.

Strict asepsis is extremely important as postoperative infection in the joint is devastating. Equally important are careful haemostasis and meticulous repair of the surgical approach through the joint capsule. The joint is usually flushed out with sterile saline at the end of the surgery, and the repair made using monofilament suture materials. Joint surgery can be very painful and good analgesia is important; some surgeons may use local anaesthetic into the joint. Seroma formation is a common postoperative complication and some veterinary surgeons will put a pressure bandage on the joint to prevent this, and to immobilize the joint for a few days. However, it is difficult to immobilize the elbow and stifle and often bandages are ineffective. Exercise is usually limited to a strict regime and it is important that the owner is given clear written instructions.

In some specialist centres, joint surgery may be carried out using **arthroscopy**. This enables access to the inside of the joint without the disadvantages and postoperative complications of the surgical approach. The arthroscope must be sterile and specialist instruments are used that are introduced into the joint via a separate hole. The joint is kept clear during surgery with a continuous high-pressure sterile fluid lavage. A sterile sleeve is used to cover the cable from the arthroscope to the viewing screen.

Arthrodesis

Arthrodesis is the surgical fusion of a joint to prevent its movement, and is used when there is intractable joint pain, chronic instability of the joint or an irreparable joint fracture. The principle is that the joint surfaces are obliterated using curettes or power-driven burrs or saws, and then the joint is fused in a normal standing position, using plates or screws to compress the surfaces together. The joint is often supported with a cast postoperatively until the arthrodesis has fully healed and can support the animal's weight. Strict asepsis is essential to the success of the procedure. Sometimes the surgery is done under tourniquet (e.g. carpal arthrodesis) to reduce blood loss and improve visibility during surgery.

Fractures

Fractures are often the result of traumatic incidents, but in small-breed dogs they can occur if the dog jumps down from a height (e.g. out of the owner's arms or off the sofa). Some fractures are pathological and are associated with bone disease or neoplasia.

In most instances, fractures are repaired surgically, though this depends on the type of fracture (see earlier). It is important that two good-quality orthogonal radiographs are obtained of the fracture prior to surgery, in order to plan the repair. Immediately postoperatively, two views are taken to assess the success of the repair and to determine the position of any implants.

Nursing the fracture patient

- Assessment and treatment of concurrent injuries
- Provision of analgesia
- Assisted walking to ensure that the animal does not slip over when taken out
- Provision of adequate dry bedding so that the animal remains dry and clean
- Monitoring for decubital ulcers
- Monitoring the temperature, pulse and respiration rate as indicators of pain, infection or distress
- Observation of the surgical wound for signs of postoperative infection
- Detailed communication with the owner over the exercise regime and prevention of excessive use of the limb during the healing process
- Regular radiography of the repaired fracture to monitor healing

Specialist orthopaedic surgery

Some orthopaedic surgery is only done in referral centres, such as tibial plateau levelling osteotomy (a treatment for cruciate rupture), total hip replacement (for chronic hip arthritis due to hip dysplasia) or very complex fractures. These procedures require detailed assessment of the animal and the surgery is done under very strict aseptic conditions. The equipment is expensive and the nursing staff must be experienced in the use and care of these instruments.

For example, when a total hip replacement is carried out, the animal is assessed for skin disease that may increase the risk of bacterial contamination at the time of surgery, obesity, and gastrointestinal disease that might cause a diarrhoea during hospitalization, as well as its orthopaedic disease.

During surgery, the surgeons may wear two pairs of gloves. Adhesive waterproof disposable drapes are used and personnel in theatre are limited to reduce aerosol contamination. Often a culture swab is taken from the surgical wound just before closure to check for any contamination in the surgical wound during surgery.

Spinal surgery

Neurosurgical procedures require certain specialized equipment and skills and are usually carried out in referral centres. Diagnosis of spinal injuries or diseases are carried out using a combination of clinical examination and neurological tests and radiographs, contrast radiography (myelography) and advanced imaging techniques (e.g. MRI or CT). Samples of spinal fluid may be taken for analysis either from between the skull and first cervical vertebra (**cisternal puncture**) or from between the lumbar vertebrae (**lumbar puncture**).

Spinal cord injury arises from any pressure on the cord within the vertebral canal. The resulting inflammatory response can result in continued injury to the nerves even after the cause of the pressure has been relieved. Recovery from spinal injuries is very slow and requires a committed and caring nursing staff. Spinal patients are at risk from:

- Pneumonia
- Decubital ulcers
- Dermatitis due to urine or faecal skin soiling
- Limb oedema
- Muscle wasting
- Urinary tract infection.

Nursing spinal injuries

Recumbent animals are at high risk of a number of complications that can be alleviated or prevented by good nursing:

- Ensure that the bladder is emptied regularly.
- Check for decubital ulcers three times daily.
- Turn the patient regularly – at last every 2 hours.
- Monitor conscious or unconscious defecation and urination.
- Monitor neurological reflexes and record improvements.
- Maintain adequate nutrition.
- Give physiotherapy for all joints to prevent stiffness and cartilage degeneration.
- Keep the skin clean and dry.
- Provide regular assisted walks and attention; move the patient into a place where it can watch general activity.

Most dedicated owners can manage small to medium-sized recumbent patients at home once the animal is urinary continent, but will need detailed written guidelines on nursing care. Regular visits help to monitor the animal's progress and to provide support to the owners that they are doing everything correctly.

Spinal fractures

Spinal fractures are usually the result of trauma, and the radiograph may not accurately reflect the degree of spinal cord damage done at the time of impact if the spinal muscles have pulled the bones back into alignment. If a spinal fracture is suspected, the patient should not be sedated or anaesthetized for radiography, as the muscles may be holding the bones in place and preventing further spinal cord damage. Some fractures are managed with cage rest if the spinal cord injury is not severe. In other cases, the vertebrae have to be stabilized using pins, plates or external fixation.

Disc disease

The intervertebral discs can cause severe spinal cord injury if they dislodge and erupt into the spinal canal, hitting the ventral aspect of the spinal cord. This classically occurs in the small-breed dogs such as Dachshunds, Pekingese and Jack Russell Terriers which have a defect in the cartilage component of the disc (Type 1). These disc protrusions can occur very suddenly and result in acute paralysis of the patient. Another disc disease syndrome is seen in ageing larger-breed dogs, which causes slow compression of the spinal cord and results in chronic nerve pain (Type 2).

Both types of disc disease are alleviated by surgery to open up the spinal canal (**laminectomy**) and to remove the fragments of disc pressing on the spinal cord. This is very specialized surgery and careful assessment of the patient is necessary to determine which part of the spinal canal is affected. Postoperatively, the patient may be slightly worse before the neurological symptoms improve and will require prolonged nursing care. Acute cases of paraplegia should be operated on as soon as possible to reduce the damage to the spinal cord.

Neoplasia

Tumours are occasionally diagnosed causing neurological symptoms secondary to slow compression of the spinal cord as they grow within the confined space of the spinal canal. Surgical removal of benign tumours of the meninges via a laminectomy can be successful, but tumours arising from the vertebrae themselves are usually inoperable.

Further reading

Anderson DM (1999) Nursing patients undergoing skin reconstruction. *Veterinary Nursing*, **14**, 52–61

Aspinall V (2003) *Clinical Procedures in Veterinary Nursing.* Butterworth-Heinemann, Oxford

Bojrab MJ (ed) (1993) *Disease Mechanisms in Small Animal Surgery, 2nd edn.* Lea & Febiger, Philadelphia

Bojrab MJ, Ellison GW and Slocum B (eds) (1998) *Current Techniques in Small Animal Surgery, 4th edn.* Williams & Wilkins, Baltimore

Coughlan A and Miller A (2006) *BSAVA Manual of Small Animal Fracture Repair and Management,* (revised reprint). BSAVA Publications, Gloucester

Ellison GW (1993) Visceral healing and repair disorders. In: *Disease Mechanisms in Small Animal Surgery, 2nd edn* (ed. MJ Bojrab), pp. 2–6. Lea & Febiger, Philadelphia

Flecknell P (1988) Developments in the veterinary care of rabbits and rodents. *In Practice*, **20**, 286–295

Harari J (ed.) (1993) *Surgical Complications and Wound Healing in the Small Animal Practice.* WB Saunders, Philadelphia

Hotston Moore A (ed) (1999) *BSAVA Manual of Advanced Veterinary Nursing.* BSAVA Publications, Cheltenham

Jeffery ND (1995) *Handbook of Small Animal Spinal Surgery.* WB Saunders, London

Moore M and Simpson G (eds) (1999) *BSAVA Manual of Veterinary Nursing.* BSAVA Publications, Cheltenham

Morgan DA (2000) *Guides for Health Care Staff, 9th edn.* Euromed Communications Ltd., Haslemere, Surrey.

Piermattei DL and Flo GL (1997) *Handbook of Small Animal Orthopedics and Fracture Repair.* WB Saunders, Philadelphia

Pope ER (1993) Skin healing. In *Disease Mechanisms in Small Animal Surgery, 2nd edn* (ed. MJ Bojrab), pp. 151–155. Lea & Febiger, Philadelphia

Seim HB and Creed JE (1998) Restraint techniques for prevention of self trauma. In: *Current Techniques in Small Animal Surgery, 4th edn* (eds MJ Bojrab *et al.*), pp. 53–62. Williams & Wilkins, Baltimore

Smeak DD (1998) Selection and use of currently available suture materials and needs. In: *Current Techniques in Small Animal Surgery, 4th edn* (eds MJ Bojrab *et al.*), pp. 19–26. Williams & Wilkins, Baltimore

Villiers E and Dunn J (1998) Collection and preparation of smears for cytological evaluation. *In Practice*, **20**, 270–377

Williams J, McHugh D and White RAS (1992) Use of drains in small animal surgery. *In Practice*, **14**, 73–81

Williams JM and Niles JD (2005) *BSAVA Manual of Canine and Feline Abdominal Surgery.* BSAVA Publications, Gloucester

Chapter 25

Reproduction, obstetric and paediatric nursing

Wendy Adams and Gary England

Learning objectives

After studying this chapter, students should be able to:

- **Understand typical behaviour and function of the reproductive system**
- **Be aware of the basic endocrine control of reproduction**
- **Be aware of the procedures involved in performing a clinical examination of the reproductive tract in males and females to enable detection of normal and abnormal function**
- **Appreciate which abnormalities are common, especially with respect to parturition**
- **Understand the unique physiology of neonatal animals so that care of the dam and neonate can be optimized at normal parturition, after assisted delivery and during the early neonatal period**

Breeding dogs and cats

Breeding of domestic pets may occur as a planned event by the experienced breeder or novice but enthusiastic owner. Commonly, pet animals also become pregnant as a result of an unintentional mating of an oestrous female. The latter situation occurs most frequently because of a lack of education on behalf of the owner. This situation is lamentable, especially considering the thousands of unwanted pets that are destroyed by humane societies every year. It is a responsibility of the veterinary profession to educate owners of new pets so that they are fully aware of the reproductive physiology and the risks of pregnancy. In the majority of cases sterilization of the puppy or kitten is recommended.

Assessment of animals for breeding

Breeding should not be undertaken lightly. Potential breeders should take advice from many sources before breeding from any animal. Both the male and female should be carefully assessed before making the decision to breed. Both potential parents should:

- Be clinically sound (in good general health and well-being)
- Be of a suitable age for reproduction (females should be skeletally mature, and both male and female should be of an age at which their temperamental and conformational qualities can be properly assessed)
- Be free from hereditary diseases (all the necessary checks for the particular breed should have been undertaken)
- Have excellent temperaments
- Be good examples of the breed (for dogs, the Kennel Club has a set of breed standards for every breed that is recognized in the UK; details of these can be obtained on www.the-kennel-club.org.uk)
- Be free from infectious disease (in the UK, but not other countries, there are no bacterial venereal pathogens in dogs and therefore routine bacteriological swabbing for the prepuce or vagina is a waste of time; however, in the cat it is important to screen for feline leukaemia virus before embarking upon breeding).

Many animals that are used at stud do not meet these criteria. Before breeding from a dog or cat, the owner should give careful consideration to the quality of their animal, the availability of homes for the potential offspring and the potential costs involved, which may include a caesarean operation if the female has parturition difficulties.

There are moral and legal responsibilities (under the Sale of Goods Act) for breeders of animals to ensure that the offspring are clinically healthy and have a sound temperament. There are many hereditary defects that should preclude animals from breeding and these are discussed in detail in other chapters. In the case of cryptorchidism, for example, the affected male and both parents should be considered to be carriers and should not be used for breeding.

Control of hereditary disease

Three schemes created in collaboration with the Kennel Club (KC) and the British Veterinary Association (BVA) aim to control the incidence of hereditary diseases (eye conditions, hip dysplasia and elbow dysplasia) in pedigree dogs (see Chapter 5). There are also several health schemes that include DNA testing (see Chapter 5). Where they exist, it is strongly recommended that both the potential sire and dam are screened before breeding is undertaken. Other schemes have been adopted by certain breed societies to monitor the level of specific diseases.

Certain breed societies have established codes of conduct that aim to control the number of litters bred per bitch and the age of first mating. The Kennel Club may not register a litter of puppies born to a bitch if she:

- Was under a year old at the date of mating
- Had already reached 8 years of age at the time of whelping
- Has whelped more than six litters.

The Kennel Club will lift the second restriction if she has previously successfully whelped at least one other litter of registered pups and there is veterinary evidence that she is in good health and a suitable candidate to whelp another litter.

Cats

The Governing Council of the Cat Fancy (GCCF) provides for the registration of cats and the production of certified certificates. In addition, it classifies breeds, licenses shows and publishes rules that control those functions. Whilst the GCCF publishes leaflets of general advice, it issues no specific guidelines regarding hereditary disease.

Male dogs and tomcats

Male dogs and tomcats are sexually active throughout the year, though a minor seasonal effect may be noted in some countries. In the cat, the testes are descended into the scrotum at birth; in the dog, they descend into the scrotum by 10 days after birth. Puppies and kittens may show sexual activity from several weeks of age, but puberty does not occur until 6–12 months in the dog and 8–12 months in the cat. For both species, **spermatogenesis** (the production of spermatozoa) commences at approximately 5 months of age.

It is preferable not to use a male at stud until he is at least 12 months of age, since it is not possible to evaluate his qualities fully until this time, and even then the occurrence of certain hereditary diseases may not be apparent. It is advisable that the first mating attempts should be with an experienced female.

The fertile lifespan of a male varies considerably and is probably related to the longevity of the breed. It is certain that average seminal quality of male stud dogs is reduced from 7 years of age onwards.

Endocrinology

The interstitial (Leydig) cells are the source of testosterone production from the testes. Luteinizing hormone (LH), a gonadotrophin hormone released from the pituitary gland, stimulates the production of testosterone. A second pituitary gonadotrophin called follicle stimulating hormone (FSH) appears to increase the process of spermatogenesis directly via the Sertoli cells. Testosterone has a negative feedback effect upon the release of FSH and LH, which is mediated by gonadotrophin-releasing hormone (GnRH) (Figure 25.1).

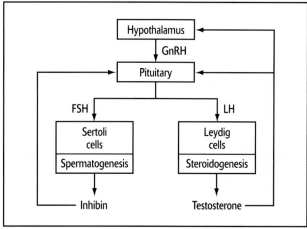

25.1 Schematic representation of the endocrine control of testicular function in the male.

Diseases of the reproductive tract

There are a variety of conditions that may affect the reproductive organs of both the tomcat and the male dog.

Endocrinological abnormalities

Primary abnormalities in the secretion of pituitary hormones may result in poor development of gonadal tissue, a condition called **hypogonadism**. This is rare but has been reported in both species.

Diseases of the testes

Cryptorchidism

An absence of the testes (**anorchia**) is very rare; in most cases the testes are retained within the abdomen. These undescended testes belong to the condition known as **cryptorchidism** (literally, 'hidden testicle'). Often the condition is unilateral, with one testicle present within the scrotum and the other retained within the abdomen. These cases are often wrongly called monorchids; **monorchidism** actually refers to an animal with a single testicle. Some cryptorchid animals are bilaterally affected and no testes are seen within the scrotum. The treatment for all cryptorchids is removal of both testes, because of the high incidence of neoplasia within the abdominal testis, and the fact that the condition is likely to be inherited.

Orchitis

This is inflammation of the testes; it is rare but may follow trauma (particularly in the tomcat) or ascending bacterial infection. In some countries (but not the UK) orchitis may be caused by the bacterium *Brucella canis*, which is a venereal pathogen transmitted at coitus.

Testicular tumours

Testicular tumours are the second most common tumour affecting the male dog but are rare in the tomcat. There are three common tumour types: those affecting the Leydig cells (Leydig cell tumour), those affecting the Sertoli cells (Sertoli cell tumour) and those affecting the germ cells (**seminoma**). Some of these tumours may be endocrinologically active and secrete female hormones (oestrogens), which produce signs of feminization.

Diseases of the accessory glands

The prostate gland in the male dog is the only accessory sex gland. The tomcat has both prostate and bulbourethral glands, but disease of either is rare.

Prostate abnormalities in the dog are common and include benign enlargement (hyperplasia), bacterial prostatitis, prostatic cysts and prostatic tumours. The clinical signs of these diseases may be similar and include difficulty urinating and defecating and the presence of blood within urine or semen.

Diseases of the penis and prepuce

It is common for there to be a creamy discharge from the prepuce of the male dog and this should be considered normal unless it is excessive. It is not seen in the tomcat.

Phimosis

This is a condition where there is inability to extrude the penis, due to an abnormally small preputial orifice. This may occur either congenitally or as a result of trauma or inflammation, and may result in pain during erection. **Paraphimosis** is a failure to retract the penis into the prepuce and may also be due to a small preputial orifice. The penis becomes dry and necrotic and urethral obstruction may result. **Priapism** refers to the persistent enlargement of the penis in the absence of sexual excitement.

Lymphoid hyperplasia

This is a relatively common condition in the male dog, where the bulbus glandis is covered with multiple nodules 2–3 mm in diameter. These are usually smooth and do not cause any significant disease, but they may be traumatized at the time of mating or semen collection.

Antisocial behaviour

In many cases, behaviour that may be normal for a male animal is considered to be antisocial by humans. These problems include territory marking, mounting inappropriate objects and aggression towards other males. They often necessitate treatment, which may include behavioural modification therapy in conjunction with drugs that inhibit male hormone production, such as progestogens. Castration may be required in certain cases.

Assessment of fertility

Male fertility may be assessed by the evaluation of semen quality. Semen may be collected by stimulating the male dog to ejaculate by hand (artificial vaginas are no longer used for this purpose). Semen collection is more difficult in the tomcat and may require general anaesthesia and electroejaculation. A special artificial vagina may be used to collect from trained tom cats. Collection equipment should be warmed before use.

Once collected, semen should be placed into a water bath at body temperature to prevent damage to the sperm. The second fraction of the dog ejaculate and the entire cat ejaculate should be used for evaluation.

1. The volume should be measured and the colour recorded. Normally the semen is white and milky in colour, and up to 2.0 ml for the dog and 0.1–0.5 ml in the tomcat.
2. After gently mixing the sample, a drop should be placed upon a warmed microscope slide and a subjective assessment made of the percentage of sperm with vigorous forward progression.

3. A small portion of the sample should be diluted with water to kill the sperm and therefore stop their movement. The spermatozoal concentration can then be measured using a haemocytometer counting chamber. The total sperm output should be calculated by multiplying this value by the volume of the sample.
4. A portion of the sample should be stained to allow the differentiation of live and dead sperm and the assessment of spermatozoal morphology. A combination of the two stains nigrosin and eosin is suitable for this purpose. Normally 4 parts of the stain are mixed with 1 part of semen, and then a smear is immediately made on to a glass microscope slide. When examined under high magnification, nigrosin appears as a background stain. The eosin is a vital stain – it stains only sperm with a damaged membrane, i.e. dead sperm (Figure 25.2). When using nigrosin and eosin, sperm are either stained pink (these are termed dead) or are unstained (these are termed live).

The semen characteristics of fertile dogs are given in Figure 25.3.

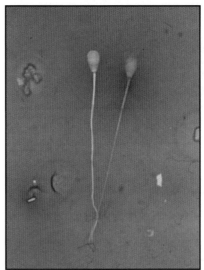

25.2 Photomicrograph of dog sperm: (left) live, and (right) dead sperm with clamped acrosome.

	Normal progressive motility (%)	Volume (ml)	Concentration (x 10^6/ml)	Total sperm output (x 10^6)
Mean	85.2	1.3	310.5	403.4
S.D.	6.2	0.4	82	120
Range	42–92	0.4–3.4	50–560	36–620

25.3 Characteristics of the second fraction of the ejaculate from 53 fertile dogs.

The bitch and queen

The oestrous cycle

The domestic bitch

In the bitch the onset of cyclical activity (puberty) is normally between 6 and 23 months of age, with most bitches having their first oestrus by the age of 12–14 months. Bitches that do not exhibit oestrous behaviour by the anticipated age are considered to have delayed puberty, but it should be remembered that many normal bitches will not cycle until they are 2 years old. The majority of bitches start to cycle about 6 months after they have reached adult height and weight, which may explain some of the variations exhibited between breeds.

Bitches generally have one or two oestrous cycles per year. As described in more detail below, each oestrus ends with spontaneous ovulation, which is followed by the luteal phase. A variable period of acyclicity (called **anoestrus**) follows the luteal phase.

The bitch is **polytocous** (produces numerous offspring in each litter) and the oestrous periods are non-seasonal. The interval between each cycle can vary between 5 and 13 months but the average is 7 months.

The end of each oestrous cycle is signified by the presence of the 'season', the onset of which is signalled by the presence of a bloody vulval discharge. During this time ovulation normally occurs, followed by the luteal phase or metoestrus (dioestrus). Each 'season' will normally last an average of 3 weeks in the domestic bitch, but they can be shorter in length or can extend to 4 weeks or more in some cases. The season length can be variable between bitches and can vary from season to season. The bitch is said to be 'out of season' once the vulval discharge has stopped.

The stages of the oestrous cycle in the bitch are pro-oestrus, oestrus, metoestrus (dioestrus) and anoestrus (Figure 25.4). The terms 'in season' or 'in heat' are both used to indicate the stage of the cycle when the bitch is receptive to the male dog, i.e. oestrus.

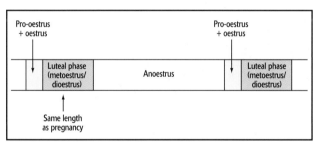

25.4 Sequence and length of various stages of the oestrous cycle of the bitch.

Late anoestrus

During late anoestrus two hormones are released from the pituitary gland: **follicle stimulating hormone (FSH)** and **luteinizing hormone (LH)**. These initiate the growth of follicles within the ovaries and cause the follicles to produce the hormone oestrogen.

Pro-oestrus

During pro-oestrus the bitch will not allow mating but may show increased receptivity to the male. Pro-oestrus is characterized by increased plasma concentrations of **oestrogen**, causing swelling of the vulva and the development of a serosangineous (bloody) vulval discharge. Oestrogens also induce the release of specific pheromones that are responsible for attracting male dogs. This period lasts for approximately 7 days. Oestrogens also cause thickening of the vaginal wall and an increase in the number of epithelial cell layers. During pro-oestrus the elevated concentrations of oestrogen have a negative feedback effect upon the release of the gonadotrophin hormones from the pituitary gland, and the concentrations of FSH and LH are reduced compared with late anoestrus.

Oestrus

During oestrus the bitch demonstrates characteristic behaviour towards the male dog including deviation of the tail and presentation of the vulva and perineum. The bitch will stand to be mated (**standing oestrus**). This period lasts for approximately 7 days. The onset of oestrus is related to a decline in the concentration of plasma oestrogen and at the same time the production of the hormone **progesterone**. The bitch is unusual in that progesterone is produced in low concentrations by luteinization of the follicle, a process that occurs before ovulation. (In many species progesterone is only produced after ovulation.) It is this decline in the concentration of oestrogen and the slight increase in the concentration of progesterone that is responsible for stimulating a surge of both FSH and LH. This surge is the trigger for the release of eggs from the ovaries (**ovulation**), which occurs spontaneously approximately 2 days later, towards the end of oestrus. It can therefore be seen that the hormonal stimulus for ovulation occurs during standing oestrus and that the release of eggs also occurs during this period. Each egg is contained within a fluid-filled structure called a **follicle**. After ovulation the follicle develops into a solid structure called a **corpus luteum**. One corpus luteum forms from each follicle that has ovulated and the corpus luteum produces progesterone. The end of standing oestrus is associated with relatively high concentrations of progesterone in the blood.

Metoestrus (dioestrus)

In many species the phase of progesterone production (the **luteal phase**) is divided into two. The early luteal phase is termed **metoestrus** and the mature luteal phase is termed **dioestrus**. In the bitch, however, the early luteal phase occurs during standing oestrus, making this terminology difficult to adopt (since metoestrus would then be occurring during oestrus). In the bitch the terms metoestrus and dioestrus are therefore often used synonymously to reflect the luteal phase of the cycle after the end of standing oestrus. This phase is characterized by the presence of the corpora lutea upon the ovaries and the presence of the hormone progesterone in the blood.

The period of metoestrus lasts whilst the corpora lutea continue to produce progesterone and is approximately 55 days in length. In the pregnant bitch the period of metoestrus is synonymous with **pregnancy**. The bitch is unusual compared with other species in that the duration of metoestrus is similar whether the bitch is pregnant or not (Figure 25.5). The birth of puppies occurs when progesterone secretion is terminated. In the non-pregnant bitch the corpora lutea persist for a similar period of time.

Towards the end of metoestrus another hormone, called **prolactin**, is released from the pituitary gland. This is responsible for the development of mammary tissue and the onset of lactation. Prolactin is produced in both the pregnant and the non-pregnant bitch and is the reason why false or **pseudopregnancy** is a common event in the bitch (see later).

The hormonal changes of the oestrous cycle are summarized in Figure 25.6.

Anoestrus

Metoestrus is followed by a period of quiescence, during which time there is effectively no hormonal activity. In the non-pregnant bitch there is no sudden decline in the concentration of progesterone but values gradually reduce and the transition to anoestrus is smooth. The situation is slightly different during pregnancy because progesterone concentrations rapidly decline, and it is this event that stimulates the onset of parturition. The length of anoestrus varies considerably between bitches, but on average it is 5 months.

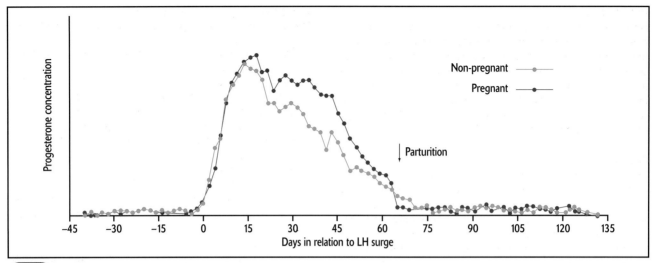

25.5 Changes in plasma progesterone concentration in the pregnant and non-pregnant bitch.

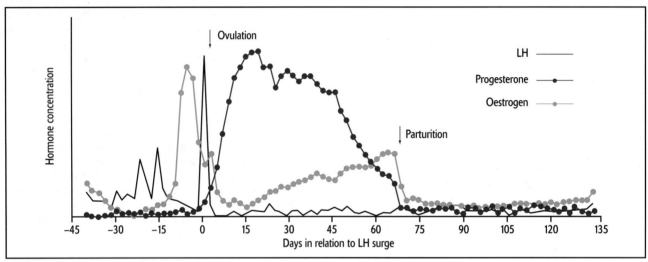

25.6 Changes in plasma hormones during the oestrous cycle of the pregnant bitch.

The domestic queen

Female cats generally exhibit their first oestrus at 6–9 months of age, but this is dependent upon photoperiod. Those that are born in the summer frequently commence cycling at the first spring; those that are born in the winter may not cycle until they are least 12 months of age.

Queens have multiple oestrous cycles each year. They are seasonally polyoestrous and typically cycle from February to September. Ovulation is induced by coitus and the interval between each oestrous cycle varies depending upon whether the queen has ovulated, or fails to ovulate either because she is not mated or because there is insufficient hormone release at mating. Unmated queens return to oestrus at intervals of 14–21 days. Queens that ovulate but do not become pregnant generally return to oestrus after approximately 45 days.

The stages of the oestrous cycle in the queen are anoestrus, pro-oestrus, oestrus and interoestrus (Figure 25.7). The terms 'in season' or 'in heat' are used to indicate the stage of the cycle when the queen is receptive to the male, i.e. oestrus. During winter there is essentially no hormone activity: the queen is in anoestrus. In springtime cyclical activity commences and, in the unmated queen, periods of sexual activity (pro-oestrus and oestrus) are interrupted by periods of non-receptivity (interoestrus). If the queen is mated and ovulation is induced, she enters metoestrus or pregnancy.

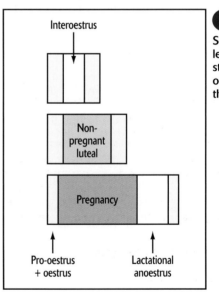

25.7

Sequence and length of various stages of the oestrous cycle of the queen.

Pregnancy follows a fertile mating; metoestrus (also called pseudopregnancy) follows a sterile mating. The duration of pseudopregnancy in the queen is shorter than that of pregnancy unlike the situation in the bitch.

Pro-oestrus

Follicular development occurs during this phase due to the release of LH and FSH. This causes the secretion of oestrogen that is responsible for the development of the signs of pro-oestrus, including attraction of the male and the changes in the vaginal epithelium similar to those seen in the bitch. Pro-oestrus in the queen is often poorly recognized unless a male is present, but during this stage the queen will not accept mating. Pro-oestrus lasts for 2–3 days.

Oestrus

The exact hormonal changes that cause the onset of standing oestrus are uncertain, but may be associated with increasing concentrations of oestrogen. The clinical signs of oestrus (also termed **calling**) include: persistent vocalization, rolling and rubbing against inanimate objects. In the presence of the male the queen may show persistent treading of the hind feet, lateral deviation of the tail and lordosis of the spine. Oestrus lasts between 2 and 10 days.

Interoestrus

In the absence of mating, or when mating does not result in ovulation, the signs of oestrus gradually decline and the queen enters a stage of non-receptivity. This period may last for between 3 and 14 days. After this time the queen returns to pro-oestrus and oestrus.

Pregnancy

Ovulation in the queen is caused by the release of LH, which is stimulated by mating. Each mating results in a surge of LH, but there appears to be a threshold value below which ovulation will not be induced. Multiple matings are therefore more likely to result in ovulation than are single matings.

Ovulation is followed by an increase in the plasma concentration of progesterone released from the newly formed corpora lutea. Peak progesterone concentrations are reached approximately 1 month after mating and are maintained for the duration of pregnancy, which varies between 64 and 68 days. It is not uncommon for queens to have an absence of cyclical activity during lactation. This has been called **lactational anoestrus**.

Metoestrus (pseudopregnancy)

Non-fertile matings result in ovulation without conception. Ovulation may also occur following stimulation of the vagina (e.g. following collection of a vaginal smear), stimulation of the perineum (which may be self-induced) or spontaneously in some queens. Ovulation results in the formation of corpora lutea and the production of progesterone in a similar manner to early pregnancy. After approximately 40 days, progesterone concentrations decline, and the queen returns to cyclical activity approximately 45 days after the previous oestrus. Should pseudopregnancy occur late in the year (autumn), the queen may not return to cyclical activity but may enter anoestrus.

Diseases of the female reproductive tract

The domestic bitch

There are several abnormalities of the reproductive tract in the domestic bitch. These may be considered under general headings of endocrinological, ovarian, uterine or external genital abnormalities.

Endocrinological abnormalities

The common endocrinological abnormalities of the bitch include:

- Delayed onset of puberty – cyclical activity is not present at 24 months of age
- Prolonged anoestrus – failure of return to cyclical activity, resulting in a prolonged interoestrus interval
- Silent oestrous cycles – normal cyclical activity, including ovulation, but without the external signs of oestrus
- Split oestrus – signs of pro-oestrus but this does not terminate in ovulation and is followed 2–12 weeks later by a normal cycle
- Ovulation failure – when bitches have apparently normal oestrous periods with an absence of ovulation; these bitches often return to oestrus with shorter than normal intervals.

Pseudopregnancy

One specific endocrinological condition frequently seen in the bitch is pseudopregnancy (false pregnancy, phantom pregnancy or **pseudocyesis**). The signs of the condition may include anorexia, abdominal enlargement, nest making, nursing of inanimate objects, mammary development and lactation. False pregnancy should be considered normal in the bitch, because the changes in plasma hormones are similar in both pregnant and non-pregnant individuals. It has been wrongly thought that pseudopregnancy is produced by either an overproduction of progesterone or abnormal persistence of the corpus luteum. The actual mechanism is related to the decline in plasma progesterone concentration during late metoestrus, which is associated with an increase in plasma concentrations of prolactin.

In many cases therapy is not required, because the signs will gradually decline. Often, removal of bedding material that the bitch is using to make a nest or removal of the toys that she is nursing will be enough to help the bitch to overcome a false pregnancy. In certain cases it may be necessary to use hormonal therapy to reduce the plasma concentrations of prolactin.

Diseases of the ovary

There are few abnormalities of the ovary. An absence of ovarian development (**agenesis**) may occur; this usually affects one side only and may affect fertility. Ovarian **cysts** are rare and may be associated with signs of persistent oestrus, but most cysts originate from the ovarian bursa and are not endocrinologically active. Ovarian **tumours** are also rare.

Occasionally bitches with both ovarian and testicular tissue are seen. These animals are termed 'intersex' and may be recognized because of the appearance of their external genitalia. The vulva may be cranially positioned and an os clitoris may develop. The gonads may be found in a normal ovarian position or within the scrotum. These animals are usually sterile.

Diseases of the uterus

Developmental problems of the uterus include **aplasia** (abnormal development) or **agenesis** (failure of development); in these cases reproductive cyclicity will be normal but the bitch may fail to become pregnant. Intersex animals may have the presence of both uterine tissue and vasa defferentia.

Cystic endometrial hyperplasia and pyometra

The most common uterine disease of the bitch is cystic endometrial hyperplasia (**CEH**), which may develop into pyometra. Hyperplasia of the endometrium occurs in response to progesterone during normal metoestrus. In young animals the hyperplasia resolves at the end of the luteal phase. This is not the case in older bitches and small cystic regions develop within the glandular tissue. The uterus in this state is probably more prone to infection than the normal uterus, and should bacteria enter during oestrus (when the cervix is open) they may proliferate. The accumulation of pus within the uterus (**pyometra**) leads to the bitch becoming unwell.

Clinical signs may include the presence of a malodorous vulval discharge, lethargy, inappetence, pyrexia, vomiting, polydipsia and polyuria. In some cases the cervix is not open and a vulval discharge is absent; these cases are called **closed pyometra**.

In all cases of pyometra the treatment of choice is ovariohysterectomy following stabilization of the patient using appropriate fluid therapy. Medical treatment (with combinations of prolactin inhibitors and prostaglandins or with progesterone receptor antagonists) has been advocated and success rates appear to be quite reasonable, but in most cases the best option is surgery.

Treatment of bitches with progestogens for the prevention or suppression of oestrus, or with oestrogens for the treatment of unwanted matings, may predispose to the development of pyometra.

Diseases of the vagina and vestibule
Congenital abnormalities of the caudal reproductive tract include segmental aplasia and hymenal or vestibular constrictions.

Vaginitis (inflammation of the vagina) is sometimes seen in prepubertal bitches and usually resolves after the first oestrus. Specific infectious causes of vaginitis include *Brucella canis* (not present in the UK) and canine herpesvirus. Many bacteria are found within the vagina as normal commensal organisms (including beta-haemolytic streptococci), which many dog breeders wrongly consider to be venereal pathogens. There is little value in routine bacteriological swabbing of the vagina before breeding, since usually only these commensal bacteria are isolated.

Diseases of the external genitalia
Congenital abnormalities such as vulval atresia and agenesis are rare. Clitoral hypertrophy may occur associated with intersexuality.

The domestic queen

Endocrinological abnormalities
Delayed puberty may be difficult to assess in the queen, since the onset of cyclical activity is related to the season of the year at birth (see above). Delayed puberty and prolonged anoestrus have been seen but they are rare.

The most common abnormality is **ovulation failure**, which often results from insufficient reflex release of LH at mating. The majority of queens will ovulate if 4–12 matings are allowed in a 4-hour period.

Pseudopregnancy also occurs in the queen. This condition is dissimilar to that seen in the bitch and usually follows a sterile mating (or occasionally spontaneous ovulation). After ovulation there is an increase in plasma progesterone (Figure 25.8), which does not occur in the absence of mating, and no return to oestrus for a further 35–40 days. The clinical signs are an absence of oestrus; treatment is not required.

Diseases of the ovary
Congenital diseases of the ovary such as ovarian agenesis and ovarian hypoplasia are rare. Ovarian cysts and neoplasms may develop similar to those seen in the bitch but are also rare.

Premature ovarian failure may be seen in queens aged 8 years and above; these animals stop cycling for an unknown reason.

Diseases of the uterus
The range of uterine abnormalities seen in the cat are similar to those seen in the bitch. Pyometra may be less common, because in the absence of mating ovulation does not occur and the luteal phase is therefore absent. Spontaneous ovulations or the common use of progestogens may cause the development of CEH and pyometra.

Diseases of the vagina, vestibule and external genitalia
Congenital abnormalities of the vagina, vestibule and external genitalia are rare but include vaginal and vulval aplasia and defects associated with intersexuality. Vaginitis is uncommon.

Control of reproduction

Male dogs and tomcats
The majority of male dogs do not cause problems if they remain entire, but there are situations where control of 'antisocial' behaviour may be necessary. The situation in the entire tomcat is rather different, because the problems of territory marking, roaming and aggression are greater than in the dog.

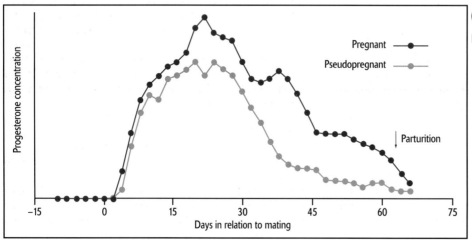

25.8 Progesterone profiles in pregnant and pseudopregnant cats.

Exogenous hormones

Chemical control of reproductive function can be achieved in both species on a short-term basis with hormones that suppress the normal release of testosterone. The most commonly used agents include the progestogens (drugs with progesterone-like activity), which may be administered daily orally (e.g. megestrol acetate) or as a depot injection (e.g. proligestone or delmadinone acetate). These drugs do not produce infertility, only a reduced libido. No single drug is commercially available as a male contraceptive agent; complicated drug regimes are required for this effect.

Surgical contraception

The most common method of regulating sexual activity is castration, which is not reversible.

Castration in the domestic dog is generally carried out at 8–12 months of age, after the dog has reached puberty. Castration before puberty may result in failure of development of the secondary sexual characteristics. In some males a change in metabolic rate may result in increased bodyweight. Castration after puberty and correct dietary control eliminate the majority of problems associated with castration.

Vasectomy is rarely performed in the dog or tomcat. It involves removal of part of the vas deferens, thus preventing ejaculation of sperm. The procedure does not interfere with sexual behaviour. Since in many cases the latter is the primary aim, vasectomy has no advantages over castration.

Vaccination

As technology advances it is becoming more likely that vaccines will be developed against components of the reproductive system. Currently, whilst some experimental vaccines are available for use in females in other species (directed against the zona pellucida), there are none available for use in the male dog or cat.

Many methods have been employed to control the reproductive cycle of the bitch and queen. These include surgical methods and medical control of cyclical activity. More recently advances have been made in the induction of oestrus and in the termination of pregnancy.

The domestic bitch

Surgical neutering

Ovariohysterectomy is the removal of both ovaries and the uterus to the level of the cervix. The term **spaying** is commonly used to describe this procedure. In some countries it is more common to remove only the ovaries (**ovariectomy**). Either technique should be considered in any bitch not required for breeding. Both have several advantages, including a reduction in the incidence of mammary tumours, elimination of the problems of false pregnancy and of pyometra as well the obvious advantages of absence of oestrous behaviour and inability to produce offspring.

There are several claimed adverse effects, including an increased incidence of incontinence, changes in coat texture and a tendency to gain weight. Whilst little can be done regarding the former two conditions, the latter may easily be controlled by correct dietary management.

Age for neutering

There is considerable discussion concerning the correct time to perform the procedure on a bitch. There is no doubt that surgery is technically easier and recovery is more rapid in young animals, and some veterinary surgeons perform surgery as early as 4 months of age.

It has been suggested that when such surgery is performed before puberty (the first oestrus) there is an increased tendency for underdevelopment of the secondary sexual characteristics and there may also be effects on the closure time of the animal's growth plates. Prepubertal neutering does significantly protect the female against the development of mammary tumours later in life. Waiting until after the first oestrus entails the risk of pregnancy and false pregnancy.

Advice from veterinary practices on the best time to neuter a bitch is variable. Whilst some practices recommend that the bitch should have her first 'season' before being neutered, many practices advise that a larger-breed bitch that is not required for breeding should be neutered at approximately 6 months of age, which would normally be before the first oestrus. In smaller breeds the advice is usually to wait until after the first oestrus, as the smaller breeds tend to have their first oestrus at a younger age, normally around 6 months.

Medical inhibition of cyclical activity

There is a variety of compounds that may be used to inhibit cyclical activity, including progesterone or progesterone-like compounds (**progestogens**), testosterone or other male hormones (**androgens**) and gonadotrophin-releasing hormone agonists and antagonists. Drugs may either be administered during anoestrus to prevent the occurrence of an oestrus (the term **prevention** is used), or be given during pro-oestrus or oestrus to abolish the signs of that particular oestrus (the term **suppression** is used).

The most commonly used compounds are the progestogens that are formulated as depot injections or as oral tablets. The depot injections may be used during anoestrus to prevent the occurrence of the next anticipated oestrus. The oral tablets may be used either during anoestrus for oestrus prevention, or during pro-oestrus to suppress the signs of that oestrus. A normal oestrus often occurs between 4 and 6 months after the administration of these hormones.

These drugs are not recommended for use before the first oestrus or in an animal that is required for breeding. The side effects of these drugs may include increased appetite, weight gain, lethargy, mammary enlargement, coat and temperament changes and the risk of inducing pyometra.

Termination of pregnancy

Unwanted matings are commonly seen in general practice. The term **misalliance** is often used to describe such cases. There are several treatment options should pregnancy termination be necessary. If the bitch is not required for breeding, an ovariohysterectomy may be performed early in metoestrus, approximately 2 weeks after the end of oestrus. Medical therapy using oestrogens on several occasions after mating or using progesterone receptor antagonists is usually successful in preventing conception. In later pregnancy it is possible to use various drugs (e.g. progesterone receptor antagonists or prolactin inhibitors and/or prostaglandins) that lower the concentration of progesterone in the blood or block its actions and therefore induce resorption or abortion.

Induction of oestrus

With the development of new drugs and new drug regimes it has become possible to induce an oestrous cycle in the bitch. The best success rates occur with prolactin inhibitors such as cabergoline. These methods may be useful in bitches that have longer than average interoestrus intervals, those that are slow to reach puberty and those that do not exhibit behavioural signs of oestrus.

The domestic queen

Surgical neutering

The indications and potential adverse effects of ovariohysterectomy and ovariectomy in the cat are similar to those in the bitch. The procedure is usually performed when the queen is 5 to 6 months of age, regardless of the onset of puberty; poor development of the external genitalia does not cause problems. In the UK the surgical procedure is frequently performed through a flank incision, but this approach is best avoided in oriental breeds where coat colour is temperature dependent and clipping of the coat may result in the growth of dark-coloured hairs.

Medical inhibition of cyclical activity

The drugs available for use in the queen are similar to those described for the domestic bitch. Long-term drug therapy is less commonly used, because queens that are not wanted for breeding are usually surgically neutered.

Termination of pregnancy

Treatment of an unwanted mating can be achieved by the administration of progestogens if the queen is still in oestrus, or progesterone receptor antagonists if she has ovulated. In many cases pregnancy termination is performed 1 month after mating using similar drug regimes to those described for the bitch.

Induction of oestrus

Various drugs may be used for the induction of oestrus and ovulation. In most cases it is important to remember that the queen is a seasonal breeder, and that her cyclicity is governed by photoperiod.

Mating

Optimum time

The domestic bitch

The determination of the time of ovulation in the bitch is important because the bitch is monoestrous and the mean interoestrous interval is 30 weeks. The clinical signs of oestrus are not always reliable indicators of the time of ovulation; in many bitches the behavioural signs do not correlate well with the changes in hormone concentration.

There are two natural methods that increase the likelihood of conception despite these potential problems. The first is the relatively long fertile period of the eggs and the second is the relatively long survival of spermatozoa within the female reproductive tract.

There are several methods by which the optimum time for mating can be detected, including clinical assessments, measurement of plasma hormone concentration and vaginal cytology.

Clinical assessments

The clinical signs of oestrus do not correlate well with the underlying hormonal events. The 'average bitch' ovulates 12 days after the onset of pro-oestrus and should be mated from day 14 onwards, when oocytes have matured. In some bitches ovulation may occur as early as day 5 or as late as day 32 after the onset of pro-oestrus, and these bitches would be unlikely to become pregnant if mated on the 12th and 14th day, which is common breeding practice.

Studies on laboratory dogs have shown that the LH surge often occurs around the same time as the onset of standing oestrus. Although there is some variation of this event, commencing mating 4 days after the onset of standing oestrus may be a suitable time in many bitches.

One clinical assessment that may be useful in the bitch is the timing of vulval softening (Figure 25.9). This often occurs during the LH surge when there is a switch from oestrogen dominance to progesterone dominance of the reproductive tract.

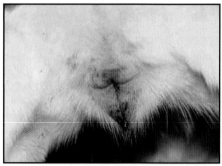

25.9

Bitch's softened vulva, just after the LH surge.

If only clinical assessments are available, the combination of the onset of standing oestrus and the timing of distinct vulval softening may be useful in the prediction of the best mating time, since each event occurs on average 2 days before ovulation.

Measurement of plasma hormone concentration

The three relevant plasma hormones are LH, oestrogen and progesterone.

- The measurement of plasma concentrations of **LH** would indicate impending ovulation; the fertile period is between 4 and 8 days after the LH surge. Unfortunately, there is no simple method by which plasma LH concentrations can be readily measured.
- There is little value in the measurement of plasma **oestrogen** concentrations because the oestrogen plateau is not predictive of the timing of ovulation.
- Plasma **progesterone** concentrations are very useful, since this hormone is absent during pro-oestrus and begins to increase at the same time as the plasma surge of LH, thus detecting a rise in the concentration of plasma progesterone is predictive of ovulation.

Progesterone can be easily measured in the practice laboratory within 30 minutes of sample collection, using a commercial enzyme-linked immunosorbent assay (ELISA) test kit. This method simply involves comparison of a colour change in the sample with the colour change in low- and high-concentration progesterone controls.

Vaginal cytology

The changes in the concentration of plasma hormone concentrations have a marked effect upon the vaginal mucosa. When the bitch is not cycling, there are approximately two or three layers of cells lining the vagina. During oestrus, the vagina develops many cell layers in order to protect itself during mating. The cells within these layers differ from each other in their shape and size. When cells are collected from the vagina (the technique called a **vaginal smear**), only the cells on the surface of the vagina are removed. Different cell types are therefore collected at the various stages of the reproductive cycle. Staining of these cells and subsequent microscopic examination allows an assessment of the underlying hormone changes to be made. Cells can be collected either by aspirating vaginal fluid using a pipette, or using a cotton swab. Once collected, cells are placed on a glass microscope slide, spread into a thin film and stained so that they can be individually examined.

- During anoestrus (Figure 25.10a) the vaginal wall is only a few cells in thickness and these cells are small and spherical in shape. Because they are positioned close to the basement membrane they are called **parabasal cells**. The anoestrus vaginal smear is characterized by the presence of these cells. There are also normally a few white blood cells (**neutrophils**), which remove cell debris and bacteria.
- During pro-oestrus (Figure 25.10b) the vaginal mucosa increases in thickness under the influence of oestrogen. The mucosa may be up to five or six cells thick. The cells further away from the basement membrane are larger in diameter than those nearer to the membrane. These cells have a large area of cytoplasm surrounding the cell nucleus and are called **small intermediate cells**. When the surface cells are collected during pro-oestrus they are therefore predominantly these small intermediate cells, though there will also be a small number of the parabasal cells present. White blood cells are also present during pro-oestrus, but numbers are reduced compared with anoestrus. This is because the increased thickness of the vaginal mucosa prevents movement of the white blood cells into the lumen of the vagina. Red blood cells are also present in the vaginal smear during pro-oestrus. These cells originate from the uterus and pass into the vagina via the cervix.

- During oestrus (Figure 25.10c) the vaginal mucosa continues to thicken and the number of cell layers increases. There may be up to 12 cell layers during oestrus. Surface cells are large and irregular in shape and are called **large intermediate cells**. Cells of this size may accumulate the material keratin and are then termed **keratinized**. The nucleus of these large keratinized cells often disappears. The cells are then called **anuclear** because of the absence of the nucleus. White blood cells are not found in the vaginal smear during oestrus because the thick vaginal wall does not allow them to penetrate. Red blood cells are present in large numbers during oestrus.
- During metoestrus (Figure 25.10d) there is sloughing of much of the vaginal mucosal epithelium. This is caused by the increasing concentrations of the hormone progesterone. The number of cell layers is reduced and the surface cells are again the small intermediate epithelial cells or parabasal cells. Several of the epithelial cells may have vacuoles within the cytoplasm, giving the cell a 'foamy' appearance. **Foam cells** and epithelial cells with cytoplasmic inclusion bodies are characteristic of metoestrus. Because of the large amount of degenerate cellular material within the vaginal lumen, there is a rapid influx of white blood cells as soon as the mucosa is thin enough to allow their penetration. Large numbers of white blood cells are therefore found in the metoestrus vaginal smear. Few red blood cells are present during metoestrus.

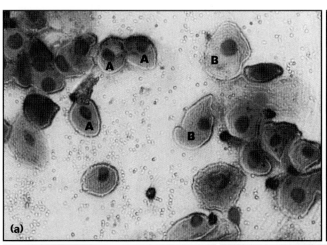

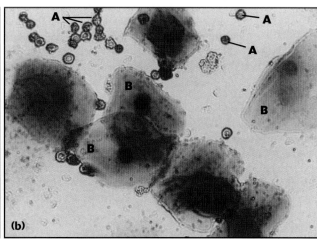

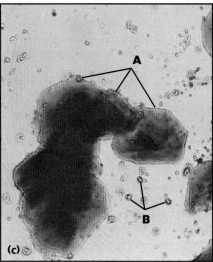

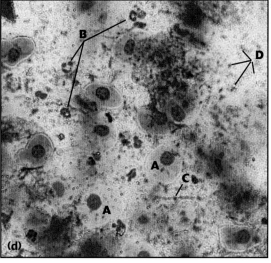

25.10

Photomicrographs of vaginal smears from a bitch.
(a) Anoestrus:
A, parabasal cell;
B, small intermediate cell.
(b) Pro-oestrus:
A, red blood cell;
B, large intermediate cell.
(c) Oestrus:
A, anuclear cell;
B, red blood cell.
(d) Metoestrus:
A, small intermediate cell;
B, white blood cell;
C, mucous strand;
D, bacteria.

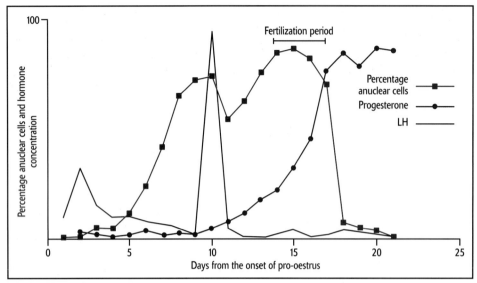

The bitch should first be mated when the percentage of anuclear cells is maximal (usually 80% or above) (Figure 25.11). There are variations from the normal: some bitches may have two peaks of anuclear cells and some have a low percentage of anuclear cells during the fertile period.

Other tests

A number of other tests have been evaluated in the past, including the measurement of electrical resistance, pH and glucose concentration in the vagina. None of these methods are reliable.

Examination of the vaginal wall using an endoscope (**vaginoscopy**) may be valuable for identifying the optimal time for breeding, as the vaginal wall undergoes specific changes around the time of ovulation.

The domestic queen

Unlike the bitch, ovulation in the queen is induced by coitus. After mating, assuming that a sufficient release of LH has occurred, follicles increase in size and ovulation follows 24–36 hours later. Mating is best planned during the peak of oestrus and vaginal cytology may be used to assess this time, but collection of the smear may itself induce ovulation. Multiple copulations should be permitted to ensure an adequate release of LH and therefore ovulation.

Normal mating behaviour

It is important that the events of natural mating are understood so that abnormalities can be recognized whilst remembering that the mating environment is often artificial. On the day of mating, bitches and queens are frequently transported large distances, are introduced to the male briefly and then expected to mate immediately. This situation eliminates the normal courtship phase associated with pro-oestrous behaviour and may result in mating problems. In addition many females are presented to males at inappropriate times, either because this is convenient for the owner or because of inexact assessment of the stage of the oestrous cycle. On such occasions sexual behaviour of both males and females may not be optimal.

Dogs

The dog and bitch will normally exhibit play behaviour when they are first introduced to each other. Generally the bitch should be taken to the designated area first. The dog can then be introduced. He should be restrained on a lead to ensure that the bitch is happy for the dog to be there and is receptive to him. Once this has been established the dog can be allowed off his lead. The dog and bitch will normally play for a few minutes (Figure 25.12a). Very experienced studs may forego this playtime and mount the bitch straight away, so it is important to establish the willingness of the bitch to be mated in the first instance. The bitch will normally settle and stand with her tail deviated to one side in order to allow mating to take place. This tail deviation is known as 'flagging'.

The dog may ejaculate a small volume of clear fluid either before mounting the bitch or whilst he is trying to gain intromission into the bitch. This fluid is the **first fraction** of the ejaculate and does not contain sperm. It originates from the prostate gland and its function is to flush any urine or cellular debris from the urethra. The dog will continue to mount, thrust and dismount (Figure 25.12b) until his position allows the penile tip to enter the bitch's vagina. This is known as **intromission** (Figure 25.12c). The dog will now achieve a full erection. The dog appears to move much closer to the bitch and the thrusting movements increase rapidly. He will now ejaculate the **second fraction** of ejaculate, which is sperm rich. Once thrusting has subsided the dog will turn through 180 degrees and dismount the bitch whilst his penis remains within the vagina. The dog and bitch will now stand tail-to-tail and this is called the **tie** (Figure 25.12d). The tie is associated with the dog ejaculating the **third fraction** of ejaculate. This is again clear fluid and prostatic in origin and its purpose is to flush the sperm forwards through the cervix into the uterus. The tie will last on average for 20 minutes but varies considerably between dogs and can be as short as 5 minutes or over an hour in length.

Once the swelling of the bulbous gland subsides, the dog and bitch will separate and the mating is finished. The bitch should be checked for any bleeding. There is normally a small amount of fluid that comes away when the tie ends; this is just the last portion of prostatic fluid and is normal. The fluid can sometimes be bloodstained, depending on the bitch's discharge. Bitches with a coloured discharge tend to have a heavier staining of this fluid. If this fluid is very heavily bloodstained, the bitch and the dog should be checked thoroughly.

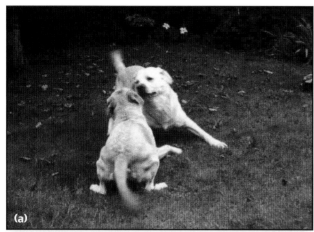

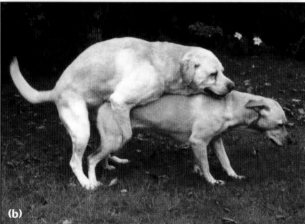

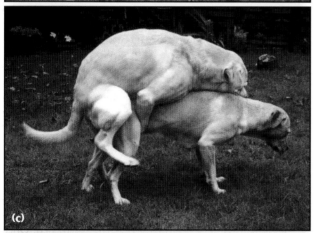

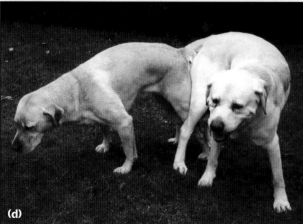

25.12 Normal mating behaviour in the dog: **(a)** playing prior to mating; **(b)** mounting prior to intromission; **(c)** intromission; **(d)** the 'tie'.

If all is normal, the bitch is taken away from the area first. The dog will usually lick at himself to help the penis re-enter its sheath. At this time the dog should be checked to ensure that his penis has returned to its sheath correctly. Occasionally, during the mating process, small blood vessels in the dog's penis will burst, resulting in a small amount of bloody discharge. This should subside quickly.

Cats

The period of sexual introduction and play is variable in the cat, depending upon the experience and aggression of the male. The normal sequence of events occurs rapidly compared with the dog. The male usually approaches the female from the side or back and grasps her neck in his mouth. Whilst maintaining this grasp he mounts the female and positions himself to align the genital regions. The queen normally lowers her chest and elevates the pelvic region whilst deviating her tail. Pelvic thrusting and ejaculation occur rapidly. During intromission the queen often emits a cry and attempts to end mating by rolling, turning and striking at the male. The female then exhibits a marked postcoital reaction consisting of violent rolling and excessive licking. She will not allow further mating at this time.

Problems in mating

Dogs

The mating of dogs and bitches always seems a straightforward process, but often there can be problems. The most common difficulty is that the dog does not 'tie' with the bitch. This is not considered a satisfactory outcome, though it is quite possible that such matings will still result in the bitch conceiving if the dog has ejaculated. The most common reason for a mating with no tie is that there is a height difference between the dog and the bitch. The dog must be able to enter the bitch as straight as possible and this could be difficult if he is too short or too tall. If the dog is too short, a step should be used to make him 'taller'; a step can be used by the bitch if the stud is too tall. Sometimes the dog will not tie because he has had an unpleasant past experience that has resulted in a loss of confidence, often causing a failure to achieve a full erection. In these instances, holding the dog and bitch together as soon as the dog's thrusting has stopped may be helpful. This is known as a **held tie**, but this in itself can be very difficult to achieve. The dog should not be allowed to mate the bitch too many times without achieving a tie. It is better to try a few times and then rest the dog until the next day.

Often the bitch's position can be a problem: she may not elevate her vulva correctly, she may not deviate her tail very well, or she may keep moving her tail from side to side. In these instances elevating the bitch's vulva to the correct position or holding her tail out of the way can help the dog. These problems are commonly associated with inexperienced bitches. **Maiden bitches** (bitches that have not been mated before) can be a little overwhelmed by the whole process and require much more support than an experienced bitch. They will often stand at first but then change their minds. In these cases, the owner must be patient. Often the bitch just requires a little more time to get used to the stud and the idea of being mated. These matings can sometimes take several hours to achieve, but the bitch should not be rushed and most certainly must not be forced to stand. This could put her off mating altogether.

Some bitches can be difficult if the stud dog is playing too much and leaping on the bitch. The more inexperienced stud will exhibit this type of behaviour. The problem is rectified by gentle restraint of the bitch, ensuring that the human presence does not upset the stud. Whenever possible a new stud dog should be put with an experienced bitch, and a new bitch with an experienced stud.

Cats

In the cat, it is frequently very difficult to be present during a mating since this puts off all but the experienced males; in most cases, it is necessary to observe from a distance. It is always best to have an experienced partner when a queen or tom is mated for the first time.

Assisted reproduction

Dogs

There are several techniques that may be used to assist reproduction in the bitch. These include the induction of oestrus (see above) and artificial insemination.

Artificial insemination

Artificial insemination is the technique of placing semen collected from a male into the reproductive tract of the female. It may involve the use of freshly collected semen, semen that has been diluted and chilled, or semen that has been frozen and then thawed. Artificial insemination has several advantages over natural mating:

- It reduces the requirement to transport animals
- It is an acceptable way of overcoming, to some extent, the quarantine restrictions that prevent the movement of animals from one country to another
- It increases the genetic pool available to an individual breed within a country
- It reduces the disease risk that is always present when unknown animals enter a kennel for mating. (In some countries the use of AI may reduce the spread of infectious diseases)
- In certain circumstances, it may be useful when natural mating is difficult (for example, bitches that ovulate when they are not in standing oestrus or bitches that have hyperplasia of the vaginal floor)
- Semen may also be collected from male animals that, due to age, debility, back pain or premature ejaculation, are unable to achieve a natural mating.

The greatest area of interest is probably the storage of genetic material by freezing semen for insemination at a future date. This may be necessary in male animals that are likely to become infertile due to castration or to medical treatments with certain hormones. The more common reason is the preservation of semen from superior animals for use in future generations.

Collected semen may be deposited easily into the vagina of the bitch using a long inseminating pipette that is gently introduced near to the cervix. When semen is placed in this position, spermatozoa must swim through the cervix, into the uterus and up the uterine horns. During a natural mating, contractions of the vagina and uterus help in transporting semen. These

contractions generally do not occur during insemination, though some may be produced by stimulating the vagina. Vaginal insemination is therefore not ideal, but usually when fresh or chilled semen is used the spermatozoa will live long enough to fertilize the eggs. In the case of frozen semen, the spermatozoa do not live for long after thawing and so vaginal inseminations are not very satisfactory.

The chance of pregnancy can be improved if the semen is placed directly into the uterus rather than into the vagina. It is very difficult to place a catheter through the bitch's cervix into the uterus (a technique that is simple in many other animals) because the vagina is long and narrow and because the cervical opening is small and at an angle to the vagina. A special insemination pipette has been developed for this purpose. Recently some research workers have been able to catheterize the cervix using an endoscope. However, in certain countries the commonest way of performing uterine insemination is surgically via a laparotomy. In the UK the ethics of this procedure have been questioned.

Because of the short lifespan of the preserved sperm, it is most important that inseminations are accurately timed in relation to ovulation. The ideal time is 2–5 days after ovulation, and this is best assessed by using the measurement of plasma progesterone concentration and the study of vaginal cytology (see above).

In the UK, puppies that are the result of artificial insemination can only be registered if the Kennel Club has given prior permission. The permission of the Kennel Club is not required before semen is imported or exported. There are specific regulations set by the Department for Environment, Food and Rural Affairs in the UK and by similar organizations in other countries, which aim to prevent the introduction of infectious diseases. Import regulations vary between countries but are particularly stringent for the UK. Import permit requirements usually include: health certification before and a set time period after semen collection; quarantine of semen until the second health examination, and various serological tests.

Cats

Whilst artificial insemination has been widely practised in the domestic cat as a research model for wild cats, the technique is not commonly used in the UK. Techniques used in the cat are further advanced than those in the dog and include the induction of ovulation, *in vitro* fertilization and embryo transfer.

Pregnancy

The domestic bitch

The length of pregnancy in the bitch is relatively consistent – at 64, 65 or 66 days from the preovulatory LH surge. However, the *apparent* length of pregnancy, assessed from the time of mating, may vary between 56 and 72 days, since both early and late matings may be fertile.

- Early matings require sperm survival within the female reproductive tract until ovulation and egg maturation; such matings produce a long apparent pregnancy.
- Late matings occur when eggs are waiting to be fertilized for some time after ovulation; such matings produce a shorter pregnancy.

The clinical signs of pregnancy might include:

- Increased bodyweight and abdominal enlargement (these signs may not be obvious if the number of puppies is small)
- A reduced food intake and a vulval discharge – these are common approximately 1 month into the pregnancy
- Enlargement and reddening of the mammary glands – may be noted especially from 40 days after mating (but may also be present in bitches with pseudopregnancy)
- Production of milk – a variable finding (some bitches produce serous fluid from day 40 and milk from day 55 onwards, whilst in others this may not occur until just before parturition).

Certain physiological changes occur during pregnancy and include the development of a normochromic normocytic anaemia and a reduction of the packed cell volume; these changes are normal.

Uterine changes during pregnancy

Under the influence of progesterone the uterus becomes prepared to accept and nourish a pregnancy. This occurs in both pregnant and non-pregnant bitches, since both have elevated concentrations of progesterone. The specific change that occurs is an increased thickness of the uterine wall (the endometrium) associated with enlargement of specific glandular regions.

Overall, the uterus increases in diameter only slightly under the influence of progesterone and it is not until approximately 21 days that there is any enlargement related to the presence of a pregnancy. At this time there is slight swelling at the site of each pregnancy. By approximately 4 weeks the uterine swellings are significant in size and can be readily detected by palpation: the swellings are approximately 4 cm x 7 cm in size at 5 weeks and 5 cm x 8 cm at 6 weeks. Normally by 7 weeks the uterus has enlarged to such a degree that the individual swellings are no longer apparent and the adjacent fetuses are in contact with one another. From here onwards the uterus is very large and the fetuses can move freely within the allantoic fluid.

Care of the bitch during pregnancy

Food intake does not increase during the first 30 days of pregnancy. After this time the absolute requirement for carbohydrate and protein increases. During the last half of pregnancy, food consumption may be doubled. Provided that diet is well balanced and contains suitable amounts of vitamins and minerals it is not necessary to provide extra supplementation, but it may be necessary to divide the food into two or three meals during the day. Supplementation with calcium and vitamin D should be avoided, since this does not prevent eclampsia and can be dangerous.

Regular exercise should be provided throughout pregnancy, limited by the amount the bitch is willing to undertake.

For the control of ascarid infections (*Toxocara*; see Chapter 8) it is necessary to administer medication during pregnancy to reduce or prevent perinatal transmission. Various drugs (benzimidazoles) and treatment regimes have been advocated for the treatment of pregnant bitches. Many veterinary practices would advise that ascarid control should be undertaken prior to mating and after parturition, normally carried out at the same time that the puppies are treated. If it does become necessary to treat the dam, then this can be done during pregnancy.

It is advisable to ensure that routine vaccination has been performed before mating. Vaccination during pregnancy is unlikely to be damaging to the fetus and therefore may be undertaken if necessary, but no live vaccine is licensed for this purpose.

Pregnancy diagnosis in the bitch

As well as observation of the clinical signs already described (noting that mammary gland development, increased weight and abdominal enlargement may be present in pseudopregnancy as well as in pregnancy), there are several methods for pregnancy diagnosis in the bitch.

Abdominal palpation

This is best performed approximately 1 month after mating, when the conceptual swellings are approximately 2.0 cm in diameter. The technique can be highly accurate but may be difficult in obese or nervous animals, and may be inaccurate if the bitch was mated early such that pregnancy is not as advanced as anticipated. After day 35 individual conceptuses cannot easily be palpated and diagnosis becomes more difficult.

Identification of fetal heart beats

In late pregnancy it is possible to auscultate the fetal heart beats using a stethoscope, or to record a fetal ECG. Both of these methods are diagnostic of pregnancy; fetal heart rate is more rapid than that of the dam.

Radiography

From day 30 it is possible to detect uterine enlargement with good-quality radiographs. This is not actually diagnostic of pregnancy, since pyometra may have a similar appearance. Pregnancy diagnosis is not possible until after day 45, when mineralization of the fetal skeleton is detectable radiographically. At this stage it is unlikely that there will be radiation damage to the fetus, but sedation or anaesthesia of the dam may be required and is a potential risk. In late pregnancy the number of puppies can be reliably estimated by counting the number of fetal skulls.

Hormone tests

Plasma concentrations of progesterone are not useful for the detection of pregnancy in the bitch. Measurement of the hormone **relaxin** is diagnostic of pregnancy, and there is now a rapid ELISA test kit that can be run within the practice laboratory to measure this hormone. Alternatively a blood sample can be sent away to a commercial laboratory.

Acute-phase proteins

The rise in the concentration of acute-phase proteins has been used as the basis of a commercial pregnancy test in the bitch. Concentrations of these proteins (including fibrinogen and C-reactive protein) increase from approximately 25 days onwards. The test is reliable although these proteins are also released in inflammatory conditions such as pyometra.

Ultrasound examination

Diagnostic B-mode ultrasonography is now commonly used for pregnancy diagnosis (Figure 25.13). The technique is non-invasive and without risk to the puppies, dam or veterinary surgeon. The bitch can be examined in the standing position with minimal restraint.

Using ultrasonography it is possible to diagnose pregnancy as early as 16 days after ovulation, but in most cases this time is not known and so it is prudent to wait until 28 days after mating. At that time the fluid-filled conceptuses can easily be imaged and embryonic tissue can be identified. It is possible to assess the number of conceptuses, though this can be inaccurate, especially when the litter size is large. Movement of the fetal heart can be seen and this confirms fetal viability. It is possible to examine the bitch at any time after day 28 to diagnose pregnancy and to confirm fetal viability and growth. With later examinations it is less easy to estimate the number of puppies.

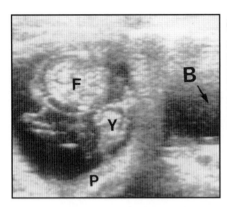

25.13

Ultrasound image of a pregnant bitch. F, fetus; Y, yolk sac; B, urinary bladder; P, placenta.

The domestic queen

The average length of pregnancy in the queen is 65 days, with a range of 64–68 days.

The clinical signs of pregnancy include increased bodyweight and abdominal enlargement (these signs are often apparent in all but young queens) and mammary development, which is obvious from approximately day 40. These changes are usually diagnostic for pregnancy, since pseudopregnancy is not common and is not usually associated with clinical signs.

During the second half of pregnancy there is an increase in food intake and in the requirement for both carbohydrate and protein. Provided that diet is well balanced and contains suitable amounts of vitamins and minerals, it is not necessary to provide extra supplementation.

Many queens continue to be active during pregnancy and the amount of exercise is best limited by the individual cat. It is advisable to ensure that routine vaccination has been performed prior to mating.

Pregnancy diagnosis in the queen

Abdominal palpation

Conceptual swellings can be palpated from approximately 21 days after mating. These are discrete until 30 days after mating but become more difficult to palpate from this time onwards.

Identification of fetal heartbeats

In late pregnancy the fetal heartbeats may be auscultated using a stethoscope. At this time it is also usually possible to palpate the fetus in all but the most obese cats.

Radiography

From day 30 it is possible to detect uterine enlargement with good-quality radiographs. Mineralization of the fetal skeleton is detectable radiographically from 40 days after mating.

Hormone tests

Plasma concentrations of progesterone are elevated in both pregnancy and pseudopregnancy, therefore measurement of this hormone is not diagnostic. Plasma relaxin concentrations are elevated from day 25; this hormone is diagnostic of pregnancy and can be measured as described for the bitch.

Ultrasound examination

Diagnostic B-mode ultrasonography may be used for pregnancy diagnosis in the cat. The pregnancy length can be assessed from mating time, unlike in the bitch. Conceptuses can be imaged from 12 days after mating and embryonic tissue can usually be seen from day 14. From this time onwards it is possible to identify pregnancy, confirm fetal viability and assess fetal growth. It is more difficult to assess the number of kittens in later pregnancy.

Embryological development

Fertilization

The **egg** (ovum) which is released at ovulation from the follicle is surrounded by a thick protective coat. The inner layer comprises glycoprotein and is called the **zona pellucida**, whilst the outer layer is made up of small follicular cells and is called the **corona radiata** (Figure 25.14).

The egg is fertilized during its passage through the uterine tube. Just before fertilization, sperm change their type of motility so that they are able to burrow through the cells surrounding the egg. During this process a reaction occurs in the head region of the sperm resulting in the release of an enzyme that starts to digest the zona pellucida. These sperm are said to be **acrosome-reacted**. The sperm is then able to penetrate into the egg (the process called **fertilization**).

The fertilized egg is frequently called a **zygote** or **conceptus** (sometimes also called an **embryo**, but this term needs to be differentiated from the embryo proper, which is the mass of cells that form the true body of the developing animal – see below).

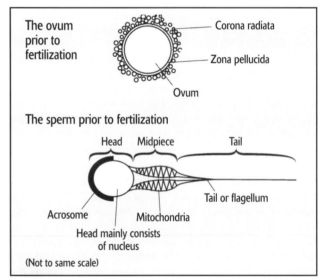

25.14 Structure of ovum and sperm.

The conceptus

After fertilization the conceptus continues to travel down the uterine tube towards the uterus and generally reaches the uterus by day 7 after ovulation. During its journey, the cells of the conceptus begin to divide (Figure 25.15). By doubling at each division the conceptus has two, then four and then eight cells, before forming a solid ball of cells called a **morula**.

The spherical morula develops a central fluid-filled cavity. The cells lining the cavity are called the **trophoblast**. Cells tend to accumulate at one end of the conceptus and are called the **inner cell mass**. This gathering of cells will eventually form the **embryo proper**. Three separate layers then develop and these will finally form specific recognizable areas of the body.

- The outer layer of the inner cell mass is called the **ectoderm** – this will form the skin and the nervous system.

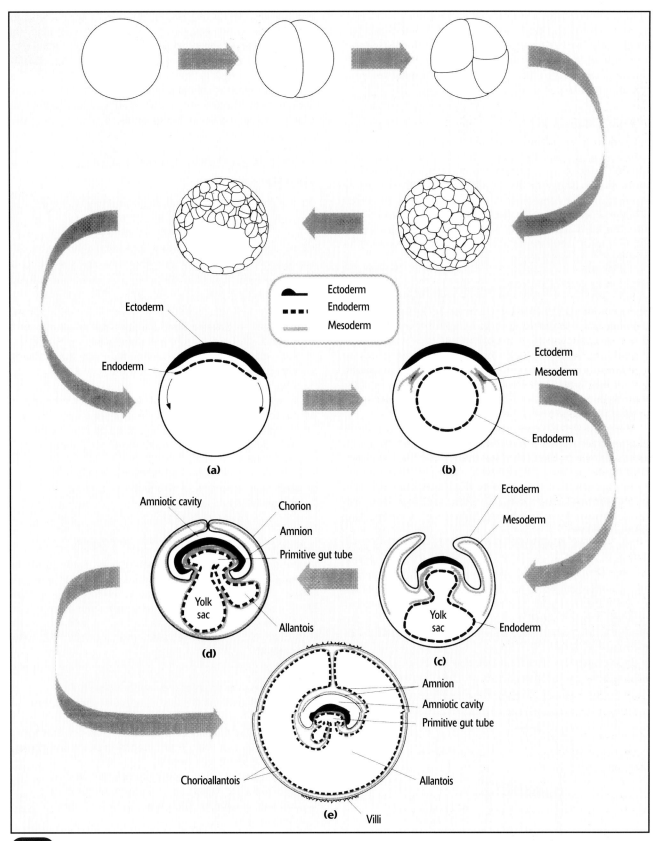

25.15 Early embryonic development.

- The middle layer of the inner cell mass is called the **mesoderm** – this will form several organ systems and the musculoskeletal system.
- The inner layer of the inner cell mass is called the **endoderm** – this will form the lining of the gastrointestinal tract and of other visceral organs.

Two long blocks of mesoderm develop. Underneath these, the endodermal cells spread out and form a lining to the trophoblast which is called the **yolk sac**. In birds (and also in reptiles) this contains a true yolk, which provides nourishment, but in mammals it is a fluid-filled sac for nutrient transfer. The two blocks of mesoderm then align themselves, one next to the ectoderm and one next to the endoderm. A cavity forms between these two layers of the mesoderm. The inner cell mass curls around and encloses the mesoderm and endoderm layers, which will then form the internal organs of the embryo. The yolk sac and the trophoblast form the **placental membranes**.

Implantation

During the period of maturation of the conceptus it has been slowly moving down the uterine tube and has entered the uterus. Usually there are multiple conceptuses, which tend to move around within the uterus and become relatively evenly spaced apart. The conceptuses lie close to the wall of the uterus and the process of **implantation** starts at approximately day 14 in the bitch and day 11 in the queen. During implantation the conceptus partly destroys an area of the uterine wall (the **endometrium**) and becomes firmly attached.

The placental membranes

The placental membranes form around the embryo and are therefore called the **extra-embryonic membranes**. There are four basic components to the extra-embryonic membranes: the yolk sac, the chorion, the amnion and the allantois.

As the gut starts to develop (from the endoderm), a specific part of this forms the **allantois**. The allantois receives urine from the kidneys via a special tube (the **urachus**) present only in the embryo and fetus (it regresses in the adult).

Whilst the allantois is developing, the trophoblast continues to expand and it spreads around the embryo as a double sheet. The outer membrane is called the **chorion** and the inner layer is called the **amnion**. Throughout the period of this development the allantois continues to be filled with fetal urine and ultimately the allantois comes into contact and then fuses with the chorion. This combined structure is called the **chorioallantois**.

The **placenta** is the thickened area of the extra-embryonic membranes that attaches the fetus to the endometrium. The placenta is an interface between the fetus and the mother that allows transmission of oxygen and nutrients to the fetus whilst ensuring the elimination of waste products. To do this the fetus develops a blood supply to the placenta (actually within the chorioallantois), which has a large surface area of contact with the maternal tissue.

In the bitch the placenta is described as having a **zonary** nature, because it forms as a broad belt around the fetus (Figure 25.16). At the edge of the placenta is the **marginal**

haematoma. This is a region where there is degeneration of the maternal endothelium with a resultant bleeding into the spaces formed by the degeneration. Substances secreted by the chorion prevent the blood from clotting, and it is thought that this blood may form a source of iron for the fetus. The fluid in the marginal haematoma is green in bitches and brownish in queens. These are the colours that are noted at the time of placental separation in these species.

Development of the canine embryo

As the cells of the inner cell mass multiply and then start to curve underneath themselves, they form the head and trunk of the embryo. Within the embryo an inner cavity forms which is called the **coelom** (the main body cavity). The coelom is divided into two separate zones by the diaphragm. The cranial zone is the thorax and the caudal zone is the abdomen.

- Generally by 3 weeks after ovulation the amnion and the allantois have formed and the embryo (in the dog) is approximately 5 mm in length. Normally the uterus itself is now slightly enlarged at the site of the placental attachment.
- By 4 weeks of age it is possible to identify the forming vertebrae and limb buds and the embryo is approaching 20 mm in length. Usually at this stage there is the first evidence of ossification (though this is not yet visible on a radiograph).
- By 5 weeks of age the eyelids, internal ears and canine teeth have started to form, and the embryo is approximately 35 mm in length.

Development of the fetus

From approximately day 35 the external features of the developing canine embryo allow it to be recognized as a dog and from this time onwards it is referred to as a **fetus**. By this time all the major internal organs have formed, and further development is characterized by an increase in size, especially elongation of the trunk and an increase in diameter of the head.

- By 6 weeks the digits and the external genitalia are well developed and the fetus is approximately 60 mm in length.
- By 7 weeks the fetus is approximately 100 mm in length and there is significant ossification of the vertebral bodies and some of the long bones.
- At 8 weeks the fetus is approximately 150 mm in length and has hair and pads. Fetuses are normally delivered at approximately 9 weeks (65 ± 1 days after ovulation).

Placental membranes at birth

During birth the chorioallantois is recognized as the outer fetal sac (often called the 'water bag') which ruptures as the fetus moves into the birth canal. The amnion, which is the inner fetal sac, is designed also to rupture and provide additional lubrication, but it does not always rupture and in some cases the fetus may be delivered within the amnion.

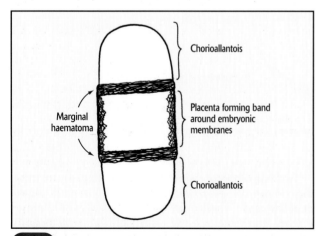

Chorioallantois

Placenta forming band around embryonic membranes

Marginal haematoma

Chorioallantois

25.16   The extra-embryonic membranes.

Abnormalities of pregnancy

Resorption and abortion

A great concern for owners is the risk of resorption or abortion during pregnancy. To understand the differences in these processes, it is necessary to define the stages of development. As explained above, in general the term **embryo** is used when the characteristics of the conceptus are not discernable. From approximately 35 days after ovulation the characteristics of a puppy become obvious and the term **fetus** is used.

- **Resorption** refers to the resorption of the entire conceptus and occurs during the embryonic stage of development.
- **Abortion** refers to the expulsion of the fetus and the fetal membranes before term (i.e. before 58 days after ovulation).
- A **stillbirth** is the expulsion of the fetus and fetal membranes after day 58 (i.e. close to term).

The incidence of resorption or abortion of the entire litter is not known, but it is certain that up to 5% of bitches and queens suffer isolated resorption of one or two conceptuses, with continuation of the remaining pregnancy.

There are many potential causes of resorption and abortion, including infectious agents, trauma, fetal defects and maternal environment.

- In the dog, the infectious agents *Brucella canis* (not present in the UK), canine distemper virus, canine herpesvirus and *Toxoplasma gondii* infection have all been implicated as causes of abortion and resorption.
- In the cat, feline herpesvirus I, feline panleucopenia virus, feline leukaemia virus, feline infections peritonitis virus and *Toxoplasma gondii* infection may produce abortion, resorption or stillbirths.

In many cases embryonic death and pregnancy loss are best assessed using real-time diagnostic B-mode ultrasound. Resorptions may be unrecognized by the owner unless associated with a period of illness. Abortion of fetal tissue may be obvious, but may not be noticed should the dam eat the aborted material. In the face of an abortion, there is little that can be administered to the patient except supportive therapy.

Hypoglycaemia

Pregnancy hypoglycaemia has been reported in the bitch and is associated with reduced blood glucose concentrations during late pregnancy. The clinical signs include weakness that may progress to coma. The condition may be confused with hypocalcaemia, which occurs at a similar time (see later).

Parturition

Preparation for parturition in the bitch

In the last few weeks of pregnancy, attempts should be made to encourage the bitch to accept a nest in a suitable place for parturition and rearing. Ideally, this should be a warm, clean, draught- and damp-proof room that can be heated. The room is best isolated from the main thoroughfare of the household, where the bitch can rest quietly, but it is beneficial for socializing the litter if noises from washing machines, radios and people talking can be heard. The room should be of a sufficient size to allow the growing litter to play and, where possible, for puppies to have access to an outside area (should the weather permit).

The room should contain a whelping bed. Ideally the bed should be large enough to allow the dam to stretch and have sufficient room for a large litter. The sides should be high enough to prevent the puppies escaping until they are approximately 4 weeks old.

In some cases, particularly in a bitch with a lot of hair, it might be useful to remove some of the hair from around the perineum and ventral abdomen, prior to the whelping. This will help the puppies gain access to the nipples and allows cleaning of the dam after parturition.

Heating

Hypothermia is a major cause of neonatal mortality and so the environmental temperature is critical. Neonates are unable to regulate their own temperature for the first week of life and rely on the dam and other neonates to keep warm. A chilled neonate will not respond normally, move properly or be able to suck, and this may result in the dam neglecting it. It is therefore recommended that the room must be able to be heated to 25–30°C for the first few days of the neonates' life. This temperature is often unbearable for the dam and so can be safely reduced to approximately 22°C after this time. It is most important that the litter is kept well away from any draughts that might chill them.

The room can easily be heated using a thermostatically controlled heater or underfloor heating. A heat lamp can be suspended over the bed, but care must be taken to ensure that the neonates do not overheat. It is recommended that perhaps only half of the bed or box is heated, so that the dam can move out of the heat if she wishes. Well protected hot-water bottles or circulating water blankets provide good alternatives.

Useful equipment

A plentiful supply of newspaper is necessary for the area. Plenty of bedding that can easily be removed when soiled should be available. Shredded paper can be used but with care, since very small neonates may get caught up in it. If using a fabric bedding material, then a least three or four of these will be needed. A supply of blankets will suffice.

A pair of weighing scales, clock and note pad are useful, to enable a record to be kept of the times of birth and weights of neonates when they have been born. A thermometer should be kept in order to record the dam's rectal temperature prior to parturition.

Sometimes dams can be clumsy at the time of parturition. If there is a large litter, it may be useful to put some of the neonates out of harm's way in a small box within the nesting bed. It is important to ensure that the neonates are kept warm whilst away from their mother. This can be achieved by wrapping a hot-water bottle in some towels and placing it in the bottom of the box.

A supply of milk substitute can be offered to the dam during parturition. No food should be offered at this time, just in case the dam gets into difficulty and requires veterinary intervention.

There should be suitable equipment to facilitate the artificial rearing of the neonates should this be required. This should include small syringes, feeding bottles and teats and substitute milk for feeding the neonates, along with cotton wool for cleaning any spilt milk off them and to aid urination and defecation if the dam is unable to care for them at all.

Stages of parturition

In the last week of pregnancy it is prudent to record the dam's rectal temperature at least twice daily. This is to detect the prepartum hypothermia that precedes the onset of parturition by 24–36 hours. This decline in body temperature is mediated by a sudden reduction in the plasma concentration of progesterone. The rectal temperature usually changes from approximately 39°C to below 37°C.

There are five stage of parturition:

1. Preparation
2. First stage (onset of contractions)
3. Second stage (propulsion of fetus)
4. Third stage (passage of placenta)
5. Puerperium (after parturition).

Preparation stage

The preparation stage is associated with the decline in plasma progesterone concentration and hence the decrease in rectal temperature. At this time the vaginal and perineal tissue will relax and the dam may show some signs of impending parturition.

She may start to prepare her nest, by shredding and ripping up the bedding. She will probably be more restless than usual. She may also show an increased mucous discharge from her vulva, which will probably be slightly more swollen. It is important to remember that some bitches may show no signs of preparation at all.

Some bitches may seek the company of others, while some will try to find solace in a quiet place on their own. Few bitches will be happy with an audience for whelping and so it is best if just one person can stay with the bitch for the birth.

Many queens will seek seclusion to give birth to their kittens, preferring not to have people around them at this time.

First stage of parturition

The first stage of parturition commences with the onset of uterine contractions and can be 1–12 hours in duration, but this is very variable. By this time, milk is usually present within the mammary glands or should appear at this stage.

With the onset of contractions the bitch might become increasingly restless, pant and/or shiver and her nesting behaviour might become more frantic. Some bitches will refuse food at this time or may vomit their last meal. Most cats will seek seclusion at this time.

The uterine contractions will push the fetus against the cervix, which has begun to dilate. This may result in the rupture of the allantochorion and so allantoic fluid may then be produced from the vulva.

Second stage of parturition

The second stage is characterized by an increase in uterine contractions and propulsion of the fetus through the cervix into the vagina. These will begin when the first fetus enters the pelvic canal. The contractions are normally quite noticeable. The bitch will appear to squeeze from her ribs towards the perineal area and then relax.

The time of the first contractions should be recorded, in case there is any delay in the whelping. The time between the onset of straining and the birth of the first fetus is variable. It can be as short as 10 minutes or up to 30 minutes or longer, particularly in maiden bitches. If the bitch continues to have contractions for more than two hours without producing a puppy, or if her waters have broken and a puppy has not been produced, veterinary advice should be sought, as this could indicate dystocia. Most bitches will be in lateral recumbency during whelping, but some prefer to stand. Delivery of the fetal head is often the most difficult part of the birth and may be associated with some pain, but once this is delivered the rest of the fetus is usually delivered rapidly.

A membrane, the amnion, surrounds the fetus and is often seen at the vulva during straining. It may appear and then disappear with the contractions, and it may rupture spontaneously or be broken by the dam. The fetus may also be born within it.

After delivery, the dam will normally commence vigorous licking, removing the membranes and clearing fluid from around the neonate's face. If the dam fails to remove the membranes immediately after the birth, it must be done for her swiftly. Occasionally young or inexperienced bitches may need help and encouragement with the immediate licking and cleaning. This can be achieved using a clean soft towel. The neonate should be given a vigorous rub with a towel to stimulate it, to help to clear the airways of any fluid and to dry it so as to avoid chilling. When rubbing a neonate it is best if the animal is held with its head lower than its bottom (to aid the drainage of fluid from its lungs) and not too high from the ground, in case it is dropped.

The birth of the fetus is usual followed by the passage of the allantochorion or placenta (**afterbirth**). Normally a dam separates the neonate from the placenta by chewing through the cord and then eating the placenta when it is expelled. It is important to ensure that the dam does not chew the umbilicus excessively, as this can cause damage to the neonate. If the dam does not sever the umbilicus, the placenta can be separated by tearing or cutting the cord using scissors. Care must be taken if the cord is to be torn. The procedure can be achieved by holding the cord an inch or so away from the neonate's abdomen and tearing the cord with the other hand. The dam should be given every opportunity to clean and fuss over the neonate before it is removed for weighing and checking etc. (see 'Examination', below).

Once all the procedures have been carried out, the neonate can be returned to the dam. The neonates are best left with their mother during the remainder of the delivery, as removing them might distress the dam, inhibiting further straining. If the dam is young, inexperienced or particularly clumsy, it can be a good idea to put a few of the neonates in a warm box, once the dam has attended to them. This will keep them safer whilst the dam continues giving birth.

Third stage of parturition

The third stage is the passage of the placenta. In the bitch and the queen the passage of the placenta occurs usually during the second stage of parturition, but occasionally one or more fetuses are delivered without their placentas, which are expelled at a later stage or delivered with subsequent fetuses. It is useful to count the number of placentas passed, as a larger number of fetuses compared with the number of placentas may indicate that the dam has retained one or more.

After a bitch has finished whelping, there is normally a dark-coloured vulval discharge. This contains a green pigment that originates from the placenta. This discharge should normally decline after about a week.

Puerperium

The puerperium is the period after parturition during which the reproductive tract returns to its normal non-pregnant state. During this time the uterus starts its involution and it is common to see a mucoid vulval discharge that may last for up to 6 weeks.

Dystocia

The term dystocia literally means difficult birth; it is used to indicate any problem that interferes with normal birth. Dystocia is rare in the queen but problems are not uncommon in the bitch, especially in brachycephalic breeds such as the Bulldog and Boston Terrier. The two main causes of dystocia are maternal factors and fetal factors.

Maternal dystocia

Maternal dystocia may be divided into two categories: poor straining efforts by the dam and obstruction of the birth canal.

Poor straining efforts of the dam

Poor straining may be the result of nervousness or pain that inhibits normal parturition, but it is more commonly the result of poor myometrial contractions, a condition that has been termed **uterine inertia**. Inertia may be primary, in which case parturition does not commence, or may be secondary to some other factor occurring during parturition.

Primary uterine inertia

This is rare in the cat but is seen not uncommonly in young bitches with only one or two puppies, or in older overweight bitches with large litters. The cause of the condition is unknown, but it may relate to poor condition of the uterine musculature in fat or debilitated animals, overstretching of the uterus when the litter size is large, poor stimulus for parturition when there are only a few fetuses or low plasma calcium concentrations.

The endocrinological events of parturition are usually normal, but subsequent uterine contractions are not fully initiated and parturition does not follow. A green vulval discharge, which indicates placental separation, may be seen some days after the expected date of parturition. In some cases the owner may have observed initial weak uterine contractions or have noted the decline in body temperature. At this stage the administration of the hormone oxytocin may stimulate uterine contractions. Some cases may respond to the intravenous administration of calcium borogluconate. Repeated doses of oxytocin may be necessary but oxytocin should only be given when it is certain that there is no obstruction to the birth canal. However, it is not possible in the bitch to assess the patency of the cervix by digital palpation (the vagina of an average 20 kg bitch is 20 cm long). In certain cases caesarean operation may be necessary.

Primary uterine inertia may be anticipated in some bitches because of a previous history of this problem or because of their age, physical condition or the number of puppies. The best assessment of the bitch is to monitor the rectal temperature twice daily during the last 7–10 days of pregnancy.

Secondary uterine inertia

This is the cessation of uterine contractions after they have started. Most commonly it is the result of uterine exhaustion following obstructive dystocia, but it may occur spontaneously during the second stage of parturition, presumably because of factors similar to those seen with primary uterine inertia. If the cause of the dystocia can be relieved, the administration of oxytocin and calcium may be suitable treatments. In some cases caesarean operation may be necessary.

Obstruction of the birth canal

Obstruction may be the result of abnormalities of the birth canal, such as:

- **Deformity of the pelvic bones** – these may be congenital malformations, developmental abnormalities or the result of previous trauma, commonly following a road accident
- **Soft tissue abnormalities** within the pelvis which press against the reproductive tract – they might include pelvic neoplasms, though these are rare in animals of breeding age
- **Abnormality of the reproductive tract** itself – for example, torsion of the uterus or congenital vaginal or uterine constrictions.

Fetal dystocia

Fetal oversize

Oversize of the fetus relative to the birth canal may be the result of:

- **Breed conformation** – dystocia may be considered almost normal for certain breeds with exaggerated physical characteristics such as a large head size
- **Actual fetal oversize** – when the litter size is small and large fetuses develop within the uterus
- **Fetal abnormalities** – including fetal monsters, resulting in relative oversize and dystocia.

In the majority of these cases caesarean operation is necessary for the delivery of the fetuses, whether normal or abnormal.

Abnormalities of fetal alignment

Variation from the normal presentation, position and posture of the fetus during delivery may result in dystocia. This may be corrected in certain cases by manipulation per vaginum; however, caesarean operation may be necessary.

Normal orientation of the fetus

- The **presentation** of a fetus is a description of the direction of its long axis in relation to the long axis of the dam (Figure 25.17). Puppies and kittens can only be delivered in longitudinal presentation (i.e. the long axis of the fetus is parallel to the long axis of the dam) but may have either anterior (fetal head delivered first) or posterior (fetus delivered backwards) presentation.
- The **position** of a fetus is a description of its dorsal axis with respect to the dorsum of the dam; this describes the degree of rotation of the fetus. Most species are normally born in dorsal position; i.e. the back of the fetus is uppermost in the same orientation as the dam.
- The **posture** of a fetus is a description of the orientation of the head and legs, which may be extended or flexed. For anterior presentation the head must be extended, and this occurs naturally during a posterior presentation.

A **breech birth** refers to a fetus delivered in posterior longitudinal presentation, usually in dorsal position with the hindlimbs flexed. This means that the fetus is presented 'bottom first' with its hindlimbs directed towards the dam's head. A fetus delivered in posterior presentation with the legs extended is not a breech presentation.

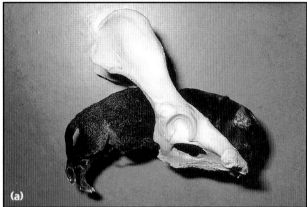

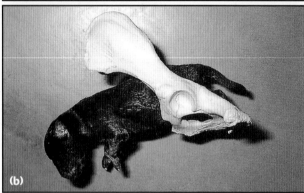

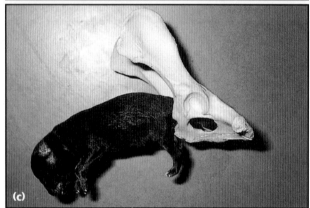

25.17 Presentation of a fetus: **(a)** normal anterior presentation; **(b)** normal posterior presentation; **(c)** breech presentation.

Recognition of dystocia

The normal events of parturition should be clearly understood so that recognition of dystocia can be achieved rapidly, thus allowing prompt intervention.

Collection of a relevant history is essential in the evaluation of a potential case of dystocia. This includes the estimation of the stage of pregnancy. Determining of the mating time is most helpful in establishing the stage of pregnancy in cats but this is not very useful in bitches, where apparent pregnancy length can vary between 56 and 72 days from mating (see above). Regular monitoring of rectal temperature is therefore essential in the bitch. It should be established whether this has been done by the owner, and if so what changes were observed.

Of particular importance is the time-course of events from the onset of parturition, e.g. the onset of behavioural changes such as restlessness, nest making and panting. The time when straining first occurred and the character of the straining efforts may also be useful as an indicator of dystocia, as will the times that any fetuses were produced.

It is not possible to give definite guidelines regarding potential cases of dystocia but examination of the patient is warranted in certain situations:

- A bitch that has exceeded 70 days from the last mating and has no signs of impending parturition.
- A cat that has exceeded 65 days from the last mating and has no signs of impending parturition.
- The dam is unsettled and strains forcefully but infrequently.
- There are signs of straining which then cease.
- There is a black/green vulval discharge with no signs of parturition.
- There has been a decline in rectal temperature and parturition has not commenced within 48 hours.
- There has been ineffectual straining for 1 hour or more.
- Several fetuses have been produced, the last more than 2 hours ago and the dam is restless.
- Several fetuses have been produced, the last more than 2 hours ago and a larger litter is expected (may not be known by the owner).

Investigation of potential cases of dystocia

In most cases it is necessary to ensure that the animal is pregnant and/or that viable fetuses remain within the uterus. This can be achieved by transabdominal palpation, auscultation of fetal heartbeats, real-time ultrasonography and radiography, as described earlier for pregnancy diagnosis.

Further investigation involves digital examination of the vagina to assess whether a fetus is present and to establish fetal alignment. This should only be performed after cleaning the vulval area thoroughly with an antiseptic solution and scrubbing the hands or wearing surgical gloves. A water-soluble lubricant should be applied to the fingers and the vestibule and vagina should be carefully examined. The presence of bone or soft-tissue abnormalities of the pelvis should be noted. The presentation, position and posture of the fetus should be established before any further intervention is contemplated.

For normal presentations delivery can be assisted using the thumb and forefinger placed in a cradle manner around the fetal head (anterior presentation) or pelvis (posterior presentation). Traction should only be applied during the straining effort of the bitch, but pressure on the roof of the vagina may be applied with the finger to stimulate straining. Sterile gauze or similar fabric may help the nurse to grip the puppy or kitten when assisting delivery. Undue force should never be applied to the feet, as these are easily damaged or deformed.

Caesarean operation

There are many reasons for performing a caesarean operation. In many cases this may be for the relief of dystocia, whilst occasionally it may be an elective procedure when there is concern over feto-maternal disproportion.

Anaesthesia

It is important to remember that there are several marked physiological changes during pregnancy that may affect the requirements for anaesthesia. These physiological changes result in decreased minimum alveolar concentrations of anaesthetic gases, an increased oxygen requirement, and commonly hypoventilation and subsequent hypoxia and hypercarbia. In addition, in cases of dystocia, the animal may be debilitated and may have recently been fed.

The general aims are to:

- Ensure adequate oxygenation (intubation and oxygen administration)
- Maintain blood volume and prevent hypotension (intravenous fluid therapy)
- Minimize depression of the fetus and dam during and after surgery (reduce the dose of anaesthetic agents used).

There are many anaesthetic regimes suitable for this procedure, including the use of volatile agents for induction and maintenance of anaesthesia and the use of rapid-acting intravenous induction agents (such as propofol) followed by maintenance of anaesthesia using a volatile inhalational anaesthetic.

Complications

There are several complications of caesarean operation in both dogs and cats. These include:

- Anaesthetic risks in the dam and the neonate
- Risks during surgery of uterine rupture and haemorrhage resulting in hypovolaemia
- Postoperative risks, including wound infection and wound breakdown
- Interference with the wound by neonates trying to suck
- Problems in the dam of accepting the litter.

Some veterinary surgeons prefer to perform the operation via a flank incision to avoid the problem of wound interference when the neonates try to suck.

The problem of rejection of the litter by a young dam after a caesarean operation may be overcome by placing the offspring with the dam as soon as possible after surgery. The mother's milk should be squeezed on to the newborn's heads if rejection is a problem. The dam should be carefully observed until she is able to coordinate sufficiently not to damage them and she must not be left unattended until successful sucking has been noted.

Postparturient care of the dam

Once the dam has finished giving birth she should be cleaned, paying particular attention to her perineum. This will make her feel more comfortable. She should also now be given the opportunity to exercise and urinate or defecate. Usually the dam will then settle with her litter during feeding. Soiled bedding should be changed for clean, fresh material.

The dam can now be offered some food. It must be remembered that, depending on the amount of afterbirths she has eaten, if any, she may be prone to gastrointestinal upset. It is therefore recommended that for the first day or so she should be offered something nutritious but 'light'. Chicken, fish, rice and pasta are all suitable. The dam should be offered her diet in five or six small meals. This can be a pre-prepared diet specifically suitable for lactation or a well balanced diet. The amount she receives should depend on the litter size. Obviously a dam with a large litter will need significantly more food than a dam with only a small litter. The dam should remain on five or six small meals per day for the first few weeks. It should also be remembered that the diet should not be altered too quickly, as this may worsen any gastrointestinal upset.

During the first 2 weeks after the birth of the litter, the dam will spend much of her time with the litter and therefore it may be preferable to feed her close to the nest bed. A readily accessible supply of fresh water should be close by. Once weaning begins the dam should be encouraged to leave the nest for increasingly longer periods.

The dam should be encouraged to exercise during lactation, but where possible this should be where she will not come into contact with other animals, due to the risk of taking infection back to the litter.

Once weaning has begun and is well underway, the demands on the dam start to reduce and therefore her relevant food intake should also gradually begin to lessen. If the dam has lost a great deal of weight through her efforts to feed the litter, then her food intake should remain high so that she can replace some of the lost bodyweight. When she has regained some weight her food intake can be reduced.

Normally a veterinary surgeon should be called to examine the dam when parturition is finished, in order to check her health and that of her newborn litter. Thereafter the dam's general health should also be closely monitored throughout lactation. Common problems to look for are signs of eclampsia (see later), mastitis (see later), pyrexia, and a foul-smelling vulval discharge. If any of these are observed, veterinary attention should be sought. The litter should also be closely monitored for fading syndrome (see later).

Lactation

The development of the mammary gland after puberty is under hormonal control. **Progesterone** from the corpus luteum causes the glands to enlarge during pregnancy; this is sometimes seen in false pregnancies. Hormones are further involved in lactation in that they are responsible for the **initiation** of milk secretion (see below). They also play a vital role in the **maintenance** of milk secretion after it has been established. The terminology used to describe the various aspects of lactation is often confused:

- **Milk secretion** refers to the synthesis of milk by the epithelial cells and the passage of milk from the cytoplasm of the cells into the alveolar lumen.
- **Milk removal** includes the passive withdrawal of milk from the cisterns and sinuses and the ejection of milk from the alveolar lumina.
- **Lactation** refers to the combined processes of milk secretion and removal.
- **Lactogenesis** is the initiation of milk secretion.
- **Mammogenesis** describes the development of the mammary gland.
- **Galactopoiesis** refers to the enhancement of established lactation.

In the bitch, there is a long luteal phase in both pregnancy and non-pregnancy. Progesterone primes the mammary glands; however, mammary gland secretion and the development of obvious clinical signs or pregnancy (and pseudopregnancy) are associated with a rise in plasma concentration of prolactin, which commences at 30–35 days after the LH surge. Prolactin is the principal luteotrophic factor in the bitch. Prolactin concentration continues to increase during late pregnancy to a plateau at approximately day 60. Prolactin concentration surges during the prepartum decline in progesterone, and reaches a peak at or shortly after parturition.

Initiation of milk secretion

The hormonal control of the initiation of lactation has not been fully explained. It is likely to be either a rise in the blood concentrations of prolactin and glucocorticoids at the time of parturition, or a decrease in the concentrations of compounds that have an inhibitory effect on the milk secretion process, namely progesterone and transcortin.

Prior to parturition, lipid and protein granules form in the epithelial cells and accumulate in the lumen of the alveolus as **colostrum**. Colostrum is the first milk produced and is a source of antibodies for the neonate. In the bitch and queen, antibodies are present in the milk for several days after parturition. Interestingly, whilst antibodies are readily absorbed on the first day after birth, the rate of absorption varies for different antibodies and the intestinal tract ceases to absorb different antibodies at different times. As a general rule of thumb, puppies and kittens should have sucked (or be given colostrum) within 8 hours of birth. Ideally they should suck within the first few hours of birth.

Oxytocin secreted by the posterior pituitary gland in the few hours around parturition enables the release or 'let down' of milk in response to sucking by the neonate. Continuation of sucking is necessary to maintain the production of milk.

Milk

Milk is the nutritious material produced after the colostrum. The composition of milk varies between species: milk produced by the bitch and queen is more concentrated and contains more protein and twice as much fat as cow's milk. The average composition of milk is shown in Figure 25.18. The basic milk sugar is lactose. A variety of milk substitutes are commercially available and these are discussed later.

Constituent	Quantity
Water	70–90%
Fat	0–30%
Protein	1–15%
Carbohydrate	3–7%
Minerals	0.5–1% calcium phosphate, magnesium, sodium, potassium and chloride. Deficient in iron and copper. Traces of iodine, cobalt, tin and silica
Vitamins	A, B2 ,B5 , E, K. Low in C and D

25.18 The average composition of milk.

Periparturient abnormalities

There are several conditions that may occur during late pregnancy or soon after parturition in both the domestic bitch and the queen. Some conditions are emergencies and prompt recognition of the clinical signs is essential to allow successful treatment.

Hypocalcaemia (eclampsia, puerperal tetany)

Low plasma concentrations of calcium are related to calcium loss in the milk and poor dietary calcium availability. The condition is most commonly seen during late pregnancy or early lactation. It is rare in the cat. The clinical signs include restlessness, panting, increased salivation and a stiff gait that may progress to muscle fasciculations, pyrexia and tachycardia. If untreated, tetany and death results. The slow administration of calcium borogluconate by intravenous injection produces a rapid resolution of the clinical signs. During administration, cardiac rate and rhythm should be monitored. Calcium supplementation may then be given orally or by subcutaneous injection to prevent recurrence of the condition.

Placental retention

The retention of placental tissue is uncommon in both the bitch and the queen, but it causes great concern for many owners. Placentas are normally delivered following each puppy or kitten and may be quickly eaten by the dam. If a placenta is retained, the clinical signs are a persistent green vulval discharge. This should be differentiated from the normal haemorrhagic discharge that may persist for 1 week after parturition (a mucoid discharge may be present for up to 6 weeks). If a retained placenta is diagnosed by either ultrasound examination or palpation, the administration of oxytocin is usually curative.

Postpartum metritis

Infection and inflammation of the uterus may occur following prolonged parturition, abortion, fetal and/or placental retention or obstetrical manipulation. The clinical signs commonly include a persistent purulent vulval discharge, lethargy and pyrexia. Treatment with broad-spectrum antimicrobial agents should be instituted immediately; fluid replacement therapy may be required.

Mastitis

Inflammation of the mammary gland is not common in the bitch or queen, but it may have disastrous results should the dam reject the litter because of pain on suckling. It is usually the result of bacterial infection following trauma (sucking). The mammary glands are tender, warm and firm upon palpation and the milk may be contaminated with blood and inflammatory cells so that it becomes yellow, pink or brown. The dam may become lethargic and anorexic if the condition is not treated. Bathing and massaging the gland with warm water and gently removing the infected fluid may be helpful, but antimicrobial agents are usually required. It should be remembered that these agents will be excreted in the milk and ingested by the neonates.

Breeding exotic pets

Small mammals

Reproductive parameters for small mammals are given in Figure 25.19.

Ferrets

The male ferret (hob) is often twice the size of the female (jill). The testicular size of the hob varies, being five to six times (or more) smaller during the non-breeding season. Neutering of hobs not required for breeding is advised, to reduce their odour.

Jills are sexually mature in the spring after their birth. The ferret breeding season in the UK stretches from February/March to September/October and the jill is in a near-permanent

	Sexual maturity	Oestrous cycle interval	Duration of oestrus	Ovulation	Gestation length	Pseudo-pregnancy	Litter size
Rat	8–10 weeks	4–5 days Non-seasonally polyoestrous	14 hours	Spontaneous	20–22 days	Approx. 14 days after non-fertile mating	6–16
Mouse	6–7 weeks	4–5 days Non-seasonally polyoestrous	14 hours	Spontaneous	19–21 days	Approx. 14 days after non-fertile mating	8–12
Syrian hamster	6–12 weeks	4 days	12 hours	Spontaneous	15–18 days	Approx. 8–10 days after non-fertile mating	4–12
Gerbil	8–10 weeks	4–6 days	12–15 hours	Spontaneous	24–26 days (42 days if delayed implantation)	Approx. 16 days after non-fertile mating	3–7
Guinea pig	1.5–3 months	16 days	1–16 hours	Spontaneous	111 days		2–6
Chinchilla	6–9 months	30–50 days		Spontaneous	59–72 days (average 63 days)		1–5
Rabbit	4–8 months	Seasonally polyoestrous	1–2 days	Induced	29–35 days (average 31 days)	Approx. 16 days after induced ovulation	4–10
Ferret	4–8 months	Seasonally polyoestrous	7 months	Induced	41–42 days	Approx. 42 days after induced ovulation	2–14

25.19   Reproductive parameters for small mammals.

(persistent) state of oestrus, as she is an induced ovulator. Jills are highly sensitive to the side effects of oestrogen and are prone to bone marrow disease if they are not mated or somehow brought out of oestrus during the season. Many ferret owners either breed their jills every year or mate them with vasectomized hobs. Alternatively, an injection of a synthetic progesterone or surgical neutering is required to prevent bone marrow suppression. Pseudopregnancy lasts approximately 42 days after induced ovulation.

The energy demand of a lactating ferret jill is 1.5–2 times normal maintenance levels.

Rabbits

Rabbits are induced ovulators and does are susceptible to uterine tumours, whether mated or not during their lifetime. It is recommended that does are surgically neutered at 5–6 months of age where possible.

After giving birth, rabbit does may be offered increasing amounts of pelleted dry foods as their energy demands increase to 3.5 times maintenance levels by peak lactation. Ad libitum feeding of dry food is often advocated but levels of food should not start to be dramatically increased until 5–7 days after parturition, as early over-feeding may lead to mastitis as a result of milk production exceeding the kits' demands.

Rodents

Female rodents have separate external orifices for their urinary and reproductive systems. This can be used for sexing the animals, in conjunction with the spacing of the urinary papilla (the nodule-like lump on the ventrum through which the urinary tract exits in the female rodent) from the anus. In females, the urinary papilla is closer to the anus and, if care is taken, the entrance to the genital tract may be seen between the urinary papilla and the caudally situated anus (Figure 25.20).

In males, the prepuce is spaced at a greater distance from the anus (Figure 25.20). There are also prominent testes in adult males, but these may be retracted into the caudal abdomen. The testes may be encouraged to descend by gently holding the male rodent vertically, with head uppermost and resting its rear on the palm of one hand.

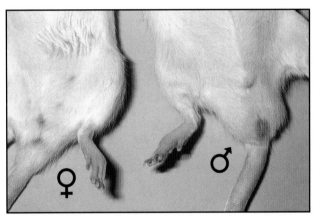

25.20   Differences in anogenital distance in rats: (left) female; (right) male. (Reproduced from *BSAVA Manual of Exotic Pets, 4th edition*)

Rodents such as rats and gerbils need dietary protein levels of 20–26% prior to and during pregnancy and lactation (compared with the more usual 16–18%).

The lactating guinea pig sow's requirement for vitamin C increases from 10 mg/kg per day to 30 mg/kg day. She also has the usual increases in demand for calcium, energy and protein. The demand for increased calories is particularly important as huge stresses are placed on the sow by her long gestation (average 63 days) and often the size of her litter (three to four piglets). If the demands are not met, pregnancy toxaemia or ketosis ensues and death can follow within 24 hours. Prevention is by avoiding obesity and sudden dietary changes.

Birds

Many bird species will breed predominantly at one time of year. Some seasonal breeders are triggered to start breeding by an initial decreasing daylength as is seen over the winter, followed by an increase as occurs in the spring. This daylength variation stimulates the pineal gland, which is connected to the pituitary gland, to alter levels of melatonin and gonadotrophin-releasing hormones that can stimulate the reproductive cycle. Other seasonal breeders are stimulated to cycle by other external

663

stimuli such as rainfall and food availability. Sexual maturity may be reached quickly in smaller species such as finches or may take several years as with many of the larger parrots.

Some bird species are sexually **monomorphic**, i.e. the two sexes look physically identical (e.g. Amazon parrots, macaws). In other species there is a distinct difference: they are sexually **dimorphic**. For example, in budgerigars the male has a blue cere and the female a brown or pinkish one. In many birds of prey, the female is up to twice the size of the male.

Mating occurs when the male mounts the female and presses his vent to the female's vent. Sperm travels down the vas deferens from the testes and drips into the cloaca of the male and so is transferred to the cloaca of the female. It then migrates into the distal portion of the female oviduct, where it may be stored for a brief while. The site of fertilization of the oocyte is the infundibulum, the portion of the oviduct adjacent to the ovary itself.

The fertilized ovum moves along the infundibulum and into the oviduct, where albumin (egg white) is deposited, and then into the isthmus, where the shell membranes are deposited. In the shell gland or 'uterus', extra water is added to the albumin (a process known as plumping) and the egg shell itself is laid down. The egg is laid by a muscular contraction of the last portion of the oviduct, the vagina. The whole process from shedding of the oocyte to laying of the egg takes roughly 2 days. The number of eggs laid in a 'clutch' varies between species.

The requirements for egg production are high, with large volumes of fat needed for the yolk, calcium for the shell and proteins for the albumin. In general, female birds (hens) will eat more food, thus removing the absolute need to increase the energy content of the diet. It is essential that the diet offered is a balanced one, with an increased protein content and a moderate increase in calcium and vitamin D3. This will ensure good calcification of eggshells and embryo and will also help to prevent egg-binding in the hen. Other compounds that help with egg production are vitamins A and B12, riboflavin and the mineral zinc.

The egg is in itself a perfect capsule of nutrients, providing all that is needed for the developing embryo. If the hen is fed a poor or deficient diet, the egg may not be fertile or there could be early embryonic death (often denoted by a blood ring left in the yolk), retarded embryonic development or deformities.

Incubation of the eggs may be performed by just the female, or just the male, or by both, depending on species. Incubation periods vary between species, as do weaning ages (Figure 25.21). For greater success in the hatching rates of cagebirds, artificial incubation is recommended. This is also preferred where hand-rearing of cage birds is required to gain a hand-tame bird. There are many commercial avian egg incubators available. If the parents are left to incubate the eggs themselves, they must not be disturbed during the hatching and weaning process as this may lead to nest or chick abandonment or even cannibalization in some species. Parent-reared birds on average take longer to wean than hand-reared ones and are usually less hand-tame.

Reptiles

Reptiles are classified as:

- **Oviparous:** these lay eggs externally
- **Ovoviviparous:** these produce live young instead of laying eggs, but the eggs are produced internally
- **Viviparous:** a form of placenta/thin-walled egg structure is produced in the reproductive system which allows the fetus to develop and live young are produced.

Reptile eggs are generally soft-shelled and more leathery than bird eggs but egg production in lizards is similar to the process in birds.

Incubation length depends upon the temperature at which the eggs are kept. Unlike birds' eggs, reptile eggs should not be moved during incubation but kept with the same side up as when they were deposited. Figure 25.22 gives an idea of some common incubation lengths, or, where the species is viviparous, the gestation length.

Species	Incubation period (days)	Weaning (days): parent-reared	Weaning (days): hand-reared	Sexual maturity
African Grey parrot	26–28	100–120	75–90	4–6 years
Amazon parrot	26–29	90–120	75–90	4–6 years
Barn owl	30–31	70–75		1 year
Budgerigar	16–18	30–40	30	6–9 months
Canary	12–14	21		< 1 year
Cockatiel	18–20	47–52	42–49	6–12 months
Cockatoo: large spp. Cockatoo: medium spp.	23–30 (depending on spp.)	60–80 45–60	95–120 75–100	5–6 years 3–4 years
Harris hawk	32	35–45 (fledging)[a]		> 3 years
Lovebird	18–24	45–55	40–45	6–12 months
Macaw: large spp. Macaw: small spp.	26–28 23–26	120–150 90–120	95–120 75–90	5–7 years 4–6 years
Peregrine falcon	29–32	35–42 (fledging)[a]		> 3 years
Pheasant	22–24	Precocial[b]		
Pigeon	16–19	35		1 year
Zebra finch	12–16	25–28		9 months

25.21 Reproductive parameters for selected bird species. [a] Fledgling refers to time when bird can first fly. [b] Self-feeding from hatchling.

Species	Method of reproduction	Incubation period (days)	Incubation temperature (°C)	Sexual maturity
Boa constrictor	Viviparous	120–240	28–32	
Burmese python	Oviparous	56–65	28–32	
Corn snake	Oviparous	55–70	28–30	
Garter snake	Viviparous	90–110	24–29.5	
Kingsnake	Oviparous	50–60	28–30	
Bearded dragon	Oviparous	65–115	28–32	1–2 years
Green iguana	Oviparous	73	25–30	2–3 years
Jackson's chameleon		90–180		
Leopard gecko	Oviparous	55–60	28–32	
Hermann's tortoise	Oviparous	85–100	30–33	7 years
Leopard tortoise	Oviparous	140–155	28–32	
Red-eared terrapin	Oviparous	59–93	28–29	
Spur-thighed tortoise	Oviparous	60	28–32	

25.22 Reproductive parameters for selected reptiles.

Chelonians

Male chelonians often have longer tails, the vent being found on the tail caudal to the edge of the carapace, in order to house the single phallus (Figure 25.23). Males of many Mediterranean species of tortoise and turtle possess a dished plastron, to make mounting the female easier, and often have a narrower angle to the caudal plastron in front of the cloaca than the egg-bearing females. Some female Mediterranean species have a hinge to the caudal part of the plastron to allow easier egg-laying. The male of the box turtle *Terrapene carolina* has red irises, whereas the female has yellow-brown ones. Females of the leopard tortoise and Indian star tortoise have longer hindlimb claws for digging than the males. The male red-eared terrapin has longer forelimb claws than the female. Some males, such as the Horsfield's tortoise, have a large hooked scale to the tip of the tail. In some there is a size difference: the female of the Indian star tortoise, the striped mud turtle and the red-eared terrapin is larger than the male when fully grown, but the reverse is true of the red-footed tortoise. The male loggerhead musk turtle has a much larger head than the female.

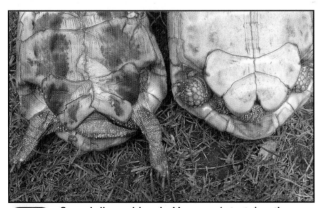

25.23 Sexual dimorphism in Hermann's tortoise: the male (left) has a longer tail and wider anal scutes than the female (right). (Courtesy of Alan Humphreys.)

In the colder northerly climes of the UK the incubation of chelonian eggs in an outside environment is not possible. It is necessary to remove the eggs from wherever they have been laid by the female and transfer them to a purpose-built incubator for hatching. Incubators may be purchased from many reptile outlets, or from commercial poultry or cagebird suppliers. Alternatively a home-made one, as described below for snakes, can be used.

Incubation temperature control is important in sex determination. For example, the spur-thighed tortoise will produce males if the eggs are kept at 29.5°C and females if kept at 31.5°C. This principle seems to apply to a large number of tortoise species, with males being predominantly produced at lower temperatures than females. If the temperature range is kept at 28–31°C, a mixture of sexes is likely to be achieved.

Lizards

Sexual identification in lizards may be performed by surgical probing as for snakes (see below); this is often the only method available for species such as the beaded lizard, some monitors and the Gila monster. In most other species there are external physical differences, including the prominent pre-femoral pores of males seen on the caudoventral aspect of the thigh in iguanids (the females possess much smaller ones). Some males have a series of pre-anal pores just cranial to the vent. Also seen are larger scales caudal to the vent in males of species such as the anoles (a small iguanid lizard). In some species the males have wider tail bases than the females, to house the large hemipenes (e.g. green iguana). Others have greater ornamentation, such as larger crests (plumed basilisks), horns (Jackson's chameleon), larger crest spines (water dragons) or a wider vent and hemipenal bulge (many male geckos).

Sexual maturity varies according to the species and also according to the husbandry provided, as poor nutrition and heat or ultraviolet light provision may lead to delays in maturation.

Lizard eggs may be incubated in vivaria. Incubation periods vary from 45–70 days in smaller lizards to 90–130 days for larger lizards (see Figure 25.22). A few species are **parthenogenetic**, i.e. females give birth to females with no need for male fertilization.

Sex determination in most lizards is dependent on genetic factors. However, in geckos sex determination is temperature-dependent: at 26.7–29.4°C 99% of eggs produce female offspring; at >32.2°C 90% of offspring are male.

Snakes

Sexing can be difficult in snakes and is best performed by surgical probing. A fine sterile blunt-ended probe is inserted through the vent and advanced just to one side of the midline in a caudal direction. If the snake is a male, the probe will pass into one of the inverted hemipenes and so will insert to a depth of 8–16 subcaudal scales. In females there are anal glands in this region and so the probe may be inserted to a depth of only 2–6 subcaudal scales. In some species, such as boas, males possess a paracloacal spur (the remnant of the pelvic limb) on either side of the body ventrally at the level of the cloaca. In very young snakes it may be possible to evert the hemipenes manually, with care, in a technique known as 'popping'.

Snakes are entirely chromosomally dependent for sex determination, as are most mammals. There is no outside influence needed, such as the temperature-dependent effects seen in chelonians.

The average incubation period in snakes is generally 45–70 days (see Figure 25.22); artificial incubation improves hatching rates. The basic components of a reptile egg incubator are:

- A plastic or toughened glass **tank**, with a plastic lid that contains aeration holes, which can be covered to regulate humidity and temperature
- **Substrate** or nesting material (e.g. loft-insulating material, vermiculite; or damp sand, sphagnum moss or peat) placed in small open **containers** within the tank. The eggs are put in slight depressions within the substrate.
- Source of **humidity** and **heat** production:
  - Egg containers may be placed on a wire mesh inside the tank above water kept at the desired temperature. This is good for species that require higher humidity
  - Alternatively, a thermostatically controlled radiant heat mat can be attached to the outside of the tank, with the inside completely filled by substrate. Regular misting and shallow containers of water can add moisture. This is good for species that require a drier atmosphere, such as desert-dwelling snakes. Humidity should not be allowed to drop below 50%.

It is important to have a thermometer and humidity gauge within the incubator. Temperatures for incubation vary from 26°C to 32°C. When eggs are retrieved from the nest site, particular care should be taken to maintain the same position of the egg in the incubator. The eggs should not be turned or touched during the incubation process, as this can cause significant fetal mortality.

Care and management of the neonate

Dogs and cats

The first essential steps after birth are to:

1. Establish a clear airway and stimulate respiration
2. Cut the umbilicus
3. Keep the neonate warm until active
4. Encourage the neonate to suck.

It is essential that a clear airway is established as soon as a fetus has been born (or delivered via a caesarean operation). This involves removal of the surrounding fetal membranes and clearing the mouth and nose of fetal fluid, using either a dry towel or a small pipette. Gentle compression of the chest usually results in the establishment of respiratory effort. If this is not the case but the heart is beating, respiratory stimulation should continue by rubbing the thorax and removal of further fluid by gently swinging the neonate in a small arc (but this should be avoided unless absolutely necessary, because of the risk of brain trauma).

In certain cases the administration of respiratory stimulant agents such as doxopram hydrochloride may be efficacious, as may the administration of oxygen. If respiration does not commence, artificial respiration can be attempted by blowing gently into the nose and mouth of the neonate. This should be done carefully to induce only slight lung expansion without overinflating the lungs. If the heart is not beating, external cardiac massage combined with artificial respiration may be attempted.

The umbilicus should be cut approximately 3 cm from the fetal abdomen; excessive bleeding can be prevented by the application of a ligature.

Once regular respiratory efforts are maintained, the neonate may be placed into a pre-warmed box or incubator until it is active, when it may be returned to the dam and encouraged to suck. Sucking normally occurs immediately after birth and at intervals of 2–3 hours for the first few days.

Examination

Once the dam is sufficiently happy for the neonate to be removed, it should be checked for abnormalities.

- The birth weight should be recorded. Normally the neonate will gain between 5% and 10% bodyweight per day; and a failure to do so may indicate poor health.
- The neonate should be checked for congenital abnormalities, such as cleft palate or harelip.
- The umbilicus should be checked for herniation. It should be clean and show no evidence of further bleeding. If the umbilicus is bleeding, this can be ligated to prevent further blood loss.
- Respiration should be regular and even. The normal respiratory rate for a neonate is 15–40 breaths per minute. There should not be excessive noise. If there is excessive noise, this may indicate that the neonate still has fluid in its lungs and the appropriate action should be taken (see second stage of parturition).
- There should be no discharge from the eyes or ears. Any other birth defects can also be recorded now as well as the neonate's colour and gender.
- The neonate's rectal temperature could also be taken and recorded at this time, but in reality this is unnecessary. The normal rectal temperature for the first week after birth should be 32–34°C.

Neonatal characteristics

Neonatal puppies and kittens are unable to stand at birth but should be quite mobile, using their limbs to crawl. Neonates need to be assessed for their general strength. The weakest must be carefully observed, since they do not feed adequately and may fail to thrive. Standing may be seen from 10 days after birth and most neonates should be able to walk at 3 weeks of age.

Puppies and kittens are born with their eyes closed; separation of the upper and lower lids with opening of the eyes should occur by approximately 10–14 days after birth. The cornea at this stage may appear slightly cloudy, but this will disappear over the first 4 weeks. Many kittens are born with strabismus, which persists until they are 8 weeks old.

Care of the litter

During the first few weeks of life the dam will take care of the needs of the litter. However, the litter need to be checked regularly for signs of problems, ensuring that all of them are receiving an adequate supply of milk from the dam and that no individual is missing out on feeding opportunities. There should be a plentiful supply of clean bedding available, so that the dam and her offspring are comfortable and not lying on soiled or wet bedding.

Normally the dam will lick the perineal region in order to stimulate the neonates to defecate or urinate and she continues to do this for the first 2–3 weeks after birth. After this time the neonates will urinate and defecate voluntarily and therefore the amount of soiling in the nest bed will increase and will require more frequent changing.

The litter should be weighed on a regular basis, usually weekly to ensure that all of them are gaining weight adequately. At 10–14 days, when the eyes of puppies and kittens should open, they will gradually be able to focus on objects. They will become stronger on their legs and begin to crawl around. At this time it is advisable to ensure that all the puppies are able to use their hind legs properly: sometimes very large or fat puppies fail to get up on their hind legs and will haul themselves around on their front legs and bellies. If this becomes apparent, the puppy should be checked to ensure that there is nothing physically wrong with the legs, and then be encouraged to use its hind legs by placing a hand under its bottom and pushing it on to its hind legs. This condition rarely persists, due to the increased competition for food, but with a small litter it may become a problem.

Once weaning commences the dam may be less inclined to clean up their mess. The litter should be encouraged to soil away from the nest so that cleaning is more easily facilitated. This may hasten toilet training.

Small mammals

It should be noted that, in pet species other than the dog and cat, there may be a tendency towards cannibalism of the litter by the dam if she is disturbed with her young in the first few weeks after parturition, or at least abandonment or abuse. For this reason female rats, mice, hamsters (in particular), gerbils and rabbits should be left alone with their litters, except for replenishing food and clearing the worst of any cage soiling.

Cannibalism is common in the hamster, though the female will also protectively place the young in her cheek pouches to move them, which may appear to be evidence of her 'eating' the young.

Neonatal characteristics in other mammalian species likely to be seen in small animal practice are described in Figure 25.24. Most small mammal species are **altricial** at birth, i.e. they are wholly dependent on the mother for nutrition and survival in the first few weeks of life. They are born blind, deaf, hairless and without teeth.

Ferrets

The average number of ferret kits in a litter is eight. They are altricial but are born with a prominent fat pad on the dorsum of the neck, which provides some calorific value during the early stages of life. They have a higher calorific requirement than adult ferrets, at 1.5–2 times adult maintenance levels

Rabbits

Rabbit does will suckle their kits for only 3–5 minutes at a time and only once or twice in a 24-hour period, though they are totally dependent on her milk up to day 21 post parturition. They will begin to take solid foods from the age of 2–3 weeks and at this time they should be weighed. Solid foods offered will increasingly be consumed and weight losses may be seen during this changeover period. Weaning occurs at around 6 weeks of age. The growing kits require higher levels of vitamin D3 and calcium than adult rabbits and should be offered a balanced diet, such as a combination of a pelleted growing-rabbit formulated food along with good-quality grass hay and some greens. The pelleted foods should be chosen carefully; many are nutritionally balanced but it is preferable to use a homogeneous pelleted diet, as rabbits are selective eaters of concentrates and will pick and choose if offered a mixed dry food. They should also be given access to unfiltered natural sunlight, even if for only 15–20 minutes a day, to ensure adequate synthesis of vitamin D.

Birds

After hatching, the chick must be supplied with high levels of energy and protein for the growth phase within 3-4 days. This delay is possible due to the remnants of the yolk sac inside the body cavity still providing some nutrition and immunity for the first few days of life. Failure to internalize the yolk sac prior

	Terminology	Precocity	Development			Weaning age
			Eyes open	Ears open	Hair and skin	
Rat	Pups	Altricial	2 weeks	4–5 days	Fur appears at 7–10 days	2–3 weeks
Mouse	Pups	Altricial	2 weeks	4–5 days	Fur appears at 10 days	2–3 weeks
Syrian hamster	Pups	Altricial	2 weeks	1½–3 days	Skin changes from pale pink to darker at 2–3 days	3–4 weeks
Gerbil	Pups	Altricial	2 weeks	4–5 days	Skin changes from pale pink to darker at 7 days with fur appearing	3–4 weeks
Guinea pig	Piglets	Precocial	At birth	At birth	Born fully furred	6 weeks (eating solids from day 1)
Chinchilla	Kits	Precocial	At birth	At birth	Born fully furred	6–8 weeks (eating solids from day 1)
Rabbit	Kits/kittens	Altricial	8–10 days	11–12 days	Fur appears 5–6 days	6 weeks (eating solids from 2–3 weeks)
Ferret	Kits	Altricial	3 weeks	10 days	Fur appears 2 days, pronounced at 3 weeks	4–6 weeks

25.24 Neonatal characteristics of small mammals.

to hatching is sometimes seen and can lead to septicaemia. Surgical removal of the non-internalized yolk sac is possible but the chick will require immediate supplementary nutritional support due to the removal of this energy/nutrient source.

When feathers are produced, a huge demand for protein occurs; there are several feather changes during the first 2 years of life. Young birds also have a large requirement for calcium and vitamin D3 for developing and mineralizing the skeleton.

It has been estimated that minimum energy requirements for small psittacine and passerine birds is five times that of adults, with young chicks nearly doubling their weights over 48 hours, with a protein level of 15–20% compared with an adult protein need of 10–14%. Diets for chicks have therefore concentrated on pre-formulated mashes with this level of protein, or the use of eggs and dairy products, which have a good broad spectrum of amino acids supplementation and 20% protein levels.

However, excessive protein supplementation (>25% of diet) has been shown to lead to behavioural problems and claw, beak and skeletal deformities, particularly if combined with a lack of calcium.

Abnormalities of the neonatal period

A number of diseases may affect puppies and kittens early in life. A certain percentage of neonates may die before weaning and it has been suggested that this can be as high as 15–20%. With good management systems (including the avoidance of hypothermia), the number of offspring lost should not be greater than 5%.

Fading puppy and kitten syndrome

The most common problem noted within the neonatal period is that of fading puppies or kittens. Most commonly neonates die when less than 1 week of age. There are numerous factors associated with this loss, but usually it is the inherent susceptibility of the newborn that results in its ultimate demise. Neonates have poor mechanisms of thermoregulation, fluid and energy balance; they are immunologically incompetent; and they may have abnormal lung surfactant composition. When combined with poor management regimes and poor mothering behaviour of the dam, the risk of neonatal mortality can be high. Approximately 50% of neonatal deaths can be attributed to either infection, maternal and management-related deficiencies, low birth weight or congenital abnormalities.

Neonatal septicaemia

The inherent vulnerability of the neonate puts it at risk of colonization by a number of bacterial agents. This may result in a rapid death with very few initial clinical signs. In some circumstances ill health results in frequent crying, restlessness and hypothermia, progressing to clinical signs of diarrhoea and/or dyspnoea with resultant dehydration or cyanosis, and ultimately death. In certain circumstances some neonates are more chronically affected and fail to grow as expected prior to the onset of obvious clinical disease.

The majority of passive immunity follows from the intake of colostrum, and gut transfer occurs only during the first 48 hours of life. It is vital, therefore, to ensure an adequate intake of colostrum at this time to protect against these organisms.

Regardless of the cause, rapid and aggressive treatment using intravenous fluid therapy, oral electrolytes, broad-spectrum antimicrobial agents and oxygen administration is essential. Despite such treatment, the mortality rate can be high.

Neonatal viral infection

Viral infections are not common in the neonate, especially when vaccination programmes are practised in the adult. Maternally derived antibody frequently provides protection for several weeks.

- Canine herpesvirus may result in the birth of congenitally infected puppies that are weak and die soon after birth.
- Feline immunodeficiency virus and feline leukaemia virus in the queen can infect kittens transplacentally as well as perinatally, and result in neonatal death after a few weeks of age.
- Neonatal deaths and the birth of kittens with cerebellar hypoplasia are not uncommon following infection with feline panleucopenia virus during pregnancy.
- Feline infectious peritonitis virus has also been implicated in cases of upper respiratory tract disease and fading kitten syndrome.

Congenital abnormalities

Congenital abnormalities are those that are present at birth. Common problems include cleft palate, where there is failure of the normal fusion of the palatine arches. The defect may occur anywhere along the length of the hard or soft palate, though most commonly it arises caudal to the incisor ridge. The defect is common in certain breeds and it has been suggested that it is a trait inherited in either a recessive or polygenic manner. In most cases euthanasia of the neonate with this problem is advisable, because of the problems of sucking and aspiration of milk.

There are many other congenital abnormalities that may affect each organ system, such as hernias, fetal monsters, hydrocephalus, microphthalmus, flat puppies (swimmers), congenital heart disease and atresia of the terminal rectum. A thorough clinical examination of each neonate after birth should allow these abnormalities to be readily detected.

Artificial rearing of neonates

In some circumstances it may be necessary to rear some or all of the litter artificially. Some instances are:

- Death of the dam
- A large litter
- A sick dam
- A dam showing no interest in her litter
- A dam with an inadequate milk supply.

Obviously, artificial rearing is best avoided where possible. In some cases it may be possible to foster the neonates on to another dam. Suitable candidates to foster orphans might include a lactating bitch or queen that has just given birth and lost her litter, or one that has a pseudopregnancy and is currently lactating, or a dam with a small litter.

In the case of an excessively large litter, it may be possible to rotate some of the neonates between artificial rearing and being reared by the dam. It has been suggested that just some neonates should be entirely artificially reared, rather than rotated, but this method is not advocated. In any case, the neonates should, where possible, remain in the nest with the dam to ensure normal socialization.

It is essential that all neonates should receive the colostrum from the dam to ensure an adequate uptake of immunoglobulins. If the dam has died, it may still be possible to express some colostrum from her, as long as it is not contaminated with drugs or toxins.

Equipment

All the equipment for artificial rearing should be readily available and where possible should be included in the equipment needed in preparation for parturition, so that it is there if needed.

Milk substitutes

There are several commercially available milk substitutes available for artificial rearing of both puppies and kittens. It is important that the neonate receives the right formulation of milk. Cow's and goat's milk are not suitable substitutes, since their composition is very different from that of the bitch or queen. It is possible to make up a milk substitute, but this must have the appropriate lactose, fat and protein content and is time consuming. It is better to make up a pre-prepared milk substitute. The milk should be warmed to body temperature (39°C) and fed according to the manufacturer's instructions, with regard to bodyweight and age.

Feeding bottles

Artificial rearing is both demanding and time consuming, especially if rearing is done entirely without the dam. The neonates normally feed every 2–4 hours during the first 5 days of life, which then reduces to every 4 hours after day 5. Feeding can be achieved by using a commercial feeding kit, which contains a bottle and teat. This encourages normal sucking, but can be more time consuming. The teat aperture should be large enough to prevent the neonate sucking in air but small enough to prevent excessive volumes of milk flowing through it.

Feeding can also be achieved using a dropper bottle or syringe feeding. A 2 ml syringe should be adequate for the first few days.

When using either of these methods, care must be taken not to rush the neonate, as this may result in inhalation of milk rather than swallowing it, which may cause pneumonia.

Orogastric tube feeding

In some cases it may be beneficial to feed neonates by means of a stomach tube (orogastric tube), especially during the first few days of life, for rapid feeding or for particularly sick neonates. The procedure is relatively simple. A small 2 mm diameter piece of soft polythene tubing should be measured against the neonate's mouth and to the end of the level of the 9th rib. This length should be marked on the tube. The outside of the tube should be lubricated with a small volume of water.

The neonate's head is held in the normal position and the mouth is held just open using a finger and thumb; if the head is extended or flexed, passage of the tube into the trachea is more likely. The tube is directed gently over the tongue into the back of the throat. Swallowing greatly assists passage into the oesophagus, but is not essential. The tube can usually be seen on the left side of the neck as it passes down the oesophagus. There is little resistance as the tube is introduced into the stomach; the length of the tube is the best guide. Once the tube is in position, the syringe can be attached and its contents slowly injected into the stomach. The tube is then gently removed.

General care

When artificial rearing has to take place entirely without the dam, the neonate is fully reliant upon its human carer.

Neonates are unable to open their bladder or bowels voluntarily and normally the dam would stimulate the pup to urinate or defecate by licking their anogenital region. This would normally be done after feeding. In the absence of the dam, this stimulation can be carried out manually by using a moistened piece of cotton wool. This should be performed every 2 hours.

Any spilt milk should be cleaned off the neonate immediately, as during the early days this might otherwise result in chilling. Once any spilt milk is allowed to dry, it will cause matting of the coat.

The orphans' only other need is to be kept warm and out of draughts. They should be maintained at an environmental temperature of 25°C.

Small mammals

Ferrets

Milk replacers for ferret kits have been adapted from puppy or kitten milk replacers, enriched with cream until the fat content reaches 20% (e.g. 3 parts puppy milk replacer to 1 part whipping cream). This can be fed on demand four to six times daily and the kits may be weaned on to adult food at 4–5 weeks of age.

Rabbits

Rabbit kits are altricial and the intestinal microflora of hand-reared kits often does not develop properly, which means that deaths from enterotoxaemia are commonplace. It may be possible to prevent this situation by transfaunation of gut flora from a healthy parasite-free adult rabbit to the kits. If hand-rearing is to be tried, a possible milk replacer formula might be 1 part whole full-fat cow's milk to 3 parts condensed milk, adding 6 g skimmed milk powder per 100 ml of the mixture. Adult foods should be offered from 2 weeks of age and weaning is attempted at 3 weeks, though a naturally reared kit would not be weaned until 6 weeks of age.

Rodents

Hand-rearing of small rodents is challenging and has a high failure rate, owing to the **altricial** nature of the young (i.e. they are totally dependent on the dam and are born blind, deaf, hairless and without teeth). The altricial rodents include rats, mice, hamsters, gerbils and chipmunks, in contrast to guinea pigs and chinchillas, which are **precocial** (born fully furred, with eyes and ears open, and able to start consuming small amounts of solid food from day 1).

All of the altricial species show evidence of poor thermoregulation and require environmental temperatures of around 35°C while they are hairless, and around 32°C once they are furred. After their eyes open, the temperature may be reduced by 2.5°C per week and a temperature gradient should be provided.

The first concern when providing supportive feeding for orphaned rodents must be to ensure hydration. Initially, oral rehydration solutions suitable for cats and dogs may be used. Once hydration is established, the orphans may be offered milk replacers such as Esbilac (PetAg) or Cimicat (Hoechst). For mice, some authors recommend using 1 part goat's colostrum mixed with 3 parts Esbilac. The milk replacer may be fed from the tip of a paintbrush, or using kitten feeders for older and larger individuals. Feeding should be once every hour during daylight and once every 2 hours overnight. Up to 35–40% of bodyweight may be fed per day. Urination and defecation must be stimulated by wiping the anogenital area with a moistened cloth.

Young guinea pigs and chinchillas are able to eat small amounts of solid food within 24 hours of birth, but they are often not hungry for the first 12–24 hours as they are able to make use of brown-fat reserves. They should not be force fed during this period. Thereafter it is important to ensure that high-fibre foods are offered preferentially (to avoid fussy eating in later life). A hand-rearing formula for guinea pigs might be 1 part condensed milk to 2 parts cooled boiled water, fed every 3–4 hours at a rate of 1–3 ml; this may be adapted for chinchillas with the addtion of 6 g skimmed milk powder to 100 ml of the formula to help to increase protein levels. Early weaning on to solid adult food is encouraged for both species, and is advised after 7–10 days.

Weaning

Weaning is a gradual process, which normally starts at about $2^1/_2$ weeks for puppies and kittens and will be complete by about 5 weeks. The neonates will still suck from their mother throughout the process, but once weaning has begun the dam will normally spend an increasing amount of time away from her offspring. She should still be allowed frequent access to them during the day and will normally still spend the night with them.

Until the weaning process begins, the neonate is reliant on the dam for all of its nutritional needs, but once weaning has begun each puppy or kitten should be closely monitored for continued weight gain. Signs associated with under-nutrition include crying, inactivity and poor weight gain.

Small quantities of food can be offered to neonates on a finger, allowing them to lick or suck the finger. The range and volume of food can be increased as the neonates get used to feeding. The food offered can be of a proprietary brand specifically designed for weaning, or cooked minced beef or rice pudding can be offered. Some animals will wean easily, taking solids and lapping straight away, whilst others may take longer. It is therefore especially important to treat each one individually and be patient.

Neonates being weaned directly from the dam will gradually increase the amount of solid food being eaten and should be on five or six feeds per day by the age of 5 weeks. Those being hand-reared will gradually have the volume of milk they receive reduced as the weaning process continues, in a similar manner to being weaned from the dam.

Further reading

England GCW (1998) *Allen's Fertility and Obstetrics in the Dog, 2nd edn.* Blackwell Scientific Publications, Oxford

England GCW (1999) Reproductive and paediatric emergencies. In: *BSAVA Manual of Canine and Feline Emergency and Critical Care*, eds L King and R Hammond, pp. 165–176. BSAVA Publications, Cheltenham

Girling SJ (2002) *Veterinary Nursing of Exotic Pets.* Blackwell Scientific Publications, Oxford

Harkness JE and Wagner JE (1995) *The Biology and Medicine of Rabbits and Rodents, 4th edn.* Lea & Febiger, Philadelphia

Harper EJ and Skinner ND (1998) Clinical nutrition of small psittacines and passerines. *Seminars I Avian and Exotic Pet Medicine*, 7(3), 116–127

Hillyer EV and Quesenberry KE (1997) *Ferrets, Rabbits and Rodents: Clinical Medicine and Surgery.* WB Saunders, Philadelphia

Hoskins JD (2001) *Veterinary Pediatrics: Dogs and Cats from Birth to Six Months, 2nd edn.* WB Saunders, Philadelphia

Jackson PGG (1995) *Handbook of Veterinary Obstetrics.* WB Saunders, London

Kelly N and Wills J (1996) *BSAVA Manual of Companion Animal Nutrition and Feeding.* BSAVA Publications, Cheltenham

Kupersmith DS (1998) A practical overview of small mammal nutrition. *Seminars in Avian and Exotic Pet Medicine*, 7(3), 141–147

Meredith A and Redrobe S (2000) *BSAVA Manual of Exotic Pets, 4th edn.* BSAVA Publications, Gloucester

Okerman L (1994) Breeding problems. In: *Diseases of Domestic Rabbits, 2nd edn* (ed. L Okerman), pp. 113–120. Blackwell Scientific Publications, Oxford

Richardson VCG (1992) The reproductive system. In: *Diseases of Domestic Guinea Pigs* (ed. VCG Richardson), pp. 15–38. Blackwell Scientific Publications, Oxford

Simpson GM, England GCW and Harvey MJ (1998) *BSAVA Manual of Small Animal Reproduction and Neonatology.* BSAVA Publications, Cheltenham

Stocker L (2000) *Practical Wildlife Care.* Blackwell Publishing, Oxford

Weber WJ (1978) *Wild Orphan Babies, 2nd edn.* Holt Rinehart and Winston, New York

Wright K (2004) Breeding and neonatal care. In: *BSAVA Manual of Reptiles, 2nd edn* (eds SJ Girling and P Raiti), pp. 40–50. BSAVA Publications, Gloucester

Chapter 26

Dentistry

Sue Vranch and Cedric Tutt

Learning objectives

After studying this chapter, students should be able to:

- **Define the terms used to describe dental disease**
- **Complete a dental chart accurately**
- **Describe how to handle an avulsed tooth**
- **List and describe the power and hand-held dental instruments used in general small animal practice**
- **List the surgical equipment required for extractions**
- **Describe the scale and polish procedure**
- **List the indications for dental radiography**
- **Instruct a client in dental homecare**
- **Describe the common dental conditions in lagomorphs and rodents**

Dental disease

Periodontal disease

Periodontal disease is one of the most common diseases seen today in small animal practice and is certainly the most common oral disease. Periodontal disease is the term used for a group of plaque-induced oral diseases. The prevention of this disease will be discussed later.

Periodontal disease usually progresses from gingivitis, though not all patients with gingivitis will go on to develop periodontitis.

- **Gingivitis**, a reversible condition, is defined as inflammation of the gingiva.
- **Periodontitis**, an irreversible condition, is inevitably a progression from gingivitis affecting the gingiva, alveolar bone, periodontal ligament and cementum of the tooth.

Aetiology

The primary cause of periodontal disease is the accumulation of dental plaque on the tooth surfaces. From the time the teeth erupt into the mouth, plaque begins to accumulate on the tooth surface. **Plaque** consists of desquamated cells, food particles and bacteria. Initially Gram-positive aerobic bacteria colonize the tooth surface and this population creates conditions that are optimum for Gram-negative anaerobic organisms to thrive. Bacterial toxins cause damage to the gingivae and oral mucosae, which results in damage to the other supporting structures of the teeth (the **periodontium** comprises gingiva, alveolar bone, periodontal ligament and cementum). Dental **calculus** is mineralized plaque, and a layer of plaque always covers the calculus. It has been shown that the surface roughness of calculus is only detrimental because of its plaque retentiveness. Therefore supra- and subgingival plaque can develop into calculus that hosts the plaque organisms, leading to persistent inflammation.

Gingivitis

Gingivitis is the earliest sign of periodontal disease. Gingivitis presents as redness of the gums and is graded depending on its severity:

- Mild gingivitis – presents as marginal redness of the gums
- Moderate gingivitis – the gums bleed when the gingival sulcus is probed
- Severe gingivitis – the gingivae are swollen and bleed spontaneously.

Gingivitis affects only the gingiva; it does not extend beyond to the deeper supporting tissues and is reversible (as there is no loss of periodontal attachment). When the gingival sulcus is gently probed (see 'Dental charting' below) the severity of gingivitis is scored according to how much bleeding there is (Figure 26.1). In patients with uncomplicated gingivitis there will be normal periodontal probing depths (with the gingival sulcus in dogs < 3 mm and in cats < 1 mm). Gingivitis is often accompanied by halitosis. However, accompanying complications to gingivitis such as gingival hyperplasia may cause additional problems (see below).

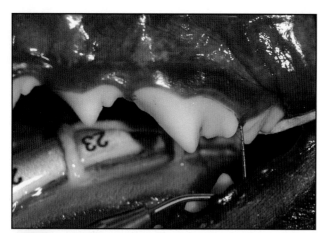

26.1   Gingivitis grade 2. The gum bleeds when gently probed during the dental examination.

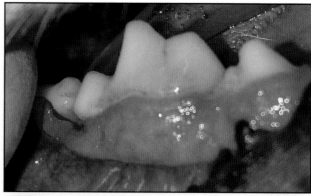

26.3   Periodontal disease. There is a deep pocket between mandibular right molars 1 and 2. It is often necessary to extract the less important tooth to save the more important tooth.

Gingival hyperplasia

This may be the result of plaque-induced inflammation (e.g. hyperplastic gingivitis); it may be idiopathic or hereditary. Boxers and, to a lesser extent, Border Collies and Labrador Retrievers show a predisposition for the condition.

The significance of gingival hyperplasia is the creation of a 'pseudo-pocket' due to the altered position of the gingival margin. This 'pocket' is formed due to the enlarged gingiva and not because of the destruction of the periodontal ligament and alveolar bone. In other words, the free gingiva has become taller, giving the impression that there is a pocket. Intraoral radiography helps to confirm the level of attachment in these cases. The presence of the hyperplastic gingiva can compromise tooth cleaning and therefore predispose to periodontitis.

Periodontitis

Periodontitis *may* develop in an individual with untreated gingivitis. The inflammation in periodontitis involves not only the gingiva but also the surrounding periodontal ligament, alveolar bone and cementum (Figure 26.2). The result of untreated periodontitis is exfoliation of the affected tooth, due to the destruction of the periodontal ligament and the alveolar bone (Figure 26.3). Periodontitis is not site-specific; it may affect one or more sites around one specific tooth or numerous teeth.

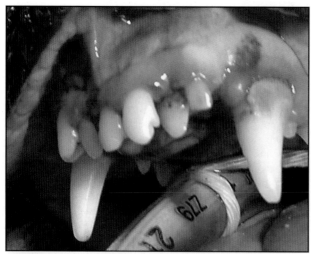

26.2   Periodontal disease. This dog has supernumerary incisors. The incisor set back in the palate has periodontal disease as a result of trapping food and other debris. There is also bony and gingival recession affecting the canine tooth.

Periodontitis is not reversible: once the alveolar bone and periodontal ligament have been destroyed it is impossible to replace them without expensive and complicated periodontal surgery. However, it can be managed with the correct treatment and home care.

Clinical signs of periodontitis include the presence of severe halitosis and large amounts of dental deposits. There may be associated ulcers, gingival recession and furcation lesions (loss of alveolar bone between the roots at the neck of the tooth) and/or loose teeth. Patients with severe oral infection develop transient bacteraemia when they eat and groom themselves. This may be associated with distant organ disease affecting the heart, liver, lungs and kidneys.

Other terms defining inflammation of oral tissues

Glossitis

Glossitis is defined as inflammation of the tongue and can be associated with plaque by-products.

Stomatitis

This is inflammation of the oral mucosal surfaces and can be further defined as:

*   Buccal stomatitis – inflammation of the cheek mucosa
*   Caudal oral stomatitis – inflammation of the caudal aspects of the oral cavity, rostral to the oropharynx.

The term 'faucitis', which is often incorrectly used to mean caudal oral inflammation, describes inflammation of the area caudal to the glossopalatine folds – the area housing the tonsils.

Generalized stomatitis is common in cats and seen periodically in dogs.

Other dental diseases and conditions

Caries

Caries, or dental decay (Figure 26.4), occurs in dogs, rabbits and chinchillas. It usually affects the molars, as these teeth have occlusal tables that can trap food that is fermented by bacteria, forming acids that induce demineralization of the hard tissues of the tooth. Extensive caries can involve tooth dentine and even invade the pulp tissue.

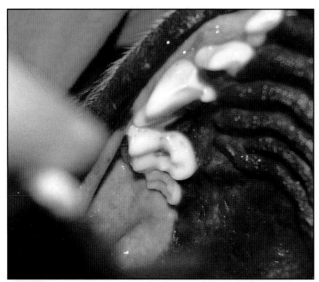

26.4 A typical site for caries in the dog is maxillary molar 1. There is a discoloured carious lesion in the occlusal surface of tooth 109.

Clinically, caries can usually be seen as craters in the enamel that may be filled with soft brown to grey material (though not all lesions are discoloured). In teeth affected by severe caries the crown may be destroyed, leaving roots exposed in the mouth. A dental explorer will stick into the softened tooth surface of caries. Teeth with carious lesions should be radiographed to reveal the extent of the problem and treatment can then be decided upon.

Teeth with caries need treatment. If the lesion is extensive, with most of the crown lost, the only treatment option is extraction. It is possible to restore a tooth with a small carious lesion and perform endodontic therapy if the lesion involves the pulp, but this will require referral to a specialist.

Teeth can become stained for a number of reasons and these lesions should not be confused with caries. Stained teeth usually have intact enamel and dentine and the surface of these lesions will be smooth when examined with a dental explorer.

Discoloured teeth

Teeth subjected to trauma, whether in the form of a blunt blow (road traffic accident), as a result of play where teeth have clashed or due to play with certain toys (tug toys), may become discoloured due to pulp inflammation and bleeding. The blood cells permeate the dentine and initially the tooth may appear pink; thereafter it will progress through the colour changes experienced in bruised soft tissue, ending up being a dull grey. Teeth with enamel defects will become discoloured due to pigments in food and also as a result of gingival bleeding. The use of tetracyclines during odontogenesis (development of the tooth – up to about 3 months of age) may cause discoloration of the tooth, as the substance chelates the calcium laid down in the dental hard tissues and becomes permanently incorporated in the tooth.

Odontoclastic resorptive lesions

Odontoclastic resorptive lesions (ORLs) are common in cats and are being seen more commonly in dogs (Figure 26.5). This is a type of idiopathic external root resorption that begins on the root surface (cementum) and can progress into the root and crown dentine and through the enamel. Often the crowns of affected teeth fracture and remnants may be visible on an oral examination. In some cases roots undergo replacement

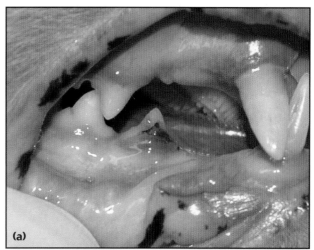

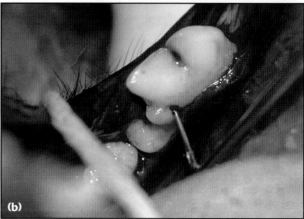

26.5 Odontoclastic resorptive lesions. **(a)** ORL affecting the mandibular right premolar 3 in a cat. **(b)** ORL affecting the mandibular left molar 1 in a dog.

resorption where the root substance is resorbed and replaced with bone-like material. It is essential to take radiographs of teeth affected by resorptive lesions to determine whether roots are still present – it makes no sense to try to extract roots that no longer exist. The aetiology of ORL is unknown; a number of possible causes are currently being investigated.

Enamel hypoplasia/dysplasia

Enamel hypoplasia or dysplasia is incomplete or absent enamel formation on the tooth crown and can be caused by systemic disease and infectious, hereditary or traumatic factors. Traumatic injuries to the face and mouth before 3 months of age can damage the enamel organ (enamel-producing and maturing cells), resulting in enamel dysplasia or hypoplasia that will be evident when the permanent teeth erupt into the mouth.

Enamel hypoplasia can affect one, several or all of the teeth; it can also affect the primary or permanent teeth (depending on when the insult occurred). Clinically the lesions can affect a part of the tooth or the whole tooth and this again depends on when the developing tooth was affected. The longer the noxious cause is present, the greater the area that will be affected (enamel is not produced over the whole crown at the same time). Distemper virus will enter the ameloblasts and destroy them, leading to enamel defects. They also affect odontoblasts, dentine production and root development.

Where enamel production has been deficient, dentine will be exposed and can become infected with plaque bacteria, leading to pulp necrosis and periapical pathology (Figure 26.6) that can lead to abscessation.

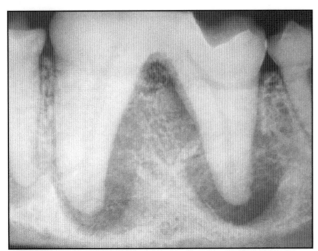

26.6 Radiograph showing periapical pathology due to enamel dysplasia. This resulted in pulpitis and pulp necrosis. (Courtesy of C Gorrel)

Other causes of enamel defects

Fractured deciduous teeth can develop periapical abscesses that can cause enamel defects in the mature teeth.

Pyrexia during amelogenesis (development of tooth enamel) will also cause enamel defects.

Traumatic tooth injuries

Fractured teeth (Figure 26.7) are common findings and may require referral to a specialist for treatment. Complicated crown fractures (the pulp is exposed) can be treated either by extraction or by endodontic therapy (root canal therapy). Uncomplicated crown fractures (pulp is not exposed) can also be treated with a restoration if necessary. Dental sensitivity often occurs after uncomplicated tooth crown fractures and therefore restoration will be required to seal the exposed dentinal tubules, eliminating pain and reducing the likelihood of pulp infection.

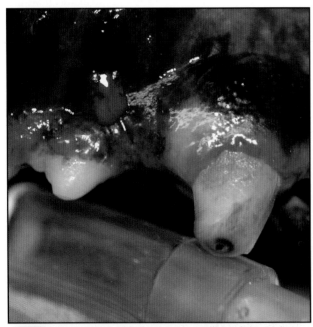

26.7 The pulp in this fractured maxillary right canine tooth has died and caused a root abscess that is draining through the sinus tract just at the mucogingival line caudal to the tooth.

Fractures that extend below the gum line will compromise the periodontium and therefore they should be evaluated by a veterinary surgeon who accepts dentistry referrals to determine whether a restoration can be placed or whether the tooth should be extracted or treated endodontically. Subgingival fractures are more plaque retentive than the normal healthy enamel surface and therefore give plaque a foothold.

Sometimes teeth are luxated or avulsed as a result of trauma. Avulsed teeth (those wrenched from the alveolus) must be handled by the crown, placed in milk at room temperature and sent to a veterinary surgeon experienced in orthodontics to be replaced in the mouth. This is a dental emergency and the patient must be attended to within hours if the tooth is to be successfully replanted in the alveolus. Luxated teeth (sometimes seen protruding from beneath the lip) also require urgent attention so that they can be reduced and stabilized.

Feline oral cavity disease

Cats with chronic gingivostomatitis are often seen. These cats are in severe pain and need immediate treatment. The aetiology of this disease complex is unknown, but affected animals should always be tested for feline leukaemia virus (FeLV), feline immunodeficiency virus (FIV), feline calicivirus (FCV) and feline herpesvirus (FHV). FCV may be isolated from the majority of cats with chronic gingivostomatitis but the association of this condition and this virus is at present unknown.

The oral examination

Dental formulae

Adult dog

$$2x \quad \frac{\text{I3 C1 PM4 M2}}{\text{I3 C1 PM4 M3}} = 42 \text{ teeth}$$

Adult cat

$$2x \quad \frac{\text{I3 C1 PM3 M1}}{\text{I3 C1 PM2 M1}} = 30 \text{ teeth}$$

(I = incisor; C = canine; PM = premolar; M = molar)

Dental charting

The oral cavity should be examined thoroughly under general anaesthesia (the conscious examination will only reveal the most superficial and obvious pathology). The animal's head shape, occlusion and each tooth should be examined and the findings recorded on a dental chart; this makes up an essential part of the patient's medical records. The lips and cheeks, tongue, hard and soft palates, oropharynx and larynx, tonsils and the oral mucous membranes should also be examined prior to intubation.

There are many types of dental chart available; examples are shown in Figure 26.8. Each chart has its own system for recording clinical findings and the choice of charting system is a matter of personal preference. Note that dental charts are viewed as if one is looking at the animal face on, i.e. the right side of the mouth is shown (and recorded) on the left of the chart.

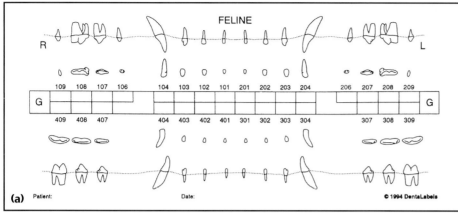

26.8 Examples of dental recording charts used in **(a)** cats; **(b)** dogs. (Reproduced by permission of John Robinson and DentaLabel.)

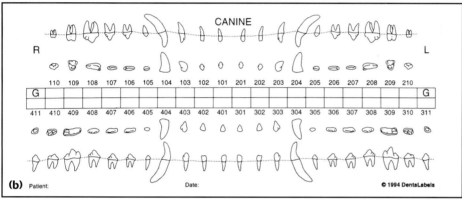

Triadan numbering system

On most of the commercially available charts the teeth are numbered using the modified three-digit Triadan numbering system. The first numeral denotes which quadrant the tooth is in and whether the tooth is part of the permanent or deciduous dentition:

Permanent dentition numeral	Quadrant	Deciduous dentition numeral
1	Right maxilla	5
2	Left maxilla	6
3	Left mandible	7
4	Right mandible	8

The second and third numbers in this system denote the tooth.

Examples

- The tooth numbered 104 would be the maxillary right canine tooth
- The tooth numbered 309 would be the mandibular left first molar
- The tooth numbered 401 would be the mandibular right first incisor.

This system is used for both the cat and the dog, even though the cat has fewer teeth – some are therefore omitted from the chart (e.g. mandibular first and second premolars and second and third molars) (Figure 26.8b).

When completing the dental charts, abbreviations are used to help record information.

Commonly used abbreviations

- **Ca** = Carious lesion
- **CCF** = Complicated crown fracture (may be recorded as '#PE')
- **ED** = Enamel defect
- **FORL** = Feline odontoclastic resorptive lesion
- **GH** = Gingival hyperplasia
- **GR** = Gingival recession
- **NAD** = No abnormality detected
- **ORL** = Odontoclastic resorptive lesion
- **PE** = Pulp exposure
- **UCF** = Uncomplicated crown fracture
- **WF** = Wear facet
- **#** = Fracture

A line is drawn on the diagram of a fractured tooth to denote the direction of the fracture. For example, if the fracture extends below the gingiva the line should be drawn correspondingly on the chart.

Missing teeth are circled. Teeth extracted are crossed through.

The examination procedure

Information to record on the charts for each individual tooth includes the following.

Calculus scores

Gross calculus should be removed prior to examining the teeth and so calculus scoring should be done first. A slight (CS), moderate (CM) and heavy (CH) scoring method is used.

Gingivitis scores

The modified Löe and Silness gingival index is generally used. It relies on visual inspection and the presence of bleeding on probing of the gingival sulcus (Figure 26.9).

Grade	Gingivitis	Mobility	Furcation
0	Healthy gingiva	No mobility	No furcation involvement
1	Marginal redness with slight thickening of marginal gingiva	Horizontal movement of 1 mm or less in one plane	Probe dips in at the furcation – little bone loss
2	Gingival margin thick and red. Bleeds on probing	Horizontal movement of 1 mm or more in two planes	Probe passes to mid furcation – significant bone loss
3	Gingiva thickened and red (to bluish). Bleeds spontaneously or when touched	Vertical as well as horizontal movement is possible	Probe passes from buccal to lingual/palatal – no furcation bone remaining

26.9 Grades of gingivitis, tooth mobility and furcation lesions.

Periodontal probing depth

The periodontal probe (see 'Dental instrumentation and equipment' below) should be inserted gently into the gingival sulcus until resistance is encountered at the base. The depth from the free gingival margin to the base of the sulcus is measured in millimetres. The normal depth of the gingival sulcus is 1–3 mm in dogs and 0.5–1 mm in cats. Measurements that exceed these values indicate the presence of pockets or pseudo-pockets. The measurement should be marked on the dental chart as close to its position on the actual tooth as possible.

Mobility

Tooth mobility can be tested by using the blunt end of a dental instrument (e.g. the handle of the mirror) in an attempt to move the tooth from its normal position. Using fingers can give a false positive movement due to the give in the finger. The grading of tooth mobility is shown in Figure 26.9.

Gingival recession

This is measured using a periodontal probe (Figure 26.10) and is the distance between the gingival margin and an imaginary line drawn across the normal gingival height at the mesial and distal edges of the tooth (or midbuccal surface, depending upon where the defect is). The gingival contour can be drawn on the dental chart.

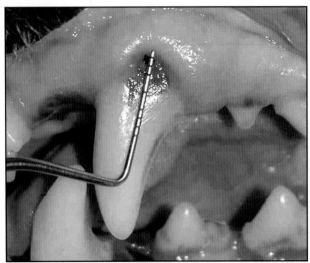

26.10 A periodontal probe is used to measure gingival and bony recession.

Furcation lesions

In patients with periodontitis the roots of multirooted teeth can become exposed and the furcation between them becomes visible. Furcation exposure is graded from 0 to 3, depending on severity (see Figure 26.9).

Gingival hyperplasia

Hyperplastic gingiva will form pseudo-pockets as there will be increased probing depth from the margin of the hyperplastic tissue to the bottom of the sulcus/pocket. In some animals with hyperplastic gingiva there may be true pockets as well in response to plaque on the tooth surface (i.e. they may have concurrent periodontitis).

Presence of traumatic injuries

This includes, for example, fractured teeth and foreign bodies. Foreign bodies may become lodged across the palate between carnassial teeth (Figure 26.11) or longitudinally along the dental arcade, and may cause the jaws to lock closed. Patients with oral foreign bodies are often presented with a chief complaint of halitosis. This is due to food and other foreign matter around the object that has become necrotic.

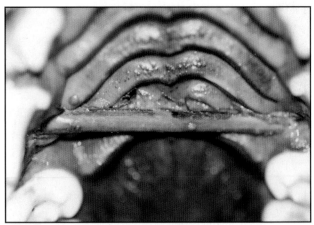

26.11 This foreign body trapped across the palate was an incidental finding in a patient that had a recent history of halitosis.

Exposed pulp

Exposed pulp is denoted on the chart by PE written adjacent to the affected tooth.

Enamel defects, abrasion and attrition

Enamel defects may be due to trauma or developmental abnormalities.

- **Abrasion** is the abnormal wear of teeth as a result of the animal's behaviour, e.g. stick or stone chewing, cage biting and playing with a tennis ball (tennis balls are inappropriate toys as they gather sand and grit and abrade the teeth each time they come in contact with them).
- **Attrition** is abnormal wear due to tooth-to-tooth contact, often seen in dogs with a malocclusion (especially dogs with a tight canine–canine–lateral incisor interlock).

Caries

Teeth affected by caries must be differentiated from those that are stained. Caries usually present as enamel craters on the tooth surface into which the dental explorer will stick when gently explored.

Stain

Teeth may be stained as a result of enamel wear and the production of tertiary dentine to protect the pulp. Arrested caries often also become stained due to the increased permeability of the enamel before remineralization occurs.

Supernumerary teeth

Supernumerary teeth (teeth in addition to the normal number) are usually smaller than their normal counterparts. Some are termed peg teeth, due to their conical shape. These teeth should be drawn on the dental chart.

Mixed dentition

The patient's dentition is considered mixed if it has deciduous and permanent teeth in the mouth at the same time (Figure 26.12). Deciduous teeth that are still present in the mouth when the adult teeth have come into occlusion are considered persistent deciduous teeth and should be extracted to prevent compromise of the permanent dentition.

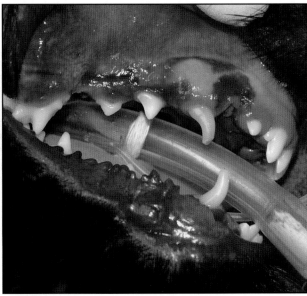

26.12 This puppy has mixed dentition: some permanent teeth have already erupted while some deciduous teeth are still present. None of the deciduous teeth in this figure would be considered persistent as they do not occupy the same location as a permanent tooth.

Retained teeth

Retained teeth are those that are found by radiographic examination after they were noted to be clinically missing from the mouth. In other words, they have not erupted and remain below the alveolar margin. This may be due to impaction where the eruption pathway is obstructed by an adjacent tooth. These teeth may be associated with other pathology (e.g. dentigerous cysts).

Soft tissue injuries

Oral soft tissue injuries should be charted. These include ulcers, lacerations secondary to tooth trauma, and degloving injuries.

Dental instrumentation and equipment

It is important that all instruments are clean, sterilized and sharpened before use on each patient. Equipment care and maintenance is of utmost importance. Equally the power equipment should be regularly maintained and serviced to ensure good working order.

The following are essential instruments used regularly in the dental operating room.

Periodontal probe

This is a blunt-ended graduated instrument (Figures 26.10 and 26.13) and is used to measure gingival sulcus and periodontal pocket depth. The periodontal probe can also be used to measure gingival recession and hyperplasia and for gingivitis scoring, as it is circumscribed around the tooth in the gingival sulcus. It can be used to grade furcation lesions, and the handle (on single-ended instruments) can be used to grade tooth mobility. The graduations on the veterinary clinic's periodontal probe should be measured so that pocket depth and other measurements are accurate.

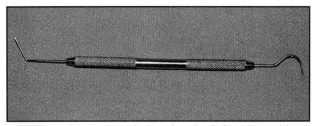

26.13 Williams 14 periodontal probe (left end) combined with a dental explorer (right end). Some clinicians prefer a double-sided instrument while others prefer individual probes and explorers.

Periodontal (dental) explorer

This is a very sharp, straight or curved instrument (see Figure 26.13) used to explore the tooth surfaces for the presence of caries or other enamel defects (e.g. enamel hypoplasia, fractured teeth, feline ORL). It is also possible to explore subgingivally using a dental explorer to examine for residual calculus after the scale and polish procedure. It is important to keep the dental explorer sharp.

Mirror

A dental mirror is commonly used in human dentistry but not necessarily in veterinary dentistry. It can be used to visualize the palatal and lingual surfaces of teeth (and distal surfaces of caudal teeth) and should be available for each procedure. It can also be used to reflect light into poorly lit areas of the mouth and to examine the nasopharynx.

Calculus-removing forceps

Calculus-removing forceps (Figure 26.14) must be correctly used by placing one beak on the gingival extent of the calculus and the other on the incisal tip of the tooth. This creates a shearing force that will dislodge the calculus from the tooth surface. Under no circumstances should the tooth surface be 'pinched' between the beaks of the forceps, or the crown may shatter. Care must also be exercised when placing the forceps at the gingival margin, or the gingiva can be damaged as well.

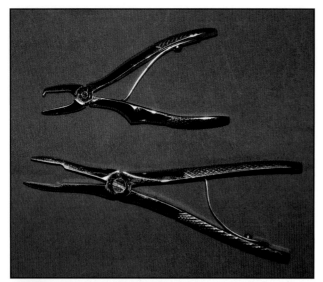

26.14 Calculus-removing forceps are available in numerous patterns. They must be used with care to prevent damage to the tooth and gingiva.

Hand scaler and curette

How to perform a dental scale and polish will be covered in a later section. The scaler and curette (Figure 26.15) are used to remove dental deposits from the tooth surfaces. They consist of a handle, shank and a working tip. The scaler has a sharp, pointed tip that should only be used supragingivally (if it is used subgingivally it can lacerate the gingival tissues). The curette has a blade that ends in a blunt rounded tip that can be used subgingivally for removal of subgingival deposits and root debridement. Both the scaler and curette should be pulled away from the gingiva towards the crown of the tooth. It is important to maintain the sharpness of these instruments for efficient use.

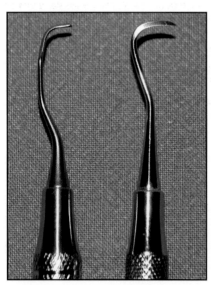

26.15
The hand curette (left) has a blunt end, while the scaler has a sharp tip and is only used above the gum line.

Ultrasonic scaler

The tip of the scaler oscillates at ultrasonic frequencies and is driven by an electromagnetic or piezoelectric handpiece. These scalers are generally used supragingivally but tips that allow minimal subgingival use are also available. Tip vibration in magnetostrictive scalers is caused by an electromagnetic field in the handpiece that surrounds a metal stack or a ferrite rod. When an electrical current is applied to the handpiece, the insert vibrates.

Piezoelectric scaler tips vibrate because of deformation of a crystal in the handpiece when an electrical current is applied to it.

Sonic scalers are available that are driven by compressed air. The tip vibration is cause by air driven through an eccentric hole in the shaft to which the tip is attached.

All electromechanical scalers have coolant water directed at their tips and this must be adjusted for optimal function. The water is also responsible for the phenomenon known as cavitation, by which very small bubbles that develop within the coolant liquid implode on the calculus, helping to dislodge it. Cavitation has also been shown to cause disruption of the cell walls of plaque bacteria.

Scalers (see Figure 26.23) must never be used with their tips perpendicular to the tooth surface, because the action of the vibrating tip will damage the tooth surface. It needs to be remembered that ultrasonic instruments were first invented to section (cut) teeth prior to extraction and that improper use will damage teeth.

The dental unit (power equipment)

Dental units are available with numerous attachments but the minimum requirements are: high-speed handpiece; slow-speed handpiece with contra-angled 'proply' attachment; (slow straight handpiece for rabbit dentistry); three way air-water syringe; and an ultrasonic scaler (the latter may be combined in the dental unit or may be a separate piece of equipment) (Figure 26.16).

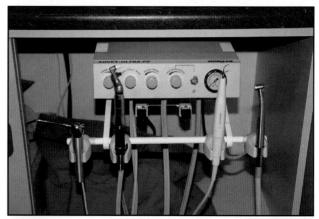

26.16 The dental unit.

High-speed handpiece

Protective eyewear must be worn by the operator and assistant when high-speed dental burs are used.

The high speed handpiece facilitates tooth extractions by allowing the operator to section multi-rooted teeth prior to extraction. The bur in the handpiece rotates at about 400,000 rpm (revolutions per minute). High-speed handpieces are more efficient at sectioning teeth but care must be exercised when using them to prevent air emboli and emphysema formation. Some high-speed handpieces have an integrated fibreoptic light that improves visibility in the work field.

Slow-speed handpiece

The slow-speed air motor on the dental unit can accept a contra-angle or straight handpiece. It also accepts the polishing head. This handpiece's rotation speed is adjustable up to 5500 rpm; it can be used for removing bone or sectioning teeth and is used for polishing teeth. When being used for sectioning teeth and alveolotomy (incision into the dental alveolus) or alveoloplasty (surgical shaping of the dental alveolus), the tooth or bone must be kept cool by applying sterile coolant to the bur and tooth or bone. This is most effectively done by an assistant squirting a gentle stream of polyionic fluid from a syringe on to the operating site.

Burs
Various burs are available (Figure 26.17). Generally, fissure burs are used to section teeth and pear-shaped or round burs are used to remove and smooth off alveolar bone.

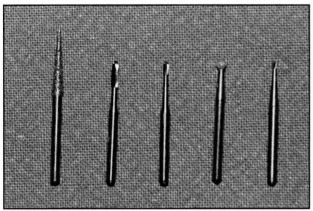

26.17 A selection of dental burs. From left: diamond fissure; round-tipped flat fissure tungsten carbide (TC); pear-shaped TC; round diamond; and small pear-shaped.

Three-way syringe
The three-way syringe (Figure 26.18) can deliver a jet of water, or a jet of water with air (effectively a water spray), or just air. It is very useful for flushing the mouth during dental procedures. A gentle puff of air will dry the tooth surface, enabling better visualization; residual calculus resembles chalk on the dry tooth surface.

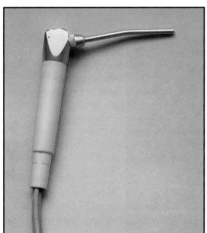

26.18 Three-way syringe.

Dental Luxator®
The dental Luxator® (Directa Dental AB, Sweden) is used for extracting teeth. It has a fine, sharp tip (Figure 26.19) that is used to cut the epithelial attachment and periodontal ligament which hold the tooth in the alveolus. An appropriately sized instrument should be used for the root in question. The Luxator® also causes condensation of the alveolar bone, creating more space that will allow insertion of the dental elevator.

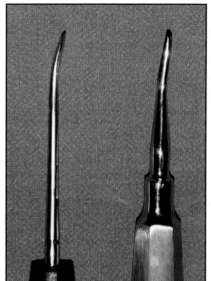

26.19 The Luxator® (left) is sharpened to a fine point, whereas elevators are sharpened to about 45 degrees.

Dental elevator
Once the gingival attachment has been severed and most of the periodontal ligament has been severed and torn and sufficient space has been created by using the Luxator®, the dental elevator (Figure 26.19) can be worked into the alveolus and used to apply rotational leverage on the root, disrupting its attachment further and leading to it being delivered from the alveolus.

Periosteal elevator
The periosteal elevator (Figure 26.20) is necessary for surgical extraction procedures. It is used to raise the mucoperiosteal flap to expose the alveolar bone. Once the gingival and alveolar mucosal incisions have been made, the periosteal elevator is inserted below the periosteum beneath the alveolar mucosa and worked along the bone surface, raising the periosteum. Once the alveolar mucosa periosteum has been raised from the bone, the instrument is worked along the bone in the direction of the alveolar margin and then under the attached gingiva. If approached via the gingival sulcus there is a risk that the periosteal elevator will puncture the flap at the mucogingival junction.

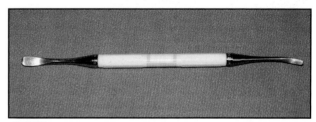

26.20 Periosteal elevator.

Extraction forceps
Extraction forceps should not be used by the veterinary surgeon without extensive training, as they can cause more harm than good. They must be used in the correct way. Incorrect use could fracture the crown of the tooth.

There are numerous extraction forceps beak patterns manufactured to fit human teeth. Most of these are inappropriate for use in veterinary dentistry.

Surgical kit

This should be readily available for surgical extractions and consists of (Figure 26.21):

- Scalpel handle and blades
- Small scissors (sharp–sharp Metzenbaum or iris scissors are ideal)
- Monofilament absorbable suture material 1 metric size (5/0)
- Small rat-toothed tissue forceps
- Periosteal elevator
- Suture cutting scissors.

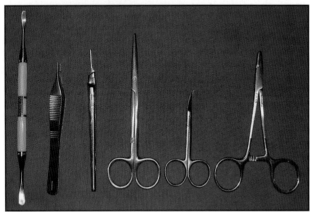

26.21 A surgical kit adequate for raising mucoperiosteal flaps. From left: periosteal elevator (Goldman Fox A&B); fine rat-toothed forceps; No.3 scalpel holder (No.15 or 15c scalpel blade not shown); Metzenbaum curved scissors; suture scissors; comfortable needle-holder able to accommodate fine suture material.

Maintenance of instruments and power equipment

When dropped, dental explorers and periodontal probes inevitably become bent. Attempts at straightening them may result in their breakage and they should therefore be replaced. Spare periodontal probes and explorers should be kept in case of emergency and replaced as necessary.

The dental unit, handpieces and instruments will require daily, weekly, monthly and annual maintenance to ensure that they remain at optimum performance. The dental unit will have instructions and a service agreement unique to it. It is recommended that the manufacturer's maintenance guidelines are adhered to.

Handpieces need to be oiled regularly prior to autoclaving and again before use. Over-lubrication can be as detrimental as under-lubrication and the manufacturer's instructions should be followed.

Sharpening instruments

Hand instruments need to be cleaned, sterilized and sharpened. Sharpening these instruments regularly not only increases their useful life but also prevents injuries to the patient and operator due to instrument slippage and takes the frustration out of this fulfilling branch of veterinary surgery.

- Hand scalers are sharpened by placing the blade of the scaler on a flat sharpening stone (Figure 26.22a). Using the fourth finger as a guide on the table surface to keep the instrument at the correct angle to the sharpening surface, it is drawn towards the operator. Both sides must be sharpened.
- Dental hand curettes are sharpened by holding the instrument in the palm grip with the scaler tip projecting from the back of the hand. A sharpening stone is held in the other hand, applied to the curette blade and drawn across it in an arc to accommodate the slight curvature of the cutting edge (Figure 26.22b).
- Luxators are sharpened on their concave surfaces. The instrument should be placed on a conical or round sharpening stone that is held firmly on a solid surface and then pushed along the stone (Figure 26.22c). This sharpens the tip without forming a 'bur' on the convex side.
- Dental elevators are sharpened on a flat sharpening stone. The convex side of the instrument is applied to the stone at the correct inclination (Figure 26.22d) and the instrument is sharpened using a back-and-forth wrist motion.

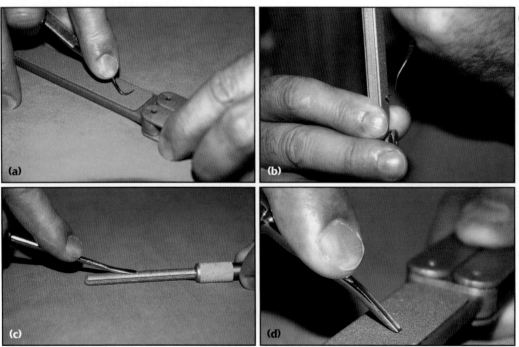

26.22 Sharpening techniques for: **(a)** scaler; **(b)** curette; **(c)** luxator; **(d)** elevator.

Health and safety considerations

Dental operating room

The dental operating room should not share airspace with the surgical preparatory room, sterile procedures room or theatres, due to aerosolized plaque and bacteria generated during the dental procedure.

Some dental chemicals contain solvents and the dental operating room should be well ventilated. Ideally it should have an air extraction system that takes the air outside so that it does not re-enter the building via the clean air supply.

There must be sufficient light in the room and this may be supplemented by an additional light source directed on to the work area. The operating light should not be excessively brighter than the room light or a dazzle effect will be created.

Operator and assistant

To reduce fatigue, both the operator and the assistant should be seated with everything within reach during the dental procedures.

Safety spectacles must be worn by the operator and assistant to prevent injury to the eye from flying debris or a fractured high-speed bur. The bur rotates at approximately 400,000 rpm and will travel at an enormous speed if it fractures. Spectacles also prevent splatter and aerosolized material from landing in the eye.

Examination gloves should be worn, as should protective clothing.

Instruments

All instruments must be kept sharp to prevent the accidents that occur when blunt instruments slip off the tooth or alveolar bone. Care must be exercised when sharpening and washing instruments and the manufacturer's instructions should be followed. Instruments should be sterilized between patients. Disposable 'sharps' must be disposed of correctly (see Chapter 1).

Handling dental instruments

- Correct handling of dental instruments is essential to prevent repetitive strain injury
- About 300 different bacteria can be cultured from the mouths of cats and dogs. Adequate disinfection of instruments must be done between patients
- Instruments must be stored in flat trays to prevent damage to the sharp edges
- Care must be exercised when cleaning dental instruments to prevent iatrogenic injury
- Hand instruments: scalers, curettes, elevators and luxation instruments must be kept sharp – regular whetting is better than infrequent sharpening

Patient safety

The patient should be placed on a soft surface that will maintain its body heat. Covering the patient with bubble wrap will help maintain body temperature. Adequate provision should be made to remove water delivered from dental equipment in order that the animal does not become wet and cold. The patient's face should be protected from the aerosolized bacteria by a towel or drape. An ocular lubricant should be placed in both eyes to prevent desiccation of the corneas.

Scaling and polishing

Tooth scaling and polishing may be performed routinely in patients that have slight calculus and mild gingivitis or may be required in the treatment of patients suffering from periodontal disease or in preparation for tooth extraction.

Intubation

Scale-and-polish procedures are performed in animals that are anaesthetized and intubated. The cuff of the endotracheal (ET) tube should be inflated to the correct pressure so as not to cause damage to the trachea or respiratory epithelial lining. Applying a thin layer of sterile water-soluble lubricant will ensure that the ET tube does not adhere to the respiratory epithelium. Inflation of the cuff does not prevent liquid from passing down the trachea and so it is important to keep the mouth lower than the pharynx, enabling liquids to flow from the mouth. It is good practice to place a pharyngeal pack into the pharynx to trap calculus and other debris and prevent blood from accumulating around the ET tube.

The cuffed ET tube ensures that the anaesthetic gases are confined to the anaesthetic circuit and disposed of via the scavenging system. It also prevents the anaesthetized animal from inhaling aerosolized bacteria, plaque and calculus.

Scaling

After the mouth has been examined and charted, gross calculus can be removed from the teeth using calculus forceps, as described earlier. The remaining calculus can then be removed using hand or electromechanical scalers. When using electromechanical scalers, the scaler tip must be applied side-on to the crown surface (Figure 26.23). If the calculus is tenacious, the operator should move on to an adjacent tooth before returning to complete scaling. This will prevent iatrogenic damage to the tooth by heating it up.

- Never use the point of the ultrasonic scaler tip against the tooth, as it will etch (engrave) the tooth surface.
- Ensure that plenty of water coolant is used to keep the scaler and tooth cool and to flush away debris.

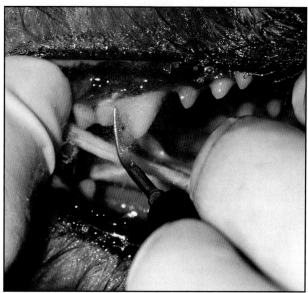

26.23 Piezoelectric scaler being used appropriately with the edge of the scaler against the tooth.

Subgingival scaling and root debridement

Short excursions may be made subgingivally to remove calculus; under ideal circumstances a subgingival scaling tip should be used for this to prevent thermal damage to the crown and gingiva. Hand curettes can be used to remove subgingival calculus and a dental explorer gently circumscribed around the subgingival crown will reveal residual calculus. Where pockets are deep it may be necessary to debride the root surface, using a curette to remove necrotic cementum.

A curette is used for both subgingival scaling and root debridement. It is inserted into the gingival sulcus; the cutting edges should then be engaged against the tooth surface and the curette pulled in a coronal direction. This should be done around the whole circumference of the tooth. An explorer can then be used to judge the smoothness of the subgingival area. Care must be exercised not to denude the root of cementum, as this will expose the dentine and may lead to dentinal hypersensitivity.

Polishing

Polishing removes the remaining plaque that is usually not visible and it helps to smooth the tooth surface. If the tooth has been scaled it must be polished, as minor scratches left on the tooth after scaling would facilitate plaque retention due to the rough surface. To minimize the amount of frictional heat generated, the prophylaxis cup or brush, used in a slow-speed contra-angle handpiece, should not rotate faster than 1000 rpm. Using prophylaxis paste and a rubber cup, the tooth surfaces can be polished. When gentle pressure is exerted on the prophylaxis cup, it flares and can pass under the gingival margin to remove subgingival plaque (Figure 26.24).

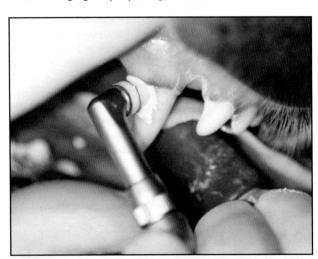

26.24 Subgingival polishing. The 'prophy cup' should be gently pressed on to the tooth to flare out and polish subgingivally.

Radiography of teeth and supportive structures

It is essential to take radiographs when performing veterinary dentistry, as the extent of pathology cannot be seen without them. Whereas the clinical examination enables visualization of the tooth crown, radiography reveals the root, which can make up about 75% the length of the tooth in deciduous canines. Radiographs also show the extent of bone loss in periodontitis and periapical pathology in teeth with inflamed or necrotic pulps.

Indications for radiography

- Missing teeth
- Fractured teeth
- Supernumerary teeth (to determine association with adjacent normal teeth)
- Prior to extraction
- Monitoring treatment progress (e.g. when retrieving root remnants)
- Teeth affected by caries
- Teeth with tertiary dentine that may have exposed pulps
- Teeth affected by periodontal disease
- Persistent deciduous teeth
- Discoloured teeth
- Teeth affected by odontoclastic resorption
- Jaw fractures
- Investigation of sinus tracts that may be associated with teeth
- Investigation of nasal discharge
- Investigation of oral masses

Good technique is vital; for the radiograph to be diagnostic it must be an accurate representation of the tooth and associated structures. It is therefore best to use intraoral radiographic film and techniques.

X-ray generators

Medical X-ray machines

Although cumbersome and usually fixed in one room, medical X-ray machines (described in detail in Chapter 20) can be used to take diagnostic dental radiographs. The focus–film distance should be adjusted to about 40 cm, either by lowering the X-ray tube head or by placing an object on top of the table on to which the patient will be placed. The kV should be set at 70 and the mAs at 15–25, depending upon the size of the patient. If dental X-ray film is not available, mammography film can be used to good effect but superimposition of structures may be problematic.

Dental X-ray machines

A dedicated dental X-ray machine has numerous advantages:

- The machine can be installed in the dental operating area (so that the anaesthetized animal does not need to be transported from the dental room to the radiography room each time a radiograph is required).
- The machine is positioned around the animal.
- The beam is well collimated, reducing scatter radiation.
- Using a dedicated dental X-ray machine frees up the radiography room for other animals to be radiographed.

Dental X-ray generators usually have a fixed kV and mA, with time being the only adjustable setting on most machines. Modern dental X-ray machines have a fixed kV of 70 and mA of 8. Time can be adjusted from 0.1 to about 2 seconds.

Dental operating room

The dental room should be planned in such a manner that the X-ray machine can be discharged from the outside to improve safety for the operator and assistant. The door to the dental operating area should be lead-lined, with a window in it permitting constant visibility of the patient.

Dental film

Dental X-ray film is available in a number of sizes. The most commonly used in veterinary dentistry are:

> Adult periapical film: 3 x 4 cm
> Occlusal film: 5 x 7 cm
> Paediatric periapical film: 2 x 3.5 cm.

These X-ray films are non-screen, single emulsion and available in two speeds:

- E (Ekta) – larger crystals, therefore faster (requiring lower exposure settings) but poorer resolution
- D (Ultra).

The dental film is packed in envelopes that are backed by a layer of lead to reduce scatter (Figure 26.25). Each film has a dot placed in one corner and is packaged in such a way that it faces the incident beam. This allows the picture to be oriented for viewing afterwards.

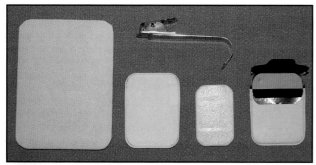

26.25 The dental X-ray films commonly used in practice are from left: occlusal, adult periapical, paediatric periapical. An opened film envelope reveals the film (green), lead backing sheet, and black protective paper. Also pictured is an X-ray film clip.

Intraoral techniques

Parallel technique

This is used for the mandibular premolars and molars caudal to premolar 2 (including this tooth in some animals). The patient is placed in lateral recumbency and the film is placed adjacent to the tooth or teeth to be radiographed (between the tongue and the teeth) and pushed down so that it becomes palpable beyond the ventral margin of the mandible (Figure 26.26). A piece of scrunched-up paper towel can be used to keep the film in the correct position. The incident beam is then directed at right angles to the long axis of the tooth and film. The tooth and film are parallel to each other and the incident beam is directed perpendicular to both.

Bisecting angle technique

This technique is used when taking radiographs of the maxillary teeth and the incisors and canines in the mandible. The film is placed as close as possible to the tooth or teeth to be radiographed. When maxillary teeth are being radiographed, the film spans the palate or is placed on the incisal tips of the canines (Figure 26.27). The tooth axis (an imaginary line joining the tip of the crown and the root tip) is determined and the angle created by this line and the film axis is bisected. The incident beam is directed perpendicular (at right angles) to the bisecting line, giving a true representation of the tooth on the radiograph. If the incident beam is close to perpendicular to the film axis, the tooth will appear short and the image is termed fore-shortened. If the beam is close to perpendicular to the tooth axis, the resultant image will be lengthened and termed elongated.

When radiographing the maxillary carnassial tooth, which has three roots (two mesially and one distally), the mesial roots are often superimposed on each other. To separate these roots on the radiograph, the incident beam must be positioned either rostrally or caudally (maintaining the same bisecting angle). On the resultant image the SLOB (Same Lingual Opposite Buccal) rule is used to identify which root is which. Using the SLOB rule, if the incident beam is moved rostrally the most mesial root will be the palatal root. If the incident beam is moved caudally, the more distal of the mesial roots will be the palatal root and the more mesial of the mesial roots will be the buccal root.

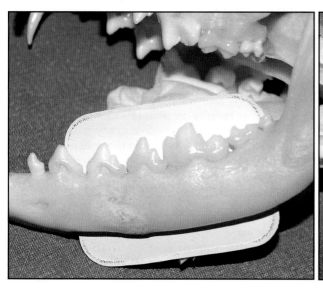

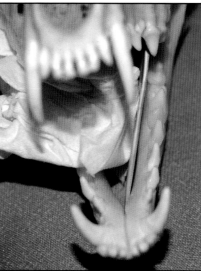

26.26

For the parallel technique, the film is placed between the tongue and teeth/mandible so that the film protrudes past the ventral margin of the mandible. The film should be parallel to the teeth and the incident beam is directed perpendicular to the teeth and film.

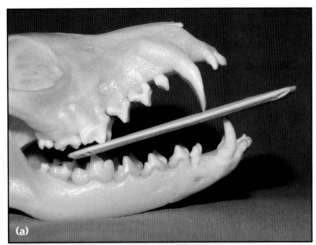

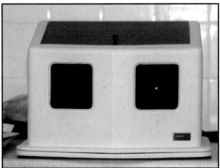

26.28 A chairside darkroom is convenient for developing dental X-ray films.

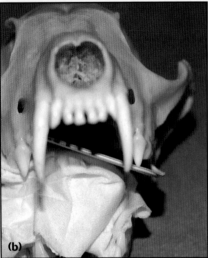

26.27 For the bisecting angle technique, the film is placed as close to the teeth as possible. **(a)** Film positioned for imaging the maxillary incisors including a rostrocaudal view of the maxillary canines. **(b)** Film positioned for imaging maxillary premolars and molars.

Positioning the patient

It may be helpful to position the patient as follows:

- Sternal recumbency for the maxillary incisors
- Lateral or sternal recumbency for the maxillary canines, premolars and molars
- Dorsal recumbency for the mandibular incisors
- Dorsal or lateral recumbency for the mandibular canines
- Lateral recumbency for the mandibular premolars and molars on each side.

When radiographing a cat's maxillary carnassials, superimposition of the zygomatic arch can be problematical. Lifting the cat's nose or tilting its head so that the dental arch is parallel to the table helps to prevent this superimposition.

Developing intraoral radiographs

Intraoral dental radiographs can be developed in a number of ways:

- In a chairside darkroom (Figure 26.28) – a purpose-made enclosure that contains three or four receptacles (developer, rinse water, fixer, rinse water) or only one receptacle, for rinse water
- In the practice darkroom – using manual processing technique
- Using an automatic film developer suited to dental film.

The film should be held at the edges to prevent fingerprint artefacts.

Intraoral radiographs are best viewed in a dark room with the viewing light only coming through the radiograph. The use of magnification is also beneficial.

Processed radiographs must be properly dried before being stored in well labelled film holders (envelopes may be used) as part of the animal's clinical records.

Digital dental radiography

Veterinary practices are increasingly investing in digital dental radiographic technology (Figure 26.29). The system not only removes the need for processing chemicals and takes less space but also requires a lower X-ray exposure and the images are visible almost instantaneously.

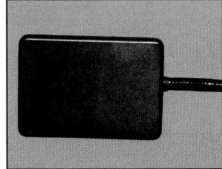

26.29 This transducer is used to take digital dental radiographs using the direct technique. The image is displayed almost immediately on a computer screen.

Maintenance of dental health and prevention of dental disease

Disease prevention is vital in the maintenance of dental health. Approximately 85% of dogs and cats older than 3 years of age suffer from early signs of periodontal disease, probably making dental disease the most common condition seen in general veterinary practice. Periodontitis almost exclusively follows on from gingivitis, a reversible condition; consequently its control is within reach. Treating gingivitis prevents most cases of periodontitis.

In the minority of cases, as a result of periapical root pathology (secondary to necrotic pulp), periodontitis may spread along the root surface in the periodontal space and eventually surface in the gingival sulcus. In these cases the gingivitis may be secondary to the periapical lesion, called an endodontic–periodontic lesion.

The causes of gingivitis have been discussed above. The treatment is routine dental scale-and-polish followed by thorough dental homecare.

Dental homecare

This consists of daily tooth brushing, feeding an appropriate diet, providing dental chews and encouraging play with tooth friendly toys. Of these routines, the most important is tooth brushing. As veterinary patients cannot be taught to brush their own teeth, reliance must be placed on the owners to institute and continue dental homecare. Thus an essential part of professional periodontal therapy is client education.

Pet owners must be aware that, whatever professional treatment is performed, it is only part of the ongoing therapy. Plaque starts to accumulate on the tooth surfaces within 24 hours of a scale-and-polish. Where homecare is not implemented, gingivitis scores 3 months after professional periodontal therapy (supra- and subgingival scaling and polishing) have been found to be the same as those prior to the treatment. The aim of dental homecare is to minimize the accumulation of plaque and therefore reduce the risk of periodontal disease developing or progressing. Continuous monitoring of dental homecare is essential, to keep owners motivated and to check on the adequacy of the oral hygiene carried out.

Tooth brushing

Tooth brushing is the most effective method of removing plaque from the tooth surfaces in the conscious animal. Daily tooth brushing can return the gingivae to health but this is not maintained if carried out less than daily. In addition an animal may require professional periodontal therapy at regular intervals, just as people need to visit the dentist on a regular basis.

The success of plaque control by tooth brushing depends on the owner's ability and the animal's cooperation. Owners should therefore start brushing their pet's teeth as early in its life as possible. Even the youngest puppies and kittens can have their teeth brushed. The primary dentition will be exfoliated but the animal will have become accustomed to the tooth-brushing process by the time the permanent dentition has erupted. It is important to brush kittens' teeth, as it is particularly difficult to introduce adult cats to the process.

Most young animals will tolerate tooth brushing as it is begun when the gingivae are healthy and the procedure is not associated with pain (which can lead to negative reinforcement). Pets that have their teeth brushed regularly enjoy increased intervals between professional dental treatments. Tooth brushing should be introduced as part of the daily routine (Figure 26.30). A treat or a walk can be the reward at the end of a tooth brushing session. In multi-pet households the added individual attention appears to appeal to pets and they will queue to have their turn.

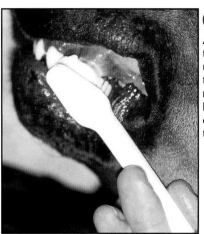

26.30
A medium toothbrush can be used to brush dog's teeth. Pet toothpaste must be used as human toothpaste can cause fluoride toxicity.

Toothbrushes and toothpaste

Pet toothbrushes are available with double-ended angled heads. A medium-texture human toothbrush can also be used. Human toothpaste must never be used, due to the high fluoride content, which can cause toxicity when pets swallow rather than rinsing and spitting. Human toothpastes usually also contain a detergent that causes foaming, a sensation apparently disliked by animals. Pet toothpastes are available in a variety of flavours and, although not essential, help to familiarize the pet with the tooth brushing process.

Toothbrushing procedure

- Ensure that the animal is comfortable before commencing and start gradually.
- Start brushing the molars and premolars and brush a few teeth each day until eventually all the teeth can be brushed in one session.
- Gentle circular motions are used to brush the teeth and gingival margin.
- Using a circular movement with the brush at an angle of 45 degrees near the gingival margin, the filaments of the brush can be made to flare slightly into the gingival sulcus, removing subgingival plaque.

Initially it is acceptable to concentrate on brushing the buccal surfaces of the teeth, but eventually it is advisable to open the mouth to brush the lingual/palatal surfaces also. It will take longer for the animal to become accustomed to this.

In patients with periodontal disease, the gums will bleed when tooth brushing is first instituted. The owners should be informed that this will happen and that they should continue brushing – less bleeding will occur as the gingivae return to health.

Diet, chews and toys

There are numerous diets formulated to be tooth friendly. Some have a structure that ensures that the food is chewed and the tooth surface is mechanically cleaned. Other diets contain minerals that prevent mineralization of plaque to calculus.

Some dental chews contain enzymes that prevent calculus formation with or without a physical cleansing effect (e.g. raw hide).

Tooth-friendly toys may have a 'window-wiper blade' effect or have projections that clean the tooth surface. Some also dispense toothpaste as the animal plays with the toy.

Dentistry for lagomorphs and rodents

Definitions

- **Brachyodont** – short crown:root ratio with a true root. The mature tooth has a closed root apex (e.g. humans, dogs, cats, ferrets).
- **Hypsodont** – tooth with a long crown and comparatively short or no true root. The subgingival part is called the reserve crown. The dentition or part thereof is radicular or aradicular:
  - **Radicular hypsodont** – true tooth root develops later in the life of the animal (e.g. horses, cattle)
  - **Aradicular hypsodont** – tooth never forms a true root with an apex and the tooth continues to grow throughout life (e.g. rabbits, hares, guinea pigs, chinchillas).

Normal dentition

Rodents have aradicular hypsodont incisors and either aradicular hypsodont or brachyodont cheek teeth. Rodents have only one pair of upper and lower incisors. Guinea pigs and chinchillas have aradicular hypsodont dentition, while rats and mice have aradicular hypsodont incisors and brachyodont cheek teeth.

Lagomorphs (rabbits and hares) have aradicular hypsodont dentition. They have four incisors in the maxillae in two rows, two large central incisors labially and two peg teeth palatally. They have no canine teeth. The teeth grow at a rate of about 2 mm per week.

The teeth of rabbits, hares, chinchillas and guinea pigs grow continuously. An abrasive diet, such as grass supplemented with hay, will keep the teeth worn to a physiological length. Commercial mixes, whilst providing a nutritionally balanced diet, do not provide the wear required for dental health.

In lagomorphs the incisors are in occlusion (touching each other) at rest and the cheek teeth are apart. This is in contrast to rodents, where the cheek teeth are in occlusion at rest and the incisors out of occlusion. Rodents gnaw with their incisors, whereas lagomorphs use their incisors in a cutting action.

Malocclusion

This is the most common dental disease. It may be caused by:

- Incorrect diet leading to lack of wear and tear and tooth overgrowth
- Congenital deformity of the maxillae – seen most commonly in brachycephalic rabbits (some dwarf rabbits)
- Tooth or mandible trauma
- Tooth root infection
- Neoplasia.

Incisor malocclusion

When this occurs the lower incisors grow into the hard palate and the upper incisors can curl around behind them, or the upper incisors can impinge on the mandible and the lower incisors protrude out of the mouth. Clinical signs include anorexia, lack of grooming and salivation. Treatment involves tooth trimming or in some cases incisor extraction.

Molar malocclusion

This may occur as a result of one of the factors listed above. An important cause of the acquired condition is lack of tooth wear. Abnormal enamel spurs will form on the crowns. Sharp projections will form, resulting in trauma to the tongue (usually by mandibular cheek teeth) and cheek tissue (usually by maxillary cheek teeth). The force exerted by the opposing cheek teeth prevents normal tooth eruption, resulting in retrograde eruption of the teeth into the mandibles and maxillae. This causes periosteal pain. Irreversible changes occur if the growth tip penetrates the jaw and the ventral mandibular margin or the orbit is perforated. Swellings may be palpated on the upper and lower jaws. There is usually secondary incisor malocclusion as a result of the molar malocclusion. Retrograde eruption of cheek and incisor teeth may cause obstruction of the nasolacrimal duct, leading to lacrimation or infection. This may progress to tooth root-associated abcessation and osteomyelits.

Selective feeding may be the initial clinical sign, progressing to anorexia, weight loss, excessive salivation and difficulty in eating. Signs of pain include slobbering (wet chin and neck), teeth grinding, aggression and depression. An animal with tooth root abcessation will present with facial swelling, by which time the prognosis is grave. Diagnosis is confirmed by a lateral extraoral radiograph of the patient's jaws and the condition can be monitored by dental radiography.

Analgesia is essential. If the ventral mandibular margin and the orbit are intact, recreating the normal occlusal surfaces is advised. Following treatment the normal abrasive diet of fresh grass or hay (less effective than fresh grass) should be fed to help to prevent recurrence. Commercial mixes do not provide the tooth wear required.

Regular weighing is an ideal method of monitoring patients that may be affected by this form of dental disease. A 10% reduction in body mass is a good indication of dental disease. Owner education is essential.

Chinchillas are often presented with advanced dental disease and euthanasia may be the only option. Radiographs should be taken to confirm the diagnosis and aid in treatment planning or the decision to euthanase the animal.

Tooth trimming

Teeth should not be clipped, as the uneven pressure applied to the tooth surfaces can cause the tooth to shatter. Clipping can cause damage to periapical tissues, affecting future tooth growth, or fissures may be produced, leading to periodontal problems and pulp infection. Sharp edges are caused, leading to oral discomfort.

The incisors are effectively trimmed using a high-speed dental fissure bur (this can be performed in the conscious animal if it is properly restrained). Care should be exercised to prevent thermal damage to the teeth. While trimming and reshaping is performed, the soft tissues should be protected by placing a tongue depressor or empty syringe case behind the incisors. The cheek teeth can be trimmed using a long-shank fissure bur in a soft tissue protective shroud or using an acrylic bur. Cheek teeth are trimmed when the animal is anaesthetized.

Extraction of malocccluding incisor teeth should be performed by an experienced veterinary surgeon.

Equipment

Lagomorphs and rodents undergoing dental treatment should be treated with analgesics to relieve postoperative pain and discomfort. Equipment for lagomorph and rodent dentistry includes the following (Figure 26.31):

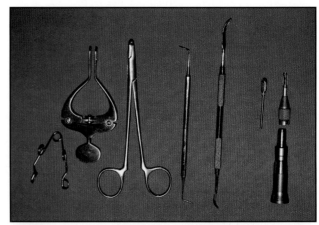

26.31 Rabbit dental kit. From left: cheek dilator; mouth opener; cheek teeth extraction forceps; cheek teeth luxators; incisor luxators; acrylic bur for shortening cheek teeth; straight surgical fissure bur and soft tissue guard with a straight slow-speed handpiece.

- High-speed handpiece and fissure burs
- Slow-speed straight handpiece with acrylic or long-shank fissure bur
- Cheek dilator
- Mouth gag
- Cheek protector
- Cheek tooth luxator
- Incisor luxator
- Molar extraction forceps.

It should be noted that damage to the temporomandibular joint (TMJ) capsule may occur if the mouth is opened maximally using the mouth gag.

Further reading

Gorrel C and Derbyshire S (2005) *Veterinary Dentistry for the Nurse and Technician*. Elsevier Butterworth Heinemann, Oxford

Hobson P (2006) Dentistry. In *BSAVA Manual of Rabbit Medicine and Surgery, 2nd edition,* eds Meredith and Flecknell, pp. 184–196. BSAVA Publications, Gloucester

Tutt C, Deeprose J and Crossley D (2007) *BSAVA Manual of Canine and Feline Dentistry, 3rd edition.* BSAVA Publications, Gloucester

Appendix 1

Dog breeds

The Kennel Club website (www.thekennelclub.org.uk) lists seven Dog Groups. Individual breeds, with their own specified Breed Standards, are placed within these Groups. (Photographs © The Kennel Club)

Hound Group

Includes: Afghan Hound, Beagle, Whippet, Wire-haired Dachshund

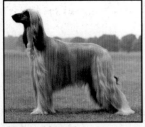

Afghan Hound

Gundog Group

Includes: English Setter, Labrador Retriever, Cocker Spaniel, Weimaraner

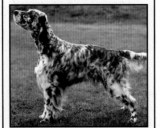

English Setter

Terrier Group

Includes: Bedlington Terrier, Norfolk Terrier, West Highland White Terrier

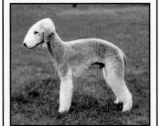

Bedlington Terrier

Utility Group

Includes: Chow Chow, Dalmatian, Shih Tzu, Standard Poodle

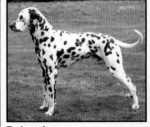

Dalmatian

Working Group

Includes: Boxer, Mastiff, Great Dane, Newfoundland, St Bernard

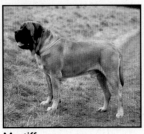

Mastiff

Pastoral Group

Includes: Border Collie, Old English Sheepdog, Pembroke Welsh Corgi

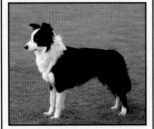

Border Collie

Toy Group

Includes: Bichon Frise, Cavalier King Charles Spaniel, Yorkshire Terrier

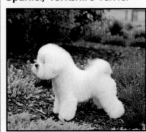

Bichon Frise

Appendix 2

Normal parameters in cats, dogs and exotic pets

Cats

Temperature (°C)	Pulse (beats/minute)	Respiration (breaths/minute)	Age at puberty	Gestation period
38.0–38.5	110–180	20–30	(Male) 8–12 months (Female) 6–9 months	64–68 days

Dogs

Temperature (°C)	Pulse (beats/minute)	Respiration (breaths/minute)	Age at puberty	Gestation period
38.3–38.7	60–80	10–30	(Male) 6–12 months (Female) average 12–14 months	64–66 days

Small mammals

	Rabbit	Ferret	Mouse	Rat	Gerbil	Syrian hamster	Chinese/ Russian hamster	Guinea pig	Chinchilla	Chipmunk
Average life expectancy (years)	5–8	8–10	1–2.5	3	1.5–2.5	1.5–2	1.5–2	4–7	10–15	3–5
Adult weight	1–10 kg (breed-dependent)	600 g (jill) 1.2 kg (hob)	20–40 g	400–800 g	70–130 g	100–200 g	20–40 g	750–1000 g	400–500 g	80–150 g
Body temperature (°C)	38.5–40	37.8–40	37–38	37.6–38.6	37–38.5	36.2–37.5[a]	36–38	37.2–39.5	37–38	37.8–39.6[a]
Heart rate (beats/minute)	130–325 (larger breeds lower rates)	200–250	500–600	260–450	300–400	280–412	300–460	190–300	120–160	150–280
Respiration rate (breaths/minute)	30–60	33–36	100–250	70–150	90–140	33–127	60–80	90–150	50–60	60–90
Age at sexual maturity	4–8 months	4–8 months	6–7 weeks	8–10 weeks	8–10 weeks	6–12 weeks		1.5–3 months	6–9 months	
Gestation length (days)	29–35 (average 31 days)	41–42	19–21	20–22	24–26 (42 days if delayed implantation)	15–18		59–72 (average 63 days)	111	
Litter size	4–10	2–14	8–12	6–16	3–7	4–12		2–6	1–5	

[a] Hibernates in the wild.

Appendix 3

Conversion tables

Biochemistry

	SI unit	Conversion	Non-SI unit
Alanine transferase	IU/l	x 1	IU/l
Albumin	g/l	x 0.1	g/dl
Alkaline phosphatase	IU/l	x 1	IU/l
Aspartate transaminase	IU/l	x 1	IU/l
Bilirubin	μmol/l	x 0.0584	mg/dl
Calcium	mmol/l	x 4	mg/dl
Carbon dioxide (total)	mmol/l	x 1	mEq/l
Cholesterol	mmol/l	x 38.61	mg/dl
Chloride	mmol/l	x 1	mEq/l
Cortisol	nmol/l	x 0.362	ng/ml
Creatine kinase	IU/l	x 1	IU/l
Creatinine	μmol/l	x 0.0113	mg/dl
Glucose	mmol/l	x 18.02	mg/dl
Insulin	pmol/l	x 0.1394	μIU/ml
Iron	μmol/l	x 5.587	μg/dl
Magnesium	mmol/l	x 2	mEq/l
Phosphorus	mmol/l	x 3.1	mg/dl
Potassium	mmol/l	x 1	mEq/l
Sodium	mmol/l	x 1	mEq/l
Total protein	g/l	x 0.1	g/dl
Thyroxine (T4) (free)	pmol/l	x 0.0775	ng/dl
Thyroxine (T4) (total)	nmol/l	x 0.0775	μg/dl
Tri-iodothyronine (T3)	nmol/l	x 65.1	ng/dl
Triglycerides	mmol/l	x 88.5	mg/dl
Urea	mmol/l	x 2.8	mg of urea nitrogen/dl

Temperature

	SI unit	Conversion	Non-SI unit
	°C	(x 9/5) + 32	°F

Haematology

	SI unit	Conversion	Non-SI unit
Red blood cell count	10^{12}/l	x 1	10^6/μl
Haemoglobin	g/l	x 0.1	g/dl
MCH	pg/cell	x 1	pg/cell
MCHC	g/l	x 0.1	g/dl
MCV	fl	x 1	μm³
Platelet count	10^9/l	x 1	10^3/μl
White blood cell count	10^9/l	x 1	10^3/μl

Hypodermic needles

	Metric	Non-metric
External diameter	0.8 mm	21 G
	0.6 mm	23 G
	0.5 mm	25 G
	0.4 mm	27 G
Needle length	12 mm	$^1/_2$ inch
	16 mm	$^5/_8$ inch
	25 mm	1 inch
	30 mm	$1^1/_4$ inch
	40mm	$1^1/_2$ inch

Suture material sizes

Metric	USP	Metric	USP
0.1	11/0	1.5	4/0
0.2	10/0	2	3/0
0.3	9/0	3	2/0
0.4	8/0	3.5	0
0.5	7/0	4	1
0.7	6/0	5	2
1	5/0	6	3

Index

Calculus (dental) 671, 675
   forceps 677, *678*
Campylobacter *119, 130*
Campylobacteriosis 501
Cancer *see* Tumours
Candida albicans 135
Candidiasis 135
Canine adenovirus 1 *127,* 491
Canine adenovirus 2 *127,* 493
Canine contagious respiratory disease 493–4
Canine coronavirus *128*
Canine distemper *490,* 491
   virus *128*
Canine herpesvirus *128*
Canine leucocyte adhesion deficiency 113
Canine parainfluenza virus *128,* 493
Canine parvovirus *490,* 492–3
Capillaria
   hepatica *142,* 149
   plica *142,* 149
Capillaries 71
Capillary refill time *230,* 355
Capnography 538
Capsid 126
Capsule history 357
Carbohydrate (dietary) 283, 299
   in disease 312
   metabolism 82
Carbon dioxide regulation 395
Carcinoma 614
Cardiac compression 359, *360,* 558
Cardiomyopathy 461, 462–3
Cardiopulmonary arrest 358, 557–9
Cardiopulmonary–cerebral resuscitation 359–60, 558–9
Cardiovascular system
   anaesthetic complications 554–5
   anatomy and physiology 68–72
   birds 98
   disease 461–5
   drugs 157
   emergencies 362–4
   emergency assessment 354–5
   ferrets 94
   fish 104
   reptiles 101–2
   surgical conditions 628
Care plans *274–5, 279*
Caries 672–3, 677
Carprofen *161,* 516, *545, 548, 551*
Carpus *52*
Cartilage 46
Castration 633, 647
Casts 609–10
Cat 'flu *see* Feline upper respiratory disease
Cataracts 618
Catgut 586
Catheters
   fluid therapy 397–8
   management 262–3, 358
   urinary 265–7
Cations 42, 388

Catteries *see* Housing
CDC group M5 134
Cells
   division 44, 107
   structure 43
Cellular immunity 122
Cellulitis 593–4
Central nervous system 58–60
   disease, anaesthesia 508–9
Central venous pressure 394
   in anaesthesia 537
Centrifuges 321
Cephalic vein, injection 253
Cerclage wire 611
Cerebrospinal fluid 60
   cytology 348–9
   sampling 327–8
Cerumen, sampling 327
Ceruminous glands 90
Cervix 89
Cestodes 142–5
Chelonians
   anaesthesia 550
   anatomy and physiology 100, 101, 102
   fluid therapy 409
   handling 190
   injection sites *252*
   nutrition 302
   radiography *454*
   reproduction 665
Chemical symbols 388
Chemicals (Hazard Information and Packaging for Supply) Amendment Regulations 1996 7
Chemosis 230
Chemotherapy 616
Chest bandage *249*
Cheyletiella *139,* 140
   diagnostics *325,*
Chinchillas
   anaesthesia 543, 544
   analgesia *545*
   body temperature *93, 233, 689*
   dental formula 94
   fluid therapy 407
   gestation *689*
   handling 186
   hand-rearing 670
   heart rate *233, 689*
   housing 219
   life expectancy *93, 689*
   litter size *689*
   nutrition 301
   PCV *405*
   reproduction *663, 667*
   respiratory rate *233, 689*
   sexual maturity *689*
   total protein *405*
   weight *93, 689*
CHIP *see* Chemicals (Hazard Information and Packaging for Supply) Amendment Regulations

injection sites 252
nutrition 303
reproduction 666
Sodium
dietary 283, 284, 285, 293, 294
levels 341
regulation 85
Soiled patients, care 257
Somatostatin 66
Somatotrophin 66
SOP *see* Standard operating procedure
Spay *see* Ovariohysterectomy
Specimens, postage 8
Specula 267–8
Spermatozoa 642, 654
storage 327
Spica bandage 250
Spinal cord 60
disease 367–8
Spinal nerves 60
Spine
fractures 638
injuries 483
radiography 439–40
contrast 446–7
surgery 638
tumours 638
Spirochaetes 130
Spleen 73
birds 99
small mammals 95
Splenectomy 630
Splints 609–10
Sponge-holding forceps *579*
Staff rest room 10
Staining procedures
Giemsa 331
Gram 334
Leishman's 331
methylene blue 334
*RAPI*DIFF® 331
Ziehl–Neelsen 334
Stainless steel sutures 587
Standard operating procedure 7
Staphylococcus 130
aureus, methicillin-resistant 119, 134, 601
intermedius 327, 486
Staples (surgical) 587, *630*
Status epilepticus 367
Steam sterilization 562–3
Steinmann pins 610–11
Stenotic nares 626
Sterilization 119, 561
cold 564–5
heat 562–4
packing supplies 565–6
of surgical equipment 566–7
Sternum 52
Steroids 159
Stifle *54*
radiography 442

Stillbirth 657
Stock control 27–9, 170
Stomach
anatomy and physiology 78–9
contrast radiography 444
surgical conditions 622–3
tumours 623
(*see also* Gastric)
Stomatitis 672
Strabismus 357
Streptococcus 130
Stress reduction 206, 228–9
in emergency patients 357–8
Struvite
crystals *345*
uroliths 315
Subcutaneous injection 253
Succinylcholine 534, 549
Sugar gliders, analgesia *545*
'Suitably qualified persons' 32
Supersession 24
Surgery
assistance 575–6
of the cardiovascular system 628
classification *617*
clothing 569, 570–2
drains 605–6
of the ears 619–21
of the endocrine system 629
of the eye 617–19
fracture repair 610–13
of the gastrointestinal tract 621–5
hernia/rupture 635
infection 561–2
prevention 617
instrumentation 576, 577–85, *680*
of the liver 629
of the musculoskeletal system 636–8
oncological 614–16
operating theatre 567–9
postoperative care 577
preoperative care 572–5
reconstructive 603–5
of the reproductive system 633–5
of the respiratory tract 625–8
scrubbing up 569–70
of the skin 619
of the spleen 630
suture materials 585–8, 603–4
suture patterns 588–9
terminology 590–1
of the urinary tract 630–3
wound closure and management 596–605
(*see also* Sterilization)
Suture materials 585–8, 603–4
Suture patterns 588–9, 603
Suture removal 599
Swabs (surgical), sterilization 567
Sweat glands 90
Sympathomimetics 157, 404–5
Synapse 58

Trachea
anatomy 74
avulsion 627
collapse 364–5, 627
disease 458–9
foreign bodies 627
Tracheostomy 627
Training
discs 199–200
obedience 200–1
(see also Learning)
Tranquillizers 158
Transcellular fluid 42, 389–90
Transporting animals 178–9
Transudates 349, 365, 593
Trauma
dental 674
emergencies 386–7
head 366
Triadan numbering system 675
Triage 352
Trichodectes canis 137, 346
Trichophyton mentagrophytes 348
Trichuris vulpis 142, 149
Trombicula autumnalis 140, 325
Trypsin 81
D-Tubocurarine 534
Tumours
adrenal 629
benign 614
biopsy 615
drugs 160–1
gastric 613
laryngeal 626
malignant 614–15
mammary 621
maxillary 621, 622
musculoskeletal 485–6
nasal 626
ocular 618
oral 621–2
ovarian 635, 645
pancreatic 629
prostatic 633
rectal 624
skin 619
spinal 638
surgery 615–16
testicular 633, 641
thoracic 460
thyroid 629
tracheal 627
urethra 632
uterine 635
vaginal 635

Ulcers
corneal 488
decubital 260, 556
ocular 618
Ulna 52

Ultrasonography
biopsy 450
Doppler 450–1
equipment 448–9
heart 450
liver 449, 450
polycystic kidney disease 450
pregnancy 653–4
principles 448
technique 449
Uncinaria stenocephala 142, 148, 149
Unconsciousness 360–1
Ureteronephrectomy 630
Ureters 85–6
avulsion 631
ectopic 631, 633
Urethra
anatomy 86
contrast radiography 446
obstruction 370, 632
rupture 632
tumours 632
Urethrostomy 632
Uric acid 99
Urinalysis 341–5
Urinary bladder
anatomy and physiology 86
contrast radiography 445–6
drugs acting on 160
manual expression 259, 271
rupture 631
surgical conditions 631
Urinary catheterization 259, 324
complications 264–5
equipment 265–8
indications for 264
preoperative 573
techniques 268–71
Urinary catheters 265–7
management 263
sterilization 567, 267
Urinary incontinence 475, 633
Urinary tract
anatomy and physiology 82–6
birds 98–9
disease 474–6
drugs acting on 160
emergencies 370
fish 104
infection 265
reptiles 102
small mammals 94
surgical conditions 630–3
Urination
inpatients 238, 259, 271
patterns 231
process 86, 160
Urine
appearance 342
calculi 344
casts 345

Index

Urine *(continued)*
    crystals 344–5
    dipsticks 343
    formation 83
    output 342, 394
        in anaesthesia 539
    sampling 324
    scalding 260, 619
    sediment 344–5
    in shock 362
        pH 343
    specific gravity 342–3, 392
Uroabdomen 362–3
Urogenital system
    birds 98–9
    contrast radiography 445–6
    fish 104
    reptiles 104
    small mammals 94
Urography 445
Urolith 344
Urolithiasis 475
    clinical nutrition 315–16
Urticaria 487
Uterus
    anatomy and physiology 89
    disorders 645, 646
    inertia 659
Uveitis 378, 488–9

Vaccination 122–4, 205, 213
    contraceptive 647
Vaccines 122–3, 163
Vacutainers 323
Vagina
    anatomy and physiology 89
    cytology 648–9
    discharge 231
    disorders 646
    hyperplasia 635
    prolapse 635
    tumours 635
Vaginitis 646
Vaginoscopy 650
Vaginourethrography 446
Vaporizers 530–1, 539
Vasectomy 647
Vasodilators 157
Vasopressin *see* Antidiuretic hormone
VAT 24
Vectors of disease 117
Vecuronium 534
Veins 71
Velpeau sling 250
Venepuncture
    cephalic, dog 180
    jugular, cat 181
Venodilators 157
Ventilation systems 217, 227
Ventricular fibrillation 360, *463*

Ventricular system 60
Vertebrae 50–2
    radiography 439–40
Vestibular disease 368
Veterinary Medicines Directorate 32, 153
Veterinary Medicines Regulations 2005 32
Veterinary Nurses Council 18
Veterinary Nurses Register 34
Veterinary nursing assistants 32
Veterinary Poisons and Information Service 383
Veterinary Surgeons Act 1966 18, 31, 36–9
Veterinary surgery, definition 31
Veterinary teams 31–2
Viraemia 117
Viral disease 127–9
    neonatal 668
Virulence 116
Viruses 125–7
    diagnostics 329
    susceptibility to disinfectants 226
Vital signs *see* Pulse, Respiration rate, Body temperature
Vitamins 286–9
    A 286–7
    B-complex 287, 288
    C 287
    D 287–8
    E 287, 288
    K 287, 288
    supplements 163
Vomiting 79, 231, 374, 468–9
    nursing care 256–7, 469
Vulva
    anatomy and physiology 89
    physical examination 231

Waste transport and disposal 2–3
Water
    balance 85, 390–1
        in geriatric patients 255
    deprivation test 481
    dietary requirement 289
    functions in the body 390
    intake 390–1
    loss 391
    (see also Body water)
Waterfowl, handling 189
Weaning 670
West Nile virus 119, 128
Whelping *see* Reproduction
Wildlife, housing 223
Wildlife and Countryside Act 1981 19
Wire forceps 581
Wood's lamp 347
Workstation risk assessment 8
Wounds
    classification 387, 595–6
    debridement 601
    dressings 601–3
    as emergencies 386–7
    healing 247, 594–7
    lavage 600–1

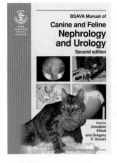 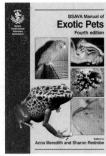 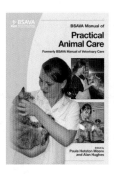 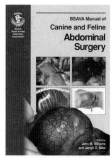 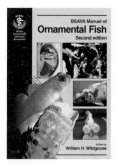 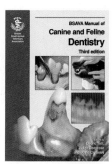
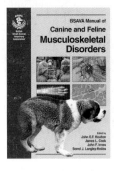 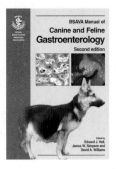 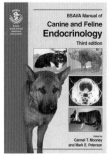 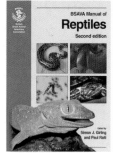 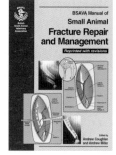 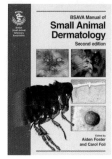
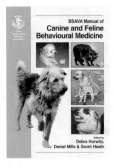 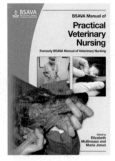 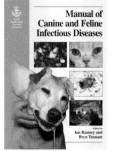 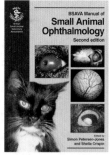 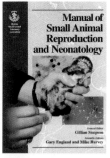 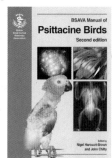
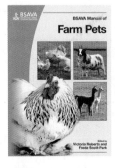 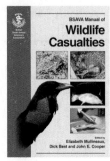 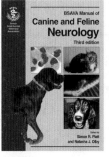 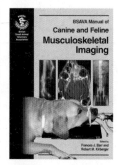 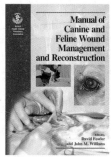 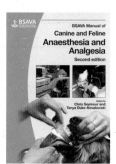
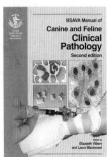 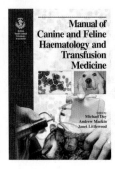 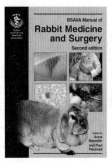 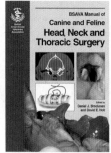 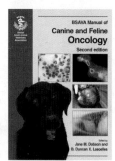 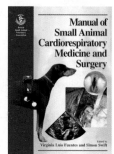